INTERVENTIONAL RADIOLOGY
Volume 1

Second Edition

INTERVENTIONAL RADIOLOGY
Volume 1
Second Edition

Edited by

Wilfrido R. Castañeda–Zúñiga, M.D., M.Sc.

Professor of Radiology
University of Minnesota Hospital and Clinic
Minneapolis, Minnesota

S. Murthy Tadavarthy, M.D.

Clinical Associate Professor of Radiology
University of Minnesota Hospital and Clinic
Cardiovascular Radiologist
Minneapolis Heart Institute
Co-Director, Cardiovascular and Interventional Radiology
Abbott-Northwestern Hospital
Minneapolis, Minnesota

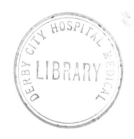

Williams & Wilkins

BALTIMORE • PHILADELPHIA • HONG KONG
LONDON • MUNICH • SYDNEY • TOKYO
A WAVERLY COMPANY

Editor: Timothy H. Grayson
Managing Editor: Marjorie Kidd Keating
Copy Editors: Janet M. Krejci, Klementyna L. Bryte
Designer: Wilma E. Rosenberger
Illustration Planner: Lorraine Wrzosek
Production Coordinator: Raymond E. Reter
Cover Designer: Wilma E. Rosenberger

Copyright © 1992
Williams & Wilkins
428 East Preston Street
Baltimore, Maryland 21202, USA

Accurate indications, adverse reactions, and dosage schedules for drugs are provided in this book, but it is possible that they may change. The reader is urged to review the package information data of the manufacturers of the medications mentioned.

Printed in the United States of America

First Edition 1988

Library of Congress Cataloging-in-Publication Data

Interventional radiology / edited by Wilfrido R. Castañeda–Zúñiga, S.
   Murthy Tadavarthy. — 2nd ed.
      p.   cm.
   Includes bibliographical references and index.
   ISBN (invalid) 0-683-01476-1
      1. Radiology, Interventional.   I. Castañeda–Zúñiga, Wilfrido R.
   II. Tadavarthy, S. Murthy.
      [DNLM: 1. Radiology, Interventional.   WN 160 I612]
   RD33.55.I58   1992
   617′.05—dc20
   DNLM/DLC
   for Library of Congress   91-18779
                                                      CIP

                                                  93 94 95
                        2   3   4   5   6   7   8   9   10

FOREWORD TO THE SECOND EDITION

It is a great personal and professional honor and privilege for me to be invited to write the Foreword to the second edition of *Interventional Radiology* by Drs. Wilfrido R. Castañeda–Zúñiga and S. Murthy Tadavarthy, both of whom I have known and admired for over a decade.

The first edition of *Interventional Radiology*, introduced in 1988, combined the disciplines of interventional radiology and angiography under a single title and is considered by many to be the most authoritative and most comprehensive single text written on these radiologic specialties. The extraordinary demand for *Interventional Radiology* attests to its reception, not only by radiologists but by other medical specialists interested in the application of interventional radiology and angiography to their academic and clinical practices. Such a reception is a clear indication of the worth of *Interventional Radiology* to the medical community. The popularity of the first edition is the more remarkable because it has become such an outstanding success in today's very competitive radiology book market in which the physician-consumer, inundated by a plethora of textbooks from which to choose, has become very discriminating in the selection process. The response to the first edition of *Interventional Radiology* is the single most important factor in the decision to prepare a new edition.

The need for a second edition having been established by the reception afforded the first edition and the extraordinary developments in this field since the completion of the first edition manuscript in 1987, Drs. Castañeda–Zúñiga and Tadavarthy and their collaborators, who comprise a majority of the world's authorities in their fields, have prepared a major revision which transforms the superb first edition into an improved, expanded, and more comprehensive second edition without altering those characteristics of the first edition which made it so popular.

The review process began with incorporation of all appropriate suggestions and constructive criticisms obtained from reviews of the first edition and from those received directly by the principle authors. The authors have retained the majority of the material that earned the first edition its enviable reputation and which remains relevant today, revised other sections to make them reflective of contemporary research and/or clinical experience in interventional radiology and angiography, and deleted those which are no longer appropriate. In this revision, the authors have incorporated the new advances that have occurred in the field of interventional radiology and angiography pertaining to both diagnosis and therapy. These additions include not only the new techniques and procedures that have become part of the "routine" angiographer-interventionist's armamentarium but also those on the leading edge of this rapidly expanding radiologic subspecialty. The new additions have been described and illustrated with the same clarity that characterized the first edition.

In the current edition, the principal authors have expanded the traditional definition of interventional radiology by the inclusion of diagnostic and therapeutic procedures of an interventional nature involving organs and organ systems not included in standard textbooks of interventional radiology, e.g., the breast. By such inclusions, this edition of *Interventional Radiology* can truly be described as "comprehensive."

The presentation of the new and revised material required a total reorganization of the text format. In the current edition, the number of chapters has been reduced from 32 to 23, with each of the new chapters dealing with a broad topic. The subject matter within the various chapters is further divided into discreet, but related, subparts to facilitate reader accessibility and to allow the reader to either review the overall chapter subject or to find very easily the subtopic of particular interest. The re-organization of this vast amount of material is masterful and is a very strong positive feature of this revision.

The extensive bibliography of the first edition has been augmented by the selective addition of the significant and substantive references from the interventional/angiographic literature published since completion of the first edition manuscript.

Because of its timeliness, the magnitude of the revision, the depth and breadth of traditional research and clinical interventional and angiographic material and the inclusion of new subject matter by virtue of the expanded definition of *Interventional Radiology* within this manuscript, and the innovative format of presentation of this enormous amount of material, I believe that *Interventional Radiology—Second Edition* is destined to become the standard text in its field against which all others will be measured.

The second edition of *Interventional Radiology* retains the unique and essential character of the first edition of being, at the same time, an eminently scholarly, encyclopedic reference source for the academic interventionist-angiographer and a comprehensive, authoritative reference source for clinical problem solving for the practicing radiologist. *Interventional Radiology—Second Edition* will be an essential addition to the library of any academic or non-academic radiologist with any interest in interventional radiology and angiography.

John H. Harris, Jr., M.D., D.Sc.

FOREWORD TO THE FIRST EDITION

It is with immense pride and pleasure that the officers and Editorial Board of Williams & Wilkins join me in introducing you, the reader, to Wilfrido R. Castañeda–Zúñiga, M.D., and S. Murthy Tadavarthy, M.D., the newest members of the distinguished group of authors in the Golden's Diagnostic Radiology Series.

Golden's Diagnostic Radiology Series was created to present authoritative, comprehensive, timely reference texts on clearly defined aspects of diagnostic radiology specifically intended for radiologists and those nonradiologists with major interest in the imaging aspects of their area of specialization.

Fulfillment of that goal demands authors and/or editors of proven stature and reputation in their field of diagnostic radiology. Candidates for authorship in the Series are identified from a rigorous selection process and are invited to become contributors to the Series. Thus, not only is the intent of the Golden's Series met and its purpose for the reader assured, but the authors are afforded an accolade available to a very select few. The unique prestige of the Golden's Series, continually enhanced by the character of its authors, has persisted for over a decade.

Drs. Castañeda–Zúñiga and Tadavarthy are uniquely qualified to author and edit *Interventional Radiology*. Both are academicians (teachers) in the true sense of the word, having spent their professional careers at the University of Minnesota. Both are direct professional descendants—or disciples—of one of the first American angiographers to expand into intervention, namely Kurt Amplatz, M.D., under whose direction both have studied, performed original bench and clinical research, and matured into respected teachers and clinicians. As disciples of Dr.

Amplatz, Drs. Castañeda–Zúñiga and Tadavarthy represent the current generation of traditional angiographer-interventionists in contradistinction to modality-oriented radiologists who perform intervention within the scope of their modality interest or radiologists who limit their intervention to the organ system of their interest. Thus, this work is the statement of the years of experience of the authors and their carefully selected contributors.

Interventional Radiology is a superb example of the intent of the Golden's Series. It is timely and comprehensive in scope yet not overbearingly encyclopedic. Its organization is logical, and the text is interesting, entirely practical, and scholarly. The volume is replete with carefully selected radiographs of excellent quality, photographs, and clean, informative drawings.

Gilbert Fletcher, M.D, in his Foreword for another Golden's Series text stated, "Writing has meaning and substance only if the authors have knowledge and conviction of the usefulness of their writing." Certainly, Drs. Castañeda–Zúñiga and Tadavarthy and their contributors have satisfied Dr. Fletcher's criteria of excellence and are to be congratulated for preparing a text that is destined to become the standard in its field.

Finally, it is an extraordinarily wonderful coincidence that *Interventional Radiology*, authored and edited by two of his students, has been published in the same year that Dr. Amplatz received the Gold Medal of the American College of Radiology for his enormous contributions to the development of interventional radiology.

John H. Harris, Jr., M.D., D.Sc.
Editor, *Golden's Diagnostic Radiology*

PREFACE

Since the first edition of *Interventional Radiology,* there have been extensive developments in different areas of the subspecialty. We attempt to describe some of these advances and have expanded the sections on vascular intervention, where most of these changes have taken place.

We have kept the same emphasis that we had in the first edition of the book, stressing mainly the general philosophy of indications, contraindications, approaches, and instrumentation, rather than specific descriptions of techniques. Contributions by several authors from the United States and Europe have also helped to make this edition a better textbook. We hope that we have included most of the new developments, but we are sure that some of them have escaped our attention and we apologize to our readers for that oversight.

Wilfrido R. Castañeda–Zúñiga, M.D.

ACKNOWLEDGMENTS

Interventional radiology has become a complex discipline. The knowledge of all the pertinent information in this field cannot be served by one or two authors; therefore, the help of a large number of contributors has been solicited. We are most grateful to these nationally and internationally known experts for their willingness to contribute, in spite of their busy professional commitments and teaching schedules.

We are indebted to our teacher, Dr. Kurt Amplatz, affectionately known as "Kurt," for training us and serving as a constant stimulus throughout our lives. His teachings, wisdom, vision, and enthusiasm in the field of cardiovascular and interventional radiology have been carried over to his residents and fellows who have directly or indirectly contributed to this book. It is difficult to find enough praise and gratitude for the excellence and motivation he has created for us.

Many of the interventional radiological procedures that we perform today were envisioned by the late Charles T. Dotter. Though we have not had the privilege or the honor to work with this "legend," we acknowledge his pioneering principles which have led to the explosion of the current interventional techniques in radiology.

We thank the present and past residents and fellows for the case material included in this book. It was the result of their hard work while training at The University of Minnesota Hospital and Clinic. A special "thank you" for David W. Hunter and Joseph W. Yedlicka, Jr. for taking on the clinical load, allowing us to complete this Second Edition on time, and to Dr. Marcos A. Herrera for the invaluable assistance provided in helping to rewrite several of the manuscripts.

The excellent quality of the artwork depicting the technicalities of the various procedures is the result of innumerable hours put in by Mr. Martin Finch, Head of Biomedical Graphics at the University of Minnesota Hospital and Clinic. We feel his artwork is second to none.

The publication of this book was only possible with the dedication and patience of Ms. Carla J. Nelson who typed innumerable revisions to the chapters of this book.

CONTRIBUTORS

John E. Abele
President, Medi-tech Incorporated
Watertown, Massachusetts

Richard N. Aizpuru, M.D.
Instructor of Radiology
Department of Radiology
University of Minnesota Hospital and Clinic
Minneapolis, Minnesota

Sandra J. Althaus, M.D.
Instructor of Radiology
Department of Radiology
University of Minnesota Hospital and Clinic
Minneapolis, Minnesota

Kurt Amplatz, M.D.
Professor of Radiology
Director, Division of Cardiovascular and
    Interventional Radiology
Department of Radiology
University of Minnesota Hospital and Clinic
Minneapolis, Minnesota

Francesco Antonucci, M.D.
Staff Radiologist
Radiologisches Institut
Kantonsspital Winterthur
Winterthur, Switzerland

Klemens H. Barth, M.D.
Professor of Radiology
Department of Radiology
Georgetown University Hospital
Washington, D.C.

John L. Bass, M.D.
Associate Professor of Pediatrics
Pediatric Cardiology
University of Minnesota Hospital and Clinic
Minneapolis, Minnesota

Gary J. Becker, M.D.
Director, Interventional Radiology
Department of Radiology
Miami Vascular Institute
Baptist Hospital
Miami, Florida

Wolfgang Beinborn, M.D.
Staff Radiologist
Department of Radiology
Aggertalklinik
Engelskirchen, Germany

Raymond E. Bertino, M.D.
Clinical Assistant Professor of Radiology
Midwest Institute for Interventional Therapy
St. Francis Medical Center
Peoria, Illinois

Heraldur Bjarnason, M.D.
Medical Fellow Specialist
Department of Radiology
University of Minnesota Hospital and Clinic
Minneapolis, Minnesota

T. J. Bowker, M.A., M.R.C.P.
Medical Registrar
The National Heart Hospital and University
    College Hospital
London, England

Terry M. Brady, M.D.
Clinical Assistant Professor of Radiology
Midwest Institute for Interventional Therapy
St. Francis Medical Center
Peoria, Illinois

Werner Brühlman, M.D.
Professor of Radiology
Department of Diagnostic Radiology
Stadtspital Triemli
Zürich, Switzerland

Peter Bub, M.D.
Associate Professor of Urology
Department of Surgery
Katharinen Hospital
Stuttgart, Germany

Dana R. Burke, M.D.
Director of Interventional Radiology
Department of Radiology
Suburban Hospital
Bethesda, Maryland

Vicente Cabrera, M.D.
Chairman of Vascular Surgery
Department of Surgery
Hospital Nuestra Señora del Pino
Las Palmas, Canary Islands, Spain

John F. Cardella, M.D.

Associate Professor of Radiology
Chief of Cardiovascular/Interventional Radiology
Department of Radiology
Milton S. Hershey Medical Center
Penn State University
Hershey, Pennsylvania

John E. Carlson, M.D.

Medical Fellow Specialist
Department of Radiology
University of Minnesota Hospital and Clinic
Minneapolis, Minnesota

C. Humberto Carrasco, M.D.

Professor of Radiology
Department of Diagnostic Radiology
The University of Texas M. D. Anderson Cancer Center
Houston, Texas

Giovanna Casola, M.D.

Associate Clinical Professor of Radiology
Department of Radiology
University of California San Diego Medical Center
San Diego, California

Flavio Castañeda, M.D.

Clinical Assistant Professor of Radiology
Midwest Institute for Interventional Therapy
St. Francis Medical Center
Peoria, Illinois

Wilfrido R. Castañeda-Zúñiga, M.D., M.Sc.

Professor of Radiology
Department of Radiology
University of Minnesota Hospital and Clinic
Minneapolis, Minnesota

Chusilp Charnsangavej, M.D.

Professor and Deputy Department Chair of Radiology
Department of Diagnostic Radiology
The University of Texas M. D. Anderson Cancer Center
Houston, Texas

Rami Chemali, M.D.

Fellow in Radiology
Service Central de Radiologie
Hôpital de Toulouse
Toulouse, France

Vincent P. Chuang, M.D.

Professor of Radiology
Department of Diagnostic Radiology
The University of Texas M. D. Anderson Cancer Center
Houston, Texas

Ralph V. Clayman, M.D.

Professor of Urology and Radiology
Department of Surgery, Division of Urology
Washington University School of Medicine
St. Louis, Missouri

Carol C. Coleman, M.D.

Associate Professor of Radiology
Chief, Cardiovascular and Interventional Radiology
Department of Radiology
Veterans Affairs Medical Center
Minneapolis, Minnesota

Frank Comhaire, M.D., Ph.D.

Associate Professor of Medicine
Department of Internal Medicine
Division of Endocrinology
State University Hospital
Ghent, Belgium

Dewey J. Conces, Jr., M.D.

Associate Professor of Radiology
Department of Radiology
Indiana University Medical Center
Wishard Memorial Hospital
Indianapolis, Indiana

Andrew H. Cragg, M.D.

Assistant Professor of Radiology
Chief of Vascular Radiology
University of Iowa Hospitals and Clinics
Iowa City, Iowa

Aracelli Cruz, M.D.

Staff Vascular Surgeon
Department of Surgery
Hospital Nuestra Señora del Pino
Las Palmas, Canary Islands, Spain

Horacio D'Agostino, M.D.

Assistant Professor of Radiology
Department of Radiology
University of California San Diego Medical Center
San Diego, California

Mariano DeBlas, M.D.

Chief, Cardiovascular and Interventional Radiology
Department of Radiology
Hospital de Guipúzcoa
Donostia-San Sebastian, Spain

Riccardo Di Segni, M.D.

Aiuto Radiologo
Reparto Centrale di Radiologia e Diagnostica per
    Immagini
Ospedale S. Giovanni
Rome, Italy

William J. Drasler, Ph.D.

Vice-President of Research and Development
Possis Medical, Inc.
Minneapolis, Minnesota

Robert G. Dutcher, M.S.

President and Chief Operating Officer
Possis Medical, Inc.
Minneapolis, Minnesota

Morteza K. Elyaderani, M.D.
Director of Radiology
Department of Radiology
Aliquippa Hospital
Aliquippa, Pennsylvania

Christopher E. Engeler, M.D.
Medical Fellow Specialist
Department of Radiology
University of Minnesota Hospital and Clinic
Minneapolis, Minnesota

Cesar Ercole, M.D.
Instructor of Surgery
Department of Urologic Surgery
University of Minnesota Hospital and Clinic
Minneapolis, Minnesota

Deborah Fein–Millar, M.D.
Staff Radiologist
Department of Radiologic Science and Diagnostic Imaging
Shadyside Hospital
Pittsburgh, Pennsylvania

José Manuel Felices, M.D.
Fellow
Vascular and Interventional Radiology
Hospital Nuestra Señora del Pino
Las Palmas, Canary Islands, Spain

Charitha C. Fernando, B.H.B., MB.ChB., D.R.A.C.R.
Consultant Radiologist
Department of Radiology
Wairau Hospital
Blenheim, New Zealand

Nikolaus L. Freudenberg, M.D.
Professor of Pathology
University of Freiburg
Freiburg, Germany

Carmen Garcia, M.D.
Fellow
Vascular and Interventional Radiology
Hospital Nuestra Señora del Pino
Las Palmas, Canary Islands, Spain

José García–Medina, M.D.
Resident
Vascular and Interventional Radiology
Hospital Nuestra Señora del Pino
Las Palmas, Canary Islands, Spain

Vladimir G. Germashev, M.D.
Research Collaborator
National Research Center of Surgery
USSR Academy of Medical Science
Moscow, USSR

José Felix Gonzalez, M.D.
Resident
Vascular and Interventional Radiology
Hospital Nuestra Señora del Pino
Las Palmas, Canary Islands, Spain

Elias Górriz, M.D.
Staff Radiologist
Vascular and Interventional Radiology
Hospital Neustra Señora del Pino
Las Palmas, Canary Islands, Spain

John N. Graber, M.D., F.A.C.S.
Staff Surgeon
Department of Surgery
Abbott Northwestern Hospital
Minneapolis, Minnesota

Wilson Greatbatch, Ph.D.
President
Chairman of the Board
Greatbatch Gen-Aid Enterprises, Inc.
Clarence, New York

Edward J. Grogan, C.C.E.
Director, Biomedical Engineering Department
The Alexandria Hospital
Alexandria, Virginia

Cayetano Guerra, M.D.
Division Head, Gastroenterology
Gastroenterology Department
Hospital Nuestra Señora del Pino
Las Palmas, Canary Islands, Spain

Masakazu Hasegawa, M.D.
Assistant Professor of Radiology
Kobe University School of Medicine
Kobe, Japan

Asuncion Hernandez, M.D.
Head, Department of Radiology
Hospital Nuestra Señora del Pino
Las Palmas, Canary Islands, Spain

Marcos A. Herrera, M.D.
Assistant Professor of Radiology
Department of Radiology
Veterans Affairs Medical Center
Minneapolis, Minnesota

David Hickok, M.D., F.A.C.S.
Staff Surgeon
Department of Surgery
Abbott Northwestern Hospital
Minneapolis, Minnesota

Shozo Hirota, M.D.
Assistant Professor of Radiology
Kobe University School of Medicine
Kobe, Japan

Robert W. Holden, M.D.
> Professor of Radiology
> Indiana University;
> Chief of Radiology
> Department of Radiology
> Wishard Memorial Hospital
> Indianapolis, Indiana

Keith M. Horton, M.D.
> Instructor of Radiology
> Department of Radiology
> University of Minnesota Hospital and Clinic
> Minneapolis, Minnesota

John C. Hulbert, M.D., F.R.C.S.
> Associate Professor of Urologic Surgery
> Department of Surgery
> University of Minnesota Hospital and Clinic
> Minneapolis, Minnesota

David W. Hunter, M.D.
> Professor of Radiology
> Department of Radiology
> University of Minnesota Hospital and Clinic
> Minneapolis, Minnesota

J. Duncan Irving, M.B., B.S., F.R.C.R.
> Consultant—Research and Development
> Cook, Incorporated;
> Emeritus Consultant Radiologist
> Guy's and Lewisham Hospitals;
> Honorary Consultant Radiologist
> Hammersmith and the Royal Free Hospitals;
> Honorary Senior Lecturer
> Royal Postgraduate Medical School
> University of London
> London, England

Mark L. Jenson, B.S.
> Senior Project Engineer
> Possis Medical, Inc.
> Minneapolis, Minnesota

William E. Jobe, M.D.
> Chairman
> Radiology Imaging Associates, P.C.;
> Swedish Medical Center;
> Porter Memorial Hospital;
> Littleton Hospital
> Englewood, Colorado

Francis Joffre, M.D.
> Professor of Radiology
> Service Central de Radiologie
> Hôpital de Toulouse
> Toulouse, France

Danna E. Johnson, M.D.
> Assistant Professor of Pathology
> Department of Pathology
> Medical College of Virginia
> Richmond, Virginia

Louis I. Juravsky, M.D., F.R.C.P.(C)
> Assistant Professor of Clinical Radiology
> Interventional Radiologist
> Department of Radiology
> Dartmouth–Hitchcock Medical Center
> Hanover, New Hampshire

Martin Kaltenbach, M.D.
> Professor of Medicine
> Abteilung für Kardiologie
> Klinikum der Universitat
> Frankfurt am Main, Germany

Keith W. Kaye, M.D.
> Clinical Associate Professor of Urologic Surgery
> University of Minnesota Hospital and Clinic;
> Twin Cities Urology, P.A.
> Minneapolis, Minnesota

Kenneth Kensey, M.D.
> Kensey Nash Corporation
> Marsh Creek Corporate Center
> Exton, Pennsylvania

Eugene C. Klatte, M.D.
> Distinguished Professor and Chairman of Radiology
> Department of Radiology
> Indiana University School of Medicine
> Indianapolis, Indiana

Jürgen Kollath, M.D.
> Professor of Medicine
> Center of Radiology
> J. W. Goethe-University Hospital
> Frankfurt, Germany

Harvey A. Koolpe, M.D.
> Clinical Associate Professor of Radiology
> Temple University;
> Department of Radiology
> Albert Einstein Medical Center
> Philadelphia, Pennsylvania

Marc Kunnen, M.D., Ph.D.
> Associate Professor of Radiology
> Department of Radiology
> State University Hospital
> Ghent, Belgium

Helmut Landgraf, M.D.
> Professor of Medicine
> Center of Internal Medicine
> J. W. Goethe-University Hospital
> Frankfurt, Germany

David Lawrence, M.D.
> Associate Professor of Radiology
> Department of Diagnostic Radiology
> The University of Texas M. D. Anderson Cancer Center
> Houston, Texas

Won J. Lee, M.D.

Associate Professor of Radiology
Section Head, Genitourinary Radiology
Department of Radiology
Long Island Jewish Medical Center
New Hyde Park, New York

Janis Gissel Letourneau, M.D.

Associate Professor of Radiology
Department of Radiology
University of Minnesota Hospital and Clinic
Minneapolis, Minnesota

Robert G. Levitt, M.D.

Staff Radiologist
Barnes County West Hospital
Creve Coeur, Missouri

Dieter Liermann, M.D.

Staff Radiologist
University of Frankfurt
Frankfurt, Germany

Deborah G. Longley, M.D.

Assistant Professor of Radiology
Department of Radiology
University of Minnesota Hospital and Clinic
Minneapolis, Minnesota

Dierk Maass, M.D.

Professor of Surgery
University of Zürich
Zürich, Switzerland

Robert D. Mackie, M.D.

Department of Radiology
Abbott Northwestern Hospital
Minneapolis, Minnesota

Manuel Maynar, M.D.

Professor of Radiology
Chief, Vascular Interventional Radiology
Department of Radiology
Hospital Nuestra Señora del Pino
Las Palmas, Canary Islands, Spain

Gordon K. McLean, M.D.

Director, Angiography and Interventional Radiology
Department of Radiology
The Western Pennsylvania Hospital
Pittsburgh, Pennsylvania

Steven G. Meranze, M.D.

Staff Radiologist
Department of Radiology
Section of Cardiovascular and Interventional Radiology
The Alexandria Hospital
Alexandria, Virginia

Richard L. Morin, Ph.D.

Assistant Professor
Department of Diagnostic Radiology
Mayo Clinic Jacksonville
Jacksonville, Florida

Amir Motarjeme, M.D.

Director of Peripheral Services
Midwest Cardiovascular Institute
Downers Grove, Illinois

Peter R. Mueller, M.D.

Associate Professor of Radiology
Division Head, Abdominal Imaging and
    Interventional Radiology
Department of Radiology
Massachusetts General Hospital
Boston, Massachusetts

Emilio Ojeda, M.D.

Staff Hematologist
Hematology Department
Hospital Nuestra Señora del Pino
Las Palmas, Canary Islands, Spain

Charles M. Orr, M.D.

Staff Cardiologist
Department of Medicine
St. Vincent's Hospital and Health Science Center
Indianapolis, Indiana

Christa Paasch, M.D.

Center of Radiology
J. W. Goethe-University Hospital
Frankfurt, Germany

Julio C. Palmaz, M.D.

Professor of Radiology
Chief, Division of Cardiovascular and Special
    Interventional Radiology
Department of Radiology
The University of Texas Health Science Center
San Antonio, Texas

Steve H. Parker, M.D.

Radiologist
Radiology Imaging Associates, P.C.;
Swedish Medical Center;
Porter Memorial Hospital;
Littleton Hospital
Englewood, Colorado

Thomas Peters, M.D.

Staff Cardiologist
Department of Medicine
St. Vincent's Hospital and Health Science Center
Indianapolis, Indiana

Joseph Pietrafitta, M.D., F.A.C.S.

Staff Surgeon
Department of Surgery
Abbott Northwestern Hospital
Minneapolis, Minnesota

Cass A. Pinkerton, M.D.

Staff Cardiologist
Department of Medicine
St. Vincent's Hospital and Health Science Center
Indianapolis, Indiana

Eugenio Ponomar–Sulepov, M.D., Ph.D.

Director of Interventional Radiology
Department of Radiology
Hospital Universitario de Oviedo
Oviedo, Spain

Zinon C. Possis, B.Mech.E.

Chairman and Chief Executive Officer
Possis Medical, Inc.
Minneapolis, Minnesota

Ingeborg Prignitz, M.D.

Staff Radiologist
Department of Radiology
Aggertalklinik
Engelskirchen, Germany

Emmanuil I. Protonotarios, M.S.

Project Engineer
Possis Medical, Inc.
Minneapolis, Minnesota

Juan M. Pulido–Duque, M.D.

Staff Radiologist
Radiologia Vascular Intervencionista
Hospital Nuestra Señora del Pino
Las Palmas, Canary Islands, Spain

Joseff E. Rabkin, M.D., Ph.D.

Professor of Radiology
Chief Roentgenologist of the USSR Ministry of Health
Head of Roentgeno-Radiology Department
National Research Center of Surgery
USSR Academy of Medical Science
Moscow, USSR

Pratap K. Reddy, M.D.

Associate Professor of Urologic Surgery
University of Minnesota Hospital and Clinic;
Chief, Urology Section
Department of Surgery
Veterans Affairs Medical Center
Minneapolis, Minnesota

Ricardo Reyes, M.D.

Staff Radiologist
Radiologia Vascular Intervencionista
Hospital Nuestra Señora del Pino
Las Palmas, Canary Islands, Spain

William R. Richli, M.D.

Associate Professor of Radiology
Department of Diagnostic Radiology
The University of Texas M .D. Anderson Cancer Center
Houston, Texas

Albert P. Rocchini, M.D.

Professor of Pediatrics
Pediatric Cardiology
University of Minnesota Hospital and Clinic
Minneapolis, Minnesota

Josef Rösch, M.D.

Professor of Radiology,
Director, Charles Dotter Memorial Institute
The Oregon Health Science University School of Medicine
Portland, Oregon

Franz Josef Roth, M.D.

Director
Department of Radiology
Aggertalklinik
Engelskirchen, Germany

Hervé Rousseau, M.D.

Professor of Radiology
Service Central de Radiologie
Hôpital de Toulouse
Toulouse, France

Masao Sako, M.D.

Associate Professor of Radiology
Kobe University School of Medicine
Kobe, Japan

Erich Salomonowitz, M.D.

Professor of Radiology
University of Vienna
Vienna, Austria

Beate Schneider, M.D.

Resident
Department of Radiology
Diakonissenkrankenhaus Karlsruhe-Rüppurr
Akademisches Lehrkrankenhaus der Universität Freiburg
Abteilung Röntgendiagnostik und Nuklearmedizin
Freiburg, Germany

Werner Schoop, M.D.

Professor of Medicine
University of Freiburg
Freiburg, Germany

Leonard Schultz, M.D., F.A.C.S.

Assistant Professor of Surgery
University of Minnesota Hospital and Clinic;
Staff Surgeon
Department of Surgery
Abbott Northwestern Hospital
Minneapolis, Minnesota

Donald E. Schwarten, M.D.

Director of Cardiovascular Laboratory
Department of Radiology
St. Vincent's Hospital and Health Science Center
Indianapolis, Indiana

J. Bayne Selby, Jr., M.D.

Assistant Professor of Radiology
Department of Radiology
University of Virginia Medical Center
Charlottesville, Virginia

John D. Slack, M.D.
Staff Cardiologist
Department of Medicine
St. Vincent's Hospital and Health Science Center
Indianapolis, Indiana

Tony P. Smith, M.D.
Assistant Professor of Radiology
Department of Radiology
University of Iowa Hospitals and Clinics
Iowa City, Iowa

Samuel K. S. So, M.B., B.S.
Assistant Professor of Surgery
Department of Surgery
Washington University School of Medicine
St. Louis, Missouri

Erhard Starck, M.D.
Professor of Radiology
Städtishche Kliniken Kassel
Akademisches Lehrkrankenhaus der Philips-Universität
    Marburg
Zentrum für Radiologie
Kassel, Germany

Ernst–Peter Strecker, M.D.
Professor and Chairman
Department of Radiology
Diakonissen-Krankenhaus Karlsruhe-Rüppurr
Akademisches Lehrkrankenhaus der Universität Freiburg
Abteilung Röntgendiagnostik und Nuklearmedizin
Freiburg, Germany

S. Murthy Tadavarthy, M.D.
Clinical Associate Professor of Radiology
University of Minnesota Hospital and Clinic;
Cardiovascular Radiologist
Minneapolis Heart Institute;
Co-Director, Cardiovascular and Interventional Radiology
Abbott Northwestern Hospital
Minneapolis, Minnesota

Robert D. Tarver, M.D.
Associate Professor of Radiology
Department of Radiology
Indiana University Medical Center
Wishard Memorial Hospital
Indianapolis, Indiana

Charles J. Tegtmeyer, M.D.
Professor of Radiology, Associate Professor of Anatomy
Director of Angiography, Interventional Radiology, and
    Special Procedures
Department of Radiology
University of Virginia Medical Center
Charlottesville, Virginia

Joseph M. Thielen
Technologist
Possis Medical, Inc.
Minneapolis, Minnesota

Patricia E. Thorpe, M.D.
Assistant Professor of Radiology
Chief, Vascular and Interventional Radiology
Department of Radiology
Creighton University Medical Center
Omaha, Nebraska

Amy S. Thurmond, M.D.
Assistant Professor of Ultrasound and Obstetrics and
    Gynecology
Department of Diagnostic Radiology
The Oregon Health Sciences University
Portland, Oregon

Ricardo Tobío, M.D.
Chief, Diagnostic Radiology
Hospital Central de la Cruz Roja
Madrid, Spain

Christian Vallbracht, M.D.
Staff Cardiologist
Department of Cardiology
J. W. Goethe-University
Frankfurt, Germany

Eric vanSonnenberg, M.D.
Professor of Radiology and Medicine
Department of Radiology
University of California San Diego Medical Center
San Diego, California

James W. VanTassel, M.D.
Staff Cardiologist
Department of Medicine
St. Vincent's Hospital and Health Science Center
Indianapolis, Indiana

Ivan Vujic, M.D.
Professor of Radiology
Department of Radiology
Medical College of South Carolina
Charleston, South Carolina

Hans–Joachim Wagner, M.D., O.A.
Staff Radiologist
Städtische Kliniken Kassel
Institute für Röntgendiagnostik
Kassel, Germany

Sidney Wallace, M.D.
Professor and Chair of Radiology
Department of Diagnostic Radiology
The University of Texas M. D. Anderson Cancer Center
Houston, Texas

Bruce F. Waller, M.D.
Staff Radiologist
St. Vincent Professional Building
Indianapolis, Indiana

Michael Westphal, M.D.
Chief, Department of Radiology
Krankenhaus Neukölln
Berlin, Germany

Mark H. Wholey, M.D.
Chairman
Department of Radiologic Science and Diagnostic Imaging
Shadyside Hospital
Pittsburgh, Pennsylvania

Hellmut R. D. Wolf, M. D.
Staff Radiologist
Department of Internal Medicine
Diakonissenkrankenhaus Karlsruhe-Rüppurr
Akademisches Lehrkrankenhaus der Universität Freiburg
Abteilung Röntgendiagnostik und Nuklearmedizin
Freiburg, Germany

Wayne F. Yakes, M.D.
Radiologist
Radiology Imaging Associates, P.C.;
Swedish Medical Center;
Porter Memorial Hospital;
Chief, U.S. Army Medical Corps
Chief, Cardiovascular and Interventional Radiology
Chief, Neuroradiology and Interventional Neuroradiology
Fitzsimons Army Medical Center
Aurora, Colorado

Joseph W. Yedlicka, Jr., M.D.
Assistant Professor of Radiology
Department of Radiology
University of Minnesota Hospital and Clinic
Minneapolis, Minnesota

Antony T. Young, F.R.A.C.R.
Radiologist
Department of Radiology
Christchurch Hospital
Christchurch, New Zealand

Heun Y. Yune, M.D.
Professor of Radiology
Department of Radiology
Indiana University Hospital
Indianapolis, Indiana

Robert M. Zeit, M.D.
Clinical Associate Professor of Radiology
Temple University;
Department of Radiology
Albert Einstein Medical Center
Philadelphia, Pennsylvania

Christoph L. Zollikofer, M.D.
Professor and Chairman
Radiologisches Institut
Kantonsspital Winterthur
Winterthur, Switzerland

CONTENTS

INTRODUCTION

INTERVENTIONAL RADIOLOGY: YESTERDAY, TODAY, TOMORROW[a]

—Wilfrido R. Castañeda–Zúñiga, M.D., M.Sc.

The origins of interventional radiology are in the angiographic Seldinger techniques developed by cardiovascular radiologists in the late 1950s and early 1960s. Using these angiographic principles, one can gain access to many organ systems by percutaneous puncture. Performance of such percutaneous radiologic procedures has been facilitated by the development of high-resolution image-intensified fluoroscopy, ultrasound (US), and computed tomography (CT). Moreover, interventional radiology has benefited from rapid developments in materials science and biotechnology.

In this brief introduction, I review the development of interventional radiology and speculate about its future and the preparation we need to make for it. In doing so, I caution that it is difficult to predict the future of such a rapidly changing field as interventional radiology.

INTERVENTIONAL CARDIOVASCULAR RADIOLOGY

As interventional radiology has its foundations in cardiovascular procedures, it is appropriate that this survey begins there.

The nonsurgical hemodynamic correction of occlusive atherosclerotic disease with the aid of coaxial Teflon dilators was first reported by Dotter and Judkins in 1964. This trial followed Dotter's incidental observation of recanalization of a totally occluded right common iliac artery by an angiographic catheter during conventional diagnostic angiography.

Because of the excessive shearing and the "snowplowing" effect produced by Dotter's coaxial techniques, modifications were devised by Staples and subsequently by Van Andel. The main disadvantage of the Teflon dilators

persisted, however; their small size limited their use to arteries no more than 4mm in diameter, because larger dilators were associated with an unacceptably high frequency of local complications. To overcome these technical limitations, Portsmann described a "caged" or "corset" balloon catheter in 1973. This catheter system employed a latex balloon enclosed in a Teflon dilator with strips cut out from the area overlying the balloon to minimize the propensity of the latex to deform with inflation in the atherosclerotic lesion. However, because of the large size of the caged catheter and its high thrombogenicity, these modifications did not change the prevailing attitude of surgeons and radiologists in the United States to the Dotter technique. In contrast, in Europe, thousands of Dotter procedures were performed at leading academic institutions, with excellent immediate and long-term results being reported by Zeitler, Portsmann, Schoop, Van Andel, and many others.

It was not until 1974 that one of Zeitler's former students, the late Andreas Grüntzig, and his colleague, Hopff, developed a nonexpandable dual-lumen balloon that produced safe, fast dilatation of narrowed vessel segments by applying radial forces against the plaque and arterial wall. In addition, the wide variety of balloon sizes available for Grüntzig catheters allowed dilatation of vessels as large as the aorta while minimizing the size of the puncture needed for catheter insertion. This catheter and its progeny are now used for dilatation procedures by many different groups. The physiopathologic changes produced by balloon angioplasty were studied extensively by University of Minnesota researchers including Amplatz, Formanek, Edwards, Zollikofer, and Laerum, who described the "controlled vascular injury" that is produced.

Cragg enriched and expanded this theory with his meticulous evaluation of the physiologic changes occurring at the cellular level. With this understanding of the physiopathologic phenomena, it has been possible to formulate more rational pharmacologic management of the acute complications of the procedure and to enhance the long-

---

[a]Excerpted from the Malcolm B. Hanson Memorial Lecture. University of Minnesota Continuing Medical Education. Radiology Annual Course, September 1986.

term patency rates of dilated vessels. The long-term results of transluminal angioplasty in properly selected patients are equivalent to the results achieved with the traditional surgical methods, often with a lower morbidity. Moreover, in most cases, angioplasty can easily be repeated if the first procedure is a failure or if the narrowing recurs. As a result, angioplasty is supplanting surgery for some diseases, such as peripheral vascular obstructions, which traditionally would be treated by the femoropopliteal bypass technique.

Five-year patency rates in peripheral angioplasty range from 90% in the iliac vessels to 60–70% for long-segment recanalization of superficial femoral artery lesions. Transluminal angioplasty is particularly useful in patients with renovascular hypertension, where the best results are obtained in patients with fibromuscular dysplasia, with patency rates between 80–90% at five years. Lower patency rates are obtained for atherosclerotic lesions, depending on the location and bilaterality of the lesion. The technique is complementary to operation in other settings such as coronary artery disease. Given these promising results, the time may have come for a more aggressive approach to patients with early symptoms of atherosclerotic vascular disease who might not be considered surgical candidates.

Perhaps in the near future one can consider removing some of these obstructive lesions rather than fracturing, remodeling, and displacing them, as is done with transluminal angioplasty. Several investigators have attempted to resolve the many problems involved with the intravascular use of laser radiation to ablate atherosclerotic lesions, with the hope that by removing the atherosclerotic plaque by the application of laser energy, a better long-term result could be obtained. In spite of the encouraging earlier reports, this has not been the case.

Despite the extensive clinical use of lasers to treat peripheral vascular disease, many fundamental questions concerning the clinical role of lasers remain unanswered. Prospective randomized studies are needed to assess whether laser-assisted angioplasty confers better patency than balloon angioplasty. Similarly, it remains to be shown whether laser recanalization of long occlusions, which cannot be treated by catheter and wire techniques, is an appropriate alternative to surgery.

It is possible that new methods of laser energy delivery, different wavelengths, larger probes, and improved guidance systems will, in the future, enable ablation of atheroma with a reduced complication rate. Lasers may allow percutaneous therapy for patients with peripheral vascular disease who are unlikely to benefit from standard techniques, but further clinical research is required before general usage can be advocated scientifically. As stated by Cragg, "Lasers may revolutionize the treatment of vascular disease some day, but until their clinical usefulness is established by rigorous scientific methods, they should remain investigational devices."

Designs for percutaneous atherectomy devices have been conceived out of frustration with the limitations of conventional angioplasty, especially with the poor long-term results obtained in the management of total arterial occlusions. The ideal atherectomy device has not been designed. Possibly, no one instrument can circumvent all the disadvantages of balloon angioplasty and provide the desired clinical and angiographic results.

With angioplasty, we attempt to restore adequate blood supply by increasing the intraluminal diameter with barotrauma. This is done by fracture of the atheromatous intima rather than by removal of the atherosclerotic plaque, as in atherectomy. Atherectomy catheters attempt to remove plaque with minimal injury to the vessel, no significant distal embolization, and a low incidence of restenosis. Atherectomy devices can be divided in two large groups: mechanical recanalization devices and percutaneous atherectomy devices.

Mechanical Recanalization Devices

The purpose of these devices is to recanalize segmental vascular obstructions. Their main indication is to help the recanalization in those cases where conventional angiographic recanalization techniques have failed. It has been demonstrated that if balloon angioplasty is attempted in patients with severe ischemia, about 90% of those lesions under 10cm long, and 70–80% of those longer than 10cm, can be crossed with a guidewire. More commonly, reported failure rates for peripheral vascular procedures fall between 10 and 20%, with most of the failures to recanalize occurring in complete occlusions. For coronary angioplasty, the failure rate ranges from 8% for stenoses to 33% for occlusions.

Several devices have been designed to try to overcome the difficulties of recanalizing vascular occlusions. Mechanical recanalizing devices are power driven. By rotation at low or high speed or by pulsating, they create a channel through an area of vascular occlusion. The following devices are included:

Low-speed recanalizing devices:
—Vallbracht slow rotational recanalizing wire;
—Zeitler pulsating wire;
—Wholey reperfusion atherolytic wire.
High-speed recanalizing atheroablating devices:
—Kensey dynamic angioplasty catheter;
—Pfeifer milling catheter;
—Auth rotational atherectomy catheter;
—Ultrasonic atherolysis.

All of these devices typically create a channel as large as the rotating part by laterally displacing or ablating atheromatous/thrombotic occlusions. Characteristically, no tissue is extracted.

Percutaneous Atherectomy Devices

Included in this group of devices are several ingenious instruments designed to excise atheromatous lesions, either stenoses or complete vascular occlusions. Among them are:

—Bard rotary atherectomy system (BRAS);
—Transluminal extraction catheter (TEC);
—Simpson directional atherectomy catheter.

Typically, these devices create a channel of a diameter equal to that of the catheter tip by excising and removing atheromatous/thrombotic material. The Simpson directional atherectomy catheter is the only atherectomy device that allows full restoration of the vessel lumen to its original dimensions.

Vascular Stents

Intense activity has been seen during the past decade in the area of vascular stents. Following the initial description by Dotter of a percutaneously implantable vascular endoprosthesis, many years passed until Palmaz described his stent. This work led to the development of several other stents, including the Wallstent, Strecker, Gianturco, Gianturco–Roubin, Wiktor, and Cordis stents, among others. Most of these stents are still in a developmental stage, with the exception of the Palmaz and the Wallstent. These two stents have been implanted in hundreds of patients, mostly in Europe, but also in the United States. Slowly, their indications, complications, and long-term results are evolving. We will see their extensive use in the near future.

Intravascular Ultrasound (IVUS)

This newly developed technology offers a unique perspective, allowing us to see through the wall of a vessel from the inside out. The exact role of IVUS in the diagnostic armamentarium of the interventionalist is evolving. It seems that its main application will be in the assessment of the results of percutaneous revascularization techniques, mostly to decide whether or not an additional procedure is necessary—for example, placement of a stent following a percutaneous transluminal angioplasty.

Cautionary Word

It should be emphasized that the different percutaneous revascularization techniques are complementary, not competitive. The best approach to a given lesion or series of lesions is a thoughtful, combined one using the technology best suited for diagnosis and treatment. Selection of a suitable sequence of devices and therapies, including thrombolysis, angioplasty, atherectomy, and stenting, requires knowledge of the strengths and weaknesses of each device,

as well as an understanding of the patient's pathology. For example, atherectomy devices have been shown to be superior in removing calcified plaque, whereas the laser is known to be very effective in penetrating organized thrombus, which is not calcified. Thus, in lieu of the perfect all-purpose instrument, the ideal approach is one which can best utilze the devices available in the angiography suite in the most suitable sequence determined by the pathology and the patient's overall clinical status. Continued application of any device should be based on careful clinical follow-up designed to evaluate how well the device or combination of devices contributes to the satisfactory outcome. The initial technical success should be correlated with the eventual clinical success or lack thereof. Such data are still forthcoming on all of the devices currently in clinical use.

Thrombolysis

Of course, not all vascular obstructions are plaques or stenoses. Some are thrombi or emboli. These, too, can be managed by the interventional radiologist. The discovery of streptokinase by Tillett and Garner in 1933 and of urokinase by McFarlane in 1946, and the subsequent understanding of the interactions of these substances with the human fibrinolytic system, resulted in a wide variety of clinical applications. In 1959, Johnson and McCarthy reported clinical lysis of clot by the intravenous administration of streptokinase. This report initiated the use of high-dose intravenous systemic infusion of thrombolytic agents to lyse thrombi and thromboemboli. In 1973, a large therapeutic trial for pulmonary embolism showed greater resolution of thrombi and a significant improvement in pulmonary artery pressures and clinical status in those patients treated with thrombolytic agents rather than with heparin. Nonetheless, the use of thrombolytic agents fell into disfavor, mainly because of the fear of systemic complications, particularly hemorrhage.

In order to avoid the hemorrhagic complications, Dotter, in 1974, suggested delivering streptokinase locally to peripheral vascular occlusions at approximately one-twentieth the systemic dose. Despite good results, this new method did not become popular. Renthrop subsequently described the use of high-dose, short-duration infusion in the coronary arterial tree in 1979, and Katzen described the use of local low-dose infusions in the peripheral vasculature in 1981. These and subsequent reports attest to the efficacy and increased popularity of local thrombolytic therapy. However, one should remember Dotter's words of caution: "Thrombolysis is not curative; it merely restores patency and helps identify a local anatomical obstruction which requires treatment" and that "even in small doses thrombolysis can cause distal systemic complications." Moreover, several challenging problems associated with thrombolytic therapy remain, including the incidence of local complications, the high cost of the drugs, and the lengthy hospitalization required for complete resolution of clots.

Some of these problems may be resolved by the development of a new generation of thrombolytic substances, particularly tissue-type plasminogen activator (tPA), which can now be abundantly produced by recombinant genetic techniques. This agent acts only on clots and thus avoids the systemic fibrinolytic effects and their associated hemorrhagic complications. Because of the localized action of tPA, nursing demands and specialized care are markedly reduced for the management of thrombolysis with this agent compared with other techniques. Some even foresee the prophylactic use of tPA by emergency medical technicians during ambulance transport of patients suffering myocardial infarction.

Mechanical Thrombectomy

Several mechanical thrombectomy devices were tested in laboratory animals in the late 1980s, and undoubtedly they will be developed further in the 1990s. Their success will undoubtedly cut into the thrombolysis caseload by providing fast, highly successful lysis of thrombi.

Inferior Vena Cava Filters

The 1980s saw a great deal of activity in the development of new vena cava filters, including the titanium Greenfield, Simon nitinol, Vena-Tech, and bird's nest filters. All of these filters offer the availability of a smaller introducer system, a high filtering capability, and a low complication rate. Longer follow-up is, however, needed to define the exact value of each one of these filters.

Embolotherapy

Whereas angioplasty and thrombolysis have been developed to resolve vascular occlusion, embolotherapy has been developed to produce vascular occlusion. As technical advances in transcatheter vascular embolization have been made, the indications for the procedure have been defined more clearly. In many situations, embolotherapy is now an alternative to the more conventional techniques of surgery, radiation, and drugs. Without the availability of controlled clinical trials, however, it is difficult to define precisely the role of embolotherapy for any given clinical situation.

Although interest in embolotherapy has been greatest in the past decade, the principle of vascular embolization dates to 1904, when Dawbain described the preoperative injection of melted paraffin (Vaseline) into the external carotid arteries of patients suffering head and neck tumors. Brooks, in 1930, introduced particulate embolization with the occlusion of a traumatic carotid cavernous fistula by the injection of a muscle fragment attached to a silver clip into an internal carotid artery. Embolotherapy was influenced greatly by a landmark 1963 paper by Nusbaum and Baum, who demonstrated the angiographic detection of gastrointestinal bleeding at 0.5ml/min. Transcatheter management of hemorrhage soon followed, first achieved with intra-arterial infusions of vasopressin. This pharmacologic success was followed, in 1972, by Rösch's report of control of acute gastric hemorrhage by embolization of the gastroepiploic artery using autologous clot.

An upsurge of interest in embolization began in the 1970s, fostered by parallel developments in catheter technology and embolic agents. The availability of a wide range of preshaped catheters and the introduction of coaxial systems allowed relatively routine superselective catheter placement and embolic agent delivery. In 1972, the tissue adhesive isobutyl cyanoacrylate was described by Zanetti and Sherman. The use of Gelfoam particles as an embolic agent was first reported by Carey in 1974, as was the use of the permanent embolic agent Ivalon in its particulate form by Tadavarthy at the University of Minnesota.

Detachable balloons were first described by Serbinenko in the USSR in 1974 for the embolization of vascular malformations and aneurysms in the cerebral circulation, and the technique was subsequently perfected by Debrun, Kerber, and White. The concept of tissue ablation by absolute ethanol was introduced by Ellman in 1980. Klatte, also in 1980, reported its efficacy for the embolization of renal tumors.

In 1982, Amplatz illustrated the efficacy of boiling contrast medium to occlude veins in laboratory animals. Because of the difficulty in finding human volunteers to test the technique, he eventually had to volunteer a vein in his forearm for hot contrast injection. The vein was subsequently removed, and light microscopy confirmed what angiography had already shown: the complete obstruction of the venous channel.

For the occlusion of larger vascular structures, Gianturco created the wool coil, a current modification of which is now in widespread use, mainly for renal artery occlusion in patients with large renal cell carcinomas. Because of the risk of pulmonary or systemic embolization in patients with large arteriovenous fistulae (AVFs), self-retaining devices to prevent pulmonary embolization were described by Castañeda and Amplatz; a barbed coil was used safely to embolize a large postnephrectomy AVF in a patient with congestive heart failure and a renal allograft. For the same purpose, a spider-like device was described by the same investigators in 1981. Large AVFs have been obliterated safely since then, not only in the abdominal area, but also in the pulmonary circulation. A detachable spider was developed subsequently by Lund to obtain better control of the release. New technology developed since the first edition of this book includes minicatheters and microcoils. These new devices have greatly facilitated the management of peripheral and neurovascular lesions.

ABSCESS DRAINAGE

The technical advances made in diagnostic and interventional cardiovascular radiology have been easily transferred to the percutaneous managment of diseases in other organ systems. For many radiologists, this means the percutaneous management of infection.

Despite the widespread use of antibiotics, abdominal abscesses not treated with additional measures carry a mortality rate of 80%. Traditional surgical treatment is associated with a mortality rate of 20–43%. Cross-sectional imaging allows earlier detection of abdominal abscesses and provides a means for guidance of percutaneous drainage procedures. With accurate detection and guidance by US and CT, percutaneous catheter drainage of abdominal abscesses can be associated with a success rate of 80–85%. Certainly, the periprocedural mortality rate of catheter drainage, 6%, compares very favorably with that of operative drainage. In addition, percutaneous drainage is less traumatic and less disruptive of the normal anatomy.

Failures of percutaneous abscess drainage usually occur in patients who are not suitable candidates. Examples of collections unsuitable for percutaneous management are multiple and multiloculated abscesses with central necrosis and poorly defined parenchymal margins, necrotic tumors, lesions with communications to the gastrointestinal tract, and diffuse microabscesses or inflammatory phlegmons. The precise role of percutaneous abscess drainage must be defined by the use of randomized trials with rigidly prescribed protocols. These trials must segregate the results of drainage in immunocompromised and nonimmunocompromised patients, because the results of treatment are different in these two groups. Until the results of these studies are available, continued significant controversy about the virtues and defects of percutaneous drainage of abdominal abscesses can be expected. Unfortunately, patient selection cannot always be ideal; many percutaneous drainages will have to be performed on patients in poor physical and hemodynamic condition because they present an unacceptably high surgical risk. These patients cannot be denied the procedure, as it may represent their only hope for survival.

PERCUTANEOUS BIOPSIES

Percutaneous biopsy of lesions has become very popular with the advent of CT and US. A wide variety of needle designs has been developed in an attempt to obtain better samples for tissue diagnosis, rather than simply procuring cells for cytologic diagnosis. The latter study is not always available because of the pathologist's dislike for cell diagnosis in place of tissue diagnosis. Newer devices to automate and standardize biopsy samples for histology have been developed based on the Biopty biopsy gun. Palestrant has simplified the technique by developing an attachment for the CT scanner to facilitate aiming and tissue sampling.

RENAL INTERVENTION

Another target for percutaneous interventional techniques is the kidney. Percutaneous nephrostomy has been refined remarkably since its original description 30 years ago by Goodwin and his colleagues as a treatment of last resort. It is currently the preferred method of relieving supravesical urinary obstruction because of its ease of performance, its low morbidity, and its minuscule mortality rate. Moreover, percutaneous nephrostomy now is often but a prelude to other interventional procedures, such as dilation of ureteral strictures, incision of infundibular stenoses and ureteropelvic junction obstructions, stenting of ureteral fistulae, retrieval of fractured or blocked stents, local infusion of various chemotherapeutic agents, and even laser ablation of renal pelvic tumors. The introduction of catheters in and around the renal pelvis is accomplished easily with the use of fluoroscopy. Cross-sectional imaging elucidates basic anatomic relations, knowledge of which helps avoid complications such as colonic, hepatic, and splenic perforations.

The feasibility of removing renal stones through a percutaneously created nephrostomy tract was initially reported by Fernström and Johannson in 1976. In 1978, Smith et al. from the University of Minnesota reported the extraction of ureteral calculi through a percutaneous nephrostomy tract from a patient with an ileal loop. The development of nephrostomy tract dilators by Amplatz in 1982 led to the development of percutaneous techniques for the removal of retained urinary stones. Since then, many reports, from both Europe and the United States, have documented the success and safety of percutaneous nephrolithotomy in thousands of patients. The success rate of percutaneous nephrostomy is 95–98% for simple decompression of obstructive uropathy, with similar success rates reported for the establishment of the more complicated nephrostomy tracts sometimes needed in patients with retained urinary stones. High success rates (98%) in the removal of stones have been reported using a combination of techniques, including ultrasonic lithotripsy and stone basketing or grasping with additional endoscopic guidance.

The University of Minnesota approach to endourology has depended on the cooperation between the radiology and urology services. Such a team utilizes the anatomic background of the radiologist in selecting a suitable puncture site in an appropriate calix by formulating a three-dimensional image from multidirectional fluoroscopic capabilities. Catheter and guidewire manipulations are also the responsibility of the radiologist. On the other hand, the urologist is primarily responsible for the management of the patient. His or her experience with rigid and flexible endoscopes and their auxiliary instruments permits stone removal. Thus, successful percutaneous nephrolithotomy is accomplished using the combined skills of radiologists and urologists.

The present technique of nephrolithotomy is associated with little postoperative morbidity and no mortality. It allows the patient to resume normal activities within several days after hospital discharge. At the University of Minnesota, the procedure has even been performed on several asymptomatic patients who had compelling reasons for having their stones removed.

However, while percutaneous stone extraction techniques were being perfected, extracorporeal shock wave lithotripsy (SWL) was being developed. This technique uses radiographic localization of the calculus and a high-wave ultrasound beam for fragmentation. SWL has restricted the use of endourologic procedures to places where SWL is not available, those cases in which SWL has failed, many cases of ureteral stones, and to those cases of several particular types of stones, such as those trapped behind an obstruction, those which are radiolucent, and those that fill much of the collecting system or are infected. Therefore, percutaneous stone extraction will continue to be a significant means of management of patients with urinary tract calculi. One warning has to be given, however, concerning the long-term effects of SWL on the kidney. We do not know what effects SWL may have, because CT or magnetic resonance imaging studies are not routinely obtained. Carefully controlled studies are a necessity!

Newer developments in stone removal include progress in ureterorenoscopy with flexible instruments through which laser tubes involving a tunable dye laser are used to break ureteral stones.

PROSTATE INTERVENTION

The early 1980s saw the birth of prostatic intervention with balloon dilatation of the prostatic urethra. Long-term follow-up has shown an overall success rate of 60–70% at two years, while in selected patients, the success rate can be as high as 92% at two years. Longer follow-up is needed to assess whether balloon dilatation is a good alternative to transurethral resection of the prostate (TURP) in the management of benign prostatic hyperplasia (BPH). Other therapeutic alternatives to TURP include the placement of stents to hold the prostatic urethra open, such as the Fabian stent (a removable stent) and the Medinvent stent (a nonremovable stent). Several other stents are being tried currently. The exact role of stents in the management of BPH remains to be defined.

Prostatic hyperthermia has been used to treat BPH either by inducing atrophy of periurethral tissue or by causing thermic necrosis of the urethra and periurethral tissues. Further experimental work is needed to define clearly the safety parameters of this promising technique.

URETHRAL INTERVENTION

Balloon dilatation of urethral strictures has not provided a significant improvement over the traditional dila-

tation techniques. A better approach may be the placement of metal stents to hold the urethra open. Encouraging results have been reported by Dick in the United Kingdom. More extensive follow-up is, however, needed before widespread use of this technique is recommended.

BILIARY INTERVENTION

Diagnostic and therapeutic biliary intervention can be carried out in a fashion analogous to that in the urinary tract.

The diagnostic technique of percutaneous transhepatic cholangiography was originally described by Burkhardt and Mueller in 1921 with injections of the gallbladder through a needle introduced through the liver. In 1937, this technique was modified by Huard and Do-Xuanhuop, who injected Lipiodol into the bile ducts. However, direct cholangiography was not routinely performed until 1952, following the reports by Carter and Leger and their coworkers, who used a large needle. In 1974, Okuda popularized transhepatic cholangiography by using a long, thin, flexible needle in 114 patients, modifying a technique described earlier by Ohto and Tsuchiya. This fine-needle technique eliminated the need for operation immediately after the procedure. Compared with techniques that utilized a large needle, there was a reduction in the rate of intraperitoneal hemorrhage by a factor of 6, of bile leakage by a factor of 3, and of the procedure-associated mortality rate by a factor of 2.6.

In 1966, Seldinger reported his experience with transhepatic cholangiography by a right costal approach using a sheathed needle that allowed decompression of the biliary system at the time of cholangiography. Ferrucci and Ring refined and popularized the technique in this country. Decompression of biliary obstruction is now performed in patients with either primary or metastatic liver tumors and in those with benign biliary strictures and fistulae. Percutaneous biliary drainage also allows access for removal of retained biliary calculi. Specialized guidewires and catheters have been developed to pass through areas of stricture or obstruction; and their aid, indwelling catheters can be placed, and combined external-internal drainage with antegrade flow of bile into the bowel can be achieved.

The principal application of percutaneous biliary decompression has been in the nonsurgical palliation of malignant biliary obstruction. The traditional treatment has been the surgical creation of a biliary-enteric anastomosis, which is associated with significant morbidity and an operative mortality rate of 5–15%. Percutaneous drainage thus permits relief of cholestasis and its sequelae with relatively low risk. The criteria that determine whether a particular patient will undergo a surgical or a percutaneous decompression are both anatomic and physiologic. Patients with high or multiple branch obstructions are also candidates for percutaneous drainage. In contrast, patients with lower common duct or periampullary obstruction presenting in stable hemodynamic condition early in the course of their disease will typically undergo surgical palliation. This preselection of more favorable patients for operation has led to statements in the surgical literature which assert that open palliation is more effective than percutaneous biliary drainage in the management of biliary obstruction. However, when similar groups of patients are treated, or when correction is made by statistical analysis, similar morbidity and mortality rates are found.

By far, progress in biliary intervention during the past few years has occurred in the gallbladder area, where we have seen the rise of gallstone dissolution, a highly effective technique, and the rise and fall of gallstone extracorporeal lithotripsy, a highly ineffective technique, which did not fulfill the high expectations created by the earlier results in Germany. Mechanical fragmentation with the Kensey–Nash lithotrite has shown great promise, but the problem of a diseased gallbladder remains. Attempts to ablate the gallbladder percutaneously have up to this moment provided mixed results. Burhenne and Coleman's results in humans have clearly failed to provide a foolproof technique to ablate the gallbladder. It seems that they way of the future in gallbladder intervention is in percutaneous cholecystectomy techniques. More refinements and further experience will doubtless lead to the development of a reliable, safe technique.

GASTROINTESTINAL TRACT

In the previous edition, we discussed several techniques in the gastrointestinal (GI) tract that have since been developed further and have seen widespread use, including percutaneous gastrostomy, percutaneous enterostomy and cecostomy, and transgastric pseudocyst drainage. Further refinements in technique and technologic advancements will undoubtedly make these procedures more popular.

THE FUTURE OF INTERVENTIONAL RADIOLOGY

Undoubtedly, the introduction of prospective pricing systems and Diagnosis-Related Groups (DRGs) in the early 1980s and the Relative Value Scale (RVS) in the late 1980s will have a strong influence on the development and utilization of interventional radiology, because, if the interest of society is to reduce medical care costs, the most effective route is to minimize hospitalization expenses. DRG and RVS reimbursement thus encourage the use of percutaneous radiologic procedures, because they typically decrease the length of the hospital stay and, therefore, minimize hospitalization expenditures.

Radiologists can rejoice in these indirect benefits but must recognize the possibility of profound alterations in practice. For example, radiologists must assume a consultative role with their clinical colleagues, provide diagnostic algorithms for the work-up of clinical problems, and establish utilization guidelines for the many new radiologic services. They must, therefore, become more directly involved in the day-to-day care of patients. *A dedicated commitment is necessary!* This approach to interventional radiology provides great rewards, because the therapeutic effects of radiologic procedures are often immediately apparent. In sum, one must leave behind the more contemplative attitude with which radiology was approached in the past.

Interventional radiology has come of age. It is here, and it should be embraced, developed, and advocated. The future is bright if technical excellence is sought. Radiologists today have been given opportunities far exceeding those granted most of their predecessors. Let us use those opportunities well.

Reference

1. Dotter CT, Judkins MP: Transluminal treatment of arteriosclerotic obstruction. *Circulation* 1964;30:654–670.

1

RADIATION PROTECTION IN INTERVENTIONAL RADIOLOGY

—Richard L. Morin, Ph.D.

Interventional radiology procedures can require substantial amounts of ionizing radiation and therefore necessitate particularly close attention to radiation protection. In this chapter, radiation units, regulations, and the fundamental principles of radiation protection are reviewed. Then the procedures and devices designed to reduce patient and staff exposure in interventional radiology are examined.

RADIATION UNITS

The fundamental interactions of x-rays with matter produce ion pairs via photoelectric and Compton interactions.[1] The *Roentgen* (SI unit: coulomb (C) per kilogram) is the unit used to measure the number of ion pairs produced by x- or γ radiation in a standard volume of air. The process of ion pair production is formally termed *radiation exposure* and is fundamental in radiation protection.

The number of ion pairs produced in air does not directly measure the amount of energy deposited in another medium because of the differences in x-ray absorption by different materials.[1] The *rad* is used as a measure of the radiation *absorbed dose* (energy deposited per unit mass). A rad is equal to 100 ergs/g (SI unit: joule per kilogram or Gray (Gy)). This unit is of fundamental importance in patient dosimetry.

Ionizing radiations other than x- and γ rays, such as α particles or neutrons, may induce a greater biologic effect for a given absorbed dose. To quantitate this observation, the *rem* (SI unit: Sievert (Sv)) is used to measure the *dose equivalent*. The rem is equal to the number of rads multiplied by a quality factor ranging from 1 to 20 that expresses the degree of biologic insult for equal amounts of different types of ionizing radiation. The quality factor for x- and γ radiation is equal to 1. This unit is most often utilized in health physics and personnel exposure measures. These radiation units are summarized in Table 1.1.

RADIATION PROTECTION FUNDAMENTALS

In order to decrease the absorbed dose to the patient and the exposure of the staff, the radiation protection principles of *time*, *distance*, and *shielding* must be considered. Radiation exposure is directly related to exposure *time*, so by halving the exposure time, one halves radiation dose. Because an x-ray beam diverges as it passes through *space*, radiation intensity decreases as the inverse square of the distance from the radiation source:

$$\frac{I_2}{I_1} = \frac{d_1^2}{d_2^2}$$

Hence, if the distance from a radiation source is doubled, the radiation intensity decreases to one-fourth its original value (Fig. 1.1). Although this relation holds strictly only for a point source, the distance principle is useful in reducing clinical radiation exposure when the patient is the principal source. The attenuation of an x-ray beam (loss of intensity as it passes through matter) is exponential ($I = I_o e^{-ux}$, where I and I_o are the initial and transmitted radiation, respectively, u is the attenuation coefficient of the material (which depends on the atomic number and density and on the energy of the photons), and x is the thickness of the attenuating material). Therefore, small amounts of attenuating *(shielding)* material can greatly reduce the intensity of an x-ray beam. For example, a 99% reduction of a diagnostic x-ray beam is obtained by using a 0.5mm Pb-equivalent material. Examples of exponential attenuation for diagnostic radiology x-ray beams are shown in Figure 1.2.

Because fluoroscopy is utilized extensively during some interventional radiology procedures, the continual observation of these fundamental principles is of far greater importance than in most areas of diagnostic radiology.

Table 1.1. Radiation Units

Radiation Quantity	Traditional Unit	SI Unit	Conversion
Exposure	Roentgen	Coulombs/kg	2.6×10^{-4} C-kg^{-1} = 1 R
Absorbed dose	rad	Gray (Gy)	10 mGy = 1 rad
Dose	rem	Sievert (Sv)	10 mSv = 1 rem

Table 1.2. Maximum Permissible Dose Equivalent (rem)[3]

Area	13 Weeks	Yearly	Cumulative
Whole body, gonads, blood forming organs, lens of eye	3		5 (*n*-18)[a]
Skin	10	30	
Hands and forearms, head, neck, feet, ankles	25	75	

[a]*n* = Age in years

RADIATION PROTECTION REGULATIONS

Unlike other areas in medicine in which ionizing radiation is used to diagnose or treat disease (e.g., therapeutic radiology, nuclear medicine), x-ray protection and use are not regulated at the federal level. No federal body analogous to the Nuclear Regulatory Commission exists to supervise the medical use of x-rays. Instead, except for the regulations concerning equipment construction,[2] this regulatory function is administered at the state level, most often within a state's department of health and human services. Although one might expect this arrangement to engender a morass of disparate regulations, the state-to-state variation actually is not great, since most states have patterned their regulations after the recommendations of the National Council on Radiation Protection and Measurements (NCRP). This body has developed an extensive set of regulatory guidelines that have become de facto standards for the safe and proper use of ionizing radiation (summarized in Table 1.2). Other sources give further details of the general philosophy of radiation protection, as well as specific recommendations for particular situations.[3-5]

Two other bodies also publish recommendations for radiation protection: the International Commission on Radiation Protection (ICRP) and the International Council on Radiation Protection and Units (ICRU). Additionally, in some instances, the regulations of the Occupational Safety and Health Administration (OSHA) govern the operation of x-ray equipment in a particular diagnostic radiology department.

The presence of these diverse recommendations is particularly important in interventional radiology, since the maximum quarterly exposure to the eyes permitted by the various recommendations differs by a factor of 6 (Table 1.3). These quarterly allowances are intended to account for sporadic or variable, not continual, exposure. Exposures should always be kept "as low as reasonably achievable" (ALARA). Although the operator's hands and forearms may be exposed during interventional radiology procedures, in general, exposure of the eyes and thyroid is of greater concern and therefore most closely monitored.

Table 1.3. Eye Exposure Limits

Regulatory/Advisory Body	Limit (rem/qtr)	Reference
ICRP	7.5	6
NCRP	3.0	3, 7
OSHA	1.25	8
NRC	1.25	9

Figure 1.1. Reduction of radiation intensity according to the inverse-square law.

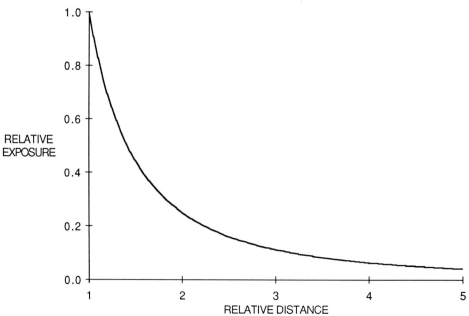

RELATIVE EXPOSURE

RELATIVE DISTANCE

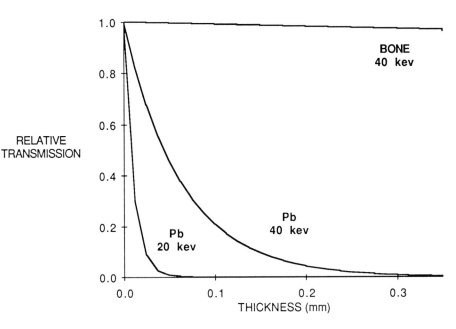

Figure 1.2. Reduction of radiation intensity with increasing thickness of lead and bone at 60 kVp *(20 kev)* and 120 kVp *(40 kev)*.

Concern is often expressed about the absorbed dose to the eye because of the risk of radiation-induced cataracts. This biologic effect appears to have a threshold, in that about 600 rads of diagnostic x-irradiation over several weeks are necessary to produce cataracts in humans.[3,10,11] It may be that absorbed doses of about 1500 rads are necessary to induce cataracts in the diagnostic radiology setting.[6,10] Nonetheless, it is prudent to monitor the staff and use all reasonable means to decrease head and neck exposures in interventional radiology. These concerns often prompt the use of helmet-like protective devices (Moti X-ray Mask; Nuclear Associates), lead-acrylic eyeglasses, and thyroid shields.

STAFF RADIATION EXPOSURE MONITORING

In general, monitoring devices must be worn if it is reasonably likely that a person could receive 25% of the maximum permissible exposure in the discharge of his or her duties. This rule most assuredly mandates exposure monitoring of the interventional radiologist, the clinical colleagues routinely involved in procedures, and the usual support staff.

The most popular method of monitoring is the film badge because it is practical and economical. Usually, each person wears one film badge beneath the lead apron and another at collar level outside the lead apron. If only one film badge is available, it can be worn at either location provided that all persons adopt the same convention. The radiation protection officer must be informed of the convention so the reports of radiation exposure can be properly interpreted. The choice of location hinges on whether the maximum exposure or the whole-body exposure is more important, a matter which has for some time been controversial in the health physics community. Usually, the choice

is made by the radiation protection officer at a particular facility.

Ring badges containing thermoluminescent dosimeters (TLD) may be worn to monitor hand radiation exposure.[10] This practice has not received overwhelming support because of technical problems with the dosimeters and the resistance of some radiologists.

A possible disadvantage of film badges and rings lies in the fact that the actual radiation exposure is not known until perhaps two months later, when the film is developed. The use of the personal ionization chamber ("pocket chamber") avoids this problem,[10] but these devices are expensive and fragile.

RADIATION PROTECTION IN FLUOROSCOPY

Radiation protection in interventional radiology using both conventional and C-arm fluoroscopy is discussed in this section. The radiation exposure of the operator is heavily dependent on imaging geometry. Typical isoexposure lines for several imaging configurations are shown in Figure 1.3; note the tremendous increase in operator exposure with configurations in which the x-ray tube is above the patient. This increase occurs for two reasons: the overall intensity of the scattered radiation beam is approximately 98% greater at the patient entrance site compared to the patient exit,[1] and there is less attenuating material (e.g., image intensifier) between the patient and the operator. As a rule of thumb, the maximum operator exposure at a given distance occurs when there is an unobstructed path between an object and the location at which the x-ray beam enters the patient. For example, maximum operator eye exposure occurs when the operator can see the beam entrance site. The "see it-beat it" radiation protection procedure consists of changing one's position if it is possible

Figure 1.3. Scatter radiation from several equipment configurations. Isoexposure lines are given in millirads/hr. **A.** Conventional fluoroscopy. **B.** Overhead tube. **C.** Posteroanterior fluoroscopy with C- or U-arm. (Courtesy of General Electric Medical Systems Division.)

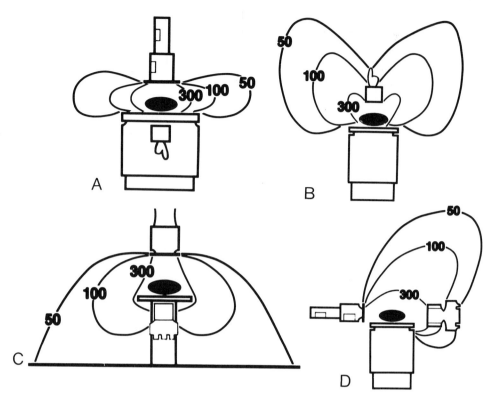

to see the beam entrance area directly. In addition to the amount of time spent in a particular area during a procedure, overall distance from the patient is also important and indeed may be a primary consideration for some staff members. For example, anthropomorphic-phantom measurements of eye exposures for individuals 5 feet 10 inches and 6 feet 4 inches tall demonstrated an exposure increase of approximately 70–115% for the shorter individual.[2] Different radiation protection considerations therefore may be necessary depending on staff members' heights. Because it is not always possible to change one's position relative to the beam, many devices have been suggested to reduce staff exposure during interventional radiology procedures.[12–17] Unfortunately, effective devices are often somewhat awkward given the usual time and space demands of interventional radiology.

In addition to time, distance, and shielding, another important radiation protection parameter is x-ray beam size. The amount of scattered radiation exposure is directly related to beam size. In addition, the patient dose and image quality are affected by changes in collimation. Hence, by limiting the beam size to the smallest necessary area, the fluoroscopist can decrease both personnel and patient exposures while improving image quality.

The recent concept of surface shielding consists of shielding the operator's line of sight from the patient's surface rather than the operator's level.[12,19] The shielding may be fabricated in strips or solid pieces from lead aprons and therefore may be sterilized for reuse. Typical radiation exposure reductions with a 0.77mm surface shield can range from 33–75% (Fig. 1.4). The use of such devices is

important to minimize staff radiation exposures and comply with regulations.

To provide perspective on the radiation exposures encountered in interventional radiology, consider the following example:

> If   Radiation exposure = 300 mR/hr,
> fluoroscopy time = 0.5 hr/exam, and
> maximum permissible exposure = 1.25
> R/quarter,
> then Allowable procedures = 8 exams/quarter!

The importance of attention to radiation protection during these procedures is apparent (Table 1.4).

In summary, to minimize personnel exposure during fluoroscopic interventional radiology, the lowest acceptable exposure rate and smallest acceptable field size should be used with the most efficacious equipment configuration.[20–22] Additionally, although the inverse-square law is not strictly maintained in fluoroscopy,[20] distance from the patient should be maximized, and, when possible, shielding material should be placed between the patient and personnel.

RADIATION PROTECTION IN CINEFLUOROGRAPHY

Because cinefluorography (cine) is an extension of fluoroscopy, all of the previous radiation protection considerations apply; however, radiation exposure is significantly

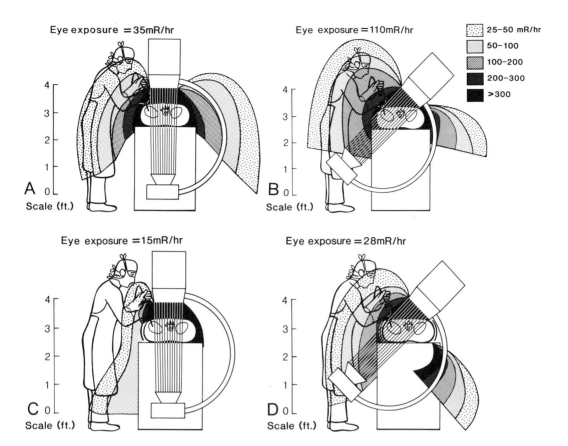

Figure 1.4. Scatter radiation reduction with surface shielding (2.8 R/min patient skin entrance exposure). **A.** Vertical fluoroscopy without shielding. **B.** Oblique (45°) fluoroscopy without shielding. **C.** Vertical fluoroscopy with a 25 × 15cm (0.75mm lead equivalent) surface shield. **D.** Oblique

(45°) fluoroscopy with surface shielding in place. (Reprinted from Young AT, Morin RL, Hunter DW, et al: Surface Shield: device to reduce personnel radiation exposure. *Radiology* 1986;159:801–803 with permission of the Radiological Society of North America, Inc.)

higher for the patient as well as the staff. Typical patient skin entrance exposures can range from 20–90 R/min,[23–25] depending on the system and image acquisition parameters—substantially higher than the typical 2–3 R/min[24,25] skin entrance exposures in fluoroscopy. The scattered radiation levels shown in Figure 1.4 were obtained with a skin entrance exposure of 2.8 R/min; to depict the cine scattered radiation exposure, the values in the figure should be multiplied by a factor of 7 to 32! Eye exposures for cine without shielding would range from 245–3520

mR/hr. The use of surface shielding would decrease these eye exposures to 105–896 mR/hr. Additionally, measurements indicate that eye exposure reductions of 84% are possible by changing the operator's position from tableside to 30cm from the table.[26] Such reductions are system-dependent and should be verified for a particular radiology suite.

From these observations, it is apparent that distance and shielding radiation protection techniques should receive increased attention when cine is used during interventional radiology procedures.

Table 1.4. Maximum Number of Fluoroscopic Procedures in a 3-Month Period without Exceeding Eye Exposure of 1.25 R/Quarter

Fluoroscopic Time per Procedure (hr)	Radiation Exposure at Eye Level (mR/hr)					
	10	25	50	100	200	300
0.10	1250	500	250	125	62	41
0.25	500	200	100	50	25	16
0.50	250	100	50	25	12	8
0.75	166	67	33	16	8	5
1.00	125	50	25	12	6	4
1.50	83	33	16	8	4	2
2.00	62	25	12	6	3	2

RADIATION PROTECTION IN COMPUTED TOMOGRAPHY

The scatter radiation distribution surrounding a computed tomography (CT) scanner is, of course, quite different from the exposure levels found in fluoroscopy, both because the beam area is much smaller during slice acquisition and because the x-ray tube gantry surrounds the patient, thereby providing shielding. Typical isoexposure lines for a CT scanner are shown in Figure 1.5.[10,27] Head and neck exposures could range from approximately 300–

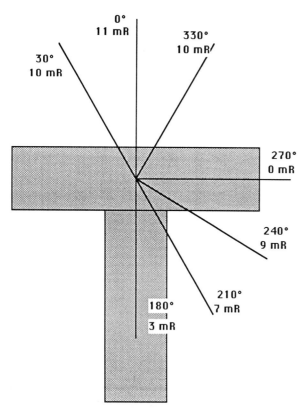

Figure 1.5. Approximate scattered radiation exposures about CT scanner. Exposures are derived from Ref. 27 for a 130-kVp, 50-mA, 10-sec, 10mm scan at a distance of 1m and a height equal to the isocenter.

900 mR for an interventional procedure involving a table-side position for 10–20 exposures. Note that movement to the side of the gantry reduces exposure greatly in comparison to that received when one stands in front of or behind the gantry. In this case, a small step dramatically reduces radiation exposure.

SUMMARY

Interventional radiology demands an increased awareness of the fundamental radiation protection principles of time, distance, and shielding. Staff exposures can be reduced through the proper use and configuration of the imaging system, as well as through the use of ancillary shielding materials such as surface shielding. These considerations should be strongly reinforced when cine is utilized. Typical patient exposures are on the order of 3 R/min during fluoroscopy and 50 R/min during cine. Staff eye exposures can range from approximately 10–100 mR/hr during fluoroscopy and from approximately 100–2500 mR/hr during cine. In general, staff exposure is markedly decreased for interventional procedures that utilize CT, with the greatest reduction if staff members step to the side of the gantry or leave the room during the slice acquisition.

References

1. Curry TS, Dowdy JE, Murry RC: *Christensen's Introduction to the Physics of Diagnostic Radiology.* Philadelphia, Lea & Febiger, 1984
2. Code of Federal Regulations, Title 21, parts 1000–1050, U.S. Government, 1985. Revision of the Radiation Control for Health and Safety Act of 1968
3. National Council of Radiation Protection and Measurements: *Basic Radiation Protection Criteria.* NCRP Report No. 39. Washington, DC, 1971
4. National Council on Radiation Protection and Measurements: *Medical X-Ray and Gamma Ray Protection for Energies up to 10 Mev.* NCRP Report No. 33. Washington, DC, 1968
5. National Council on Radiation Protection and Measurements: *Structural Shielding Design and Evaluation for Medical Use of X-Rays and Gamma Rays of Energies up to 10 Mev.* NCRP Publication No. 49. Washington, DC, 1976
6. Recommendations of the International Commission on Radiological Protection: *Radiation Protection.* ICRP Publication 26. Oxford, Pergamon Press, 1977
7. National Council on Radiation Protection and Measurements: *Review of the Current State of Radiation Protection Philosophy.* NCRP Report No. 43. Washington, DC, 1975
8. Code of Federal Regulations, Title 29, part 16, chapter 17, section 1910.96. Washington, DC, U.S. Government Printing Office, 1971
9. Code of Federal Regulations, Title 10, part 20, chapter 1, section 20.102. Washington, DC, U.S. Government Printing Office, 1971
10. Bushong SC: *Radiologic Science for Technologists: Physics, Biology, and Protection.* St. Louis, CV Mosby, 1984
11. Pizzarello DJ, Witcosfski RC: *Medical Radiation Biology.* Philadelphia, Lea & Febiger, 1982
12. Rusnak B, Castañeda–Zúñiga WR, Kotula F, et al: Radiolucent handle for percutaneous puncture under continuous fluoroscopic monitoring. *Radiology* 1981;141:538
13. Gertz EW, Wisneski JA, Gould RG, et al: Improved radiation protection for physicians performing cardiac catheterization. *Am J Cardiol* 1982;50:1283
14. Allsion JD, Teeslink CR: Special procedures screen. *Radiology* 1980;136:233
15. Thomson KR, Brammall J, Wilson BC: "Flagpole" lead-glass screen for radiographic procedures. *Radiology* 1982;143:557
16. Gilula LA, Barbier J, Totty WG, Eichling J: Radiation shielding device for fluoroscopy. *Radiology* 1985;147:882
17. Miotto D, Feltrin G, Calamosca M: Radiation protection device for use during percutaneous transhepatic examinations. *Radiology* 1984;151:799
18. Young AT, Morin RL, Hunter DW, et al: Surface shield: device to reduce personnel radiation exposure. *Radiology* 1986;159:801
19. Miller DL, Vucich JJ, Cope C: A flexible shield to protect personnel during interventional procedures. *Radiology* 1985;155:825
20. Linos DA, Gray JE, McIlrath DC: Radiation hazard to operating room personnel during operative cholangiography. *Arch Surg* 1980;115:1431
21. Jacobson A, Conley JG: Estimation of fetal doses to patients undergoing diagnostic x-ray procedures. *Radiology* 1976;120:683
22. Bush WH, Jones D, Brannen GE: Radiation dose to personnel during percutaneous renal calculus removal. *AJR* 1985;145:1261

23. Webster EW: Quality assurance in cineradiographic systems, in Waggener RG, Wilson CR (eds): *Quality Assurance in Diagnostic Radiology: Medical Physics Monograph No. 4*. New York, American Institute of Physics, 1980

24. Gray JE, Winkler NT, Stears J, Frank ED: *Quality Control in Diagnostic Imaging*. Baltimore, University Park Press, 1983

25. American Institute of Physics: *Evaluation of Radiation Exposure Levels in Cine Cardiac Catheterization Laboratories*. AAPM Report No. 12. New York, American Institute of Physics, 1984

26. Jeans SP, Faulkner K, Love HG, Bardsley RA: An investigation of the radiation dose to staff during cardiac radiological studies. *Br J Radiol* 1985;58:419

27. Picker International, Inc: *Typical Drawings and Specifications for Synerview 1200 SX/600S*. Cleveland, Picker International, Inc, 1982

VASCULAR EMBOLOTHERAPY

Part 1. Embolotherapy: Agents, Equipment, and Techniques

—Antony T. Young, M.D., S. Murthy Tadavarthy, M.D., Joseph W. Yedlicka, Jr., M.D., David W. Hunter, M.D., Gary J. Becker, M.D., Marcos A. Herrera, M.D., Flavio Castañeda, M.D., Kurt Amplatz, M.D., and Wilfrido R. Castañeda–Zúñiga, M.D., M.Sc.

Transcatheter vascular embolization has become an important aspect of the burgeoning field of interventional radiology and promises to increase in popularity as the indications for embolization are clarified and the techniques refined. Nonetheless, at present, when examining the considerable volume of literature on the subject, it should be recognized that many of these reports are anecdotal and written to demonstrate that a certain technique might be possible rather than to show the technique to be safe or as effective as traditional therapy by comparison with an adequate control group. Because of this failing, it is difficult to define the relative roles of embolotherapy and the conventional techniques of surgery, radiotherapy, drugs, and endoscopy for any given clinical situation. However, it seems likely that, although embolotherapy is now often used as a last resort when conventional therapy has failed, it eventually will assume a more prominent place in the treatment of hemorrhage and neoplasia. The challenge is to continue developing new techniques, to demonstrate the efficacy of embolotherapy, and to show that it can be reliable and safe.

HISTORICAL ASPECTS

Although it has been only in the last decade that there has been much interest in embolotherapy, the principle of vascular embolization is not new; it dates back to 1904, when Dawbain described the preoperative injection of melted paraffin-petrolatum into the external carotid arteries of patients suffering head and neck tumors.[1] Brooks, in 1930, introduced particulate embolization when he described occluding a traumatic carotid-cavernous fistula by injecting a fragment of muscle attached to a silver clip

into the internal carotid artery.[2] Similarly, Lussenhop and Spence, in 1960, injected spheres of methyl methacrylate into the surgically exposed common carotid artery of a patient suffering from an arteriovenous malformation (AVM) fed by the middle cerebral artery, achieving clinical improvement.[3]

In 1963, Baum and Nusbaum, in a landmark paper, demonstrated that bleeding at rates as low as 0.5ml/min could be detected angiographically.[4] This report set the stage for the transcatheter management of hemorrhage, which was first achieved with selective infusions of vasopressin. In 1972, Rösch, Dotter, and Brown reported controlling acute gastric hemorrhage by embolization of the gastroepiploic artery with autologous clot.[5]

The tremendous upsurge of interest in embolization that began in the 1970s was fueled by parallel developments in catheter technology and embolic agents. The availability of a wide range of preshaped catheters and the introduction of coaxial systems allowed radiologists to place catheters subselectively, making possible highly selective delivery of embolic agents. Lin et al., in 1974, introduced the concept of injecting soft silicone tubing through lumens only slightly larger than itself,[6] and this was followed in 1974 by the report of Serbinenko from the Soviet Union of the use of detachable balloon catheters for embolization.[7] White, Debrun, and their colleagues borrowed from these researchers and produced an injectable flow-directed catheter with a detachable silicone balloon for permanent vascular occlusion.[8,9] Similarly, Kerber developed a silicone calibrated-leak balloon that allows highly selective flow-directed placement and then balloon occlusion angiography or embolization using the low-viscosity tissue adhesives.[10]

The tissue adhesive isobutyl 2-cyanoacrylate (IBCA; Bucrylate) was introduced as an embolic agent in the United States by Zanetti and Sherman in 1972.[11] The use of Gelfoam particles as an embolic agent was first described by Carey and Grace in 1974.[12] Polyvinyl alcohol (Ivalon) was initially used as a plug for closure of a patent ductus arteriosus by Portsmann et al. in 1971.[13] This led to research on its use in particulate form by Tadavarthy and coworkers.[14,15] In 1975, Gianturco and his colleagues created the wool coil, a modification of which is currently in widespread use.[16]

The concept of tissue ablation with absolute ethanol was introduced in 1981 by Ellman et al., who used it for infarction of kidneys.[17] In 1982, Amplatz and his colleagues demonstrated the efficacy of boiling contrast medium by publishing photomicrographs of an occluded vein from his own forearm.[18,19] Sodium tetradecyl sulfate (Sotradecol) has been similarly used as a sclerosing agent.[20]

It is difficult to predict developments in a rapidly changing field such as interventional radiology. It may well be that the authors have overlooked what will turn out to be milestones and, for that, they apologize. Transcatheter electrocoagulation,[21,22] the guidance of emboli by external magnetic forces (Chapter 2, Part 7),[23] and embolization with capsules of drugs or radioactive particles[24] may well be such milestones.

PATIENT CARE

Preoperative Management

Embolization is a major procedure, and it is imperative that the radiologist be fully aware of the clinical status of the patient. When taking the history, inquiry should be made into any previous operations. For example, previous surgery around the stomach may have destroyed the rich collateral blood supply to this organ, so that left gastric artery embolization, which is normally a relatively benign procedure, may lead to severe gastric ulceration or infarction.[25] Informed consent is obtained after a full and frank discussion of the benefits and risks of the procedure, including the possibility of unintentional embolization of nontarget areas and pain both during and after the procedure. Relevant laboratory values and previous radiologic studies should be reviewed.

Before embolization, the patient should be well hydrated, both because of the potential need for large volumes of contrast medium and because of the possibility of acute renal failure, which can follow embolization of large soft tissue tumors as a result of hyperuricemia. Antibiotics are used preoperatively and for two or three days after embolization. A cephalosporin is a common choice. Other premedication consists of an intramuscular sedative such as secobarbital and a narcotic analgesic such as meperidine (Demerol), or midazolam (Versed) given intravenously during the procedure.

The intended puncture site should be shaved immediately before the procedure, preferably in the radiology suite, in order to reduce the superficial skin irritation with infection caused by shaving.

Intraoperative Care

During embolization procedures, the authors prefer to have a nurse anesthetist monitor the patient and administer drugs as necessary. Most embolizations are performed using local anesthesia and intravenous sedation. However, in children, when embolization is likely to be painful (for example, during embolization in a limb), general anesthesia may be chosen. Oxygen is delivered by nasal prongs; this may help to protect any tissues unintentionally embolized until collaterals develop. In all patients, proper fluid balance must be maintained.

Postoperative Care

Postoperatively, a high fluid input is important to reduce the likelihood of acute urate nephropathy. This is particularly true after embolization for liver tumors. Adequate analgesia should also be given, not only for the patient's comfort but also to reduce the risk of complications.[5] For example, abdominal pain may impair breathing motion, which may, in turn, lead to atelectasis and pneumonia. Antibiotics are continued for two to three days in most cases, and for up to one week after splenic embolization to decrease the risk of splenic abscess. Postembolization measurement of serum creatinine concentration is advisable as an assessment of renal function.

GENERAL PRINCIPLES OF EMBOLIZATION

The effects of embolization on any organ are specific to that organ, and this fact makes generalization about the techniques of embolization difficult. For example, proximal occlusion of the main renal artery is likely to cause infarction of the kidney, whereas occlusion of the common hepatic artery rarely results in hepatic necrosis because of the collateral blood supply of the liver and of the portal circulation, which provides approximately 75% of the blood flow to the liver and 50% of its oxygen requirement. The effects of embolization also depend on the clinical status of the patient. For example, hypotensive shock and infusions of vasopressin reduce portal venous flow and render the liver more susceptible to ischemic necrosis. Previous operations around the stomach and vasopressin infusion reduce the collateral supply, again increasing the susceptibility of the organ to necrosis following embolization. Concurrent disease such as atherosclerosis or vasculitis may also leave an organ more susceptible to ischemic necrosis. Age is another factor: occlusion of the common femoral artery in a child is usually well tolerated, although it often leads to later growth disturbance in the limb, whereas occlusion of the common femoral artery in an adult often leads to severe ischemia.

Proximal occlusion of an artery carries less chance of tissue necrosis because of the potential for collateralization into the distal circulation. Such occlusion may, however, alter the hemodynamics sufficiently to stop a hemorrhage. Inducing the development of collaterals may be the purpose of the procedure. For example, when infusion of chemotherapy into the liver is complicated by the existence of an anomalous arterial supply to the right or left lobes, embolization of one of the major arteries results in the blood supply to the entire liver arising from the other vessel via existing collaterals that open up almost immediately.[26] Chemotherapy may then be given more efficiently.

Distal occlusion of vessels with minute particles or liquid agents carries a higher likelihood of tissue necrosis, which may well be the purpose of the procedure—for example, in renal ablation with ethanol.[17] Distal embolization reduces the possibility of blood being supplied to the tissues from collaterals, which may be desired, e.g., in embolization of an arteriovenous malformation (AVM). Such lesions almost invariably recur unless embolization is performed beyond the inflow from any collateral branches.

Generally, catheters should be placed as selectively as possible in order to avoid embolization of normal tissues. Reliance on the increased flow in a bleeding artery to guide the emboli is not only unsafe but particularly dangerous.

Reflux of emboli from the catheterized artery must be avoided. Delivery of particulate materials should be stopped once flow is severely reduced; no attempt should be made to occlude the vessel totally distal to the catheter with particulates, as these are likely to reflux. Balloon occlusion catheters have been advocated to avoid reflux, although their value for this task is unproven.

Where a large organ or lesion is to be embolized, performing the procedure in separate stages is advisable in order to prevent widespread tissue necrosis, to allow time for normal tissues to recover, and to permit early detection of complications. Great care must be taken when embolizing with liquids such as silicone, IBCA, or absolute ethanol, because neurologic damage, both of peripheral nerves and of the spinal cord, necrosis of the bile ducts and of bronchi, and gastrointestinal perforation have all occurred.

MATERIALS FOR EMBOLIZATION

The radiologist performing embolization procedures should know well the physical, chemical, and biologic characteristics of the different embolic agents and devices currently available, as well as the best technique for their delivery. The embolic agent is selected on the basis of whether temporary or permanent occlusion is wanted; whether proximal or peripheral occlusion is desirable; and the individual vascular anatomy. Only if the proper choice is made will permanent success be achieved.

Embolic materials can be classified as absorbable (used for temporary occlusion) and nonabsorbable (used for permanent occlusion):

Absorbable materials:
  a. Autologous blood clot;
  b. Modified autologous blood clot;
  c. Oxycel (oxidized cellulose);
  d. Gelfoam (surgical gelatin sponge).
Nonabsorbable materials:
  a. Particulate agents:
    —Autologous fat or muscle;
    —Ivalon (polyvinyl alcohol (PVA) sponge);
    —Silastic spheres and Silastic with steel balls;
    —Stainless-steel pellets;
    —Ferromagnetic microspheres;
    —Acrylic spheres;
    —Methyl methacrylate spheres.
  b. Injectable (fluid) embolic agents:
    —IBCA;
    —IBCA modifications (tissue glues);
    —Silicone rubber;
    —Ethibloc (amino acid occlusion gel).
  c. Sclerosing agents:
    —Absolute ethanol;
    —Boiling contrast medium;
    —Sodium morrhuate;
    —Sotradecol.
  d. Nonparticulate agents:
    —Stainless-steel coils;
    —Stainless-steel coils with barbs;
    —Silk streamers;
    —Plastic brushes;
    —Detachable balloons.
Electrocoagulation (endovascular diathermy).

Embolic materials can either be radiopaque by themselves or be made radiopaque by the addition of various chemical compounds containing barium, tantalum, bismuth, tin, or other metals. However, with good fluoroscopy, even nonopaque emboli such as Ivalon can be seen if suspended in dilute contrast medium, particularly Pantopaque. Recently, techniques for radionuclide labeling of Gelfoam have been described that allow nonradiographic external location of the emboli with a γ camera.[27,28]

Specific Embolic Agents and Techniques

AUTOLOGOUS MATERIALS

Various autologous materials, such as fragments of skeletal muscle, dura, and fat, have been used for embolization.[3,29,30] The duration of vessel occlusion with these agents is not known for certain but is probably several weeks to several months. The main disadvantage of these materials is that they need to be harvested from the patient, which necessitates a further procedure.

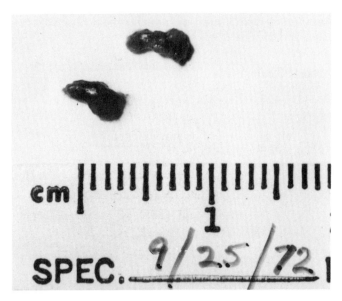

Figure 2.1.1. Autologous blood clot.

The most widely used autologous material has been blood clot (Fig. 2.1.1). The duration of vessel occlusion in swine, which have a fibrinolytic system similar to that of human beings, is >48 hr. After two weeks, approximately one-half of the vessels will be recanalized.[5]

The technique of injecting blood clot is as follows. Blood is drawn from the patient and allowed to clot in a sterile container. Once a solid clot has formed, some of it is aspirated into a 1ml syringe and injected into the catheter. Because the clot conforms to the size of the catheter, it is easy to inject. Mixing the clot with additives has been proposed as a way to prolong vessel occlusion,[31] but the addition of thrombin or ε-aminocaproic acid to clot does not retard fibrinolysis, although it will help produce a firmer clot in patients with coagulation abnormalities.[31-33] Oxycel, which is made from oxidized cellulose, has also been added to clot; in dogs, this significantly retards clot lysis.[31,33,34] Because patients undergoing embolization for hemorrhage have impaired coagulation as a result of either their underlying disease or multiple transfusions, platelets and thrombi have been added to clots.

The advantages of autologous clot are its low cost and lack of toxicity. Its major disadvantage is its rapid lysis, which makes it unsuitable for uses other than treatment of hemorrhage and fistulae. Autologous clot has been said to be the embolic material of choice for severe bleeding after biopsy of the kidney, because the rapid dissolution may prevent renal infarction.[32]

Autologous blood clot is increasingly being superseded by Gelfoam and the more permanent embolic materials.

THROMBIN

Thrombin (Thrombostat; Parke–Davis, Morris Plains, NJ) is a physiological protein, a product of the conversion of prothrombin into thrombin by activated tissue thromboplastin in the presence of calcium chloride. Thrombin, then, reacts with circulating fibrinogen to form fibrinogen complexes that eventually form a firm clot. Thrombin fails to clot only in those cases where the primary clotting defect is the absence of fibrinogen itself.

Thrombin (Thrombostat) is of bovine origin and is supplied as sterile powder. It is packaged by the manufacturers as 5, 10, and 21mg vials that contain 5,000, 10,000, and 20,000 units of thrombin, respectively. When mixed with the enclosed isotonic saline, the chemical is ready to be used.

Thrombin has been used as a stand-alone[35] or as an adjunct embolic agent along with blood clots treated with aminocaproic acid,[36] steel coils,[37-40] and detachable balloons.[40]

The success of thrombin as a thrombostatic agent depends on its concentration and the flow rate in an aneurysm.[35] Thrombin may not be effective in coagulopathies or in high flow states because of the dilutional effects of blood flow.[35,37] In surgery, it has been extensively used as a topical agent on the cut surfaces of skin, liver, and spleen, either by itself or in combination with Gelfoam.

The thrombogenic effect of the Gianturco coils can be enhanced by soaking them in a thrombin solution prior to their introduction.[37]

The coils preloaded in their introducing cartridges are dropped into a medicine cup that contains 10,000 units of thrombin reconstituted with 10ml of solvent. The coils are then injected in the usual fashion.

The injected dose of thrombin varies upon the anatomical problem present, the flow rate, and the presence or absence of other occluding agents. Doses as small as 300 units[36] and as high as 5000 units[38] have been used for effective thrombosis.

Extreme caution has been advised to avoid reflux into the nontargeted blood vessels.[37] Thrombin can be injected through a catheter or directly into an aneurysm through a percutaneously placed 21-gauge needle.[35] According to Cope, if it is judiciously used, it has no untoward thrombotic or allergic manifestations, even though the extract is of bovine origin.[35]

GELFOAM

Gelfoam (The Upjohn Co., Kalamazoo, MI) is an absorbable sponge derived from gelatin that was introduced in 1945 as an aid to hemostasis in surgical procedures. Light and Prentice showed that, when Gelfoam is implanted in various locations in the cranium, the maximum tissue reaction is reached within 12 days, with complete disappearance of the material by 45 days.[40] In 1967, Ishimori introduced pledgets of Gelfoam into the surgically exposed internal carotid artery for embolization of carotid-cavernous fistulae.[41] Carey and Grace, in 1974, controlled hemorrhage from a duodenal ulcer.[12]

Gelfoam embolization causes a severe form of panarteritis characterized by infiltration of leukocytes into all layers of the vessel wall, as well as by disruption of the intima and

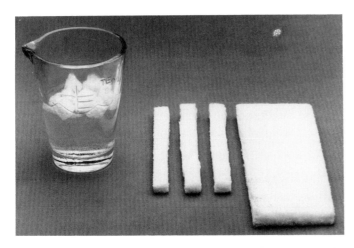

Figure 2.1.2. Gelfoam emboli cut with scissors into small fragments.

elastic tissues. This panarteritis usually resolves completely within four months.[34,42,43] The occlusion lasts from a few days to a few weeks.

Gelfoam is commercially available in sheets or in powder. The sheets may be cut into suitable sizes with a scalpel or scissors (Fig. 2.1.2). The powder form consists of particles of $40-60\mu m$ in diameter.

To prepare Gelfoam for injection, appropriate size particles are mixed thoroughly with 30% iodinated contrast medium. The Gelfoam is ready when it is clear and jelly-like. A 10ml syringe is used to aspirate one or several particles, depending on the target vascular bed. Because Gelfoam floats, the syringe should be held nozzle up while the particles are injected into a transparent tube connected to the angiographic catheter after the stopcock is removed. The loaded syringe is replaced with a syringe containing normal saline, and the contents of the connecting tube are carefully injected into the catheter. It is important not to inject too fast to avoid causing reflux of emboli from the target artery. The particles of Gelfoam usually can be seen as filling defects within the half-strength column of contrast medium.

After the emboli have been injected, careful test injections of full-strength contrast medium are made to determine the flow patterns. Once all the branch arteries have been occluded and blood flow is severely reduced, no more emboli should be injected. No attempt should be made to fill the main artery with Gelfoam, as there is a high risk of reflux of particles because of the turbulence produced by the fast injection of additional emboli into the stagnant column of blood.[44] Greenfield et al. advocate Gelfoam embolization with the aid of balloon occlusion to prevent reflux.[45] Even if balloon occlusion is used, the target vessel should not be filled with Gelfoam because of the risk of reflux once the balloon is deflated. Test injections into the artery should be gentle, because otherwise they may dislodge fragments.

Fragments of Gelfoam as large as 4mm in diameter can be injected through angiographic catheters as small as 3Fr.

There is evidence that the Gelfoam pledgets fragment in the catheter, making the injected particles smaller than intended.[45,46]

Gelfoam powder occludes vessels of $100-200\mu m$. As the particles measure $40-100\mu m$, they apparently clump to some extent. These particles travel more distally than do the larger fragments of Gelfoam, so there is a much higher incidence of ischemic complications when Gelfoam powder is used, particularly with embolization of the gastrointestinal tract.[47] Gelfoam powder should not be used for embolization of large arteriovenous communications, because the particles may pass into the lung.

Gelfoam promotes clot formation, so thrombosis commonly propagates distal to the embolization site, but intact Gelfoam fragments are seldom found more than 24–48 hours postembolization. The duration of vascular occlusion averages three to four months, and recanalization usually follows.[34,42]

Gelfoam is commonly used for one of two purposes: nonpermanent occlusion, such as for preoperative embolization or control of hemorrhage,[48,49] and, in combination with a nonabsorbable substance such as a coil or tissue adhesive, for complete permanent vascular occlusion. A minor disadvantage of Gelfoam is its rapid contamination with bacteria when left exposed to room air, even in the operating room.[46]

Conroy et al. label Gelfoam with radionuclides so that the destination of the emboli can be determined.[27] The present authors have also found this useful.

Oxycel

This cotton-like material is made from oxidized cellulose (Parke–Davis, Detroit, MI). When added to blood, it makes a clot firmer. For introduction, the Oxycel-clot preparation is cut into small fragments with a blade or scissors. The fragments are aspirated with a 10ml syringe, injected into the clear plastic tubing connected to the angiographic catheter, and flushed into the vessel with dilute contrast medium. Because of the harder nature of this embolic agent and the fact that recanalization commonly occurs within four months,[34] it is seldom if ever used now.

Ivalon

Ivalon is a biologically inert polyvinyl alcohol sponge with the unique property of being compressible when wet and of re-expanding to its original shape and size when a dried piece is placed in an aqueous solution such as blood (Fig. 2.1.3).[15] This property makes Ivalon particularly attractive for the occlusion of large vessels,[13,14,50] in which it produces a permanent occlusion.[15,50,51] Histologically, Ivalon is initially invaded by fibroblasts, with subsequent dense fibrous connective tissue formation around the sponge and a moderate inflammatory reaction around the area of thrombosis that involves the wall of the arteries. Organization of the thrombus then takes place, with fibro-

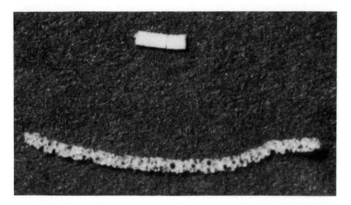

Figure 2.1.3. Ivalon plug in compressed *(top)* and re-expanded *(bottom)* forms.

sis of the arterial wall and disappearance of the inflammatory infiltrate (Fig. 2.1.4). Recanalization of the thrombus does not occur, and partial occlusion of the vessel wall by an organized thrombus is commonly found beyond the site of the initial occlusion.[51]

Delivery Techniques

Plug Delivery via a Catheter

From compressed Ivalon sponge, plugs of the proper size are cut and placed in plastic tubing connected to the catheter, from which they are flushed into the vessel.[15,52,53] Catheters should not have tapered tips and therefore require introduction through a sheath.

Delivery with a Wire

Ivalon plugs also can be delivered by means of a wire.[50] The Ivalon is compressed around a stainless-steel mandrel in a vise (Figs. 2.1.5 and 2.1.6), and the resulting plugs are delivered through the catheter to a preselected site (Fig. 2.1.7). The plug and wire are left in place until the sponge re-expands to its original size. The plug is then stripped off either against a stainless-steel spring coil that fits over the mandrel or against the catheter tip. Small and medium-sized vessels can be occluded with one plug (Fig. 2.1.8). Some flow through the meshwork of the expanded plug may occur during the first 10 to 20 minutes until all pores become filled with fibrin. If flow is still apparent after 20 minutes, a second plug can be placed to complete the obliteration. Since it is friction against the vessel wall which holds the swollen plug in place, the plug should always be larger than the lumen of the vessel to be embolized, particularly in high-flow arteries, to prevent distal dislocation.

This method is especially helpful for exact placement of the plug at a predetermined site. Also, the site can be tested by advancing a similar wire without an attached plug. The main advantage of this technique is that the plug is passed rapidly through the catheter lumen, eliminating the intra-catheter expansion of the plug that is so often a problem with transcatheter delivery of compressed Ivalon plugs because of their high friction coefficient. To retard the re-expansion of the compressed sponge, it is coated with a thin layer of 75% dextran solution, which keeps the plug in its compressed state for 60–90 seconds after it makes contact with blood. This period is adequate for safe positioning of the plug at the desired site in the vessel. The 4 or 5mm diameter plugs can be introduced through a 7Fr non-tapered catheter; 9mm plugs need a 9Fr thin-wall catheter (Formocath; Becton Dickinson).

Shavings

Ivalon shavings are small particles produced from an uncompressed block (Fig. 2.1.9) with a metal saw blade (Fig. 2.1.10), blender,[54] or motor-driven rotating grasp (Fig. 2.1.11).[54,55] After the particles have been separated by size in a vibrating sieve (Fig. 2.1.12), shavings of similar size (0.25mm, 0.5mm, 1mm, and larger) are packaged in plastic bags and sterilized with ethylene oxide (Fig. 2.1.13).

The Ivalon suspension is prepared at the beginning of the procedure by mixing 20ml of Rheomacrodex (dextran 40,000; Pharmacia, Piscataway, NJ), 10ml of 60% diatrizoate, and 5ml of albumin with 1 teaspoonful (about 5ml) of Ivalon particles in a glass beaker (Fig. 2.1.14A). This mixture prevents aggregation of the Ivalon particles resulting from their surface charge (Fig. 2.1.14B). That is, albumin, because of its bipolar charge, probably is adsorbed onto the surface of the particles, so that each Ivalon particle exerts a repellent force. Dextran probably increases the viscosity, delaying sedimentation of the particles. To facilitate delivery, a special cone-shaped syringe is used for injection (Fig. 2.1.15). This design eliminates peripheral stagnation of the particles at the distal end of the syringe.[54]

A simpler preparative method has been described by Kerber et al.[53] After being sorted by size, particles are placed in 50ml bottles with saline and sterilized. For injection, the particles are passed back and forth between two syringes connected by plastic tubing through a partially closed stopcock after the air has been expelled. When the particles are uniformly suspended, they are transferred to a syringe containing contrast medium for injection through the angiographic catheter.[53]

Ivalon is nonradiopaque, and complications can occur because of the inability of the angiographer to localize the injected particles that might have inadvertently entered the non-target organs such as the lungs and the brain. Ivalon is supplied by the commercial manufacturers in three different sizes that range from 150–250-micron, 250–590-micron, and 590–1000-micron particles, respectively.

In one of the commercial preparations, because of the inhomogeneity, there are smaller particles that range from 2 to 20 microns. It was determined that in vials of 5ml containing particles of 150–250 microns in size, there were 85,000,000 particles that were in the 2–20 microns range in size and 2,000,000 particles larger than 45 microns.[56] The smaller 20 micron size particles not only can pass through AVMs but also through normal capillary vessels. Two infants that were embolized with this commercial

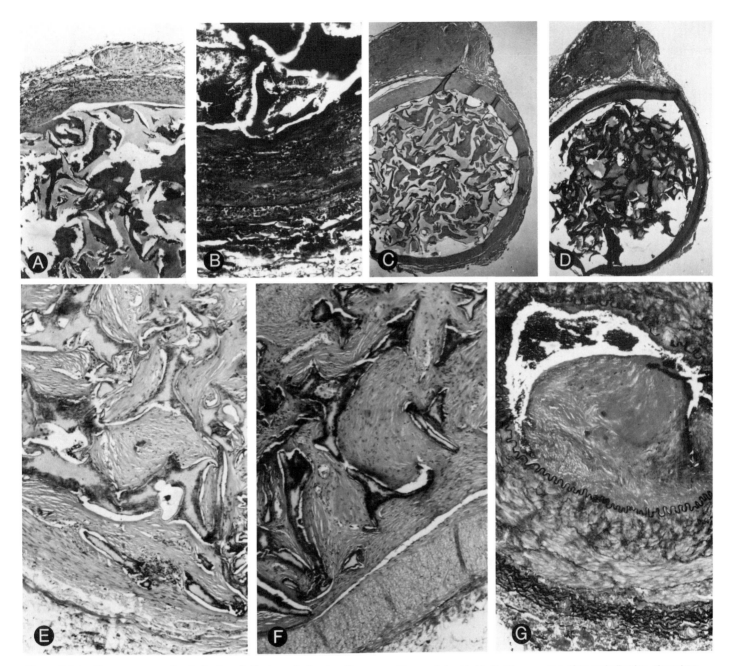

Figure 2.1.4. Consequences of embolization. **A.** Canine splenic artery 3 days after embolization. Ivalon fragments fill vessel lumen, and clotted blood is present between fragments. Arterial wall is unremarkable. H & E; × 40. **B.** Splenic artery soon after embolization. Plastic fragments fill lumen. Note blood clot between fragments. Wall of artery is intact. × 250. **C.** Splenic artery of dog sacrificed 15 days after embolization. Thrombus has a histologic appearance similar to that in previous figure panel, but wall of artery appears to be infiltrated by polymorphonuclear leukocytes. Intimal division has disappeared. H & E; × 80. **D.** Artery 15 days after embolization, showing disruption of intima, disarranged elastic tissue, and wall with marked inflammatory infiltrate. Elastic tissue stains black with van Gieson stain. × 44. **E.** Nine months after embolization, thrombus appears fibrous and seems to be in continuity with vessel wall. Plastic fragments appear partially coated by calcium *(dark areas).* H & E; × 100. **F.** Arterial wall appears detached from thrombus and well preserved. H & E; × 100. **G.** Organized thrombus distal to main embolus does not contain plastic fragments. Note that lamina elastica is fragmented in one small area. van Gieson stain; × 125. (Reproduced from Castañeda–Zúñiga WR, Sanchez R, Amplatz K: Experimental observations on short- and long-term effects of arterial occlusion with Ivalon. *Radiology* 1978;126:783–785.)

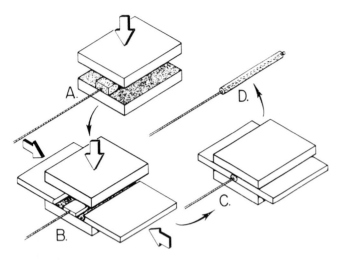

Figure 2.1.5. Schematic representation of compression of Ivalon plug around a wire. (Reproduced from Zollikofer C, Castañeda–Zúñiga WR, Galliani C, Rysavy JA, Formanek A, Amplatz K: Therapeutic blockade of arteries using compressed Ivalon. *Radiology* 1980;136:635–640.)

preparation died as a result of massive embolization of Ivalon particles into their lungs and other systemic organs secondary to a patent foramen ovale.[56] (Since the publication of this report, the manufacturers have corrected the inhomogeneity of the particle size.)

Because it is very difficult to determine which particle size will be safe in any given AVM, a new protocol has been initiated that allows the angiographer to monitor the location of the particles.[57,58] The Ivalon particles are tagged with [99mTc] sulfur colloid.

A small amount of tagged Ivalon with [99mTc] sulfur colloid is injected as the first step of embolization and the smallest particle that does not shunt through the AVM into the lungs is used for the embolization.[58] In this manner, during the embolization procedure, the particles can be localized with a portable γ camera.

The use of this technique allows the angiographer to recognize the inadvertent pulmonary embolism and a corrective action can be taken to avoid complications.

Uses

The disadvantage of Ivalon is that it is cumbersome to prepare and introduce. Furthermore, a relatively high injection pressure is needed to eject the particles into the blood vessel, increasing the risk of reflux of the embolus. Therefore, delivery of shavings through balloon occlusion catheters has been recommended.[44,45] On the other hand, because of the readily adjustable size of this material, prac-

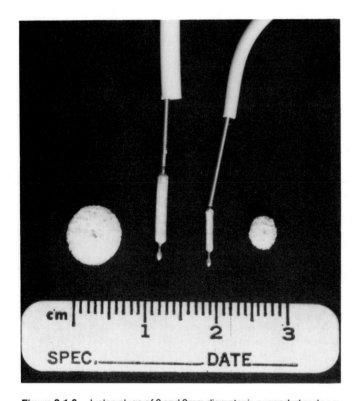

Figure 2.1.6. Ivalon plugs of 8 and 3mm diameter in expanded and compressed form around stainless-steel wire. The 8mm compressed plug passes through 9Fr thin-wall Formocath nontapered catheter; the 3mm compressed plug passes through 7Fr wire mesh catheter with tapered tip cut off. (Reproduced from Zollikofer C, Castañeda–Zúñiga WR, Galliani C, Rysavy JA, Formanek A, Amplatz K: Therapeutic blockade of arteries using compressed Ivalon. *Radiology* 1980;136:635–640.)

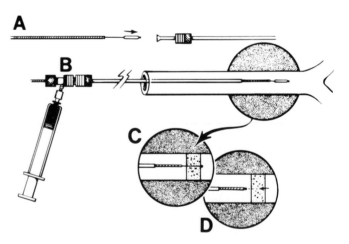

Figure 2.1.7. Schematic representation of mechanism of delivery of compressed Ivalon plugs over wire. **A.** Compressed Ivalon plug on wire is advanced through angiographic catheter after removal of Tuohy–Borst adapter. **B.** Compressed Ivalon plug on wire is advanced to preselected site for arterial occlusion; Tuohy–Borst adapter has been tightened around wire to prevent blood loss during wait for Ivalon re-expansion. Flushing can be performed through sidearm of adapter. **C.** Ivalon plug has re-expanded to its original dimensions after contact with blood. **D.** Stainless-steel wire is pulled back gently from within re-expanded, slightly oversized Ivalon plug, which remains in place without migration because of pressure it exerts on arterial wall. (Reproduced from Zollikofer C, Castañeda–Zúñiga WR, Galliani C, Rysavy JA, Formanek A, Amplatz K: Therapeutic blockade of arteries using compressed Ivalon. *Radiology* 1980;136:635–640.)

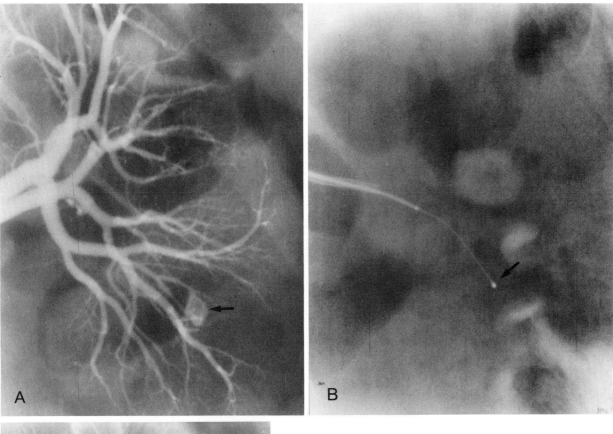

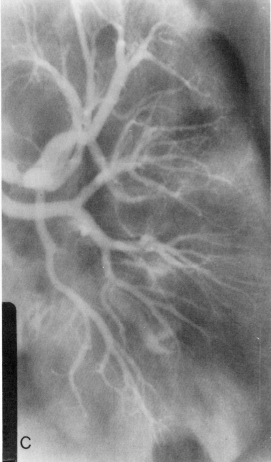

Figure 2.1.8. Management of AV fistula. **A.** Left renal arteriogram in patient with postbiopsy AV fistula and recurrent hematuria; false aneurysm of branch of anterior division of artery *(arrow).* **B.** A 3mm compressed Ivalon plug has been advanced beyond tip of catheter into branch with abnormality *(arrow).* **C.** Complete obliteration of lower branch is noted 10 minutes after release of plug.

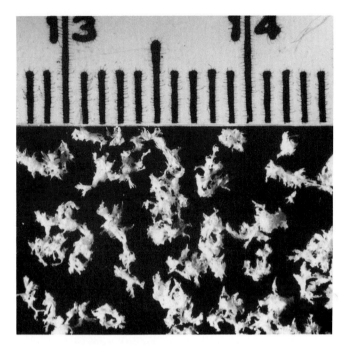

Figure 2.1.9. High-power view of Ivalon particles produced by saw blade. Observe extreme variability in size, which makes separation of the particles by graduated sieves a necessity.

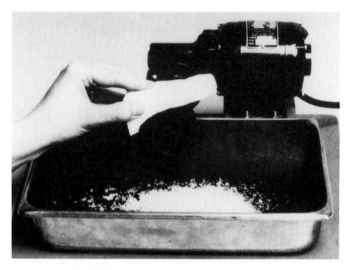

Figure 2.1.11. Rotating grasp for mechanical production of Ivalon particles. (Reproduced from Herrera M, Rysavy J, Kotula F, Castañeda–Zúñiga WR, Amplatz K: Ivalon shavings: a new embolic agent. *Radiology* 1982;144:638–640.)

tically all types of embolization can be performed. The small particles are ideal for peripheral embolization of AVMs and for tumor ablation,[15,54,59] while, in combination with metal devices that secure it in the lumen, an Ivalon plug can be used for occlusion of larger arteries.[60,61] For example, compression in a vise of the Ivalon plug around the straightened end of a stainless-steel spring coil (coilon) (Fig. 2.1.16*A,B*) or on a wire attached to a spider (spiderlon) (Fig. 2.1.17*A,B*) was reported by Zollikofer and Castañeda and their coworkers.[60,61] The advantages of these

devices are, first, that total occlusion is achieved in one stage at the chosen site and, if needed, an additional Ivalon plug can be safely placed behind the coilon or spiderlon. In addition, a large Ivalon plug occludes the vessel more rapidly than does a woolly or Dacron-tailed coil. Finally, the same technique can be used in the venous system simply by changing the location of the Ivalon plug: pulmonary embolization is prevented by placing the steel coil upstream from the plug (Fig. 2.1.18*A*). For placement, the coilon is mounted over a special introducer from which it is stripped by advancing the spring coil over the mandrel (Fig. 2.1.19).

Attempted occlusion of large AV fistulae with Gianturco coils, Gelfoam, Ivalon, or other embolic agents can lead to pulmonary embolization (Fig. 2.1.20) because of the larger

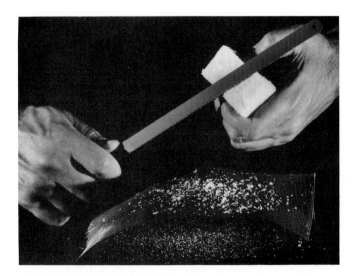

Figure 2.1.10. Manual production of Ivalon particles by using saw blade to shave surface of block. A wire mesh of known dimension is used to separate particles.

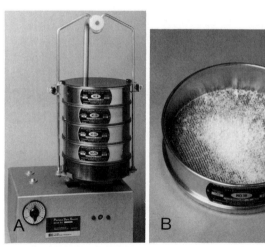

Figure 2.1.12. Sorting of Ivalon particles. **A.** Vibrating sieve used to sort Ivalon particles by size. **B.** Individual container from sieve, showing collected particles.

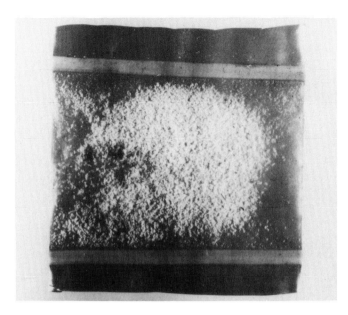

Figure 2.1.13. Ivalon particles packed in sterile plastic container for storage. (Reproduced from Herrera M, Rysavy J, Kotula F, Castañeda–Zúñiga WR, Amplatz K: Ivalon shavings: a new embolic agent. *Radiology* 1982;144:638–640.)

caliber and rapid flow in the vessel.[62] To prevent this complication, two devices have been developed. The first is a barbed stainless-steel coil, whose sharp barbs are embedded in the vascular wall upon leaving the catheter (Fig. 2.1.21), so that the coil forms a baffle behind which additional Gianturco coils or Ivalon plugs can be deposited (Fig. 2.1.22).[63] On the venous side, dislodgment of the embolic agent may result from pressure changes such as coughing or because the veins become larger toward the heart. The other device is a stainless-steel spider with a design similar to the Mobin–Uddin-type vena caval filter (Fig. 2.1.23).[64] The spider can be modified by attaching a piece of stainless-steel wire to its cone head, over which an Ivalon plug is compressed.[61] For introduction, the spider is mounted on an introducer wire (Fig. 2.1.24) and placed in the catheter with the prongs oriented in the direction of the blood flow and the Ivalon plug trailing. As the prongs emerge from the catheter tip, they open immediately, piercing the vessel wall and preventing migration and pulmonary embolization (Fig. 2.1.25). Once the prongs engage the vessel wall, the introducing wire is removed.[61,64]

Ivalon has been used as a plug after percutaneous

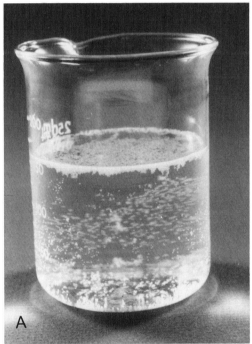

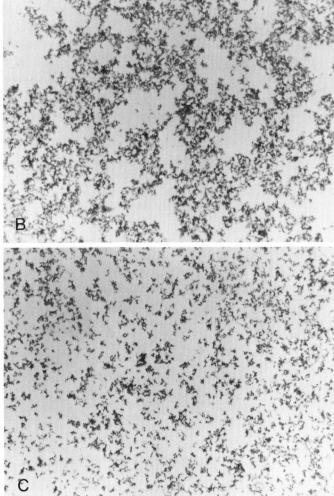

Figure 2.1.14. Preparation of Ivalon particles for injection. **A.** Ivalon suspension in crystal container ready for injection. **B.** Particles suspended in contrast medium; note agglutination. **C.** Particles suspended in solution of contrast medium and Rheomacrodex; note lack of agglutination. (Reproduced from Herrera M, Rysavy J, Kotula F, Castañeda–Zúñiga WR, Amplatz K: Ivalon shavings: a new embolic agent. *Radiology* 1982;144:638–640.)

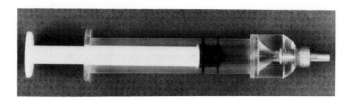

Figure 2.1.15. Cone-shaped syringe for injection of Ivalon particles facilitates central flow.

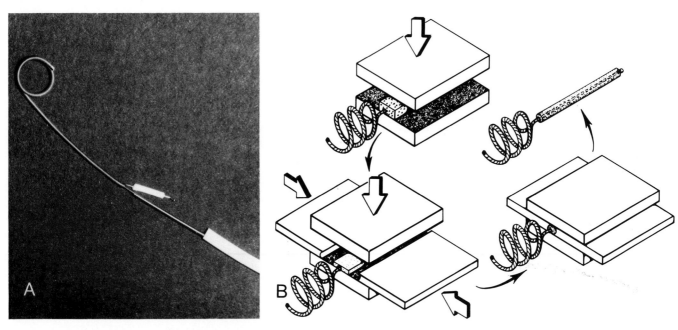

Figure 2.1.16. Embolization devices. **A.** Coilon for arterial embolization loaded over coil introducer. **B.** Ivalon plug mounted over wire attached to spring coil during compression in a vise. (Reproduced from Zollikofer C, Castañeda–Zúñiga WR, Galliani C, et al: A combination of stainless steel coil and compressed Ivalon: a new technique for embolization of large arteries and arteriovenous fistulas. *Radiology* 1981;138:229–231.)

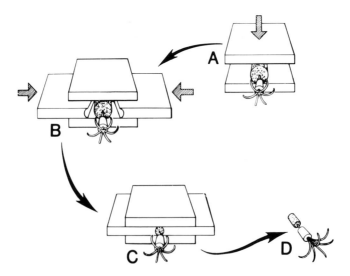

Figure 2.1.17. Ivalon plug mounted over wire attached to a spider during compression in a vise (**A–C**). Spiderlon (**D**). (Reproduced from Castañeda–Zúñiga WR, Galliani CA, Rysavy J, Kotula F, Amplatz K: "Spiderlon": a new device for simple, fast arterial and venous occlusion. *AJR* 1981;136:627–628. © by American Roentgen Ray Society, 1981.)

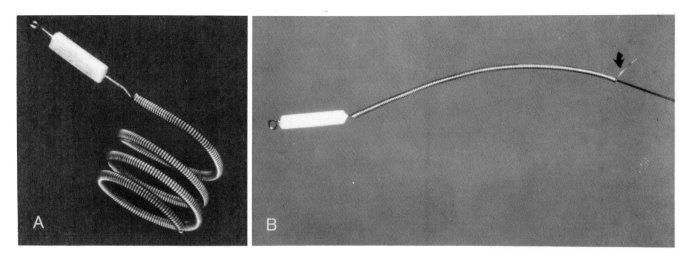

Figure 2.1.18. Coilons. **A.** Spring embolus with compressed Ivalon plug on wire for venous obliteration. **B.** Coilon for venous embolization loaded over introducer. Observe modification of proximal end of spring by straightening to facilitate fixation of device in vein and so prevent migration *(arrow)*.

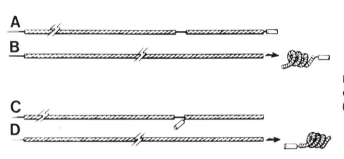

Figure 2.1.19 Schematic representation of delivery of venous (**A,B**) and arterial (**C,D**) coilon using coil introducer.

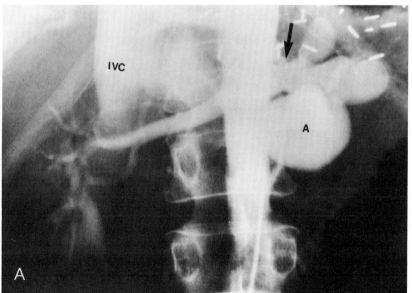

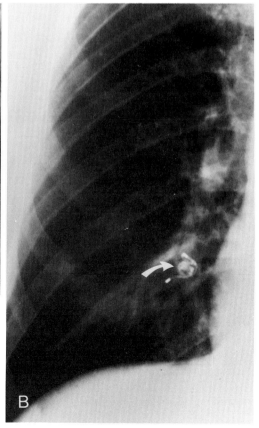

Figure 2.1.20. Inappropriate embolization of occluding device in high-flow fistula. **A.** Abdominal aortogram reveals extensive AV shunting through stump of left renal artery postnephrectomy *(arrow)*. *IVC* = inferior vena cava; *A* = aneurysm. **B.** Attempts to obliterate fistula with Gianturco–Wallace–Chuang (GWC) spring coil resulted in pulmonary embolization of occluding device *(arrow)*. (Reproduced from Mazer MJ, Baltaxe HA, Wolf GL: Therapeutic embolization of the renal artery with Gianturco coils: limitations and technical pitfalls. *Radiology* 1981;138:37–46.)

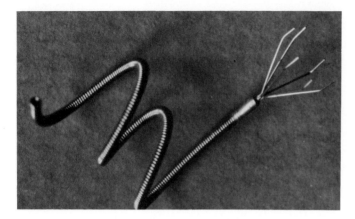

Figure 2.1.21. Spring coil with barbed ends used for embolization of large AV fistulae. (Reproduced from Castañeda–Zúñiga WR, Tadavarthy SM, Beranek I, Amplatz K: Nonsurgical closure of large arteriovenous fistulas. *JAMA* 1976;236:2649–2650. Copyright 1976, American Medical Association.)

splenoportography to tamponade the tract,[65] as well as for occlusion of any other tubular structure. Generally, Ivalon is used in diluted contrast medium, but the particles also can be made radiopaque by adding 60% barium sulfate or tantalum powder.[52,53]

OTHER NONABSORBABLE PARTICULATE MATERIALS

Microspheres of different materials such as stainless[66] or ferromagnetic[23,67] steel, acrylic,[68] methyl methacrylate,[3] Silastic, and silicone[69–71] are inert and available in a great variety of sizes. Most of them are radiopaque, allowing

detection by radiography. Microspheres are commonly used to occlude AVMs of the nervous system.

One of the specific advantages of Silastic or silicone spheres is a specific gravity that lets them float and consequently have a flow-guided distribution. This makes them advantageous for occluding lesions with strong flow, such as hypervascular tumors or AVMs.[72]

ISOBUTYL 2-CYANOACRYLATE

IBCA (Ethicon; Braum–Melsungen, etc.) is a rapidly hardening plastic adhesive chemically similar to Superglue. It has been used surgically since the 1960s[73] and radiologically since 1972.[11] The rationale behind its use is the possibility of directly and selectively depositing the embolic agent in the desired location. The liquid plastic is readily injectable, even through very small (3Fr) catheters, and polymerizes almost immediately upon contact with ionic fluids such as blood or vascular endothelium. This polymerization leaves the plastic solid.[74] By modifying the introducing technique or the polymerization process, localized obstruction or casts of the vascular tree can be obtained (Fig. 2.1.26).

A coaxial technique is used, utilizing a 6.5Fr or 7Fr catheter for catheterization of the desired vessel. Once a suitable position has been reached, a 3Fr Teflon catheter is introduced through the larger catheter and advanced beyond its tip. The inner catheter is then flushed with glucose solution through a three-way stopcock to clear it of blood or contrast medium. The previously opacified IBCA is injected through the inner catheter after changing the

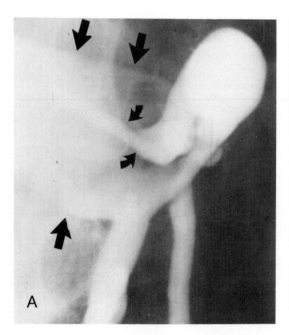

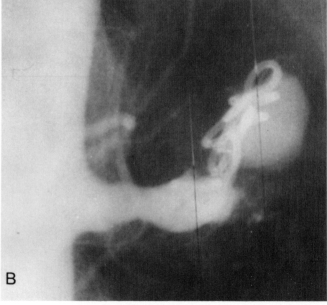

Figure 2.1.22. Postnephrectomy AV fistula in patient with renal allograft and severe high-output congestive heart failure. **A.** Selective injection of stump of left renal artery *(small arrows)* reveals extensive AV shunting through stump of renal vein, which is severely dilated *(large arrows)*. **B.** After placement of barbed coil, additional GWC spring embolus and silk streamers were placed to cause complete thrombosis of fistula. (Reproduced from Castañeda–Zúñiga WR, Tadavarthy SM, Beranek I, Amplatz K: Nonsurgical closure of large arteriovenous fistulas. *JAMA* 1976;236:2649–2650. Copyright 1976, American Medical Association.)

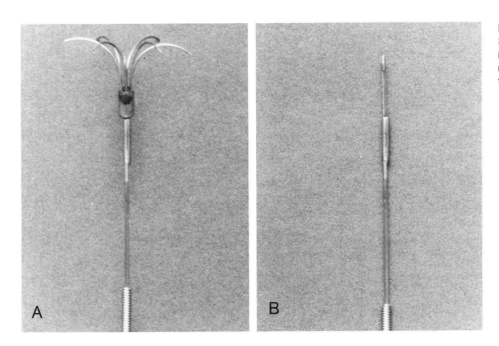

Figure 2.1.23. Stainless-steel spider. **A.** Spider mounted on introducer. **B.** Tip of introducer is of smaller diameter than the remainder of stylet to allow its placement through hollow core of spider.

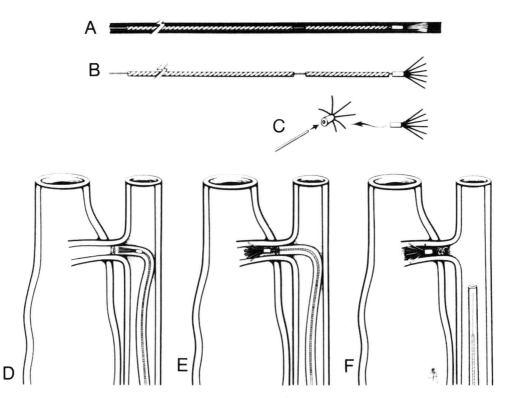

Figure 2.1.24. Spider delivery system. **A.** Schematic representation. **B.** Folded spider is being advanced with legs forward through angiographic catheter. **C.** Upon exiting from angiographic catheter, legs of spider expand and engage arterial wall. **D.** Diagram of AV communication between stump of renal artery and inferior vena cava with selective catheterization of arterial stump by angiographic catheter, through which spider is being advanced. **E.** Spider has been released beyond catheter tip. **F.** With spider secured, angiographic catheter has been removed. (Reproduced from Castañeda–Zúñiga WR, Tadavarthy SM, Galliani C, Laerum F, Schwarten D, Amplatz K: Experimental venous occlusion with stainless steel spiders. *Radiology* 1981:141;238–241.)

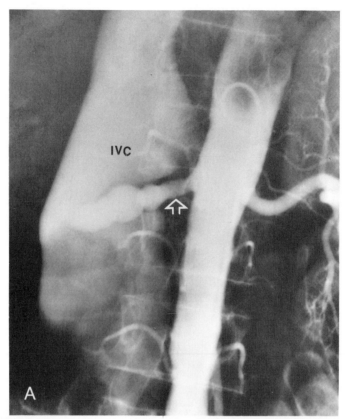

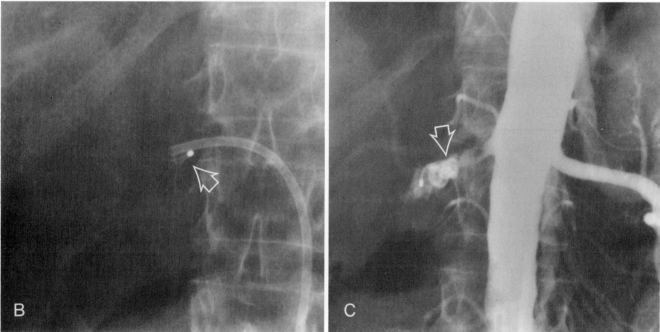

Figure 2.1.25. Postnephrectomy AV fistula of left kidney. **A.** Abdominal aortogram shows large fistula between stump of right renal artery *(open arrow)* and inferior vena cava (*IVC*). **B.** A spider has been placed within stump of artery *(arrow).* **C.** Aortogram reveals complete thrombosis of arterial stump *(arrow)* after placement of two GWC spring emboli behind spider. (Reproduced from Castañeda-Zúñiga WR, Tadavarthy SM, Galliani C, Laerum F, Schwarten D, Amplatz K: Experimental venous occlusion with stainless steel spiders. *Radiology* 1981:141;238–241.)

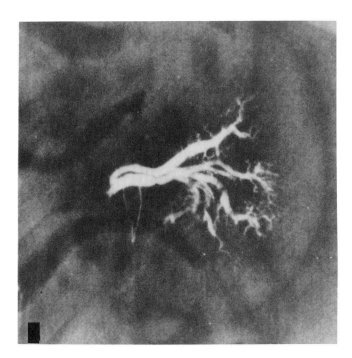

Figure 2.1.26. Cast of renal artery produced with IBCA made radiopaque by addition of tantalum powder.

position of the stopcock. The forward progress of the adhesive should be carefully monitored so the injection can be stopped as soon as the desired occlusion has been obtained; at this moment, the stopcock is switched and the inner catheter is flushed with glucose solution, to prevent the catheter tip from being glued to the blood vessel.[75,76] Balloon occlusion of the vessel has been recommended to help localize the obstruction.[75]

Modification of the polymerization process is required when a cast of the vascular tree is desired, as for AVMs or for organ ablation. Goldman et al. recommend mixing the adhesive with Ethiodol.[75]

Abroad, IBCA is the most popular tissue adhesive. In the United States, however, it is not approved for clinical use except for experimental purposes.

Because of the rapid polymerization of the plastic upon contact with ionic substances, a coaxial catheter technique and considerable skill are required for IBCA use.[75,77] It is not radiopaque by itself, but it can be readily mixed with tantalum powder,[75,78] ethiodized oils,[78] or iophendylate.[79] Addition of these oily substances or of nitrocellulose[80] also slows the polymerization of the plastic, making it easier to handle. Prefilling of the catheter and flushing of the entire system with 50% glucose solution permit clinical application without risk of the catheter tip becoming glued to the vessel.[76]

This occlusive material can be introduced through small catheters, yet larger vessels can be occluded.[75] One of the principal applications is in AVMs because the instant hardening of the plastic can prevent the pulmonary embolization that is often a problem in such lesions with other

agents.[52,77] A disadvantage of IBCA is the severe inflammatory local reaction it engenders, which is predominantly a foreign body-type reaction with multinucleated giant cells migrating around the particles.[73,81] Use of IBCA should be undertaken with great caution in the gastrointestinal tract, since peripheral embolization of the adhesive can cause ischemic changes.[81,82] The use of IBCA is discussed further in Chapter 2, Part 2 on embolotherapy in the treatment of male subfertility.

SILICONE RUBBER

Silicone rubber (Dow–Corning) is a convenient biocompatible material for vascular embolization. The substance can be made radiopaque by adding tantalum powder but is also available from the manufacturer as a radiopaque preparation. A silicone rubber mixture consists of Silastic elastomers that are vulcanized by catalysts.[83] The catalysts are mixed with liquid prior to injection, and the amount of catalyst can be altered in order to control the speed of polymerization.[83,84] To decrease the viscosity of the silicone rubber mixture, a specific fluid can be added in various proportions.[84] Thus, selective injection of vessels of any size can be achieved.

Silicone rubber seems to be an ideal substance for creating complete vascular casts.[83,84] Cessation of blood flow facilitates the injection, so the use of double-lumen balloon catheters is advantageous.[84] For safe delivery of the substance and to prevent spillover, a highly selective injection is desired. The disadvantage of silicone rubber is that it does not have adhesive properties. Thus, the vascular bed must be completely filled to keep the substance in place (Fig. 2.1.27). No reaction between the elastomer and the vessel wall is apparent macroscopically or microscopically.[83]

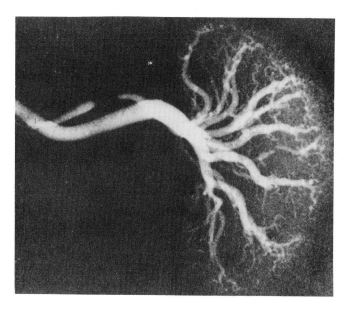

Figure 2.1.27. Cast of renal artery has been formed with silicone mixture made radiopaque by addition of heavy metals.

ETHIBLOC

Ethibloc (Ethicon) is an amino acid occlusion gel said to be specifically appropriate for preoperative embolization of renal tumors.[85] The substance is made radiopaque with iodine. Ethibloc has a low viscosity and comes premixed in a plastic syringe. It penetrates deep into the vascular tree, apparently without risk of pulmonary embolization.[85,86]

MICROFIBRILLAR COLLAGEN

Microfibrillar collagen (MFC) is a hemostatic agent derived from bovine hide. Its mechanism of action is thought to involve platelet aggregation and activation.[87] When mixed with methylglucamine diatrizoate, MFC forms a radiopaque suspension that can be injected easily through an angiographic catheter as small as 3Fr. Two weeks after embolization, there is a severe granulomatous arteritis, which subsides by three months, with fibrosis replacing inflammation. Histologically, MFC occludes large and medium vessels as well as small end arteries. This last feature, although desirable in the preoperative or palliative embolization of tumors or in the nonsurgical management of AVMs, where a distal occlusion is important to prevent recurrences,[88] is undesirable in other applications such as control of bleeding in the gastrointestinal tract, where it could cause tissue necrosis by reducing collateral flow.[89]

MFC is available in sterile 1g and 5g containers as a dry, finely shredded substance that is mixed with contrast medium to produce a suspension. Small amounts of the suspension are injected, and the catheter is immediately flushed with 3–5ml of saline to prevent blockage. The use of an introducer sheath is recommended for catheter exchange purposes. A coaxial technique has also been used for delivery, as has a balloon occlusion method to prevent reflux of the embolic agent into peripheral vessels, which has been one of the complications of MFC use.[88]

ABSOLUTE ETHANOL

Recently, absolute ethanol was added to the list of sclerosing agents for transvascular embolization. It has aided in the obliteration of gastroesophageal varices and is able to produce organ ablation.[17,90] Absolute ethanol is presumed to have a direct toxic effect on the endothelium that activates the coagulation system on the dehydrated endothelial layers. Vascular occlusion, therefore, is not achieved instantly but rather in days to weeks.[17] The toxic effect extends into the perivascular tissues, and use of absolute ethanol has caused perivascular necrosis.[91]

Depending on the size of the vessel to be occluded and on the velocity of blood flow, the amount of absolute ethanol needed differs. Several injections may be required to occlude major feeders. The use of double-lumen balloon catheters is recommended. Absolute ethanol can also be delivered through tiny flow-guided balloon catheters, which is a distinct advantage of this substance. It is naturally sterile and is diluted quickly after injection, which reduces the direct toxic effect. No clinically important systemic toxic effects have been reported. Use of this agent is discussed in more detail later in this chapter.

HOT CONTRAST MEDIUM

Contrast medium heated to 100°C has been used successfully at the University of Minnesota in experimental animals for obliteration of spermatic veins.[18,19] Both toxic[92] and heat[18,19] damage was seen in the vessels, and permanent occlusion of veins was achieved after injection of as little as 2ml (Fig. 2.1.28A–C). Thrombosis was not immediate; thrombi usually appeared in the lumen and vasa vasorum after one to five days. In all cases, the thrombi were well organized at the end of two weeks, with no evidence of perivascular damage.[18] The occlusion becomes permanent by the invasion of fibroblasts, which turn the vessel into a fibrous cord (Fig. 2.1.28D).

The technique requires transmission of heat through an angiographic catheter 80–100cm long. Fortunately, minimal heat loss occurs during transit through the catheter, probably due to the poor thermal conduction properties of plastics and the high specific heat of the contrast medium. Heated contrast medium is preferred to heated saline or glucose solutions for two reasons. First, contrast medium can be seen fluoroscopically, so the length of the thermal injury can be controlled. Second, the hypertonicity of contrast medium may cause cumulative damage to the vascular endothelium. An advantage of heated contrast medium over other sclerosing agents is that heat is rapidly dissipated by mixing with blood, whereas thrombosis caused by the effects of other sclerosing agents cannot be prevented by blood.[93] Thus, the extent of thermal injury is governed by heat dissipation, the capacity of the treated vessel, and the diluting effect of blood flow.

Clinically, this method has been successful for obliterating the spermatic vein in subfertile men with varicoceles.[94] The method has been unsuccessful in obliterating AVMs, probably due to too rapid dissipation of heat by the inflow of blood from additional feeding vessels during hot contrast medium injection into the main vessel.

GIANTURCO COILS

Gianturco and Wallace introduced steel coils for permanent vascular occlusion of major arteries.[16,95] The devices have been used mainly for preoperative embolization of renal cell carcinomas and bleeding tumors. They also have been used for complete organ ablation as an alternative to surgical intervention, although, because of the persistence of distal flow beyond the coil from collateral parasitic vessels, particulate or fluid embolic agents generally are preferred for palliative purposes when no operation is contemplated.

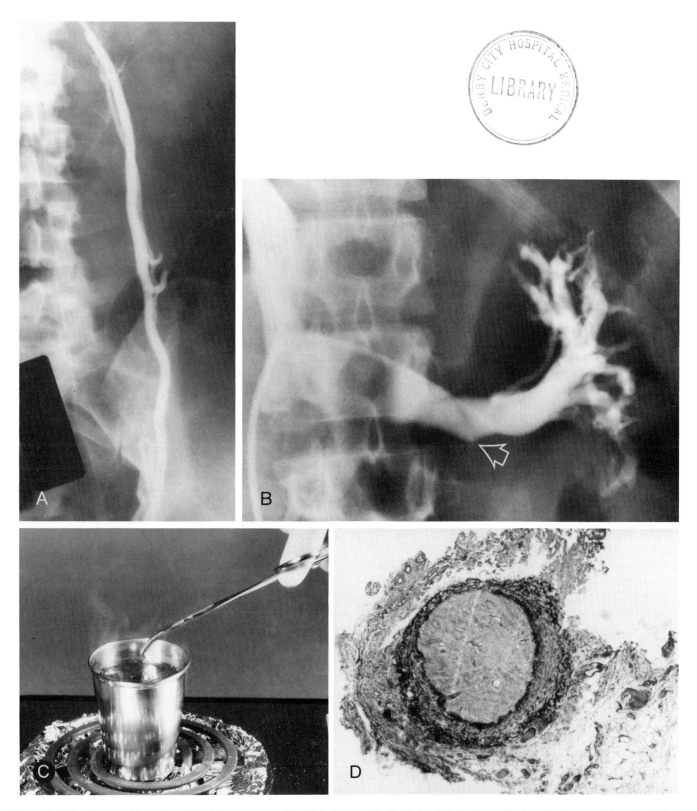

Figure 2.1.28.   Venous obliteration with boiling contrast medium. **A.** Left spermatic venogram in patient with incompetent valves after failure of surgical ligation. Observe distal reflux of contrast medium, with two venous channels opacified. **B.** Follow-up venogram after obliteration of left spermatic vein with hot contrast medium shows complete occlusion of vein at its origin *(arrow)*. **C.** Boiling contrast medium is removed from hot plate with the help of Kelly clamp. **D.** Organized venous thrombosis three months after injection of boiling contrast medium in human volunteer. (Reproduced from Cragg A, Castañeda–Zúñiga WR, Amplatz K, et al: Embolization of the spermatic vein with hot contrast medium. *Radiology* 1983;148:683–686.)

There is experimental as well as clinical evidence that permanent vascular occlusion occurs after coil placement.[81] The coils do not occlude the vessel lumen completely but rather induce thrombosis. To increase thrombogenicity, wool strands ("tails") were attached to the coils, but because of the severe granulomatous arteritis induced by these woolly tails, which extended into and beyond the adventitia, the wool was replaced by Dacron in subsequent designs. The result of embolization with these devices is similar to surgical ligation, although if complete control of hemorrhage or complete organ infarction is desired, combined use of a more peripheral occluding agent plus a coil placed more proximally is recommended. The principal indications for the use of spring coils currently are obliteration of large AV fistulae,[96] occlusion of large vessels after trauma,[97] preoperative embolization of renal tumors,[16,95] obliteration of esophageal varices,[98] and occlusion of systemic-pulmonary shunts accompanying congenital heart disease.[99] Steel coils are available in many sizes (Fig. 2.1.29*A,B*) and may be introduced through small catheters—e.g., the 4mm diameter coil through an untapered 5Fr polyethylene catheter.[100]

PLATINUM COILS

Platinum wire has been tried as a thrombogenic material. The material was initially obtained from the distal tips of coronary-type 0.014-inch guidewires.[101] They can be injected through 2.2Fr coaxial Tracker catheters. These microcatheters have been recently developed for superselective catheterization of small vessels. Platinum wires are highly thrombogenic, radiopaque, and biocompatible.[101]

Platinum wires in simple and complex shapes have been tested with and without silk or synthetic fibers to increase their thrombogenicity in experimentally created aneurysms (Hilal Microcoil; Cook, Inc., Bloomington, IN; Target Therapeutics, Santa Monica, CA).

It has been proven beyond doubt that thrombogenicity is primarily related to the added silk and/or synthetic fibers and without them the coils produce only an incomplete occlusion.[102,103] The main advantages of platinum coils are that they do not reflux as the liquid embolic agents, they do not migrate, and when deposited in aneurysms, they do not deflate like the detachable balloons do.[103]

The platinum microcoils are available commercially in straight, curved, and complex helical (Fig. 2.1.29*C*) (Flower) forms.[104] The straight forms can be simply delivered into target vessels by saline flush, but the complex forms require advancement by specially designed coil pushers. The advantages of a complex shape is that since it is multilobular upon expansion, it reduces the dead space evident in the single helical coil design.

The complications of steel coil use, both immediate and delayed, have been discussed in detail by Mazer and coworkers[62] and will be summarized here.

Immediate Complications of Coil Use

Misplacement during Insertion of the Coil through a Noncustomized Catheter

Minicoils are designed for insertion through a 5Fr polyethylene, tapered-tip, nontorquable catheter with a floppy-tip 0.035-inch guidewire as a pusher. A common mistake is attempting to pass a minicoil through a 6Fr or 7Fr preshaped torque-control catheter; but when this is done, the minicoil tends to buckle inside the larger lumen (Fig. 2.1.30), allowing the pusher to wedge through it and hinder coil advancement. Switching to a more rigid mechanical pusher may only produce additional complications such as proximal catheter perforation.[62] A coil wedged within a catheter can be safely withdrawn by removing the catheter, but a coil that is partially dangling outside the catheter and cannot be extruded further is a more difficult dilemma. If the coil is not washed off the catheter by the blood current, it is likely to be expelled from the tip as the catheter is withdrawn from the puncture site. Thus, a second puncture is needed for the introduction of a snare to trap and remove the coil (Fig. 2.1.31).

The obvious solution is not to pass a coil through a catheter that it is not meant to go through. A coil introducer has been described for a safest introduction (Fig. 2.1.32).[105]

Improper Selection of Coil Size

Too small. A coil of a diameter too small for the arterial lumen in which it is deposited will not wedge into position effectively at that site and could potentially be washed back into the aorta by forceful flushing or be carried distally into a segmental renal artery branch. The AV communications in a renal cell carcinoma have the dimensions of a small distal vessel, and it is inconceivable that even the smallest coil carried distally could pass through such an opening into the inferior vena cava. However, this complication is certainly possible in AV communications at a more proximal level (Fig. 2.1.20). Simultaneous balloon occlusion of the renal vein has been used to diminish blood flow to allow better placement and stabilization of a coil deposited from the arterial side. However, there is a risk that, when the balloon is deflated, the coil and the formed thrombus will produce an even greater embolic compromise of the pulmonary arteries.

Therefore, if angiographic occlusion is to be attempted, a modification of the coil system is desirable. Stainless-steel barbs are attached to the proximal end of a large coil in an inverted-umbrella configuration (Fig. 2.1.21). The distal tips of these barbs are curved slightly inward to permit this retracted, inverted umbrella to be pushed ahead of the coil through the catheter without embedding its barbs in the catheter wall. Once extruded into the proximal portion of the AV fistula, the steel barbs spring open and embed themselves in the aneurysmal vessel wall to provide an

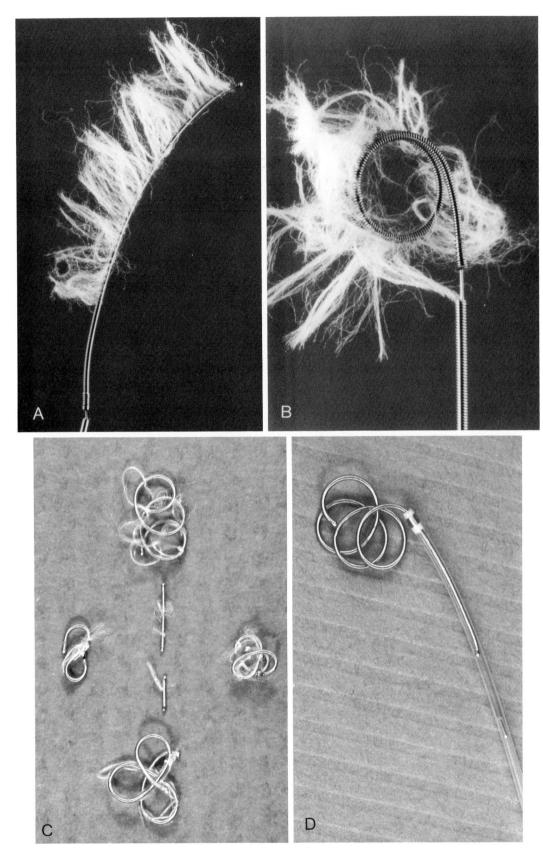

Figure 2.1.29.   GWC minicoil. **A.** Mounted over introducer wire. **B.** Partially extruded from introducer wire. **C, D.** Platinum microcoils of varied designs: straight, curved, and helical. (Reproduced from Castañeda–Zúñiga WR, Zollikofer C, Barreto A, Formanek A, Amplatz K: A new device for the safe delivery of stainless steel coils. *Radiology* 1980;136:230–231.)

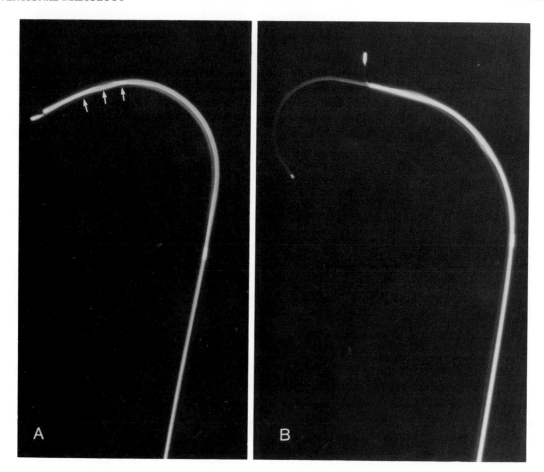

Figure 2.1.30. Problem with minicoil insertion. **A.** Minicoil is stuck within angiographic catheter due to buckling of thinner shaft of the device around curve of catheter *(arrows).* **B.** Thinner wire placed alongside stuck minicoil during attempts to deliver occluding device.

effective mechanical baffle and to prevent venous embolization of the proximally attached coil.[63] Additional coils or other embolizing agents can then be added proximal to the baffle without fear of distal embolization (Fig. 2.1.22). Alternatively a spider can be used to create a baffle (Fig. 2.1.23) behind which additional embolic agents can be placed (Fig. 2.1.25). A detachable coil is also available for the obliteration of large AV fistulae (Fig. 2.1.33). If the fistula is larger than the diameter of the coil, this can be retracted into the introducer catheter.

Too large. A coil that is too large for the main renal artery or segmental branch into which it is inserted will remain elongated and be less effective. If this occurs in the main renal artery, the proximal segment of the elongated coil could protrude from the arterial orifice into the abdominal aorta. The entire coil might then be dragged into the aorta by the downstream blood current. More likely, a marginal thrombotic nidus could develop at this site and become a potential source of recurrent peripheral vascular emboli. An analogous complication is mentioned by Anderson et al. after closure of carotid-jugular AV fistulae with steel coils in experimental animals.[106] Distally, an elongated large coil in a smaller segmental renal arterial branch can act like a stiletto, repeatedly traumatizing the intima during the up-and-down movement of the kidney with breathing. Frank perforation of the vessel wall may ensue, or a false aneurysm may develop.[62]

Too Many Coils Inserted

Sometimes, too many coils are inserted. For example, backing up coils extruded from the distal main renal artery to incorporate the take-off of a proximal bifurcating branch is particularly tempting, but in this situation one coil too many is invariably added, with extrusion of the most proximal coil into the aorta. When there is a large proximal branch vessel that contributes to the vascular supply of the superior portion of a renal cell carcinoma, a solution safer than complete embolization is initial selective occlusion of this vessel either with a minicoil[100] or with Gelfoam inserted by subselective catheterization with a routine diagnostic catheter. The distal main renal artery can then be occluded with a minimum of appropriately sized coils.

Improper Proximal Coil Placement

A tortuous aorta or a sharply angulated take-off of the renal artery can cause instability of the delivery catheter within the renal artery. In such a situation, passage of the pusher may result in sudden catheter recoil at the moment of coil expulsion, accidentally depositing the coil directly

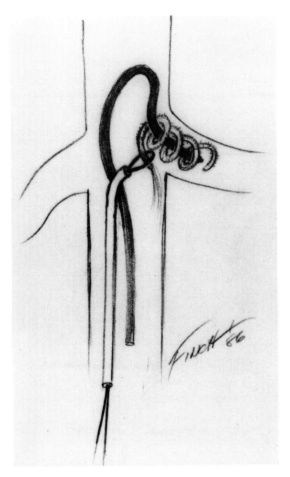

Figure 2.1.31. Diagram of percutaneous removal of misplaced spring coil embolus with the help of vascular snare.

into the aorta or into an unsatisfactory position at the renal artery orifice that would hinder surgical ligation of the renal pedicle during subsequent nephrectomy.[107–109] Therefore, if a tortuous catheter course is noted, trial passages of the pusher through the catheter are advisable before the coil is deposited in the catheter. A less rigid pusher or a less tortuous catheter approach downstream via the left axillary artery may be necessary.

Piston-like Coil Reflux due to Contrast Injection

After satisfactory placement of coils in the distal main renal artery, it is common to inject contrast medium through the delivery catheter to document the occlusion. In some cases, the most distal coil is the main cause of arterial occlusion, and a more proximal coil, particularly if it is slightly smaller than the artery, can reflux into the aorta in the washout turbulence created by the injection (Fig. 2.1.34).[62] If documentation of occlusion is desired, an aortogram performed with the catheter sideholes positioned just above the origin of the embolized vessel is recommended. When there is fear of pulmonary embolization following a venous embolization, to prevent central migration of Gianturco–Wallace–Chuang (GWC) spring embolus after spermatic embolization, the coils can be modified by straightening their distal end, to form a sharp prong which can engage the venous wall, anchoring the device (Fig. 2.1.35).

Delayed Complications of Coil Use

Failure of Vessel Occlusion

The occlusive action of coils is dependent on the patient's clotting mechanism. Therefore, in patients with poor clotting, including those receiving anticoagulants, the use of cast-forming embolic agents (silicone, IBCA) is preferable to the use of coils.[110]

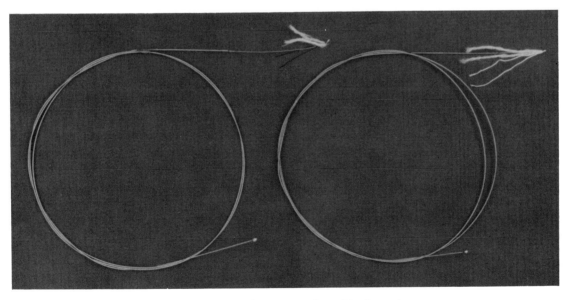

Figure 2.1.32. GWC coil mounted over introducer wire.

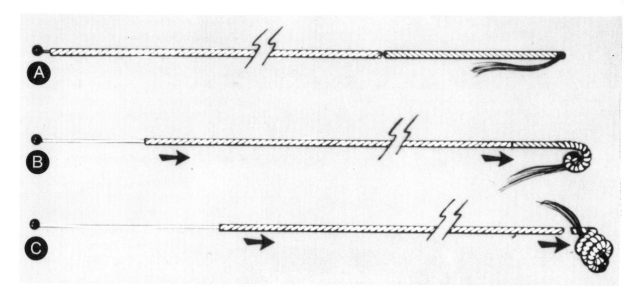

Fig. 2.1.33 Introduction of detachable coil. **A.** Introducer with GWC coil loaded, ready for advancement through angiographic catheter. **B.** In order to release spring embolus, movable core of introducer is pulled back while keeping outer sheath in place. **C.** After stylet has been completely removed from spring embolus, this resumes its coiled shape and is released.

SILK TUFTS ("STREAMERS")

Silk has been used extensively in surgery, and its biocompatibility has been proved. Since the original report,[62] it has been used in combination with coils for rapid, permanent occlusion of large vessels and malformations and of post-traumatic (including postbiopsy) AV communications and for tumor ablation (Fig. 2.1.36A,B).

BRISTLE BRUSHES

Small nylon brushes are safe and effective for transcatheter occlusion of large arteries both experimentally and clinically. They are particularly suitable for occlusion of larger AV communications. Brushes rapidly occlude the artery by mechanical blockage and induce secondary formation of a firmly adherent thrombus.[111] Histologic examination of the artery wall reveals only a mild inflammatory reaction in all three layers without destruction. Brushes create a less obvious density on x-ray films than do coils but have no other particular disadvantages.

DETACHABLE BALLOONS

Detachable balloons (Becton Dickinson; Surgimed; Ingenoor; and others) are available for occlusion of vessels as large as 6mm in luminal diameter (Fig. 2.1.37).[8] They have the advantage of being carried by the blood to a superselective location, where they can be detached.[7–10,112] The effect of vessel occlusion can be tested before detaching the balloon. For the occlusion of AVMs, detachable balloons appear ideal; there is no danger of influx or reflux leading to pulmonary embolism. The disadvantages are the considerable cost of these devices and their tendency to deflate after several weeks, which may lead to recanalization and migration. Also, the introduction system can be difficult to handle.

ELECTROCOAGULATION (DIATHERMIC VASCULAR OCCLUSION)

Blood clots can be produced in vivo by electrocoagulation with an indifferent electrode applied to the body, a conducting wire extending through a selectively placed catheter, and a direct current.[21] The method is the same as that of the electrocautery used in surgery. The blood coagulates at the intravascular electrode, but this takes as long as 30 minutes or even one hour. With an electrode designed primarily to cauterize the vascular wall with a diathermic current, there is higher probability of vascular occlusion.[22] Because of the high current density at the electrode, localized heat is produced, resulting in thrombus formation and local necrosis of the vascular wall. With an endothelial lesion, the thrombi cause permanent vascular occlusion. At present, this technique is experimental.[22]

ANGIOGRAPHIC TECHNIQUES AND CATHETER SELECTION

The appropriate catheters for angiography and embolization depend on the embolic substance that will be used and on the vascular structure that will be embolized.

Introducer Sheaths

An introducer sheath is almost invariably used during transcatheter embolization, principally because it permits catheter exchange. Catheters may become blocked during injection of particulate materials, especially Ivalon, or of tissue adhesives or Gianturco coils. In this last situation, the presence of the sheath may allow a partially extruded coil to be removed safely from the artery, whereas without

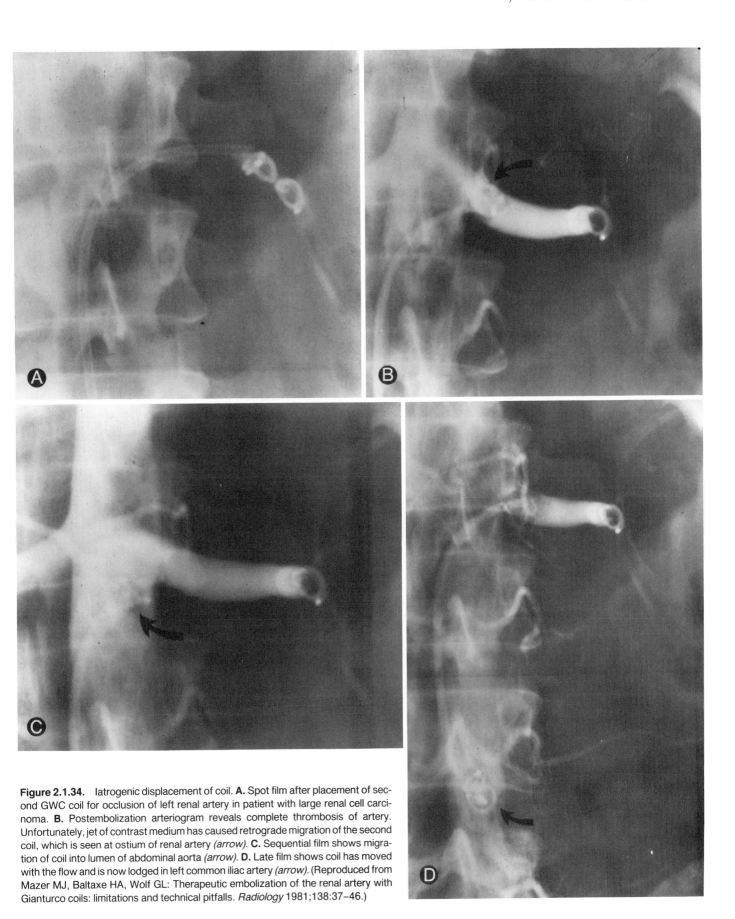

Figure 2.1.34. Iatrogenic displacement of coil. **A.** Spot film after placement of second GWC coil for occlusion of left renal artery in patient with large renal cell carcinoma. **B.** Postembolization arteriogram reveals complete thrombosis of artery. Unfortunately, jet of contrast medium has caused retrograde migration of the second coil, which is seen at ostium of renal artery *(arrow)*. **C.** Sequential film shows migration of coil into lumen of abdominal aorta *(arrow)*. **D.** Late film shows coil has moved with the flow and is now lodged in left common iliac artery *(arrow)*. (Reproduced from Mazer MJ, Baltaxe HA, Wolf GL: Therapeutic embolization of the renal artery with Gianturco coils: limitations and technical pitfalls. *Radiology* 1981;138:37–46.)

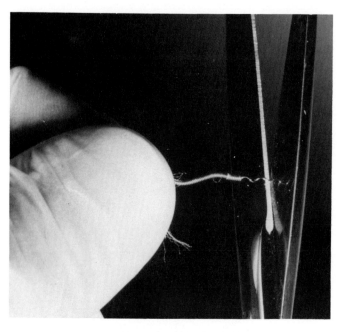

Figure 2.1.35. GWC coil being modified by partial straightening of distal spring, which is subsequently trimmed with scissors.

a sheath, it probably would pull free as the catheter is pulled back through the arteriotomy. Sheaths also simplify routine catheter exchanges and allow insertion of balloon catheters (Fig. 2.1.38).

Sheaths are available with and without a sealing diaphragm. The advantage of a diaphragm is that there is no blood loss once the catheter has been removed. The disadvantage is that balloons may be dislodged by the diaphragm, as may partially extruded coils. Sheaths without diaphragms may be fitted with adapters such as the Tuohy–Borst, or Iris diaphragm, which may be tightened to provide a watertight seal around a smaller catheter yet be loosened to allow safe withdrawal of balloon catheters.

Catheters

Depending on the embolizing agent selected and the vascular structure to be embolized, the available angiographic catheters include:

A tapered catheter with an end hole (used for spring coils, Gelfoam, Ivalon particles, and fluid embolic agents);

Figure 2.1.36. Silk streamers. **A.** Streamers with different numbers of silk threads. **B.** Streamer loaded in Teflon tubing and connected to syringe loaded with dilute contrast medium for flushing.

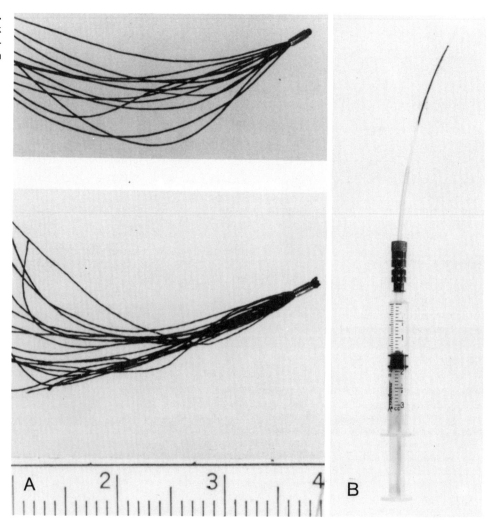

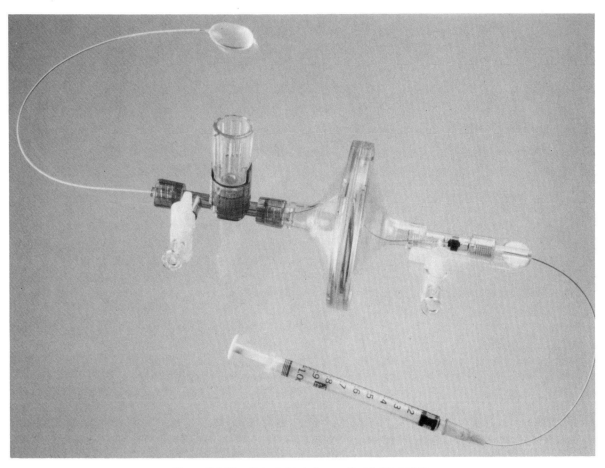

Figure 2.1.37. Detachable balloon with delivery system.

Coaxial systems (used for fluids such as IBCA or MFC or for small particulate agents);
Nontapered Teflon catheters (used for spider placement or delivery of compressed Ivalon);
A balloon catheter (used to prevent reflux during delivery of particulate media and fluid agents).

Each of these will be reviewed.

TAPERED CATHETERS

Most embolization techniques can be performed through regular tapered angiographic catheters. The authors prefer to use 5Fr catheters with a 45° curve at the tip, which can be easily reshaped with steam. Occasionally, larger French-size catheters are used, such as the 7Fr reinforced polyurethane catheters, which have a much better torque control than the 5Fr catheters.

COAXIAL CATHETERS

A safe and effective embolization can only be achieved by advancing the catheters as near as possible to the selected site. The standard 5.0 and 6.5Fr diagnostic catheters commonly cannot be advanced very far because of their stiffness. Because of this, coaxial catheters are becoming increasingly popular, particularly when a highly selec-

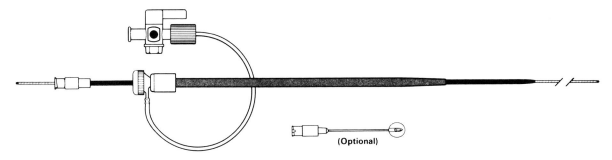

(Optional)

Figure 2.1.38. Introducer sheath with check-flow valve and sidearm for intermittent flushing. (Courtesy of Cook, Inc.)

tive catheter placement is required. The first commercially available coaxial catheter was developed at the Massachusetts General Hospital.[113] It is a 3.0Fr Teflon catheter and accommodates a 0.025-inch guidewire (Cook, Inc., Bloomington, IN). This catheter has been used coaxially, introducing it through a guiding catheter (commonly a conventional angiographic catheter), fitted with a Y-connector to allow irrigation around the 3Fr catheter. Because the catheter is made of Teflon material, it is relatively stiff. Another drawback of this catheter is its lack of radiopacity. Because of this, the catheter is commonly preloaded with a platinum-tipped 0.016-inch, high-torque floppy guidewire (ACS).[114,115] The guidewire provides visibility and facilitates the catheterization of small arterial branches. Placement of the guidewire beyond the catheter tip and advancing the catheter over the wire is the safest method of introduction of Teflon catheters.

It has been used for delivery of 0.64mm coils,[114] Gelfoam pledgets, and liquid plastic polymers such as IBCA.[113-115]

TRACKER COAXIAL INFUSION CATHETERS

The second-generation coaxial infusion catheter, widely known as the Tracker System (Target Therapeutics, Los Angeles, CA), was recently introduced and has several advantages over the Massachusetts General Teflon catheter.[116-120] The Tracker catheter has been used extensively, both in peripheral and neuroangiography. The interventional neuroangiographers primarily rely on this system for interventional procedures, and several publications support this fact. The catheter shaft has a composite construction from extruded high- and low-density polyethylene, to provide a graded shaft stiffness ranging from a highly flexible tip to a semi-rigid proximal segment.[116] It is fitted with a Luer-Lok adaptor in the proximal end and the distal end is highly visible because of the presence of a platinum marker. The Standard Tracker-18 catheter is graded from a highly flexible distal end of 2.7Fr to a stiffer proximal end of 3.0Fr (1mm). The length of the distal flexible end can be: 6, 12, and 18cm. Recently, a new Tracker-18 Hi-Flow infusion and Tracker-18 LF infusion systems were added for the easier injection of diagnostic and therapeutic agents. Apparently, the platinum coil transition zone in the Tracker-18 LF system protects the inner luminal surface from substantial guidewire manipulations and reduces the likelihood of kinking.

The newer Tracker-18 Unibody infusion catheter is a molded one-piece design, with balanced shaft positions. This benefits the angiographer because of its increased pushability, trackability and the decreased potential for kinking. The Tracker-18 and the Tracker-18 LF are compatible with guiding catheters that accept an 0.038-inch guidewire. The Tracker-18 Hi-Flow infusion catheter requires guiding catheters which accept 0.042-inch guidewires. The Tracker-18 catheter system accepts a guidewire diameter of 0.018 inch. A variety of torque guidewires that range from 0.014- to 0.018-inch diameter with excellent torque transition and different flexibilities are available for usage along with the Tracker-18 system. The inner diameter of the Tracker Hi-Flow catheter is 0.533mm; therefore, it can accept Ivalon particles up to 500 microns in size.[120]

Clinical experience indicates that occlusion of the lumen is seen more frequently when Ivalon particles are injected through the Tracker-18 LF than with the Tracker-18 or the Tracker-18 Hi-Flow.

The next larger system, Tracker-25, requires a guiding catheter with an inner diameter of 0.054 inch. The proximal outer diameter is 4.0Fr and the distal end is 3.6Fr. It accepts microcoils as big as 0.025 inch.

The largest Tracker-38 infusion system proximally measures 5.3Fr and the distal end is 4.7Fr. Standard and torque guidewires with diameters of 0.035 and 0.038 inch can be used. It can deliver larger coils of 0.035 and 0.038 inch as well as larger Gelfoam pledgets and particulate emboli. It is primarily used as a guiding catheter for the Tracker-18 system.

HIESHIMA MICRO CATHETER

This is another coaxial catheter based on the technology of single-tapered polyethylene extrusion without any internal steps (Microvena Corporation, Vadnais Heights, MN). The proximal end is stiffer and measures 3.0Fr in its outer diameter, and the distal end measures either 2.0 or 2.3Fr. The 2.0Fr distal tip catheter accepts 0.014-inch guidewires, and the 2.3Fr distal end accepts 0.016- and 0.018-inch torque wires.

The distal end of the catheter tapers down to a smaller diameter over a 10–15cm transition area resulting in a softer distal segment. There is a recess radiopaque marker at the distal end for easy identification. Because of its recent introduction, it has not been tried as widely as the Tracker-18 systems.

The coaxial system has greatly enhanced the capabilities of angiographers and interventionalists to reach smaller distal vessels safely and precisely. Superselective embolization minimizes the likelihood of complications, as a minimum amount of embolic material is required for effective devascularization.[119]

OPEN-ENDED GUIDEWIRE CATHETERS

The concept of an open-ended guidewire by removing its mandril to develop a catheter infusion system for small vessels, has brought a new dimension to the field of embolization and infusion techniques.[121-124] The Sos wire is constructed of stainless steel with a Teflon jacket and an inner removable mandrel wire. It is available in 0.035-inch and 0.038-inch outer diameters, with an inner lumen of 0.021 and 0.018 inch, respectively[121] (USCI Radiology Products; Division of C. R. Bard, Bellerica, MA; Medi-tech, Inc.,

Watertown, MA). A variety of inner mandrel wires with a variable stiffness and distal tapers transforms the open-ended outer jacket either to a flexible or heavy-duty wire. Open-ended wires have been used to monitor intravascular pressures, to inject various fluids, to infuse chemotherapeutic agents, and to inject embolic material. Supraselective placement of open-ended guidewires can be achieved by steering them with a steerable wire of 0.014 or 0.018 inch.[123] They are relatively inexpensive compared with the newer generation of coaxial infusion systems.

Open-ended wires have been utilized for the injection of liquid embolic agents such as isobutyl 2-cyanoacrylate (IBCA) (Ethicon, Inc., Somerville, NJ) or ethanol.[123] Soaked gelatin sponges that were cut into 1–2mm pledgets have been safely injected through open-ended wires.[124]

Ivalon particles with a size range of 149–250 microns can also be injected.[122] A tuberculin syringe generates more pressure as compared to a 3ml syringe during injection through the open-ended guidewire, and, therefore, better propulsion of embolic agents is achieved.

A second generation of an open-ended guidewire with a large inner diameter was developed by Cragg.[125] The inner diameter of the Cragg wire is 0.027 inch which compares to the inner diameter of the Sos wire of 0.021 inch.[125]

The luminal area of the new injectable wire is 65% larger than that of the Sos wire. It is constructed from flat wire with a coating of polyvinyl and Teflon.[125] Ivalon particles and minicoils that measure 0.025 inch are easily injected through the Cragg wire. The flow rate of contrast is 8.5ml/sec, consistently higher than the flow obtained through the Sos open-ended wire and the Tracker-18 infusion system.

A similar design to the one used in the Sos open-ended guidewire has been used in the Schneider infusion wire.

SUPPLE CATHETERS

A supple, flexible catheter has been developed and tested in humans to selectively catheterize second- and third-order branches of the hepatic arteries, as well as other vessels with difficult anatomy.[126] It is made from radiopaque silicone and polyurethane. The catheter is available in two sizes with an outer diameter of 1.0 and 1.3mm (Balt Montmorency, France; Japan Mallinckrodt, Tokyo). The corresponding inner diameters are 0.6 and 0.9mm. The maximum rate of injection is 4ml/sec; however, 1ml/sec is recommended to avoid catheter recoil. The catheter tip is shaped into a ball by heating it with a soldering iron and injecting air from the other end until the desired size of the ball is attained. A slit is made with a surgical scalpel.

The desired artery is initially catheterized with a conventional catheter and a guidewire, preferably a plastic-coated guidewire (Terumo, Inc., Tokyo, Japan), is advanced into the proximal vessel. After removal of the conventional catheter, the supple catheter is advanced over the guidewire through a sheath introducer, a guiding catheter is not necessary. Once the catheter is in the desired vascular

lumen, the guidewire is removed, and the catheter is slowly advanced to allow the blood to propulse the ball tip distally. Vessel spasm or intimal damage has seldom been noted. The catheter has been successfully placed in branches of the hepatic artery in 47 of 49 patients.[126]

NONTAPERED CATHETERS

Nontapered wide-lumen catheters are useful as guiding catheters in the coaxial systems for introduction of large baffle-forming devices such as barbed coils[63] and spiders[64] and for the introduction of one-step occluding devices such as coilons,[60] spiderlons,[61] detachable balloons,[7-10,112] and compressed Ivalon.[50]

BALLOON OCCLUSION CATHETERS

The balloon occlusion catheters in current use are constructed with either double or single lumens.

Double-lumen Balloon Catheters

The double-lumen balloon occlusion catheters have the advantage of allowing distal injection after occlusion of an artery. They are used to prevent reflux during embolization with particulate materials, such as Gelfoam and Ivalon, or with liquids such as ethanol. Proximal occlusion of the vessel allows the introduction of polymerizing plastics, because the control of blood flow by the balloon prevents passage of the material into the capillaries or the venous circulation before it polymerizes. The injection of contrast medium prior to the injection of liquid embolic agents provides a measure of the total capacity of the arterial circulation distal to the inflated balloon. By eliminating dilution with unopacified blood, balloon occlusion arteriography provides exquisite detail, even in the presence of torrential flow through an AV fistula.

These catheters are available in sizes of 5Fr to 8Fr with balloons up to 4cm in diameter fully inflated. They are available preshaped (Cordis, Inc.) (Fig. 2.1.39) or may be custom shaped using steam. Care should be taken not to heat the junction between catheter and balloon for fear of weakening this area.

Single-lumen Balloon Catheters

The simplest single-lumen balloon catheter is the Fogarty, which is commonly used for arterial embolectomy and for temporary intraoperative occlusion—for example, occlusion of a carotid-cavernous sinus fistula[127] or traumatized pelvic vessels.[128] These catheters are made of polyvinyl chloride and require insertion through a coaxial catheter.

In 1976, Kerber described an elegant single-lumen catheter with a controlled-leak balloon[10] that allows occlusion of the vessel with a balloon and distal injection of contrast medium or embolic material. The shaft of the catheter and the balloon are both made from silicone, which creates a very soft flexible catheter. Silicone catheters may be

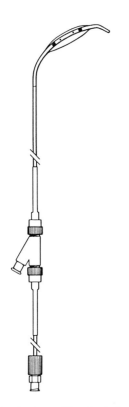

Figure 2.1.39. Angiographic cobra balloon catheter.

passed through a larger coaxial catheter and are excellent for flow direction. Similarly, Pevsner developed a controlled-leak balloon mounted on a polyethylene shaft.[129] This catheter is not propelled by injection as in the Kerber system, but it does allow a degree of flow direction.

The other single-lumen balloon catheters are used solely for embolization. Contrast medium must be injected either through a separate catheter or through the larger coaxial guiding catheter. Such catheters were described by Debrun et al. in 1975,[9] Pevsner in 1977,[129] DiTullio et al. in 1978,[130] and White et al. in 1979[131] and will be discussed more specifically in a subsequent section.

X-RAY EQUIPMENT

High-quality fluoroscopy is a sine qua non of most interventional radiologic procedures, and this is particularly true of transcatheter embolization. Facilities for video recording and playback are also desirable. For embolization in the central nervous system, including the spinal cord, high-quality photographic subtraction is essential. This is also true of embolization of intercostal or lumbar arteries, the reason being that small reticular branches may not be seen on the regular films, and embolization in such a situation has led to disastrous complications. Digital subtraction angiography has similar advantages and allows to speed up the procedure.

The portable γ camera has been useful in determining the destination of injected emboli. Conroy, Endert, and their colleagues labeled Gelfoam particles with radionuclide and were then able to pinpoint their final resting place.[27,28]

BRONCHIAL ARTERY EMBOLIZATION

Hemoptysis is one of the most impressive and alarming manifestations of tracheobronchial or pulmonary disease. In most acute episodes, the blood loss is of moderate volume and ceases spontaneously. The less common cases of severe hemoptysis are life-threatening emergencies, not because of the volume of blood lost (500–600ml) but because the continuous bleeding floods the tracheobronchial tree, with subsequent asphyxiation, which accounts for as many as 80% of the deaths.[132–134] Common causes of significant hemoptysis in the United States include cystic fibrosis, neoplasm, and bronchiectasis. In most other countries, pulmonary tuberculosis accounts for a larger percentage of cases.[135]

Anatomy

The bronchial arteries usually originate from the aorta at the level of the T_5 and T_6 vertebrae, although there is considerable variation. The classic work of Caldwell et al. in 1948 described four major vascular patterns[136]:

1. Two arteries on the left and one on the right as a common trunk with the intercostal suprema;
2. One artery trunk on the left and one on the right;
3. Two arteries on the left and two on the right;
4. One artery on the left and two on the right.

In a series published by Cohen et al., there are one or more aberrant bronchial arteries in 35% of cases (7 out of 20 patients). These arteries have originated from: 1) thyrocervical trunk; 2) internal mammary artery; 3) costocervical trunk; 4) lower intercostal artery.[137,138] They have been also reported to originate from the arch of aorta between the left carotid and left subclavian arteries.[138]

The interventionalists should be aware of the above-cited anomalous origins if one cannot find the bronchial arteries from the descending thoracic aorta.

First-class bronchial arteriography is a must, with subtraction or digital subtraction films to study the anterior and posterior radicular arteries, which can originate from the intercostal arteries and supply collaterals to the spinal cord. Therefore, the presence of an anterior spinal artery arising from the cervicointercostal trunk,[139] from an intercostal artery,[140] or from the common intercostobronchial trunk[141] should be considered an absolute contraindication to therapeutic embolization; several instances of transverse myelitis have followed intercostal or bronchial arteriography[140–142] or embolization in such cases.[135,140,143,144]

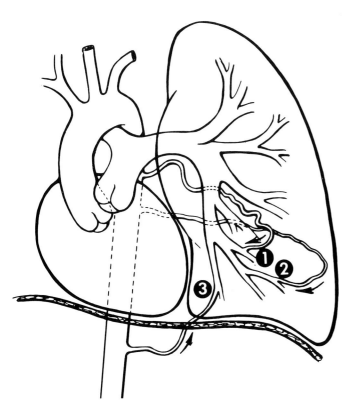

Figure 2.1.40. Diagram of sources of transpleural collateralization of left pulmonary artery in patient in Figure 2.1.51. (Reproduced from Tadavarthy SM, Klugman J, Castañeda–Zúñiga WR, Nath PH, Amplatz K: Systemic to pulmonary collaterals in pathologic states: a review. *Radiology* 1982;144:75–76.)

Extensive collateralization from mediastinal arteries and transpleural collaterals may be found, particularly after thoracotomy or in chronic inflammatory processes of the lung. Collateralization can be so strong as to reverse blood flow in the pulmonary artery (Fig. 2.1.40).[145–147] Consequently, a complete study of the bronchial circulation should include a thoracic aortogram to exclude the presence of this type of collaterals, particularly in patients with recurrent bleeding after successful embolization of bronchial arteries.[146,147]

A recent paper has emphasized the recognition of nonbronchial vessels as a source of hemoptysis.[146] The shunts between the systemic vessels and the pulmonary circulation increase the blood pressure that may account for hemoptysis. They have emphasized the systemic collaterals from the internal mammary artery and the branches of the subclavian artery.[146]

Technique

Except in patients with cystic fibrosis, bronchial arteriography is performed first on the side where there is bronchoscopic evidence of bleeding. Catheterization is usually performed with a Simmons catheter. Digital subtraction arteriography is particularly useful, because it allows eval-

uation of the existence of radicular branches while minimizing the amount of contrast medium needed, thus decreasing the risk of neurotoxicity.

After the presence of radicular branches has been ruled out, the catheter tip is advanced deeper into the artery, and embolization is performed, usually with Gelfoam or Ivalon particles.

If one elects to use Ivalon particles, the size of the particles used should be no less than 500 microns in size. The smaller size Ivalon particles can presumably occlude the smaller esophageal and bronchial branches leading to ischemia and fistula formation.[148] Particles of this size are particularly too large to enter smaller spinal feeders and the complications of spinal cord injury are therefore avoided.[137] Embolization with IBCA and alcohol have been tried and are not popular because of the associated complications.[149]

Embolization should be as distal as possible to reduce the chances of recurrence due to distal collateralization. Care should be taken, however, to avoid reflux of the embolic agent into the aorta.

The recent introduction of coaxial open-ended (Sos, Cragg wires) and the 0.018-inch Tracker infusion catheters have been a tremendous help in these patients. These catheters or guidewires can be advanced through the 5.0Fr guiding catheters as far distally as possible for safe embolization.

Although every attempt should be made to avoid embolization of bronchial arteries with spinal feeders, their presence may not be an absolute contraindication.[137] The embolic agent is preferentially carried to the bleeding site because of the sump effect. The coaxial infusion catheters or the open-ended guidewires can be advanced beyond the spinal artery, and relatively safe embolization can be accomplished.

A postembolization angiogram is obtained to assess the results. If the opposite side was considered to be free of problems, a thoracic aortogram is performed to evaluate the existence of other systemic influx into the bronchial circulation. If other sources of collateral inflow are present, they also are embolized (Fig. 2.1.41). This is particularly important in the patient with recurrent bleeding after an initially successful embolization.

In patients with cystic fibrosis, selective bronchial arteriography and embolization are performed bilaterally.

Indications

The marked improvement in the diagnosis and pharmacotherapy of pulmonary tuberculosis and of other granulomatoses and infectious diseases that used to be the cause of bronchiectasis has left cystic fibrosis as the leading cause of hemoptysis in the teenager and young adult. Malignant tumors are the most common cause in the elderly.

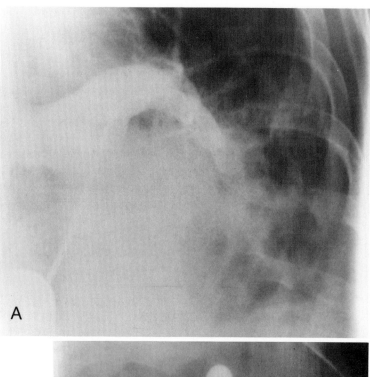

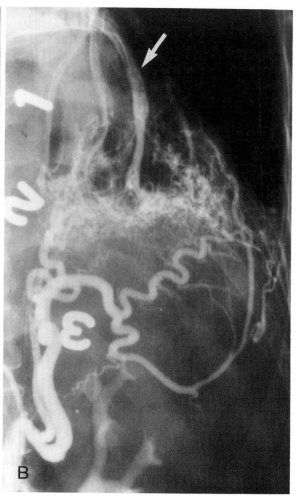

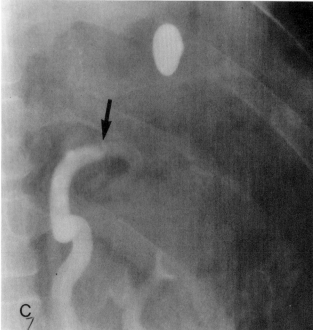

Figure 2.1.41. After embolization of phrenic artery with small Ivalon shavings, there was complete thrombosis *(arrow).* (Reproduced from Tadavarthy SM, Klugman J, Castañeda-Zúñiga WR, Nath PH, Amplatz K: Systemic to pulmonary collaterals in pathologic states: a review. *Radiology* 1982;144:75–76.)

CYSTIC FIBROSIS

Among the many factors that contribute to the production of hemoptysis in cystic fibrosis are:

Destruction of lung parenchyma;
Erosion of blood vessels;
Hyperemia with enlarged, tortuous bronchial arteries in the areas of bronchiectasis[150,151];
The existence of bronchopulmonary arterial anastomoses,

with concomitant development of a systemic-pulmonary shunt[152];
Development of pulmonary hypertension.[152]

Fellows and coworkers treated 13 patients with cystic fibrosis by embolization. Seven patients had no recurrence of hemoptysis, and five had only a minor recurrence (loss of 60ml or less). One of the main advantages of embolization is that vigorous treatment for cystic fibrosis can be reinstated within 24–48 hours, with consequent shortening of the hospital stay.[153]

In another recent series, control of hemoptysis was achieved in 19 of 20 cystic fibrosis patients with repeat embolization in eight of them.[137]

Unresectable Malignant Tumors, Either Pulmonary or Metastatic

Embolization is an alternative to radiation or chemotherapy for these otherwise terminally ill patients.[135,154]

Tuberculosis and Other Granulomatous or Occupational Diseases (Pneumoconioses)

Embolization can be used for palliation while more conventional therapy controls the primary disease.[135,154]

Other indications of bronchial artery embolization are:

Post-thoracotomy bleeding (in these patients, reoperation has a high mortality rate due to associated complications such as sepsis and renal failure)[155];
Bilaterally for advanced bronchopulmonary disease when no bleeding site can be identified by bronchoscopy[156];
Patients who refuse operation.[156]

In the polytraumatized patient, embolotherapy of a bleeding bronchial artery can be a life-saving maneuver.[155]

The complications from bronchial artery embolizations include:

1. Chest pain, dysphagia, and fever that may require narcotics and analgesics for 5–7 days.[137]
2. Left main bronchial stenosis from devascularization of bronchus has been reported.[149]
3. Left main bronchoesophageal fistula has been also reported as another complication of embolization.[148]
4. Transverse myelitis is the most dreaded complication and in the past has been reported with diagnostic angiography utilizing ionic contrast medium. The incidence has fallen sharply and, if it occurs, there is partial recovery with time.[154]

Vascular Trauma

The recognition of serious vascular trauma in a wound from which blood is spurting is simple, but recognition of the same problem in the chest, abdomen, or extremities when there is no blood visible, particularly after blunt trauma, is sometimes difficult. Any patient who is in shock or who has a penetrating injury or severe blunt trauma must be considered to have a serious vascular injury until proved otherwise.

Blunt abdominal trauma may cause particularly difficult diagnostic problems. The principal findings are shock and hemoperitoneum, which may be confirmed by peritoneal tap. Retroperitoneal hemorrhage is particularly difficult to diagnose and requires extensive evaluation.

Proper assessment of the severely injured patient requires a fast, complete diagnostic evaluation. Abdominal computed tomography and angiography provide the most accurate and precise diagnostic information on the location and extent of injury. However, proper surgical care should not be delayed in the unstable patient in whom major vascular or organ injury is suspected.[157] Frequently, it is in the treatment of postoperative complications—delayed bleeding, abscess, etc.—that interventional radiology is particularly important.

Extremities

Vascular injury in the extremities is commonly caused by penetrating injuries, rarely by blunt trauma. Preoperative evaluation is commonly performed only where a stable lesion is suspected since if the patient is bleeding severely, immediate operation is indicated. Significant arterial injury can be present even when peripheral pulses are present.[158,159]

Adequate angiographic evaluation can prevent delays in surgical repair. It demonstrates to best advantage the precise location and extent of the vascular injury, providing a road map for surgical repair or for therapeutic embolization, particularly in patients in critical condition or in injuries where surgical hemostasis is difficult, as in the thigh or buttocks.[160] Catheterization should be as selective as possible without extending the exploration time unduly. Steel coils are commonly used, since they produce a fast and permanent occlusion, but agents such as Gelfoam or Ivalon can also be used. Embolization should not be attempted when the vascular lesion is in such a location that arrest of blood flow would endanger limb viability.

If untreated, these vascular lesions can lead to the formation of post-traumatic AV fistulae (Fig. 2.1.42), 85% of which occur in the extremities.[161]

Pelvis

Deaths after pelvic fracture are due to blood loss in 60% of cases.[162] Ligation of the hypogastric artery has been used to control bleeding.[158] Selective catheterization to demonstrate the source of bleeding, followed by embolization of the hypogastric artery with autologous blood clot, was used by Kerr et al. to stop the bleeding in three patients.[163]

Due to the extensive pelvic collateral arterial network, a proximal occlusion of the hypogastric artery crossing the midline can help maintain extravasation at the site of vascular injury distal to the proximal occlusion. This leakage can be prevented by using Gelfoam or Ivalon particles to accomplish a distal embolization beyond the bleeding point. In addition, bleeding following pelvic trauma is frequently diffuse due to the transection of innumerable small peripheral vessels (Fig. 2.1.43). Often, this type of bleeding can be stopped only by bilateral peripheral embolization of

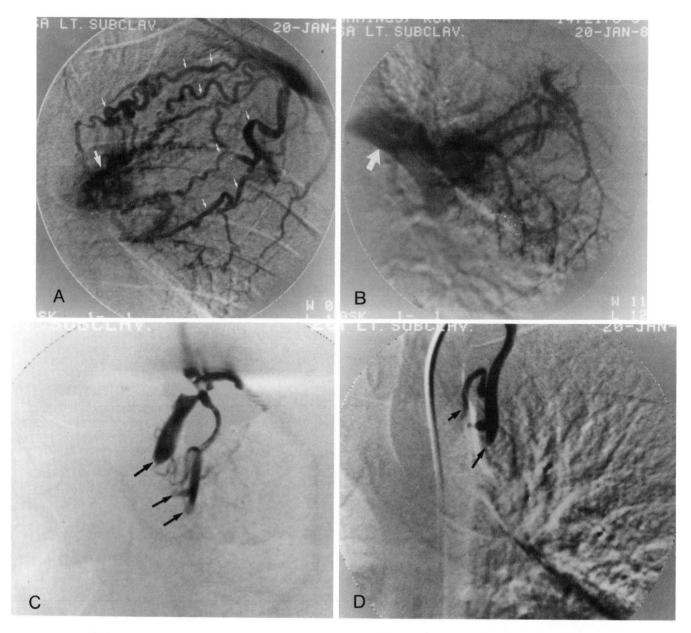

Figure 2.1.42. A 21-year-old man with left-sided sternal murmur and hemoptysis after motor vehicle accident. **A.** Selective left subclavian arteriogram shows numerous fistulous communications between branches of intercostal arteries *(small arrows)* and right upper pulmonary artery *(large arrow)*. **B.** Opacification of pulmonary veins on late films *(arrow)*. **C,D.** After embolization with Ivalon and Gelfoam plugs, complete thrombosis of feeding arteries is apparent *(arrows)*.

the hypogastric artery. In one study, branches of the anterior division of the hypogastric artery were involved in 66% of the cases, whereas posterior division branches were involved in only 33%. Many patients had only one site of bleeding in spite of multiple fractures.[164] The early angiographic evaluation in patients with major pelvic trauma prevents the development of serious renal, pulmonary, and hepatic complications of shock and of multiple transfusions.

Retroperitoneum

RENAL TRAUMA

Renal vascular injuries are due to iatrogenic trauma in almost 50% of the cases, with renal biopsy accounting for the largest percentage.[131,165–175] Recently, injuries secondary to percutaneous nephrostomy also have become important.[176–178] Penetrating wounds account for a smaller percentage of cases.[179]

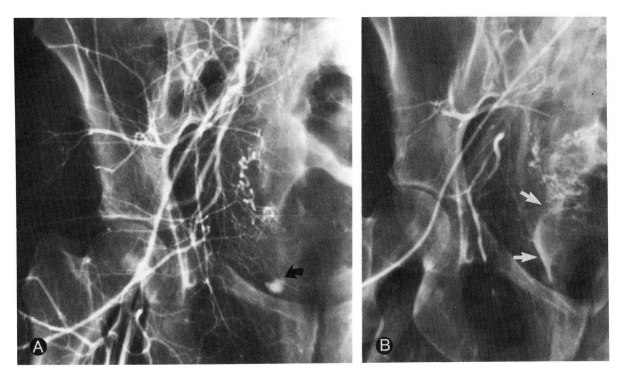

Figure 2.1.43. Post-traumatic bleeding. **A.** Right common iliac arteriogram in patient with history of pelvic trauma and falling hematocrit. Observe extravasation of contrast medium from branches of anterior division of hypogastric arteries *(arrow)* and fracture of ischion. **B.** Late phase shows extensive extravasation of contrast medium *(arrows)*. Because of midline location of extravasation, bilateral occlusion would probably be necessary for adequate control.

Arteriovenous fistula formation is a relatively common complication of percutaneous renal biopsy, occurring in as many as 36% of hypertensive patients.[140] Hypertension and nephrosclerosis are the most important predisposing factors.[180–182] The use of large-bore cutting needles and the performance of the biopsies without radiologic guidance (fluoroscopy, ultrasound, CT) to minimize the number of attempts have also been blamed for the relatively high incidence of postbiopsy fistulae (Fig. 2.1.44).[183–186]

Approximately 70% of these fistulae close spontaneously. Therefore, in the absence of life-threatening symptoms, conservative management is generally fol-

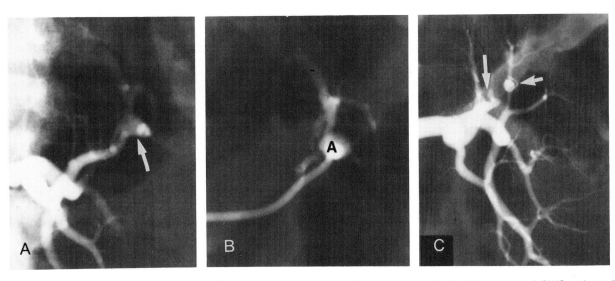

Figure 2.1.44. Control of postbiopsy AV fistula. **A.** Selective left renal arteriogram in patient with postbiopsy fistula and persistent hematuria reveals AV communication from a branch of upper pole *(arrow)*. **B.** Superselective catheterization of involved arterial branch with tip of catheter within false aneurysm *(A)*. **C.** After release of GWC spring coil *(small arrow)* within false aneurysm, observe complete thrombosis of branch artery *(large arrow)*.

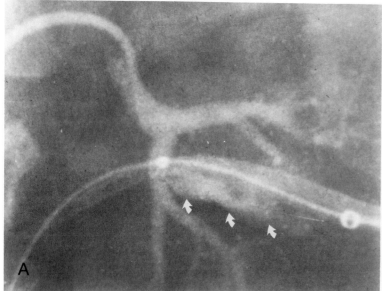

Figure 2.1.45. Hemorrhage during tract creation for nephrostolithotomy. **A.** Selective renal arteriogram shows extensive extravasation of contrast medium from lobar branch *(arrows).* **B.** Angioplasty balloon in tract tamponades bleeding site *(arrows).*

lowed.[180–182] The most common complications are hematuria, hypertension, decreased renal function, and congestive heart failure.[63,180–182] Percutaneous obliteration of a postbiopsy renal AV fistula was reported by Bookstein and Goldstein.[165] Subsequently, several reports of successful embolization confirmed the benignity of the procedure.[131,166–173] Various embolic agents have been used: autologous clot, fat, Gelfoam, IBCA, and spring coils. Short-acting, absorbable embolic agents are preferred to minimize the size of the areas of ischemia produced by the vascular occlusion, since too extensive ischemia could lead to hypertension.

Nephrostomy-induced vascular trauma is usually associated with arteriovenous lacerations (Fig. 2.1.45A), false aneurysm formation (Fig. 2.1.46), or an AV fistula.[176–178] Many of these vascular lesions heal spontaneously after tamponade of the nephrostomy tract with a large-bore drainage catheter. The remaining cases require selective arterial embolization to obliterate the bleeding site (Fig. 2.1.45B). The lower incidence of vascular complications after percutaneous nephrostomy in comparison with that of renal biopsy is probably due to the use of an approach through the relatively hypovascular posterolateral margin of the kidney for nephrostomy and to the use of fluoroscopy.

The choice between conservative versus surgical treatment in patients with noniatrogenic renal trauma is a difficult one. In general, the treatment is conservative. In the patient with multiple injuries and hematuria, renal evaluation is commonly limited to an intravenous urogram (IVU). Occasionally, ultrasound or CT is performed just prior to an emergency surgical exploration. Exploration of

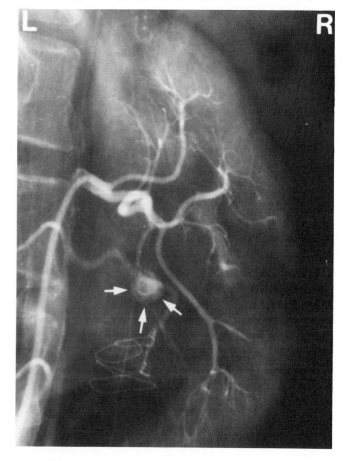

Figure 2.1.46. Hemorrhage two weeks after percutaneous renal stone removal. Selective renal arteriogram shows large false aneurysm of lobar artery *(arrows).*

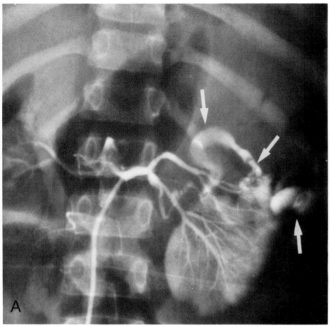 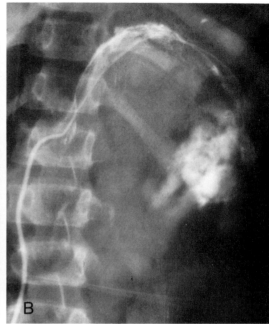

Figure 2.1.47. An 18-year-old victim of a motor vehicle accident. **A.** Selective left renal arteriogram shows fracture of kidney with extensive extravasation from branches of renal artery *(arrows)*. **B.** After embolization of artery with Gelfoam plugs, persistence of extravasation of contrast medium was noted on an aortogram. Selective injection of capsular artery slows extravasation of contrast medium. Observe displacement of capsular branches by large hematoma. (Courtesy of A. Waltman, M.D., Massachusetts General Hospital.)

the renal fossa is usually performed in those patients with gross hematuria with a large retroperitoneal hematoma or nonfunctioning kidneys on an IVU.[187]

More definite diagnostic information is provided by selective renal arteriography to demonstrate the source of bleeding.[188-193] Therapeutic embolization is an excellent alternative in the management of renal trauma, because bleeding commonly is from a single lobar branch (Fig. 2.1.47).[189] Furthermore, the absence of a dual vascular supply enhances the success rate of embolization. Superselective embolization is recommended to minimize ischemic damage.

Angiography is superior to surgical exploration both as a diagnostic and as a therapeutic modality, since during surgical exploration, the presence of a large retroperitoneal hematoma and the continuous extravasation of blood make examination of the surgical field extremely difficult. Not uncommonly, heminephrectomy or total nephrectomy is the only answer to the problem, yet with arteriography some of these kidneys or parts thereof might be salvaged.

OTHER RETROPERITONEAL VASCULAR TRAUMA

If renal injuries are excluded from this group, the most commonly affected vascular structures are the lumbar arteries[192,194-197] and less often, the duodenal and pancreatic arteries.[198] Angiography with selective embolization of the injured vessel commonly controls the problem (Fig. 2.1.48).

Liver Trauma

Liver injuries caused by blunt or penetrating trauma are second only to small bowel injuries in incidence.[199] Liver trauma is commonly associated with severe injuries to the pancreas, spleen, stomach, bowel, or diaphragm.[200]

Liver injuries can be divided anatomically into three categories: lacerations, linear fractures, and deep stellate fractures.[200] Many injuries (70%) stop bleeding spontaneously and require surgical drainage and debridement of devitalized structures.[199] The remaining 30% of cases require extensive surgical manipulation for control of bleeding and bile leakage, resection of devitalized tissues, etc. Angiography is usually required only in the stable patient with persistent hemobilia,[200-203] AV fistula, or extravasation of blood.[204-206] It is also indicated postoperatively for recurrent bleeding causing subcapsular or intrahepatic hematomas[207,208] or severe hemobilia[202-205] or for the control of large hepaticosystemic fistulae causing hemodynamic disturbances.[209]

The angiographic evaluation of these patients includes imaging of the hepatic arterial and portal circulation, commonly by aortography and celiac and hepatic artery injections. Superior mesenteric artery (SMA) injections are needed to study the replaced right hepatic artery arising from the SMA. Adequate confirmation of an intact, physiologically normal portal circulation is needed before attempting embolization of the hepatic artery, inasmuch as 80% of hepatic perfusion is provided by this system and

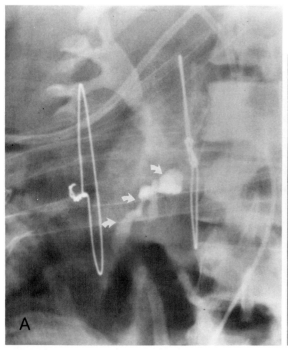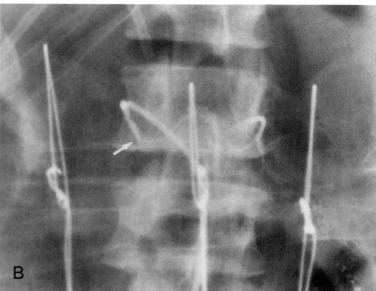

Figure 2.1.48. A 16-year-old boy with severe retroperitoneal bleeding three weeks after gunshot injury. **A.** Selective lumbar arteriogram shows extensive extravasation from second right lumbar artery *(arrows)*. **B.** Arteriogram after embolization of bleeding artery with Gelfoam shows complete thrombosis *(arrow)*. (Courtesy of A. Waltman, M.D., Massachusetts General Hospital.)

embolization of the hepatic artery in a patient with an occluded portal vein or in the presence of portal hypertension would be catastrophic.[209–211]

Superselective catheterization of the injured hepatic artery branch is ideal, although a more central embolization is acceptable if selective catheterization is difficult or if the bleeding is life threatening (Fig. 2.1.49). In these instances, embolization of the cystic artery may result in gallbladder necrosis.[212,213] Different embolic agents have been used, including Gelfoam, Ivalon, IBCA, and coils.

Iatrogenic injuries are commonly caused by percutaneous liver biopsy or percutaneous biliary drainage procedures. The most common lesions are AV fistulae[214–224] and hemobilia.[202–205] Small peripheral AV communications and arteriobiliary communications tend to close spontaneously.[225] When bleeding persists or when systemic manifestations of the hepatic shunt such as congestive heart failure are evident, therapeutic embolization can be accomplished easily. Again, a superselective embolization of the involved hepatic artery branch is desired to minimize parenchymal damage.

Splenic Trauma

The spleen is the organ most frequently injured in blunt abdominal trauma.[226] An angiographic classification of splenic trauma was developed by Fisher et al.[227] with therapeutic implications. According to this study, severe splenic injuries, including fragmentation of the parenchyma (Fig. 2.1.50) and transection of major arterial branches (Fig. 2.1.51), mandate emergency splenectomy. Patients in the intermediate group (major injuries including parenchymal lacerations (Fig. 2.1.52) and intraparenchymal, subcapsular, and extrasplenic hematomas (Figs. 2.1.53 and 2.1.54) may require splenic operation. This is the group in which therapeutic embolization can be useful, either to help stabilize the patient or to control extravasation. Patients with minor injuries, including small lacerations and small intraparenchymal hematomas (Fig. 2.1.55), can usually be managed conservatively.[227]

The late sequelae of splenectomy, particularly in children, namely overwhelming infection and rapid death, are well documented.[228–232] Because of these problems, there is a growing consensus in favor of splenic preservation. To preserve splenic function, a central embolization has been advocated by Sclafani[230,231]; this technique avoids the extensive infarction commonly caused by peripheral particulate embolization.[59,233] The rationale of Sclafani's technique is that the decrease in splenic artery flow and pressure allows thrombus to form around the site of injury, stopping the extravasation, while at the same time flow to the remainder of the spleen is preserved via collaterals beyond the site of occlusion.[230,231]

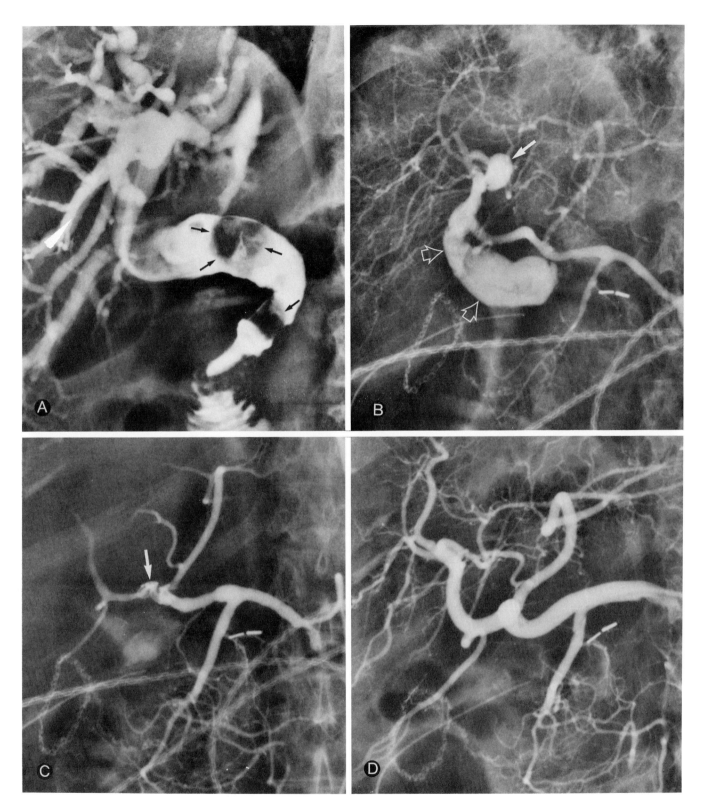

Figure 2.1.49. A 77-year-old woman with massive hemorrhage from a percutaneous transhepatic tract, manifested by hemobilia and hematemesis. **A.** Transhepatic cholangiogram demonstrates marked dilatation of the biliary tree with multiple stones in the common bile duct *(arrows).* **B.** Selective celiac arteriogram because of persistent hemobilia reveals the presence of a large arterial biliary fistula *(white arrow)* in central part of the right lobe of the liver with massive opacification of the common bile duct *(open arrows).* Diffuse vasoconstriction of the arterial system is due to hypovolemic shock. **C.** Follow-up hepatic arteriogram 15 minutes after the placement of two GWC spring coils in the origin of the right hepatic artery *(arrow)* demonstrates minimal flow through the right hepatic artery with no evidence of opacification of the fistula. **D.** Follow-up hepatic arteriogram six days after transcatheter embolization reveals good flow in the right hepatic artery with no evidence of opacification of the false aneurysm. (Courtesy of J. Rösch, The Oregon Health Science University School of Medicine.)

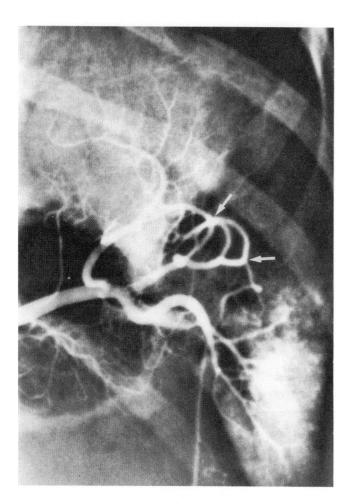

Figure 2.1.50. Fragmentation pattern: selective splenic arteriogram three days after blunt abdominal trauma. The spleen is fragmented at the center, with the two parts being held together by a large clot. The arterial branches are patent and are seen embedded in the clot *(arrows)*. There is no evidence of active bleeding. Punctate hemorrhages are also present in the lower pole (regional snowstorm pattern). (Reproduced from Fisher RG, Foucar K, Estroda R, Ben-Menachem Y: Splenic rupture in blunt trauma. *Radiol Clin North Am* 1981;19:141–166.)

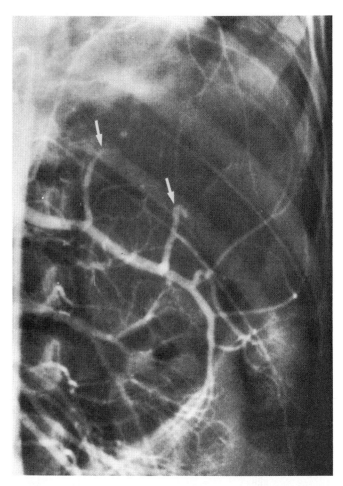

Figure 2.1.51. Transection of the major arterial branches: detail of the early arterial phase of a celiac arteriogram shows absence of blood flow in the major branches of the splenic artery *(arrows)*. Note splaying of parenchymal branches around large hematoma. (Reproduced from Fisher RG, Foucar K, Estroda R, Ben-Menachem Y: Splenic rupture in blunt trauma. *Radiol Clin North Am* 1981;19:141–166.)

ORGAN ABLATION

Spleen

Surgical removal of the spleen is a well established procedure in a number of hematologic disorders, including various types of hemolysis and thrombocytolysis, when splenic destruction of peripheral blood cells is especially rapid and replacement and drug therapy prove inadequate. On the other hand, the absence of the spleen impairs the body's ability to produce antibodies[232] and to eliminate encapsulated microorganisms from the bloodstream[234] and increases the susceptibility to fulminant sepsis.[235] From studies on laboratory animals, Van Wyck and Witte suggested that a critical mass of spleen (more than one-third) is needed to maintain host resistance to lethal blood-borne infection from encapsulated microorganisms.[236] Although these problems have been more common in children, overwhelming infection apparently can appear in all patients, regardless of age.[237] Vulnerability to infection seems to be higher in children under five years of age and in patients undergoing splenectomy for secondary hypersplenism caused by disease affecting the reticuloendothelial system such as Hodgkin's disease, Cooley's anemia, Gaucher's disease, and histiocytosis[237–239] as well as in renal allograft recipients.[240]

INDICATIONS

The indications for splenic embolization are:

Post-traumatic splenic bleeding[33,241];
Control of variceal bleeding in portal hypertension[242–246];
Hypersplenism in portal hypertension[55,233];
Thalassemia major[233];
Variceal bleeding in splenic vein thrombosis[233];
Thrombocytopenia[55,246,247];
Gaucher's disease[247];
Hodgkin's disease.[247]

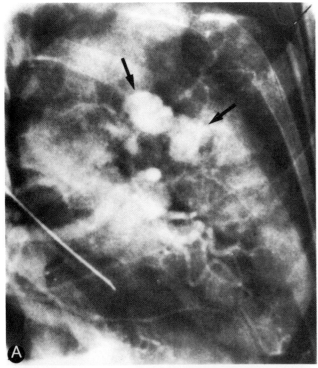

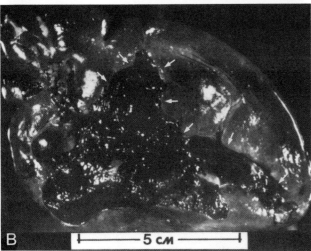

Figure 2.1.52. **A.** Large intrasplenic bleeding in the upper portion of the splenic hilum is evident *(arrows)* without angiographic indication of a laceration. **B.** A specimen of the spleen of another patient shows a large hematoma *(arrows).* The hematoma occupies the entire splenic hilum. (Reproduced from Fisher RG, Foucar K, Estroda R, Ben-Menachem Y: Splenic rupture in blunt trauma. *Radiol Clin North Am* 1981;19:141–166.)

METHOD

Initial attempts to embolize the spleen by proximal occlusion of the splenic artery were unsuccessful because of the inadequate hemodynamic response produced. The failure to respond was attributed to the abundant collateral circulation available through the short gastric and gastroepiploic arteries, which re-establish the blood supply to the spleen around the occluded segment of the splenic artery (Fig. 2.1.56).[55,248,249] Nevertheless, the hemodynamic

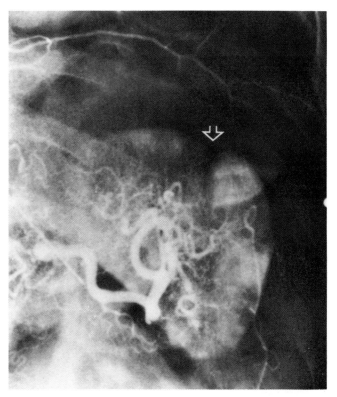

Figure 2.1.53. Extrasplenic hematoma. The hallmark of this splenic injury is the displacement of the spleen from the diaphragm and abdominal wall by a massive extrasplenic clot. A cleavage point on the surface of the spleen *(arrow)* is part of a fetal lobulation. A relatively avascular line can be traced from this point downward representing the continuation of the cleavage line of the lobulation. Slight arterial irregularity and small branch occlusions along this line, as well as the presence of an extrasplenic hematoma, indicate laceration of the spleen along the line. (Reproduced from Fisher RG, Foucar K, Estroda R, Ben-Menachem Y: Splenic rupture in blunt trauma. *Radiol Clin North Am* 1981;19:141–166.)

effects of embolization in the patients with thrombocytopenia, although temporary, improve the patient's status sufficiently to permit surgical splenectomy with a lower risk.[250]

Because of the need for a more enduring and effective hematologic or hemodynamic response, total infarction of the organ was attempted with particulate materials in either one or two steps (Fig. 2.1.57) with adequate hemodynamic results.[55,247,251] Unfortunately, in a high percentage of patients, severe complications developed, including severe unrelenting bronchopneumonias,[233,246,252] splenic abscess,[55,233,246,251–253] and splenic vein thrombosis.[253] This high incidence of complications reflects experimental data in animals, where the larger the infarcted splenic mass, the more serious the complications and secondary effects of the procedure.[55]

It has been suggested that widespread infarction of splenic parenchyma predisposes to growth of anerobic microorganisms in the hypoxic, devitalized tissues. Other factors mentioned include a decrease in the immunologic response of the patient, introduction of exogenous bacteria with the catheter[219] or embolic agents,[231] and contami-

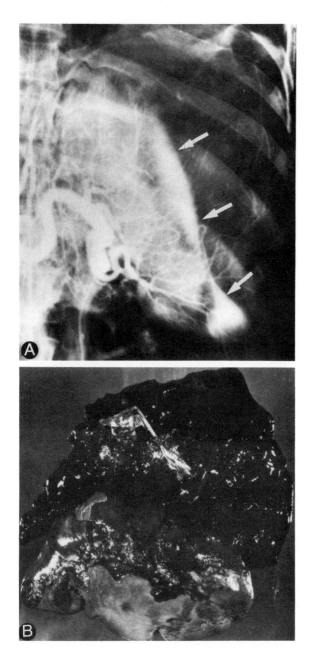

Figure 2.1.54. Subcapsular hematoma. **A.** Massive subcapsular hematoma is indicated by the severe compression of the splenic pulp *(arrows),* the concavity of the splenic outline, and extension of the stretched branches of the splenic artery well beyond the visible splenic parenchyma. These three findings should help to distinguish subcapsular hematomas from extrasplenic ones. **B.** The massive size of this subcapsular clot is clearly depicted; the capsule has been partially sliced to show the contents of the hematoma. Subcapsular hematomas are not necessarily as large as this one, and are sometimes discernible only on microscopic examination. (Reproduced from Fisher RG, Foucar K, Estroda R, Ben-Menachem Y: Splenic rupture in blunt trauma. *Radiol Clin North Am* 1981;19:141–166.)

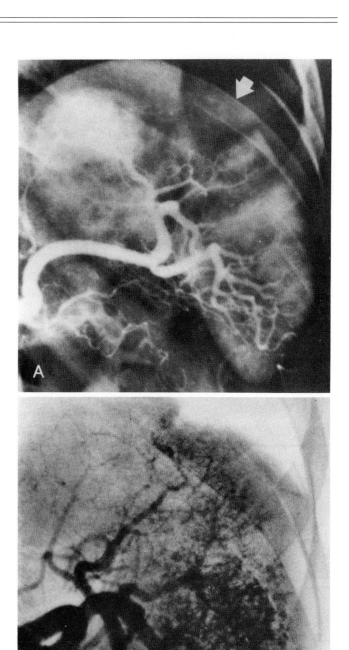

Figure 2.1.55. **A.** Large avascular areas as in this patient can be interpreted as clots filling the base of a laceration, with or without a capsular tear *(arrow).* **B.** Widespread snowstorm extravasation. Typical fluffy appearance of snowstorm hemorrhages. This is a fairly benign injury. (Reproduced from Fisher RG, Foucar K, Estroda R, Ben-Menachem Y: Splenic rupture in blunt trauma. *Radiol Clin North Am* 1981;19:141–166.)

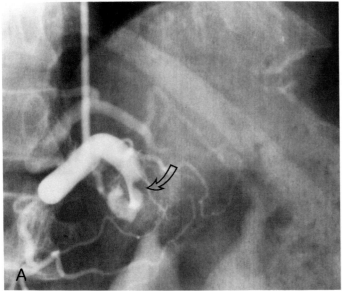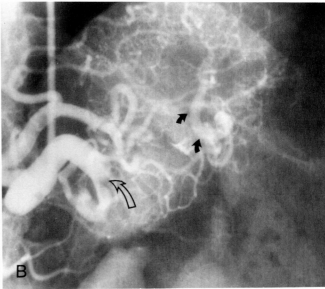

Figure 2.1.56. A 50-year-old man with immune thrombocytopenia and platelet count of 44,000/ml. **A.** Splenic angiogram after proximal occlusion of splenic artery with large Ivalon plugs; observe complete thrombosis of vessel in its midsegment *(arrow)*. **B.** Repeat splenic arteriogram four days later shows complete thrombosis of medial segment of vessel *(open arrow)*. However, left gastric artery is markedly enlarged, with extensive collateralization to distal splenic artery and to peripheral splenic artery branches *(black arrows)*. Initially, transient rise in platelet count to 104,000/ml occurred, but count returned to 74,000/ml within 24 hr because of the extensive collateralization through left gastric artery as a consequence of proximal occlusion of splenic artery. Surgically removed spleen showed only segmental infarct with peripheral organization despite splenic artery thrombosis. (Reproduced from Castañeda–Zúñiga WR, Hammerschmidt DE, Sanchez R, Amplatz K: Nonsurgical splenectomy. *AJR* 1977;129:805–811. © by American Roentgen Ray Society, 1977.)

nation of the ischemic vascular bed with intestinal organisms by retrograde flow of portal blood secondary to an inversion of portal vein flow due to the splenic ischemia.[233,247,249,254]

Because of these overwhelming complications, Spigos et al. adopted a modified strict protocol including the use of local and systemic antibiotics, careful aseptic techniques, and effective pain control, and accomplished a 30–70% partial embolization of the organ in 87% of their patients, with a remarkably low incidence of complications: one case each of splenic abscess and pancreatitis, pleural effusion in two, and pneumonia in five, with no deaths.[233] However, other investigators who followed a similar protocol have not been able to reproduce the results. In one series, three abscesses were the result of partial splenic embolization in three patients.[251] It is conceivable that patients with terminal liver disease react differently to splenic embolization[251,253] than do patients in better hemodynamic condition such as those in the Spigos series, virtually all of whom were transplant recipients or were in chronic renal failure.

Spigos Protocol

The steps of the Spigos technique are as follows[233]:

1. Systemic antibiotics: broad-spectrum antibiotics (gentamicin-penicillin G-cefoxitin) are started 8–12 hours before the procedure and continued for one to two weeks;

2. Local antibiotics: a suspension of 32,000 units of penicillin G and 12mg of gentamicin in 100ml of normal saline is used for suspending the embolic particles (Ivalon or Gelfoam) and for flushing the embolic agent toward the spleen;

3. Local care: either wide scrubs or whole-body baths with povidone-iodine;

4. Superselective catheterization, preferably with the tip of the catheter beyond the dorsal pancreatic artery, to decrease the chances of pancreatitis. Careful fluoroscopic control of the extent of infarction is a must to limit the total to approximately 60%;

5. Effective pain control with narcotics, or, as Spigos has done, with epidural block for 48 hours to prevent splinting of the hemidiaphragm and pleuropulmonary complications;

6. If needed, repeat embolization at a subsequent date;

7. Postembolization white blood cell and platelet count to evaluate the hematologic response.

Kidney

INDICATIONS

In patients with end-stage renal disease or renovascular hypertension and in renal allograft recipients with native kidneys in situ, for whom unilateral or bilateral nephrectomy has been chosen as an elective treatment, renal ablation is a useful alternative. Its principal advantage is the

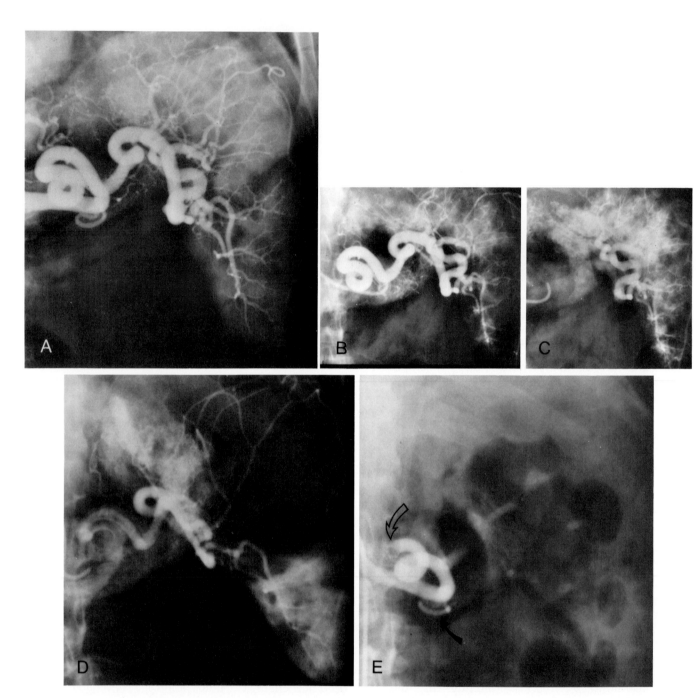

Figure 2.1.57. A 49-year-old man admitted for renal transplant with diagnosis of immune thrombocytopenic purpura. **A.** Splenic arteriogram reveals markedly enlarged spleen. **B,C.** After partial distal embolization of spleen with small Ivalon particles, multiple peripheral infarcts are seen throughout the organ. **D.** Angiogram 10 days after first embolization reveals extensive infarction of spleen, with slow clearance of contrast medium and large capsular arteries. **E.** Angiogram after second embolization shows complete infarction of spleen, with complete occlusion of splenic artery *(open curved arrow)* and persistence of large pancreatic branch of splenic artery *(black arrow)*. Adequate platelet response fol-

lowed procedure, reaching maximum of 511,000/ml on 16th day. Patient was discharged eight days after the second procedure with normal platelet count. Two months later, fever and left upper quadrant abdominal pain developed, and on admission a large, tender, nonpulsatile, left upper quadrant mass was palpable. Cardiac arrest occurred, and during resuscitation attempts, the abdominal mass disappeared. The patient died. At autopsy, abscess of lesser omental sac and splenic necrosis were found. (Reproduced from Castañeda–Zúñiga WR, Hammerschmidt DE, Sanchez R, Amplatz K: Nonsurgical splenectomy. *AJR* 1977;129:805–811. © by American Roentgen Ray Society, 1977.)

substantially lower morbidity and mortality rates for the percutaneous method in comparison with the surgical technique.[255,256]

Renal ablation as a treatment for severe, uncontrollable hypertension was first described by Goldin et al. in 1974.[257] Subsequently, the technique has been successful in ablating kidneys in patients with end-stage renal disease on dialysis,[257,258] the native kidneys in allograft recipients,[259] and in nephrotic syndrome.[260] The rationale behind both surgical nephrectomy and percutaneous renal ablation in patients with drug-resistant hypertension is that the ischemic renal parenchyma continues to produce renin; the function of the renin-angiotensin system is preserved long after the diseased kidneys have lost all their excretory capacity.[261]

TECHNIQUE

Abdominal aortography is the initial screening procedure, with either standard or digital intra-arterial technique (Fig. 2.1.58A,B). In patients with an occluded renal artery, delayed films are taken to evaluate the degree of reconstitution of the renal circulation via collaterals. Selective renal arteriography is commonly needed for a more precise delineation of the renal artery anatomy and the number of vessels and their contribution to total blood flow.

In subjects with nonoccluded renal arteries, a Simmons I or II catheter is preferred for selective catheterization, because it can easily be wedged into the renal artery for embolization (Fig. 2.1.58C). For patients with occluded renal arteries, a technique of recanalization angioplasty of the occluded segment with subsequent embolization was described by Eliscu et al.[262] and Denny et al.[265] Embolization can be done in the same sitting or it can be delayed to evaluate the function in the involved kidney and the effects of reperfusion on blood pressure.[263]

The purpose of embolization in these patients is to ablate the juxtaglomerular apparatus and therefore prevent renin production. This can be accomplished only by performing a distal embolization at the arteriolar level or beyond.[86] Small particulate agents such as Gelfoam powder and Ivalon shavings (250–500μm) or liquid agents such as ethanol or IBCA should be used (Fig. 2.1.58D). The catheter is wedged in the renal artery, and, under fluoroscopic control, small amounts of the particulate embolic agent suspended in contrast medium are injected, with great care to avoid reflux into the aorta. If a liquid embolic agent is to be used, the total capacity of the renal vascular bed is determined by injecting contrast medium through the catheter until complete opacification of the vascular bed is documented fluoroscopically. Subsequently, an equal amount of the embolic agent is injected through the wedged catheter, and this is repeated until the flow is decreased significantly. Embolization beyond this point would predispose to reflux into the aorta and concomitant complications. The completeness of embolization is verified by follow-up selective arteriography (Fig.

2.1.58C). If residual renal parenchyma is detected, it is embolized.

Postinfarction syndrome with severe pain is common after the percutaneous procedure and may be attributable in part to an immunologic response to the necrosing tissue. It is managed by the administration of narcotics and subsides in 48–72 hours. No infectious complications have been reported. Delayed reperfusion of segments or of the entire kidney has been seen after apparently complete embolizations.[260] Embolization can easily be repeated, usually with a long-lasting result.[260]

Selective segmental infarction of the kidney was proposed by Reuter et al. for patients with segmental renal artery stenosis causing hypertension.[264] Today, these lesions can best be treated by transluminal angioplasty.

EMBOLIZATION IN CANCER

Embolotherapy has been used for both primary and metastatic tumors. The reasons for embolization can be classified into two large groups:

1. Preoperative embolization of primary tumors;
2. Palliative embolization of unresectable tumors to:
   a. Alleviate symptoms, e.g., pain, bleeding, fever, hypercalcemia;
   b. Minimize further dissemination;
   c. Enhance the response to chemotherapy or radiation.

Kidney Tumors

Renal carcinoma is the most common malignancy of the urinary tract, accounting for approximately 3% of all malignancies. The tumor occurs with a 3:1 male:female ratio. In adults, 85–90% of renal tumors are adenocarcinomas (renal cell carcinomas), with the remainder being sarcomas and lymphoblastomas. Most tumors of the renal pelvis are transitional cell carcinomas.[265,266] Approximately one-fourth (25–27%) of the patients have metastases at the time of diagnosis.[267,268] Renal cell carcinoma is characterized by a remarkably extensive variety of presentations, systemic effects, and prognoses.[269] Radical nephrectomy has been the conventional therapy, particularly for relatively localized disease (Stages I–III).[270,271]

Attempts to modify the progression of renal carcinoma by embolization were initially reported by Lang, who used radioactive gold seeds in 20 patients, reportedly with a decrease in the size of the tumor.[271] Almgard et al. reported reduced tumor vascularity, widespread necrosis, shrinkage, and easier resection after tumor embolization with autologous muscle.[272] In a prospective study in 1981, Wallace et al. reported a 36% response rate in patients with known metastases.[273] In a similar study, Kaisary et al. confirmed that surgery is technically easier, but they could not confirm any changes in the response to delayed hypersen-

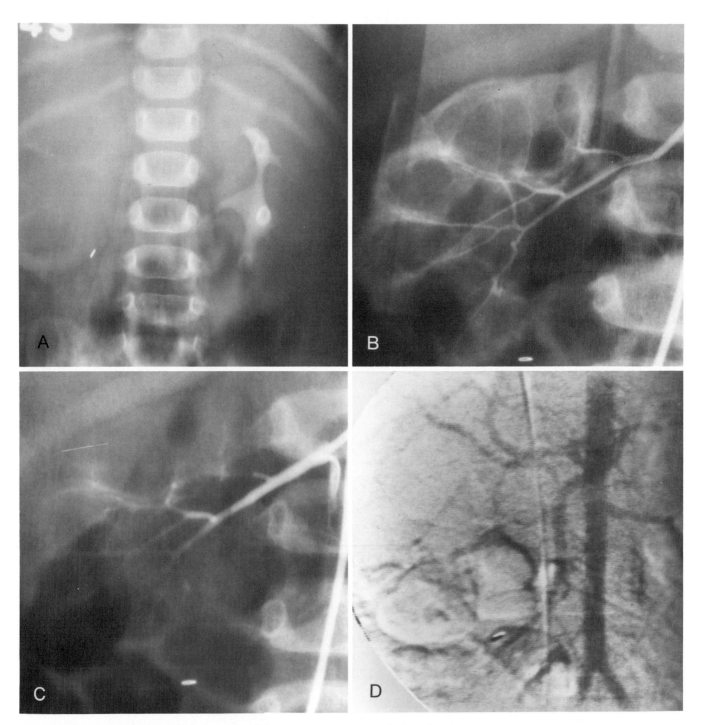

Figure 2.1.58. Five-year-old boy with hypertension. **A.** Intravenous urogram reveals normal collecting system on left and excretion of contrast medium from hydronephrotic right kidney. **B.** Selective right renal arteriogram reveals marked hydronephrosis of kidney with splaying of renal artery branches around hydronephrotic sacs. **C.** Arteriogram after injection of 1.5ml of absolute ethanol shows marked reduction in flow through right kidney. **D.** Intravenous digital subtraction study three months after embolization shows no flow through right renal artery. Blood pressure normalized.

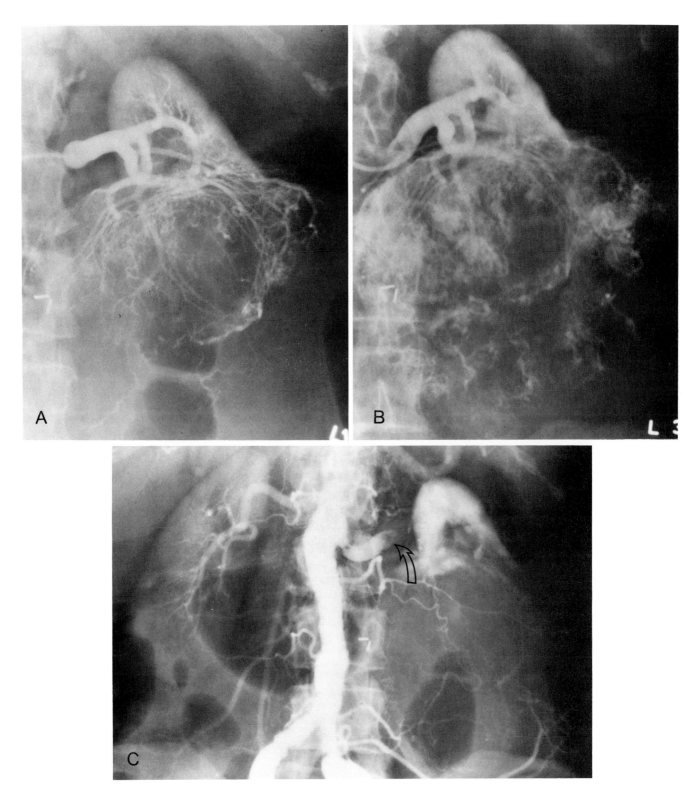

Figure 2.1.59. Large renal cell carcinoma of left kidney. **A.** Early phase of balloon occlusion selective left renal arteriogram shows large vascular mass in lower pole. **B.** Late phase of balloon occlusion arteriogram after deflation of balloon shows to better advantage the large mass with irregular margins. It is highly vascular but with areas of hypovascularity, probably representing areas of necrosis within tumor. **C.** Aortogram after embolization of left renal artery with Gelfoam plugs during balloon occlusion of artery. Observe complete thrombosis *(arrow)*.

sitivity skin testing or any significant regression of the primary or metastatic tumor after embolization alone, or with nephrectomy and hormonal/chemotherapeutic treatment in those patients who underwent embolization alone.[274] Sandoval Parra et al. obtained an average of 78.2% tumor necrosis with dextran and 53–64% with Gelfoam and Gelfoam-aluminum. Only 5 of the 81 patients required a second embolization.[275]

INDICATIONS

The principal indications for embolization are:

1. Preoperative: Dilated, tortuous veins commonly cover the surface of large hypervascular tumors. Regional tumor extension into the renal hilum can make dissection of this area difficult. Embolization in these cases will shrink the tumor and minimize blood loss, facilitating the operation. Tumors unresectable because of their size and local extension can be made operable by tumor embolization (Fig. 2.1.59).[273,274] Preoperative embolization is not indicated for small tumors, oncocytomas, or cancers of the renal pelvis.[275]
2. Palliation: In patients with metastatic disease, mean sur-

vival is 6 months if there are pulmonary metastases, 15 months with bone metastases, and 2–3 months with cerebral and hepatic metastases. Because of this dismal prognosis, embolization is used only as a palliative measure for control of pain and hematuria (Figs. 2.1.60 and 2.1.61).[273]

TECHNIQUE

Because of the severe pain commonly induced by the procedure, premedication with atropine and morphine is useful. These drugs are commonly supplemented by the administration of additional narcotics during and after the procedure.

Because of the frequent presence of a parasitic blood supply to the tumor, an extensive angiographic evaluation, including aortography and selective hepatic and bilateral selective renal arteriography, is performed to delineate the tumoral vascular anatomy. Peripheral obliteration of as many vascular sources as possible is necessary for successful tumor ablation; a proximal or partial vascular embolization will not sufficiently reduce the tumor's blood supply. A distal obliteration is particularly important in

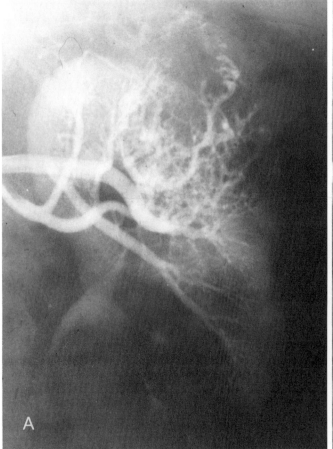

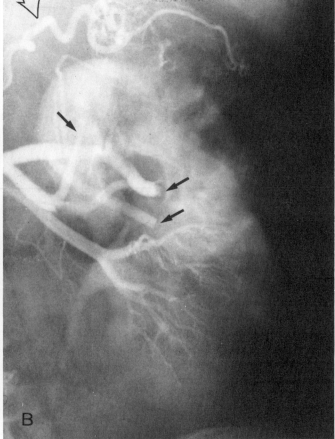

Figure 2.1.60. Tumor embolization for palliation in patient with extensive metastatic disease. **A.** Selective left renal arteriogram shows large hypervascular mass lesion in upper pole with perirenal extension. **B.** After distal embolization of branches feeding tumor with small Ivalon fragments *(arrows)*, observe increase in diameter of capsular artery providing parasitic blood supply *(open arrow)*. This vessel was selectively embolized.

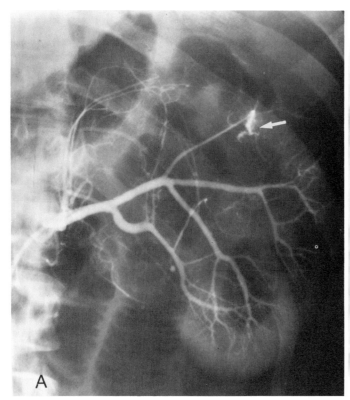

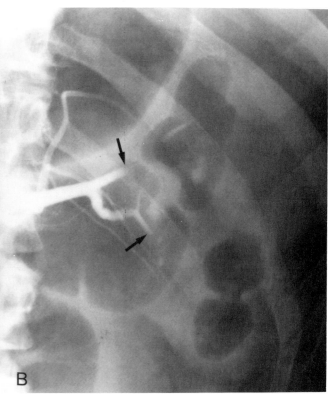

Figure 2.1.61. Twenty-year-old man with primary bone carcinoma with metastases to kidney and lung, presenting with severe hematuria. **A.** Selective left renal arteriogram shows splaying of renal artery branches by large mass in hilum. Note extravasation of contrast medium from periph- eral branch of renal artery *(arrow)*. **B.** Arteriogram after embolization of the left renal artery with Gelfoam shows complete occlusion *(arrow)* with ces- sation of extravasation. (Courtesy of A. Waltman, M.D., Massachusetts General Hospital.)

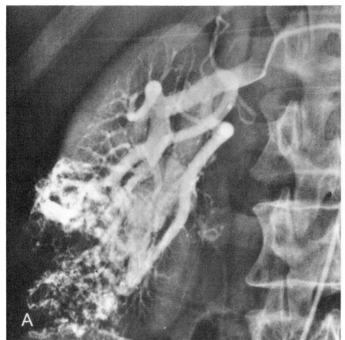

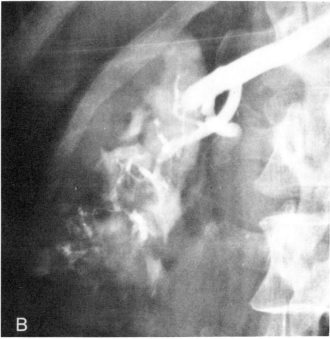

Figure 2.1.62. Palliative embolization in metastatic renal cell carcinoma. **A.** Hypervascular mass in lower pole of right kidney. **B.** Selective right renal arteriogram after embolization with ethanol shows occlusion of the renal artery. (Reproduced from Becker GJ, Holden RW, Klatte EC: Ther- apeutic embolization with absolute ethanol. *Semin Intervent Radiol* 1985;1:118–129.)

patients in whom embolization is planned as the sole treatment because they have extensive metastatic disease or medical contraindications to surgery (Fig. 2.1.62).

Several embolic agents have been used: radioactive gold seeds, emulsified autologous muscle, Gelfoam, IBCA, spring coils, and ethanol. Of these, distal Gelfoam embolization complemented with spring coils for proximal occlusion[275] and ethanol[276] are most commonly used at present. Gelfoam is cut into small (2 X 2mm) pieces that are suspended in contrast medium for small vessel embolization. Larger pieces (2 X 3 X 20mm) are used for more proximal occlusion.[273] Once a substantial decrease in blood flow is visible angiographically, one or two spring coils are deposited in the renal artery to complete the obliteration, preventing the vascular recanalization that occurs one week to four months after deposition of Gelfoam alone.[31]

Balloon occlusion of the renal artery has been recommended during embolization with Gelfoam[44] and ethanol[276] to prevent reflux of the embolic agent and systemic embolization.

COMPLICATIONS

The most common complications are the postembolization syndrome, consisting of fever, nausea, vomiting, and pain, which occurs in nearly all patients and can last one to five days. Narcotics and intravenous fluids are needed for pain control and fluid replacement.[273] Transient hypertension has been reported by Wallace et al., and prolonged hypertension (four to seven days) was reported by Mazer et al. in patients who underwent palliative embolization for inoperable tumors.[62,273] This condition probably is related to high plasma renin levels after renal parenchymal embolization, as reported by Cho et al.[277] Renal failure is commonly related to the use of large amounts of contrast medium.[273] Undetected coil embolization to the contralateral kidney has been reported by Mazer et al. as an unusual cause of renal failure after preoperative renal embolization.[62]

Because of the possible development of a renal abscess after embolization, patients with chronic calculous disease or recurrent or concurrent urinary infections should receive antibiotics before, during, and after embolization.[62,273]

Poor technique and lack of understanding of blood flow characteristics are the common denominators in all systemic complications involving embolization of the agent to undesired sites. Although this complication most commonly occurs with particulate or liquid embolic agents, it has also been reported with coils.[62] A good-quality image intensifier and proper positioning of the catheter are the first steps in prevention. Injection of particulate and liquid embolic agents should be interrupted immediately when the blood flow can be seen to have slowed markedly; insisting on completing the obliteration beyond this point will only cause reflux of the embolic agent. The use of occlusion balloons has been recommended to prevent reflux.[44]

Pelvic Malignancy

As in other parts of the body, therapeutic embolization is frequently indicated in patients with neoplasia of the pelvic organs. Common indications include control of bleeding, palliation of pain, shrinkage of the tumor, and minimizing of blood loss during resection of large vascular tumors.

Typically, in bleeding from genital or vesical tumors, bilateral embolization of the hypogastric artery is performed, because unilateral occlusion is not sufficient to control the hemorrhage due to the crossover circulation from the contralateral hypogastric artery.

The embolizations should be limited to the anterior division of the hypogastric arteries, reflux into the posterior division can lead to ischemic paresis. At times, the subselective catheterization is not possible, in those situations, the emboli delivered from the main hypogastric artery will reach the hemorrhagic region preferentially by sump effect.

BLADDER HEMORRHAGE IN RADIATION CYSTITIS

Control of intractable hemorrhage from the bladder by embolization was first reported in 1974 by Hald and Mygind, who used fragments of muscle.[278] Commonly, the preembolization angiographic study fails to demonstrate extravasation of contrast medium (Fig. 2.1.63A,B). Bilateral embolization of the anterior division of the hypogastric artery is usually needed to accomplish hemostasis (Fig. 2.1.63C). The excellent collateral network in the bladder muscularis assures an acceptable capillary blood flow to the areas where the main vascular blood supply has been obliterated, thus preventing tissue necrosis. In spite of this collateral flow, the procedure is effective, because the reduced pressure gradient in the embolized vascular system permits clot formation at the level of the diffuse mucosal bleeding.[279]

BLADDER TUMORS

Adequate staging and topographic localization of the tumor by CT and arteriography are important factors in determining whether unilateral or bilateral embolization should be undertaken in patients with primary or metastatic tumors of the bladder.[279] As with hemorrhagic cystitis, the bleeding site is frequently not identified in these cases; and in those patients in whom the tumor is not lateralized, both hypogastric arteries have to be embolized to control the bleeding.[279,280] Unilateral embolization can, however, control the bleeding from bladder carcinoma, as in two patients in Lang's series.[279] When possible, superselective catheterization of the vesical arteries should be attempted to limit embolization to the affected area. An axillary or brachial artery approach is particularly suitable for bilateral superselective catheterization. In emergencies due to severe bleeding or in critically ill patients, central occlusion

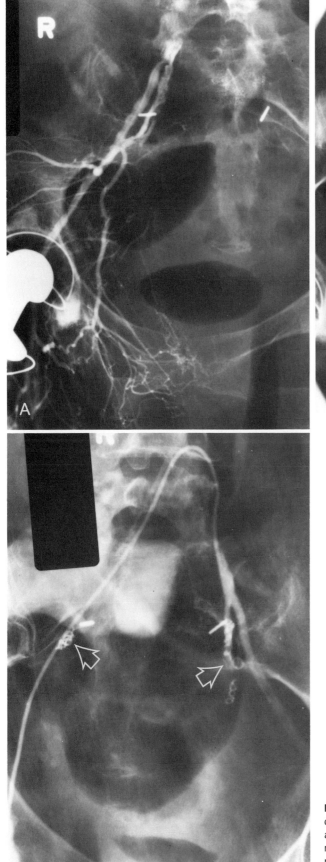

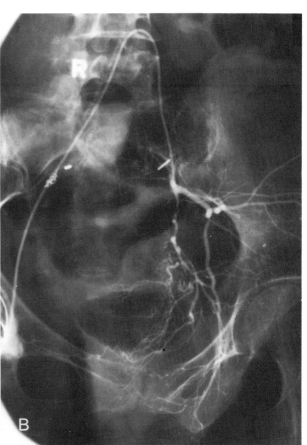

Figure 2.1.63. Patient with recurrent severe bladder hemorrhage secondary to postradiation cystitis. **A,B.** Selective right and left hypogastric artery arteriograms show no evidence of extravasation of contrast medium from arterial branches. **C.** Arteriogram after embolization of anterior division of both hypogastric arteries with small Ivalon particles and occlusion of proximal trunk with GWC coils shows complete occlusion of both arteries *(arrows)*.

of the anterior division is adequate to control the hemorrhage.

PROSTATE CANCER

Massive postoperative bleeding from the prostate in three patients and postbiopsy with a Vim–Silverman needle in another were successfully controlled by the uni- or bilateral embolization of the hypogastric artery.

GYNECOLOGIC TUMORS

Ligation of the hypogastric arteries is the established surgical approach for control of hemorrhage in gynecologic and small malignant genital tumors. Embolization of the hypogastric artery, usually bilaterally, provides a more than satisfactory alternative (Fig. 2.1.64).[279–282] Other indications for embolization include pain control, tumor shrinkage, and reduction of intraoperative blood loss.[280] As is the case with bladder tumors, the bleeding site may not be identified. Nonetheless, hemorrhage is almost immediately controlled by bilateral embolization of the hypogastric artery.[280] Lack of extravasation in the presence of active bleeding has been explained as chronic capillary bleeding from a broad surface of hypervascular granulation tissue formed in response to radiation or from hypervascular neoplastic tissue.[283]

Transcatheter embolizations of hypogastric arteries has been carried out by Pisco in 108 patients with pelvic malignancies.[284] The most common malignancies in this series include cancers of the urinary bladder in 50 patients, uterus in 39, ovary in 16, and prostate in 3. Complete hemorrhagic control was achieved in 74 patients, partial control in 23, and the technique was ineffective in 4 patients. The initial few patients were embolized with Gelfoam. In subsequent patients, Ivalon replaced Gelfoam in order to achieve a permanent occlusion. Seventy-seven patients exhibited postembolization syndrome that included nausea, vomiting, pain, and fever.[284]

Unilateral embolization was only performed when the preembolization arteriogram demonstrated a localized source of bleeding. Although not uncommonly bilateral hypogastric embolization would be required, due to the extensive collateral network from the external iliac, common femoral, and inferior mesenteric arteries.[285]

Bone Tumors

Preoperative embolization has been used to reduce blood loss from vascular bone tumors, which can total 1–3 liters,[286–291] during resection of the tumor or during orthopedic maneuvers such as hip replacement[291] or internal fracture fixation.[291] There is no evidence that embolization retards healing at the fracture site. Callus formation, restoration of function, and resolution of pain were observed within the first two weeks after embolization in a series reported by Rowe et al.[292] Embolization has also been used as the primary treatment for benign tumors, particularly when resection would require a crippling major operation or when the tumor is in a poorly accessible part of the body such as the spine. Such use was reported by Keller et al. in two patients with aneurysmal bone cysts and another with a giant cell tumor of the sacrum.[291,293,294]

The embolization of recurrent aneurysmal bone cyst has been carried out in three postoperative cases with relief of pain and reformation of bone as a result of embolization.[295] Embolization of the aneurysmal bone cyst has been carried out as the primary therapy for relief of pain and remineralization.[296,297]

Embolization of bone tumors has been applied primarily for relief of pain.[286,290,291,293,298] The mechanism by which the procedure relieves pain is unknown. Although Wallace and Chuang have hypothesized that the fastest growing portion of the tumor is the more vascular area and that vascular occlusion decreases the tumor growth rate, thereby reducing the pressure on the periosteum, with consequent decrease or disappearance of pain.[290,293] An additional beneficial side effect of a successful embolization is the shrinkage of tumor mass, particularly when nonabsorbable embolic agents are used (Fig. 2.1.65).

Embolic Agents

Depending on whether embolization will be followed immediately by surgical resection, an absorbable embolic agent, such as Gelfoam, or a nonabsorbable agent, such as Ivalon particles or IBCA, should be used. Gelfoam produces a temporary occlusion, with subsequent recanalization of the vessels, so proximal vascular occlusion with 2–3mm Gelfoam pieces might be adequate as an immediate preoperative measure designed to minimize blood loss.[286–290] However, if the surgical procedure is delayed, recanalization of the occluded vessel, development of parasitic peripheral blood flow, or both will ensue if Gelfoam is used, negating the embolization procedure. If embolization is carried out for palliation (e.g., pain relief, tumor shrinkage, fracture fixation) or as the primary treatment for benign tumors, permanent embolic agents should be used. The agent used in these cases should be able to inhibit the development of collaterals beyond the site of vascular occlusion to prevent revascularization of the tumor. Embolic fluid agents, with the possible exception of ethanol (because of the ischemic complications it can cause[292]), and Ivalon microparticles are the best agents to create this type of embolization.

Superselective catheterization is desirable to confine infarction to the tumor. If an ideal superselective catheter position is not attainable, protection of the noninvolved distal vessels with coils has been used in the pelvic area.[291]

Complications

A postembolization syndrome of pain, fever, numbness, and paresthesia of the affected area has been described[290,295]; it usually subsides within 48–72 hours.

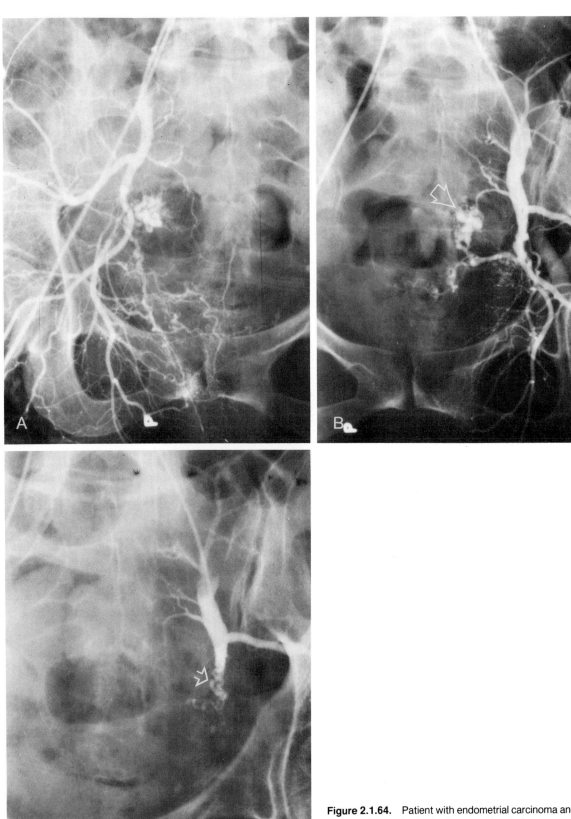

Figure 2.1.64. Patient with endometrial carcinoma and recurrent bleeding. **A,B.** Bilateral selective hypogastric arteriograms reveal extravasation of contrast medium from left uterine artery *(open arrow).* **C.** After bilateral embolization of anterior division of hypogastric artery with Ivalon particles, observe complete thrombosis of this vessel *(arrow).*

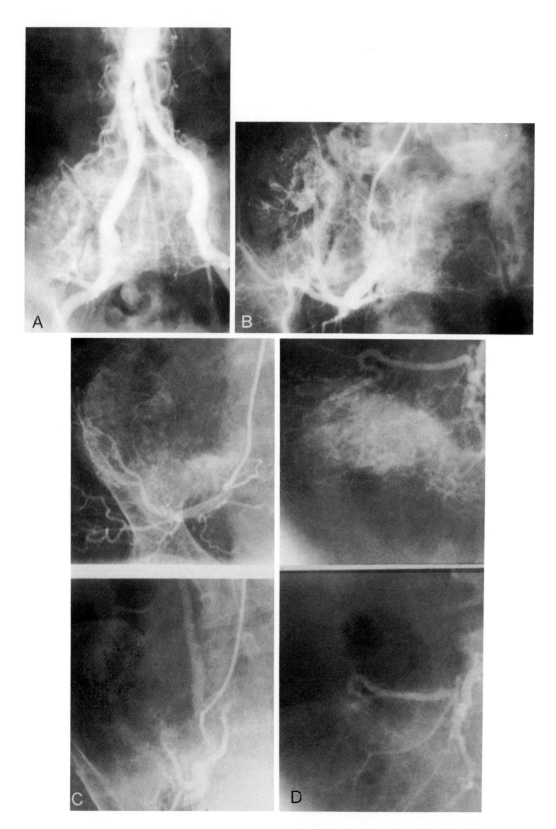

Figure 2.1.65. Metastatic colon carcinoma to iliac. **A.** Highly vascular mass fed by branches of the right internal iliac artery and fifth right lumbar artery. **B.** Selective catheterization of right hypogastric artery confirms presence of hypervascular mass. **C.** Post-Ivalon embolization hypogastric angiogram reveals adequate devascularization. **D.** Pelvic arteriogram. Persistent opacification of tumor through fifth right lumbar artery.

Unintentional embolization of normal vessels is the greatest risk, and skin breakdown[293] and ischemic neuropathy[292] have been reported after otherwise successful embolizations. Protection by occlusion of noninvolved contiguous vessels[292] with GWC coils, particularly careful angiographic evaluation before the embolization to select the target vessels, superselective distal catheterization, and avoidance of overzealous injections of the embolic agent are the best means of avoiding these complications.

EMBOLIZATION OF ANEURYSMS

Embolization of true aortic aneurysms, peripheral arterial pseudoaneurysms, and visceral artery aneurysms has been accomplished under certain clinical and anatomical situations, either through a catheter or by direct puncture.

TRUE ATHEROSCLEROTIC AORTIC ANEURYSMS

The conventional treatment for abdominal aneurysms is aneurysmectomy with interposition of a bypass graft and carries a mortality rate of 2–5%.[299] In patients with severe cardiac, pulmonary, and renal disease, the mortality of surgery can be as high as 60%. An alternative surgical treatment that consists of placing an axillo-bifemoral bypass graft with ligation of the iliac and hypogastric arteries has been described. The outflow obstruction of the iliac vessels induces retrograde thrombosis of the aneurysm.[299] This type of procedure minimizes blood loss, causing less tissue trauma and fewer respiratory difficulties in comparison to the abdominal operation. Seventeen patients underwent nonresective treatment; in 4 out of the 17, the aneurysm remained patent because of the persistent flow through the hypogastric arteries.[299–301] The outflow of the aorta was interrupted by the percutaneous injection of a tissue adhesive, (Bucrylate) through a catheter into the distal abdominal aorta and iliac vessels.[300,301]

Prior to embolization, abdominal aortography should be obtained for identification of three potential problems.[299]

A. The location of the main or accessory renal arteries. Since if they are located at a lower level, retrograde thrombosis of the aorta can infarct the kidney(s).
B. A patent enlarged inferior mesenteric artery can potentially maintain flow to the aneurysm. Bowel infarction can be anticipated, if this is the main supply to the bowel in cases of celiac and superior mesenteric artery occlusions.
C. The flow to the hypogastric arteries should be determined, if patent, plans should be made for occlusion by transcatheter embolization.

In the earlier attempts with Bucrylate embolization, one patient died of aneurysm rupture because of incomplete thrombosis. A second patient experienced muscle necrosis, secondary to gluteal artery thrombosis. The second and third patients had an excellent outcome.[299–301]

In a group of four patients, thrombosis of the aneurysm was accomplished by placing strips of Gelfoam and Gianturco coils in the hypogastric, external and common iliac arteries. Prior to embolization, all four patients underwent axillo-femoral bypass procedure.[302] Figure 2.1.66 illustrates the technique.

Transcatheter embolization of saccular aneurysms of the thoracic and abdominal aorta has also been attempted utilizing Gianturco coils.[303] Although maximum packing of the aneurysmal sacs with coil was obtained, persistent antegrade flow allowed the continuous growth of the aneurysm.[303]

Reflux embolization during the procedure was prevented by placing a balloon catheter across the neck of the aneurysm. The angiographic follow-up revealed displacement of coils towards the periphery of the enlarging aneurysm. The authors concluded that thrombosis of saccular aneurysms is not possible without the obstruction of the parent artery.[303]

A thoracic aneurysm was treated by proximal and distal ligation and bypass of the vessel. In spite of ligation, the thoracic aorta remained patent. Occlusion was obtained by straddling 8 and 15mm Gianturco coils across the incompletely ligated sites.[304] Overall results of the technique have been satisfactory provided the outflow vessels are adequately occluded.

EMBOLIZATION OF PERIPHERAL PSEUDOANEURYSM AND VISCERAL ARTERIES

Pseudoaneurysms are secondary to trauma and infection. They represent the contained blood leakage at the site of blood vessel disruption. The conventional treatment involves surgery and is recommended to prevent catastrophic ruptures. In certain anatomical situations, like when pseudoaneurysms are not accessible, or when the overwhelming sepsis prevents surgery, transcatheter embolization offers a nonsurgical alternative. A limited number of case reports have been published, over the past few years, in the radiology literature.[305–315]

The pseudoaneurysms reported involved the subclavian, renal, hepatic, pancreatic-duodenal, iliac, and the common and deep femoral arteries. The embolic agents used in these cases include Gianturco coils, detachable balloons, thrombin, Gelfoam, isobutyl 2-cyanoacrylate.[305–317]

The advantages of transcatheter embolization over surgery are that: 1) it requires only local anesthesia; 2) collaterals are preserved and 3) surgical dissection may be difficult in areas of infection or hemorrhage.[313]

If the vessels to the pseudoaneurysms cannot be catheterized, direct puncture of the aneurysm with a 22-gauge needle and injection of thrombin have been accomplished with successful outcome.[312,317]

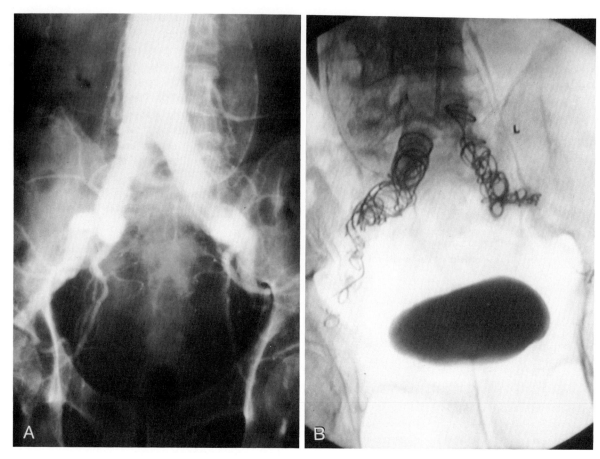

Figure 2.1.66. Large aneurysm of abdominal aorta post axillofemoral bypass graft and ligation of both external iliac arteries. **A.** Because of the patency of both hypogastric arteries, there is no evidence of thrombosis of the aneurysm. **B.** Follow-up aortogram after embolization with GWC coils of both common iliac arteries. Stasis and retrograde thrombosis of the abdominal aorta occurred.

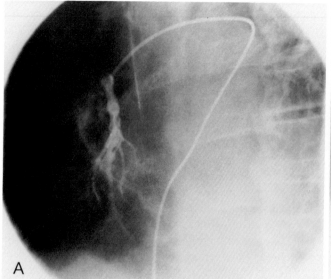
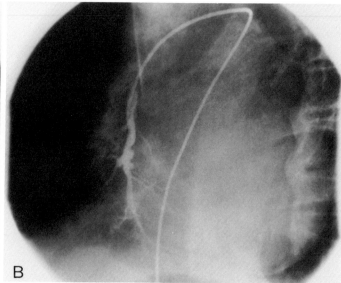

Figure 2.1.67. Massive hemoptysis post-Swan–Ganz catheter placement. **A.** Selective pulmonary arteriogram reveals presence of pseudo-aneurysms of a right lower lobe pulmonary artery branch *(arrow).* **B.** Post-GWC coil embolization. No antegrade flow is present.

Catheter-induced Pulmonary Artery Hemorrhage

The introduction of flow-directed, balloon-tipped catheters by Swan et al. was extremely helpful in managing critically ill patients.[318] The majority of complications related to catheter insertion are minor and are easily treatable. One of the rare, but catastrophic, complications is pulmonary hemorrhage with an incidence of 0.06 to 0.2%.[319,320] The mortality rate ranges from 45 to 65%.[321–323] The pulmonary hemorrhage may be immediate or delayed (Fig. 2.1.67A). Hemoptysis is the hallmark of pulmonary artery rupture and may present as small or massive hemoptysis leading to rapid death.

A number of mechanisms have been proposed and the potential risk factors include:

1. Patients above 60 years of age.
2. Pulmonary artery hypertension. The degenerative changes in the vessel wall increase the risk of perforation. The vessels are less compliant and aneurysmal. In patients with pulmonary hypertension, the pressure gradient across the balloon may drive the catheter distally and perforate the weakened wall.[324,325]
3. Balloon overdistension of a pulmonary artery may rupture the vascular wall as has been documented in human cadavers.[326]
4. The balloon tip may protrude beyond an eccentrically inflated balloon and further propulsion might drive the tip into the vascular wall.[324]
5. Peripheral migration of a stiff catheter tip in patients undergoing cardiopulmonary bypass might perforate the vascular wall.[325]
6. Anticoagulation has been also frequently cited as one of the risk factors for pulmonary artery rupture.[319,324,327]

The delayed rupture of pulmonary hemorrhage has been so far reported in eight patients.[325] The diagnosis can be made by pulmonary angiography. The pseudoaneurysms are manifested as eccentric pouches from the vascular wall.[325]

A multitude of treatments have been proposed and they include endotracheal intubations with a single- or double-lumen catheter[328] and application of positive and expiratory pressure (PEEP) to reduce the pulmonary artery pressure and flow to a minimum.[329]

The other modalities that have been proposed are Swan-Ganz and Fogarty catheter balloon inflation of the traumatized pulmonary vessel.[325] Surgically, pulmonary artery hemorrhage has been controlled by banding of the vessel,[330] and by pneumonectomy or lobectomy.[321]

The seriously ill patient may not be able to tolerate an extensive surgical procedure such as a lobectomy or pneumonectomy. A relatively simple method of controlling hemorrhage by transcatheter embolization has been recently proposed and successfully implemented.[325,331–333] This should be preceded by immediate resuscitation by establishing an airway with a double-lumen tube and correction of coagulation deficiencies induced by anticoagulants.

The pulmonary artery can be easily embolized with appropriate size detachable balloon or by Gianturco–Wallace coils (Fig. 2.1.67B).

References

1. Dawbain G, Lussenhop AJ, Spence WT: Artificial embolization of cerebral arteries: report of use in a case of arteriovenous malformation. *JAMA* 1960;172:1153–1155
2. Brooks B: The treatment of traumatic arteriovenous fistula. *South Med J* 1930;23:100–106
3. Lussenhop AJ, Spence WT: Artificial embolization of cerebral arteries: report of use in a case of arteriovenous malformation. *JAMA* 1960;172:1153–1155
4. Baum S, Nusbaum M: The control of gastrointestinal hemorrhage by selective mesenteric arterial infusion of vasopressin. *Radiology* 1971;98:497–505
5. Rösch C, Dotter CT, Brown MJ: Selective arterial embolization. *Radiology* 1972;102:303–306
6. Lin SR, LaDow CS, Tatoian JA, Go EB: Angiographic demonstration and silicone pellet embolization of facial hemangiomas of bone. *Neuroradiology* 1974;17:201–204
7. Serbinenko FA: Balloon catheterization and occlusion of major cerebral vessels. *J Neurosurg* 1974;41:125–145
8. White RI, Barth KH, Kaufman SL, DeCaprio V, Strandberg JD: Therapeutic embolization with detachable balloons. *CardioVasc Intervent Radiol* 1980;3:229–241
9. Debrun G, Lacour P, Caron JP, Hurth M, Comoy J, Keravel Y: Inflatable and released balloon technique experimentation in dog: application in man. *Neuroradiology* 1975;9:267–271
10. Kerber C: Balloon catheter with a calibrated leak. *Radiology* 1976;120:547–550
11. Zanetti PH, Sherman FE: Experimental evaluation of a tissue adhesive as an agent for the treatment of aneurysms and arteriovenous anomalies. *J Neurosurg* 1972;36:72–79
12. Carey LS, Grace DM: The brisk bleed: controlled by arterial catheterization and Gelfoam plug. *J Can Assoc Radiol* 1974;25:113–115
13. Portsmann W, Wierny L, Warnke H, Gerstberger G, Romaniuk PA: Catheter closure of patent ductus arteriosus: 62 cases treated without thoracotomy. *Radiol Clin North Am* 1971;9:203–218
14. Tadavarthy SM, Knight L, Ovitt TW, Snyder C, Amplatz K: Therapeutic transcatheter arterial embolization. *Radiology* 1974;112:13–16
15. Tadavarthy SM, Moller JH, Amplatz K: Polyvinyl alcohol (Ivalon): a new embolic material. *AJR* 1975;125:609–616
16. Gianturco C, Anderson JH, Wallace S: Mechanical devices for arterial occlusion. *AJR* 1975;124:428–435
17. Ellman BA, Parkhill BJ, Curry TS, Marcus PB, Peters PC: Ablation of renal tumors with absolute ethanol: a new technique. *Radiology* 1981;141:619–626
18. Rholl KS, Rysavy JA, Vlodaver Z, Cragg AH, Castañeda-Zúñiga WR, Amplatz K: Transcatheter thermal venous occlusion: a new technique. *Radiology* 1982;145:333–337
19. Cragg AH, Rosel P, Rysavy JA, Vlodaver Z, Castañeda-Zúñiga WR, Amplatz K: Renal ablation using hot contrast medium: an experimental study. *Radiology* 1983;148:683–686
20. Cho KJ, Williams DM, Brady TM, et al: Transcatheter embolization with sodium tetradecyl sulfate: experimental and clinical results. *Radiology* 1984;153:95–99

21. Thompson WM, Johnsrude IS: Vessel occlusion with transcatheter electrocoagulation. *CardioVasc Intervent Radiol* 1980;2:244–255

22. Cragg AH, Galliani CA, Rysavy JA, Castañeda–Zúñiga WR, Amplatz K: Endovascular diathermic vessel occlusion. *Radiology* 1982;144:303–308

23. Fingerhut AG, Alksne JF: Thrombosis of intracranial aneurysms: an experimental approach utilizing magnetically controlled iron particles. *Radiology* 1966;86:342–347

24. Lang EK: Superselective arterial catheterization as a vehicle for delivering radioactive infarct particles to tumors. *Radiology* 1971;98:391–399

25. Prochaska JH, Flye MW, Johnsrude IS: Left gastric artery embolization for control of gastric bleeding: a complication. *Radiology* 1973;107:521–522

26. Chuang VP, Wallace S: Hepatic arterial redistribution for intra-arterial infusion of hepatic neoplasms. *Radiology* 1980;135:295–299

27. Conroy RM, Lyons KP, Kuperus JH, Juler GL, Joy I, Pribram HFW: New technique for localization of therapeutic emboli using radionuclide labeling. *AJR* 1978;130:523–528

28. Endert G, Ritter H, Schumann E: ^{99m}Tc-Markierung von Gelantineschwamm für die Katheterembolisation. *Fortschr Röntgentstr* 1979;131:600–603

29. Cunningham DS, Paletta FX: Control of arteriovenous fistula in massive facial hemangioma by muscle emboli. *Plast Reconstr Surg* 1970;46:305–308

30. Bryan WM, Maull KI: Arteriovenous malformations of the mandible. *Plast Reconstr Surg* 1975;55:690–696

31. Bookstein JJ, Cholasta EM, Foley D, Walters JS: Transcatheter hemostasis of gastrointestinal bleeding using modified autogenous clot. *Radiology* 1974;113:227–231

32. Meaney TF, Chicatelli PD: Obliteration of renal arteriovenous fistula by transcatheter clot embolization: case report and experimental observations. *Cleve Clin Q* 1974;41:33–38

33. Chuang VO, Reuter SR: Experimental diminution of splenic function by selective embolization of the splenic artery. *Surg Gynecol Obstet* 1975;140:715–720

34. Barth KH, Strandberg JD, White RI Jr: Long-term follow-up of transcatheter embolization with autologous clot, Oxycel, and Gelfoam in domestic swine. *Invest Radiol* 1977;12:273–280

35. Cope C, Zeit R: Coagulation of aneurysms by direct percutaneous thrombin injection. *AJR* 1986;147:383–387

36. Bookstein JJ, Chlosta GM, Foley D, et al: Transcatheter hemostasis of gastrointestinal bleeding using modified autogenous clot. *Radiology* 1974;133:277

37. McLean GK, Stein EJ, Burke DR, Meranze SG. Steel occlusion coils: pretreatment with thrombin. *Radiology* 1986;158:549–550

38. Fedullo LM, Meranze SG, McLean GK, Burke DR. Embolization of a subclavian artery aneurysm with steel coils and thrombin. *Cardiovasc Intervent Radiol* 1987;10:134–137

39. Walker TG, Geller SC, Brewster DC: Transcatheter occlusion of profunda femoral artery pseudoaneurysm using thrombin. *AJR* 1987;149:185–186

40. Lammert GK, Merine D, White RI Jr, et al: Embolotherapy of a high-flow false aneurysm by using an occlusion balloon, thrombin, steel coils, and a detachable balloon. *AJR* 1989;152:382–384

41. Ishimori S: Treatment of carotid-cavernous fistula by Gelfoam embolization. *J Neurosurg* 1967;27:315–319

42. Goldstein HM, Wallace S, Anderson JH, Bell RL, Gianturco C: Transcatheter occlusion of abdominal tumors. *Radiology* 1976;120:539–545

43. Page RC, Larson EJ, Siegmund E: Plastic sponge occludes arteriovenous defect. *JAMA* 1976;236:1335–1338

44. Levin DC, Beckmann CF, Hillman B: Experimental determination of flow patterns of Gelfoam emboli: safety implications. *AJR* 1980;134:525–528

45. Greenfield AJ, Athanasoulis CA, Waltman AC: Transcatheter embolization: prevention of embolic reflux using balloon catheters. *AJR* 1978;131:165–168

46. Greenfield AJ: Transcatheter vessel occlusion: selection of methods and material. *Cardiovasc Intervent Radiol* 1980;3:222–228

47. Rösch J, Keller FS, Kozak B, Niles N, Dotter CT: Gelfoam powder embolization of the left gastric artery in treatment of massive small gastric bleeding. *Radiology* 1984;151:365–370

48. Jander HP, Russinovich NAE: Transcatheter Gelfoam embolization in abdominal, retroperitoneal, and pelvic hemorrhage. *Radiology* 1980;136:337–344

49. Richman SD, Green WM, Kroll R, Casarella WJ: Superselective transcatheter embolization of traumatic renal hemorrhage. *AJR* 1977;128:843–844

50. Zollikofer C, Castañeda–Zúñiga WR, Galliani C, Rysavy JA, Formanek A, Amplatz K: Therapeutic blockade of arteries using compressed Ivalon. *Radiology* 1980;136:635–640

51. Castañeda–Zúñiga WR, Sanchez R, Amplatz K: Experimental observations on short- and long-term effects of arterial occlusion with Ivalon. *Radiology* 1978;126:783–785

52. Berenstein A, Kricheff II: Catheter and material selection for transarterial embolization. Technical considerations II: materials. *Radiology* 1979;132:631–639

53. Kerber CW, Bank WO, Horton JA: Polyvinyl alcohol foam: prepacked emboli for therapeutic embolization. *AJR* 1978;130:1193–1194

54. Herrera M, Rysavy J, Kotula F, Castañeda–Zúñiga WR, Amplatz K: Ivalon shavings: a new embolic agent. *Radiology* 1982;144:638–640

55. Castañeda–Zúñiga WR, Hammerschmidt DE, Sanchez R, Amplatz K: Nonsurgical splenectomy. *AJR* 1977;129:805–811

56. Repa I, Moradian GP, Dehner LP, Tadavarthy SM: Mortalities associated with use of a commercial suspension of polyvinyl alcohol. *Radiology* 1989;170:395–399

57. Sirr SA, Johnson TK, Stuart DD, Stanchfield WR, Cardella JF, duCret RP, Boudreau RJ: An improved radiolabeling technique of Ivalon and its use for dynamic monitoring of complications during therapeutic transcatheter embolization. *J Nucl Med* 1989;30:1399–1404

58. duCret RP, Adkins MC, Hunter DW, Yedlicka JW Jr, Engeler CM, Castañeda–Zúñiga WR, Amplatz K: Therapeutic embolization: enhanced radiolabeled monitoring. *Radiology* 1990;177:571–575

59. Chuang VP, Soo CS, Wallace S: Ivalon embolization in abdominal neoplasms. *AJR* 1981;136:729–733

60. Zollikofer C, Castañeda–Zúñiga WR, Galliani C, et al: A combination of stainless steel coil and compressed Ivalon: a new technique for embolization of large arteries and arteriovenous fistulas. *Radiology* 1981;138:229–231

61. Castañeda–Zúñiga WR, Galliani CA, Rysavy J, Kotula F, Amplatz K: "Spiderlon": new device for simple, fast arterial and venous occlusion. *AJR* 1981;136:627–628

62. Mazer MJ, Baltaxe HA, Wolf GL: Therapeutic embolization of the renal artery with Gianturco coils: limitations and technical pitfalls. *Radiology* 1981;138:37–46

63. Castañeda–Zúñiga WR, Tadavarthy SM, Beranek I, Amplatz K: Nonsurgical closure of large arteriovenous fistulas. *JAMA* 1976;236:2649–2650

64. Castañeda–Zúñiga WR, Tadavarthy SM, Galliani C, Laerum F, Schwarten D, Amplatz K: Experimental venous occlusion with stainless steel spiders. *Radiology* 1981;141:238–241

65. Probst P, Rysavy J, Amplatz K: Increased safety of spleno-portography by plugging the needle tract. *AJR* 1978;131:445–449

66. Doppman JL, DiChiro G, Ommaya A: Obliteration of spinal-cord arteriovenous malformations by percutaneous embolization. *Lancet* 1968;1:477–486

67. Meyers PH, Cronic F, Nice CM Jr: Experimental approach in the use and magnetic control of metallic iron particles in the lymphatic and vascular system of dogs as a contrast and isotopic agent. *AJR* 1963;90:1068–1077

68. Loop JW, Foltz EL: Applications of angiography during intracranial operation. *Acta Radiol [Diagn]* 1966;5:363–376

69. Fleischer AS, Kricheff I, Ransohoff J: Postmortem findings following the embolization of an arteriovenous malformation. *J Neurosurg* 1972;37:606–609

70. Lin SR, LaDow CS, Tatoian JA, Go EB: Angiographic demonstration and silicone pellet embolization of facial hemangiomas of bone. *Neuroradiology* 1974;7:201–204

71. Longacre JJ, Benton C, Unterthiner RA: Treatment of facial hemangioma by intravascular embolization with silicone spheres. *Plast Reconstr Surg* 1972;50:618–621

72. Kricheff I, Madayag M, Braunstein P: Transfemoral catheter embolization of cerebral and posterior fossa arteriovenous malformations. *Radiology* 1972;103:107–111

73. Matsumoto T: *Tissue Adhesives in Surgery.* New York, Medical Examination Publishing Co, 1972

74. Dotter CT, Goldman ML, Rösch J: Instant selective arterial occlusion with isobutyl-2-cyanoacrylate. *Radiology* 1975;114:227–230

75. Goldman ML, Philip PL, Sarrafizadeh MS: Bucrylate, a liquid tissue adhesive for transcatheter embolization. *Appl Radiol* 1984;Nov/Dec:89–94

76. Thelen M, Bruehl P, Gerlach F, Biersack HJ: Katheteroembolisation von metastasierten Nierenkarzinomen mit Butyl-2-Cyanoacrylat. *Fortschr Röntgenstr* 1976;124:232–235

77. Freeny PC, Bush WH, Kidd R: Transcatheter occlusive therapy of genitourinary abnormalities using isobutyl-2-cyanoacrylate. *AJR* 1979;133:647–656

78. Papo J, Baratz M, Merimsky E: Infarction of renal tumors using isobutyl-2-cyanoacrylate and Lipiodol. *AJR* 1981;137:781–785

79. Cromwell LD, Kerber CW: Modification of cyanoacrylate for therapeutic embolization: preliminary experience. *AJR* 1981;137:781–785

80. Salomonowitz E, Gottlob R, Castañeda–Zúñiga WR, Amplatz K: Transcatheter embolization with pro-celloidin cyanoacrylate. *Radiology* 1983;149:445–448

81. White RI, Strandberg JV, Gross GS, Barth KH: Therapeutic embolization with long-term occluding agents and their effects on embolized tissues. *Radiology* 1977;125:677–687

82. Goldman ML, Land WC Jr, Bradley EL III: Transcatheter therapeutic embolization in the management of massive upper gastrointestinal bleeding. *Radiology* 1976;120:513–521

83. Doppman JL, Zapol W, Pierce J: Transcatheter embolization with a silicone rubber preparation: experimental observations. *Invest Radiol* 1971;6:304–309

84. Berenstein A: Flow-controlled silicone fluid embolization. *AJR* 1980;135:1213–1218

85. Buecheler E, Hupe W, Klosterhalfen J, Altenaehr E, Erbe W: Neue Substanz zur therapeutischen Embolization von Nierentumoren. *Fortschr Röntgenstr* 1976;124:232–235

86. Kauffman GW, Rassweiler J, Richter G, Hauenstein HK, Rohrbock R, Friedburg H: Capillary embolization with Ethibloc: new embolization concept test in dog kidneys. *AJR* 1981;137:1163–1168

87. Abbott WM, Austen WG: The effectiveness and mechanism of collagen induced hemostasis. *Surgery* 1975;78:723–729

88. Diamond NG, Casarella WJ, Bachman DM, Wolff M: Microfibrillar collagen hemostat: a new transcatheter embolization agent. *Radiology* 1979;133:775–779

89. Kaufman SL, Strandberg JD, Barth KH, White RI: Transcatheter embolization with microfibrillar collagen in swine. *Invest Radiol* 1978;13:200–204

90. Mineau DE, Miller FJ, Lee RG, Nakashima EN, Nelson JA: Experimental transcatheter spenectomy using absolute ethanol. *Radiology* 1982;142:355–359

91. Ekelund L, Jonsson N, Trugut H: Transcatheter obliteration of the renal artery by ethanol injection: experimental results. *Cardiovasc Intervent Radiol* 1981;4:1–7

92. Doppman JL, Popovsky M, Girton M: The use of iodinated contrast agents to ablate organs: experimental studies and histopathology. *Radiology* 1981;138:333–340

93. Seyferth W, Jecht E, Zeitler E: Percutaneous sclerotherapy of varicocele. *Radiology* 1981;139:335–340

94. Hunter DW, Castañeda–Zúñiga WR, Young A, et al: Spermatic vein embolization with hot contrast medium or detachable balloons. *Semin Intervent Radiol* 1984;1:163–169

95. Wallace S, Gianturco C, Anderson JH, Goldstein HM, Davis LJ: Therapeutic vascular occlusion utilizing steel coil technique: clinical applications. *AJR* 1976;127:381–387

96. Anderson JH, Wallace S, Gianturco C: Transcatheter intravascular coil occlusion of experimental arteriovenous fistulas. *AJR* 1977;129:795–798

97. Formanek A, Probst P, Tadavarthy SM, Castañeda–Zúñiga WR, Amplatz K: Transcatheter embolization in the pediatric age group. *Ann Radiol* 1979;22:150–158

98. Widrich WC, Robbins AJ, Johnson WC, Nasbeth DC: Pitfalls of transhepatic portal venography and therapeutic coronary vein occlusion. *AJR* 1978;131:637–640

99. Fuhrman BP, Bass JL, Castañeda–Zúñiga WR, Amplatz K, Lock JE: Coil embolization of congenital thoracic vascular anomalies in infants and children. *Circulation* 1984;70:285–289

100. Anderson JH, Wallace S, Gianturco C: "Mini" Gianturco stainless steel coils for transcatheter vascular occlusion. *Radiology* 1979;132:301–303

101. Yang PJ, Halbach VV, Higashida RT, Hieshima GB: Platinum wire: a new transvascular embolic agent. *AJNR* 1988;9:547–550

102. Graves VB, Partington CR, Rufenacht DA, Rappe AH, Strother CM: Treatment of carotid artery aneurysms with platinum coils: an experimental study in dogs. *AJNR* 1990;11:249–252

103. Hilal SK, Khandji AG, Chi TL, Stein BM, Bello JA, Silver AJ: Synthetic fiber-coated platinum coils successfully used for the endovascular treatment of arteriovenous malformations, aneurysms and direct arteriovenous fistulas of the CNS. *AJNR* (abstr) 1988;9:1030

104. Morse SS, Clark RA, Puffenbarger A: Platinum microcoils for therapeutic embolization: nonneuroradiologic applications. Technical note. *AJR* 1990;155:401–403

105. Castañeda–Zúñiga WR, Zollikofer C, Barreto A, Formanek A, Amplatz K: A new device for the safe delivery of stainless steel coils. *Radiology* 1980;136:230–231

106. Anderson JH, Wallace S, Gianturco C: Transcatheter intravascular coil occlusion of experimental arteriovenous fistulas. *AJR* 1977;129:795–798

107. Wallace S, Gianturco C, Anderson JH, et al: Therapeutic vascular occlusion utilizing steel coil technique: clinical applications. *AJR* 1976;127:381–387

108. Tisnado J, Beachley MC, Cho SR: Peripheral embolization of a stainless steel coil. *AJR* 1979;133:324–326

109. Chuang VP: Nonoperative retrieval of Gianturco coils from abdominal aorta. *AJR* 1979;132:996–997

110. Freeny PC, Busch WH Jr, Kidd R: Transcatheter occlusive therapy of genitourinary abnormalities using isobutyl-2-cyanoacrylate (Bucrylate). *AJR* 1979;133:647–656

111. Gomes AS, Rysavy JA, Spadaccini CA, Amplatz K: The use of the bristle brush for transcatheter embolization. *Radiology* 1978;129:354–360

112. Hieshima GBM, Grinnell VS, Mehringer CM: A detachable balloon for therapeutic transcatheter occlusion. *Radiology* 1981;138:227–228

113. Waltman AC: Catheter systems used in therapeutic angiogram and methods of superselective vessel catheterization, in Athasouilis CA, Pfister RC, Greene RE, Roberson GH (eds): *Interventional Radiology*, 1982, 14–21

114. Olliff S, Thomas S, Karani J, Walters H. Superselective embolization using a coaxial catheter technique. *Br J Radiol* 1990;63:197–201

115. Meyerovitz MF, Levin DC, Boxt LM: Superselective catheterization of small-caliber arteries with a new high-visibility steerable guide wire. *AJR* 1985;144:785–786

116. Kikuchi Y, Strother CM, Boyer M: New catheter for endovascular interventional procedures. *Radiology* 1987;165:870–871

117. Chuang VP: Superselective hepatic tumor embolization with Tracker-18 catheter. *J Intervent Radiol* 1988;3:69–71

118. Matsumoto AH, Shuocki PV, Barth KH: Superselective Gelfoam embolotherapy using a highly visible small caliber catheter. *Cardiovasc Intervent Radiol* 1988;11:303–306

119. Okazaki M, Higashihara H, Koganemaru F, et al: A co-axial catheter and steerable guidewire used to embolize branches of the splenic arteries. *AJR* 1990;155:405–406

120. Coldwell DM: Hepatic arterial embolization utilizing a coaxial catheter system. Technical note. *Cardiovasc Interv Radiol* 1990;13:53–54

121. Sos TA, Cohn DJ, Srur M, Wengrover SI, Saddekni S: A new open-ended guidewire/catheter. *Radiology* 1985;154:817–818

122. Coldwell DM: Hepatic embolization with an open-ended guide wire. *Radiology* 1987;165:285–286

123. Jungreis CA, Berenstein A, Choi IS: Use of an open-ended guidewire: steerable microguidewire assembly system in surgical neuroangiographic procedures. *AJNR* 1987;8:237–241

124. Encarnacion CE, Kadir S, Malone RB: Subselective embolization with gelatin sponge through an open-ended guide wire. *Radiology* 1990;174:265–267

125. Barnhart W, Snidow JJ, Smith TP, Castañeda F, Nakagawa N, Cragg AH: New guide wire for high-flow infusion. *Radiology* 1990;174:1058–1059

126. Hori S, Matsushita M, Narumi Y, Fujita M, Tomoda K: Hepatic arterial catheterization with use of a supple catheter with a ball tip. *Radiology* 1989;171:860–861

127. Wholey MH, Kessler L, Boehnke M: A percutaneous balloon catheter technique for the treatment of intracranial aneurysms. *Acta Radiol [Diagn]* 1972;13:286–292

128. Paster SB, Van Houten FX, Adams DF: Percutaneous balloon catheterization. *JAMA* 1975;230:573–575

129. Pevsner PH: Micro-balloon catheter for superselective angiography and therapeutic occlusion. *AJR* 1977;128:225–230

130. DiTullio MC, Rand RW, Frisch E: Detachable balloon catheter: its application in experimental arteriovenous fistulae. *J Neurosurg* 1978;48:717–723

131. White RI, Kaufman SL, Barth KH, DeCaprio V, Strandbert JD: Embolotherapy with detachable silicone balloons: technique and clinical results. *Radiology* 1979;131:619–627

132. Wagner RB, Baeza OR, Stewart JE: Active pulmonary hemorrhage localized by selective pulmonary arteriography. *Chest* 1975;67:121–122

133. Garzon A, Cerruti M, Gourin A: Pulmonary resection for massive hemoptysis. *Surgery* 1970;67:633–638

134. Thoms NW, Wilson RF, Puro HE: Life-threatening hemoptysis in primary lung abscess. *Ann Thorac Surg* 1972;14:347–358

135. Remy J, Arnaud A, Fardou H, Giraud R, Voisin C: Treatment of hemoptysis by embolization of bronchial arteries. *Radiology* 1977;122:33–37

136. Caldwell EW, Siekert RG, Lininger RE: The bronchial arteries: an anatomic study of 150 human cadavers. *Surg Gynecol Obstet* 1948;86:396–415

137. Cohen AM, Doershuk CF, Stern RC: Bronchial artery embolization to control hemoptysis in cystic fibrosis. *Radiology* 1990;175:401–405

138. McPherson S, Routh WD, Nath H, Keller FS: Anomalous origin of bronchial arteries: potential pitfall of embolotherapy for hemoptysis. *JVIR* 1990;1:86–88

139. Di Chiro G: Unintentional spinal cord arteriography: a warning. *Radiology* 1974;112:231–233

140. Kardjiev V, Symeonov A, Chankov I: Etiology, pathogenesis and prevention of spinal cord lesions in selective angiography of the bronchial and intercostal arteries. *Radiology* 1974;112:81–83

141. Botenga ASJ: *Selective Bronchial and Intercostal Arteriography.* Leiden, The Netherlands, HE Stenfert Kroses, 1970

142. Milne E: *Bronchial Arteriography*, ed. 2. Boston, Little, Brown & Co, 1971, pp 567–577

143. Remy J, Marache P, Lemaitre ML: Accidents de l'embolisation dans le traitment des hemoptysies. *Nouv Presse Med* 1978;7:4306–4310

144. Vujic I, Pyle R, Parker E, Mithoefer J: Control of massive hemoptysis by embolization of intercostal arteries. *Radiology* 1980;137:617–620

145. Tadavarthy SM, Klugman J: Castañeda–Zúñiga WR, Nath PH, Amplatz K: Systemic to pulmonary collaterals in pathologic states: review. *Radiology* 1982;144:75–76

146. Jardin M, Remy J: Control of hemoptysis: systemic angiography and anastomoses of the internal mammary artery. *Radiology* 1988;168:377–383

147. Lois JF, Gomes AS, Smith DC, Laks H: Systemic-to-pulmonary collateral vessels and shunts: treatment with embolization. *Radiology* 1988;169:671–676

148. Munk PL, Morris C, Nelems B: Left main bronchial-esophageal fistula: a complication of bronchial artery embolization. *Cardiovasc Intervent Radiol* 1990;13:95–97

149. Girard P, Baldeyrou P, Lemoine G, Grunewald D: Left main-stem bronchial stenosis complicating bronchial artery embolization. *Chest* 1990;97:1246–1248

150. Liebow AA, Hales MR, Lindskog GE: Enlargement of the bronchial arteries and their anastomoses with the pulmonary arteries in bronchiectasis. *Am J Pathol* 1949;25:211–225

151. Mack JF, Moss AJ, Harper WW, O'Loughlin BJ: The bronchial arteries in cystic fibrosis. *Br J Radiol* 1965;38:422–431

152. Moss AJ, Desilets DT, Higashino SM, Ruttenberg HD, Mar-

cano BA, Dooley RA: Intrapulmonary shunts in cystic fibrosis. *Pediatrics* 1968;41:438–447

153. Fellows KE, Shaw KT, Schuster S, Shwachman H: Bronchial artery embolization in cystic fibrosis: technique and long-term results. *J Pediatr* 1979;95:959–963

154. Stoll JF, Bettman MA: Bronchial artery embolization to control hemoptysis: a review. *Cardiovasc Intervent Radiol* 1988;11:263–269

155. Wholey MH, Chamorro HA, Gopal R, Ford WB, Miller WH: Bronchial artery embolization for massive hemoptysis. *JAMA* 1976;236:2501–2504

156. Harley JD, Killien FC, Peck AG: Massive hemoptysis controlled by transcatheter embolization of the bronchial arteries. *AJR* 1977;128:302–304

157. Ben-Menachem Y, Handel SF, Ray RD, Childs TL III: Embolization procedures in trauma: a matter of urgency. *Semin Intervent Radiol* 1985;2:107–117

158. Seavers R, Lynch K, Ballard R, Jernigan S, Johnson J: Hypogastric artery ligation for uncontrollable hemorrhage in acute pelvic trauma. *Surgery* 1964;55:516–525

159. Margolies MN, Ring EJ, Waltman AC: Arteriography in the management of hemorrhage from pelvic fractures. *N Engl J Med* 1972;287:317–321

160. Fisher RG, Ben-Menachen Y: Embolization procedures in trauma: the extremities—acute lesions. *Semin Intervent Radiol* 1985;2:118–124

161. Rich NM, Hobson RW, Collins GJ: Traumatic arteriovenous fistulas and false aneurysms: a review of 558 lesions. *Surgery* 1975;78:817–825

162. Hauser CW: Initial treatment of pelvic fractures. *Lancet* 1966;86:285–286

163. Kerr WS Jr, Margolies MN, Ring EJ, Waltman AG, Baum SN: Arteriography in pelvic fractures with massive hemorrhage. *J Urol* 1973;109:479–485

164. Matalon T, Athanasoulis CA, Margolies MN, Waltman AC, Novelline RA: Hemorrhage with pelvic fractures: efficacy of transcatheter embolization. *AJR* 1979;133:859–867

165. Bookstein JJ, Goldstein HM: Successful management of post biopsy arteriovenous fistula with selective arterial embolization. *Radiology* 1973;109:535–536

166. Rizk GK, Atallah NK, Bridi GI: Renal arteriovenous fistula treated by catheter embolization. *Br J Radiol* 1973;46:222–223

167. Chuang VP, Reuter SR, Walter J, Foley WD, Bookstein JJ: Control of renal hemorrhage by selective arterial embolization of renal arteriovenous fistula. *AJR* 1975;125:300–306

168. Goldman ML, Fellner SK, Parrott TS: Transcatheter embolization of renal arteriovenous fistula. *Urology* 1975;6:386–388

169. Silber SJ, Clark RE: Treatment of massive hemorrhage after renal biopsy with angiographic injection of clot. *N Engl J Med* 1975;292:1387–1388

170. Barbaric FL, Cutcliff WB: Control of renal arterial bleeding after percutaneous biopsy. *Urology* 1976;8:108–111

171. Kerber CW, Freeny PC, Cromwell L, Margolis MT: Cyanoacrylate occlusion of renal arteriovenous fistula. *AJR* 1977;128:663–665

172. Rosen RJ, Feldman L, Wilson AR: Embolization for postbiopsy renal arteriovenous fistula: effective occlusion using homologous clot. *AJR* 1978;131:1072–1073

173. McAlister DS, Johnsrude I, Miller MM, Clap J, Thompson WM: Occlusion of acquired renal arteriovenous fistula with transcatheter electrocoagulation. *AJR* 1979;132:998–1000

174. Pontes JE, Parekh N, McGuckin JT, Banks MD, Pierce JM: Percutaneous transfemoral embolization of arterio–infundibular-venous fistula. *J Urol* 1976;116:98–100

175. Maxwell DD, Frankel RS: Wedged catheter management of a bleeding renal pseudoaneurysm. *J Urol* 1976;116:96–97

176. Coleman CC, Kimura Y, Reddy P, et al: Complications of nephrostolithotomy. *Semin Intervent Radiol* 1984;1:70–74

177. Clayman RV, Surya V, Hunter DW, et al: Renal vascular complications associated with percutaneous removal of renal calculi. *J Urol* 1984;132:228–230

178. Clayman R, Castañeda–Zúñiga WR: Nephrostolithotomy: percutaneous removal of renal calculi. *Urol Radiol* 1984;6:95–112

179. Fisher RG, Ben-Menachen Y: Embolization procedures in trauma: the abdomen—extraperitoneal. *Semin Intervent Radiol* 1985;2:148–157

180. Silverberg DS, Dossetor JB, Eid TC, Mant MJ, Miller JDR: Arteriovenous fistula and prolonged hematuria after renal biopsy: treatment with epsilon aminocaproic acid. *Can Med Assoc J* 1974;110:671–672

181. Ekelund L, Gothlin J, Lindholm T, Lindstedt E, Mattsson K: Arteriovenous fistulas following renal biopsy with hypertension and hemodynamic changes. *J Urol* 1972;108:373–376

182. O'Brien DP, Parott TS, Walton KN, Lewis EL: Renal arteriovenous fistulas. *Surg Gynecol Obstet* 1976;118:1305–1311

183. Iverson P, Brun C: Aspiration biopsy of the kidney. *Am J Med* 1951;11:324–328

184. Bartels ED, Jorgensen HE: Experiences with percutaneous renal biopsy. *Scand J Urol Nephrol* 1972;15(suppl 6):57–65

185. Bolton WK: Localization of the kidney for percutaneous biopsy: a comparative study of methods. *Ann Intern Med* 1974;81:159–164

186. Zeis PM: Ultrasound localization for percutaneous renal biopsy in children. *J Pediatr* 1976;89:263–268

187. Morrow JW, Mendez R: Renal trauma. *J Urol* 1970;104:649–653

188. Kalish M, Greenbaum L, Silber SJ: Traumatic renal hemorrhage: treatment by arterial embolization. *J Urol* 1978;112:138–141

189. Grace DM, Pitt DF, Gold RE: Vascular embolization and occlusion by angiographic techniques as an aid or alternative to operation. *Surg Gynecol Obstet* 1976;143:469–482

190. White RI Jr: Arterial embolization for control of renal hemorrhage. *J Urol* 1976;115:121–122

191. Richman SD, Green WW, Kroll R, Casarella WJ: Superselective transcatheter embolization of traumatic renal hemorrhage. *AJR* 1977;128:843–844

192. Chang J, Katzen BT, Sullivan KP: Transcatheter Gelfoam embolization of post-traumatic bleeding pseudoaneurysms. *AJR* 1978;131:645–650

193. Blackwell JE, Potchen EJ, Laidlaw WW, Paul LH: Traumatic arteriocaliceal fistula: effective occlusion using homologous clot. *AJR* 1978;129:633–634

194. Haydu P, Chang J, Knox G, Nealson TF Jr: Transcatheter arterial embolization of a traumatic lumbar artery false aneurysm. *Surgery* 1978;84:288–291

195. Fankuchen EI, Martin EC, Karlson KB, Mattern RF, Casarella WJ: Small coils for large hemorrhages. *AJR* 1981;136:816–818

196. Stock JR, Athanasoulis CA: Musculoskeletal trauma: control of bleeding with transcatheter embolization, in Athanasoulis CA, Pfister RC, Greene RE, Roberson GH (eds): *Interventional Radiology.* Philadelphia, WB Saunders Co, 1982, pp 174–195

197. Scalfani SJA, Shaftan GW, Mitchell WG, Nayaranaswamy TS, McAuley J: Interventional radiology in trauma victims: analysis of 51 consecutive cases. *J Trauma* 1982;22:353–360

198. Ben-Menachem Y: Interventive and guidance procedures,

in Ben-Menachem Y (ed): *Angiography in Trauma: A Work Atlas.* Philadelphia, WB Saunders Co, 1981, pp 411–452

199. Trunkey DD, Shires GT, McClelland R: Management of liver trauma in 811 consecutive patients. *Ann Surg* 1974;179:722–728

200. Heinbach DM, Ferguson GS, Harley JD: Treatment of traumatic hemobilia with angiographic embolization. *J Trauma* 1978;18:221–224

201. Hirsch N, Avinoach I, Keynan A: Angiographic diagnosis and treatment of hemobilia. *Radiology* 1982;144:771–772

202. Scenoy SS, Bergsland J, Cerra FB: Arterial embolization for traumatic hemobilia with hepatoportal fistula. *Cardiovasc Intervent Radiol* 1981;4:206–208

203. Walter JF, Paaso BT, Cannon WB: Successful transcatheter embolic control of massive hematobilia secondary to liver biopsy. *AJR* 1976;127:847–849

204. Aldrete JS, Halpern NB, Ward S: Factors determining mortality and morbidity in hepatic injuries. *Ann Surg* 1979;189:466–474

205. Lambeth W, Rubin BE: Non-operative management of intrahepatic hemorrhage and hematoma following blunt trauma. *Surg Gynecol Obstet* 1979;148:507–511

206. Rubin BE, Katzen BT: Selective hepatic artery embolization to control massive hepatic hemorrhage after trauma. *AJR* 1977;129:253–256

207. Bass EM, Crosier JH: Percutaneous control of post-traumatic hepatic hemorrhage by Gelfoam embolization. *J Trauma* 1977;17:61–63

208. Jander HT, Laws HL, Kogget MS: Emergency embolization in blunt hepatic trauma. *AJR* 1977;129:249–252

209. Sclafani SJA, Shaftan GW, McAuley J: Interventional radiology in the management of hepatic trauma. *J Trauma* 1984;24:256–262

210. Struyven J, Krener M, Pirson P, et al: Post-traumatic bilhemia: diagnosis and catheter therapy. *AJR* 1982;138:746–747

211. Reuter SR, Palmaz JC, Berk RV: Hepatic artery injury during the portocaval shunt surgery. *AJR* 1980;134:349–353

212. Doppman JL, Girton M, Vermass M: The risk of hepatic artery embolization in the presence of obstructive jaundice. *Radiology* 1982;143:37–43

213. Kuroda C, Iwaski M, Tanaka T: Gallbladder infarction following hepatic transcatheter arterial embolization. *Radiology* 1983;149:85–89

214. Levinson JD, Olsen G, Terman JW, Cleaveland CR, Graham CP, Breen KJ: Hemobilia secondary to percutaneous liver biopsy. *Arch Intern Med* 1972;130:396–400

215. Viranuvatti V, Plengvanit U, Kalayasiri C, Bhamarapravati N: Needle liver biopsy with particular reference to complications. *Am J Gastroenterol* 1964;42:529–536

216. Attiyeh FF, McSweeney J, Fortner JG: Hemobilia complicating needle liver biopsy. *Radiology* 1976;18:559–560

217. Walter JF, Paaso BT, Cannon WB: Successful transcatheter embolic control of massive hematobilia secondary to liver biopsy. *AJR* 1976;127:847–849

218. Terry R: Risks of needle biopsy of the liver. *Br Med J* 1952;1:1102–1105

219. Debray D, Leymarios E, Martin E, Hernandez CI, Carayon J, Coste F: Fistules arterioveineuses hepatico-portale consecutive a une ponctionbiopsie du foie. *Presse Med* 1968;76:737–740

220. Preger L: Hepatic arteriovenous fistula after percutaneous liver biopsy. *AJR* 1976;101:619–620

221. Walter JF, Paaso BT, Connon WB: Successful transcatheter emboli control of massive hematobilia secondary to liver biopsy. *AJR* 1976;127:847–849

222. Merino–de Villasante J, Alvarez–Rodriquez RE, Hernandez–Ortiz J: Management of post biopsy hemobilia

with selective arterial embolization. *AJR* 1977;121:668–671

223. Perlberger RR: Control of hemobilia with angiographic embolization. *AJR* 1977;128:672–673

224. Dunnick NR, Doppman JL, Brereton HD: Balloon occlusion of segmental hepatic arteries: control of biopsy induced hemobilia. *JAMA* 1977;238:2524–2525

225. Scalfani SJA, Nayaranaswamy T, Mitchell WG: Radiologic management of traumatic hepatic artery–portal vein arteriovenous fistulae. *J Trauma* 1981;21:576–580

226. Fitzgerald JB, Crawford ES, DeBakey ME: Surgical considerations of nonpenetrating abdominal injuries: an analysis of 200 cases. *Am J Surg* 1960;100:22–41

227. Fisher RG, Foucar K, Estroda R, Ben-Menachem Y: Splenic rupture in blunt trauma. *Radiol Clin North Am* 1981;19:141–166

228. King H, Schumaker MB Jr: Splenic studies: susceptibility to infection after splenectomy performed in infancy. *Ann Surg* 1951;136:239–242

229. Robinette CD: Splenectomy and subsequent mortality in veterans of 1939–45 war. *Lancet* 1977;2:373–381

230. Sclafani SJA: Angiographic control of intraperitoneal hemorrhage caused by injuries to the liver and spleen. *Semin Intervent Radiol* 1985;2:138 147

231. Sclafani SJA: Angiographic hemostasis: its role in the salvage of the injured spleen. *Radiology* 1981;141:645–650

232. Rowley DA: The formation of circulatory antibody in the splenectomized human after injection of heterologous erythrocytes. *J Immunol* 1950;65:515–521

233. Spigos DG, Jonasson O, Mozes M: Partial splenic embolization in the treatment of hypersplenism. *AJR* 1979;132:777–782

234. Leung LE, Szal GJ, Drachman RH: Increased susceptibility of splenectomized rats to infection with *Diplococcus pneumoniae. J Infect Dis* 1972;126:507–515

235. Singer DB: Postsplenectomy sepsis, in Rosenberg JS, Bolande RP (eds): *Perspectives in Pediatric Pathology.* Chicago, Year Book Medical Publishers, 1973, p 285

236. Van Wyck DB, Witte MH: Critical splenic mass for survival from experimental pneumococcemia. *J Surg Res* 1980;28:14–17

237. Boles TE Jr: The spleen, in Ravich MM, Welch KJ, Benson CDM, Aberdeen E, Randolph JC (eds): *Pediatric Surgery*, vol 2, ed 3. Chicago, Year Book Medical Publishers, 1979, pp 878–883

238. Krivit W, Giebink GS, Leonard A: Overwhelming postsplenectomy infections. *Surg Clin North Am* 1979;59:223–235

239. Pearson JA: Disorders of the spleen, in Cellis SS, Kagan BM (eds): *Current Pediatric Therapy*, ed 9. Philadelphia, WB Saunders Co, 1980, pp 286–287

240. Schroter GPJ, West JC, Weil R: Acute bacteremia in asplenic renal transplant patients. *JAMA* 1977;237:2207–2208

241. Guilford WB, Scatliff JH: Transcatheter embolization of the spleen for control of splenic hemorrhage and in situ splenectomy: an experimental study using silicone spheres. *Radiology* 1976;119:549–553

242. Bucheler E, Thelen M, Schirmer G: Katheter Embolization der Milzarterien zum Stop der akuten Varizenblutung. *Fortschr Röntgenstr* 1975;122:539–546

243. Günther R, Bohl J, Klose K, Anger J: Transkatheterembolisierung der Milz mit Butyl-2-Cyanoacrylat. *Fortschr Röntgenstr* 1980;133:158–163

244. Maddison F: Embolic therapy of hypersplenism. *Invest Radiol* 1973;8:280–295

245. Zannini G, Masciariello S, Pagano G, Sangiulo P, Zotti G: Percutaneous splenic artery occlusion for portal hypertension. *Arch Surg* 1983;118:897–900

246. Witte CL, Ovitt TW, Van Wyck DB, Witte MH, O'Mara RE: Ischemic therapy in thrombocytopenia from hypersplenism. *Arch Surg* 1976;111:1115–1121
247. Wholey MH, Chamorro HA, Rao G, Chapman W: Splenic infarction and spontaneous rupture of the spleen after therapeutic embolization. *Cardiovasc Radiol* 1978;1:249–253
248. Thanopoulos BD, Frimas CA: Partial splenic embolization in the management of hypersplenism secondary to Gaucher disease. *J Pediatr* 1982;101:740–742
249. Anderson JH, VuBan A, Wallace S, Hester JP, Burke JS: Transcatheter splenic arterial occlusion: an experimental study in dogs. *Radiology* 1977;125:95–102
250. Levy JM, Wasserman P, Pitha N: Presplenectomy transcatheter occlusion of the splenic artery. *Arch Surg* 1979;114:198–199
251. Vujic I, Lauver JW: Severe complications from partial splenic embolization in patients with liver failure. *Br J Radiol* 1981;54:492–495
252. Alwmark A, Bengmark S, Gullstrand P, Joelsson BO, Lunderquist A: Evaluation of splenic embolization in patients with portal hypertension and hypersplenism. *Ann Surg* 1982;196:518–524
253. Owman T, Lunderquist A, Alwmark A, Borjesson B: Embolization of the spleen for treatment of splenomegaly and hypersplenism in patients with portal hypertension. *Invest Radiol* 1979;14:457–464
254. Tsapogas MJ, Peabody RA, Karmody AM: Pathophysiological changes following ischemia of the spleen. *Ann Surg* 1973;178:179–183
255. Matas AJ, Simmons RL, Buselmeier TJ, Najarian JS, Kjellstrand CM: Lethal complications of bilateral nephrectomy and splenectomy in hemodialized patients. *Am J Surg* 1975;129:616–620
256. Yarimizu SN, Susan LP, Straffon RA, Stewart BM, Magnusson MO, Nakamoto SS: Mortality and morbidity in pretransplant bilateral nephrectomy: analysis of 305 cases. *Urology* 1978;12:55–58
257. Goldin AR, Naude JH, Thatcher GN: Therapeutic percutaneous renal infarction. *Br J Urol* 1974;46:133–135
258. Powischer G, Wolf A, Eyre G: Kidney embolization with collagen fluids in malignant hypertension, in Anacker V, Burotta V, Rupp N (eds): *Percutaneous Biopsy and Therapeutic Vascular Occlusion*. Stuttgart, Georg Thieme, 1980, pp 169–172
259. Fletcher EWL, Thompson JF, Chalmers DHK, Taylor HM, Wood RFM, Morris PS: Embolization of host kidneys for the control of hypertension after renal transplantation: radiology aspects. *Radiology* 1984;57:279–284
260. McCarron DA, Rubin RJ, Barnes BA, Harrington JT, Millan VG: Therapeutic bilateral renal infarction and end-stage renal disease. *N Engl J Med* 1976;294:652–660
261. Leenen FHH, Galla SJ, Geyshes GG, Murdaugh HV, Shapiro AP: Effects of hemodialysis and saline loading on body fluid compartments, plasma renin activity and blood pressure in patients on chronic hemodialysis. *Nephron* 1977;18:93–100
262. Eliscu EH, Haire HM, Tew FT, Newton LW: Control of malignant renovascular hypertension by percutaneous transluminal angioplasty and therapeutic renal embolization. *AJR* 1980;134:815–817
263. Denny DF, Perlmutt LM, Bettmann MA: Percutaneous recanalization of an occluded renal artery and delayed ethanol ablation of the kidney resulting in control of hypertension. *Radiology* 1984;151:381–382
264. Reuter SR, Pomeroy PR, Chuang VP, Kyung JC: Embolic control of hypertension caused by segmental renal artery stenosis. *AJR* 1976;127:389–392
265. Bennington JL, Beckwith JB: Tumors of the kidneys, renal pelvis and ureter, in *Atlas of Tumor Pathology*, 2nd series, fasc 12. Washington DC, Armed Forces Institute of Pathology, 1975, pp 25–29
266. Bennington JL: Cancer of the kidney—etiology, epidemiology, and pathology. *Cancer* 1973;32:1017–1029
267. Skinner DG, Colvin RB, Vermillion CD: Diagnosis and management of renal cell carcinoma: a clinical and pathologic study of 309 cases. *Cancer* 1971;28:1165–1177
268. Lokich JJ, Harrison JH: Renal cell carcinoma: natural history and chemotherapeutic experience. *J Urol* 1975;114:371–374
269. Robson CJ, Churchill BM, Anderson W: The results of radical nephrectomy for renal cell carcinoma. *J Urol* 1969;101:297–302
270. Hulten L, Rosencrantz M, Seeman T: Occurrence and localization of lymph node metastases in renal carcinoma: a lymphographic and histopathological investigation in connection with nephrectomy. *Scand J Urol Nephrol* 1969;3:129–133
271. Lang EK: Superselective arterial catheterization as a vehicle for delivering radioactive infarct particles to tumors. *Radiology* 1971;98:391–399
272. Almgard LE, Fernström I, Haverling M: Treatment of renal adenocarcinoma by embolic occlusion of the renal circulation. *Br J Urol* 1973;45:474–479
273. Wallace S, Chuang VP, Swanson D, Bracken B, Hersch EM: Embolization of renal carcinoma. *Radiology* 1981;138:563–570
274. Kaisary AV, Williams G, Riddle PR: The role of preoperative embolization in renal cell carcinoma. *J Urol* 1984;131:641–646
275. Sandoval Parra R, Wingartz Plata HF, Gonzalez Gonzalez HJ, et al: Renal embolization: experience in 81 cases. *World Urol Update Ser* 1983;11(3):2–7
276. Becker GJ, Holden RW, Klatte EC: Therapeutic embolization with absolute ethanol. *Semin Intervent Radiol* 1985;1:118–129
277. Cho KJ, Nichiyama RH, Shields JJ: Functional, angiographic and histologic studies in experimental renal infarction. Presented at the 27th Annual Meeting of the Association of University Radiologists, Rochester, NY, May 1979
278. Hald T, Mygind T: Control of life-threatening vesical hemorrhage by unilateral hypogastric artery muscle embolization. *J Urol* 1974;112:60–63
279. Lang EK, Deutsch JS, Goodman JR, Barnett TF, Lanasa JA Jr, Duplessis GH: Transcatheter embolization of hypogastric branch arteries in the management of intractable bladder hemorrhage. *J Urol* 1979;121:30–36
280. Bree RL, Goldstein HM, Wallace S: Transcatheter embolization of the internal iliac artery in the management of neoplasms of the pelvis. *Surg Gynecol Obstet* 1976;143:597–601
281. Miller FJ Jr, Mortel R, Mann WJ, Jahshan AE: Selective arterial embolization for control of hemorrhage in pelvic malignancy: femoral and brachial catheter approaches. *AJR* 1976;126:1028–1032
282. Athanasoulis CA, Waltman AC, Barnes AB, Herbst AL: Angiographic control of pelvic bleeding from treated carcinoma of the cervix. *Gynec Oncol* 1976;4:144–150
283. Higgins CB, Bookstein JJ, Davis GB, Galloway DC, Barr JW: Therapeutic embolization for intractable chronic bleeding. *Radiology* 1977;122:473
284. Pisco JM, Martins JM, Correia MG: Internal iliac artery: embolization to control hemorrhage from pelvic neoplasms. *Radiology* 1989;172:337–339
285. Mitchell ME, Waltman AC, Athanasoulis CA, Kerr WS Jr, Dretler SP: Control of massive prostatic bleeding with angiographic techniques. *J Urol* 1976;115:692–695

286. Feldman F, Casarella WJ, Dick HM, Hollander BA: Selective intra-arterial embolization of bone tumors: a useful adjunct in the management of selected lesions. *AJR* 1975;123:130–139

287. Hilal SK, Michelsen JW: Therapeutic percutaneous embolization for extra-axial vascular lesions of the head, neck and spine. *J Neurosurg* 1975;43:275–287

288. Dick HM, Bigliani LU, Michelsen WJ, Johnston AD, Stinchfield FE: Adjuvant arterial embolization in the treatment of benign primary bone tumors in children. *Clin Orthop* 1979;139:133–144

289. Channon GM, Williams LA: Giant-cell tumour of the ischium treated by embolization and resection: a case report. *J Bone Joint Surg (Br)* 1982;64:164–165

290. Chuang VP, Wallace S, Swanson D, et al: Arterial occlusion in the management of pain from metastatic renal carcinoma. *Radiology* 1979;133:611–614

291. Keller FS, Rösch J, Bird CB: Percutaneous embolization of bony pelvic neoplasms with tissue adhesive. *Radiology* 1983;147:21–27

292. Rowe DM, Becker GJ, Rabe FE, et al: Osseous metastases from renal cell carcinoma: embolization and surgery for restoration of function. *Radiology* 1984;150:673–676

293. Wallace S, Granmayeh M, deSantos LA, et al: Arterial occlusion of pelvic bone tumors. *Cancer* 1979;43:322–328

294. Murphy WA, Strecker WB, Schoenecker PL: Transcatheter embolization therapy of an ischial aneurysmal bone cyst. *J Bone Joint Surg (Br)* 1982;64:166–168

295. Radanovic B, Simunic S, Stojanovic J, Orlic D, Potocki K, Oberman BB: Therapeutic embolization of aneurysmal bone cyst. *Cardiovasc Intervent Radiol* 1990;12:313–316

296. Suby-Long T, Bos GD, Rösch J: Biopsy proven eradication of an aneurysmal bone cyst treated by superselective embolization: a case report. *Cardiovasc Intervent Radiol* 1988;11:292–295

297. Cory DA, Fritsch SA, Cohen MD, Mail JT, Holden RW, Scott JA, DeRosa GP: Aneurysmal bone cysts: imaging findings and embolotherapy. *AJR* 1989;153:369–373

298. Chiang V, Soo C–S, Wallace S, Benjamin R: Arterial occlusion: management of giant-cell tumor and aneurysmal bone cyst. *AJR* 1981;136:1127–1130

299. Leather RP, Shah D, Goldman M, Rosenberg M, Karmody AM: Nonresective treatment of abdominal aortic aneuysms. *Arch Surg* 1979;114:1402–1408

300. Goldman ML, Sarrafizadeh MS, Philip PK, Karmody AM, Leather RP, Parikh N, Powers SR: Bucrylate embolization of abdominal aortic aneurysms: an adjunct to nonresective therapy. *AJR* 1980;135:1195–1200

301. Goldman ML: Bucrylate, silicones, and Ivalon as agents for intravascular embolization, in Abrams H (ed): *Angiography.* Boston, Little, Brown and Co., pp 191–220

302. Carrasco H, Parry CE: Transcatheter embolization of abdominal aortic aneurysms. *AJR* 1982;138:729–733

303. Rao VR, Mandalam RK, Joseph S, Satija V, Gupta VK, Gupta AK, Jain SK, Unni MN, Rao AS: Embolization of large saccular aneurysms with Gianturco coils. *Radiology* 1990;175:407–410

304. Mori H, Fukuda T, Ishida Y, Hayashi N, Hayashi K, Maeda H: Embolization of a thoracic aortic aneurysm: the straddling coil technique: technical note. *Cardiovasc Intervent Radiol* 1990;13:50–52

305. Fedullo LM, Meranze SG, McLean GK, Burke DR: Embolization of a subclavian artery aneurysm with steel coils and thrombin. *Cardiovasc Intervent Radiol* 1987;10:34–137

306. Lammert GK, Merine D, White RI Jr, Fishman EK, Porterfield JK: Embolotherapy of a high-flow false aneurysm by using an occlusion balloon, thrombin, steel coils, and a detachable balloon. *AJR* 1989;152:382–384

307. Hall CL, Cumber P, Higgs CM, Chalmers AH: Life threatening hemorrhage from a mycotic renal pseudoaneurysm treated by segmental renal artery embolization. *Br Med J* 1987;294(6586):1526

308. Uflacker R: Transcatheter embolization of arterial aneurysms. *Br J Radiology* 1986;59:317–324

309. Rosen RJ, Rothberg M: Transhepatic embolization of hepatic artery pseudoaneurysm following biliary drainage. *Radiology* 1982;145:532–533

310. Uflacker R, Mourao GS, Piske RL, Souza VC, Lima S: Hemobilia: transcatheter occlusive therapy and long-term follow-up. *Cardiovasc Intervent Radiol* 1989;12:136–141

311. Teich S, Tsangaris N, Giordano J, Druy E: Mycotic aneurysm of the inferior pancreaticoduodenal artery: successful nonoperative management. *South Med J* 1989;82(2):267–269

312. Cope C, Zeit R: Coagulation of aneurysms by direct percutaneous thrombin injection. *AJR* 1986;147:383–387

313. Glanz S, Gordon D, Selafani JA: Percutaneous coil embolization in the management of peripheral mycotic aneurysms. *Cardiovasc Intervent Radiol* 1987;10:198–201

314. Sharma RP, Shetty PC, Burke TH, Shepard AD, Khaja F: Treatment of false aneurysm by using a detachable balloon. *AJR* 1987;149:1279–1280

315. Walker TG, Geller SC, Brewster DC: Transcatheter occlusion of a profunda femoral artery pseudoaneurysm using thrombin. *AJR* 1987;149:185–186

316. Kadir S, Athanasoulis CA, Ring EJ, Greenfield A: Transcatheter embolization of intrahepatic arterial aneurysms. *Radiology* 1980;134:335–339

317. Rothbarth LJ, Redmond PL, Kumpe DA: Percutaneous transhepatic treatment of a large intrahepatic aneurysm. *AJR* 1989;153:1077–1078

318. Swan HJC, Ganz W, Forrester J, Marcus H, Diamond G, Chonette D: Catheterization of heart in man using a flow directed balloon tipped catheter. *N Engl J Med* 1970;283:447–451

319. Shah KB, Rao TLK, Laughlin S, El-Etr AA: A review of pulmonary artery catheterization in 6245 patients. *Anesthesiology* 1984;61:271–275

320. McDaniel DD, Stone JG, Faltas AN, et al: Catheter-induced pulmonary artery hemorrhage: diagnosis and management in cardiac operations. *J Thorac Cardiovasc Surg* 1981;82:1–4

321. Kelly TF Jr, Morris GC Jr, Crawford ES, Espada R, Howell JF: Perforation of the pulmonary artery with Swan–Ganz catheters: diagnosis and surgical management. *Ann Surg* 1981;193:686–692

322. Paulson DM, Scott SM, Sethi GK: Pulmonary hemorrhage associated with balloon flotation catheters: report of a case and review of the literature. *J Thorac Cardiovasc Surg* 1980;80:453–458

323. Klibaner MI, Hayes JA, Dobnick D, McCormick JR: Delayed fatal pulmonary hemorrhage complicating use of a balloon flotation catheter. *Angiology* 1985;36:358–362

324. Barash PG, Nardi D, Hammond G, et al: Catheter-induced pulmonary artery perforation: mechanisms, management and modifications. *J Thorac Cardiovasc Surg* 1981;82:5–12

325. Carlson A, Hilley HD, Meuten DJ, et al: Catheter-induced delayed recurrent pulmonary artery hemorrhage. *JAMA* 1989;261(13):393–397.

326. Hardy JF, Morissette M, Taillefer J: Pathophysiology of rupture of the pulmonary artery by pulmonary artery balloon-tipped catheters. *Anesth Analg* 1983;62:925–930

327. Hannan AT, Borwn M, Bigman O: Pulmonary artery catheter-induced hemorrhage. *Chest* 1984;85:128–131

328. Stein JM, Lisbon A: Pulmonary hemorrhage from pulmo-

nary artery catheterization treated with endobronchial intubation. *Anesthesiology* 1981;55:698–699

329. Scuderi PE, Prough DS, Price JD, Comer PB: Cessation of pulmonary artery catheter-induced endobronchial hemorrhage associated with the use of PEEP. *Anesth Analg* 1983;62:236–238

330. Stone JG, Faltas AN, Khambatta HJ, Hyman AI, Malm JR: Temporary unilateral pulmonary artery occlusion: a method for controlling Swan–Ganz catheter-induced hemoptysis. *Ann Thorac Surg* 1984;37:508–510

331. Davis SD, Neithamer CD, Schreiber TS, Sos TA: False pulmonary artery aneurysm induced by Swan–Ganz catheter: diagnosis and embolotherapy. *Radiology* 1987;164:741–742

332. Dieden JD, Friloux LA III, Renner JW: Pulmonary artery false aneurysm secondary to Swan–Ganz pulmonary artery catheters. *AJR* 1987;149:901–906

333. Carlson TA, Goldenberg IF, Murray PD, Tadavarthy SM, Walker M, Gobel FL: Catheter-induced delayed recurrent pulmonary artery hemorrhage. *JAMA* 1989;261(13):1943–1947

Part 2. Nonsurgical Cure of Varicocele by Transcatheter Embolization of the Internal Spermatic Vein(s) with a Tissue Adhesive (Histoacryl Transparent)

—Marc Kunnen M.D., Ph.D., and Frank Comhaire, M.D., Ph.D.

Varicocele is the most common detectable cause of male infertility. It is caused by a disturbance of the efflux of venous blood from the testicle(s) due to inversion of blood flow in the internal spermatic vein(s). Impairment of testicular and epididymal function probably results from countercurrent exchange of noradrenaline from the refluxing venous blood into the testicular arterial blood, at the level of the pampiniform plexus. The latter causes chronic vasoconstriction of the intratesticular arterioles and decreased tissue perfusion with degeneration of the Sertoli cells and, finally, decreased production of spermatozoa.[1]

Varicoceles may cause local discomfort and are associated with prostatovesiculitis as well as sexual inadequacy. Although Ahlberg et al.[2] showed in 1966 that varicoceles could be detected by retrograde phlebography, this technique was rarely used, whereas many investigators performed ascending phlebography during varicocelectomy.[3,4]

In 1976, the authors described a method for selective venography of the internal spermatic vein(s),[5,6] which was claimed to be safe and suitable for routine use. At present, this method is in practice throughout the world.

In 1979, Kunnen developed a new method for nonsurgical cure of varicocele disease, namely, transcatheter embolization with the tissue adhesive isobutyl 2-cyanocrylate (IBCA, Bucrylate from Ethicon/Somerville).[7-10] As Bucrylate was withdrawn from the market in 1985, Kunnen replaced it successfully by *n*-butyl cyanoacrylate (NBCA), Histoacryl Transparent (Braun-Melsungen, Germany). To date, more than 900 patients have been treated with this technique. The procedure will be described and the results presented.

GENERAL INFORMATION

Diagnostic Venography

The catheterization is performed from the right groin under local anesthesia and according to a strict protocol, using coaxial catheters exclusively. Diagnostic venography should always precede the therapeutic procedure.

One starts with the cobra catheter, which is the outer part of the Kunnen Left Spermatic Set (No. 833010, Meadox-Surgimed, Denmark) (Fig. 2.2.1*A*). At first, the right renal and internal spermatic veins are examined. The right renal vein is catheterized, probing the segmentary veins with a J-tipped 0.038-inch guidewire with a movable core. The venogram has to show the segmentary veins clearly. Connecting collaterals to the spermatic vein or a direct connection between the renal and the spermatic veins (Figs. 2.2.3 and 2.2.4) have to be searched for. If these are not found, and if the outlet of the right internal spermatic vein is not easily catheterized from the inferior caval vein, or if it shows a competent valve, the right-sided venography is regarded as negative.

Right-sided venography is positive in 30% of the patients presenting with a left-sided varicocele.

The catheter is placed in the left renal vein and probing is done with a J-tipped 0.038-inch guidewire. The renal venogram has to show the renal segmental veins (Fig. 2.2.5*A*), together with the presence or absence of perirenal collaterals (Fig. 2.2.6), as well as the competence of (Fig. 2.2.7*A*) or insufficiency (Fig. 2.2.6*A*) of the venous valve at the outlet of the left internal spermatic vein.

If the left renal venography is positive; i.e., retrograde

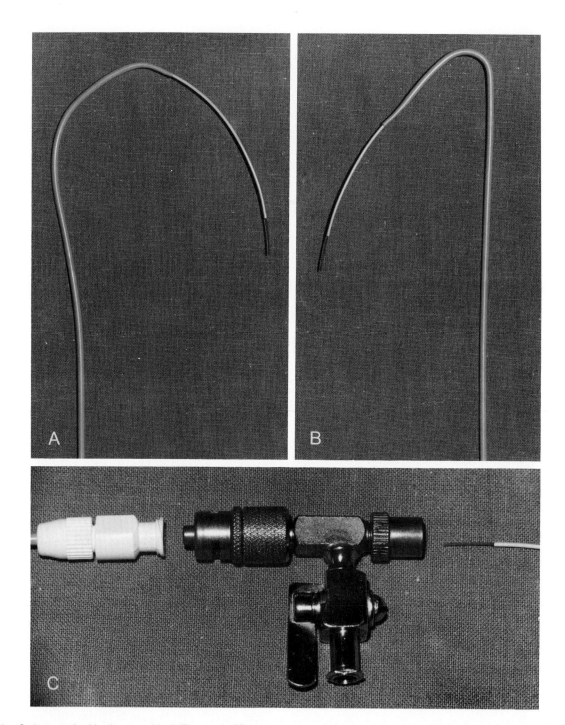

Figure 2.2.1. Catheter and guidewire assembly. **A.** The coaxial 3Fr inner catheter fitted with a small guidewire is advanced through the 7Fr cobra catheter. **B.** The coaxial inner catheter fitted with a small guidewire is advanced through the 7Fr hooked catheter. **C.** T-adapter (Cook sidearm design, catalog no. SOWS-PCF-MLL-RA-TO) for moistening catheters with 5% glucose.

opacification of the left spermatic vein is seen, this vein should be catheterized coaxially, opacified superselectively, and embolized with NBCA. The occlusion should be monitored by means of a follow-up selective spermatic venogram.

If the right-sided venography is positive, the cobra catheter is exchanged for a hooked catheter—outer part of the Kunnen Right Spermatic Set (No. 833015, Meadox-Sur-

gimed, Denmark) (Fig. 2.2.1B)—for easier coaxial catheterization of the right internal spermatic vein. Superselective venography of the right internal spermatic vein, followed by embolization with NBCA and follow-up selective venography to monitor the occlusion, are the final steps of the procedure.

It should be noted that the pre-embolization venography must be carried out carefully in order to demonstrate

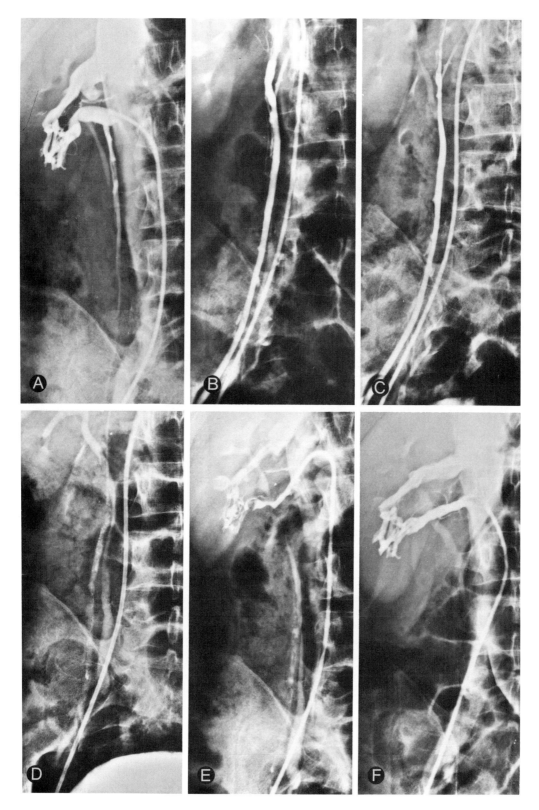

Figure 2.2.2.   Typical embolization procedure in the right internal spermatic vein with the right spermatic set. **A.** Diagnostic venography with injection into the caudal segment of the right renal vein using a cobra catheter. Right internal spermatic vein is connected directly with the renal vein and displays pathologic reflux. **B.** After examination (and possibly embolization) of the left side with the cobra catheter, the hooked catheter is introduced into the orifice of the right spermatic vein, and a selective venography is performed. **C.** The coaxial catheter is introduced into the spermatic vein through the outer hooked catheter. Superselective venography reveals valves of connecting vessels and bifurcation at the level of the sacroiliac joint. **D.** X-ray picture taken during injection of embolus above the bifurcation. **E.** Follow-up renal venogram 10 minutes after embolization shows no reflux. **F.** Control renal venogram 15 months after embolization shows integrity of renal veins and absence of reflux. The embolus is no longer visible.

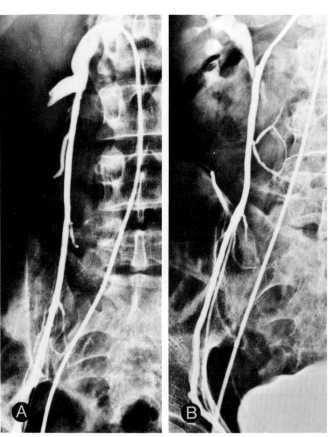
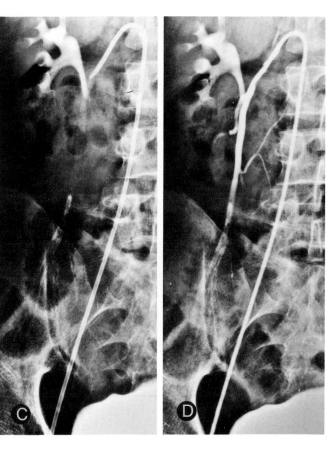

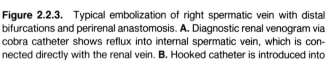

Figure 2.2.3. Typical embolization of right spermatic vein with distal bifurcations and perirenal anastomosis. **A.** Diagnostic renal venogram via cobra catheter shows reflux into internal spermatic vein, which is connected directly with the renal vein. **B.** Hooked catheter is introduced into the spermatic vein; top of coaxial catheter is located at the junction of the perirenal anastomosis with bifurcated distal branches. **C.** NBCA embolus opacified with Lipiodol Ultrafluoride. **D.** Selective control venogram demonstrating total occlusion.

not only the retrograde filling of the internal spermatic vein(s), but also all the accompanying, connecting, or collateral veins. Superselective venography by means of the small, straight coaxial catheter yields more precise information on the most suitable site for embolization.

Also, if one fails to obtain a good venogram of the right renal vein when using the cobra catheter, the examination should be interrupted on this side; the procedure is continued on the left side, and after exchange of catheters the right venography is repeated using the hooked catheter. This, however, rarely occurs.

Superselective Coaxial Catheterization and Embolization

The outer cobra-shaped catheter (for the left side; Fig. 2.2.6) or the hooked catheter (for the right side; Fig. 2.2.2) is placed in the orifice of the internal spermatic vein. The thin inner catheter, fitted with the small (0.021 inch) guidewire included in the left spermatic set, is pushed through the outer catheter to enter the spermatic vein. The catheters are moistened with 5% glucose through a T-adapter (Fig. 2.2.1).

Under fluoroscopic control, the tip of the catheter is

brought to the exact site selected for embolization. This site should be inferior to the lowermost anastomosis between the spermatic vein and the (peri)renal venous plexus and preferably superior to any bifurcations (Fig. 2.2.6C). The catheter moves more easily when the patient coughs. The guidewire is removed, and the exact location of the catheter is determined by injecting nonionic Omnipaque 240 (iohexol, 240mg of iodine/ml). The patient is examined on a remote-controlled tilting table, with 2°–10° anti- Trendelenburg, in order to stop the circulation in the internal spermatic vein completely. The latter is controlled by injecting a small bolus of contrast medium (Fig. 2.2.6D). This procedure is extremely important because it excludes accidental thrombosis of the renal vein as well as injection into the pampiniform plexus.

A tuberculin syringe is filled with 1ml of 10% glucose and connected to the plastic three-way stopcock of the embolization catheter, which is filled with 5% glucose (Fig. 2.2.8A,B). The glucose solution slows down the polymerization of the tissue adhesive. In a second syringe, 0.2–0.3ml of Lipiodol Ultrafluide is mixed with 0.4–0.6ml of NBCA (Histoacryl Transparent), just prior to the embolization (Histoacryl Blue should be avoided, as it polymerizes much too rapidly). One should never use more than one

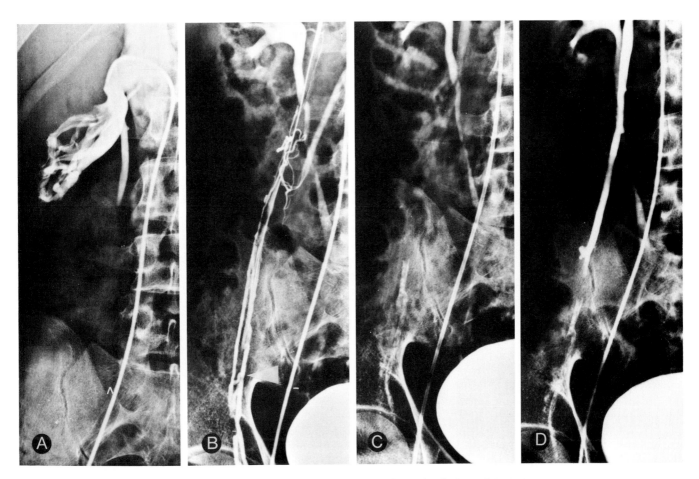

Figure 2.2.4. Embolization of right spermatic vein with bifurcated vessels in distal segments. **A.** Diagnostic renal venogram via cobra catheter shows slight reflux into the internal spermatic vein, which is connected directly to the renal vein. **B.** Via hooked outer catheter placed at the orifice of the spermatic vein, the coaxial catheter is placed into the medial bifur-cated vessel at the level of the distal connection with a contralateral vein *(arrowhead)*. **C.** Embolic agent is seen in both vessels. **D.** Control selective venogram reveals total occlusion and anastomosis with perirenal venous plexus superior to the embolus.

ampule (0.6 ml) of NBCA. The contrast medium is used not only to delineate the nonopaque bolus of NBCA on the TV monitor and the x-ray films, but also to slow down the polymerization; once the NBCA is in contact with the Lipiodol, one must proceed quickly. The second syringe with the embolus is connected to the stopcock (Fig. 2.2.8*C*), and the embolic material is injected into the coaxial catheter (Fig. 2.2.8*D*) and flushed into the spermatic vein with the contents of the first syringe; i.e., 0.5ml of 10% glucose from the first syringe is injected in order to flush the embolic material completely into the spermatic vein (Fig. 2.2.8*E*). The coaxial embolization catheter is immediately pulled back 2–3cm, and the remaining 0.5ml of 10% glucose from the first syringe is injected to remove all NBCA from this catheter (Fig. 2.2.8*F*).

The inner catheter is withdrawn from the outer one, which is pulled back into the vena cava, where blood is aspirated (Fig. 2.2.6*E*). If it is not possible to aspirate blood, the caval wall may adhere to the tip of the catheter; this can be avoided by placing the tip of the catheter in the left common iliac vein.

Whenever aspiration of blood remains impossible,

occlusion of the outer catheter by a residue of NBCA should be suspected, and the outer catheter should be withdrawn and replaced by a new outer catheter. (In these rare cases, one can cut the external part of the catheter obliquely, introduce a 7Fr sheath over it, and withdraw and replace the catheter by the new one fitted with an 0.038-inch guidewire.)

As soon as the tissue adhesive comes in contact with blood, it polymerizes to form a permanent occlusion. The embolus is seen on the x-ray pictures (Figs. 2.2.6*E–G* and 2.2.2*D,E*). A follow-up venogram is performed ten minutes postembolization through the outer catheter. First, the renal vein is injected without a Valsalva maneuver in order to check its integrity. The renal vein is then injected during a Valsalva maneuver (Figs. 2.2.6*F* and 2.2.2*E*), and finally the thrombosed spermatic vein is selectively opacified (Fig. 2.2.6*G*) to confirm the absence of residual reflux.

During the whole procedure, 5% glucose is used as a moistening and rinsing solution. Physiologic saline is absolutely *contraindicated*, because it will cause premature polymerization of the NBCA.

Never try to perform more than one embolization through the

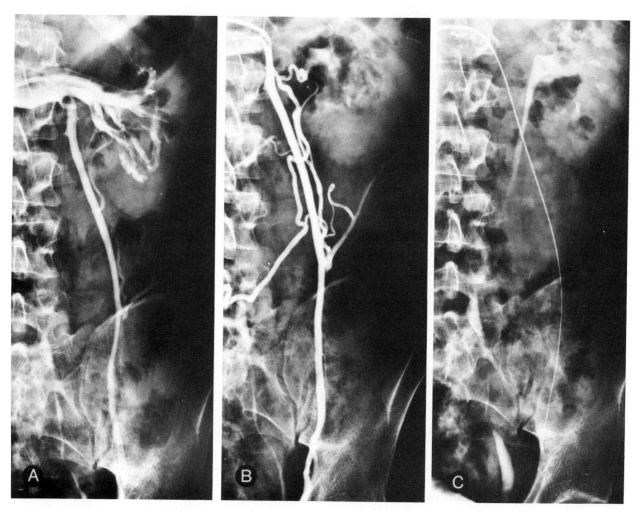

Figure 2.2.5.   Typical embolization at the level of the lowest anastomosis between perirenal plexus and left spermatic vein. **A.** Reflux in left spermatic vein during injection of contrast medium into renal vein. Some connecting vessels are visible. **B.** Selective spermatic venogram shows these vessels better. **C.** The coaxial catheter fitted with the guidewire is introduced into the spermatic vein. **D.** Superselective injection of small amount of contrast medium at the level of the lowest anastomosis shows the different branches and also the caudal lateral accompanying vein, which were not clearly seen on selective venograms. **E.** Since flow of contrast is evident through the tortuous cranial collateral, remote-controlled table has to be tilted a few more degrees upward, in order to stop the blood flow in the spermatic venous system completely. **F.** The embolic agent enters all vessels, but only for a few centimeters. **G.** No blood could be aspirated through the cobra catheter when pulled back to the vena cava because the caval wall adhered to the tip of the catheter. The catheter is therefore pulled back into the left iliac vein, and blood is aspirated. The catheter may be used for follow-up venograms. **H.** Follow-up renal venogram during Valsalva maneuver ten minutes after embolization; slight filling of spermatic vein. **I.** Selective follow-up venogram shows total occlusion of the spermatic venous system.

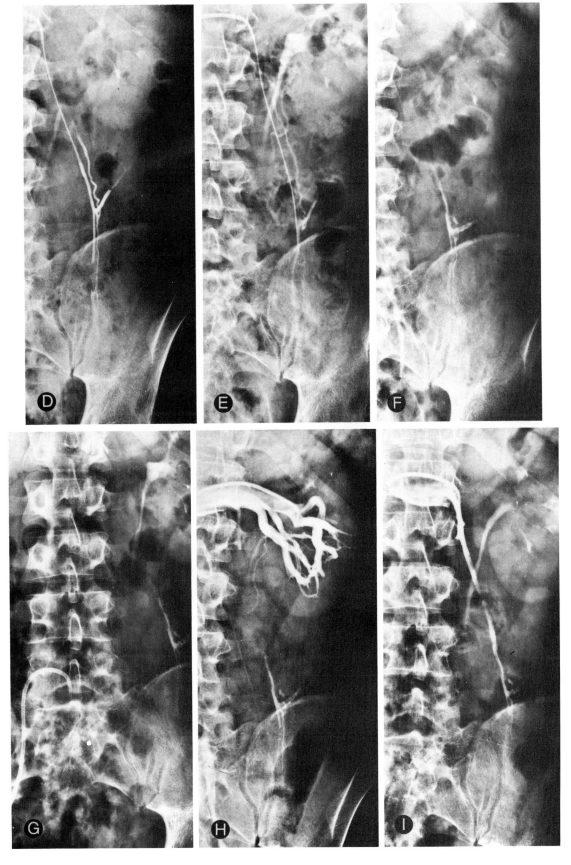

Figure 2.2.5 (D–I).

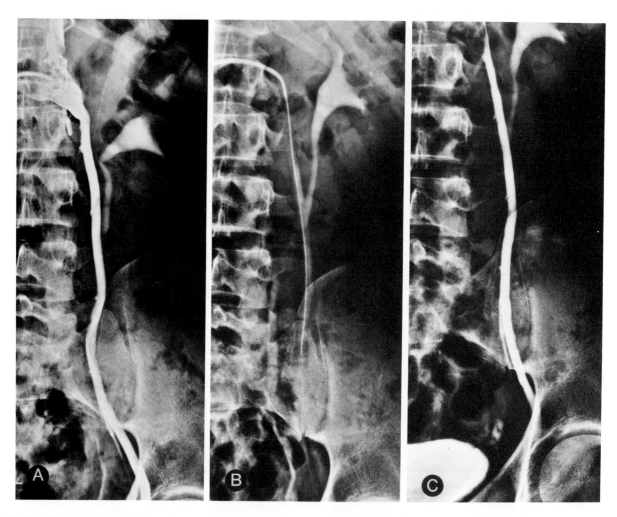

Figure 2.2.6. Typical embolization procedure in left internal spermatic vein with the left spermatic set. **A.** Selective venogram with cobra catheter in the outlet. The vessel presents a bifurcation at the level of the sacroiliac joint. **B.** The thin inner catheter fitted with 0.021-inch guidewire is advanced through the outer catheter into spermatic vein. **C.** Superselective venography through the thin catheter clearly defines the anatomic details. Note the bifurcation and competent valves of connecting vessels. The exact site for embolization is selected just superior to the bifurcation. **D.** Tip of the thin catheter is placed at the embolization site, the guidewire is removed, and the exact location is monitored by injecting small quanti-

ties of Omnipaque 240. The tilting table is moved so as to stop the blood flow in the spermatic vein completely. **E.** After the tissue adhesive is injected, the inner catheter is immediately withdrawn, and the outer catheter is pulled back into the vena cava. Blood is aspirated to assure absence of adhesive in the cobra catheter lumen. The embolus is clearly visible at the level of the left sacroiliac joint. **F.** Ten minutes later, control venogram is performed with the cobra catheter; renal vein injection during Valsalva maneuver shows incomplete filling of the spermatic vein. **G.** Selective spermatic venogram during Valsalva maneuver confirms complete occlusion.

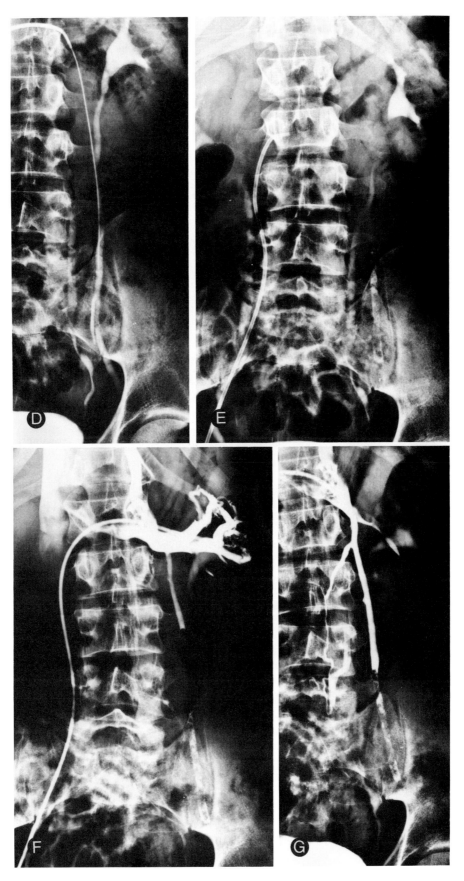

Figure 2.2.6 (D–G).

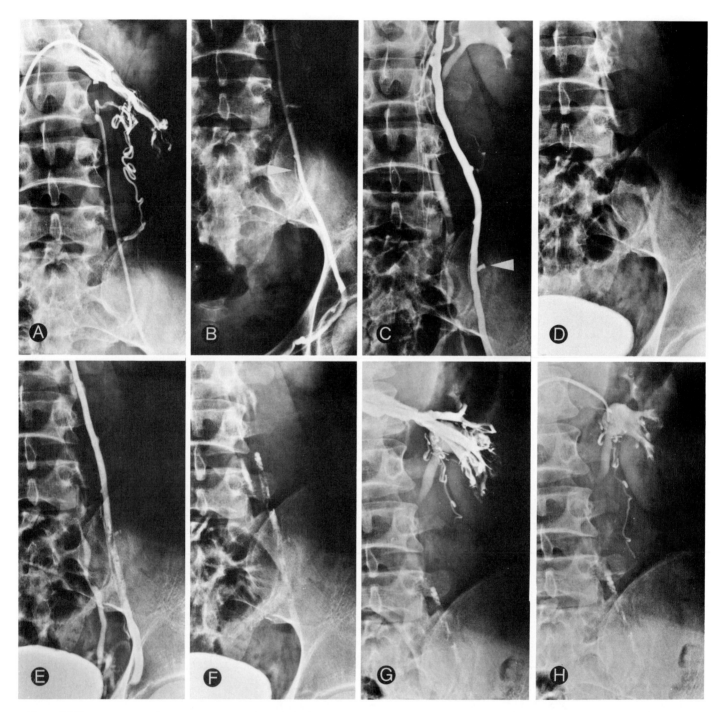

Figure 2.2.7. Association of competent outlet valve with bypassing peri-renal collaterals, compelling application of two emboli for anatomic reasons. **A,B.** Diagnostic renal venography shows competent spermatic outlet valve together with bypassing anastomosis. There is a distal bifurcation and a small medial branch (*arrowhead* in **B**). **C.** Superselective venography reveals connection of a low anastomosis at the level of the sacroiliac joint *(arrowhead)*. **D.** First embolus is placed at the level of the lower anastomosis. **E.** Superselective control venography shows that the medial bifurcated branch is not occluded. **F.** Use is made of a new 3Fr straight catheter, while the cobra catheter is reused. A second embolus is placed at the site of bifurcation (compare **D**). **G,H.** Control venography after complete embolization. Only one collateral is filled; the contrast medium is blocked at the level of the connection with the spermatic vein.

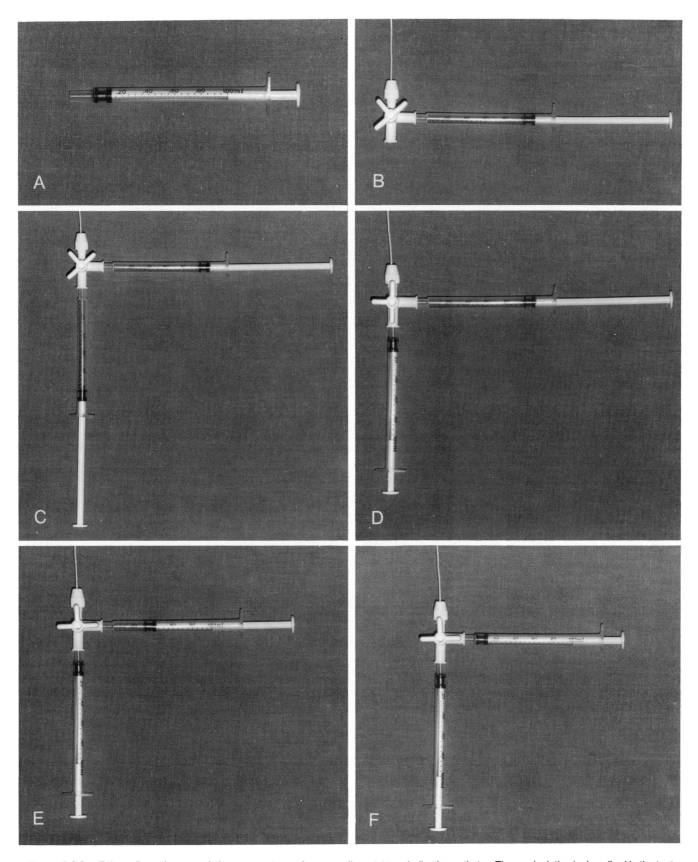

Figure 2.2.8. Tuberculin syringes and three-way stopcock on small straight embolization catheter. The manipulation is described in the text.

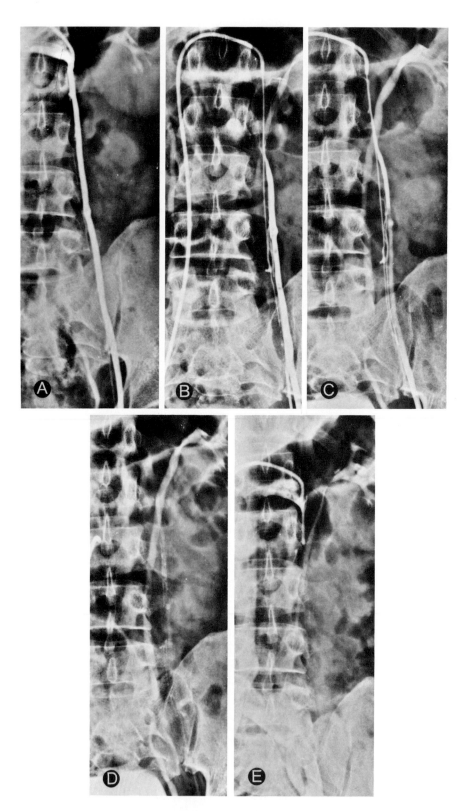

Figure 2.2.9. Embolization via small branch of bifurcation situated in the cranial segment with distal connections. **A.** Selective injection of incompetent spermatic vein with small medial collateral vein. **B.** Upon coaxial catheterization, the coaxial catheter enters the medial vein and reveals a bifurcation in the cranial segment. Connections to the principal vein are shown by superselective venography, which reveals a lateral valve at the level of L4, suggesting the presence of a renospermatic bypass. **C.** During further injection of contrast medium, definite runoff is shown and another distal accompanying vessel revealed. After the vessels have been cleared with 5% glucose, NBCA is injected, flushed by 1ml of 10% glucose. **D.** Embolus is clearly visible in the two small branches and in the principal vessel. **E.** Follow-up venogram shows complete occlusion with superior limit at the level of L2/3.

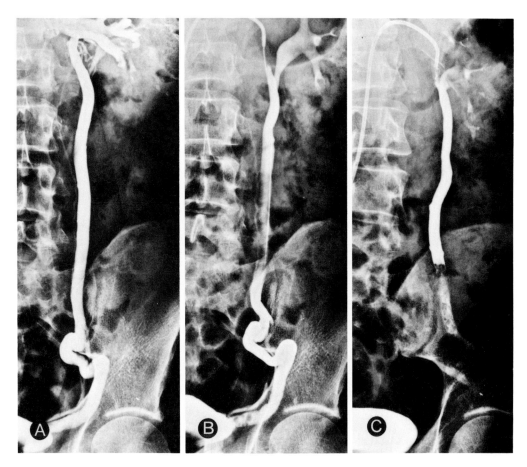

Figure 2.2.10. Embolization of large (9mm) left spermatic vein. **A.** Renal venography reveals massive reflux into the spermatic vein, which presents distal bifurcation as well as a small medial accompanying vein. **B.** Tip of coaxial catheter is just above bifurcation. Small medial accompanying vein is found to be connected to the main spermatic vein immedi- ately above the bifurcation. Embolus is concentrated on this spot. **C.** Follow-up selective venogram shows total occlusion. Embolus is clearly seen; it is large and rather short. Accompanying vein is blocked at its junction.

same inner catheter! However, the outer catheter can be used for a second embolization.

Examples of the Technique

In Figure 2.2.5, another example of a typical left spermatic venous embolization is shown. The embolus is placed at the level of the lowest anastomosis between the perirenal plexus and the spermatic vein (also called the renospermatic bypass). The liquid embolic agent enters the different connecting vessels and occludes them all in one procedure (Fig. 2.2.5*F*); this is one of the major advantages of the authors' technique over the methods in which detachable balloons or coils are used. On the other hand the embolus will never move further than a few centimeters, as NBCA polymerizes rapidly when it is in contact with blood. Hence, there is no danger of damaging surrounding tissues, unlike the situation when large amounts of sclerosing agents are used (sclerotherapy).

In Figure 2.2.3, an embolization is shown in a patient with bifurcations of the caudal part of the right internal spermatic vein together with an anastomosis with the peri- renal plexus. The NBCA embolus is located at the junction of these vessels, near the level of the right sacroiliac joint. Figure 2.2.4 demonstrates how several distal branches are occluded with a single embolus, which is injected at the site of their distal connections.

If the spermatic vein has high bifurcations but no renospermatic bypass, one can embolize the superior part of the vein. One must completely stop the spermatic circulation as usual by tilting the table and monitoring the circulation with small contrast injections. If, on the contrary, there is an anastomosis with the perirenal plexus, as suggested by the presence of a lateral valve (Fig. 2.2.9), embolization of the cranial segment is to be avoided. In this case, the embolization catheter did enter the small medial branch of the bifurcation. One can embolize via the small vessel, as shown here, and expect occlusion of the whole system by one embolus if contrast injections have revealed runoff through the connections. If there is no evident runoff, or if the catheter is located more than 10cm deep into such a small accompanying vein, the authors advise against using this procedure, because the catheter may be trapped in the embolic material.

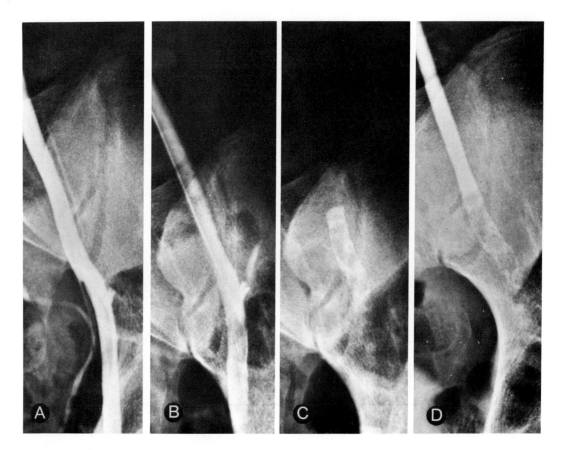

Figure 2.2.11. Embolization of large (8mm) left spermatic vein at level of its lowermost anastomosis with the perirenal plexus and at the level of the connection with the medial-caudal and lateral-superior accompanying veins. **A.** Selective venography shows medial-caudal and lateral-superior accompanying veins connected to the main spermatic vein at the level of the sacroiliac joint. (Projection may differ as a function of the position of the patient—erect or horizontal position—and the performance of Valsalva maneuver.) Slight filling of renal anastomosis. **B.** The embolization catheter is placed distal to the connection of this anastomosis, which is clearly visible now. **C.** Large and rather short "concentrated" embolus. **D.** Selective follow-up venogram demonstrates total occlusion of all vessels.

Large veins are also easily occluded, usually with one single embolization. A slightly different technique is used, in so far as the embolus is pushed into the vessel with the entire 1ml volume of 10% glucose in order to concentrate all the NBCA in one single spot. Figure 2.2.10 shows embolization of a left spermatic vein 9mm in diameter just above its distal bifurcation. Figure 2.2.11 shows the occlusion of an 8mm diameter vessel at the level of the lowermost renospermatic bypass and of the connections with medial-caudal and lateral-superior accompanying veins.

Procedures in More Complex Anatomic Conditions

PERIRENAL ANASTOMOSIS CONNECTED TO BIFURCATED DISTAL PART OF SPERMATIC VEIN

In the cases shown in Figures 2.2.12 and 2.2.13, the lateral branch of a bifurcated distal part of the spermatic vein is connected to the lowest perirenal anastomosis on a slightly lower level than the bifurcation. The embolization catheter must be placed in the lateral branch, and the embolus should be injected at the site of the perirenal anas-

tomosis. Usually, the embolic agent will reflux into the bifurcation after the initially injected embolic agent begins to polymerize in the collateral vessel, and it will occlude all the branches and anastomoses. In the majority of cases, this can be achieved with the use of the straight guidewire of the spermatic set. If this procedure is unsuccessful, one should exchange the wire for a steerable J-wire manufactured for coronary angioplasty (Fig. 2.2.14), which is useful in negotiating eccentric connections and in selectively entering small branches. The flexible J-tip can be steered by rotating the guidewire around its axis. As shown in Figure 2.2.13, one can even reach the perirenal anastomosis itself.

If one were to occlude only the medial vein, the varicocele would persist as a result of the bypassing anastomosis and the lateral branch. The latter would now be unreachable for nonsurgical cure! If, after embolization of the lateral vein, the medial one would not be occluded, one has only to inject a second bolus of embolic agent. This will always be the case if the distance between the bifurcation and the renospermatic bypass is important (Fig. 2.2.7).

The authors stress that one should always first embolize

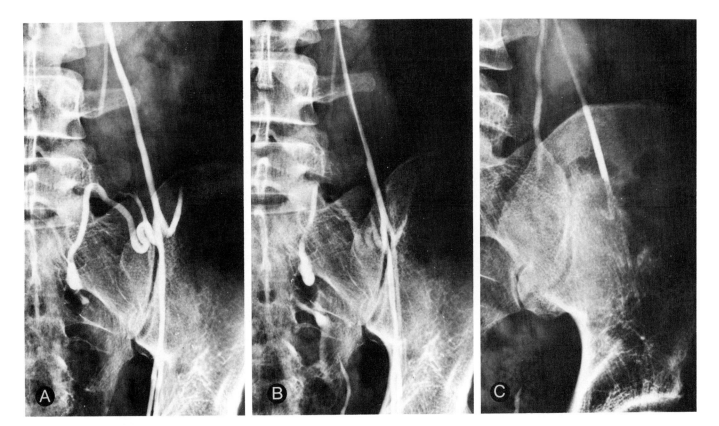

Figure 2.2.12. Embolization of bifurcated left spermatic vein with a perirenal anastomosis connected to the lateral branch. **A.** Selective spermatic venography shows medial collateral and renospermatic bypass. A bifurcation can be suspected. **B.** Coaxial catheterization of lateral branch of bifurcation shows that this branch is connected with the renospermatic bypass. Embolization is performed at the level of this connection. **C.** Follow-up venogram shows embolus in the different vessels; occlusion is complete.

the more distal connections and be aware of the fact that it is easy to put a second embolus higher up when necessary, whereas once a particular vessel is embolized, it is impossible to reach the more distal parts.

Perirenal anastomoses can never be coaxially catheterized in the caudal direction but only in the cranial direction from the spermatic vein.

REFLUX THROUGH BYPASSING COLLATERAL IN CASES WITH COMPETENT OUTLET VALVES

In a relatively large proportion of patients with a varicocele (in the authors' series, more than 30%), renal venography reveals one or even several competent valves in the cranial part of the internal spermatic vein. However, reflux occurs through one or more bypassing renospermatic anastomoses. It is clear that these patients can be treated nonsurgically only if the spermatic vein is occluded distal to these renospermatic bypasses. The correct site for embolization can be reached only after catheterization through the competent valves. With the authors' coaxial technique, they generally succeed in passing these valves, which is another advantage of this procedure. Usually, they place the appropriate catheter in, or just above, the competent outlet valve and pass the valve with the guidewire reaching slightly out of the thin catheter, just as in cases

without outlet valves. The trick consists of bringing the patient to a Trendelenburg position, which opens the valves as blood effluxes. If this procedure fails, the patient is asked to cough or to perform a Valsalva maneuver. Once the ideal site for embolization is reached, i.e., the distal part of the spermatic vein, they proceed as described above. The completeness of the occlusion is checked by a follow-up renal venogram, which should demonstrate lack of filling or the opacification of only the cranial part of the collaterals without further reflux.

In Figure 2.2.15, an example of this situation is demonstrated. The competent valves are clearly seen. They are bypassed by several short collaterals (Fig. 2.2.15B) and by long renospermatic anastomoses (Fig. 2.2.15B,C,E). The tip of the catheter is placed at the level of the sacroiliac joint, where the lower part of the embolus is injected (Fig. 2.2.15F). The embolus also fills the distal part of the renospermatic bypass. Upon control venography with injection of the renal vein, the collaterals are no longer filled (Fig. 2.2.15G). Moreover, the outlet valve remains competent (Fig. 2.2.15H).

In the case shown in Figure 2.2.16, the competent outlet valve is bypassed by a hooked medial collateral vessel. This collateral is used for selective venography before (Fig. 2.2.16C) and, again, after the embolization (Fig. 2.2.16F),

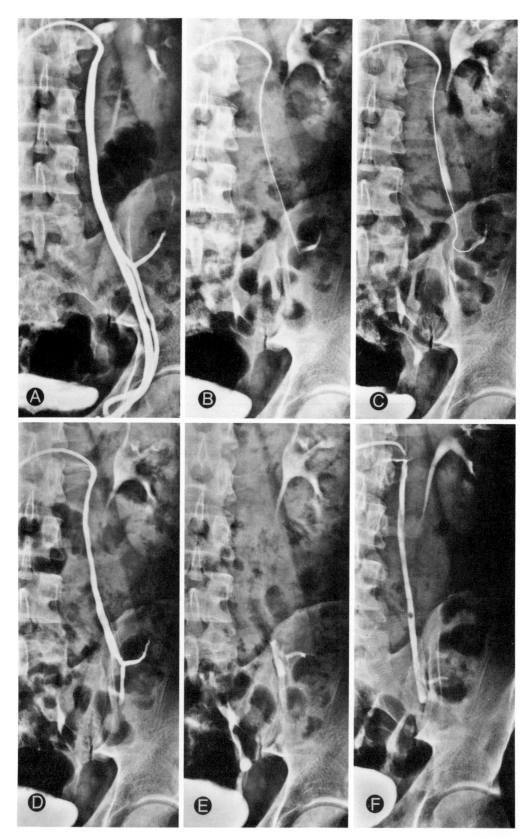

Figure 2.2.13. Use of steerable J-guidewire to reach perirenal anastomosis connected to the lateral branch of a bifurcated spermatic vein. **A.** Selective venography in incompetent spermatic vein which is bifurcated and shows renospermatic bypass connected to its lateral branch that ends below the level of the bifurcation. **B.** Coaxial catheterization. **C.** The J-wire is pushed into the anastomosis. **D.** Coaxial catheter is advanced into the anastomosis. **E.** Embolus fills part of branches, including the bypass. **F.** Follow-up selective venogram shows complete occlusion.

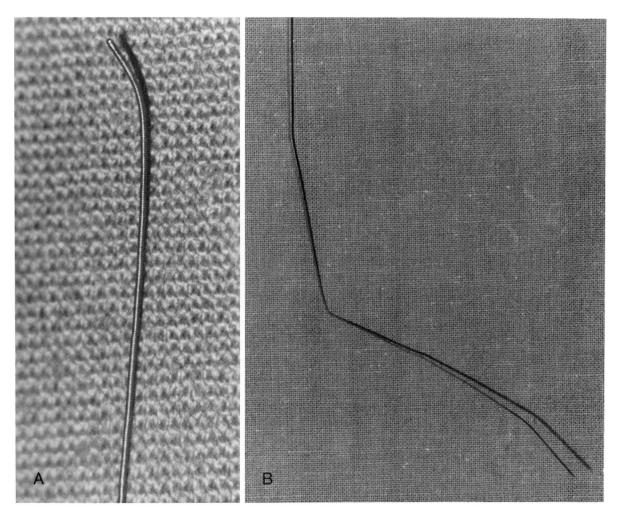

Figure 2.2.14. Steerable J-guidewire designed for coronary angioplasty. **A.** Direction of flexible J-tip can be steered by rotating the shaft (**B**) of guidewire around its axis.

whereas the competent valve is passed coaxially (Fig. 2.2.16D,E) to achieve the embolization. Also shown is the right side of the same patient (Fig. 2.2.16G–J). The right spermatic vein shows a typical outlet in the vena cava but, in addition, a direct communication with the right renal vein (Fig. 2.2.16G). The latter remained open (Fig. 2.2.16J) after embolization through the thin catheter, which was brought to the site via a cobra catheter passing through a small lateral accompanying vein (see the *arrow* in Fig. 2.2.16H). Control venography performed from the vena cava demonstrated total occlusion of the spermatic vein at the site selected for embolization (Fig. 2.2.16I).

In some cases, such as that illustrated in Figure 2.2.17, the upper part of the spermatic vein is very narrow. Nevertheless, it can be catheterized coaxially to permit embolization in the distal part of the spermatic system. In Figure 2.2.7, an association of a competent outlet valve and renospermatic bypasses is illustrated. Treatment consisted of two applications of NBCA for anatomic reasons.

An example is presented of the few cases with competent outlet valves and bypassing collaterals in which the

coaxial catheter could not be passed through the valve via a cobra catheter because the spermatic vein was situated too medially. By using a 7Fr catheter with a curve of 180° (F-curve; No. 833114, Meadox-Surgimed, Denmark; Fig. 2.2.18), the authors succeeded in catheterizing and embolizing this spermatic vein also (Fig. 2.2.19).

It should be admitted that, despite all of these procedures, the authors do not succeed in passing competent valves in a few cases. These are the only technical failures of this technique.

TREATMENT OF PERSISTENT VARICOCELES

Most varicoceles that persist after either surgical or nonsurgical treatment can be cured by coaxial embolization with NBCA.

Persistence after Surgery

According to Weissbach et al., the failure rate after surgical treatment of varicocele ranges from 0.2 to 25%.[11] The

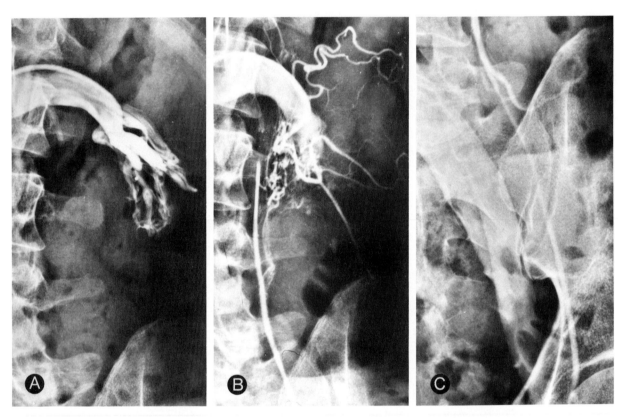

Figure 2.2.15. Embolization in a typical case with a competent valve at the level of the spermatic venous outlet, with evidence of reflux through a bypassing collateral. **A.** Diagnostic renal venography, early phase. Contrast outlines the proximal segment of the internal spermatic vein and is then stopped by a competent valve. **B.** Via several and tortuous collaterals, the distal, incompetent spermatic vein is filled. A long renospermatic bypass is also filled. **C.** Contrast medium in one of these anastomoses reaches the spermatic vein at the level of L4/5. **D.** The tip of the cobra catheter is placed above a competent valve. **E.** Competent valve is passed by coaxial catheter fitted with 0.021-inch guidewire. Superselective venography reveals a second renospermatic anastomosis, which is situated more caudally and is connected to the spermatic vein halfway to the level of the sacroiliac joint. This site must be included in the occlusion. **F.** Embolus is clearly visible; its lower limit occludes the distal anastomosis and its upper part occludes cranial one. **G.** Control renal venogram shows that the anastomoses no longer fill because they are occluded more distally. **H.** Selective spermatic venography shows a competent valve, which has not been damaged by the procedure.

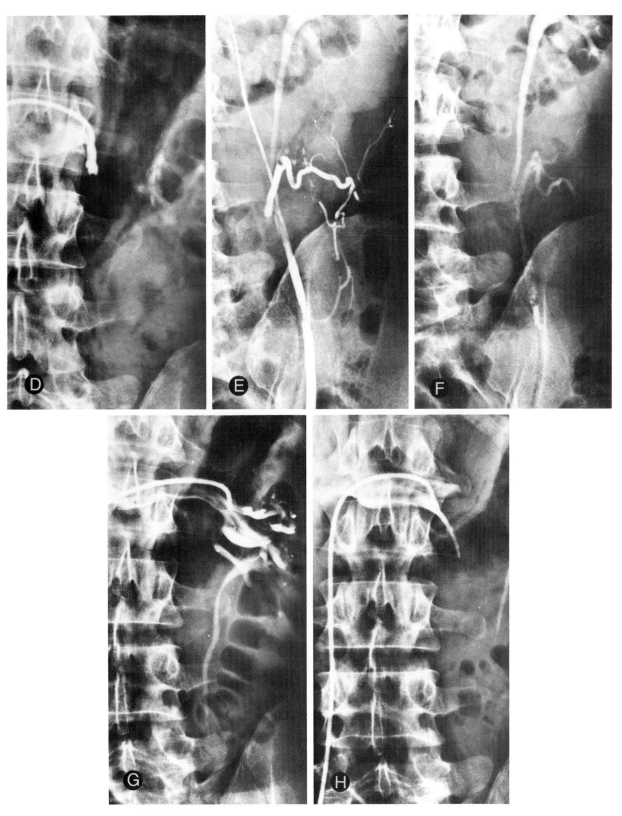

Figure 2.2.15 (D–H).

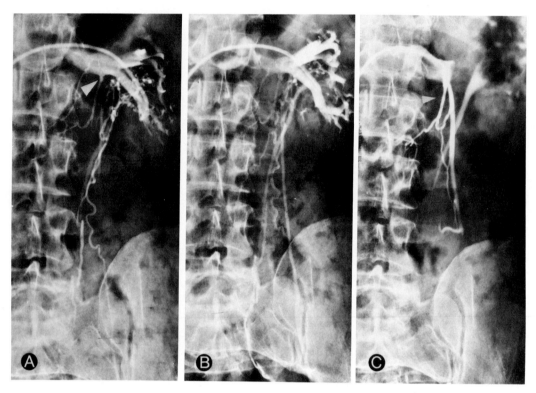

Figure 2.2.16. This patient presented with bilateral varicoceles with a competent valve and bypassing collaterals on the left side and an outlet to the vena cava as well as a direct connection to the renal vein on the right side. Bilateral embolization is performed with the left spermatic set (cobra catheter). On the *left,* the catheter was introduced through the competent valve; on the *right,* the catheter was introduced via the renal vein and a small collateral. **A.** Diagnostic left renal venography, early phase. Competent outlet valve *(arrowhead)* is bypassed by a medial collateral and by several short tortuous and one long renospermatic bypass. There is opacification of a small upper and a larger lower segment of the main spermatic vein. **B.** Same injection as in **A,** one second later. Outlet valve is more clearly visible. Main spermatic vein is almost completely opacified; only the upper 2cm are not visible. **C.** When the medial hooked bypass is injected *(arrowhead),* the upper part of the main vein and the renal vein are opacified. Accompanying veins are disclosed. **D.** Coaxial catheter is advanced through the competent outlet valve. **E.** Superselective venogram reveals additional branches and distal bifurcation. All vessels are connected at the level of the iliac crest. **F.** Follow-up venogram through the medial anastomosis reveals total occlusion after embolization at the level of the iliac crest. **G.** Right renal diagnostic angiography via cobra catheter. Right spermatic vein has two outlets, one into the vena cava and one into the renal vein; the communication stands out clearly. **H.** Superselective catheterization was performed with a left spermatic set passing from the renal vein through a small accompanying vein *(upper arrowhead).* Embolization must be performed at the site of cranial bifurcation *(lower arrowhead).* **I.** Control venogram with cobra catheter in caval outlet of right spermatic vein. Total occlusion is achieved at level of bifurcation. **J.** Control venogram with cobra catheter in renal outlet of right spermatic vein. As planned, these vessels are free of embolus.

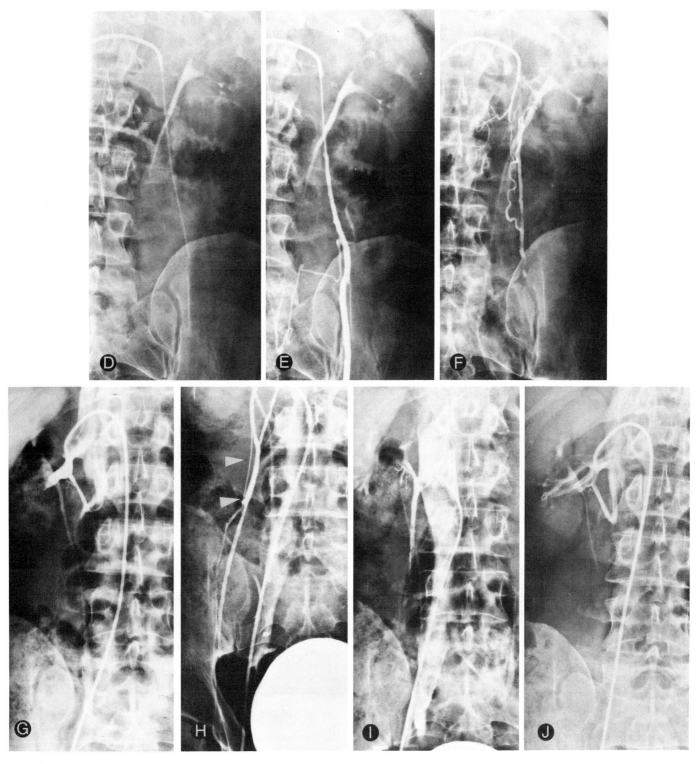

Figure 2.2.16 (D–J).

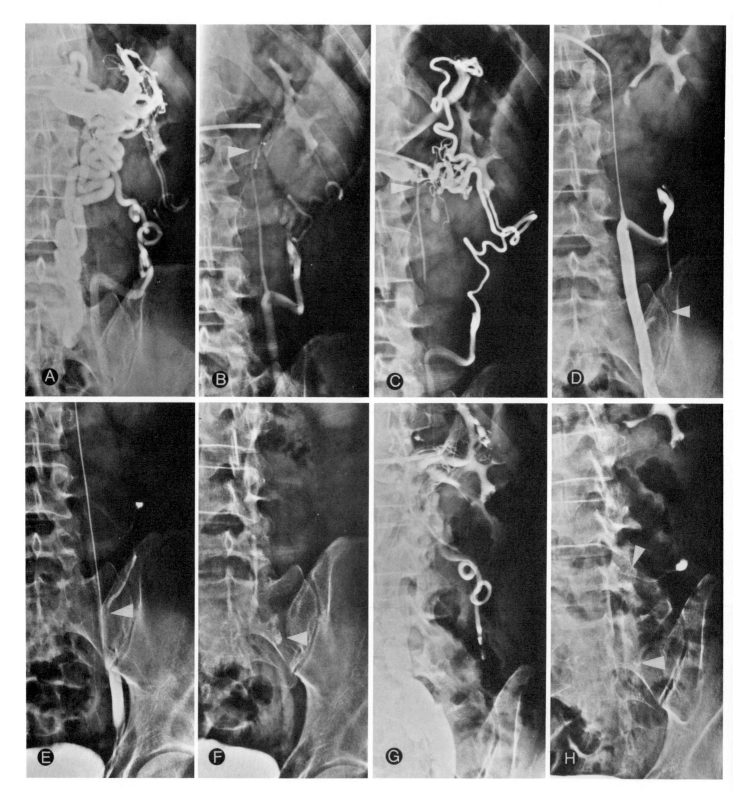

Figure 2.2.17. Association of competent outlet valve with hypoplastic cranial segment of spermatic vein and renospermatic anastomoses. **A.** Diagnostic renal venography. Large periureteral varices are of no importance for the varicocele, since they do not drain into the pampiniform plexus. Note presence of tortuous lateral perirenal anastomosis bypassing to large diameter distal segment of the spermatic vein. **B.** The hypoplastic upper segment of the spermatic vein opacifies in antegrade fashion; competent valve is indicated by the *arrowhead.* **C.** Selective injection of perirenal plexus clearly shows anastomosis but also reveals small anas-

tomosis just below a competent valve *(arrowhead).* **D.** Hypoplastic upper part of spermatic vein is passed coaxially. Superselective venography reveals an additional anastomosis ending at the level of the sacroiliac joint *(arrowhead).* **E.** Small injection shows tip of embolization catheter situated distal to lowest anastomosis *(arrowhead).* **F.** Lower limit of embolus *(arrowhead)* is distal to outlet of lower anastomosis. **G.** Control venography, injecting perirenal plexus (compare **C**). **H.** Anastomoses fill very slowly and are all occluded at their connection with spermatic vein *(arrowheads).*

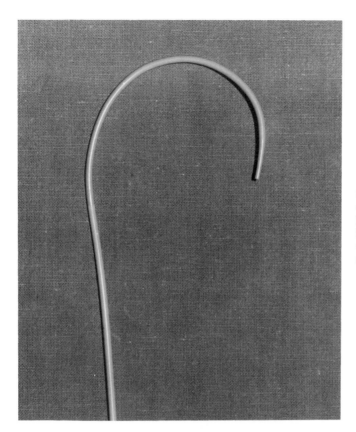

Figure 2.2.18. A 7Fr catheter with F-curve of 180° (Meadox–Surgimed, catalog no. 833114) used for coaxial catheterization of competent valves in cases where outlet of left spermatic vein is situated close to the vena cava.

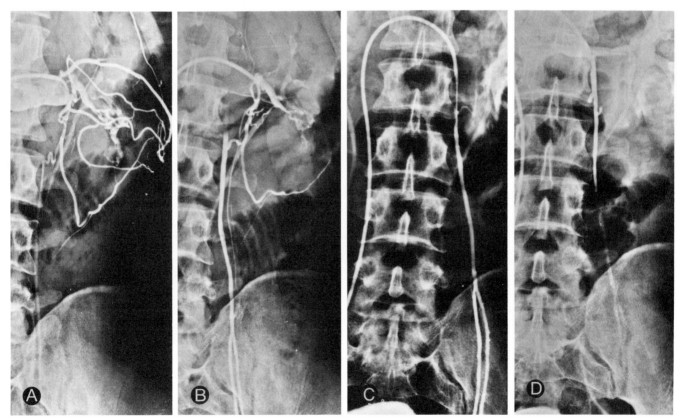

Figure 2.2.19. Coaxial catheterization and embolization using F-curve instead of cobra catheter in patient with competent outlet valve and medially situated left spermatic vein. **A.** Diagnostic venography, early phase. Perirenal anastomoses bypass to distal part of spermatic vein, which is incompetent. **B.** A few seconds later, distal bifurcation and cranial lateral accompanying branch are revealed. The competent outlet valve could not be passed because distance from vena cava to outlet of spermatic vein was too small and tip of cobra catheter cannot be properly seated ("streamlined") in the outlet valve. During each attempt to bypass the valve with the coaxial catheter, the cobra catheter recoiled. With F-curved catheter, 3Fr straight catheter, and 0.021-inch wire of the left spermatic set, a competent valve is passed rather easily. **C.** Superselective venography via F-curve and coaxial catheter. Embolization is performed at the junction of all the branches (iliac crest). **D.** Control venography via F-curve catheter shows total occlusion of spermatic venous system at level of L4/5.

95

persistence of varicoceles after ligation has stimulated the authors to examine such cases by selective venography and to treat them by embolization. In general, these patients had been operated on by a low ligation, and therefore the vessels could be catheterized and embolized according to the authors' standard procedure. It usually proved that one or more contributing vessels had not been ligated, and it was not uncommon to find no ligation at all. One patient presented with persistent bilateral varicoceles after bilateral surgery. He had competent outlet valves on both sides and bypassing perirenal anastomoses. His disease was cured by bilateral embolization.

Persistence after Coil Embolization

This problem commonly results from embolization performed in the cranial segment of the spermatic vein, leaving the accompanying veins or renospermatic anastomoses open. Moreover, coil-treated vessels may also remain open or become partly patent later.

The presence of coils may render distal coaxial catheterization of the spermatic vein and correct embolization with NBCA impossible. All these factors were noticed in a patient presenting with primary infertility due to persistent bilateral varicoceles. Two years previously, this patient had undergone operation on the left side. Because surgery was unsuccessful, he was subsequently treated on the same side by coil embolization at the level of L4. Because of the lack of improvement, two additional coils were placed at the level of L3 in a subsequent session. At the same time, an embolization with two coils was performed in the caval outlet of the right spermatic vein. All of this treatment remained ineffective, and the patient was referred to the authors for further treatment.

Upon right-sided renal venography, an insufficient branch of the right spermatic vein was detected, which connected to the higher segmental renal vein. Furthermore, selective venography showed a bifurcation of the distal spermatic vein. The coaxial catheter was advanced as caudally as possible until its tip was situated at the level of the sacroiliac joint. By means of superselective venography a renospermatic bypass was revealed. The blood flow was monitored by injecting a small amount of contrast medium which filled the different branches over a few centimeters. An embolus of NBCA was injected according to the authors' standard procedure. On follow-up renal venography, no further reflux in the spermatic system on the right side was found. The embolus reached from the sacroiliac joint almost as high as the coils. Left renal venography revealed a large renospermatic anastomosis connecting with the insufficient caudal part of the spermatic vein bypassing the coils (Fig. 2.2.20). In addition, the superiorly placed coils seemed to be unable to block the blood flow, whereas the inferior coil was located in a collateral branch (Fig. 2.2.20A–D). Unfortunately, the superior coils prevented passage of the tip of the coaxial guidewire, and a

fortiori, NBCA embolization of the distal spermatic vein was impossible. For this reason, the patient was operated on through a suprainguinal incision on the left side. Three months later, a successful pregnancy was reported.

Persistence after NBCA Embolization

FALSE PERSISTENCE

In the authors' first series of patients, they commonly embolized only the left side, rarely the right side. As a matter of fact, they experienced difficulties in catheterizing the right spermatic vein coaxially with the cobra catheter, because its tip struck the vessel wall at too steep an angle. As a result, they observed six patients with bilateral varicoceles who were embolized only in the left spermatic vein and presented with clinical persistence of left-sided varicocele. Upon follow-up venography, the occlusion was found to be complete on the left side and absolutely unchanged (Fig. 2.2.21). In all these cases, however, intrascrotal connections filled the left-sided varicocele from the right spermatic vein. Embolization of the right spermatic vein cured these patients.

The same situation was found in seven patients after left-sided surgical ligation.

TRUE PERSISTENCE

Of the 926 patients the authors have embolized to date, clinical persistence was observed in only 15 patients in whom a residual reflux was detected on the embolized side. In 14 of these, the embolized vessel was still occluded, but additional insufficient vessels were found that had not been detected at the initial venography. All but one of the patients with persistence were treated by repeat embolization. Since only three of these cases occurred among the 393 patients treated in the last five-year period, the authors concluded that superselective systematic venography has dramatically improved the results, with less than 1% true persistence.

The authors registered only one patient with true persistence where the embolized vessel was found to be patent upon follow-up venography. Repeat embolization of the same vessel cured the patient. Thus, persistence after NBCA embolization is rare and "recanalization" of the embolized vessel seems to be exceptional.

COMPLICATIONS AND TECHNICAL RESULTS

By using coaxial catheters and stopping the blood flow in the spermatic venous system, it is ensured that the embolic agent cannot reach the general circulation and that contact with the testicle will not occur. Pain, thrombophlebitis, or hydrocele did not occur in this series.

Only two complications have occurred. In one case, the coaxial catheter was not pulled back immediately, and after a few minutes, it was found to be trapped in the embolus. In a 12-year-old boy who had already been operated on

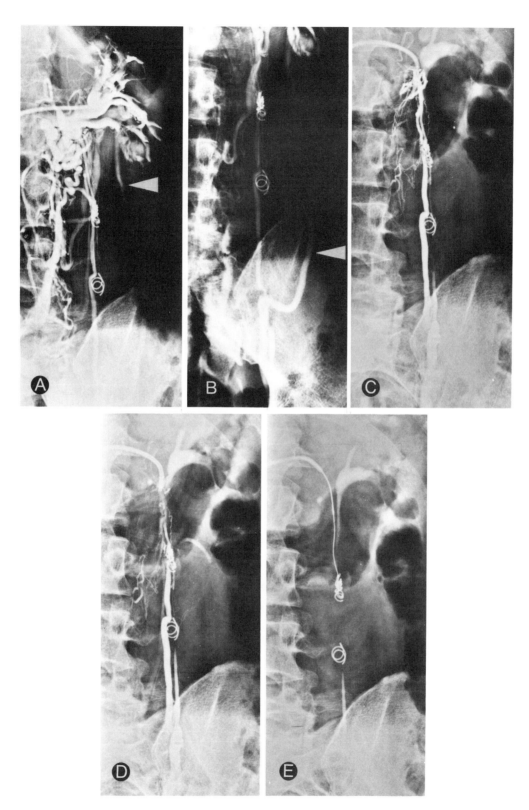

Figure 2.2.20. Postoperative persistence of varicocele after surgical ligation and two sessions of coil embolization. **A,B.** Diagnostic renal venography reveals large renospermatic anastomosis *(arrowheads)* that bypasses to the incompetent caudal part of the spermatic vein. **C,D.** Superior coils (two or three at level of L3) are unable to stop the blood flow. Inferior coil (L4) is placed in a lateral, smaller branch of a bifurcation, leaving a major medial branch open. **E.** Superior coils blocks passage of coaxial catheter.

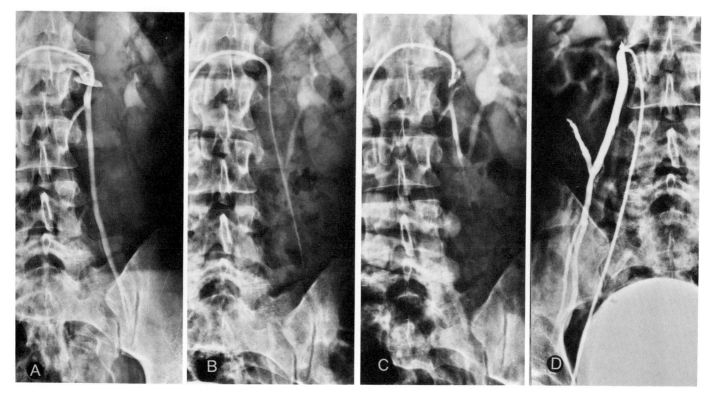

Figure 2.2.21. In this patient, clinical persistence of left-sided varicocele after left-sided embolization is due to an incompetent right spermatic vein together with intrascrotal collaterals. **A.** Diagnostic left venography shows distal bifurcations. **B.** Tip of coaxial catheter at site of superior bifurcation. **C.** Control venography after embolization shows complete occlusion at level of L3. **D.** Diagnostic right-sided venogram via cobra catheter clearly reveals reflux through bifurcated right spermatic vein, as well as presence of perirenal anastomosis. Right spermatic vein was not treated during the first session (see text). **E.** Control left venography four months later because of clinical persistence shows that occlusion is unchanged (*arrowhead* indicates spermatic occlusion). Lumbar ascending vein is opacified. **F–H.** Right-sided venography with hooked catheter confirms the findings in *D* and shows right-sided varicocele with intrascrotal connections that fill left pampiniform plexus. Normally, the testicles are x-ray shielded with 1mm lead and varicoceles are not depicted. **I.** Upon coaxial superselective venography, all branches are found to be connected at the level of the iliac crest. **J.** Embolization is performed at this level. **K.** Right venography shows complete occlusion.

without success on the left side, the authors first embolized the persistent varicocele. Because reflux through the right spermatic vein was also detected, this side was embolized as well. The right spermatic venous system consisted of at least four small, interconnected branches. The coaxial catheter was placed distally, partly wedged in one of the branches. During the injection of contrast medium, there was no clear runoff. Immediately after injection of the embolus, the catheter could not be removed because it was trapped in the embolus. At present, the authors consider such wedging with poor run-off to be a contraindication to the injection of NBCA, and a better site for embolization must be selected or superselective sclerotherapy performed. Both patients were immediately operated on and recovered uneventfully. In the last nine years no catheter trapping occurred.

The high accuracy of this embolization method is emphasized by the results achieved in the last five-year period, during which 420 patients were treated. Twenty-four of these had normal selective venograms. Of the 396 patients with abnormal venograms, 14 of whom had been operated on without success, only 3 patients (0.75%) could not be cured by embolization. All three had a left reno-spermatic bypass and a competent spermatic outlet valve that could not be passed by the coaxial catheter. Such a valve was found in 33% of the cases with left-sided varicoceles and could be passed in 98% of these. Thirty percent of the patients presented with bilateral varicoceles, but only five had a unilateral right-sided varicocele (1.2%). All 123 right-sided varicoceles could be embolized. Sixteen of these patients had a renospermatic bypass together with a competent outlet valve.

The authors have obtained the same high success with superselective sclerotherapy using the same coaxial catheterization method.[12] Instead of NBCA, 5ml of a 3% sodium tetradecyl sulfate solution (Thrombovar from Lepetit/France; Sotradecol, U.S.A.) is injected superselectively in the spermatic vein. Provided the blood flow is arrested by tilting the examination table and the prescribed dosage is adhered to, the authors seldom observed pain or scrotal swelling. Once the sclerosant is injected, the inner catheter is pulled back 10cm. Flushing of the spermatic vein is avoided, and a follow-up venogram is obtained 30 minutes later. A clear drawback is the fact that this control venogram must be postponed for at least 30 minutes after the injection of the sclerosing agent.

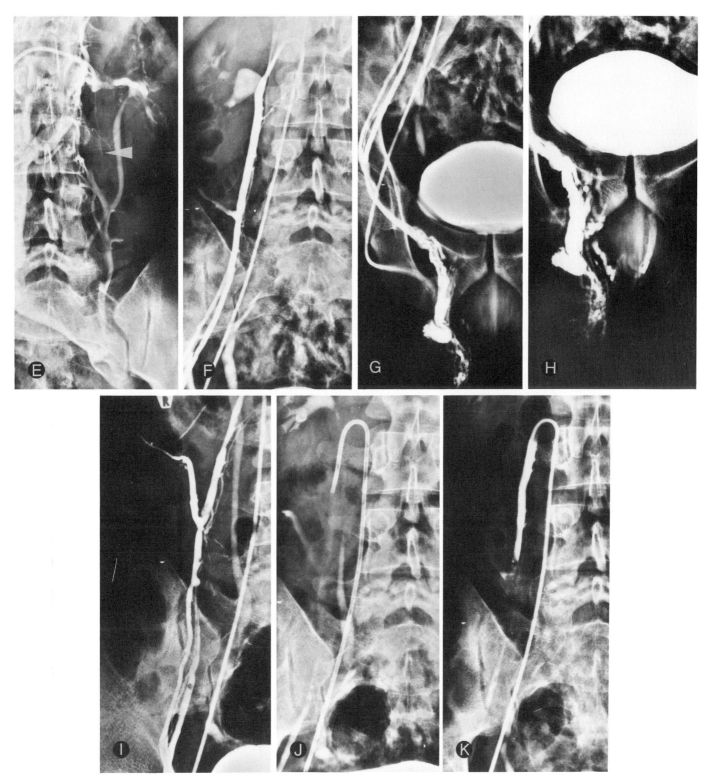

Figure 2.2.21 (E–K).

In the last five-year period, 282 patients with abnormal venograms were successfully treated by superselective sclerotherapy. Fifty-five patients presented with bilateral varicoceles and two patients had a unilateral right varicocele. All these varicoceles were successfully catheterized coaxially, in spite of the possible presence of a competent spermatic vein valve. The latter occurred in 39% of the left and in 14% of the right spermatic veins. A complete occlusion was obtained after one superselective administration of sodium tetradecyl sulfate in 65% of the varicoceles. The remainder required a second dose, injected through the same coaxial catheter. No single case of clinical persistence was observed.

EFFECT OF VARICOCELE TREATMENT ON SEMEN AND PREGNANCIES

Treatment of varicocele aims at repair of testicular function, namely recovery of fertility and normalization of androgen production. The latter was indeed observed in most of the men consulting the authors for subfertility and who presented with subnormal plasma testosterone concentration.[13] Slightly more than half of the couples who consulted for varicocele-associated infertility achieved pregnancy. The probability of success was 4% per cycle (Fig. 2.2.22). This is significantly better than the expected treatment-independent pregnancy rate, which is estimated to be no more than 1.5% per cycle. The causal relationship between varicocele treatment and the occurrence of pregnancies is further substantiated by the observation that no significant improvement of semen quality occurred in men who were unsuccessful in impregnating their wives, whereas those who were successful did present a significant improvement.

The success rate of varicocele treatment was 60–80% in men with normal testicular volume, below-average serum follicle-stimulating hormone (FSH) concentrations, and moderate impairment of spermatogenesis. The success rate was moderate (20–50%) in men combining varicocele with other pathology that may influence fertility and in patients with below-normal testicular volume and/or above-average serum FSH concentrations. The probability of conception was <20% if serum FSH concentration was grossly elevated, if testicular volume was severely reduced, if circulating sperm antibodies were present, or if there was azoospermia (absence of spermatozoa in his ejaculate). The latter patients stand such poor chances of success that treatment probably should not be offered to them.[14,15]

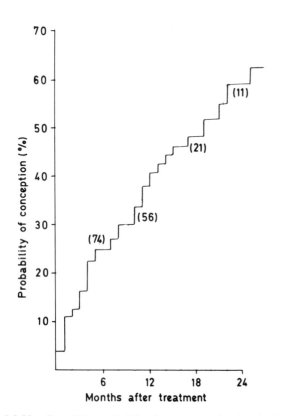

Figure 2.2.22. Cumulative probability of pregnancy related to the time elapsed after treatment in a group of 100 couples with varicocele-associated infertility. The *numbers in parentheses* indicate the number of couples under follow-up at 6, 12, 18, and 24 months.

References

1. Comhaire F, Simons M, Kunnen M, Vermeulen L: Testicular arterial perfusion in varicocele: the role of rapid sequence scintigraphy with technetium in varicocele evaluation. *J Urol* 1983;130:923
2. Ahlberg NE, Bartley O, Chidekel N, Fritjofson A: Phlebography in varicocele scroti. *Acta Radiol[Diagn]* 1966;4:517
3. Brown JS, Dubin L, Hotchkiss RS: The varicocele as related to fertility. *Fertil Steril* 1967;18:46
4. Hiel JT, Green NA: Varicocele: a review of radiological and anatomical features in relation to surgical treatment. *Br J Surg* 1977;64:747
5. Comhaire F, Kunnen M: Selective retrograde venography of the internal spermatic vein: a conclusive approach to the diagnosis of varicocele. *Andrologia* 1976;8:11
6. Comhaire F, Kunnen M: The value of scrotal thermography as compared with selective retrograde venography of the internal spermatic vein for the diagnosis of "subclinical" varicocele. *Fertil Steril* 1976;27:694
7. Kunnen M: Neue Technik zur Embolisation der Vena spermatica interna: intravenöser Gewebekleber. *Fortschr Röntgenstr* 1980;133:625
8. Kunnen M: Traitement des varicocèles par embolisation l'iso-butyl-2-cyanoacrylate. *Ann Radiol* 1981;64:406
9. Kunnen M: Nonsurgical cure of varicocele by transcatheter embolization of the internal spermatic vein with Bucrylate, in Zeitler E, Jecht E (eds): *Varicocele and Male Infertility (Recent Advances in Diagnostic and Therapy)*. Berlin, Springer–Verlag, 1982, p 153
10. Kunnen M, Comhaire F: Transcatheter embolization of the internal spermatic vein(s) with Bucrylate: further improvements. *Ann Radiol* 1984;27:303
11. Weissbach L, Thelen M, Adolphs HD: Treatment of idiopathic varicoceles by transfemoral testicular vein occlusion. *J Urol* 1981;126:354
12. Kunnen M: Treatment of varicocele by transcatheter embolization with tissue adhesive. 1987; Proc 10th Annual Con-

gress of the Phlebology Society of America. October 10–11, 1986, New York, p 70

13. Comhaire F, Vermeulen A: Plasma testosterone in patients with varicocele and sexual inadequacy. *J Clin Endocrinol Metab* 1975;40:824

14. Comhaire F, Kunnen M: Factors affecting the fertility out-come after treatment of subfertile men with varicocele by transcatheter embolization with Bucrylate. *Fertil Steril* 1985;43:781

15. Kunnen M, Comhaire F: Fertility after varicocele emboliza-tion with bucrylate. *Ann Radiol* 1986;29:169

Part 3. Embolization of the Internal Spermatic Vein with Mechanical Devices for the Treatment of Varicocele

—Marcos A. Herrera, M.D., Riccardo Di Segni, M.D., Keith W. Kaye, M.D., Wilfrido R. Castañeda–Zúñiga, M.D., M.Sc., Cesar Ercole, M.D., David W. Hunter, M.D., Joseph W. Yedlicka, Jr., M.D., Flavio Castañeda, M.D., and Kurt Amplatz, M.D.

The term "varicocele" originally described the visible enlargement of veins of the pampiniform plexus, nearly always on the left. The relationship between this condition and male subfertility was suspected as early as 1929 and was confirmed by the frequent improvement in semen quality after operative correction of this condition.

In the past several years, spermatic studies with Doppler sonography, thermography, scintigraphy, and venography have shown that classical varicoceles result from absent or inadequate valves in the internal spermatic veins. Such studies also have proved that valvar inadequacy can also be present without being clinically apparent, a condition known as subclinical varicocele.[1] Although subclinical var-icocele is most often encountered on the right side in patients with obvious varicocele on the left, it can also be bilateral. Its lack of signs and symptoms does not mean that it can be ignored in the evaluation of the subfertile man, because the size of the varicocele does not correlate with the extent of testicular and epididymal dysfunction asso-ciated with it.[2,3] Eight to nine percent of patients are found to have bilateral varicocele, and in a few patients (1–22%) only a right varicocele is detected.[4] Interestingly enough, varicocele is present in 17% of fertile males.[5] Bilateral var-icocele in infertile men can be as high as 60%, as shown by Amelar during open varicocelectomy in 870 patients.[6] Narayan showed a 60% incidence of bilateral varicoceles by spermatic venography.[7] Overlooked right side varicocele could be the cause of failure to obtain clinical improve-ment following left varicocelectomy.[6]

WHICH VARICOCELES SHOULD BE CORRECTED?

For the purposes of this discussion, two kinds of vari-coceles can be distinguished: those large enough to be a nuisance to the patient and those in men complaining of subfertility.

Annoying Varicoceles

If a varicocele is large enough to interfere with the patient's activities, it may be ablated. Although this can be achieved by a traditional Ivanissevitch operation, this approach usually requires general anesthesia and fails in many cases because not all of the contributing vessels are ligated.

It must be mentioned that an evident varicocele appear-ing for the first time in a middle-aged or older man often indicates tumor invasion of the veins upstream.

Varicocele Associated with Subfertility

The past few years have seen an enormous increase in the sophistication of understanding of male subfertility.[8] Unfortunately, this development has not been accompa-nied by an equal increase in the ability to correct the prob-lems that have been identified. One problem that can be corrected is varicocele. Correction of varicocele in an infertile patient offers the most encouraging results among all therapeutic options. Increasingly, venous embolization is the method of choice, because it can be carried out, together with venography to identify small collateral ves-sels as well as unusual venous anatomy so common in these patients,[9] as an outpatient procedure using only local anes-thesia.[10] In nearly all patients, a significant improvement in sperm count and motility index follows.[10]

SPERMATIC VENOGRAPHY AND EMBOLIZATION

Therapeutic embolization is indicated in men with clin-ical or subclinical varicoceles who have been infertile for at least two years and who have oligoasthenospermia and no other apparent cause of infertility. A coagulation profile should be obtained one or two days before admission.

For outpatient venography and embolization, the

patient is admitted early in the morning, and the radiologist discusses the procedure with the patient. The procedure itself can be performed via the femoral vein, but an approach via the right internal jugular vein generally makes catheterization of the internal spermatic veins easier.[11] Local anesthesia suffices.

Method of Venography

Two approaches to spermatic vein catheterization and embolization have been used in the authors' institution: femoral and jugular. The standard femoral approach is adequate for routine venography, although it is difficult to advance a catheter deep into either the right or the left spermatic vein if embolization is to be attempted. It is, however, adequate for the injection of sclerosing agents or detachable balloons. A jugular approach facilitates deep catheterization of both spermatics; thus the authors use this technique whenever embolization is planned.

FEMORAL APPROACH

The femoral vein is punctured using the Seldinger technique, and a gently curved 7Fr or 8Fr modified headhunter No. 1 or cobra catheter is advanced over a guidewire into the inferior vena cava. Under fluoroscopic control, the left renal vein is selectively catheterized and its inferior surface

probed until the left spermatic vein is engaged; usually the orifice is 2–3cm from the junction of the renal vein and vena cava. In a high percentage of cases, the spermatic vein has a common origin with lumbar veins that arise from the inferior surface of the renal vein, just to the left of the lumbar vertebral bodies. In a small number of cases, the left spermatic vein arises from intrarenal venous branches or from elsewhere in the vena cava.[12,13]

Once the orifice of the left spermatic vein has been engaged, a test injection is made to determine the competence of the valves (Fig. 2.3.1*A,B*). If they are incompetent, a wire is advanced deep into the spermatic vein, and the catheter is passed over the wire. It is frequently difficult to advance the catheter, since it tends to buckle as it enters the renal vein, pulling the wire out of the spermatic vein. Exchange of the rigid torque control catheter for a soft 5Fr polyethylene catheter may facilitate this maneuver. Both venograms and embolization procedures can be carried out once deep catheterization of the vein has been accomplished. Usually, venography will demonstrate a common collateral channel at the level of the iliac crest communicating with lumbar veins (Fig. 2.3.2).

The right spermatic vein is difficult to catheterize from the femoral approach. A 7Fr sidewinder II catheter is used to probe the anterolateral surface of the inferior vena cava, just caudal to the orifice of the right renal vein. When the

Figure 2.3.1.   A,B. Left renal venogram: Incompetence of venous valves in left spermatic veins with marked reflux of contrast medium to level of the testicle. Small accessory channels are seen alongside large left spermatic vein *(arrows).*

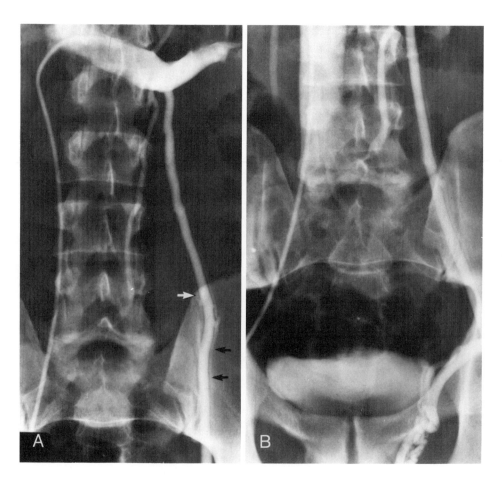

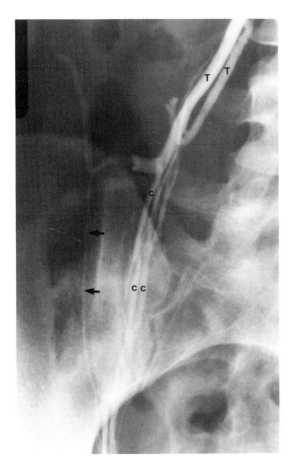

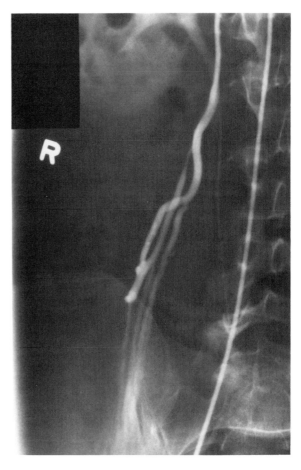

Figure 2.3.2. Right spermatic venogram: Multiple venous channels within pelvis *(c)* with two large common trunks *(T)* in most proximal segment. Collaterals to retroperitoneal veins are present *(arrows)*.

Figure 2.3.3. Multiple large communicating veins joining to form a common trunk before entering the inferior vena cava. Large or multiple veins such as these contain enough blood moving fast enough to cool hot contrast medium below temperature needed to damage vessel wall.

catheter tip engages the orifice of the right spermatic vein it is pulled down into the vein (Fig. 2.3.3). The right spermatic vein enters the right renal vein in 10% of cases. In this situation, the sidewinder can be used to probe the inferior surface of the right renal vein.

Jugular Technique

Because deep catheterization of both spermatic veins is difficult using the femoral route, the authors have developed a transjugular approach that greatly facilitates catheterization and embolization.[11] The patient's head is turned 45° to the left, and the carotid artery 5–6cm above the level of the clavicle is palpated. Local anesthesia is administered just lateral to this point, and a 19-gauge needle is directed to a point approximately 5cm lateral to the sternoclavicular joint. (A 19-gauge needle is used to minimize trauma during localization of the vein.) Once venous blood has been aspirated, the needle is withdrawn, and a larger needle is inserted in the same direction. Puncture of the vein is aided by having the patient perform a Valsalva maneuver.

Catheterization can usually be accomplished with a

modified headhunter catheter for the left spermatic vein (Fig. 2.3.4*A,B*) and a modified cobra catheter for the right (Fig. 2.3.5*A,B*). Deep catheterization of both veins is easily accomplished by advancing the catheter over a wire once the spermatic vein has been entered.

Venograms are obtained by the manual injection of 20–30ml of contrast medium. Four to six exposures are generally made in order to demonstrate the proximal and distal segments of the spermatic vein. Alternatively, digital subtraction studies may be obtained. It is particularly important to demonstrate all collaterals present, because occlusion of all of them is needed in order to prevent recurrence. Digital subtraction angiography provides a useful technique to demonstrate the anatomy while using limited amounts of contrast medium (Fig. 2.3.6).

Anatomic variations in the spermatic system are common (Fig. 2.3.7). Anastomoses of the internal spermatic veins with other retroperitoneal veins (capsular, periureteral (Fig. 2.3.8), internal iliac (Fig. 2.3.9), and femoral (Figs. 2.3.10 and 2.3.11)) are frequently seen.[8,9] Such collateral anastomoses make the precise placement of occluding devices imperative.

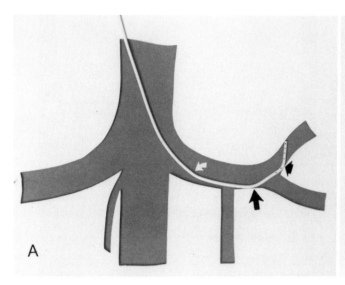

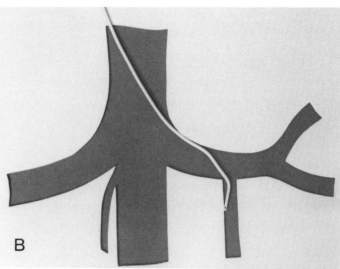

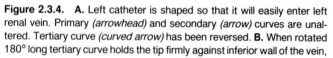

Figure 2.3.4. **A.** Left catheter is shaped so that it will easily enter left renal vein. Primary *(arrowhead)* and secondary *(arrow)* curves are unaltered. Tertiary curve *(curved arrow)* has been reversed. **B.** When rotated 180° long tertiary curve holds the tip firmly against inferior wall of the vein, entering easily into the spermatic vein. (Reproduced from Hunter DW, Castañeda–Zúñiga WR, Coleman CC, et al: Spermatic vein embolization with hot contrast medium or detachable balloons. *Semin Intervent Radiol* 1984;1(2):163–169.)

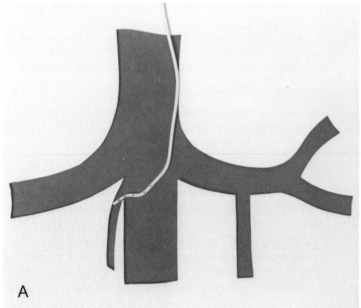

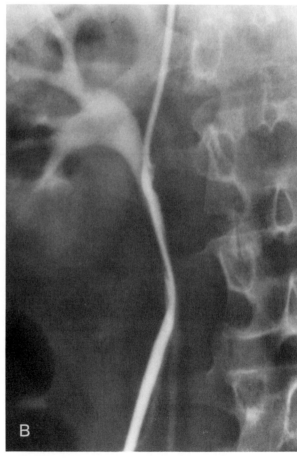

Figure 2.3.5. Catheterization of right side. **A.** Right-sided catheter tip points inferiorly. No other changes are made to convert a left catheter into a right. **B.** Right spermatic vein most commonly originates from inferior vena cava anterior and inferior to right renal vein at a steep downward angle.

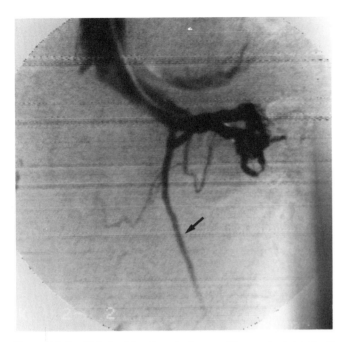

Figure 2.3.6. Digital subtraction studies provide excellent detail with minute doses of dilute (20%) contrast medium injected into the left renal vein; reflux into spermatic vein *(arrow)*.

TREATMENT
Surgery

The traditional treatment of varicocele has been high ligation of the left internal spermatic vein at the level of the internal inguinal ring. Although the technique has recently been performed under local anesthesia,[14] thus increasing its appeal, it still has a failure rate of 5% caused by incomplete ligation of all branches of the spermatic vein.[15]

Nonsurgical Spermatic Vein Occlusion

COILS, SPIDERS, IVALON

Transcatheter embolization of the spermatic veins can be carried out at the time of venography. Stainless-steel coils, compressed Ivalon plugs, and detachable spiders[1,16,17] can be passed through a thin-walled, 9Fr polyethylene catheter. If coils are used, their diameter should be slightly larger than that of the spermatic vein and their ends should be modified to prevent dislodgment (Fig. 2.3.12).[18] The introduction of a spider in a proximal portion of the vein reduces the possibility of coil or Ivalon plug embolization (Fig. 2.3.13). A spider combined with an Ivalon plug (spiderlon) can be used for a one-step embolization (Fig. 2.3.14). Because duplication and collateralization of the

Figure 2.3.7. Diagram showing anatomic variations of spermatic veins. *ISV* = Internal spermatic vein.

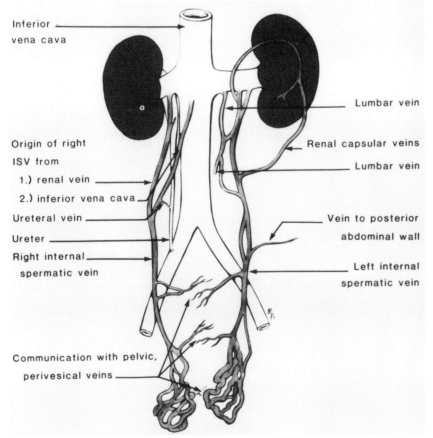

Inferior vena cava

Origin of right ISV from

1.) renal vein

2.) inferior vena cava

Ureteral vein

Ureter

Right internal spermatic vein

Communication with pelvic, perivesical veins

Lumbar vein

Renal capsular veins

Lumbar vein

Vein to posterior abdominal wall

Left internal spermatic vein

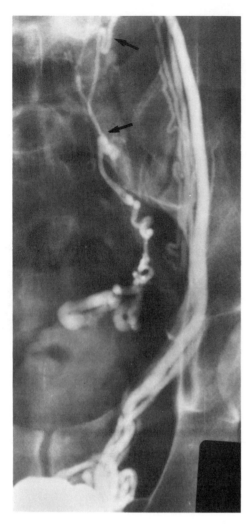

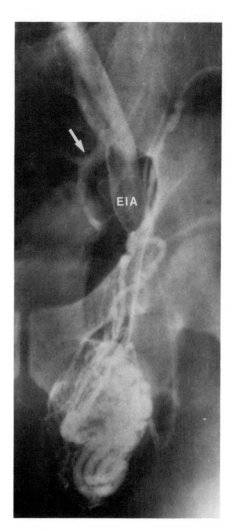

Figure 2.3.8. Left spermatic venogram; one large venous channel with multiple accessory channels. Note also collaterals to retroperitoneal venous channels *(arrows)*.

Figure 2.3.9. Incompetent left spermatic vein: Observe collaterals to hypogastric artery *(white arrow)*. *EIA* = External iliac artery.

Figure 2.3.10. **A.** Left spermatic venogram; incompetence of venous valves with reflux of contrast medium down to the testicle. **B.** Collaterals are seen below level of inguinal ligament to common femoral vein *(arrows)*.

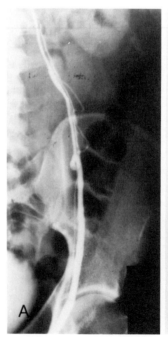

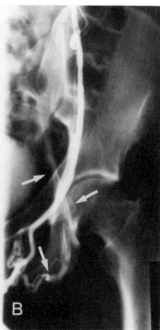

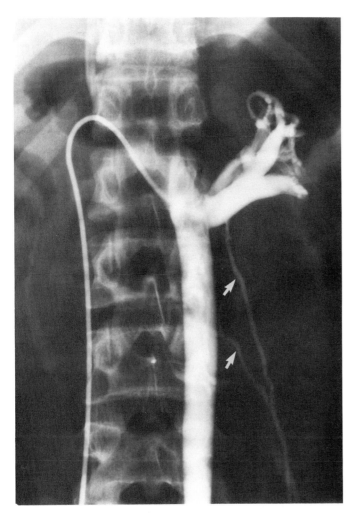

Figure 2.3.11. Persistent left inferior vena cava to which left renal vein is connected. Two left spermatic veins are seen, one arising from left renal vein and one from left inferior vena cava *(arrows).*

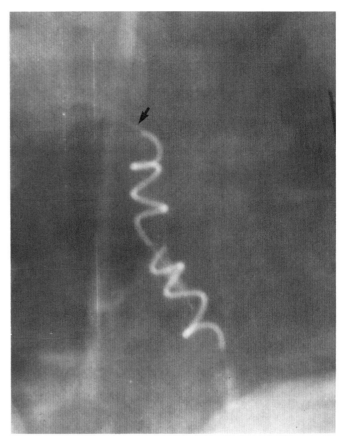

Figure 2.3.12. Spot film showing position of two coilons within left spermatic vein in patient with infertility due to large left-sided varicocele. Observe that proximal end of most proximal coilon has been modified *(arrow)* for better fixation within the venous wall to prevent migration.

internal spermatic vein system are common (Fig. 2.3.15), embolic devices are usually placed at the level of the pelvis and also as near as possible to the level of the renal vein (Fig. 2.3.16).

The advantage of this technique is that precise occlusion of the spermatic vein relative to collateral vessels is achieved. The disadvantages are those associated with placement of a foreign body and the attendant risk of embolization. It is also often difficult to pass embolic devices when the spermatic vein has been catheterized by the femoral route. For this reason, the authors recommend a jugular approach when embolization with particulate material or mechanical devices is attempted.

TISSUE GLUE

Cyanoacrylate-based tissue glue has been used to occlude the spermatic veins.[19] Isobutyl 2-cyanoacrylate is a rapidly polymerizing agent that hardens immediately on contact with an ionic solution such as blood. The glue is injected through a 3Fr catheter placed coaxially through a 7Fr or 8Fr catheter. The advantage of tissue glue is that an immediate selective vessel occlusion is obtained. In addition, it may be easier to introduce from a femoral route than are other embolic agents. Unfortunately, there are numerous drawbacks associated with the technique. The catheter system must be flushed with a nonionic solution such as glucose to prevent polymerization of the glue in the catheter. If the agent is flushed too rapidly, it may reflux and embolize the renal vein or lung. Considerable experimental skill should be obtained in the laboratory before this agent is used clinically.

SCLEROTHERAPY

The first transvenous occlusion of the spermatic vein was accomplished by injection of a sclerosing agent directly into the vein.[20] Since that time, numerous reports have been made of the efficacy of this technique.[21-24] The most popular sclerosing agent is Varicocid 5%, the salt of a fatty acid of cod liver oil,[24] which has been successfully used in Europe. This product is not available in the United States. Other agents include 80% iothalamate sodium, 3% ethoxysclerol, and 3% sodium tetradecyl sulfate (Sotradecol 3%).

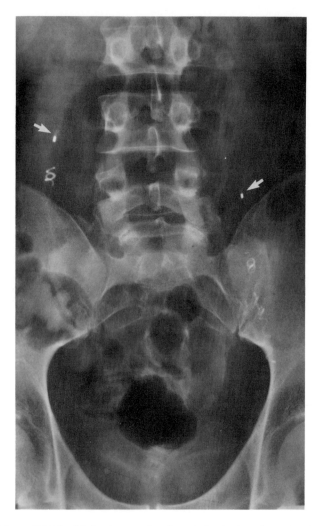

Figure 2.3.13. Bilateral spermatic vein embolization in patient with infertility and bilateral varicoceles. Spider has been placed on left side proximal to a GWC spring embolus to prevent migration *(arrow)*. Spider has been placed on right side proximal to spring coil *(arrow)*.

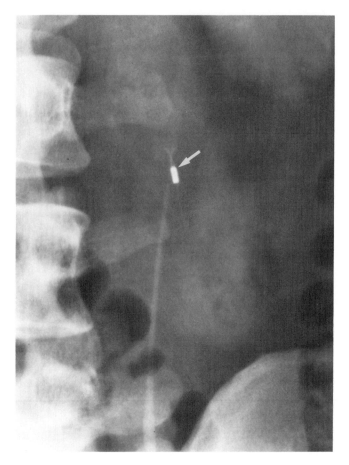

Figure 2.3.14. Spiderlon in left spermatic vein.

DETACHABLE BALLOONS

Selective occlusion of the spermatic vein has also been achieved with detachable balloons.[27] Depending on the size of the spermatic vein, 1 or 2mm Mini-Balloons are passed through an untapered 9Fr polyethylene catheter placed in the spermatic vein. The balloons usually are inflated with isosmotic contrast medium diluted with equal parts of sterile water (not saline) (Isoviev 300 (Squibb), contrast medium and sterile water), and a test injection is made through the introducing catheter to determine if the balloons are optimally placed in relation to any collateral vessels. When detached, the balloons are supposed to remain inflated for 30 days or longer.

The advantages of detachable balloons are the same as with other mechanical occluding agents, primarily selective occlusion of the spermatic vein relative to collaterals. An additional advantage not shared by other embolic agents is the ability to determine the optimal balloon position by a test inflation prior to detachment. Detachable balloons can be used in conjunction with sclerosant agents. Disadvantages of detachable balloons include their high cost and the possibility of their embolization to the lung if too small a balloon is selected or if the balloon is placed while the vein is in spasm.[25] A "sandwich" technique was described by Halden and White, using two detachable balloons: one

Approximately 3ml of a sclerosing agent is introduced into the distal third of the spermatic vein, left in place for 5–15 minutes, and then aspirated. The patient is instructed to perform a Valsalva maneuver during injection of the sclerosant to facilitate its passage down the spermatic vein. Venography is repeated 15 to 30 minutes after the procedure, and, if necessary, sclerosing is repeated.

The advantages of sclerotherapy include ease of delivery, minimal patient discomfort (80–98%), higher success rate when compared with other modalities, and ability to occlude collateral vessels that may be the cause of persistent or recurrent varicocele (Fig. 2.3.17). Disadvantages include possible reflux of the agent into the renal vein and testicular thrombophlebitis when the sclerosing agent is allowed to fill the pampiniform plexus.[21,22,24] Bach reported a recurrence rate of only 3.3% at 6–18 months following sclerotherapy with Varicocid in 314 patients.[25] Wilms reported the use of an open-ended guidewire to inject sclerosing agent into the distal spermatic vein.[26]

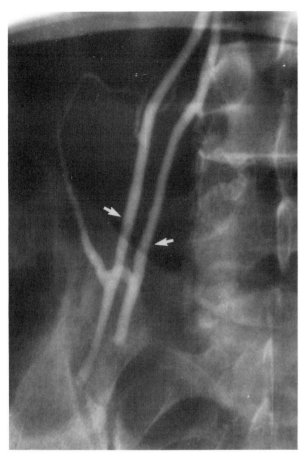

Figure 2.3.15. Right spermatic venogram reveals incompetent venous valves and dual venous trunk *(arrows)*.

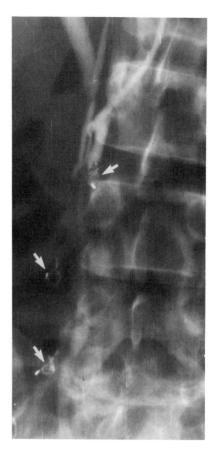

Figure 2.3.16. Both venous channels have been obliterated with GWC spring embolus *(arrows)*. The postembolization venogram reveals complete thrombosis of both channels.

placed distally and one proximal to all collaterals, injecting a sclerosing agent between the balloons.[28]

THERMAL VESSEL OCCLUSION

The authors have recently developed a new, as yet experimental, technique, transcatheter thermal vessel occlusion, that may obviate many of the disadvantages of present techniques.[29-31] The injection of 3–6ml of boiling contrast medium into canine spermatic veins produces complete long-term occlusion without evidence of collateralization or systemic effects. Ionic contrast media are inexpensive and readily available and can be injected through small catheters. A femoral rather than a jugular approach can be used, since deep catheterization of the spermatic vein is not necessary. Hot contrast medium produces thermal sclerosis of both the spermatic vein and its collaterals, which may decrease the rate of varicocele recurrence associated with mechanical occluding devices provided the anatomy is suitable (Fig. 2.3.13). In addition, hot contrast medium may be superior to sclerosing agents because it is rapidly converted to a nontoxic substance by cooling. (Clinical trials are underway.)

In the authors' institution during a study over a five-year period, venography follow-up after spermatic vein terminal occlusion in 81 patients showed successful obliteration up to 91% and pregnancy of 40.5%.[32]

Complications were reported in 5 of the 81 patients; four complained of anesthesia of the anterior thigh, lasting one to six months, but all patients recovered. One of the patients became aspermic following the procedure. The disadvantages of hot contrast medium obliteration are pain, which lasts only 5 to 20 seconds and can be avoided with appropriate sedation, and damage to the testicles if medium is refluxed in the pampiniform plexus.

Postembolization Management

Repeat venograms are obtained 10–30 minutes after the procedure. After removal of the catheter, light pressure is maintained over the neck or groin for five minutes, and the patient is then monitored for two to four hours before discharge. Follow-up angiography is generally not needed. Varicocele regression can be monitored clinically at the time that spermiograms are checked, usually every three months for one year.

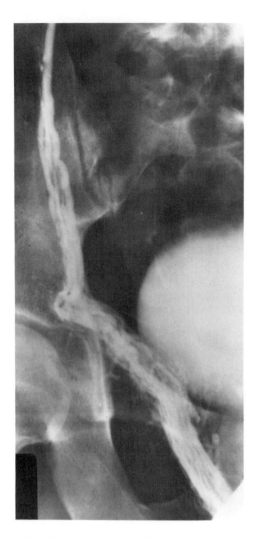

Figure 2.3.17. Multiple small venous channels are seen within the inguinal canal extending into the pelvis and finally forming a common trunk at the level of the iliac crest.

RESULTS

Catheterization of the spermatic veins is difficult in many cases, perhaps due to anatomic abnormalities so often associated with varicocele. In 3–40% of patients, the spermatic vein cannot be embolized[11,21,22,24]; therefore, both nonsurgical occlusion and traditional operative interruption of the spermatic vein have a place. The importance of right spermatic vein incompetence has recently been stressed.[1,11] If treated surgically, bilateral spermatic vein ligation would, of course, require two separate incisions.

The fact that interruption of the spermatic veins causes regression of varicoceles and improvement in semen characteristics in a significant number of patients is well documented.[1,10,11] Semen quality is improved in 55–85%, and impregnation has been reported in 25–55% for those treated.[10,11,33] Results with both surgical and nonsurgical techniques appear to be similar, although long-term follow-up of patients treated nonsurgically is not yet available. Whether transcatheter spermatic vein occlusion is more

effective than operation in preventing varicocele recurrence is also not yet known. Theoretically, the ability to place embolic devices selectively should eliminate the surgical problem of incomplete ligation of the spermatic vein and its collaterals. In addition, by also causing thrombosis of existing collaterals, sclerotherapy may decrease the rate of varicocele recurrence.

Complications associated with transcatheter spermatic vein occlusion are infrequent and usually self-limiting. The most significant complication is embolization of a mechanical occluding device to the lung. Other, less serious, complications include extravasation, contrast reactions, testicular thrombophylytitis from sclerosing agents, pain, venous spasm, accidental puncture of femoral artery, and hematoma at the puncture site.

References

1. Gonzalez R, Narayan P, Castañeda–Zúñiga WR, Amplatz K: Transvenous embolization of the internal spermatic veins for the treatment of varicocele scroti. *Urol Clin North Am* 1982;9:177–184
2. Verrstoppen GR, Steeno OP: Varicocele and the pathogenesis of the associated subfertility: a review of the various theories. 1: Varicocelogenesis. *Andrologia* 1977;9:133–140
3. Coolsaet BRRA: The varicocele syndrome: venography determining the optimal level for surgical management. *J Urol* 1980;124:833–841
4. Tjia TT, Rumping WJM, Landman GHM, Cobben JJ. Phlebography of the internal spermatic vein (and the ovarian vein). *Diagn Imaging* 1982;51:8–18
5. Kursh ED. What is the incidence of varicocele in a fertile population? *Fertil Steril* 1987;48:510
6. Amelar RD, Dubin L: Infertility in the male, in Kendall R, Karifin L (eds): *Practice of Surgery (Urology)*, Volume 2, Philadelphia, Harper and Row, 1984, p 43
7. Narayan P, Amplatz K, Gonzalez R. Varicocele and male subfertility. *Fertil Steril* 1981;36:92
8. Ross LS: Diagnosis and treatment of infertile men: a clinical perspective. *J Urol* 1983;130:847–859
9. Narayan P, Amplatz K, Gonzalez R: Varicocele and male subfertility. *Fertil Steril* 1981;36:92–96
10. Castañeda–Zúñiga WR, Gonzalez R, Amplatz K: Spermatic vein embolization in the treatment of infertility, in Kaye KW (ed): *Outpatient Urologic Surgery*. Philadelphia, Lea & Febiger, 1985, pp 165–172
11. Formanek A, Rusnak B, Zollikofer C, et al: Embolization of the spermatic vein for treatment of infertility: a new approach. *Radiology* 1981;139:315–321
12. Comhaire F, Kunnen M: Selective retrograde venography of the internal spermatic vein: a conclusive approach to diagnosis of varicocele. *Andrologia* 1976;8:11–24
13. Johnsen SG, Agger P: Quantitative evaluation of testicular biopsies before and after operation for varicocele. *Fertil Steril* 1978;29:58–63
14. Ross LS, Lipson S, Dritz S: Surgical treatment of varicocele. *Urology* 1982;19:179–180
15. Palomo A: Radical cure of varicocele by a new technique: preliminary report. *J Urol* 1979;61:604
16. Thelen M, Weibback L, Franken T: Die Behandlung der idiopathischen Varikozele durch transfemorale Spiralokklusion der vena testicularis sinistra. *RöFo* 1979;131:24–29
17. Zollikofer C, Castañeda–Zúñiga WR, Galliani C, et al: Ther-

apeutic blockage of arteries using compressed Ivalon. *Radiology* 1980;136:635–640

18. Castañeda–Zúñiga WR, Tadavarthy SM, Gonzalez R, Rysavy J, Amplatz K: Single barbed stainless steel coils for venous occlusion: a simple but useful modification. *Invest Radiol* 1982;17:186–188

19. Kunnen M: Traitment des varicoceles par embolization a l'isobutyl-2-cyanoacrylate. *Ann Radiol* 1981;24:406–409

20. Lima SS, Castro MP, Costa OF: A new method for the treatment of varicocele. *Andrologia* 1978;10:103–106

21. Riedel P, Lunglmayr G, Stackl W: A new method of transfemoral testicular vein obliteration for varicocele using a balloon catheter. *Radiology* 1981;139:323–325

22. Iaccarino V: A nonsurgical treatment of varicocele: transcatheter sclerotherapy of gonadal veins. *Ann Radiol* 1980;23:369–370

23. Zeitler E, Jecht E, Richter EI, Seyferth W: Selective sclerotherapy of the internal spermatic vein in patients with varicocele. *Ann Radiol* 1980;23:371–373

24. Seyferth W, Jecht E, Zeitler E: Percutaneous sclerotherapy of varicocele. *Radiology* 1981;139:335–340

25. Bach D, Bahren W, Gall H, Altwein JE: Late results after sclerotherapy of varicocele. *Eur Urol* 1988;14(2):115–119

26. Wilms G, Oyen R, Casselman J, Baert AL: Percutaneous sclerotherapy of the internal spermatic vein for varicocele through an open ended guide wire. *RöFo* 1987;147(2):168–170

27. White RI Jr, Kaufman SL, Barth KH, Kadir S, Smyth JW, Walsh PC: Occlusion of varicoceles with detachable balloons. *Radiology* 1981;139:327–334

28. Halden W, White RI Jr: Outpatient embolotherapy of varicocele. *Urol Clin North Am* 1987;14(1):137–144

29. Cragg AH, Galliani CA, Rysavy JA, Castañeda–Zúñiga WR, Amplatz K: Endovascular diathermic vessel occlusion. *Radiology* 1982;144:303–308

30. Rholl KS, Rysavy JA, Vlodaver Z, et al: Transcatheter thermal venous occlusion: a new technique. *Radiology* 1982;145:333–337

31. Rholl KS, Rysavy JA, Vlodaver Z, et al: Spermatic vein obliteration using hot contrast medium. *Radiology* 1983;148:85–87

32. Hunter DW, Cragg AH, Darcy MD, et al: Spermatic vein occlusion using hot contrast material: clinical results. Presented at the RSNA Annual Meeting, Chicago, IL, 1990

33. Greenberg SH: Varicocele and male fertility. *Fertil Steril* 1977;28:699–706

Part 4. Extracranial Embolotherapy with Detachable Balloons

—Klemens H. Barth, M.D.

Balloon embolotherapy has received most of its developmental impetus through neurovascular applications, with the pioneering work having been reported by Serbinenko in 1974.[1-6] Now, detachable balloons are the preferred device for embolization where precise placement and a high margin of safety are required.

Detachable balloon embolization, as any other transcatheter embolization, is fluoroscopically guided; however, unlike other techniques, it uses the bloodstream to advance the occluding device to its destination remote from the introducing catheter. Control over balloon position is maintained via a catheter on which the balloon is mounted. This catheter serves the function of a "leash," and needs to be both strong enough to retain the balloon at any distance, and needs to be flexible enough not to impede balloon travel through curved vessels and branch angles. A competent balloon-catheter connection is a crucial element in the delivery system, and this aspect proved to be most difficult during the development of various systems. For this and other reasons, only four balloon embolization systems have, to the author's knowledge, reached broader practical application, and only one of those[7] has been approved to date by the U.S. Food and Drug Administration (FDA) for marketing (Mini-Balloon; Bard–Parker Division of Becton Dickinson Inc., Lincoln Park, NJ). Two systems, among them the first one introduced, have latex balloons[2,6]; the other systems have silicone balloons.[7,8]

GENERAL PRINCIPLES OF BALLOON EMBOLIZATION SYSTEMS

To embolize a flow-directed balloon, a specific delivery system is required, in contrast to embolization with particles, steel coils, or ethanol, which can be pushed or injected through standard tapered angiographic catheters. Three components are essential to deliver a balloon embolus: the balloon itself, the delivery (balloon) catheter to which the balloon is attached, and the catheter through which the balloon catheter is introduced or injected (introducer catheter) (Fig. 2.4.1). Some systems also include a coaxial catheter that is passed over the balloon catheter for balloon detachment.[8,9] None of the available balloons is radiopaque, although one system has a silver clip in the balloon tip to make it visible fluoroscopically.[2]

Silicone is a semipermeable membrane that preserves balloon volume when inflated with a liquid isosmolar to blood (285mosm/liter) but which expands when filled with a hyperosmolar liquid and contracts when filled with a hyposmolar liquid.[8,10-12] Therefore, use of a hyperosmolar liquid leads to balloon overdistention and rupture, whereas use of a hyposmolar liquid causes balloon shrinkage and potential dislodgment. For convenience, silicone balloons are filled with isosmolar angiographic contrast material.[8,10-12] Because most ionic contrast media used for angiographic procedures have osmolalities much higher

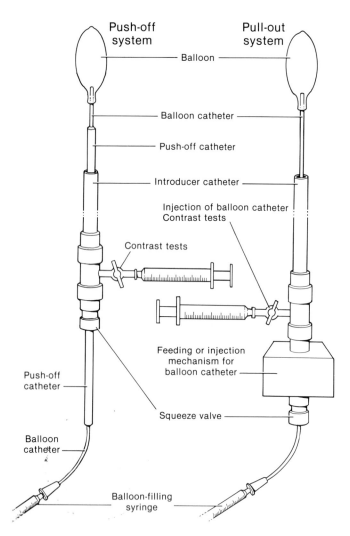

Figure 2.4.1. Available detachable balloon embolization systems. Injection of the balloon is possible only with pushoff catheter (pullout detachment).

than blood (>1000mosm/liter), the required dilution would greatly reduce visibility.[11] Before low-osmolality contrast medium became available, a popular solution was 52% iodipamide meglumine (Cholografin; Squibb) mixed 1:1 with water, which was radiopaque and only slightly hyperosmolar (430mosm/liter).[7] Isosmolar ioliesol (Omnipaque; Winthrop) (175mg of iodine/ml), has been found suitable,[11] as weak as an isosmolar dilution of the ionic dimer ioxaglate meglumine sodium (Hexabrix; Mallinckrodt).

Ultrastructurally, latex is a coarse lattice that leaks liquid over time. Therefore, detachable latex balloons do not remain inflated very long with contrast medium[13]; the most appropriate long-term balloon filler is a hardening liquid such as medical grade silicone. Silicone is obtainable as two components (one of which is a catalyst) that are mixed in a 1:1 ratio for each application (Ingenol; Ingenor Co., Paris, France). To render the mixture radiopaque without interfering with the vulcanization process, tantalum powder can be added. The vulcanization time of the mixture (10–15 minutes) is monitored individually by observing the setting of a sample in vitro at body temperature.

It is important to realize that the silicone compound does not completely replace the nonsolidifying liquid (contrast) used for test inflation because of the dead space of the catheter. Since the dead space of the catheter is fixed, the smaller the balloon, the larger the percentage of dead space. Silicone filling is not effective if the dead space is over 50% of the balloon volume.[13] The problem can be solved by using a double-lumen balloon catheter, but this catheter is larger and more rigid than the usual balloon catheter.[13] The dead space problem exists for any exchange of two nonmiscible balloon fillers; it is irrelevant when using contrast medium only.

Limits in the tensile strength of the balloon determine its maximum inflated size and the vessel lumen it can occlude. For present silicone balloons filled with liquid, the expansion limit is about four times the uninflated diameter,[10] whereas it is about six times for latex balloons. The internal pressure of a balloon detached in an artery may be >200mm Hg (lower in a vein) and represents a combination of the inflation pressure and the counterpressure of the vessel wall. Barth et al.'s in vivo experiments have shown that the chronic pressure exerted by the balloon on the vessel wall leads to intimal fibrosis (collagen deposition) and thinning of the muscle layer (Fig. 2.4.2).[11] Interestingly, there is little foreign body reaction in the vessel wall adjacent to a silicone balloon, in contrast to the response to other embolization agents.[11] The embolic occlusion produced by the balloon was short, with just a cover of organized thrombus on both ends of the balloon (Fig. 2.4.2).[11] Therefore, balloon embolization can be considered to produce a vascular occlusion similar to that of a surgical ligation.

As mentioned earlier, the catheter-balloon connection is an important element. Pressure cuffs and miter valves are the principal designs.[4,6–8,13] One system (Mini-Balloon) uses an interconnecting metal cannula between the balloon pressure cuff and the catheter,[10] allowing pullout detachment (described below). The miter valve of the other silicone balloon system (Hieshima) allows both pullout and pushoff detachment.[8] The latex balloon (Debrun) is designed for pushoff detachment with a coaxial catheter (Figs. 2.4.1 and 2.4.3).[2,13] The other latex balloon system, developed by Taki and coworkers and not yet available in the U.S., uses a twist-off detachment mechanism and a vinyl polymer for permanent filling.[6]

None of the existing balloon systems is completely safe from premature detachment, particularly when the balloon is exposed to rapid flow. This becomes an important consideration for embolization of arteriovenous fistulae (AVFs). Conversely, resistance to balloon detachment may be encountered occasionally and cannot be detected until the balloon has been inflated and detachment is attempted. Under no circumstances should the detachment force lead to overstretching of the balloon catheter.

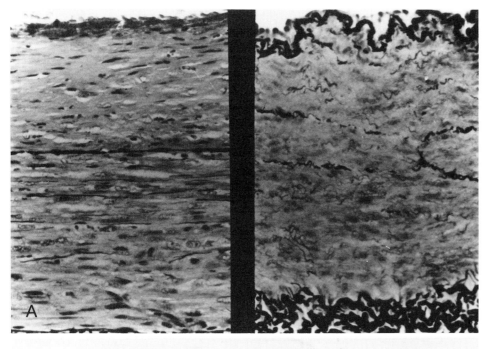

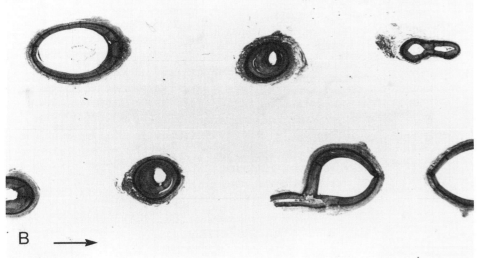

Figure 2.4.2. Histologic effects of embolization balloons. **A.** Cross-section of intima and adjacent muscle layer of canine deep femoral artery through site of balloon embolization *(left)* or of normal vessel *(right)*. Note stretching of elastic fibers and thickening of intima by collagen deposits. There is also thinning and stretching of muscle layer. No giant cells or other evidence of foreign body reaction is apparent. van Gieson trichrome stain; × 40. **B.** Serial cross-sections at low power of canine deep femoral artery between proximal and distal limits of balloon occlusion (in direction of *arrow*). Immediately proximal and distal to balloon, intramural thrombus is present. Balloon did not match caliber of artery and overdistended it; this was done to investigate reactive changes in vessel wall as seen in **A.**

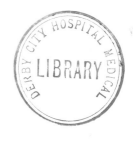

AVAILABLE BALLOON EMBOLIZATION SYSTEMS (TABLE 2.4.1)

Detachable Latex Balloon System (Pushoff Type)

This balloon system, developed and introduced clinically by Debrun,[2] features a radiolucent latex balloon that is available in a variety of sizes and shapes with or without a silver clip in its distal end to ease radiologic observation (Ingenor).[9,13] This balloon is hand-tied by latex strings to the tip of a 2Fr Teflon catheter, a procedure that requires practice (Fig. 2.4.4A). Recently, balloon cuffs have been shaped to fit rather tightly around the 2Fr catheter so that tying with latex strings is required only if the risk of accidental detachment is considerable, as in AVFs. For balloon

detachment, a 4.5–5Fr polyethylene catheter is advanced coaxially over the balloon catheter to "push" the balloon off. (Actually, this catheter is advanced until it contacts the balloon, then held in position while the 2Fr catheter is pulled out.) This coaxial catheter assembly is inserted, not injected, through an 8.8Fr or 9Fr thin-walled, nontapered introducer catheter (Fig. 2.4.4B).

The advantage of the latex balloon system is the availability of assorted balloon sizes and shapes, allowing embolization of small aneurysms and vessels with lumens ≤14mm. Its disadvantages are the need for considerable practice to tie the balloon correctly to the catheter, the need for a pushoff catheter, the limited shelf-life of latex balloons, the need to fill the balloon with a hardening liquid (silicone) to maintain long-term occlusion, the inability to use silicone in small balloons because of dead space (see

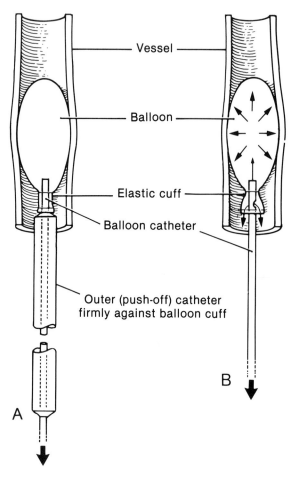

Figure 2.4.3. Technique of balloon detachment.

above), and, finally, the latex membrane itself, which, unlike silicone rubber, is not an established medical implant material.

Detachable Silicone Balloon System (Pushoff/Pullout Type)

This system, developed by Hieshima,[8] remains an investigational device. Several balloon sizes have been developed. The balloon is connected to a 2Fr polyethylene catheter via a miter valve. The pushoff detachment mechanism is similar to that of Debrun's system; however, the balloon can also be detached by pullout (Fig. 2.4.5). Balloons are filled with blood-isosmolar angiographic contrast material. Intracranial and extracranial (particularly renal) embolizations have been described by Hieshima and coworkers. Filling with an inert polymerizing agent is being tested as a means of expanding the balloon beyond the 4:1 ratio considered safe for long-term occlusion with liquid fillers. The problem of dead space again becomes a limitation for smaller balloons when a nonmiscible hardening liquid is used.

Detachable Silicone Balloon System (Pullout Type)

This is the only detachable embolization balloon system approved for intravascular use by the FDA and will be described in some detail. It has been applied for several types of extracranial embolizations.[7,8,10;−12]. It is marketed under the trade name Mini-Balloon (Bard–Parker). Unfortunately, at the time of this writing the manufacturer has stopped product supply. Product transfer to another manufacturer is in progress. Only two balloon sizes are available. The smaller balloon, with an outer diameter (OD) of about 1mm (0.039 inch), passes through a 0.044-inch lumen introducer catheter (4.9Fr thin-walled, nontapered

Table 2.4.1.   Comparison of Detachable Balloon Embolization Systems

Origin	Balloon Material	Balloon Filler	Detachment Mechanism	Catheter Outer Diameter (F) and Material[a]			Balloon Diameter/ Length (mm)			
				Balloon	Pushoff	Introducer	Uninflated	Volume (ml)	Inflated Maximum	Maximum Expansion
Bard	Silicone	Isosmolar iodinated contrast	Pullout	2/PU		4.9/PE	1/5	4/14	0.15	4×
						8.8/PE	2/8	8.8/17	0.60	
Ingenor (Debrun)	Latex	2-component silicone elastomer	Pushoff	1.8/Te	3.3/PE	6/PE	0.8/2	4.5/8.5	0.12	
						7/PE	1.1/2.4	6.0/10	0.4	
						8/PE	1.3/2.5	7.8/14	0.5	6–7×
							1.6/6	10/20	1.5	
						9/PE	2.3/2.2	13/12	1.3	
							2/5	14/25	3.0	
Heishima	Silicone	Isosmolar iodinated contrast	Pushoff/ pullout	2/PE	4/PE		1.3/5	5/9	0.16	
							1.5/6	7/14	0.26	4×

[a]PU = polyurethane; Te = Teflon; PE = polyethylene.

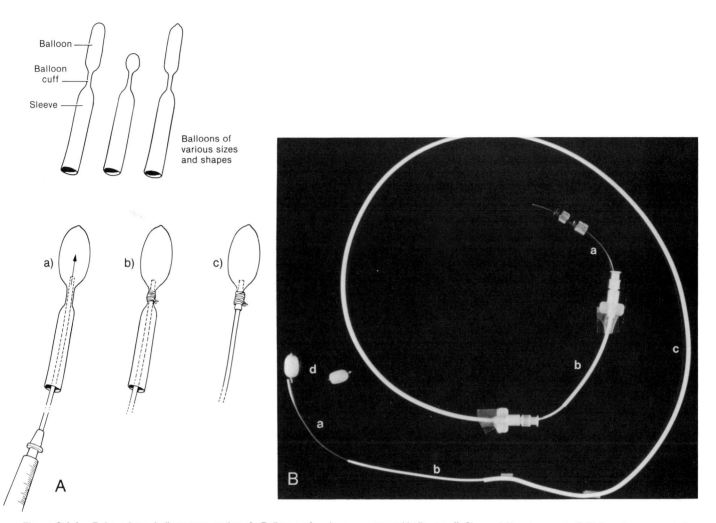

Figure 2.4.4. Debrun latex balloon preparation. **A.** Balloons of various sizes and shapes are available. After balloon catheter has been inserted through sleeve *(a)*, fluid injection distends balloon cuff and allows advancement of catheter into balloon. Latex tie *(b)* is placed under tension around balloon cuff. Sleeve *(c)* has been cut off. Balloon is now ready for use. **B.** Coaxial catheter assembly for detachable Debrun latex balloon, showing catheter *(a)* passed through pushoff catheter *(b)*, introducer catheter *(c)*, and two detached silicone-filled balloons 12mm in diameter *(d)*.

Figure 2.4.5. Hieshima balloon system.

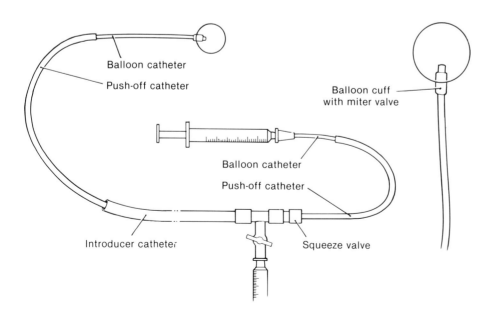

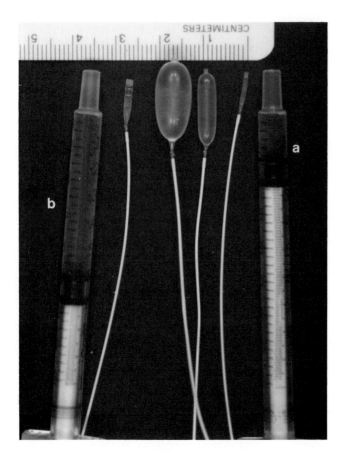

Figure 2.4.6. Side-by-side comparison of inflated and uninflated diameters of 1mm and 2mm silicone balloons (Mini-Balloons) with filling volume indicated by 1ml syringes: 0.15ml for 1mm balloon *(a)* and 0.6ml for 2mm balloon *(b)*.

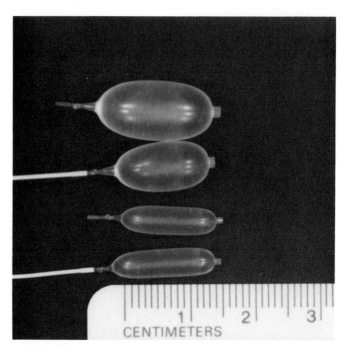

Figure 2.4.7. Side-by-side comparison of inflated dimensions of 1mm and 2mm silicone Mini-Balloons.

polyethylene catheter (Bard–Parker) or 6.5Fr reinforced-wall, nontapered catheter (Cook, Inc)). The larger 2mm OD (0.079-inch) balloon passes through a 0.096-inch (8.8Fr) thin-walled nontapered polyethylene catheter (Cook) (Fig. 2.4.6). The thin-walled catheters can be shaped over steam to the appropriate configuration for selective catheterization; the reinforced-wall torque catheters are preshaped.

The balloon is mounted on a 2Fr radiopaque polyurethane catheter. Catheter and balloon are connected via a metal cannula. The balloon has a pressure cuff over the cannula that seals upon detachment (Fig. 2.4.7).

The detachment mechanism is activated as the balloon pressure rises sharply when the expanding balloon encounters counterpressure from the vessel wall during filling (Fig. 2.4.8A). The cuff portion loosens slightly around the cannula, permitting fluid to exit through side-holes in the cannula (Fig. 2.4.8B). At this time, the cannula can be retracted, whereupon the excess pressure in the cuff is released momentarily, and the cuff collapses to seal the balloon (Fig. 2.4.8C). The polyurethane catheter is strong enough to transmit the necessary pullout force, which is best described as a quick manual tug on the catheter while filling pressure is maintained on the balloon. The

detachment force can be transmitted around vascular curves; however, tight curves, such as in the carotid siphon, may present an obstacle to this detachment mechanism. Under no circumstances should the pulling force lead to stretching of the balloon catheter. If this occurs, the balloon cannot be detached safely and should be deflated and repositioned. Since successful detachment with this system requires firm engagement of the balloon in the vessel, the angiographer judges the time for detachment by observing the size and shape of the balloon in the vessel, slightly tugging on the balloon catheter to see if it can be pulled out of its position and observing the amount of filler injected, which should not exceed 0.15ml for the 1mm balloon and 0.6ml for the 2mm balloon (Figs. 2.4.6 and 2.4.7). Once these criteria are met, the detached balloon can be expected to remain inflated for an indefinite time. The maximum expanded diameter of the 1mm balloon is 4mm and of the 2mm balloon up to 9mm (Fig. 2.4.6). These balloons are cylindrical to maximize contact between their surface and the embolized vessel (Fig. 2.4.7). The balloon remains cylindrical in arteries, whereas in veins with thinner walls, such as the spermatic vein, the balloon may assume an oval shape.

If the tests described above do not wedge the balloon firmly within the vessel, the balloon cannot be safely detached. Either the next larger size must be used or the procedure must be abandoned. The angiographer should therefore carefully measure the lumen of the vessel to be occluded on a conventional cut-film angiogram with allowance for magnification (usually 15–20%) before the procedure is started.

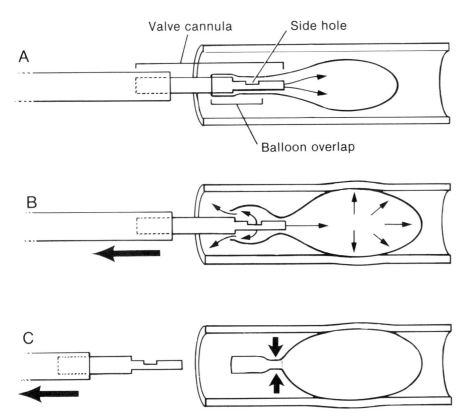

A — Valve cannula — Side hole — Balloon overlap

B

C

Figure 2.4.8. Technique of pullout Mini-Balloon detachment. **A.** Balloon expanding with liquid filler *(arrows)* within vessel lumen. Metal cannula connects balloon catheter to balloon; fluid passes through end hole of cannula into balloon. **B.** Having been filled adequately, balloon is subject to counterpressure from vessel wall, increasing intraluminal pressure, which allows fluid to exit through sidehole of valve cannula *(arrows)*. This flow widens balloon cuff and allows pullout of catheter with cannula. **C.** Detached balloon with cuff collapsed after cannula *(arrows)* has been pulled out.

The balloon filler is blood-isosmolar contrast medium, as described above. Hardening silicone liquid cannot be used, since it would soften the balloon membrane and also interfere with the detachment mechanism.

The manufacturer supplies the balloon catheter threaded through an injection port in line with a coaxial valve and an injection chamber with a Tuohy–Borst valve at its end through which the end of the catheter extends (Fig. 2.4.9). The injection chamber has a filling port for heparinized saline. Before the balloon is used, the residual air is removed from it and the catheter by filling the balloon halfway with isosmolar contrast medium and allowing the air, which is pushed ahead of the contrast medium, to diffuse out. This diffusion process requires about 10–15 minutes. Thereafter, the balloon is allowed to deflate without aspiration by letting the contrast drip out of the end of the catheter. This way, complete collapse of the balloon is avoided. It is necessary to keep the balloon in a cylindrical shape with a residual volume for proper injection and flow direction. If the balloon is totally collapsed, it tends to fold backward during injection, impairing filling and emptying.

After the balloon has been prepared, the catheter is coiled in the fluid-filled coiling chamber until only the balloon protrudes from the injection port. The balloon is covered with a protective plastic cap before the entire assembly is connected to the hub of the introducer catheter (Fig. 2.4.10). A final check of the position of the introducer catheter is made to be certain the tip will be free in the vascular lumen. The balloon is now ready for injection into the vessel to be embolized.

Injection of the balloon is carried out after opening the coaxial valve between the injection port and the coiling chamber with a half turn (Fig. 2.4.9); then, 5–10 ml of heparinized saline is injected quickly, propelling the balloon catheter through the introducer catheter. The balloon may travel a considerable distance from the tip of the introducer catheter and will then need to be pulled back into the desired position. To permit the balloon catheter to be pulled back into position, the coaxial valve is opened, and the squeeze valve at the end of the coiling chamber is loosened (Fig. 2.4.9). If the balloon needs to be further advanced, enough of the catheter is coiled within the coiling chamber, the squeeze valve is tightened, and injection is performed as described. Flow-guided balloon advancement is facilitated by partial balloon inflation. Once the balloon is in the proper position, a test inflation is carried out, followed by contrast injection through the introducer catheter to check the occlusion. This step can be repeated as often as necessary. Before final balloon inflation, it is recommended that the balloon be evacuated completely in order to determine exactly the filling volume at the time of detachment.

After the balloon catheter has been injected, the coiling chamber can be detached from the coaxial valve for ease of handling. However, the author prefers to leave it attached so that he is ready to reinject the balloon at any time. Air that has leaked into the coiling chamber during balloon catheter movements can be vented by injecting flushing solution through the filling port while holding the detached chamber upright (Fig. 2.4.11).

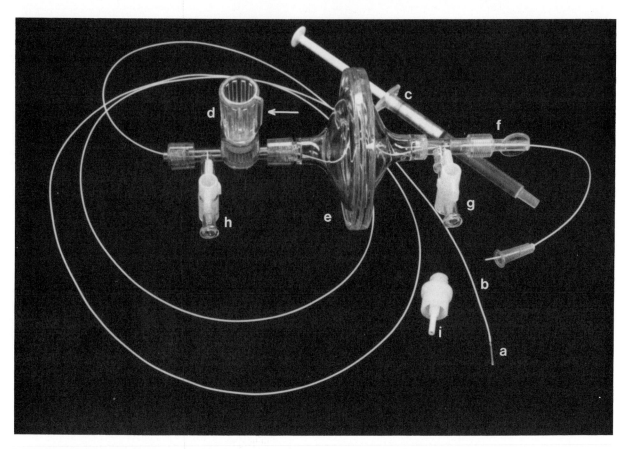

Figure 2.4.9. Mini-Balloon assembly as supplied by the manufacturer: balloon *(a)*, balloon catheter threaded through coaxial valve and coiling chamber *(b)*, 1ml syringe for balloon filling *(c)*, coaxial valve in open position *(arrow) (d)*, coiling chamber *(e)*, winged squeeze valve to hold balloon catheter in place *(f)*, filling port *(g)*, injection port *(h)*, protective cap for balloon (balloon guide) *(i)*.

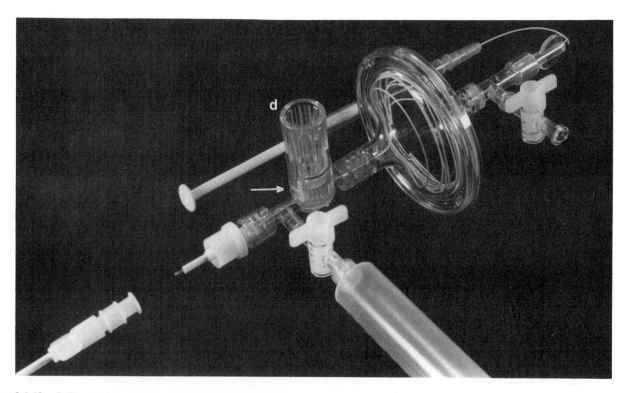

Figure 2.4.10. Balloon delivery system ready to attach to introducer catheter. Note that protective cap (balloon guide) is fitted over balloon to ease passage through hub of introducer catheter and prevent backfolding. Note coaxial valve *(d)* in closed position *(arrow)*.

118

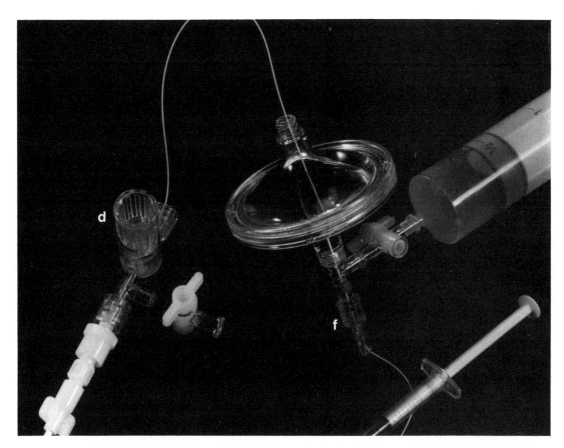

Figure 2.4.11. Purging air from coiling chamber. Winged squeeze valve *(f)* tight around balloon catheter; coiling chamber upright to push air ahead of fluid. Thereafter, chamber is ready for reconnection with coaxial valve *(d)*.

INDICATIONS FOR BALLOON EMBOLIZATION

Because the detachable balloon provides only a short occlusion, its application to most tumor embolizations and embolization of extensive arteriovenous (AV) malformations is limited. However, it is a superior tool and an agent of choice in the occlusion of AVFs and false aneurysms of medium size and larger arteries. Other short occlusion agents such as steel coils are cheaper and simpler to use and are therefore preferred when the specific advantages of a detachable balloon are not required.

In order to define a rational indication for balloon embolotherapy, the following pros and cons need to be weighed. The advantages include flow directability to vessels far distal to the introducer catheter and correctability of the occlusion, increasing the precision of embolic occlusion. These advantages must be balanced against the disadvantages, including the need for nontapered catheters and introducer sheaths, 9Fr introducer catheters for the occlusion of vessels >4mm in diameter, the complexity of the embolization system, and its cost.

If, for example, embolization of an AVF is required, the advantages of the balloon system outweigh those of the alternative methods. If, however, rerouting of hepatic artery blood flow is to be accomplished, e.g., for chemotherapy infusion, by occluding either the origin of the gas-

troduodenal artery or the left hepatic artery branch of the left gastric artery, coil occlusion is preferred as long as the catheter can be placed in the branch origin. If the vessel to be occluded cannot be selectively catheterized, flow-directable balloon embolization becomes a reasonable alternative.[14] Balloons can also be used conveniently as reliable proximal occluders after distal embolization with particles, especially since steel coils are not necessarily permanent large-vessel occluders.[15]

Once the balloon system is mastered, the radiologist is usually inclined to employ rational criteria for its use, rather than settling for technical ease with a compromise in safety and efficiency. The following are considered specific indications for balloon embolotherapy and will be discussed in detail:

1. Pulmonary AV malformations or AVFs;
2. Systemic false aneurysms and AVFs;
3. Certain systemic AV malformations;
4. Artificially created shunts;
5. Varicocele.

Secondary applications are those already mentioned in which balloon occlusion may either be combined with use of embolic particles, such as Ivalon, or with ethanol or when other methods turn out to be ineffective. Nonvascular balloon embolizations have been reported for ureters

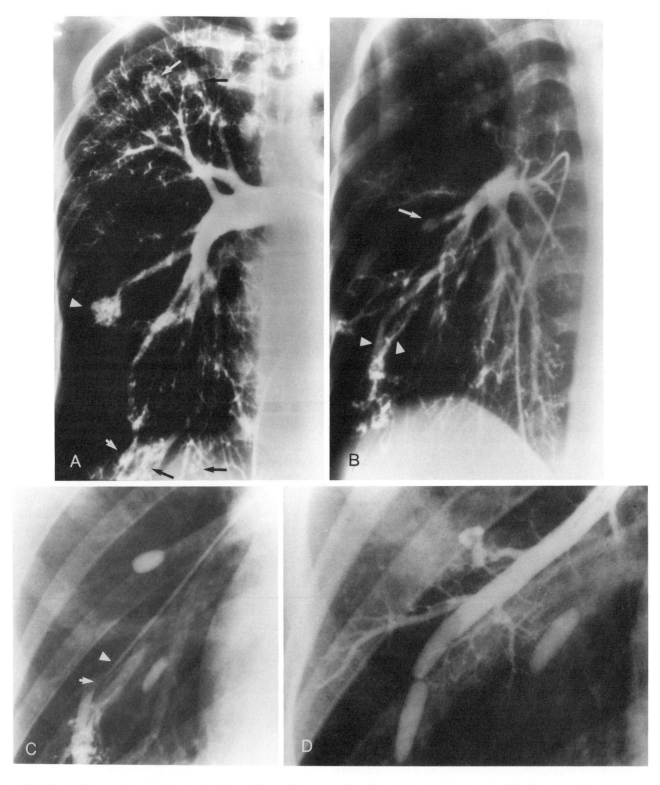

Figure 2.4.12. A 26-year-old man with chronic fatigue; PO_2 = 40mm Hg; hematocrit = 59%. Several nodules were visible on chest radiograph. **A.** Right pulmonary survey arteriogram shows several small AV malformations in basilar portion of lower and upper *(arrows)* lobes and medium-sized malformation *(arrowhead)* in lower lobe. **B.** Selective right lower lobe pulmonary arteriogram after balloon embolization of feeder artery *(arrow)* to larger AV malformation with 2mm balloon better delineates feeder arteries to smaller malformation *(arrowheads)*. **C.** A 5Fr introducer catheter in feeding artery *(arrowhead)* with balloon catheter in malformation *(arrow)* after embolization of two adjacent lesions. **D.** Immediately after embolization with 1mm balloon. **E.** After embolization, right lower lobe pulmonary arteriogram shows occlusion of all embolized lesions. In one session, PO_2 rose to 60mm Hg.

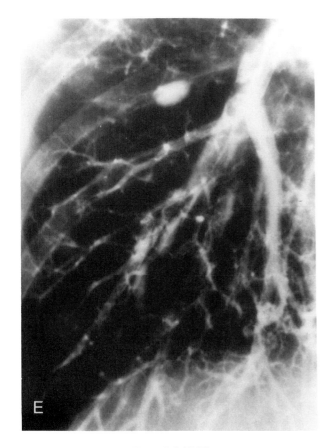

Figure 2.4.12 (E).

signs. Other clinical presentations include systemic embolization and brain abscess in approximately 10% of patients and, infrequently, severe hemoptysis.

Surgical removal has been successful for solitary or even multiple fistulae as long as the extent of loss of functioning lung tissue can be tolerated. Lobectomy or segmental resections are the usual surgical procedures.[18–20] In contrast, surgical management of patients with multiple AV malformations, in particular those with hereditary hemorrhagic telangiectasia, has limited usefulness because the natural history of this condition includes progressive development of new pulmonary AV malformations.[18,21,24]

In recent years, successful transcatheter embolization of pulmonary AV malformations has been reported.[21,22] After selective catheterization of the feeding artery, an embolic device that safely occludes the fistula is inserted. Coils have been successful in some patients.[21,22,27] However, because coils are generally not retrievable, vessel caliber and coil diameter must be estimated accurately before embolization. Even if this is done, there is still no assurance that the coil will not embolize through the fistula. Therefore, the author considers detachable balloons the embolic agent of choice for pulmonary AV malformations.[23–26] Since it is frequently impossible to occlude all the AV connections in patients with Osler–Weber–Rendu disease, the strategy is to occlude the largest lesion first. Oximetry data indicating a satisfactory increase of blood oxygen usually determine the end of the embolization procedure.

TECHNIQUE

Pulmonary arteriography must demonstrate the location, size, and inflow and outflow vessels of single or multiple pulmonary AV malformations. Cut-film studies are important for direct caliber measurements; however, rapid flow through the malformation frequently superimposes arterial and venous channels, masking the best point for embolic occlusion (Fig. 2.4.12).[29] Angled high-speed digital subtraction arteriography (DSA) (15–30 films/sec) complements cut-film arteriograms.[29] Baseline blood oximetry and pulmonary artery pressure measurements are obtained.

The caliber of the feeding artery to be embolized determines the choice of the appropriate embolization balloon(s). If the caliber of that feeding artery exceeds 9mm (the largest Mini-Balloon), latex balloons, with sizes up to 14mm, must be considered (Fig. 2.4.13). The potential use of latex balloons, an experimental device, should be specifically discussed with the referring physician, as well as with the patient, and be considered only in specific circumstances by a radiologist thoroughly familiar with this balloon system.

The embolization procedure is performed under full heparinization, with placement of an introducer catheter into the lobar or, if feasible, the segmental artery feeding the AV malformation (Fig. 2.4.12). If more than one AV malformation is to be embolized, the catheter required for

and enteric fistulae.[15,16] Because the Mini-Balloon is generally available, the following discussion is based on the use of this system unless otherwise noted.

Embolization for Pulmonary Arteriovenous Malformations and Fistulae

GENERAL CONSIDERATIONS

As do other AV malformations, pulmonary AV malformations originate from abnormal capillary development. These lesions may be single or multiple and enlarge with time.[17–20] Patients with multiple pulmonary AV malformations are likely to have hereditary hemorrhagic telangiectasis (Osler–Weber–Rendu disease).[18] Pulmonary AV malformations are located predominantly in the lower lobes and near the pleural surface.[19,20] Their important anatomic features are their almost universal development from low-pressure pulmonary, rather than systemic, arteries and the frequency of a single artery to single vein connection.[18–28] The less common type consists of multiple arterial feeders to a network of small tortuous AV connections.[28] Since the symptomatology of pulmonary AV malformations is directly related to the magnitude of the right-to-left shunting, these lesions are often referred to as pulmonary AVFs.[18–20,24] Shunt-related cyanosis and fatigue caused by progressive hypoxemia are the most frequent

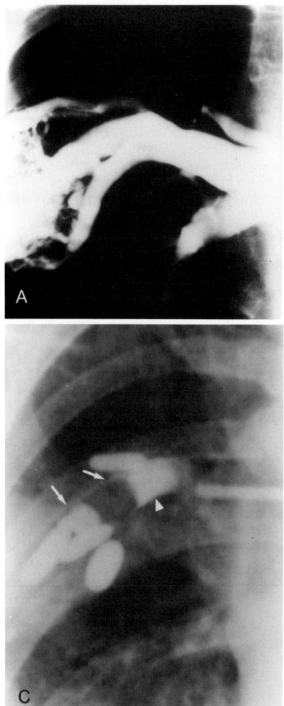

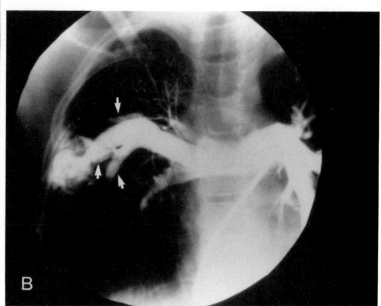

Figure 2.4.13. A 9-year-old girl with cyanosis and digital clubbing; hematocrit = 59%; right pleural-based mass seen on chest radiograph. **A.** Right pulmonary arteriogram shows several feeder arteries to large malformation in anterior segment of right upper lobe. **B.** After occlusion of smaller feeder branches with 2mm silicone balloons *(arrows)*; largest branch remained open and necessitated placement of 12mm latex balloon. **C.** In separate procedure, 12mm latex balloon was placed in largest feeder *(arrows)* and filled with silicone polymer. Contrast stasis *(arrowhead)* indicates total occlusion of AV malformation.

the largest occlusion balloon is chosen. The femoral vein is the preferred entry site, starting with placement of a self-sealing sheath to accommodate the largest catheter. The thin-walled balloon introducer catheters, particularly the 9Fr size, cannot be placed directly. Therefore, negotiation of the right side of the heart and the pulmonary bifurcation with a regular angiographic catheter or a balloon-tipped catheter, followed by exchange for the balloon introducer over a guidewire, is recommended (Fig. 2.4.14).[26–28]

Guidewire exchange is performed with the intention of placing the tip of the introducer catheter as close to the AV malformation as possible, and this requires advancing the guidewire far into the periphery for good anchoring. For the 9Fr catheter, guidewire anchoring may be insufficient. In this situation, the 9Fr catheter can be loaded over a long 5Fr balloon-tipped catheter, which must extend sufficiently beyond the 9Fr catheter to allow free negotiation through the heart and proximal pulmonary arteries.[26] The

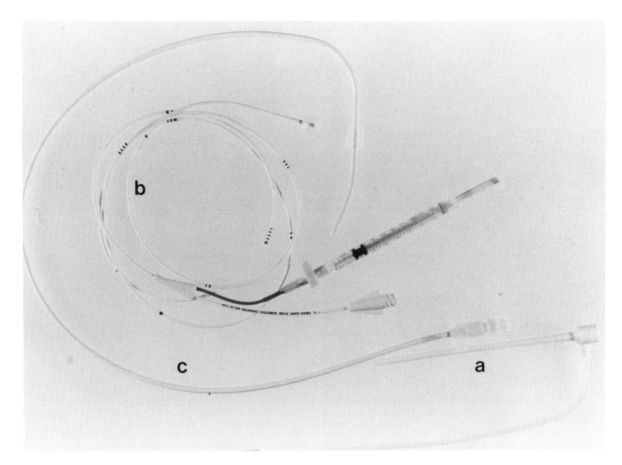

Figure 2.4.14. Introducer system for pulmonary balloon embolization. Percutaneous introducer sheath for femoral vein entry *(a)*; Swan–Ganz or Berman-type balloon catheter *(b)*; 5Fr or 8.8Fr nontapered introducer catheter *(c)*.

balloon tip is advanced as peripherally as possible, and the balloon is inflated to anchor the advancing introducer catheter (Fig. 2.4.14). Sometimes, a large-curvature (15mm) deflector wire will help position the tip of the introducer catheter in individual segmental branches. Tightly curved deflector wires are to be avoided because of the risk of kinking or other damage to the thin-walled catheter.

Once the introducer catheter is in place, definitive exploration of the embolization site is carried out, including videotape recording with freeze-framing or DSA road-mapping.[29] The latter is most useful, since it allows superimposition of the pre-embolization anatomy over the course of the embolization balloon; it also reduces substantially the amount of contrast medium required for test injections, which is particularly critical if several AV malformations are to be embolized in a single session. Oximetry and pulmonary pressure recording are repeated at this time. Meanwhile, the proper-sized embolization balloon has been prepared and is now injected to the site chosen for embolization. Sometimes, the balloon will travel through the fistula and must be retracted to the proper position; in other cases, it may stop short of the occlusion site. Then, partial inflation is applied to further flow-direct the balloon. If the balloon enters the wrong branch artery,

it is partially retracted and reinjected and the above maneuvers are applied. During these manipulations, it is of the utmost importance to avoid any air accumulation in the embolization system because of the risk of systemic, in particular cerebral, embolization.

With the balloon in the intended embolization position, a test inflation is performed to demonstrate complete occlusion. Firm fit of the balloon can be tested by slight tugging on the balloon catheter. The balloon position should be adjusted until a site is found that avoids as many side branches to normal pulmonary parenchyma as possible (Fig. 2.4.15). If a firm fit cannot be achieved, a larger balloon needs to be selected (Fig. 2.4.13). However, before this decision is made, one needs to consider that the smallest caliber of the feeding artery is usually found close to its junction with the usually much larger venous portion of the AV malformation.

Once the definitive embolization position has been found, the balloon is completely emptied as described and then filled to the required volume. Immediately before it is detached, it is observed carefully for any dislodgment while the pullout force is increased and the injection pressure on the balloon is maintained. Sometimes, the pulling force may move the artery slightly with the balloon. To differentiate this from loosening of the balloon, a test injection

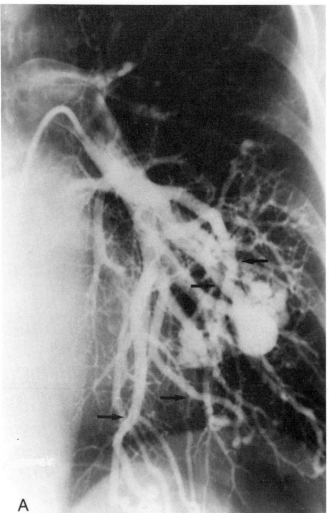

A

B

Figure 2.4.15 Embolization of lower lobe pulmonary AV malformation. **A.** Several single-feeder malformations *(arrows)*. **B.** Selective emboliza-

tion with 1mm silicone balloons *(arrows)* spared most of normal pulmonary artery branches.

is made through the introducer catheter. Once the balloon is detached, a documentation angiogram is obtained, followed by repeat oximetry and pulmonary pressure recording.

Several pulmonary AV malformations can be embolized in one session, with each individual embolization being carried out as described.[26,29] The limitations are maximum contrast dose and the total amount of time required as related to operator fatigue and the ability of the patient to cooperate. A high degree of alertness is required of the operator throughout the procedure, and it may be better to resume the embolization in a subsequent session (Fig. 2.4.13). All these procedural details should be discussed with the patient when presenting the treatment plan.

In the author's experience with embolization of multiple pulmonary AV malformations, as many as six separate procedures have been carried out to complete the embolization and to reach the therapeutic goal, which was to raise the patient's blood oxygen saturation to 90% (a par-

tial arterial oxygen pressure of 60mm Hg).[24–26,29] Definitive oximetry readings should be obtained with the patient sitting or standing in room air, since changes in blood flow distribution between the upper and lower lobes must be considered.

COMPLICATIONS

A significant risk of embolotherapy of pulmonary AV malformations is inadvertent systemic embolization, for which the detachable balloon technique provides, in the author's opinion, the best possible prevention compared to particles or steel coils. Among the author's earlier patients, there was one instance in which a balloon dislodged into a pelvic artery after passing through the AVF; this was the result of poor visibility of the occlusion point because of the juxtaposition of several AV malformations in the lower lobe region. Another risk is occlusion of normal pulmonary arteries, which may lead to a pulmonary infarction. This happened to the author in two separate procedures but was judged unavoidable due to the closeness of a normal artery branch to the most appropriate point of occlusion.[26-29] Both patients suffered transient pain and slight fever without significant morbidity.

Although the treatment of pulmonary AV malformations, particularly of multiple lesions, may present a time-consuming and demanding task for all persons involved, its successful completion is gratifying and benefits an often severely incapacitated patient whose working ability may be restored and whose life expectancy may be increased.

Systemic False Aneurysms and Arteriovenous Fistulae

These spontaneous or post-traumatic lesions may occur anywhere and may be an indication for balloon embolotherapy unless surgical repair is simpler, as it is in many extremity AVFs. Balloon embolization of lesions in the abdomen and in the retroperitoneum, which often present technical problems, will be discussed here, but this is not to say the technique is not equally effective elsewhere.[30,31]

HEPATIC ARTERY EMBOLIZATION

Among lesions in the liver, post-traumatic AVFs and false aneurysms are prime targets for balloon embolization. Hemobilia as a result of arteriobiliary fistula from iatrogenic trauma such as operation, needle biopsy, percutaneous cholangiography, and biliary drainage, is a well recognized entity.[32] The fistula is usually located near the porta hepatis (Fig. 2.4.16). Hepatic artery mycotic aneurysms may necessitate embolization to control acute rupture,[33,34] as in other areas.[35,36] Infantile hepatic hemangioendothelioma can be a rare indication for emergency embolotherapy when large-volume transhepatic shunting

leads to high-output cardiac failure. Most of these tumors regress spontaneously if the child survives. Several emergency transcatheter embolizations have been reported, including balloon embolization.[25,37,38]

The technical aspects of hepatic artery balloon embolization include careful angiographic mapping with exact localization of the false aneurysm or AVF to determine the most appropriate balloon size and catheterization approach. Flow directed balloons will not seek false aneurysms as readily as AVFs for obvious reasons, so subselective placement of the introducer catheter is frequently necessary (Fig. 2.4.16). In most instances, the 1mm silicone balloon will suffice. This will allow use of a 5Fr introducer catheter. Although the 5Fr thin-walled catheter does not offer a great deal of torque, it is adequate for catheterization from the axillary or brachial artery, analogous to placement of hepatic artery infusion catheters. An introducer catheter with a shallow double curve (H1H) serves best to enter the celiac axis downstream, aided by a steerable guidewire which will help advancing the introducer catheter into the proper hepatic artery. From there, the balloon can be floated toward the embolization site if the right hepatic artery branches are to be embolized. For left hepatic artery embolization, it is necessary to place the introducer catheter directly in the origin of the left hepatic artery; this is best accomplished again by steerable guidewires. Flow direction of the balloon may be compromised by vasospasm, which needs to be eliminated by a combination of slight catheter retraction and injection of a vasodilator such as 15–20mg of papaverine. To position the balloon, repeated partial inflations, deflations, and reinjections may be required.

In this setting, one must be aware of the balloon folding

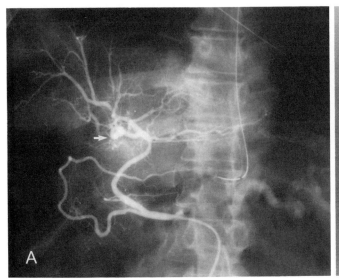
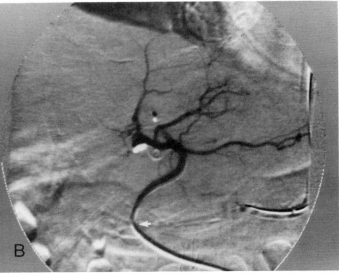

Figure 2.4.16. A 58-year-old man suffered hemobilia when stent was removed after surgical hepaticojejunostomy for benign biliary stricture. **A.** Common hepatic arteriogram shows false aneurysm of proximal right hepatic artery *(arrow)*. **B.** Digital subtraction arteriogram with balloon inflated in false aneurysm before detachment. Introducer catheter tip *(arrow)* in proper hepatic artery; all right hepatic artery branches distal to balloon are occluded. (Courtesy of Steven L. Kaufman, M.D., Johns Hopkins Hospital, Baltimore, MD.)

back over its catheter (see Ref. 29 for pictorial display), preventing adequate inflation and emptying. This problem should be suspected any time the balloon does not drain spontaneously after partial filling. The balloon will unfold, either after the balloon catheter has been pulled back or, if this does not readily occur, after the balloon has been partially filled to give it more drag to fold back in downstream flow. The latter maneuver is not advisable in low-flow situations, because the balloon may not move with the blood flow and may become impacted. If these maneuvers fail, the backfolded balloon should not be pulled into the introducer catheter, since this may shear it off. Instead, the entire assembly, including the introducer catheter, should be retracted as a unit. As soon as the balloon is in a larger vessel (common hepatic artery, celiac axis), it will spontaneously unfold. Since backfolding is most frequently encountered during maneuvering in a tight space, the need to relieve vasospasm should be appreciated.

SPLENIC ARTERY EMBOLIZATION

Lesions of splenic artery branches also can be treated. The tip of the introducer catheter can be left in the proximal splenic artery and the balloon flow directed distally.

RENAL ARTERY EMBOLIZATION

Balloon embolization of renal artery lacerations and AVFs may be one of the most common applications of small balloons.[34,39,40] Virtually any embolization technique known today has been used to treat traumatic renal hemorrhage; however, from the standpoint of tissue preservation, selective balloon embolotherapy is preferable.

Traumatic lesions include those complicating biopsy, nephrostomy, percutaneous stone extractions, anatrophic lithotomies, and nephrectomies. Most smaller branch artery lacerations obliterate spontaneously; however, interlobar or hilar branches may continue to bleed or create AVFs requiring treatment. Stump AVFs following nephrectomies may not be detected until high-output cardiac failure appears.

For balloon embolotherapy, the introducer catheter must be placed in the main renal artery or the bifurcation (Figs. 2.4.17 and 2.4.18). The balloon will, in most instances, float directly toward the lesion. Thin-walled 5Fr introducer catheters or torque catheters may be used as described above. The 1mm balloon is the size usually required; infrequently, the 2mm balloon is needed. Diagnostic arteriography in any obliquity is necessary before

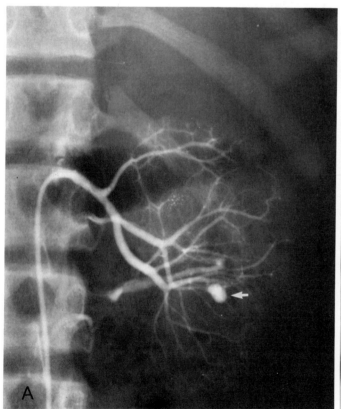
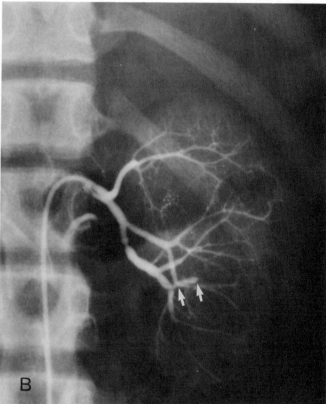

Figure 2.4.17. An 11-year-old girl with chronic glomerulonephritis; intermittent hematuria occurred eleven days after needle biopsy of left kidney. **A.** Left renal arteriogram shows AV fistula of lower pole branch *(arrow).* **B.** After embolization of branch artery with 1mm silicone balloon *(arrows),* fistula is occluded. Introducer catheter remained at renal artery bifurcation. Note spasm ring in lower pole artery.

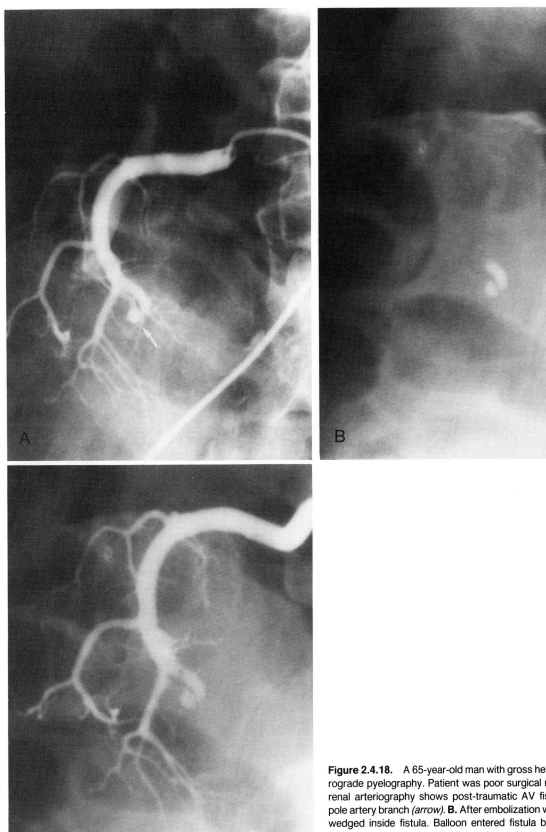

Figure 2.4.18. A 65-year-old man with gross hematuria after retrograde pyelography. Patient was poor surgical risk. **A.** Selective renal arteriography shows post-traumatic AV fistula from lower pole artery branch *(arrow)*. **B.** After embolization with 1mm balloon wedged inside fistula. Balloon entered fistula by flow direction; introducer catheter remained in main renal artery *(arrowhead)*. **C.** Postembolization arteriogram via introducer catheter shows occlusion of fistula and some adjacent renal artery branches.

embolization to demonstrate the course of the artery and the position of the side branches to the lesion. For a larger AVF, it is important to know that the lesion is no larger than the largest balloon available.

Unlike low-pressure pulmonary AV malformations, flow through systemic AVFs can exert a tremendous pulling force on the balloon during inflation, resulting in spontaneous detachment and pulmonary embolization. It is important to realize that spontaneous detachment occurs before the balloon is able to reach its fully inflated size and occlude the fistula. Therefore, blood flow needs to be reduced before balloon embolization. In the author's experience, this is definitely required in AVFs larger than 3mm. Flow reduction is accomplished by placing a nondetachable balloon catheter upstream and impeding the flow just enough to allow flow direction and determination of balloon occlusion. Alternatively, a stainless-steel spider can be placed first, to form a baffle for the balloon behind it.

In postnephrectomy stump AVFs (renal artery to renal vein or inferior vena cava), the arterial stump may not allow flow reduction maneuvers, so it may be impossible to treat such fistulae with a detachable balloon. Surgical ligation can be helped by leaving a nondetachable occlusion balloon in place until the surgeon is ready to place the ligature, at which time the radiologist deflates the balloon and pulls the catheter out.[41] In this way, potentially serious intraoperative bleeding can be avoided.

As previously indicated, embolization of AVFs with detachable balloons should always be carried out under full heparinization. The AVFs of interlobar or smaller branch arteries are readily embolized with the 1mm balloon which, in most instances, will readily follow the flow and can be detached close to or in the fistula, occluding a minimum of parenchymal branches (Fig. 2.4.18).

RETROPERITONEAL AND PELVIC ARTERY EMBOLIZATION

In the retroperitoneum and pelvis, a balloon embolization for arterial lesions is approached first with a standard diagnostic catheterization technique, for which the 6.5Fr torque catheters are most suitable. In lumbar and intercostal arteries, some lesions may be closer than 1cm to the origin of the aorta; in such cases, available balloons are too long to fit into the proximal limb. Pre-embolization arteriography should therefore include oblique views to reveal the true length of the lumbar artery, which curves posteriorly from its origin on the aorta. One may need a suitably shaped latex balloon or a shorter Hieshima silicone balloon (Table 2.4.1). Lesions in the more distal distribution of these arteries are reached through flow direction, which can negotiate even sharp turns (Fig. 2.4.19).[36]

Post-traumatic pelvic AVFs usually require flow reduction. For this purpose, crossover nondetachable balloon occlusion of the proximal internal iliac artery is preferred; however, circumstances may call for temporary crossover or ipsilateral retrograde occlusion of the common iliac

artery. Alternatively, as previously discussed, a steel spider may be placed in the fistula in front of the balloon.[42]

Systemic Arteriovenous Malformations

An AV malformation can be treated only by excluding the nidus from the circulation; otherwise collateral channels will develop promptly. A particularly complex situation exists in pelvic AV malformations, where multiple feeders are the rule and numerous potential collaterals are present.[25,43] These lesions become clinically apparent through bleeding, local pain, or high-output cardiac failure. Embolotherapy with detachable balloons is indicated only as a palliative procedure to close large AV shunts[25]; embolizing with multiple balloons in an attempt to eradicate the lesion is futile. Before balloon embolization, the same careful diagnostic mapping is required as for other areas to determine the approach to, and the diameter of, the AVF to be occluded.

Should a balloon detach prematurely despite flow reduction measures and embolize to the lung, an attempt can be made either to rupture it by percutaneous thin-needle puncture or to retrieve it with a basket. One should consider, however, that in otherwise normal lungs even a 5mm balloon will in all likelihood not cause symptoms if left untouched.[44]

Embolization of the Internal Spermatic Vein for Varicocele

GENERAL CONSIDERATIONS

Balloon embolization is one of several methods for nonoperative occlusion of the internal spermatic vein in patients with varicocele (Chapter 2, Part 3).[45-49] The clinical presentation, pathology, and pathophysiology of varicocele have been described in several articles[50-52]; the present discussion is limited to the technical aspects of balloon embolotherapy. Briefly, the purpose of treatment is prevention of retrograde blood flow in the right or left internal spermatic vein and its branches, which interferes with spermatogenesis and is often associated with a clinically evident varicocele.

Left-sided varicoceles are found more frequently than bilateral ones or isolated right-sided varicoceles. The left internal spermatic vein always enters the left renal vein (Fig. 2.4.20), although duplications of the left renal vein and circumaortic rings will occasionally be encountered.[53-55] The left spermatic vein is best approached by selective catheterization with a wide "U"-shaped catheter. The catheter tip searches the inferior aspect of the renal vein for the orifice of the left internal spermatic vein, which enters at a variable distance from the vena cava. Anatomic variations are frequent (summarized in Ref. 56). The closer the inferior vena cava runs to the paraspinal lumbar veins, the more likely are direct communications with those

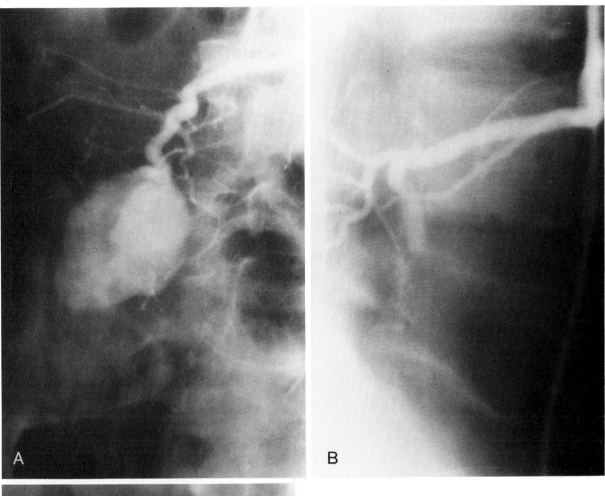

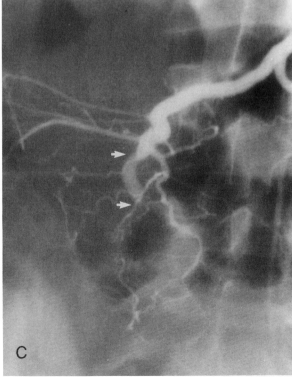

Figure 2..4.19. A 27-year-old male renal allograft recipient with severe right flank pain radiating to groin with swelling of groin. There was no history of trauma. **A.** Selective right fourth lumbar arteriogram reveals enlargement of artery and large bleeding false aneurysm. **B.** Lateral view shows typical angled course of lumbar artery, with introducer catheter remaining in arterial orifice. Flow carried balloon into neck of false aneurysm, occluding it. **C.** Antero-posterior view shows 1mm silicone balloon (*arrows*) occluding aneurysm.

Figure 2.4.20. Internal spermatic vein with insufficiency of valves on both left *(LISV)* and right *(RISV)*, producing bilateral varicocele. Region between arrows on RISV and LISV is most common single-channel site for embolization with single balloon. Left *(LESV)* and right *(RESV)* external spermatic vein.

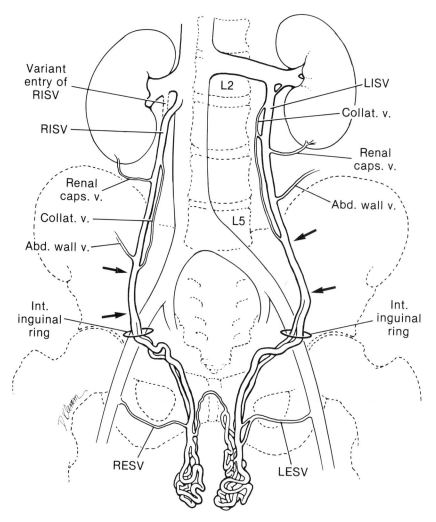

veins.[54] Two consistent branch veins of the spermatic vein, one to the renal capsule and one to the left abdominal wall, are found in the mid to lower lumbar region.[54] The mid-iliac portion of the spermatic vein is the most common single-channel segment.[45,55] Above the inguinal canal, the vein usually divides into two or three branches; therefore, the preferred place for balloon embolotherapy is the single-channel segment in the mid-iliac region (Fig. 2.4.20).

TECHNIQUE

To gauge the venous caliber properly and to determine the anatomy, a single-film venogram is obtained, which, in a typical insufficient spermatic vein, should show the vein and collaterals from the left renal vein down to the inguinal area. There is no need to film or to observe fluoroscopically the spermatic vein distal to the pubic ramus.[47] The testicle is shielded by a leaded wrap throughout the procedure.

In most patients with clinically evident varicoceles, an insufficient vein 5–8mm in diameter will have to be occluded; this requires the 2mm balloon. The angiographer needs to study carefully all collateral channels and place the balloon distal to any communication that could allow collateral retrograde flow (Fig. 2.4.21).

For balloon embolotherapy, the introducer catheter

must be firmly placed within the orifice of the spermatic vein, although it does not have to be introduced any further distally (Figs. 2.4.21 through 2.4.23). Since the initial diagnostic catheter is exchanged for the 8.8Fr introducer catheter in most instances, the guidewire will have to be advanced well into the vein to allow sufficient anchoring for the advancing introducer catheter. This introducer catheter should have a gentle (180°) curve. Frequently, despite careful maneuvering, venospasm results during the exchange. It should be allowed to resolve before balloon injection and embolization, because, in the author's experience, the complication of pulmonary balloon embolization occurred only after the balloon was placed into a spastic spermatic vein.[47] The best method to brake spasm, in the author's experience, has been slow infusion of body temperature saline into the vein. When spasm has resolved, the embolization balloon can be injected and usually travels down to the inguinal canal. It is positioned and test inflated as described previously (Fig. 2.4.22). In the venous system, the balloon may assume an oval shape due to the more compliant venous wall. Expect movement of the vein when tugging on the balloon to test firm fit. The venous occlusion site is documented on a photospot film.

The right internal spermatic vein typically enters the

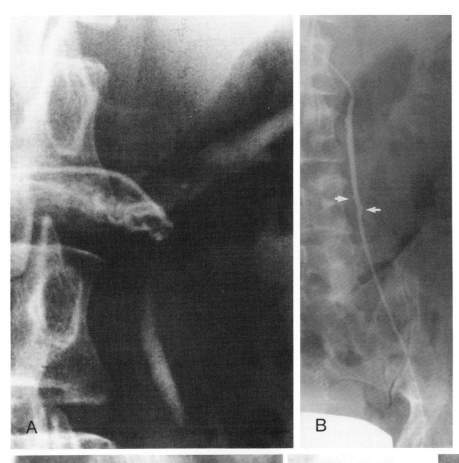

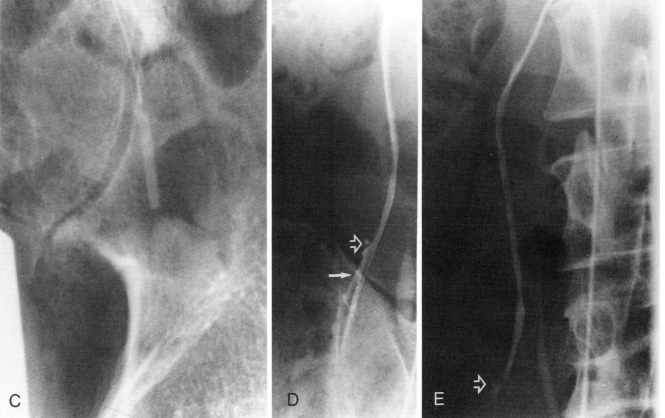

Figure 2.4.21. A 31-year-old subfertile man with small varicoceles bilaterally. **A.** Semiselective left-sided internal spermatic venogram shows narrow orifice and reflux; there is no proximal valve. **B.** Selective left-sided internal spermatic venogram via 5Fr introducer catheter shows valveless vein with retrograde flow. Small protrusions from lumen *(arrows)* indicate branch and collateral venous entries, which could cause recurrence if occlusion balloon is placed proximally. Note testicular shield over symphysis. **C.** A 1mm silicone balloon in intrapelvic portion of vein for definitive occlusion. **D.** Selective right-sided internal spermatic venogram shows reflux to level of iliac crest in single-channel vein. Occluding agent needs to be placed in each branch vein or above bifurcation *(arrow)* and below branch vein entry *(open arrow)*. **E.** After embolization of each of two small-caliber branch veins twice with 0.2ml of ethanol through open-end guidewire; occlusion at level of bifurcation and below branch vein entry *(open arrow)*.

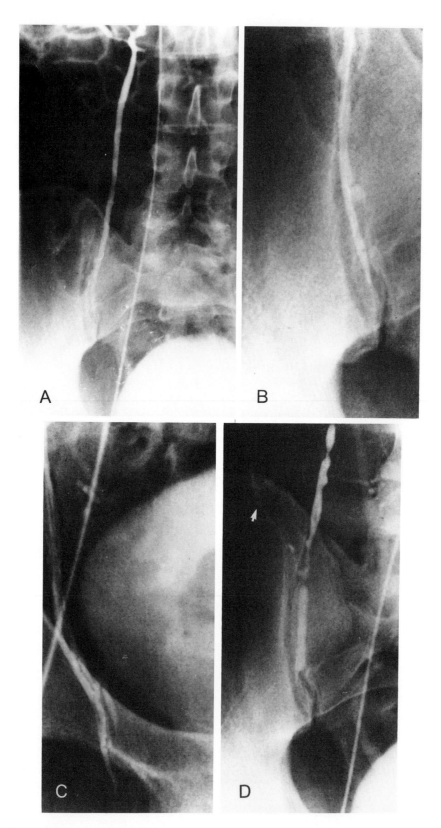

Figure 2.4.22. A 26-year-old man with recurrent right-sided varicocele along with decreased sperm count after bilateral suprainguinal internal spermatic vein ligation. **A.** Right single channel internal spermatic vein arising from lower pole renal vein is valveless with slow retrograde flow. **B.** Severe spasm after insertion of open-end guidewire into distal internal spermatic vein, preventing reflux; this reaction should not be misread as effective distal ligation. **C.** After relief of spasm, distal filling shows suprainguinal bifurcation of vein. **D.** Occlusion of internal spermatic vein after embolization with 1mm silicone balloon in typical area proximal to bifurcation and distal to renal capsular vein *(arrow)*.

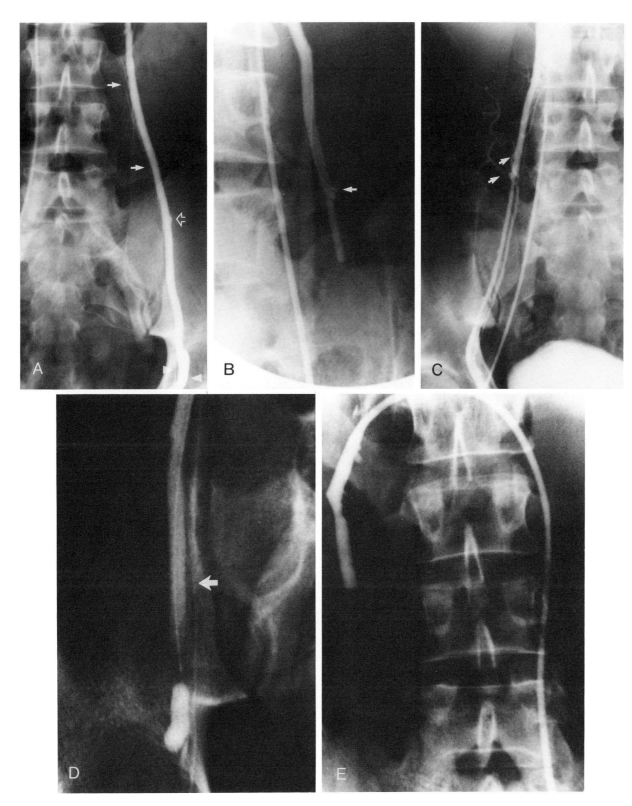

Figure 2.4.23.   A 28-year-old man with bilateral varicoceles and subfertility. **A.** Left-sided internal spermatic venogram via 8.8Fr introducer catheter in vein orifice shows typical valveless vein with retrograde flow. Small proximal collateral vein *(arrows)*. Branch vein entry below iliac crest *(open arrow)*; bifurcation above inguinal canal and distal collateral vein *(arrowheads)*. **B.** Balloon distal to branch vein inflow *(arrow)*. **C.** Right-sided internal spermatic venogram shows smaller caliber right-sided vein with several collateral channels and renal capsular branches *(arrows)*. **D.** Balloon distally does not occlude collateral channel *(arrow)*, which could allow recurrence. **E.** Proximal placement of balloon to occlude collateral inflow. This balloon alone would not have prevented retrograde flow from renal capsular veins, which is blocked by distal balloon. (Courtesy of Steven L. Kaufman, M.D., Johns Hopkins Hospital, Baltimore, MD.)

anterolateral aspect of the inferior vena cava caudad to the right renal vein. In about 10% of patients, however, the vein enters the right renal vein or a lower pole branch vein. Collateral veins and variations are at least as common, if not more so, on the right side than on the left.[55]

Even in patients with clinically evident right-sided varicocele, the right spermatic vein is usually smaller than the left. Therefore, a nontapered, preshaped high torque catheter should be used initially to enter the vein which is in many instances sufficient to carry out embolization with the 1mm balloon. In this way, vasospasm associated with catheter exchange can be avoided. As on the left side, the preferred place for right-sided balloon embolization is in the mid-pelvic region, where most of the collaterals will have re-entered the main channel (Fig. 2.4.21).

Collateral veins occasionally require separate embolization and may be difficult to catheterize. Any collateral veins that could bypass the balloon need to be embolized during the initial procedure in order to prevent recurrence by progressive enlargement of these channels (Figs. 2.4.21 through 2.4.23). If the balloon introducer catheter cannot enter these veins, an open-ended guidewire with a steerable tip can be advanced into the collateral vein, which is then embolized with ≤5ml of ethanol (Fig. 2.4.21). During alcohol injection, the patient will experience pain, which relents within 10–15 minutes; during this time, intravenous analgesics should be given. Otherwise, the embolization procedure is largely painless except during periods of vasospasm, when a dull lumbar pain may be felt. The entire embolization procedure is carried out on an outpatient basis, and the patient is allowed full physical activity after 24 hours.

Despite careful embolization technique, 5–7% of patients have recurrences, usually through collaterals that have not appeared on initial and postembolization venography.[49,57,58] Repeat venography and embolization are usually successful in these instances. Balloon embolization may not be required; ethanol or small coils may suffice to occlude these collateral channels.

Effective treatment of varicocele may not improve spermatogenesis enough to generate offspring, which is, after all, the most frequent reason for the treatment. However, for patients with fertility problems, treatment of varicocele may be the only chance for improvement, and, given the minimal invasiveness of embolotherapy, this procedure appears to present an acceptable risk. With shielding applied throughout the procedure, total radiation exposure to the testicle should not exceed 50 mrem.[58]

References

1. Serbinenko FA: Balloon catheterization and occlusion of major cerebral vessels. *J Neurosurg* 1974;41:125–145
2. Debrun G, Lacour P, Caron JP, et al: Inflatable and released balloon technique: experimentation in dog—application in man. *Neuroradiology* 1975;9:267–271
3. Kerber C: Balloon catheter with a calibrated leak. *Radiology* 1976;120:547–550
4. Laitinen L, Servo A: Embolization of cerebral vessels with inflatable and detachable balloons. *J Neurosurg* 1978;48:307–308
5. DiTullio MV, Rand RW, Frisch E: Detachable balloon catheter: its application in experimental arteriovenous fistula. *J Neurosurg* 1978;48:717–723
6. Taki W, Handa H, Yamagata S, et al: Embolization and superselective angiography by means of balloon catheters. *Surg Neurol* 1979;12:7–14
7. White RI Jr, Kaufman SL, Barth KH, et al: Embolotherapy with detachable silicone balloons: technique and clinical results. *Radiology* 1979;131:619–627
8. Hieshima GB, Grinnell VS, Mehringer CM: A detachable balloon for therapeutic transcatheter occlusions. *Radiology* 1981;138:227–228
9. Debrun G, Lacour P, Caron JP, et al: Detachable balloon and calibrated-leak balloon techniques in the treatment of cerebral vascular lesions. *J Neurosurg* 1978;49:635–649
10. White RI Jr, Ursic TA, Kaufman SL, et al: Therapeutic embolization with detachable balloons: physical factors influencing permanent occlusion. *Radiology* 1978;126:521–523
11. Barth KH, White RI Jr, Kaufman SL, Strandberg JD: Metrizamide, the ideal radiopaque filling material for detachable silicone balloon embolization. *Invest Radiol* 1979;14:35–40
12. Kaufman SL, Strandberg JD, Barth KH, et al: Therapeutic embolization with detachable silicone balloons: long term effects in swine. *Invest Radiol* 1979;14:156–161
13. Debrun G: Balloon catheter techniques in neuroradiology, in Athanasoulis CH, et al (eds): *Interventional Radiology*. Philadelphia, WB Saunders, 1983, pp 707–730
14. White RI Jr: Embolotherapy with detachable balloons. In Abrams HA (ed): *Interventional Techniques*. Philadelphia, WB Saunders, 1983, pp 2211–2222
15. Jhaveri HS, Gerlock AJ, Ekelund L: Failure of steel coil occlusion in a case of hypernephroma. *AJR* 1978;130:556–557
16. Gunther R, Klose K, Alken P: Transrenal ureteral occlusion with a detachable balloon. *Radiology* 1982;142:521–523
17. Pace R, Rankin RN, Finley RJ: Detachable balloon occlusion of bronchopleural fistula in dog. *Invest Radiol* 1983;18:504–506
18. Dines DE, Arms RA, Bernatz PE, Gomes MR: Pulmonary arteriovenous fistulas. *Mayo Clin Proc* 1974;49:460–465
19. Lindskog GE, Laebow A, Hausel H, Janzen A: Pulmonary arteriovenous aneurysm. *Ann Surg* 1959;132:591–610
20. Gomes MR, Bernatz PE, Dines DE: Pulmonary arteriovenous fistulas. *Ann Thorac Surg* 1969;7:582–593
21. Castañeda–Zúñiga WR, Epstein M, Zollikofer C, et al: Embolization of multiple pulmonary artery fistulas. *Radiology* 1980;134:309–310
22. Jonsson K, Hellekant C, Olsson O, Holen O: Percutaneous transcatheter occlusion of pulmonary arteriovenous malformation. *Ann Radiol* 1980;23:335–337
23. White RI Jr, Barth KH, Kaufman SL, Terry PB: Detachable silicone balloons: results of experimental study and clinical investigations in hereditary hemorrhagic telangiectasia. *Ann Radiol* 1980;23:338–340
24. Terry PB, Barth KH, Kaufman SL, White RI Jr: Balloon embolization for treatment of pulmonary arteriovenous fistulas. *N Engl J Med* 1980;302:1189–1190
25. Kaufman SL, Kumar AAJ, Roland JMA, et al: Transcatheter embolization in the management of congenital arteriovenous malformations. *Radiology* 1980;137:21–29
26. Barth KH, White RI Jr, Kaufman SL, et al: Embolotherapy

of pulmonary arteriovenous malformations with detachable balloons. *Radiology* 1982;149:599–605

27. Taylor BG, Cockerill EM, Manfredi F, Klatte EC: Therapeutic embolization of the pulmonary artery in pulmonary arteriovenous fistula. *Am J Med* 1978;64:360–365

28. Knudson RP, Alden ER: Symptomatic arteriovenous malformation in infants less than six months of age. *Pediatrics* 1979;64:238–241

29. White RI Jr, Mitchell SE, Barth KH, et al: Angioarchitecture of pulmonary arteriovenous malformations: an important consideration before embolotherapy. *AJR* 1983;140:681–686

30. Dublin AB, Lantz BMT, Link DP: Video dilution technique evaluation of an arteriovenous fistula: monitoring detachable balloon embolization. *AJR* 1981;137:1249–1250

31. Barth KH, Kumar AJ, Kaufman SL, White RI Jr: Therapeutic embolizations in the extracranial head and neck region using a new detachable balloon system. *Fortschr Röntgenstr* 1980;133:409–415

32. Franklin RH, Bloom WF, Schoffstall RO: Angiographic embolization as the definitive treatment of posttraumatic hemobilia. *J Trauma* 1980;20:702–705

33. Porter LL, Houston MC, Kadin S: Mycotic aneurysms of the hepatic artery: treatment with arterial embolization. *Am J Med* 1979;67:695–701

34. Marshall FF, White RI Jr, Kaufman SL, Barth KH: Treatment of traumatic renal arteriovenous fistulas by detachable silicone balloon embolization. *J Urol* 1979;122:237–239

35. Renie WA, Rodeheffer RJ, Mitchell S, et al: Balloon embolization of a mycotic pulmonary artery aneurysm. *Am Rev Respir Dis* 1982;126:1107–1110

36. Stewart JR, Barth KH, Williams GM: Ruptured lumbar artery pseudoaneurysm: an unusual cause for retroperitoneal hemorrhage. *Surgery* 1983;93:592–594

37. Stanley P, Grinnell VS, Stanton RE, et al: Therapeutic embolization of infantile hepatic hemangioma with polyvinyl alcohol. *AJR* 1983;141:1047–1051

38. Burrows PE, Rosenberg HC, Chuang HS: Diffuse hepatic hemangiomas: percutaneous transcatheter embolization with detachable silicone balloons. *Radiology* 1985;156:85–88

39. Kadir S, Marshall FF, White RI Jr, et al: Therapeutic embolization of the kidney with detachable silicone balloons. *J Urol* 1983;129:11–13

40. Grinnell VS, Hieshima GB, Mehringer CM, et al: Therapeutic renal artery occlusion with a detachable balloon. *J Urol* 1981;126:223–237

41. Kadir S, Kaufman SL, Barth KH, White RI Jr: *Selected Technique in Interventional Radiology*. Philadelphia, WB Saunders, 1982

42. Grinnell VS, Flanagan KG, Mehringer MC, Hieshima GB: Occlusion of large fistulas with detachable valved balloons and the spider. *AJR* 1983;140:1259–1261

43. Palmaz JC, Newton TH, Reuter SH, Bookstein JJ: Particulate intraarterial embolization in pelvic arteriovenous malformations. *AJR* 1981;137:117–122

44. Florentine M, Wolfe RR, White RI Jr: Balloon embolization to occlude a Blalock-Taussig shunt. *J Am Coll Cardiol* 1984;3:200–202

45. Kunnen M: New technique for embolization of the internal spermatic vein: intravenous tissue adhesive. *Fortschr Röntgenstr* 1980;133:625–629

46. Formanek A, Rusnak B, Zollikofer C, et al: Embolization of the spermatic vein for treatment of infertility: a new approach. *Radiology* 1981;139:315–321

47. White RI Jr, Kaufman SL, Barth KH, et al: Occlusion of varicoceles with detachable balloons. *Radiology* 1981;139:327–334

48. Seyferth W, Jecht E, Zeitler E: Percutaneous sclerotherapy of varicocele. *Radiology* 1981;139:335–340

49. Barth KH, Kaufman SL, Kadir S, White RI Jr: Treatment of varicoceles by embolization with detachable balloons, in Jecht EW, Zeitler E (eds): *Varicocele and Male Infertility*. Berlin, Springer, 1982

50. MacLeod J: Further observations on the role of varicocele in human male infertility. *Fertil Steril* 1969;20:545–563

51. Klosterhalfen H, Schirren C, Wagennecht LV: Pathogenesis and therapy of varicocele. *Urologe* 1979;18:187–192

52. Cockett ATK, Takihara H, Cosentino MJ: The varicocele. *Fertil Steril* 1984;41:5–11

53. Lien HH, Kolbenstvedt A: Phlebographic appearances of the left renal and left testicular veins. *Acta Radiol [Diagn]* 1977;18:321–332

54. Riedl P: Selective phlebography and catheter sclerosation of the spermatic vein in primary varicocele. *Wien Klin Wochenschr* 1979;91(Suppl 99):3–20

55. Comhaire F, Kunnen G, Nahoum C: Radiological anatomy of the internal spermatic vein(s) in 200 retrograde venograms. *Int J Androl* 1981;4:379–387

56. Gonzalez R, Narayan N, Castañeda–Zúñiga WR, Amplatz K: Transvenous embolization of the internal spermatic vein for the treatment of varicocele scroti. *Urol Clin North Am* 1982;9:177–184

57. Kaufman SL, Kadir S, Barth KH, et al: Mechanisms of recurrent varicocele after balloon occlusion or surgical ligation of the internal spermatic vein. *Radiology* 1983;147:435–440

58. Walsh PC, White RI Jr: Balloon occlusion of the internal spermatic vein for the treatment of varicoceles. *JAMA* 1981;246:1701–1702

Part 5. Ablation with Absolute Ethanol

—Gary J. Becker, M.D., Robert W. Holden, M.D., Heun Y. Yune, M.D., and Eugene C. Klatte, M.D.

The current body of knowledge concerning absolute ethanol as an embolic agent derives largely from uncontrolled clinical applications. However, laboratory work in animals by several investigators has begun to elucidate important basic information, particularly regarding the mechanisms of action.[1–11] A large body of clinical information about other embolic agents[12–17] has been applied to the development of techniques for clinical use of absolute ethanol. This chapter encompasses the indications, contraindications, methods of administration, results, and complications of the use of absolute ethanol in interventional radiology. References to animal work are included to enlighten the reader about current understanding of the mechanisms of action of this embolic agent.

RENAL EMBOLIZATION
Animal Studies

The use of particulate embolic agents, autologous clot, and coils is complicated by difficulties in handling the agents, incomplete infarction of target tissue, vascular recanalization, and inadvertent reflux that occludes nontarget vessels. These problems, which are discussed in Chapter 2, Part 1 of this volume, led Ellman et al. to study the potential for transcatheter therapeutic infarction of the kidney with absolute ethanol.[1] In their canine study, transcatheter injection of high concentrations of ethanol into the renal artery produced complete renal infarction. This dramatic result was attributed to the protein-denaturing property of ethanol administered in high concentration and to vascular thrombosis attributable to endothelial damage. Low concentrations (10%) did not damage the kidney, and reflux of ethanol into the aorta in concentrations as high as 10% produced no damage.

In a study of therapeutic renal infarction in eight rabbits and one pig, Ekelund et al. found absolute ethanol easy to administer, reliable in producing complete renal infarction with renal artery thrombosis, and entirely safe despite a small amount of reflux into the aorta that may occur with slow renal artery injection. Indeed, they injected 2ml of absolute ethanol directly into the abdominal aorta in one animal and found no injury.[2] For canine renal artery embolization, Buchta et al. infused 0.2ml/kg of absolute ethanol at rates of 1–2ml/sec. Angiograms showed complete vascular occlusion.[3] Light and electron microscopic studies showed glomerular necrosis, a proteinaceous precipitate in Bowman's capsules, and vascular congestion without thrombosis, changes that were thought to represent the effect of direct toxicity to the cells rather than thrombosis-induced hypoxia. The 1ml/sec injection rate produced necrosis in approximately 50% of the glomeruli, whereas the 2ml/sec injection produced necrosis in all glomeruli.

Recently, Ellman et al. studied more thoroughly the light and electron microscopic changes in the kidney as a function of the rate of injection of absolute ethanol.[11] In this series of elegant experiments, the authors made a number of pertinent negative and positive findings, of which the following are most important:

1. Renal artery spasm, which had been thought important in producing vascular occlusion after ethanol injection, was not demonstrable radiographically when animals were given a metrizamide-ethanol mixture.
2. Renal infarction can be produced without vascular thrombosis in heparinized kidneys made bloodless with an occlusion balloon inflated and saline infused for three minutes before ethanol administration. Vasculitis with marked pruning is found angiographically, while parenchymal necrosis and vascular injury with endothelial sloughing are demonstrable histologically.

3. With slow (<0.5ml/sec) ethanol injection, there is a high likelihood of acute major vascular occlusion, because the ethanol interacts with blood components, particularly red cells, creating denatured protein debris that embolizes within the renal vasculature. Extensive parenchymal necrosis is also observed.
4. Rapid (> 0.5ml/sec) ethanol infusion produces angiographic evidence of vasculitis without vascular occlusion, as well as histologic evidence of severe endothelial injury, and extensive parenchymal necrosis. Vascular occlusion occurs late and is a secondary phenomenon.

Human Experience

RENAL TUMORS
Published Reports

Transcatheter renal devitalization using particulate emboli, steel coils, and other agents for renal cell carcinoma has been practiced widely. Although probably not effective as primary therapy, it has proved a useful adjunct to operation and an excellent means of palliation in cases of inoperable advanced and metastatic disease.[18–22] However, when particulate agents or steel coils are used, there may be incomplete infarction of the kidney,[22] unintentional embolization of nontarget organs,[23–27] and difficulty in handling and administering the agent.[26] Greenfield et al. were the first to describe prevention of reflux of embolic materials and prevention of unintentional embolization by using a balloon occlusion catheter.[28] This technique, originally used with particulate embolic agents, has proved useful for embolization with absolute ethanol.

Klatte first reported clinical use of absolute ethanol for transcatheter renal artery occlusion in renal cell carcinoma in 1980. Subsequently, Rosenkrantz et al. reported three patients who underwent prenephrectomy embolization with absolute ethanol.[29] Following the lead of Wallace and colleagues, Rosenkrantz et al. left at least a two-day interval between the diagnostic angiogram and the embolization in an effort to minimize the risk of renal failure. They used epidural anesthesia and an ethanol dose of 0.2ml/kg of body weight, a dose that did not produce systemic toxicity in animal studies. Ethanol injection rates approximated rates of contrast injection which did not produce reflux from the renal artery into the aorta at angiography. As others did before them, Wallace and colleagues delayed nephrectomy for 10 days in an effort to maximize the potential immune response.[22] (Importantly, there are insufficient data to prove the enhanced immune response hypothesis, as discussed below.) Each embolization procedure resulted in a relatively bloodless nephrectomy. Angiographic and pathologic findings in all cases were similar to those of early animal studies: complete renal necrosis and tumor necrosis, with no evidence of thrombosis in the renal arteries. This finding is to be expected with relatively high (>0.5ml/sec) injection rates of ethanol according to the work of Ellman et al. The highest blood ethanol level attained in any of the patients was 0.07% by volume, well below legal intoxication levels. Patients experienced a postembolization syndrome similar to that which follows renal artery occlusion with other agents,[22] with nausea, vomiting, pain, and fever that generally lasted one to five days. Narcotic analgesia, antipyretics, antiemetics, and intravenous fluids were often indicated. It was this pain that led Rosenkrantz et al. to give their patients epidural anesthesia for 36–72 hours after ethanol transcatheter embolization or until patients were able to tolerate oral analgesics with minimal symptoms.

Gas was found in the tumors by computed tomography (CT) after embolization. Although this finding may appear alarming, seeming to indicate infection, Bernardino et al. have attributed it to tumor necrosis.[30] Furthermore, the experimental findings of Carroll and Walter indicate that some of the gas might actually be introduced during the embolization procedure.[31]

Ellman et al. reported successful renal ablation with absolute ethanol in six patients, two preoperatively and four palliatively, with good results and only mild postembolization syndromes.[32]

Rabe et al. infarcted 15 renal cell carcinomas and 1 angiomyolipoma with absolute ethanol.[33] Embolizations were performed for palliation of symptoms in metastatic disease (10 patients, 9 of whom improved), preoperatively to reduce blood loss during radical nephrectomy (3 patients, all of whom were alive and well without further evidence of disease 1–26 months postoperatively), or as primary therapy in 2 patients. One of these two had earlier undergone a right nephrectomy for renal cell carcinoma, so the carcinoma of the left lower pole necessitated a limited approach, which culminated in a selective lower pole embolization with absolute ethanol. The patient was alive and well four months after embolization. The second patient in whom embolization was the primary treatment was a young woman who presented with a large retroperitoneal hemorrhage due to rupture of an aneurysm in a left lower pole angiomyolipoma. After surgical evacuation of the hematoma and a second severe hemorrhage, she underwent transcatheter embolization of the tumor. The patient returned three weeks later with a large perinephric abscess, the only complication of the series. She had not been given antibiotics before embolization, had been receiving corticosteroids for an unrelated condition, and had undergone the aforementioned operation. Any or all of these factors could have contributed to the formation of the abscess. Although there is no conclusive evidence of the need for antibiotic prophylaxis, Rabe et al. recommend that broad-spectrum antibiotics be administered to all patients beginning the night before embolization and continuing for five days afterward.

Injection of ethanol through a balloon occlusion cath-

eter positioned in the midportion of the main renal artery, now universally accepted, is the technique that was used by Rabe et al. The balloon was inflated immediately before ethanol injection, remained inflated for 2 minutes, and was deflated during a 10-minute waiting period, after which the catheter was aspirated to remove residual ethanol and then cleared with saline. A repeat angiogram was performed. Although the endpoint in each case in this series was total occlusion of the main renal artery, the reader is reminded that the aforementioned study of Ellman et al. indicates that total renal infarction can be achieved without angiographic evidence of thrombus in the main or interlobar renal arteries, particularly with slow injection rates. Rabe et al. cited several potential benefits of balloon occlusion: interruption of renal blood flow, thus prolonging the contact of the ethanol with the endothelium; prevention of unintended reflux into the aorta; and effective infarction achieved by injection of ethanol into the main renal artery. The latter obviates the segmental renal artery injections frequently required with particulate embolic agents in cases requiring total renal infarction and so reduces the procedure time. Patients treated before the advent of the balloon occlusion method commonly required a subsequent embolization procedure, the need for which was determined by either ^{99m}Tc red blood cell dynamic and static imaging of renal blood flow or by contrast-enhanced CT scanning. Figures 2.5.1 and 2.5.2 are examples of renal cell carcinoma treated by transcatheter injection of absolute ethanol.

The importance of balloon occlusion became certain when Cox et al. reported two cases of left colon infarction following renal embolization with ethanol using conventional catheters.[34] The authors postulated that any ethanol that refluxed into the aorta during injection layered because of the differences in density and viscosity of ethanol and blood and that laminar flow in the aorta prevented dilution of the layered ethanol by blood. Consequently, the concentration of ethanol in the blood entering the inferior mesenteric artery must have been considerably higher than would have been expected following a midstream aortic injection (such as that used in the animal study of Ekelund et al.).[2] Clearly, one cannot simply use a standard angiographic catheter without an occlusion balloon, determine the rate of flow of contrast medium that does not produce fluoroscopic evidence of reflux, and then attempt to reproduce that injection rate for safe transcatheter renal ablation with ethanol. Balloon occlusion catheters must be used. Uflacker reported in 1986 another case of left colonic infarction, two cases of skin necrosis, and two cases of gastrointestinal bleeding, with an overall complication rate of 18%.[35]

Recently, several additional clinical series have been published.[36–39] Ekelund et al. reported 20 patients with renal cell carcinoma: 14 with locally advanced disease or distant metastases underwent embolization with ethanol for palliation of pain or hematuria, and 6 underwent

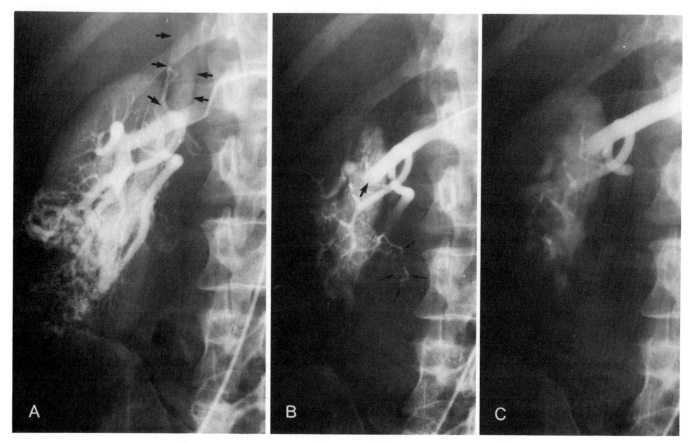

Figure 2.5.1. Patient with metastatic right renal cell carcinoma and flank pain. **A.** Selective right renal arteriogram. In addition to the neoplasm, early opacification of right renal vein and inferior vena cava *(arrows)* provides evidence of rapid shunting through tumor bed. **B.** Selective right renal arteriogram after 10ml of absolute ethanol shows occlusion of main renal artery *(large arrow)* and minimal residual tumor vascularity *(small arrows)*. **C.** After another 5ml of ethanol has been injected, there is no residual tumor vascularity. Flank pain resolved after embolization. This patient also had a metastasis in the right proximal humerus, which was managed with transcatheter Ivalon and surgical fixation.

postembolization nephrectomy.[36] Those authors found that intraprocedural pain was diminished when lidocaine was administered through the catheter before the ethanol. This has been true in the present authors' experience as well. Ekelund's group also found the postembolization syndrome to be milder with ethanol ablation than with other methods of embolization. Although some other investigators also believe this to be true, the experience has not been common to all series. Ekelund et al. found gas in the kidney and tumor on CT to be common after embolization and suggested that it probably arose from carbon dioxide from anaerobic metabolism or the release of oxygen from oxyhemoglobin.

To investigate the hypothesis that in vivo necrosis enhances the patient's immune response to the tumor, the authors evaluated the natural killer (NK) cell activity of circulating monocytes in seven of their patients before and after embolization. All patients had low baseline NK activity. After embolotherapy, NK activity increased in four patients, decreased in two, and was unchanged in one. Although the mean cytotoxicity increased, the increase was not statistically significant. Thus, these investigators found no support for the immunity enhancement hypothesis.

Klimberg et al. reported 34 patients who underwent renal ablation, 25 for renal cell carcinoma, with a balloon occlusion catheter and an average absolute ethanol dose of 15ml.[37] Of these, 21 underwent transabdominal radical nephrectomy several hours to 57 days after renal ablation. At operation, tumor was confined to the renal capsule in six patients (Stage I); had penetrated into perinephric fat but not beyond Gerota's fascia in four (Stage II); involved the renal vein, vena cava, or regional nodes in nine (Stage III); and had metastasized in two (Stage IV). The mean tumor mass was 830g and the median blood loss was 725ml. The authors were convinced that dissection had been greatly facilitated, particularly in the large vascular tumors, but this contrasts with two recent reports in which the authors question the value of preoperative angioinfarction for renal cell carcinoma.[38,39] Thus, MacErlean et al. believe that the usefulness of preoperative angioinfarction for renal carcinoma is limited to cases involving large hypervascular tumors.[38] Also, in the series of Teasdale et al., 28 patients underwent transcatheter renal embolization, 26 as prenephrectomy procedures, and the authors question the value of embolization largely because histologic examination did not demonstrate complete infarc-

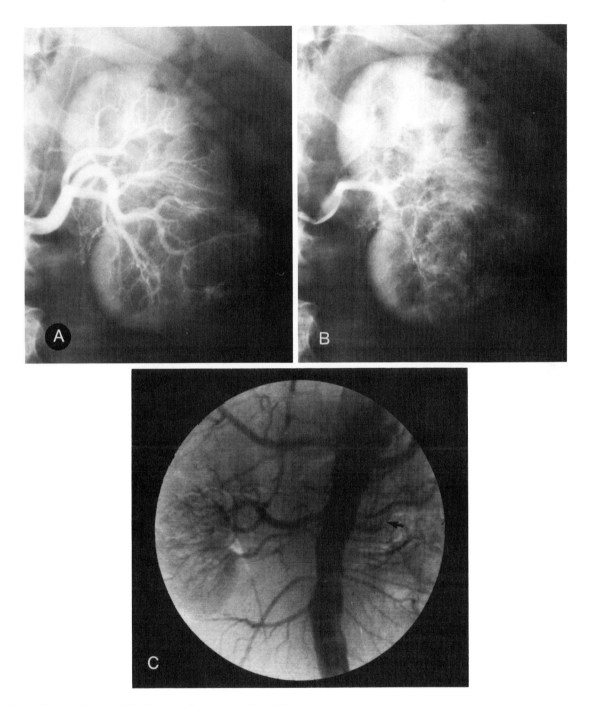

Figure 2.5.2. A 57-year-old man with left renal cell carcinoma. Early (**A**) and late (**B**) arterial phases of selective left renal arteriogram reveal moderately vascular left lower pole neoplasm. **C.** Intra-arterial digital subtraction angiography after transcatheter ethanol embolotherapy reveals occluded stump of left renal artery *(arrow)*.

tion of the tumor in 24 of the embolized kidneys, in eight of which it appeared that the tumor had completely escaped infarction.[39] However, these embolizations had been performed using gelatin sponge, stainless-steel coils, or both. Importantly, in the series of both Ekelund et al. and Klimberg et al., extensive tumor necrosis was found at histopathologic examination after transcatheter absolute ethanol renal ablation.[36,37] In both series, balloon occlusion catheters were used. Klimberg et al. also found the post-embolization syndrome to be milder with the ethanol

method than with other agents and the immediate pain of renal infarction to be diminished with pre-embolization transcatheter injection of 2ml of lidocaine. They concluded that ethanol is the embolic agent of choice in renal cell carcinoma, not only for these reasons, but also because it is inexpensive, readily available in sterile form, greatly simplifies angioinfarction, and decreases the procedure time.

Mebust et al., in their experience with 46 patients who underwent transcatheter angioinfarction for renal cell carcinoma, concluded that no reduction in operative blood loss or operating time could be documented in patients who underwent preoperative embolization.[40] However, only five of their patients had transcatheter ethanol angioinfarction, the other procedures being done with gelatin sponge or Gianturco coils. Two of their patients suffered left colon infarction after embolotherapy, but balloon occlusion was not used, and it would appear that reflux into the aorta was involved, as in the previously described cases.

Recently, Earthman et al. used subselective ethanol embolotherapy to treat two patients with a total of three hemorrhaging angiomyolipomas. They also reviewed the world literature and concluded that the method is one of the best for achieving safe, permanent, and complete ablation.[41]

Technical Guidelines

The following guidelines, derived from the collective experience of many investigators including the present authors,[42,43] should aid angiographers who use absolute ethanol embolotherapy for renal tumors.

The indications for transcatheter absolute ethanol devitalization of renal tumors are:

1. Immediate preoperative devascularization of the tumor to facilitate surgical resection. Since available data do not strongly support the enhanced immune response hypothesis, there is no need to delay the operation for 10–14 days after embolization; rather, a period of 1–6 hours is recommended, since the shorter delay decreases the duration of symptoms of the postembolization syndrome. Case selection need not be limited to patients with renal cell carcinoma; palliation and preoperative devascularization may be useful also in benign lesions such as angiomyolipoma;
2. Palliation of hematuria, fever, and other tumor-related problems such as secondary polycythemia;
3. Primary therapy in selected cases, such as subselective tumor embolization in a solitary kidney.

Pre-embolization broad-spectrum antibiotics are used by some radiologists to prevent abscess formation in the devitalized renal and tumor tissue. Those who use them tend to continue administration for approximately five days after the procedure. Most interventionalists agree that antibiotics should be used in patients with ureteronephrolithiasis or urinary tract infection.

Most investigators believe it is wise to delay the embolization procedure for at least two days after diagnostic angiography to minimize the risk of renal failure.

Pre-embolization parenteral analgesia is essential. Although epidural anesthesia may be used, the shortened postembolization syndrome attending the author's recommendations should reduce the need for it.

The technique is as follows:

1. The standard transfemoral approach should be used to position a balloon occlusion catheter in the midportion of the main renal artery beyond the origins of the inferior adrenal and gonadal arteries. (See below under "Adrenal Ablation" for an explanation of the potential ill effects of transcatheter adrenal ablation with ethanol.) To reiterate, one should avoid using a diagnostic angiographic catheter without an occlusion balloon and simply estimating the proper ethanol injection rate by fluoroscopic monitoring of an injection of contrast medium; such estimation can cause reflux of ethanol into the aorta and inferior mesenteric artery, with left colon infarction.
2. Parenteral analgesics should be used during the procedure, because the pain of renal infarction is often severe. Morphine is probably the drug of choice. In the authors' experience, as well as in that of others, 3–5ml of 2% lidocaine given through the catheter after inflation of the occlusion balloon and before ethanol administration also help reduce pain.
3. The occlusion balloon should be inflated immediately before ethanol injection and remain inflated during and for two minutes after the injection in order to increase the endothelial contact time by eliminating or markedly reducing renal blood flow. This maneuver also prevents reflux of ethanol into the aorta. Furthermore, balloon occlusion provides more effective total renal necrosis with a main renal artery injection, thereby eliminating the need for segmental injections and dramatically reducing the procedure time.
4. As much as 0.2ml of absolute ethanol (95% ethyl alcohol)/kg of body weight may be administered on the first (and often only) injection. Injection rates from <0.5ml/sec to 2.0ml/sec can be justified by available evidence, and it is likely that either of these extremes will provide the desired extensive tumor necrosis, albeit by different mechanisms.[11] These doses and rates produce total renal necrosis without creating toxic ethanol levels in either animals or humans. Importantly, the authors have used as much as 0.4ml/kg in thromboembolotherapy for gastroesophageal varices in average-sized adults without creating signs of systemic toxicity. They also frequently exceed 0.2ml/kg in patients undergoing renal ablation with ethanol when a second injection is required to complete the embolization. The authors have not measured the ethanol levels in these patients.
5. The balloon is deflated after 2 minutes, and the catheter is left undisturbed for another 10 minutes. The catheter is then aspirated to remove residual ethanol and any particulate debris and flushed with heparinized saline.
6. A repeat angiogram is obtained. In the past, the authors believed that total renal artery occlusion was the only desirable endpoint, but they now know that this angiographic picture is most likely to result from very slow ethanol injection rates (<0.5ml/sec), whereas more rapid injections (≤2ml/sec) are more likely to result in an immediate postembolization angiographic pattern of severely pruned intrarenal vessels, stasis of contrast

medium in the pruned renal artery branches, absence of the nephrographic picture obtained at diagnostic angiography, and no evidence of contrast washout.[11] It is likely that long-term follow-up of patients with the latter angiographic appearance will usually show renal artery occlusion. In any event, both of these angiographic pictures indicate that the desired result probably has been achieved. If the maximum ethanol dose has not been administered on the first attempt and the desired result has not been obtained, then the procedure may be repeated.

On follow-up CT, ultrasound, or plain film examination, gas in the infarcted kidney and tumor is to be expected. It probably is the result of tissue necrosis, air injected during the embolization procedure, or postembolization accumulation of carbon dioxide from anaerobic tissue metabolism or of oxygen from oxyhemoglobin dissociation. It should not be misconstrued as a sign of abscess. If, however, increasing gas, or gas associated with a soft tissue mass, is found, particularly in association with continued pain, tenderness, and fever, one should consider the possibility of a renal or perinephric abscess.

In the follow-up of patients not undergoing nephrectomy, continuation or recurrence of the symptoms for which the embolization was originally performed may herald the need for repeat embolization. An increase in tumor size may indicate the same. In these instances, verification of continued blood flow to the tumor may be accomplished with either a contrast-enhanced CT scan or [44m]Tc red blood cell dynamic and static images of renal blood flow.

Other possible complications include transient elevation of both systolic and diastolic blood pressure for two to four hours after embolization, temporary or irreversible renal failure, and pulmonary, or even systemic, embolization of nontarget tissues with high concentrations of ethanol.

Hypertension and Other Complications of End-stage Renal Disease

Nanni et al. reported five patients who underwent renal ablation with ethanol for uncontrolled hypertension.[45] Although the present authors do not consider renal ablation for just any case of uncontrolled hypertension, one must remember that 80% of patients with end-stage renal failure develop systemic hypertension and that those who do not respond to antihypertensive drugs or dialysis typically have elevated renal vein renin concentrations.[46] Surgical nephrectomy has been used, but given the current effectiveness of transcatheter "medical nephrectomy" with absolute ethanol, one must consider the newer technique seriously. Before embolization, Nanni et al. demonstrated elevated renal vein renin concentrations in four of their patients. Using a technique similar to the one described above, they injected smaller quantities of ethanol. Of the two patients with functioning renal allografts at the time of embolization, one eventually developed a sec-

ond acute rejection, the only complication in the small series. No hypothesis was offered to explain this occurrence. In each of the five embolized patients, the result was normotension on either no drugs or on reduced doses. Since the original publication, this series has expanded to nine patients.

Recently, Denny et al. reported a patient with severe hypertension despite a multiple-drug antihypertensive regimen and renin lateralizing to the left kidney who had a completely occluded left renal artery and only collateral flow to the left kidney at angiography.[47] After recanalization using a curved catheter and a straight guidewire, percutaneous transluminal angioplasty was performed. When this procedure failed to control the patient's hypertension, the poorly functioning kidney was embolized with ethanol. The result was normotension on a two-drug regimen. A renal scan six months later showed no flow to the left kidney.

Keller et al. recently reported their experience with renal ablation in eighteen kidneys of 10 patients with end-stage renal disease.[48] Embolic material varied from isobutyl 2-cyanoacrylate to sodium tetradecyl sulfate-soaked gelatin sponge pledgets to Gianturco spring coils to ethanol. Since 1978, ethanol has been used in all renal ablations (seven patients, thirteen renal ablations). Indications included nephrotic syndrome with massive protein loss (7 patients, 13 kidneys), poorly controlled post-transplantation, hypertension in the absence of transplant renal artery stenosis (two patients, three kidneys), and diabetic nephropathy with persistent urine leak from ureterocutaneous fistulae following pelvic irradiation (one patient, two kidneys). Desired clinical results were achieved in all cases.

Iaccarino reported results in 15 patients, with all patients improving and five being cured at 24.8 months follow-up. Permanent renal ablation was confirmed by DSA in 14 patients. No complications were reported (49).

The proper indications and potential complications of this treatment method need to be more fully elucidated. For the present, suffice it to say that some patients with complications of end-stage renal disease appear to be good candidates for renal ablation with transcatheter ethanol.

PERCUTANEOUS TRANSHEPATIC SCLEROSIS OF ESOPHAGEAL VARICES

Published Reports

Patients with bleeding esophageal varices due to cirrhosis continue to frustrate gastroenterologists, surgeons, and interventional radiologists. The involvement of interventional radiology stems from the availability of the transhepatic approach for catheterization of the portal vein, with selective catheterization and obliteration of the coronary (left gastric) and short gastric veins that are tributary to the varices.[50–55] Widrich et al., who used primarily autologous clot, balloon occlusion, and gelatin sponge soaked in sodium tetradecyl sulfate, helped to pioneer this temporizing treatment.[54] Many of their important experiences and observations are applicable to transcatheter coronary vein sclerosis with absolute ethanol. Therefore, some of their concepts are included below the recommended technique.

The aforementioned problems with particulate embolic agents led to investigation with ethanol. Ethanol provides the following additional advantages: easy handling, shortened procedure time, and apparent permanence as a vaso-occlusive agent. It is also inexpensive and readily available in sterile containers.

The first report of a series was by Yune et al. and encompassed 12 cirrhotic patients.[56] This series has now been expanded to 50 patients,[57] 13 of whom were Child Class B and 37 Class C.[58] The etiologies of the cirrhosis were alcoholic in 22, postnecrotic in 9, primary biliary in 2, and unknown in 2. All patients had endoscopic confirmation of esophageal varices within the 24 hours preceding treatment, with documentation of active or recent bleeding. The latter was suggested by the presence of fresh blood clot on the surface of prominent varices. All had varices treated by transhepatic selective catheterization and embolization with absolute ethanol via a balloon occlusion catheter whenever possible. Gelatin sponge pledgets and stainless-steel Gianturco coils were used adjunctively in several cases. Technical failure due to one or more of the following was encountered in 13 instances: severe ascites, small rigid liver, cavernous transformation of the main portal vein, and severe coagulopathy. Of these failures, 12 were in patients in Child Class C. Of the 37 patients initially treated successfully, 13 had recurrent hemorrhage, and 9 of these were Child Class C. Rebleeding, which was fatal in five of the nine patients, was due to recanalization of previously thrombosed veins in two. Nine patients died of other medical conditions despite successful variceal obliteration with ethanol. Of the 24 patients (48%) who have survived 6–36 months after the initial procedure with or without recurrent hemorrhage, only 1 was an initial technical failure. The authors concluded that patients in Child Class B are better candidates than those in Class C for this form of therapy. In addition, they concluded that Class C patients with extensive ascites and severely contracted and rigid livers pose a difficult technical challenge, which is overcome to the point of control of bleeding in only one-third of cases. Most of the long-term survivors had lessening of signs and symptoms.

Transient pain upon ethanol injection was experienced by all patients. Death due to sepsis occurred in two patients with adult respiratory distress syndrome. One patient died three days after the procedure of small bowel infarction, the cause of which was not determined. Portal vein thrombosis with cavernous transformation developed in three patients. These patients, who experienced recurrent hemorrhage as early as 3 weeks and as late as 2.5 years after initial thrombotherapy with ethanol, were treated with transendoscopic sclerotherapy or conservative medical management.

In the initial series report, Yune et al. stated that ethanol can coagulate blood cells and plasma and thus is able to occlude small branch vessels. In addition, they assumed that there is instantaneous physical injury to the vascular endothelium upon contact with ethanol which accounts for the permanent occlusion.

Fifteen patients (13 in Child Class C and 2 in Class B) reported by Keller et al. had acute hemorrhage from gastroesophageal varices which was managed by transhepatic sclerosis with absolute ethanol.[59] All were uncontrolled by Sengstaken–Blakemore tube, intravenous vasopressin, or both, and all underwent pre-embolization endoscopy, to document variceal bleeding, as well as arterial portography, to document the patency of the portal venous system. Although initial control and angiographic success were achieved in 13 patients, 2 died within 48 hours from unrelated causes. All experienced chest pain at the time of embolization and an average initial rise in portal venous pressure of 10.6mm Hg. Of the 11 with initial control who survived, 7 rebled 1 week to 13 months after embolization. Of the four who did not rebleed, two died four weeks and six months after embolization. Only two were alive (at 14 and 16 months) after embolization without evidence of rebleeding. The authors expressed their dislike for the radiolucency of ethanol and the seemingly long procedure times. They also reported a 20% frequency of portal vein thrombosis, which may have resulted from unintended reflux of ethanol into the portal vein or from the catheterization procedure itself. The problem of radiolucency is readily handled by mixing the ethanol with nonionic contrast media, which the present authors have done in a few cases. Unfortunately, these media are expensive. The ionic media cannot readily be mixed with absolute ethanol, because this often produces a precipitate that can occlude the catheter. In the present authors' experience, the problems of reflux and of procedure time are best handled by using balloon occlusion catheters. More recently, other investigators have begun to use them and have noted a decrease in the volume of ethanol needed to produce complete coronary venous occlusion.

In Uflacker's series of 11 patients with variceal bleeding treated with transhepatic ethanol, 5 had alcoholic cirrhosis, 5 had postnecrotic cirrhosis, and 1 had portal hypertension and varices of unknown cause.[60] Six were treated with ethanol alone; three with ethanol and gelatin sponge; and two with ethanol, gelatin sponge, and coils. Two patients died of recurrent hemorrhage and two died without rebleeding. The remaining seven had had no rebleeding 13–19 months after embolization. The hypothesis that distal embolic occlusion of the varices occurs with ethanol thrombotherapy could not be substantiated in those who died. Since this initial report, Uflacker has treated six more patients. Of three who rebled, two had angiographically documented portal or splenic vein thrombosis, adding to the experience of Keller and his colleagues and to our experience. All three died. The three patients who survived without rebleeding had endoscopic re-examination that showed a decrease in the size and number of varices. Of potential importance regarding Uflacker's frequency of portal vein thrombosis is the fact that he reports inserting a catheter as far as possible into the coronary vein in each instance in order to avoid reflux of ethanol into the portal vein. He did not use balloon occlusion catheters.

Using transhepatic cineportography, Sano and Kuroda demonstrated macrofistulous portopulmonary venous anastomoses in 10 of 40 cirrhotic patients with esophageal varices.[61] In most instances, the communication between the gastroesopheageal and pulmonary veins was easily identified at the level of the seventh thoracic vertebra, with drainage into the left atrium by way of the left lower lobe pulmonary veins. Portopulmonary anastomoses also occurred on the right. A serious implication of this finding is that particulate embolic materials used to obliterate varices may enter the systemic circulation. To avoid this complication, Sano and Kuroda recommend one further diagnostic study to aid in case selection: they used contrast-enhanced left atrial echocardiography, in which the fistulous communications were easily demonstrated by the real-time sonographic appearance of microbubbles in the left atrium after transcatheter injection of saline into the portal or splenic vein. Imaging of these microbubbles, cineportography, or both should help interventional angiographers identify patients unsuitable for embolization with particulate agents. The authors believe that ethanol thrombotherapy in patients with macrofistulous portopulmonary venous anastomoses may not be as fraught with the problems of systemic embolization because of the dilution that follows injection of absolute ethanol. However, it has not been proved that the concentration of ethanol reaching the left atrium and systemic circulation in these patients is harmless.

Widrich et al. described collateral pathways of the left gastric vein in portal hypertension.[62] In their study of 347 portal venograms, the authors identified portopulmonary anastomoses in a small percentage of patients and believed that, had cineportography been performed on all patients, the recognized frequency of this finding would have been much higher. They also reported a high frequency of multiple coronary veins with intercommunication and other tributaries to gastroesophageal varices, all of which, the authors emphasize, need to be properly mapped with splenic venography if thromboembolotherapy is planned.

Technical Guidelines

The following recommendations for transcatheter ethanol embolotherapy in gastroesophageal varices have been listed in two previous publications.[42,43] They derive from the present authors' experience and that of other investigators.

1. Before considering embolization, the interventional radiologist must consult with the gastroenterologist and vascular surgeon. Referring practices for such cases vary from one community to another. Alternative treatment modalities, including distal splenorenal shunt[63-65] and transendoscopic variceal sclerosis with 5% sodium morrhuate, must be considered.[66]

2. Verification of the patency of the portal vein is necessary before attempting the percutaneous transhepatic approach. Keller et al. used arterial portography[59]; the present authors advocate the use of real-time ultrasound to determine the patency of the portal vein and its intrahepatic radicles. They also obtain a depth measurement with the transducer positioned at the desired entry site. This simple procedure is extremely helpful in gaining access to the portal vein and in minimizing the number of passes with the sheathed needle. Portal vein thrombosis and cavernous transformation of the portal vein can be detected by ultrasound.[67,68]

3. Intravenous or intramuscular analgesia and local anesthesia should be used.

4. A 5mm skin incision that exposes subcutaneous fat is needed. The optimal location of the incision is generally on the right side of the chest wall between two of the lowest ribs laterally or anterolaterally. An anterior approach should be avoided in order to reduce irradiation of the examiner's hands. Fluoroscopic control should be used to avoid puncturing the pleura; real-time ultrasonography should have already aided the angiographer in avoiding the gallbladder and the hepatic flexure of the colon.

5. A sheathed 19- or 18-gauge needle is used to enter the liver and portal vein. One should use a sheath made of stiff material; thin-walled polyethylene sheaths are inadequate, as they tend to kink or "accordion" in cirrhotic livers. A large amount of ascites can prevent successful entry into the liver and portal vein, particularly if the liver is hard; for this reason, some angiographers consider tense ascites a contraindication to transhepatic variceal obliteration. The needle puncture should be made during mid-exhalation, as should the initial sonogram for portal vein location, because if the patient is asked to hold his breath in deep inhalation or exhalation during needle puncture, but then necessarily breathes quietly throughout the remainder of the procedure, one often finds that the skin entry point is remote from the liver entry point, sometimes as much as 5-10cm cephalocaudal, so that the entire procedure is hampered by the uneven catheter tract to the portal vein. Once the sheath and guidewire are in the vein, the sheath is advanced along the guidewire to gain optimal position in the portal venous system. The guidewire may then be advanced into the splenic vein, and the sheath may be replaced with an angiographic catheter. The authors usually attempt to use a C-1 catheter (7.0Fr Cordis with occlusion balloon), because subselection of the coronary vein will be nec-

essary and balloon occlusion will be desired. If this C-1 or a 6.5Fr or 7Fr Cook catheter cannot be advanced all the way into the splenic vein because of ascites or resistance in the liver, the authors frequently use an exchange wire and a straight Teflon catheter with a tapered tip. The latter can usually be advanced into the portal vein and will follow a guidewire into the splenic vein. This catheter dilates the liver parenchyma and thereby facilitates subsequent selective catheterization. On occasion, use of a sheath is desirable or necessary to bridge the distance between the parietal peritoneum and the portal vein. This space contains a variable amount of ascites and, typically, rather firm liver substance, with much resistance. Once the sheath enters the portal vein, all subsequent selective catheter manipulations are relatively easy. Care should be taken in selecting a sheath with sufficient length to enter the portal vein. However, if the sheath is too short but a guidewire remains in place throughout all exchanges, access to the portal system will not be lost, and a catheter can be re-introduced.

6. After the portal venous pressure has been measured, a portal venogram should be performed. The authors most frequently inject contrast medium at 12ml/sec for a total volume of 36ml of a 76% mixture of meglumine diatrizoate and sodium diatrizoate or iohexol (350mg of iodine/ml) and use an angiographic film sequence of two films/sec for three seconds, one film/sec for three seconds, and one film every two seconds for six seconds. Once the portal venous anatomy is understood, the proper embolization procedure can be planned.

7. Selective coronary venography should be performed to identify the varices, intercommunications with other variceal tributaries, portopulmonary venous anastomoses (one must film over the lung fields for this, preferably with cineportography), and portosystemic shunts.

8. After balloon occlusion, 10–12ml of absolute ethanol are injected into the coronary vein at a rate of approximately 2ml/sec. After a 10-minute waiting period, a repeat venogram is performed to search for continued flow into the varices. If there is flow, the procedure is repeated. If balloon occlusion is not possible, the angiographer may consider using particulate emboli to retard blood flow prior to ethanol administration. Gelfoam or sodium tetradecyl sulfate-soaked Gelfoam pledgets may be used for this purpose.

9. After coronary vein occlusion, a repeat portal venogram should be performed to document the occlusion and to search for other pathways to the varices that become visible after the initial procedure. If no accessible pathways are found, the procedure is complete. The portal venous pressure is measured again; it is usually higher than before the embolization.

10. As the catheter is removed from the liver, Gelfoam pledgets are placed in the catheter tract. The catheter is removed when blood return is minimal or absent.

11. Potential complications include infection, pleural effusion, pneumothorax, arteriovenous fistula, renal failure, hemorrhage, subcapsular hematoma, and portal vein-splenic vein thrombosis with or without recurrent hemorrhage. The latter may occur at higher frequency with ethanol thromboembolotherapy, but it is likely that this problem can be minimized by using balloon-occlusion catheters. To minimize the risk of infection, caps, gowns, masks, and gloves are used for these procedures.

Figures 2.5.3 and 2.5.4 are examples of patients with cirrhosis and esophageal varices managed by transcatheter ethanol thromboembolotherapy.

Each of the remaining interventional applications of absolute ethanol is either entirely experimental or has been used only on a limited basis clinically.

HEPATIC ARTERIAL EMBOLIZATION

Hepatic arterial embolization has been used extensively for palliation in patients with liver neoplasms.[69–73] Interest in this method has evolved because of evidence that hepatic neoplasms are supplied principally by the hepatic arterial circulation rather than by the portal venous circulation.[74,75] In the hope of deriving the same advantages of absolute ethanol over the particulate embolic agents and steel coils described earlier in this chapter, investigators have begun to study the potential application of this agent in hepatic neoplasms.

Animal Studies

Stridbeck et al. reported on segmental hepatic arterial ethanol administration in pigs.[7] Using 4–5ml of ethanol manually injected at approximately 0.5ml/sec, they produced angiographically demonstrable acute segmental hepatic arterial occlusion in all of their eight animals. Liver enzyme concentrations rose transiently to moderately high levels. Follow-up angiography at various times up to three months after embolization disclosed occlusions in all animals and common hepatic-artery occlusions in half. All animals had reconstitution of intrahepatic arterial branches by way of intrahepatic collaterals; some also had prominent extrahepatic collaterals. They were killed at various times after embolization, and the gross evidence of liver infarction was seen to be inversely related to the length of the observation (survival) period. Only four animals underwent microscopic examination. In the earliest specimen (four days after embolization), there was midzonal necrosis similar to that seen with hepatotoxic agents, inflammation, edema, and bile duct proliferation. Necrosis was found in the walls of hepatic artery branches, which were also occluded by fresh thrombi. In longer survivors, the areas of necrosis were less extensive and were demarcated by

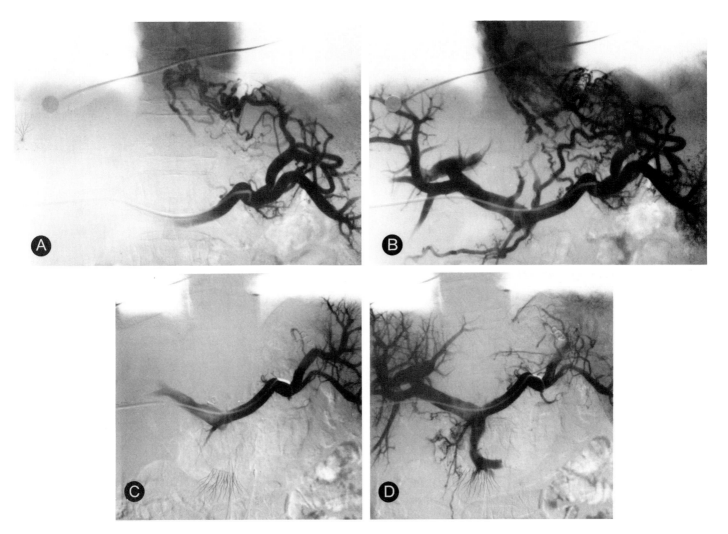

Figure 2.5.3. A 53-year-old alcoholic man with cirrhosis and bleeding esophageal varices. Early (**A**) and late (**B**) phases of percutaneous transhepatic portal venogram reveal large esophageal varices. Note: one does not ordinarily identify a bleeding site on these studies. After subselective catheterization of the coronary and short gastric veins and obliterative therapy with absolute ethanol and Gianturco coils, early (**C**) and late (**D**) phases of transhepatic portal venogram show no evidence of varices.

granulation tissue. The thrombi were more organized, and there was more bile duct proliferation. For unknown reasons, no macroscopic or microscopic abnormalities were found in the animal killed three months after embolization. The authors concluded that ethanol produces effective and permanent occlusion of injected vessels in the liver, but that the occluding effect is counteracted by the development of collaterals.

O'Riordan et al. studied proper hepatic arterial administration of ethanol in dogs in doses ranging from 0.3 to 1.0ml/kg (4.5–20ml total).[9] Doses were given through a standard angiographic catheter over a 20-second period. All animals had significant pain requiring analgesia within 24 hours. One animal died of pancreatitis, presumably secondary to reflux of ethanol into the pancreaticoduodenal arterial supply during the procedure. Although this study also showed effective occlusion of target hepatic vessels, collaterals did develop. Only one animal had recanalization of a major vessel. Dogs experienced leukocytosis, serum enzyme elevation (alanine aminotransferase and alkaline phosphatase), and hyperbilirubinemia (which occurred in only two dogs). At microscopic examination, vessel intimas were split, thrombi were present, hemorrhage and coagulative necrosis were found in the involved parenchyma, and inflammatory infiltrate with polymorphonuclear leukocytes was identifiable throughout the liver. In animals killed at four weeks, the pathologic changes had regressed, but there was marked perisinusoidal fibrosis. The authors emphasized that arteriograms taken 15 minutes after embolization with absolute ethanol do not indicate the true extent of infarction, since the changes tend to progress over at least one week, as demonstrated by angiography, leukocyte count, liver enzyme alterations, and histopathologic analysis.

In a study of six adult rhesus monkeys, Doppman and Girton tested the hypothesis that absolute ethanol is an ideal transarterial embolic agent for liver lesions because portal venous flow should protect normal hepatocytes by

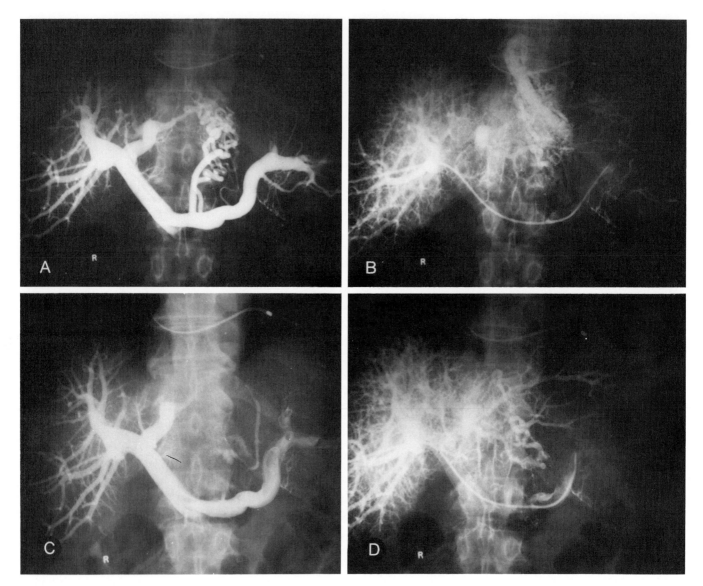

Figure 2.5.4. A 68-year-old man with alcoholic cirrhosis and bleeding esophageal varices. Middle (**A**) and late (**B**) phases of transhepatic portal venogram reveal esophageal varices. After subselective catheterization of all identifiable tributaries and obliterative therapy with absolute ethanol, mid (**C**) and late (**D**) phases of repeat portal venogram show no evidence of esophageal varices. Several small varices not in direct communication with portal or splenic vein are seen in **D**.

dilution.[8] Although they found that injury to hepatocytes was minimal, they also discovered that absolute ethanol perfuses the peribiliary plexus (the plexus of vessels surrounding the bile ducts in the portal tracts[76,77]) and produces scarring of the bile ducts, resulting in a cholangiographic pattern similar to that of sclerosing cholangitis. The authors recommend that continued careful investigation into the role and effects of ethanol in hepatic embolization be undertaken before clinical trials of this treatment are contemplated.

Ekelund et al. examined the blood supply of experimental liver tumors in rats after intra-arterial embolization with Gelfoam powder in some animals and ethanol in others.[10] They studied the remaining vascular supply in these experimental and in other control animals by postmortem

Microfil perfusion. Filling of tumor lakes from the portal venous supply was seen in only 20% of control animals but in 50% of the animals embolized with Gelfoam and in 85% of those embolized with ethanol. The authors explain that histologic studies have shown tumor lakes to be abnormally dilated blood vessels. Their study with Microfil showed that tumor lakes can be filled from either arterial or portal venous routes. They further remind us that there are numerous routes of arterioportal communication within the liver,[78,79] including direct arterioportal connections in the sinusoids, as well as the vasa vasorum of the portal vein and the peribiliary arterial plexus, all of which may provide supply in the event of arterial occlusion. Other investigators have not overlooked the potential importance of the portal-venous supply to the tumor.[80–82] Ekelund et al. postulate that transcatheter arterial occlusion combined with intraportally administered chemotherapeutic agents may prove more effective in the treatment of hepatic neoplasms than an entirely arterial approach. Of importance with respect to studies involving transarterial ethanol hepatic embolization is the fact that one can expect to witness increased portal venous supply to regions treated with arterial occlusion therapy.

Human Experience

Of 325 patients who underwent transarterial therapy for hepatic neoplasms, Wallace and his colleagues treated 20 with 1–5ml of absolute ethanol alone or in combination with Ivalon (5ml of absolute ethanol with 100mg of Ivalon, 150μm particles).[83,84] Injections were not made in wedged positions, nor was balloon occlusion used. Their longest follow-up has been two years without evidence of biliary obstruction, but the biliary tract has not been imaged for evidence of sclerosing cholangitis.[85] These investigators have been able to demonstrate the development of arterial collaterals on follow-up angiography that have been significant enough to necessitate sequential hepatic artery embolizations. Wallace and colleagues have summarized both their assessment of current animal data and their own clinical experience by stating that the optimal indications for the use of ethanol in hepatic artery embolization have yet to be established. Shiina reported in 30 patients with hepatocellular carcinoma treated with ethanol injections, 18 with single and 12 with multiple lesions. The tumor was completely necrotic in six cases and 90% necrotic in two cases and 70% necrosis was found in the remainder. The technique was more effective in patients with single lesions, eight of whom had complete tumor resolution by angiography.[86] A case of focal nodular hyperplasia was treated by Rasuli et al., resulting in shrinkage of a 10 × 14cm tumor, to a 1.5cm calcified nodule over an 18-month period.[87]

TRANSCATHETER SPLENIC EMBOLIZATION

Animal Studies

Mineau et al. reported a study of artery embolization with absolute ethanol in swine and dogs.[6] Importantly, three of the five pigs treated in this study developed gastric perforation without evidence of peritonitis. The work of Spigos and his colleagues outlines the need for controlled segmental splenic infarction, and Mineau et al. were mindful of this in their animal work. There were 11 successful splenic infarctions in 14 attempts, and 2 of those successes involved flow-directed balloon catheters to guide segmental infarction. Although these results are promising, the gastric perforations are of great concern, and the technique must still be viewed as experimental.

Human Experience

Many of the indications, techniques, and complications of splenic artery occlusion in place of surgical splenectomy have been described.[88–91] The many indications include thrombocytopenia, other signs of hypersplenism, and hemorrhage due to trauma. Spigos et al. described partial splenic embolization for hypersplenism as a means of treating the patient while preserving splenic function.[92] All human series have involved particulate embolic material, stainless-steel coils, or both. Risks and complications include pain, fever, leukocytosis, abscess formation (low incidence), left pleural effusion (in approximately one-half the patients), transient hyperkalemia, transient hyperamylasemia, and splenic rupture. Another potential complication is overt pancreatitis or pancreatic infarction. Because these techniques are complex, often requiring a staged approach for completion, the reader is advised to consult the references before attempting treatment in any given case. To the authors' knowledge, ethanol has not been used clinically to produce a transcatheter splenectomy.

ADRENAL ABLATION

Doppman and Girton investigated unilateral adrenal ablation in rhesus monkeys by direct injection of absolute ethanol into the adrenal veins as a means to ablate functioning neoplasms and hyperplasia.[5] The investigators found that the injections resulted in severe hypertensive crises due to torrential catecholamine release. Postmortem histologic studies showed residual viable glandular tissue. Because of this residual viable tissue and the severe hypertensive episodes, the authors concluded that the technique was both dangerous and ineffective. Some of the animals premedicated with sympathetic blocking agents exhibited less severe or absent hypertensive responses. It should be noted that although the investigators wedged the catheters into the veins before injection, balloon occlusion was not used. Balloon occlusion might have helped induce more effective organ ablation.

Recently, Fink et al. reported that transcatheter injection of 0.4ml of ethanol into the adrenal artery in each of three rhesus monkeys resulted in a mean increase of 60mm Hg in systolic pressure and 50mm Hg in diastolic pressure within two minutes after injection.[93] The injections also caused cardiac arrhythmias, and the authors postulated that all of the ill effects were due to catecholamine release upon embolization. In the same study, inferior phrenic artery embolization with Gelfoam powder produced only mild (6mm Hg systolic, 10mm Hg diastolic) increases in blood pressure in an additional three monkeys. The authors are aware of no studies involving ethanol adrenal ablation in humans. Although these methods may eventually prove useful, the current experimental evidence is not promising. Injection of absolute ethanol into any vessel for adrenal ablation must be regarded as dangerous.

BRONCHIAL ARTERY EMBOLIZATION

Naar et al. used absolute ethanol embolization of a bronchial artery to control severe hemoptysis in a patient with a small bronchial artery orifice and a catheter too tenuously positioned at the orifice to allow particulate embolization.[94] Other authors have reported embolization for hemoptysis using other agents.[95,96] Absolute ethanol is considered to be vaso-occlusive at the level of minute vessels, as is isobutyl 2-cyanoacrylate. One month after the report of Naar et al., Grenier et al. reported using the latter agent to embolize the bronchial arteries in 14 patients.[97] Bookstein criticized the use of capillary occlusive agents for bronchial artery embolization, citing the theoretically greater tendency of such agents to produce injury to bronchial, mediastinal, and spinal structures.[98] Subsequently, Ivanick et al. reported infarction of the left mainstem bronchus as a complication of bronchial artery embolization with ethanol.[99] The present authors agree with Bookstein and therefore strongly discourage the use of ethanol for bronchial artery embolization.

ARTERIAL EMBOLIZATION FOR GASTROINTESTINAL BLEEDING

In keeping with the above-mentioned complications and risks, as well as concern about the capillary occlusive potential of ethanol, the authors strongly discourage its use for bleeding Mallory–Weiss tears, gastric or duodenal ulcers, or bleeding small bowel or colon lesions. They are not aware of any reports of these uses of ethanol in humans.

CONTROL OF BLOOD LOSS FROM NONVISCERAL SOURCES

McLean et al. reported successful use of ethanol to manage bleeding from an internal mammary artery.[100] The hemorrhage was from a chest wall ulcer due to carcinoma of the breast. The authors emphasized that the internal mammary artery was functioning as an end vessel in this instance, and that no clinically apparent necrosis followed embolization. It is important to note that because of the potential for necrosis in the distribution of the feeding vessel, applications of the type described by McLean and his colleagues are limited.

TREATMENT OF ARTERIOVENOUS MALFORMATIONS AND VASCULAR TUMORS OF THE EXTREMITIES

Arteriovenous malformations are difficult to manage, and surgical ligation of feeding arteries is fraught with the long-term problems of reconstitution of the lesion by smaller vessels, which are more difficult to manage. Because of these problems, good transcatheter embolization techniques using particulate materials have evolved, as discussed in Chapter 2, Part 1.[101–103] Use of transcatheter absolute ethanol in the treatment of these lesions is contraindicated in certain instances. As has been stated above, the potential for complete capillary obliteration and tissue necrosis with absolute ethanol is significant. In one patient whose only other option was hemipelvectomy, the technique was used to embolize a vascular sarcoma of the pelvis. Inadvertent total occlusion of the superior gluteal artery, probably at the capillary level, resulted in marked tissue necrosis, with external breakdown together with necrosis of the sciatic nerve. Another lesion that might cause similar problems is a vascular renal cell carcinoma metastasis to an extremity; in one such case, a patient sloughed a small patch of skin from the lower leg after ethanol embolotherapy for a metastasis in the proximal tibia.[44]

Some investigators feel that superselective catheter position allows embolization of renal cell carcinoma osseous metastases with absolute ethanol or other capillary occlusive agents. Indeed, at the authors' institution this procedure has repeatedly been performed successfully and safely in lesions involving the vertebrae. However, they have recently witnessed a case of postembolization sympathectomy in a woman whose distal femur renal cell carcinoma metastasis was superselectively embolized with ethanol.[35] Fortunately, this complication resolved within three weeks.

Although some lesions of this type may be amenable to transcatheter vaso-occlusion with absolute ethanol, the angiographer must be careful not to occlude end vessels supplying the capillary beds of muscle, skin, and other nontarget tissues. There are other agents available that cause sufficient small vessel occlusion to devascularize such lesions without inducing complete tissue necrosis in nontarget areas.

INTERVENTIONAL THERAPY OF NEUROVASCULAR LESIONS

Transcatheter ablation of neurovascular lesions with absolute ethanol in humans must be viewed as entirely experimental. Pevsner et al. recently reported their experience with selective alcohol injection into the middle cerebral artery in six rhesus monkeys using a flexible version of the Pevsner Mini-Balloon catheter coaxially positioned through a 5Fr catheter.[4] Thrombus was identified in a short segment of vessel beyond the catheter tip but not in the more distal branches. Although the initial results appear promising, the technique is not ready for human application.

NONANGIOGRAPHIC USES OF ETHANOL IN INTERVENTIONAL RADIOLOGY

Ablation of Renal Cysts

Bean reported transcatheter ablation at the time of ultrasound-guided diagnostic aspiration of 34 benign renal cysts in 29 patients.[104] Knowing that most renal cysts are benign and that only a few cause hypertension or pyelocaliectasis, he still argued in favor of this form of therapy. Bean ablates the cysts with ethanol at the time of diagnostic aspiration, because, in his experience, the incidence of complications from treatment is no higher than that of diagnostic aspiration alone. Hence, he stated, one can treat the cysts in order to prevent complications. Bean recommends placement of a small pigtail catheter in the cyst before ethanol injection to prevent extracystic injections of ethanol, which can occur if the injection is made through a sharp needle. Bean also emphasized the need for injection of contrast medium into the cyst before the therapeutic procedure in order to ensure intracystic location. Confusion can arise otherwise, since there is a morphologic similarity between benign cysts and diverticula. After the injection, ethanol inactivates the secreting cells rapidly (within three minutes). Ethanol is withdrawn through the pigtail catheter, which is removed. No leakage of ethanol occurred in Bean's series, and only about one-eighth of the volume of the cyst had to be injected to inactivate epithelial cells. Only one cyst recurred.

Parathyroid Tumor Ablation

Solbiati et al. recently reported 12 uremic patients with secondary hyperparathyroidism, in whom 13 parathyroid tumors were detected by sonography and confirmed by fine needle aspiration biopsy.[105] These patients were treated by percutaneous injection of absolute ethanol into the tumors under ultrasound guidance for a variety of indications, including recurrence after previous subtotal resection, high surgical risk, and refusal of operation. In the large glands, volume decreased after ablative therapy; in most cases of single hyperplastic glands, therapeutic clinical and biochemical effects were obtained. Maximum volume reductions were noted by sonography at six months following treatment.

Three treatments were unsuccessful. In two of these the injected alcohol diffused anterior to the gland, and in one the lesion had partially calcified walls, which prevented adequate intraglandular injection. Complications included 24 hours of dysphonia in one patient after fine needle aspiration biopsy and a small hematoma in one gland after injection with ethanol. The latter sometimes occurs with needle biopsy alone. After considering the structural, clinical, and biochemical results of their series, Solbiati et al. concluded that percutaneous ethanol ablation of enlarged parathyroid glands can be used in certain cases of secondary hyperparathyroidism and that it can improve responsiveness to medical therapy and delay the need for operation. Kostrup reported on the percutaneous sonographically guided injection of ethanol in 12 patients with primary hyperparathyroidism. Success was achieved in eight patients who became normocalcemic. Unilateral vocal cord paralysis occurred in one patient.[106] Charboneau reported ablation of an occult adenoma using ultrasound guidance.[107]

Thyroid

Livraghi et al. reported eight patients with autonomous thyroid nodules 2.4–4.3cm in diameter, treated with ethanol under ultrasound guidance. At two months' follow-up, symptoms subsided and hormonal levels returned to normal.[108]

SUMMARY

Transcatheter absolute ethanol embolization is indicated in many instances of primary renal tumor, in some instances of complicated end-stage renal disease, in the management of gastroesophageal varices, and in a few other instances. In most cases of arteriovenous malformation and vascular metastasis to an extremity, ethanol-mediated ablation is contraindicated. In these instances, extensive capillary damage can result in widespread myonecrosis and necrosis of other nontarget tissues. The techniques are exciting but fraught with real and potential complications. The interventional radiologist should be familiar with all aspects of absolute ethanol embolization prior to attempting it in any case.

References

1. Ellman BA, Green EC, Elgenbrodt E, Garriott JC, Curry TS: Renal infarction with absolute ethanol. *Invest Radiol* 1980;15:318–322
2. Ekelund J, Jonsson N, Treugut H: Transcatheter obliteration of the renal artery by ethanol injection: experimental results. *Cardiovasc Intervent Radiol* 1981;4:1–7
3. Buchta K, Sands J, Rosenkrantz J, Roch WD: Early mechanism of action of arterially infused alcohol U.S.P. in renal devitalization. *Radiology* 1982;145:45–48
4. Pevsner PH, Klara P, Doppman J, George E, Girton M: Ethyl alcohol: experimental agent for interventional therapy of neurovascular lesions. *AJNR* 1983;4:388–390
5. Doppman JL, Girton M: Adrenal ablation by retrograde venous ethanol injection: an ineffective and dangerous procedure. *Radiology* 1984;150:667–678
6. Mineau DE, Miller FJ Jr, Lee RG, Nakashima EN, Nelson JA: Experimental transcatheter splenectomy using absolute ethanol. *Radiology* 1982;142:355–359
7. Stridbeck H, Ekelund L, Jonsson N: Segmental hepatic arterial occlusion with absolute ethanol in domestic swine. *Acta Radiol [Diagn]* 1984;25:331–335

8. Doppman JL, Girton ME: Bile duct scarring following ethanol embolization of the hepatic artery: an experimental study in monkeys. *Radiology* 1984;152:621–626

9. O'Riordan D, McAllister H, Sheahan BJ, MacErlean DP: Hepatic infarction with absolute ethanol. *Radiology* 1984;152:627–630

10. Ekelund L, Lin G, Jeppsson B: Blood supply of experimental liver tumors after intraarterial embolization with Gelfoam powder and absolute ethanol. *Cardiovasc Intervent Radiol* 1984;7:234–239

11. Ellman BA, Parkhill BJ, Marcus PB, Curry TS, Peters PC: Renal ablation with absolute ethanol: mechanism of action. *Invest Radiol* 1984;19:416–423

12. Harley JD, Killien FC, Peck AG: Massive hemoptysis controlled by transcatheter embolization of the bronchial arteries. *AJR* 1977;128:302–304

13. Gianturco G, Anderson JH, Wallace S: Mechanical device for arterial occlusion. *AJR* 1975;124:428–435

14. Reuter SR, Chuang VP, Bree RL: Selective arterial embolization for control of massive upper gastrointestinal bleeding. *AJR* 1975;125:119–126

15. Gomes AS, Rysavy JA, Spadaccini CA, Probst P, D'Souza V, Amplatz K: The use of the bristle brush for transcatheter embolization. *Radiology* 1978;129:345–350

16. Tadavarthy SM, Moller JHJ, Amplatz K: Polyvinyl alcohol (Ivalon)—a new embolic material. *AJR* 1975;125:609–616

17. White RI, Kaufman SL, Barth RH, Kadir S, Smyth JW, Walsh PC: Occlusion of varicoceles with detachable balloons. *Radiology* 1981;139:335–340

18. Lalli AF, Peterson N, Bookstein JJ: Roentgen-guided infarctions of kidneys and lungs: a potential therapeutic technic. *Radiology* 1969;93:434–435

19. Lang EK: Superselective arterial catheterization as a vehicle for delivering radioactive infarct particles to tumors. *Radiology* 1971;98:391–399

20. Almgard LE, Fernström I, Haverling M, et al: Treatment of renal adenocarcinoma by embolic occlusion of the renal circulation. *Br J Urol* 1973;45:474–479

21. Lang EK, Sullivan J, de Kernion JB: Work in progress: transcatheter embolization of renal cell carcinoma with radioactive infarct particles. *Radiology* 1983;147:413–418

22. Wallace S, Chuang VP, Swanson D, et al: Embolization of renal carcinoma: experience with 100 patients. *Radiology* 1981;138:563–570

23. Woodside J, Schwarz H, Gergreen P: Peripheral embolization complicating bilateral renal infarction with Gelfoam. *AJR* 1976;126:1033

24. Chuang VP: Nonoperative retrieval of Gianturco coils from the abdominal aorta. *AJR* 1979;132:996–999

25. Mukamel E, Hadar H, Nissenkorn I, Servadio C: Widespread dissemination of Gelfoam particles following occlusion of renal circulation. *Urology* 1979;14:194

26. Mazer MJ, Baltaxe HA, Wolf GL: Therapeutic embolization of the renal artery with Gianturco coils: limitations and technical pitfalls. *Radiology* 1981;138:37–46

27. Kuntslinger F, Brunelle F, Chaumont P, Doyon D: Vascular occlusive agents. *AJR* 1975;136:151–156

28. Greenfield AJ, Athanasoulis CA, Waltman AC, LeMoure ER: Transcatheter embolization: prevention of embolic reflux using balloon catheters. *AJR* 1978;138:651

29. Rosenkrantz H, Sands JP, Buchta KS, Healy JF, Kmet JP, Gerber F: Renal devitalization using 95 percent ethyl alcohol. *J Urol* 1982;127:873–875

30. Bernardino ME, Chuang VP, Wallace S, Thomas JL, Soo CS: Therapeutically infarcted tumors: CT findings. *AJR* 1981;136:527–532

31. Carroll BA, Walter JF: Gas in embolized tumors: an alternative hypothesis for its origin. *Radiology* 1983;147:441–444

32. Ellman BA, Parkhill BJ, Curry TS III, Marcus PB, Peters PC: Ablation of renal tumors with absolute ethanol: a new technique. *Radiology* 1981;141:619–626

33. Rabe FE, Yune HY, Richmond BD, Klatte EC: Renal tumor infarction with absolute ethanol. *AJR* 1982;139:1139–1144

34. Cox GG, Lee KR, Price HI, Gunter K, Noble MJ, Mebust WK: Colonic infarction following ethanol embolization of renal cell carcinoma. *Radiology* 1982;145:343–345

35. Uflacker R, Paolini RM, Nobrega M: Ablation of tumor and inflammatory tissue with absolute ethanol. *Acta Radiol [Diagn] (Stockh)* 1986;27(2):131–138

36. Eklund L, Ek A, Forsberg L, et al: Occlusion of renal arterial tumor supply with absolute ethanol: experience with twenty cases. *Acta Radiol [Diagn]* 1984;25:195–201

37. Klimberg I, Hunter P, Hawkins IF, Drylie DM, Wajsman Z: Preoperative angioinfarction of localized renal cell carcinoma using absolute ethanol. *J Urol* 1985;133:21–24

38. MacErlean DP, Owens AP, Bryan PJ: Hypernephroma embolization: is it worthwhile? *Clin Radiol* 1980;31:297

39. Teasdale C, Kirk D, Jeans WD, Penry JB, Tribe CT, Slade N: Arterial embolization in renal carcinoma: a useful procedure? *Br J Urol* 1982;54:616–621

40. Mebust WK, Weigel JW, Lee KR, Cox GG, Jewell WR, Krishnan EC: Renal cell carcinoma—angioinfarction. *J Urol* 1984;131:231–234

41. Earthman WJ, Mazer MJ, Winfield AC: Angiomyolipomas in tuberous sclerosis: subselective embolotherapy with alcohol, with long-term follow-up study. *Radiology* 1986;160:437–441

42. Becker GJ, Holden RW, Klatte EC: Absolute ethanol in interventional radiology. *Rev Interam Radiol* 1984;9:31–39

43. Becker GJ, Holden RW, Klatte EC: Therapeutic embolization with absolute ethanol. *Semin Intervent Radiol* 1984;1:118–129

44. Rowe DM, Becker GJ, Rabe FE, et al: Osseous metastases from renal cell carcinoma: embolization and surgery for restoration of function. *Radiology* 1984;150:673–676

45. Nanni GS, Hawkins IF Jr, Orak JK: Control of hypertension by ethanol renal ablation. *Radiology* 1983;148:51–54

46. Vertes V, Cangiano JL, Berman LB, Gould A: Hypertension in end stage renal disease. *N Engl J Med* 1968;280:978–981

47. Denny DF, Perlmutt LM, Bettmann MA: Percutaneous recanalization of an occluded renal artery and delayed ethanol ablation of the kidney resulting in control of hypertension. *Radiology* 1984;151:381–382

48. Keller FS, Coyle M, Rösch J, Dotter CT: Percutaneous renal ablation in patients with end stage renal disease: alternative to surgical nephrectomy. *Radiology* 1986;159:447–451

49. Iaccarino V, Russo D, Niola R, Muto R, Testa A, Andreucci VE, Porta E: Total or partial percutaneous renal ablation in the treatment of renovascular hypertension: radiological and clinical aspects. *Br J Radiol* 1989;62(739):593–598

50. Lunderquist A, Vang J: Transhepatic catheterization and obliteration of the coronary vein in patients with portal hypertension and esophageal varices. *N Engl J Med* 1974;291:646–649

51. Scott J, Dick R, Long RG, Sherlock S: Percutaneous transhepatic obliteration of gastroesophageal varices. *Lancet* 1976;2:53–55

52. Pereiras R, Viamonte M Jr, Russell E, LePage J, White P, Hutson D: New techniques for interruption of gastroesophageal venous bloodflow. *Radiology* 1977;124:313–323

53. Viamonte M Jr, Pereiras R, Russell E, LePage J, Hutson D: Transhepatic obliteration of gastroesophageal varices:

results in acute and nonacute bleeders. *AJR* 1977;129:237–241

54. Widrich WC, Robbins AH, Nabseth DC, Johnson WC, Goldstein SA: Pitfalls of transhepatic portal venography and therapeutic coronary vein occlusion. *AJR* 1978; 131:637–643

55. Pereiras R, Schiff E, Barkin J, Hutson D: The role of interventional radiology in disease of the hepatobiliary system and the pancreas. *Radiol Clin North Am* 1979;17:555–605

56. Yune HY, Klatte EC, Richmond BD, Rabe FE: Absolute ethanol in thrombotherapy of bleeding esophageal varices. *AJR* 1982;138:1137–1141

57. Yune HY, O'Conner KW, Klatte EC, Olson EW, Becker GJ, Strickler SA: Ethanol thrombotherapy of esophageal varices: further experience. *AJR* 1985;144:1049–1053

58. Child CG III: *Hepatic Circulation and Portal Hypertension.* Philadelphia, WB Saunders, 1954

59. Keller FS, Rösch J, Dotter CT: Transhepatic obliteration of gastroesophageal varices with absolute ethanol. *Radiology* 1983;146:615–619

60. Uflacker R: Percutaneous transhepatic obliteration of gastroesophageal varices using absolute alcohol. *Radiology* 1983;146:621–625

61. Sano A, Kuroda Y: Cine-portographic characteristics of porto-pulmonary venous anastomosis in portal hypertension. Presented at the 83rd Annual Meeting of the American Roentgen Ray Society, Atlanta, GA, 1983

62. Widrich WC, Srinivasan M, Semine MC, Robbins AH: Collateral pathways of the left gastric vein in portal hypertension. *AJR* 1984;142:375–382

63. Galambos JT, Warren WD: Surgery for portal hypertension. *Clin Gastroenterol* 1979;8:525–541

64. Adson MA, van Heerden JA, Ilstrup DM: The distal splenorenal shunt. *Arch Surg* 1984;119:609–614

65. Langer B, Rotstein LE, Stone RM, et al: A prospective randomized trial of the selective distal splenorenal shunt. *Surg Gynecol Obstet* 1980;150:45–48

66. Allison JG: The role of injection sclerotherapy in the emergency and definitive management of bleeding esophageal varices. *JAMA* 1983;249:1484–1487

67. Merritt CRB: Ultrasonographic demonstration of portal vein thrombosis. *Radiology* 1979;133:425–427

68. Kauzlaric D, Petrovic M, Barmeir E: Sonography of cavernous transformation of the portal vein. *AJR* 1984;142:383–384

69. Clouse ME, Lee R, Duszlak E, et al: Peripheral hepatic artery embolization for primary and secondary hepatic neoplasms. *Radiology* 1983;147:407–413

70. Lunderquist A, Ericsson M, Nobin A, Sanden G: Gelfoam powder embolization of the hepatic artery in liver metastases of carcinoid tumors. *Radiologe* 1982;22:65–73

71. Nakamura H, Tanaka T, Hori S, et al: Transcatheter embolization of hepatocellular carcinoma: assessment of efficacy in cases of resection following embolization. *Radiology* 1983;147:401–409

72. Wallace S, Chuang VP: The radiologic diagnosis and management of hepatic metastases. *Radiologe* 1982;22:56–66

73. Soo C–S, Chuang VP, Wallace S, Charnsangavej C, Carrasco H: Treatment of hepatic neoplasm through extrahepatic collaterals. *Radiology* 1983;147:45–48

74. Breedis C, Young G: The blood supply of neoplasms in the liver. *Am J Pathol* 1954;30:969–981

75. Lien WM, Ackerman NB: The blood supply of experimental liver metastases: a microcirculatory study of the normal and tumor vessels of the liver with the use of perfused silicone rubber. *Surgery* 1970;68:334–337

76. Grisham JW, Nopanitaya W: Scanning electron microscopy of casts of hepatic microvessels: review of methods and results, in Lautt WW (ed): *Hepatic Circulation in Health and Disease.* New York, Raven Press, 1981, pp 87–95

77. Ohtani O: The peribiliary portal system in the rabbit liver. *Arch Histol Jpn* 1979;42:153–159

78. Cho KJ, Lunderquist A: Experimental hepatic artery embolization with Gelfoam powder. *Invest Radiol* 1983;18:189–193

79. Bookstein JJ, Cho KJ, Davis GB, Dail D: Arterioportal communications: observations and hypotheses concerning transsinusoidal and transvasal types. *Radiology* 1982;142:581–590

80. Honjo I, Matsumura H: Vascular distribution of hepatic tumors: experimental study. *Rev Int Hepatol* 1965;15:681–690

81. Honjo I, Suzuki T, Ozawa K, Takasan H, Kitamura O, Ishikawa T: Ligation of a branch of the portal vein for carcinoma of the liver. *Am J Surg* 1975;130:296–302

82. Nilsson LAV, Zettergren L: Effect of hepatic artery ligation on induced primary liver carcinoma in rats: preliminary report. *Acta Pathol Microbiol Scand* 1967;71:187–193

83. Chuang VP, Wallace S, Soo C–S, Charnsangavej C, Bowers T: Therapeutic Ivalon embolization of hepatic tumors. *AJR* 1982;138:289–294

84. Carrasco CH, Chuang VP, Wallace S: Apudomas metastatic to the liver: treatment by hepatic artery embolization. *Radiology* 1983;149:79–83

85. Wallace S, Charnsangavej C, Carrasco CH, Bechtel W: Ethanol for hepatic artery embolization. *Radiology* 1984;152:821–822

86. Shiina S, Yasuda H, Muto H, Tagawa K, Unuma T, Ibukuro K, Inoue Y, Takanashi R. Percutaneous ethanol injection in the treatment of liver neoplasms. *AJR* 1987;149:949–952.

87. Soucy P, Rasuli P, Chou S, Carpenter B: Definitive treatment of focal nodular hyperplasia of the liver by ethanol embolization. *J Pediatr Surg* 1989;10(24):1095–1097.

88. Castañeda–Zúñiga WR, Hammerschmidt DE, Sanchez R, Amplatz K: Nonsurgical splenectomy. *AJR* 1977;129:805–811

89. Wholey MH, Chamorro HA, Rao G, Chapman W: Splenic infarction and spontaneous rupture of the spleen after therapeutic embolization. *Cardiovasc Radiol* 1978;1:249–253

90. Witte CL, Ovitt TW, Van Wyck DB, Witte MH, O'Mara RE, Woolfenden JM: Ischemic therapy in thrombocytopenia from hypersplenism. *Arch Surg* 1976;111:1115–1121

91. Yoshioka H, Kuroda C, Hori S, et al: Splenic embolization for hypersplenism using steel coils. *AJR* 1985;144:1269–1274

92. Spigos DG, Honasson O, Mozes M, Capek V: Partial splenic embolization in the treatment of hypersplenism. *AJR* 1979;132:777–782

93. Fink IJ, Girton M, Doppman JL: Absolute ethanol injection of the adrenal artery: hypertensive reaction. *Radiology* 1985;154:357–358

94. Naar CA, Soong J, Clore F, Hawkins IF Jr: Control of massive hemoptysis by bronchial artery embolization with absolute ethanol. *AJR* 1983;140:271–272

95. Wholey MH, Chamorro HA, Rao G, Ford WB, Miller WH: Bronchial artery embolization for massive hemoptysis. *JAMA* 1976;236:2501–2504

96. Uflacker R, Kaemmerer A, Neves C, Picon P: Management of massive hemoptysis by bronchial artery embolization. *Radiology* 1983;146:627–634

97. Grenier P, Cornud F, Lacombe P, Via UF, Nahum H: Bronchial artery occlusion for severe hemoptysis: use of isobutyl-2-cyanoacrylate. *AJR* 1983;140:467–471

98. Bookstein J: Editorial comment. *AJR* 1983;140:471
99. Ivanick MJ, Thorwarth W, Donohue J, Mandell V, Delany D, Jaques PF: Infarction of the left main-stem bronchus: a complication of bronchial artery embolization. *AJR* 1983;141:535–537
100. McLean GK, Mackie JA, Hartz WH, Freiman DB: Percutaneous alcohol injection for control of internal mammary artery bleeding. *AJR* 1983;141:181–182
101. Gomes AS, Mali WP, Oppenheim WL: Embolization therapy in the management of congenital arteriovenous malformations. *Radiology* 1982;144:41–49
102. Stanley RJ, Cubillo E: Nonsurgical treatment of arteriovenous malformations of the trunk and limb by transcatheter arterial embolization. *Radiology* 1975;115:609–612
103. Kaufman SL, Kumar AAJ, Roland JA, et al: Transcatheter embolization in the management of congenital arteriovenous malformations. *Radiology* 1980;137:21–29
104. Bean WJ: Renal cysts: treatment with alcohol. *Radiology* 1981;138:329–331

105. Solbiati L, Giangrande A, De Pra L, Bellotti E, Cantu P, Ravetto C: Percutaneous ethanol injection of parathyroid tumors under US guidance: treatment for secondary hyperparathyroidism. *Radiology* 1985;155:607–610
106. Karstrup S, Holm HH, Glenthoj A, Hegedus L: Nonsurgical treatment of primary hyperparathyroidism with sonographically guided percutaneous injection of ethanol: results in a selected series of patients. *Amer Roentgen Ray Soc* 1989;154:1087–1090.
107. Charboneau JW, Hay ID, van Heerden JA: Persistent primary hyperparathyroidism: Successful ultrasound-guided percutaneous ethanol ablation of an occult adenoma. *Mayo Clin Proc* 1988;63:913–917.
108. Livraghi T, Paracchi A, Ferrari C, Bergonzi M, Garavaglia G, Raineri P, Vettori C: Treatment of autonomous thyroid nodules with percutaneous ethanol injection: preliminary results. *Radiology* 1990;175:827–829.

Part 6. Diagnosis and Management of Vascular Anomalies

—Major Wayne F. Yakes, M.D., and Steve H. Parker, M.D.

INTRODUCTION

Vascular anomalies constitute some of the most difficult diagnostic and therapeutic enigmas that can be encountered in the practice of medicine. The clinical presentations are extremely protean and can range from an asymptomatic birthmark to fulminant life-threatening congestive heart failure. Attributing any of these extremely varied symptoms that a patient may present with to a vascular malformation can be challenging to the most experienced clinician. Compounding this problem is the extreme rarity of these vascular lesions. If a clinician sees one patient every few years, it is extremely difficult to gain a learning curve to diagnose and optimally treat them. Typically, these patients bounce from clinician to clinician only to experience disappointing outcomes, complications, and recurrence or worsening of their presenting symptoms.

Vascular anomalies were first treated by surgeons. The early rationale of proximal arterial ligation of arteriovenous malformations (AVMs) proved totally futile as the phenomenon of neovascular recruitment reconstituted arterial inflow to the AVM nidus. Microfistulous connections became macrofistulous feeders. Complete extirpation of an AVM nidus proved very difficult and extremely hazardous necessitating suboptimal partial resections. Partial resections could cause an initial good clinical response, but with time the patient's presenting symptoms recurred or worsened at follow-up.[1–3] Because of the significant blood loss that frequently accompanied surgery, the skills of interventional radiologists were eventually employed to embolize these vascular lesions preoperatively. This allowed more complete resections; however, complete extirpation of an AVM was still extremely difficult and rarely possible. As catheter delivery systems and embolic agents improved, embolotherapy has since emerged as a primary mode of therapy in the management of vascular anomalies. In many cases, vascular malformations are anatomically in surgically difficult or inaccessible areas. This has led to increased reliance on the sophisticated endo-surgical skills of the interventional radiologist and interventional neuroradiologist in the management of these problematic patients.

Because the clinical and angiographic manifestations can be extremely varied, hemangiomas and vascular malformations are always difficult to classify. Moreover, a vast array of descriptive terms have been given to impressive clinical examples in the hopes of distinguishing them as distinct syndromes. This has resulted in significant confusion in the categorization and treatment of these complex vascular lesions. Some of the confusing terms include congenital arteriovenous aneurysm, interosseous arteriovenous malformation, cirsoid aneurysm, serpentine aneurysm, capillary telangiectasia, angioma telangiectaticum, angioma arteriale racemosum, angioma simplex, angioma serpingiosum, nevus angiectoides, hemangioma simplex, lymphangioma, hemangiolymphangioma, naevus flammeus, verrucous hemangioma, capillary hemangioma, cavernous hemangioma, and venous angioma. Based on the landmark research of Mulliken et al.,[4–9] a rational classification of hemangioma and vascular malformations has evolved that should be incorporated into modern clinical practice. This classification system, based on endothelial cell characteristics, has removed much of the confusion in terminology that is present in the literature today. Once all clinicians understand and utilize this important classification system, ambiguity and confusion will be removed as all clinicians will speak a common language.

Theoretical Embryologic Origins

In the embryo, the primitive mesenchyme is nourished by an interlacing system of blood spaces without distinguishable arterial and venous channels. As the embryo matures, the interlacing system of blood spaces becomes more differentiated by partial resorption of the primitive vascular spaces and the formation of mature arterial and venous vascular spaces with an intervening capillary bed. The classically outlined sequence of events includes: (a) the undifferentiated capillary network stage; (b) the retiform developmental stage, characterized by coalescence of the original equipotential capillaries into large interconnecting plexiform vascular spaces without an intervening capillary bed; and (c) the final developmental stage, characterized by the resorption of the primitive vascular elements and the formation of mature arterial, capillary, and venous elements.[10-13]

Arrests in development or the failure of orderly resorption of embryologic primitive vascular elements results in persistence of immature vascular anomalies. Retention of vascular elements from the undifferentiated embryonal capillary network stage reveal a strong structural similarity to pediatric hemangiomas. Failure of resorption of vascular elements from the retiform developmental stage result in the retention of interconnecting channels of immature arteries and veins without an intervening capillary bed. Microfistulous and/or macrofistulous AVMs correspond to this embryologic stage of vascular development. Other errors in embryologic morphogenesis during the retiform plexus stage could result in other types of vascular malformations. Retention or sequestration of primitive retiform elements in post-capillary venous vascular channels results in congenital venous malformations. Another example would be retention of primitive capillary elements which would explain capillary malformations found in port wine stains. Arteriovenous fistulae (AVF) could result if there was faulty vascular morphogenesis during the later retiform stage. However, due to the constant breakdown and formation of vascular spaces in the embryo, there can be overlap of these distinct stages. This can lead to retained mixed vascular lesions that are complex and contain multiple combinations of these early stages of vascular morphogenesis. As Reid has stated, "In view of the common development on each side of the vascular tree, and in view of the enormous constructive and destructive changes necessary before the final pattern of the vascular tree is reached, it is a marvel not that abnormal congenital communications occasionally, or rarely, occur, but that they do not occur more often."[12]

Classification of Hemangiomas and Vascular Malformations

Pediatric cutaneous vascular lesions (hemangiomas) and vascular malformations have been classified by Mulliken, Glowacki, and coworkers, after research into endothelial cell characteristics, numbers of mast cells present, and endothelial cell in vitro characteristics.[4-9] Most pediatric hemangiomas are not present at birth, clinically manifest within the first month of life, and exhibit a rapid growth phase in the first year. More than 90% of pediatric hemangiomas spontaneously regress to near complete resolution by five to seven years of age. Hemangiomas occur with a reported incidence of 1–2.6%.[14] Hemangiomas in the proliferative phase are characterized by rapid growth, significant endothelial cell hyperplasia forming syncytial masses, thickened endothelial basement membrane, ready incorporation of triated thymidine into the endothelial cells, and the presence of large numbers of mast cells.[4-6] After this period of rapid expansion in the proliferative phase, hemangiomas can stabilize and grow commensurately with the child. Because of the complex nature of hemangiomas, the proliferative phase may continue as the involutive phase slowly begins to dominate. Involuting hemangiomas show diminished endothelial cellularity and replacement with fibrofatty deposits, exhibit a unilamellar basement membrane, demonstrate no uptake of triated thymidine into endothelial cells, and have normal mast cell counts.[4-6]

Vascular malformations are vascular lesions that are present at birth and grow commensurately with the child. Trauma, surgery, hormonal influences caused by birth control pills, and the hormonal swings during puberty and pregnancy may cause the lesion to expand hemodynamically. Vascular malformations demonstrate no endothelial cell proliferation, contain large vascular channels lined by flat endothelium, have a unilamellar basement membrane, do not incorporate triated thymidine into endothelial cells, and have normal mast cell counts. They may be formed from any combination of primitive arterial, capillary, venous, or lymphatic elements with or without direct arteriovenous (AV) shunts. Vascular malformations are true structural anomalies resulting from inborn errors of vascular morphogenesis.

Vascular malformations are categorized into arterial, capillary, and venous malformations (with or without AVF), and lymphatic malformations. The term hemangioma should be solely reserved for the previously described pediatric cutaneous lesions which are not present at birth, become manifest within the first month of life, exhibit a rapid proliferative phase and slowly involute to near complete resolution by five to seven years of age. The old terms describing adult conditions such as "cavernous hemangioma," "hepatic hemangioma," "extremity hemangioma," "vertebral hemangioma," "facial hemangioma," etc., should be replaced with the term "venous malformation."

The term "intramuscular hemangioma" should be replaced with "intramuscular venous malformation." The typical port wine stain, composed of dilated capillary-like vessels, previously incorrectly termed "capillary hemangioma," should instead be termed "capillary malformation." The old terms "simple capillary lymphangioma," "cavernous lymphangioma," "lymphangioma," and "cystic hygroma," should instead be termed "lymphatic malformations." The old term "hemangio-lymphangioma" should be replaced with "mixed venous-lymphatic malformation." The old terms "arteriovenous hemangioma," "arterial angioma," "arteriovenous aneurysm," "cirsoid aneurysm," "red angioma," and "serpentine aneurysm," should be replaced with "arteriovenous malformation."

Eponyms have further clouded and confused the nomenclature of hemangiomas and vascular malformations in the literature. Maffuci's syndrome (or Kast syndrome) has been defined as a condition whereby the patient has multiple enchondromas and coexistent hemangiomatosis.[15] In the current classification system, "hemangiomatosis" should be termed "venous malformation." The Riley–Smith syndrome is previously characterized by macrocephaly, pseudopapilladema, and multiple hemangiomas.[16] The term "hemangioma" should be replaced with "venous malformation." Capillary malformations and lymphatic malformations may also be present with the Riley–Smith syndrome. The Riley–Smith syndrome, the Proteus syndrome, and Bannayan's syndrome are probably a spectrum of similar congenital vascular anomalies.[16–19] Gorham syndrome, Gorham–Stout syndrome, and Trinquoste syndrome are similar entities described as osteolysis (disappearing bone disease) caused by an underlying hemangiomatosis.[20] The term "hemangiomatosis" should be replaced by intraosseous vascular malformation (usually venous).

Another confusing group of eponyms (Klippel–Trenaunay syndrome, naevus vasculosus osteohypertrophycus, naevus verrucosus hypertrophycans, osteohypertrophic naevus flammeus, angioosteohypertrophy syndrome) all describe a congenital entity characterized by unilateral lower limb hypertrophy, cutaneous capillary malformations, lymphatic malformations, a normal, hypoplastic, or atretic deep venous system, occasional extension of the vascular malformation into the trunk, a lower extremity retained embryonic lateral venous anomaly (Servelle's vein), and increased subcutaneous fat in the affected limb.[21–23] A similar group of eponyms (Parkes–Weber syndrome, Klippel–Trenaunay–Weber syndrome, Klippel–Trenaunay–Weber–Rubashov syndrome, giant limb of Robertson) represent a similar clinical entity, that has the same features of the Klippel–Trenaunay syndrome with the coexistence of multiple arteriovenous fistulae (Fig. 2.6.1).[24] The Klippel–Trenaunay syndrome and Parkes–Weber syndrome usually occur in the lower extremity, but occasionally can affect the upper extremity. In the upper extremity, the Parkes–Weber syndrome is more commonly

seen, although the Klippel–Trenaunay syndrome is much more common overall.

These examples are but a few of the confusing terms used in the literature and in clinical practice. Utilizing this modern classification system, the current confusion can be eliminated and all clinicians can finally speak the same language. Accurate terminology will lead to precise identification of clinical entities and to enhanced patient care. The remainder of this chapter will utilize this modern classification system originated by Mulliken, Glowacki, and coworkers.

CONCEPTS IN PATIENT MANAGEMENT

Vascular malformations are congenital lesions that are present at birth, whether or not evident clinically, and grow commensurately with the child. Arteriovenous malformations (AVMs), congenital arteriovenous fistulae (AVF), capillary malformations, venous malformations, lymphatic malformations, and mixed malformations are grouped under the collective term vascular malformations. Post-traumatic AVF are different in that they are acquired lesions.

A thorough clinical exam and history can usually establish the diagnosis of hemangioma or vascular malformation. Hemangiomas are usually not present at birth and initially have a bright scarlet color that gradually deepens. Vascular malformations have a persistent color, depending on the dominant arterial, capillary, venous, or lymphatic component. Evaluating for skeletal abnormalities, abnormal veins, arterial abnormalities, pulsatility or nonpulsatility of a lesion, if the lesion swells when dependent and flattens when elevated, disparity of limb size, if reflex bradycardia occurs in the Nicoladoni–Branham test of inflow arterial occlusion, neurologic evaluation, and a good history can frequently diagnose a hemangioma or categorize a vascular malformation.

Color Doppler imaging (CDI) is an essential tool in the diagnostic work-up of vascular malformations. Both high flow lesions (AVMs, AVF) and low flow lesions (venous malformations) can be accurately diagnosed. Furthermore, CDI is also an important noninvasive imaging modality to follow patients undergoing therapy. Documentation of decreased arterial flow rates in high-flow malformations and persistent venous malformation thrombosis can be accurately assessed.[25]

Computed tomography (CT), although also helpful in the diagnostic work-up, is less useful than magnetic resonance (MR) imaging. Unlike CT, MR easily distinguishes between high-flow (AVMs, AVF) and low-flow (venous malformations) vascular malformations. Furthermore, the anatomic relationship of the vascular malformation to adjacent nerves, muscles, tendons, organs, bone, and subcutaneous fat allows a total assessment. MR is also an excellent noninvasive imaging modality to follow patients to

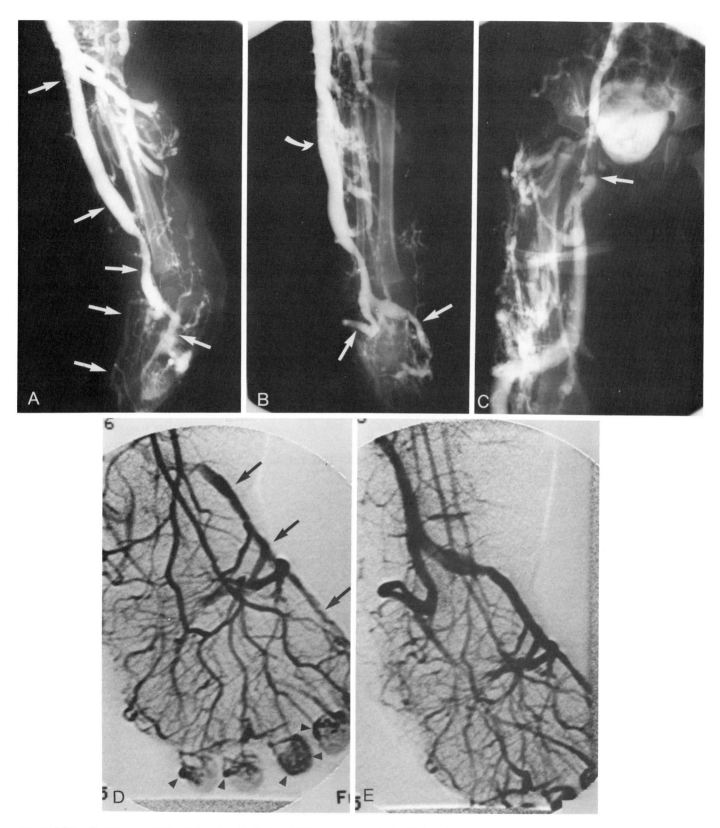

Figure 2.6.1. Twenty-two-month-old female with Parkes–Weber syndrome affecting the right lower extremity. **A.** Lateral right lower extremity venogram. Note retained primitive veins over dorsum of foot and anterior leg *(arrows)*. Also note significant amount of dysplastic soft tissues and fat in the leg and foot. **B.** AP venogram. Note hypoplasia of normal deep veins and dominance of retained primitive veins in the foot *(arrows)*, and Servelle's vein *(curved arrow)*. **C.** Note cross-over of Servelle's vein to anterior thigh and anastomosis near the common femoral vein *(arrow)*. Note primitive venous structures in the lateral thigh. Note more normal appearing right external iliac and common iliac vein. **D.** Right foot DSA. Note AV shunting into primitive dorsal foot vein in early arterial phase *(arrows)*. Note multiple AVF in the toes *(arrowheads)*. **E.** Late phase DSA. Note anomalous veins over dorsum of the foot and compare with **B**.

155

determine the efficacy of therapy, many times obviating repetitive arteriography and venography.[26]

After the diagnosis is established, the next major hurdle is to determine whether therapy is warranted. Multiple surgical specialists familiar with vascular anomalies must be in place, despite the fact that the interventional radiologist should primarily plan and direct the patient's care. According to D. Emerick Szilagyi, M.D., editor for the *Journal of Vascular Surgery*, "... with few exceptions, their (vascular anomalies) cure by surgical means is impossible. We intuitively thought that the only answer of a surgeon to the problem of disfiguring, often noisome, and occasionally disabling blemishes and masses, prone to cause bleeding, pain, or other unpleasantness, was to attack them with vigor and with the determination of eradicating them. The results of this attempt at radical treatment were disappointing."[2] Indeed, of 82 patients seen in this patient series, only 18 patients were deemed operable. And of these 18 patients operated on, 10 patients were improved, 2 were the same, and 6 were worse at follow-up.[2]

This patient series points to the enormity of the problem posed by vascular malformations. Vascular malformations are best treated in medical centers where the patients are seen regularly. The interventional radiologist who occasionally evaluates a patient every year or so will never gain a significant learning curve or enough experience to manage these challenging lesions. All too frequently, the patient ultimately pays for the interventional radiologist's initial enthusiasm, inexperience, folly, and lack of necessary clinical back-up. To optimally treat these patients, a vascular malformation team should be in place. Headed by the interventional radiologist/interventional neuroradiologist, the various surgical and medical specialties function together, much like the tumor board team of specialists. When patients are seen and treated regularly, then experience can be gained, rational decisions can be made, and patient care is then optimized. It cannot be emphasized enough that, as a group, vascular anomalies pose one of the most difficult challenges in the practice of medicine. A cavalier approach to their management will always lead to significant complications and dismal patient outcomes.

Many endovascular occlusive agents are currently in use to treat vascular malformations. With the use of intravascular ethanol, pain control is a significant problem. Anesthesiologists can greatly aid in solving this problem. Whether the anesthesiologist performs general anesthesia or deep intravenous (IV) sedation during the procedure, this is one less burden the interventional radiologist assumes so that he/she can concentrate on the case at hand. In pediatric patients, general anesthesia is usually a requirement. In adults, an interventional radiologist may consider standard IV sedation with the patient awake to perform provocative testing in nonintracranial sensitive neural areas with lidocaine. Amytal is used for intracranial provocative testing because lidocaine causes seizures.

After provocative testing has been performed and no neural deficits are identified, IV sedation can be administered prior to ethanol injection.

ENDOVASCULAR ABLATIVE AGENTS

Endosurgical vascular ablation (embolotherapy) has evolved as one of the cornerstones of modern interventional radiology. The extensive array of catheters, guidewires, endovascular ablative agents (embolic materials), and imaging systems are a tribute to the hard work, insight, and imagination of the many dedicated investigators in this area. Because of significant laboratory research, clinical research, and extensive clinical experience, the judicious use of endosurgical vascular ablative therapy is common in modern clinical practice. Now that it is firmly established as an essential therapeutic tool, its role will only continue to grow.

Endosurgical vascular ablative therapy began in the 1930s with the work of Brooks when he used muscle to treat a traumatic carotid-cavernous fistula.[27] There are now many endovascular ablative agents that are utilized in various clinical scenarios. The choice of agent depends upon several factors: the vascular territory to be treated, the type of abnormality being treated, the possibility of superselective delivery of an occlusive agent, the goal of the procedure, and the permanence of the occlusion required. The following is a list of occlusive agents that have been used to treat vascular anomalies.

Gelfoam (The Upjohn Company, Kalamazoo, MI). Autologous clot was the first widely used particulate agent, but subsequently Gelfoam (gelatine sponge) has become the much more popular transcatheter embolic agent. Initially used for surgical hemostasis, Gelfoam is readily available, inexpensive, and easy to use. Gelfoam is packaged in sheets that can be cut into pledgets of any size required by the interventional radiologist. Gelfoam induces mild-to-moderate tissue reactivity which enhances its thrombogenic effects. Gelfoam is not a permanently occluding agent with regard to vascular malformations. Recanalizations usually occur within 7–30 days of the procedure.

Gelfoam powder (The Upjohn Company, Kalamazoo, MI). Gelfoam is available as a powder with the individual particles measuring approximately 40–60 microns in size. Because of this small particle size, deep penetration can be expected. In high flow vascular malformations, shunting to the pulmonary arterial bed will occur. It possesses the same properties as the gelatin sponge sheets. Because of its small particle size, small vessel occlusion is possible. Therefore, its use in the pelvis, head, and neck regions, and paraspinal area, should be with extreme caution to prevent possible denervation of nerves by occluding the vasa nervorum.[28] If superselective positioning of the embolizing catheter cannot be achieved, then the use of Gelfoam powder should probably be avoided in sensitive neural territories. Other more suitable larger particle agents could be used which will decrease the chance of neuropathy. Its use is limited in the management of vascular malformations because recanalizations always occur.

Avitene (Alcon Laboratories, Fort Worth, TX). Avitene (microfibrillar collagen hemostat) is similar to Gelfoam in that it is inexpensive, readily available, and easy to use. It also is a nonpermanent occluding agent. Because of the small particles (~200 microns) that are present in the mixture, the potential complications that can occur with Gelfoam powder are also possible with Avitene. Avitene is prepared from denatured bovine collagen and is, therefore, potentially antigenic. Animal and human studies have shown no significant effects, however. A solution of Avitene with 33% ethanol has shown promise as a good embolic agent in a pig model.[29] However, this has not been attempted in humans.

Angiostat (Regional Therapeutics, Santa Monica, CA). Angiostat (GAX) is a collagen-based embolic agent that has characteristics similar to Gelfoam and Avitene in that it is not a permanently occluding agent. As opposed to a particle, Angiostat is a fiber measuring 5 × 75 microns.[29]

Polyvinyl alcohol foam (Contour, Interventional Therapeutics Corp., South San Francisco, CA; PVA, Biodyne Inc., El Cajon, CA; PVA, Ingenor Medical, Paris, France). Polyvinyl alcohol foam (PVA), formerly known as Ivalon, is formed by the reaction of polyvinyl alcohol foam with formaldehyde. It is biologically inert and provokes a mild inflammatory reaction. Initially thought to be a permanently occluding agent, PVA is now known to recanalize when treating vascular malformations. PVA is usually supplied in suspensions in sizes of 150–300, 300–500, 500–700, 700–1000, 1000–1500, 1500–2000, and 2000–2500 microns.[30] Its greatest utility is in the endovascular management of neural axis vascular malformations (Fig. 2.6.2).

Coils (Cook Inc., Bloomington, IN; Target Therapeutics, Los Angeles, CA). Metallic coils with or without attached cotton or Dacron fibers have long been used to induce vascular occlusion. Many coils have been developed which will pass through standard 5Fr and 6.5Fr catheters, as well as the new mini 2.2Fr catheter systems. These occluding spring coil emboli function similarly to an arterial ligation in that they occlude the artery where the coil is released and do nothing to the capillary bed distally.[31,32] Coil emboli have their greatest utility in the management of congenital and post-traumatic AVF.

"Glues" (Bucrylate, Ingenor Medical, Paris, France; Avacryl, CRX Medical, Durham, NC). Isobutyl 2-cyanoacrylate (Bucrylate, IBCA) and *N*-butyl cyanoacrylate (Avacryl, NBCA) belong to a class of tissue adhesives that are used for endosurgical vascular ablation. Bucrylate is no longer in use. Avacryl has replaced Bucrylate and is used to treat arteriovenous malformations and arteriovenous fistu-

lae.[33–35] These "glues" remain in the liquid state until contact occurs with an ionic solution such as contrast material, saline, or blood, whereby it polymerizes from its monomeric form to its polymeric form. In this polymerization process, the cyanoacrylates generate heat which may contribute to some level of histotoxicity in the adjacent area and angionecrosis. Tantalum powder is used to opacify the embolic mixture so it can be visualized fluoroscopically and on plain films. Pantopaque or acetic acid has been used to retard the polymerization time of the mixture so that it can effectively reach the embolization target and then solidify. The cyanoacrylates were initially thought to be permanent occluding agents; however, it is now well documented that recanalizations do occur.[33,36] Once solidified intravascularly, the cyanoacrylates incite a mild inflammatory response. In the management of head and neck vascular malformations the cyanoacrylates cause a rock hard mass that is extremely undesirable cosmetically. Furthermore, white tantalum powder should be used in caucasian patients and black tantalum powder should be used in black patients to minimize unwanted subcutaneous discoloration.

98% ethyl alcohol (dehydrated alcohol injection USP, Abbott Laboratories, North Chicago, IL). Ethanol is a well known sclerosing agent that induces significant thrombosis from the capillary bed backward. This results in total tissue devitalization. Ethanol induces thrombosis by denaturing blood proteins, dehydrating vascular endothelial cells and precipitating their protoplasm, denuding the vascular wall of endothelial cells, and segmentally fracturing the vessel wall. In the treatment of vascular malformations, ethanol has demonstrated its curative potential as opposed to palliation seen with other embolic agents.[37–44] As with Gelfoam powder, extreme caution and superselective catheter placement are requirements when using ethanol as an endovascular occlusive agent. Ethanol can induce significant pain when injected intravascularly. Proper anesthesia such as deep IV sedation or general anesthesia may be required to minimize patient discomfort. Postembolization edema always occurs with the use of ethanol. Extreme caution must be taken with its use to minimize the possibility of nontarget embolization of normal tissues to prevent tissue necrosis and neuropathy.

Sotradecol (sodium tetradecyl sulfate, Elkins–Sinn Inc., Cherry Hills, NJ). Sotradecol is another sclerosing agent available in a 1 or 3% aqueous solution. Its properties are similar to ethyl alcohol and it contains 2% benzyl alcohol.[45–47] The same caveats apply to the use of Sotradecol as to the use of ethyl alcohol and Gelfoam powder in neurologically sensitive areas.

Detachable balloons (Becton Dickinson balloon, Franklin Lakes, NJ; Debrun balloon and Balt balloon, Ingenor Medical, Paris, France; Hieshima balloon, Interventional Therapeutics Corp., South San Francisco, CA). Since first introduced by Serbinenko in 1974,[48] several detachable

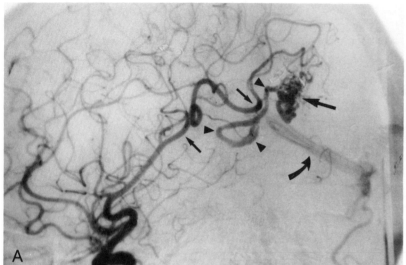

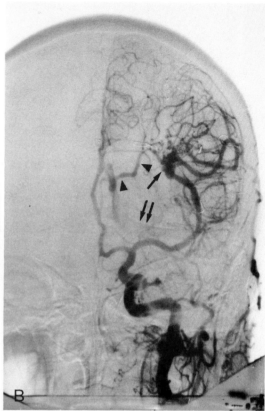

Figure 2.6.2. Thirty-six-year-old male with postoperative recurrence of AVM deep in the left occipital lobe white matter. Because the patient already had a visual field cut, endosurgical vascular ablative therapy was performed instead of a second operation that would require dissection into the deep white matter and potentially worsen his field cut. **A.** Lateral left common carotid arteriogram, arterial phase. Note hypertrophied angular artery *(arrows)* supplying AVM *(large arrow).* Note draining vein *(arrowheads)* to vein of Galen. Note shunt into the straight sinus *(curved arrow).* **B.** AP left common carotid study. Note AVM *(arrow),* draining vein *(arrowheads),* and transverse sinus *(paired arrows).*

balloons have been developed[49] and they have been used to endovascularly treat carotid-cavernous fistulae, head and neck aneurysms, varicocele, and arteriovenous fistulae.[49–55]

Ethibloc (Ethnor Laboratories, Ethicon, 8 rue Bellini, Paris, France). Ethibloc is a prolamine protein derived from corn which is mixed with ethanol, amidotrizoic acid, and oleum papaveris. Prior to its use for endosurgical vascular ablation, Ethibloc may be mixed with 10% ethyl alcohol additionally, but it is always mixed with an oil-based contrast agent for opacification such as Ethiodol (Savage Laboratories, Melville, NY) or Duroliopaque (Guerbet Laboratories, Paris, France). Ethibloc is degraded within the body enzymatically into glutamic acid, leucine, proline, and alanine. Because Ethibloc is a protein, a strong concern is the potential for antigenic anaphylaxis, although none has been reported. Ethibloc has a slow rate of solidification (10–15 minutes) and is mainly recommended for venous malformation sclerotherapy[56]; however, it was successfully used to acutely occlude a facial congenital AVF (Fig. 2.6.3). Ethibloc is approved for human use in Europe, but not in the United States. Ethibloc always produces acute swelling, as does ethanol, and may cause prolonged pain in the treated area, unlike ethanol.

SPECIFIC VASCULAR ANOMALIES
Pediatric Hemangioma

It must be plainly stated that the vast majority of hemangiomas should not be treated to allow the natural history of involution to occur. On hemangiomas that ulcerate or occasionally bleed, local compression and dressings will suffice. There are rare conditions that may warrant therapy, however. Upper eyelid hemangioma can cause refractive errors and amblyopia.[57] Subglottic hemangioma may be a cause of chronic respiratory stridor.[58] The combination of cutaneous and hepatic hemangiomas or isolated giant skin hemangiomas may cause congestive heart failure and systemic clotting changes.[59] Systemic steroid therapy has usually proven successful in the medical management of these clinical problems.[57–60] Because hepatic arteriovenous malformation in the newborn can present with the identical clinical picture of high output failure, the differential diagnosis must be made because steroids do not affect AVMs. If two weeks of steroid therapy fails to improve the high output failure caused by pediatric hemangioma, then angiography should be performed prior to endovascular abla-

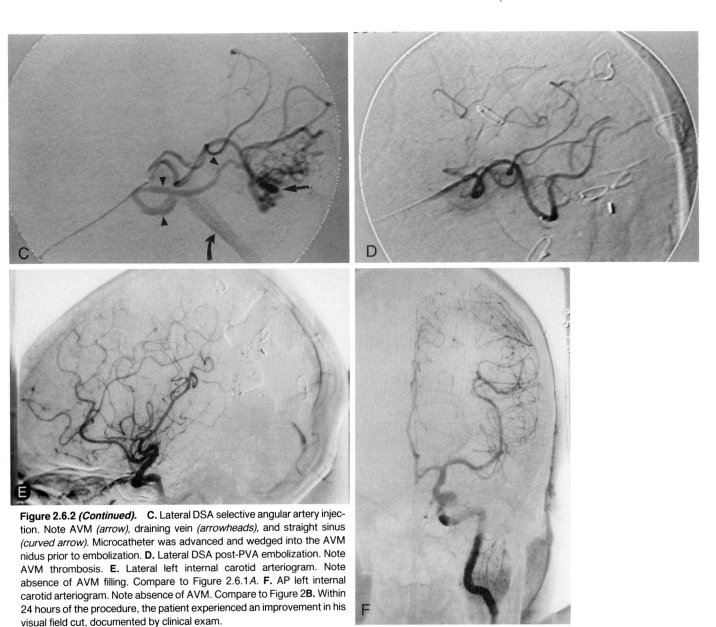

Figure 2.6.2 (Continued). C. Lateral DSA selective angular artery injection. Note AVM *(arrow)*, draining vein *(arrowheads)*, and straight sinus *(curved arrow)*. Microcatheter was advanced and wedged into the AVM nidus prior to embolization. **D.** Lateral DSA post-PVA embolization. Note AVM thrombosis. **E.** Lateral left internal carotid arteriogram. Note absence of AVM filling. Compare to Figure 2.6.1A. **F.** AP left internal carotid arteriogram. Note absence of AVM. Compare to Figure 2B. Within 24 hours of the procedure, the patient experienced an improvement in his visual field cut, documented by clinical exam.

tion or surgery. Frequently, endovascular ablation is useful to control the high output shunt until the natural involution of the hemangioma occurs.[60]

The Kasabach–Merritt syndrome is usually a self-limited condition of consumptive coagulopathy secondary to platelet trapping that may not require therapy.[61,62] If treatment is needed, a trial of steroid therapy is indicated.[61–63] If the hemangioma fails to respond to steroid therapy, then a trial of cyclophosphamide,[64] aminocaproic acid and cryoprecipitate,[65] or endovascular ablative therapy should be instituted.[60]

Arteriovenous Malformations

AVMs are congenital vascular anomalies typified by hypertrophied inflow arteries shunting through a primitive

vascular nidus into tortuous dilated outflow veins (Fig. 2.6.4). No intervening capillary bed is present. Symptoms are usually referable to the anatomic location of the AVM. The larger and the more central anatomically an AVM is, the greater the likelihood for high-output cardiac consequences. Other presenting symptoms can include pain, progressive nerve deterioration or palsy, disfiguring mass, tissue ulceration, hemorrhage, impairment of limb function, limiting claudication, etc.

The baseline imaging workup prior to any therapy includes extensive arteriography, CDI, and MR scanning. Selective and superselective arteriography defines the AVM's angioarchitecture and identifies any dangerous anastomoses to normal structures, any aneurysms within the lesion, the venous drainage, and the potential routes of access for endosurgical vascular ablative therapy. Further-

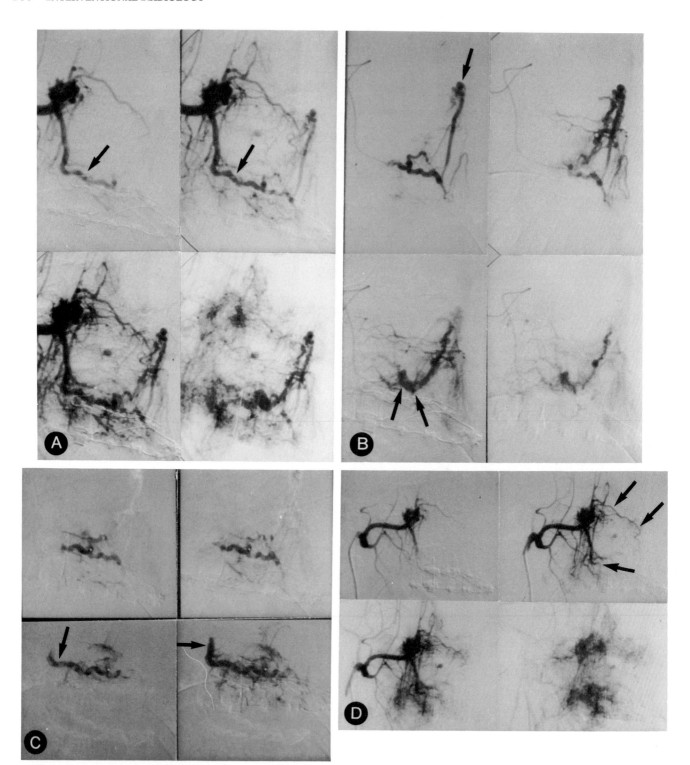

Figure 2.6.3. Example of use of Ethibloc to treat a maxillary AVF. Case was performed at the Academic Medical Center in Amsterdam, the Netherlands by Professor F. L. M. Peters, M.D. and W. F. Yakes, M.D. Thirteen-year-old female presented with recurrent gingival hemorrhage. **A.** Lateral external carotid DSA. Note hypertrophy of the distal internal maxillary artery and the greater palatine artery *(arrow)*. Note hyperemia in the maxillary area. **B.** Lateral selective greater palatine artery DSA, pre-therapy. Note AVF in anterior aspect of maxilla *(arrow)*. Note vein aneurysm *(arrows)*. **C.** Lateral greater palatine artery DSA post-Ethibloc embolization. Note the acute arterial occlusion with retrograde flow *(arrows)*. **D.** Lateral internal maxillary DSA post-Ethibloc embolization. Note the closure of the AVF and occlusion of the greater palatine artery distally *(arrow)*. Note patency of the infraorbital artery *(arrows)* and that it does not reconstitute the AVF, further documenting its complete closure. The patient suffered no complication and was discharged the following day.

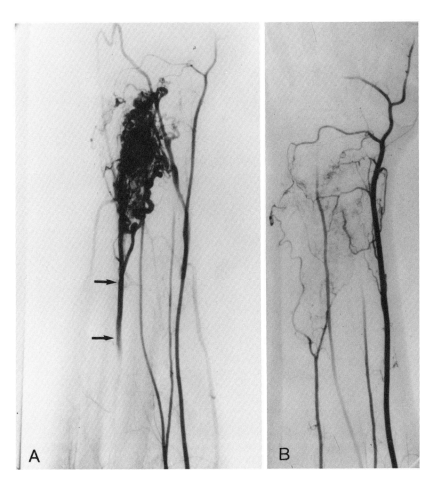

Figure 2.6.4. Twenty-six-year-old male with right dorsal wrist AVM. **A.** AP left hand arteriogram. Note AVM nidus fed by retained primitive arterial branch arising from the brachial artery *(arrows)*. **B.** AP left hand arteriogram four months post-therapy. Note obliteration of AVM. (From Yakes WF, Parker SH, Gibson MD, et al: Alcohol embolotherapy of vascular malformations. *Semin Intervent Radiol* 1989;6:146–161. Reprinted with permission.)

more, these baseline studies are compared to follow-up studies to determine the efficacy of therapy.

Many endovascular occlusive agents have been used to treat AVMs.[30–35,47,53,66–69] Most agents produce excellent palliative results; however, follow-up procedures are required as recanalizations and neovascular recruitment stimulate renewed symptoms. We have currently treated 25 patients with AVMs using absolute ethanol as the sole endovascular occlusive agent. With the use of ethanol, recanalizations and neovascular recruitment have not been observed. Furthermore, untreated inflow arterial feeders have decreased in size in response to the decreased AV shunt. CDI has provided physiologic data documenting decreased flow rates through arterial feeders at follow-up as well.[25]

In treating AVMs, superselective catheter placement is absolutely essential (Fig. 2.6.4). When this is not possible, then direct percutaneous puncture techniques should be used to circumvent catheterization obstacles (Fig. 2.6.5). If superselective placement at the AVM nidus is not possible, then the use of ethanol must be avoided. Frequently, inflow occlusion is required to induce vascular stasis to maximize the thrombogenic properties of ethanol. This can be achieved through the use of occlusion balloon catheters, blood pressure cuffs, tourniquets, etc. We empirically utilize occlusive techniques for at least 10 minutes.

The amount of ethanol used in each endosurgical vascular ablative procedure is tailored to the flow-volume characteristics of the individual lesion. No predetermined volume of ethanol is ever considered.

Endovascular ablation of AVMs with ethanol has ushered in a new era in the therapy of these problematic anomalies. Cures and permanent partial ablations have been documented in our patient series resulting in symptomatic improvement. Because neovascular recruitment and recanalizations have not been observed, permanent partial ablations have led to long-term symptomatic improvement obviating the need for further treatment. Despite the success that is possible with ethanol, it must be remembered that it is an extremely dangerous intravascular sclerosant that can cause tissue necrosis and neuropathy. The occasional embolizer should refrain from treating AVMs, especially with ethanol. We have observed a 15% complication rate in our AVM patient series and a 0.6% death rate. The death was not directly attributable to an endovascular therapeutic procedure; however, because it occurred within 30 days of a procedure, it must be claimed as a death in our series as per standard surgical protocols (Fig. 2.6.6).

In small AVMs, a single procedure may be sufficient. Treatment of large, complex lesions should be staged for several reasons. In a protracted procedure, contrast limits can be exceeded and an interventionalist can become

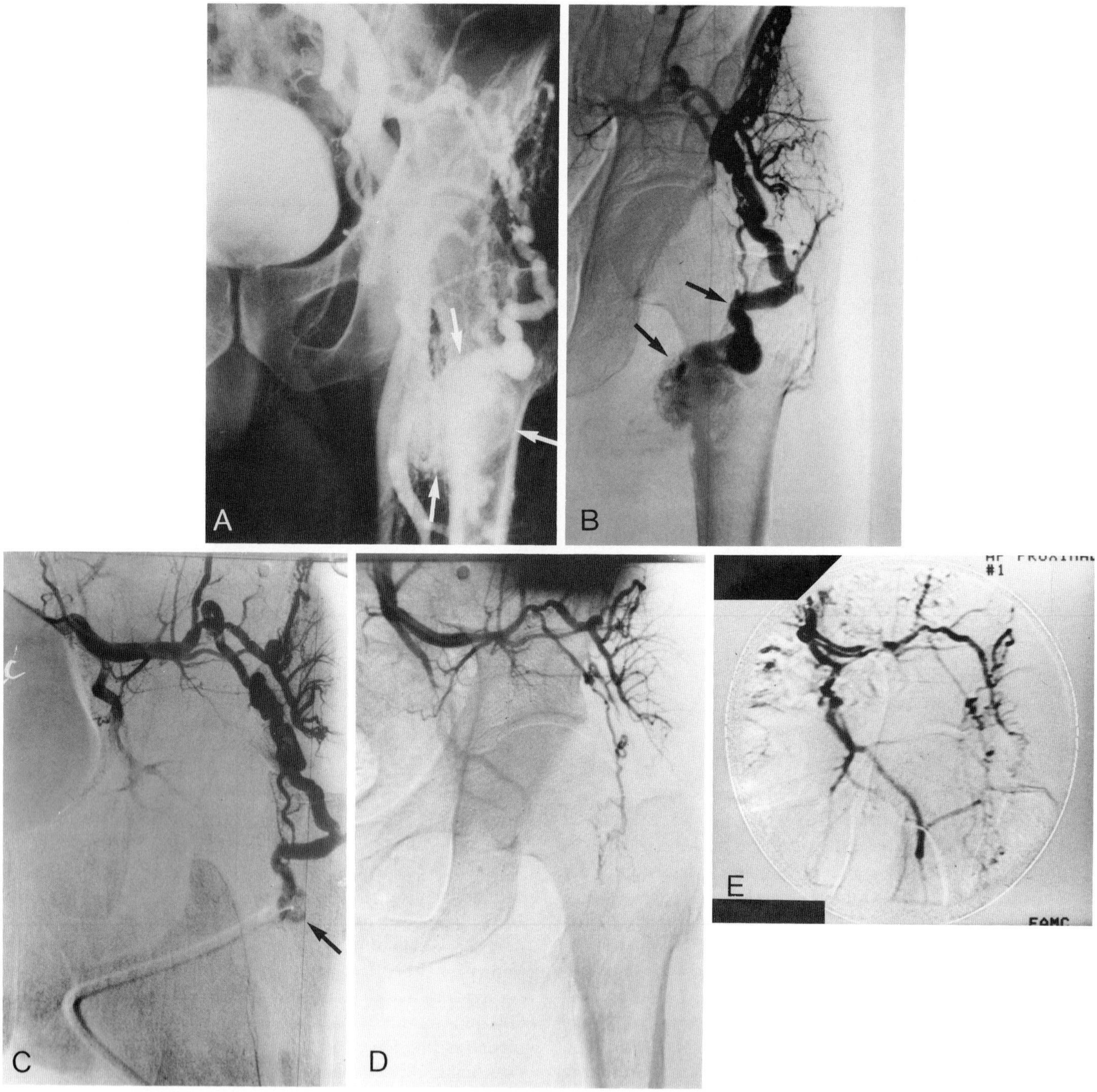

Figure 2.6.5. **A.** AP left common iliac arteriogram. Note hypertrophied arterial system and filling of AVM nidus *(arrows)*. **B.** AP left superior gluteal arteriogram (LSGA), pre-therapy. Note hypertrophied branch supplying superior aspect of AVM nidus *(arrows)*. **C.** AP LSGA, post-ethanol ablation. Film was obtained 5 seconds post-contrast injection. Note stasis in feeder vessel to point where direct puncture ethanol injection was performed *(arrow)*. Note thrombosis of this portion of AVM nidus. **D.** AP LSGA, 6 months post-therapy. Note back thrombosis of entire inflow arterial pedicle secondary to stasis. **E.** AP LSGA DSA, 25 months post-therapy. Vascular pedicle remains thrombosed with no evidence of recanalization or neovascular recruitment. (From Yakes WF, Persner PH, Reed MD, et al: Serial embolizations of an extremity arteriovenous malformation with alcohol via direct percutaneous puncture. *AJR* 1986;146:1038–1040. Reprinted with permission.)

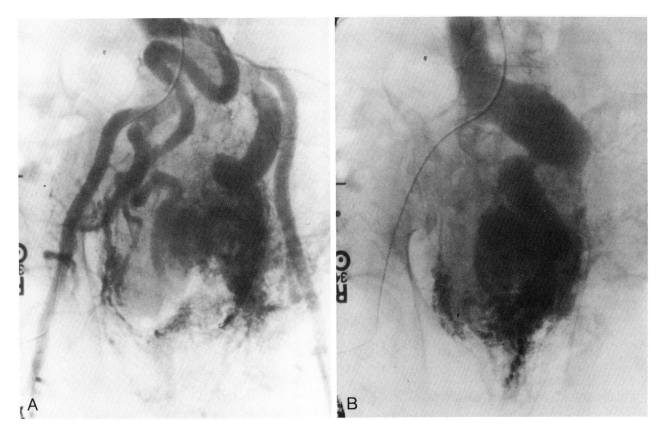

Figure 2.6.6. A 65-year-old male presented with intractable chest pain at rest. **A.** AP pelvis arteriogram showing massive pelvic AVM with enlarged iliac and superior hemorrhoidal branches. **B.** AP pelvis arteriogram, venous phase. Note dilated left common iliac vein and IVC.

fatigued, thereby increasing the probability of a judgment error or technical mishap. Most importantly, serial treatments reduce the risks of too extensive an ablation, thereby decreasing the risk of tissue injury, AVM rupture, or potential complications arising from post-thrombosis edema.

ILLUSTRATIVE CASES

Figure 2.6.4. A 26-year-old right-handed male presented with a seven-month history of progressive swelling over the dorsum of the right wrist. It was painful to palpation and any motion of the wrist and hand. Essentially, the patient had a painful, useless right hand. One endosurgical vascular ablative procedure was performed. A small skin blister appeared six hours post-procedure that led to no sequelae. Follow-up arteriography was performed four months later which demonstrated complete obliteration of the AVM. The painful mass completely shrank and the patient regained full function of his right hand. At three year clinical follow-up, the patient has continued excellent use of his hand without deterioration, and has no evidence of recurrence of the painful mass.

Figure 2.6.5. A 34-year-old male presented with a 10-year history of worsening claudication secondary to an anterior left thigh AVM. At the time of presentation, the

patient's left lower extremity was useless. Prior standard embolotherapy resulted in clinical pulmonary emboli documented on perfusion lung scan imaging. The only surgical alternative was amputation and hemipelvectomy. After four endosurgical vascular ethanol ablative procedures, the patient has suffered no permanent complication, and at six-year clinical follow-up has maintained excellent function of his left lower extremity. No further therapy has been required despite the fact that portions of his AVM remain.

Figure 2.6.6. A 65-year-old male presented to the cardiology service with debilitating resting angina resulting from increased cardiac output secondary to a massive pelvic AVM. Cardiac catheterization revealed an astonishing 16 liters/min cardiac output and high grade stenoses of his left main coronary artery and left anterior descending coronary artery. Coronary artery angioplasty could not be performed because dissection of his left main coronary artery would kill him instantly. Coronary artery bypass could not be performed because no cardiac bypass pump in the world can keep up with a cardiac output of 16 liters/min; hepatorenal failure and severe cerebral ischemia would result. Due to the patient's extremely debilitated and bedridden state, pulmonary embolism was considered a real danger. Because the inferior vena cava measured 3.5cm, a Kimray–Greenfield filter could not be placed. The

Figure 2.6.6 *(Continued).* **C.** AP DSA left internal iliac artery branch prior to treatment. **D.** AP DSA immediately post-therapy. Significant thrombosis occurred. (From Yakes WF, Haas DK, Parker SH, et al: Symptomatic vascular malformations: ethanol embolotherapy. *Radiology* 1989;170:1059–1066. Reprinted with permission.)

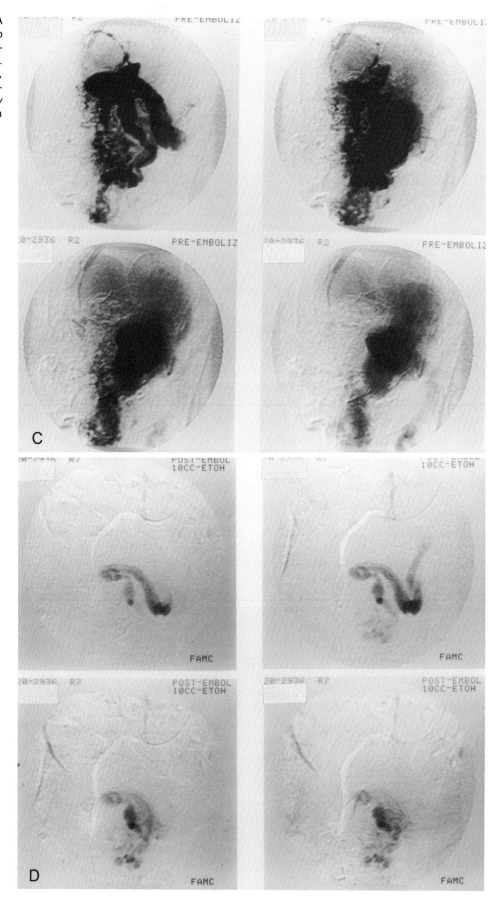

patient was, therefore, placed on heparin therapy despite the fact that it could potentially interfere with the planned endosurgical ethanol ablative procedures. Because of the patient's debilitated status, procedures were performed every four days. After three procedures, the patient's cardiac output was reduced to 12 liters/min documenting the efficacy of therapy. One day after the fourth procedure, a small hematocrit drop was identified. A pelvic CT scan showed a small left pelvic hematoma. Heparin therapy was discontinued and the patient's hematocrit remained stable. Three days after the discontinuation of the heparin therapy the patient suffered a pulmonary embolus, could not tolerate this added insult, and died.

Arteriovenous Fistulae

Congenital and post-traumatic AVF are similar to AVMs in that they are high-flow vascular malformations. AVF are characterized by an artery connected to a draining vein without an intervening capillary bed. Post-traumatic AVF are usually secondary to blunt or penetrating trauma, with injury to an artery and adjacent vein. Fistulization between the artery and vein is stimulated by preferential vascular shunting through the AVF from the high-pressure arterial system to the low-pressure venous system. Chronic AVF may be confused with AVMs at arteriography because multiple enlarged inflow arteries can simulate an AVM nidus near the AV connection.[70,71]

The natural history of AVF can be extremely varied. AVF can remain clinically silent and well tolerated by the patient as can be seen in the iatrogenic dialysis fistula patient or the asymptomatic renal AVF incidently found at aortography. If the shunt through an AVF is large, hemodynamic consequences such as cardiomegaly, increased cardiac output, and intermittent bouts of congestive heart failure can occur. Pain and swelling may also be a presenting complaint. Vascular steal alone may cause ischemic symptoms in the tissues or organs adjacent to the AVF as well.

Treatment of AVF requires complete occlusion of the AV connection. As in treating AVMs, proximal arterial ligations and/or distal venous ligations are doomed to failure (Fig. 2.6.7).[44,71] Surgical ligations are not only futile, they remove possible vascular access routes for endosurgical vascular ablative therapy. Various vascular occlusive devices, such as autologous muscle, spring coil emboli, detachable balloons, PVA, silk suture, and tissue adhesives (IBCA) have been successful in occluding AVF.[27,30,32,49,53-55,71] Recanalizations and recurrences have been reported with the use of IBCA[44] and detachable balloons.[72] Ethanol has proven extremely successful in closing renal AVF,[37] and recurrent peripheral and neural axis AVF.[44] Thus, a great armamentarium exists for the successful endovascular management of AVF. Again, only interventional radiologists skilled in endovascular occlu-

sive techniques should attempt these procedures with the appropriate clinician back-up.

We have treated eight patients with AVF. Five patients had congenital AVF. Three patients had post-traumatic AVF. Two patients had single AV connections and one patient had numerous AVF secondary to a high velocity bullet injury to the thigh (Fig. 2.6.8). One patient was treated using Ethibloc as the endovascular occlusive agent (Fig. 2.6.3) and the other seven patients were treated with ethanol.[44] Our total complication rate is 9% in treating problematic AVF, of which four patients underwent failed prior surgeries and two patients had failed prior embolization procedures.

ILLUSTRATIVE CASES

Figure 2.6.7. A 34-year-old male presented with pain and claudication in the anterior aspect of his left lower extremity (shin) where he had suffered a knife injury 18 years earlier. Surgery was performed but the AVF recurred within 30 days. Because the anterior tibial artery (the feeding artery) was ligated proximally and distally, transfemoral vascular access was lost. Direct percutaneous access to the ligated anterior tibial artery stumps proximally and distally as well as the draining anterior tibial vein was required. After endovascular exclusion of the proximal and distal anterior tibial artery stumps to protect the anterior tibial nerve, ethanol ablation of the AV connection through the anterior tibial vein catheter was successfully performed. The patient suffered no complication and his symptoms were immediately relieved. At one year arteriographic and CDI follow-up, the AVF remains thrombosed and the patient remains symptom-free.

Figure 2.6.8. A 30-year-old male was referred to our service from Texas to treat his multiple AVF secondary to a high velocity bullet injury to his right thigh. His symptoms included intermittent significant pain and marked exercise intolerance due to a massive 18 liters/min cardiac output. Multiple surgeries had failed to relieve the patient's symptoms. Multiple endovascular ablative therapies with various agents failed to effect permanent closure and had no clinical effect. Particulate arterial embolization caused significant multiple pulmonary emboli that caused the patient to become comatose for nine days. A prominent vascular surgeon recommended bilateral lower extremity amputation and a right hemipelvectomy because all therapies had failed to obliterate the AV connections or reduce his massive cardiac output. At our institution, the patient has undergone 21 endosurgical ethanol vascular ablative procedures with successful and permanent closure of all AVF treated documented at follow-up angiography. Furthermore, after 15 procedures, his 18 liters/min cardiac output has been reduced to 8 liters/min with resultant increased exercise tolerance and discontinued use of all cardiac medications. The patient has suffered two small areas of skin necrosis in the posterior thigh, successfully

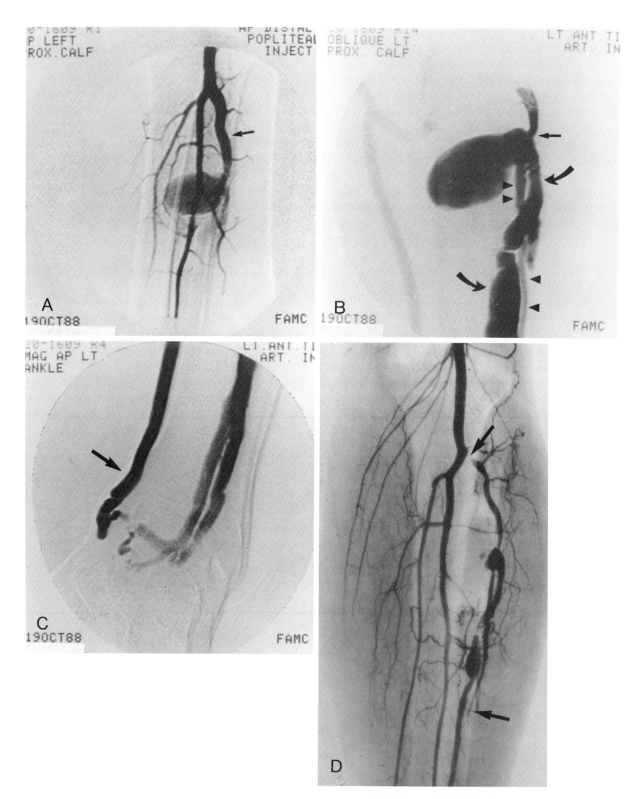

Figure 2.6.7. **A.** AP left popliteal DSA. Note enlarged anterior tibial artery *(arrow)* supplying pseudo-aneurysm and AVF. **B.** AP selective left anterior tibial DSA. Note transected anterior tibial artery proximally *(arrow)* and distally *(arrowheads)*. Note the pseudoaneurysm at the AVF. Note the enlarged anterior tibial vein draining the AVF inferiorly *(curved arrows)*. **C.**

DSA at left ankle. Note inferiorly draining anterior tibial veins coursing medially to drain into the superficial saphenous venous system *(arrow)*. **D.** AP popliteal arteriogram 1 month after surgery. The AVF has recurred, but the pseudoaneurysm has thrombosed. Note ligation of the anterior tibial artery proximal and distal to the fistula *(arrows)*.

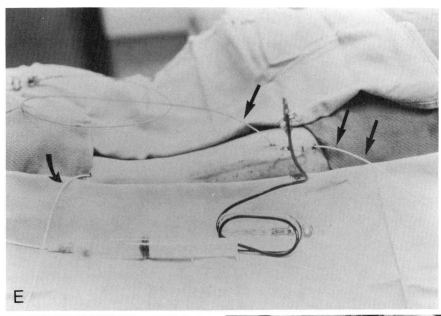

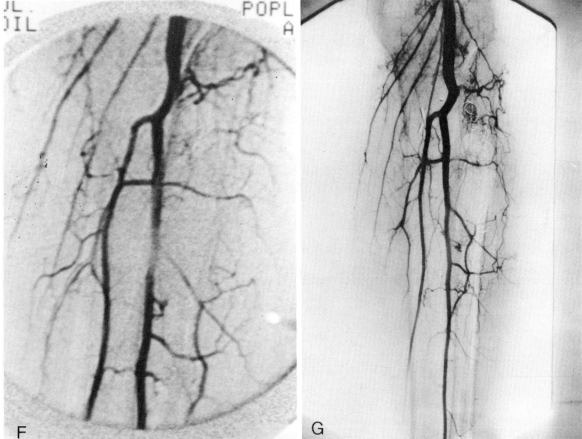

Figure 2.6.7 (Continued). **E.** Direct puncture access catheters in proximal *(arrow)* and distal *(arrows)* anterior tibial artery stumps as well as retrograde anterior tibial vein catheter *(curved arrow)*. Note surgical scar on leg. **F.** AP popliteal DSA immediately post-ethanol ablation. Note closure of AVF. **G.** AP popliteal arteriogram obtained 12 months after ethanol embolotherapy. The AVF remains thrombosed with no evidence of recanalization. (From Yakes WF, Luethke JM, Merland JJ, et al: Ethanol embolization of arteriovenous fistulas: a primary mode of therapy. *JVIR* 1990;1:89–96. Reprinted with permission.)

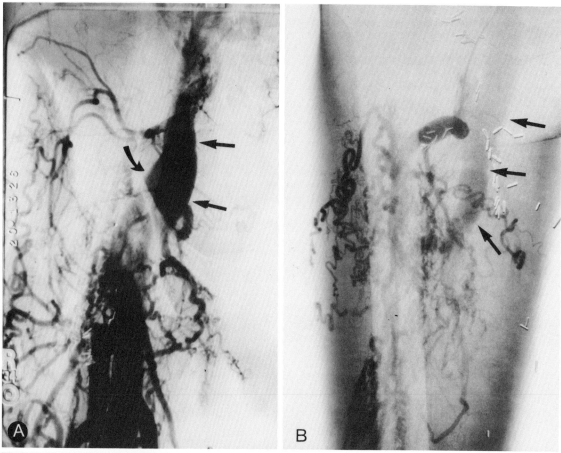

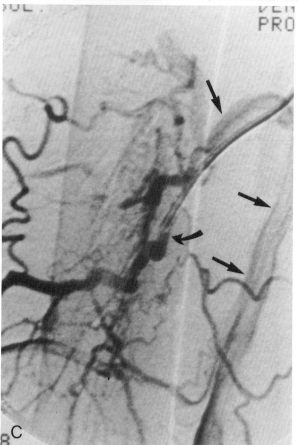

Figure 2.6.8. **A.** AP pelvis arteriogram demonstrating rapid AV shunting with demonstration of the right iliac arterial system *(curved arrow)* and concurrent filling of the right iliac veins *(arrows)*. **B.** AP right profunda femoris arteriogram demonstrating arterial hypertrophy with multiple AVF rapidly shunting into the femoral veins *(arrows)*. **C.** AP retrograde DSA at one fistulous AV connection, pre-therapy. Note multiple arterial channels. Catheter tip at AVF *(curved arrow)*. Note vein opacification *(arrows)*.

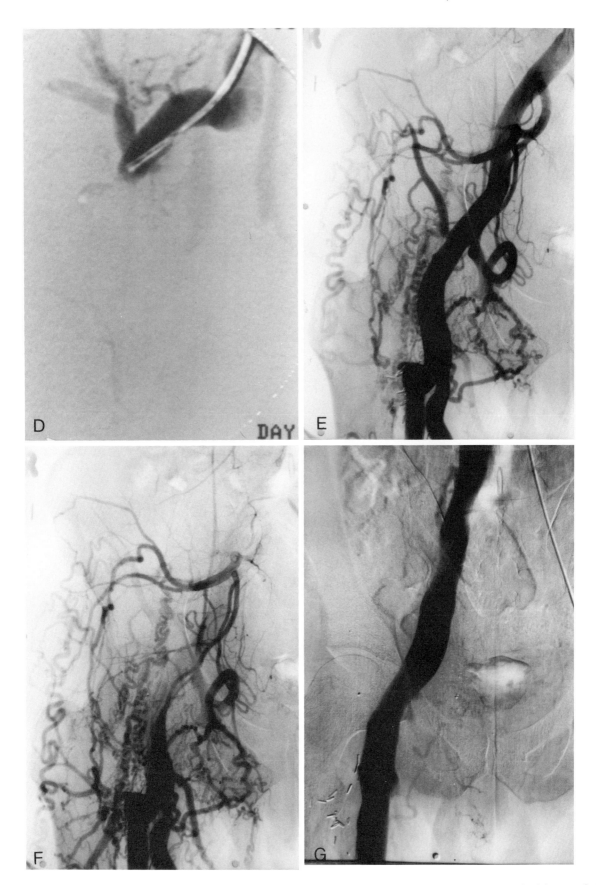

Figure 2.6.8 *(Continued).* **D.** AP retrograde DSA post-ethanol ablation. Note thrombosis at AVF. Only veins are opacified at this point. **E.** AP right iliac arteriogram mid-arterial phase. Note absence of filling of right iliac veins. Compare to **A.** This study was performed after 20 endosurgical ablative procedures. **F.** Same study, late arterial phase. Note that the right iliac veins are still not filling, indicative of a marked decrease in AV shunting. **G.** Same study, late venous phase. Note that right iliac vein is finally seen well past the arterial phase. (From Yakes WF, Luethke JM, Merland JJ, et al: Ethanol embolization of arteriovenous fistulas: a primary mode of therapy. *JVIR* 1990;1:89–96. Reprinted with permission.)

treated with local wound care and antibiotics. No skin grafts or myocutaneous grafts were required.

Venous Malformations

Vein anomalies may occur anywhere in the body but are most often seen in the superior vena cava (SVC), inferior vena cava (IVC), portal vein, and peripheral veins. The SVC may be duplicated, left-sided, or demonstrate anomalous systemic venous return. The IVC may be duplicated, left-sided, have continuation into the azygous and hemiazygous veins, or be atretic. The portal vein may be duplicated, have a congenital portosystemic connection, or may be atretic. Peripheral veins may be atretic, hypoplastic, duplicated, demonstrate avalvulosis, or have retained embryologic remnants. Vein aneurysms are rare anomalies (Fig. 2.6.9).

Venous malformations are congenital vascular malformations arising from abnormal vein morphogenesis. On plain x-ray films, calcified phleboliths may be present. Inflow arteries are of normal size because there is a normal intervening capillary bed. In the late arterial phase, contrast pooling in the postcapillary dilated abnormal venous structures occurs because of slow stagnant flow within the

malformation. Venous malformations are usually incompletely opacified by arteriography alone. Closed system venography[73] or direct puncture venography[74] better demonstrate the extent of the abnormal postcapillary vascular spaces.

The work-up of venous malformation includes CDI, MR scanning, closed-system venography and/or direct puncture venography, and arteriography. CDI is an excellent noninvasive imaging modality to document the presence of a slow-flow venous malformation and distinguish it from a high-flow AVM or AVF. MR is superior to CT to noninvasively diagnose the presence of a venous malformation and to fully evaluate its relationship to adjacent anatomic structures. MR also easily distinguishes venous malformations from AVMs and AVF. Furthermore, CDI and MR posttherapy follow-up studies can be compared to the baseline studies to determine the efficacy of any therapy performed, many times obviating the need for repetitive venography. Because of the imaging sophistication of CDI and MR to noninvasively diagnose the presence of a venous malformation and distinguish it from other types of malformations, venography and arteriography are required only when therapy is indicated.

Venous malformations may be asymptomatic, cosmeti-

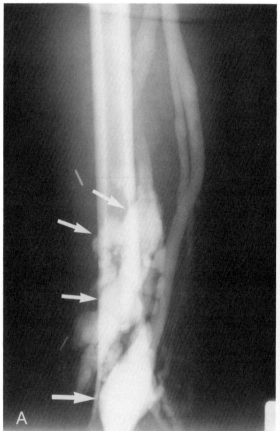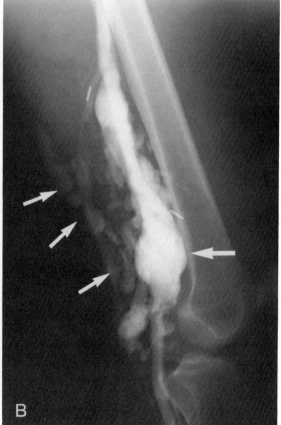

Figure 2.6.9.   Closed system left lower extremity venogram. **A.** AP view. Note popliteal vein aneurysm *(large arrow)*. Also note filling of the abnormal vascular mass of the venous malformation *(arrows)*. **B.** Lateral vein.

Again note popliteal vein aneurysm *(large arrow)* and venous malformation opacification *(arrows)*.

cally deforming, cause pain, induce neuropathy, ulcerate, hemorrhage, induce changes of abnormal bone growth, cause pathologic fractures, and have mixed venous-lymphatic components. Once it is decided that therapy is warranted, then arteriography and venography should be performed. Venography best identifies the extent of the abnormal vascular mass.[73,74] Arteriography usually shows no arterial abnormality; however, occult AVF may be present in mixed lesions and need to be documented prior to therapy. After scrutinizing all baseline studies, an appropriate treatment plan can be presented to the patient and the referring clinician.

We have treated 31 patients with venous malformations in all anatomic locations (Figs. 2.6.10 and 2.6.11). All patients were treated by percutaneous puncture to directly access the abnormal venous vascular elements. Transarterial ablation with ethanol is never performed. Ethanol will thrombose from the capillary bed backward in the arterial system, thus sparing the venous malformation and result in tissue devitalization. Direct puncture techniques directly attack the venous malformation, thus the inflow arterial system and capillary bed is not affected and tissue loss should be minimized. We are experiencing a 10% complication rate with the use of ethanol in treating venous malformations in all anatomic locations.

Illustrative Cases

Figure 2.6.10. A 24-year-old male initially presented with a small venous malformation on the ventral aspect of the wrist. After six surgical procedures which failed to control the lesion, the venous malformation became more aggressive after each surgery, expanded hemodynamically, and threatened to engulf the patient's distal forearm, wrist, and hand. The vascular mass surrounded the median nerve and was causing its degeneration. The patient was then referred to our service and 11 procedures were performed with significant reduction of the abnormal vascular mass at follow-up. After the second procedure, the patient experienced decreased tactile sensitivity of the index finger which has not recovered.

Figure 2.6.11. A 28-year-old male presented with a left facial venous malformation that was cosmetically deforming. The patient has undergone five ethanol ablative procedures without complication. This has resulted in a significant decrease in the size of the abnormal vascular mass and a significant improvement cosmetically. His therapy is ongoing.

Intramuscular Venous Malformations

Intramuscular venous malformations (IVMs), previously incorrectly termed "intramuscular hemangioma," comprise an uncommonly seen subgroup of venous malformations. These venous malformations are largely contained within a muscle and may extend from the affected muscle into surrounding tissues. Although histologically identical, IVMs have a different clinical presentation than nonintramuscular venous malformations. The age of presentation of patients with IVMs is 20–30 years of age, but occasionally may present earlier. IVMs most commonly occur in the extremities and all patients present with a growing palpable mass with or without pain.[75-77]

We have treated six patients with IVMs. If the affected muscle can be resected and the limb function can remain intact, then surgery should be undertaken. However, preoperative transarterial PVA embolization of all feeding arterial pedicles should be performed to minimize surgical blood loss (Fig. 2.6.12). In IVMs in which the muscle cannot be resected without functional loss, direct puncture endosurgical ethanol ablative therapy can be performed to decrease symptoms by shrinking the abnormal vascular mass (Fig. 2.6.13).

Illustrative Cases

Figure 2.6.12. A 26-year-old male presented with a six month history of a painless enlarging mass in his left temporalis fossa. CT documented enhancement within an enlarged left temporalis muscle. Arteriography was then performed which revealed a hypertrophied left internal maxillary artery and deep temporal artery, a dense venous phase stain, and no AV shunts. After superselective catheterization of the left deep temporal artery with a Tracker catheter (Target Therapeutics, Los Angeles, CA), PVA embolization was performed. Five days later, the temporalis muscle was completely excised and the histologic diagnosis was IVM.

Figure 2.6.13. A 21-year-old female presented with a painful enlarging mass in her medial gastrocnemius muscle. Operative excisional biopsy confirmed the diagnosis of IVM. Because the patient did not want surgery, ethanol ablative therapy was performed. After seven treatments, the vascular mass decreased in size and the pain symptoms resolved. At two-year clinical follow-up, the patient remains asymptomatic.

Neural Axis Vascular Malformations

General Concepts

The modern beginnings of cerebral vascular ablative procedures first employed in 1960 by Luessenhop and Spence,[78,79] and later adapted to a transfemoral approach by Kricheff et al.,[80] have undergone significant modifications over the last 30 years. Technological advances in fluoroscopic equipment, C-arm, digital subtraction angiography (DSA), "road mapping" capability, current catheter and microcatheter systems, a vast array of embolic materials, sophisticated angiographic techniques, and the increased knowledge and understanding of neurovascular anatomy and physiology have led to ever-increasing applications of these surgical neuroangiographic procedures. In the last decade particularly, a mushrooming of proce-

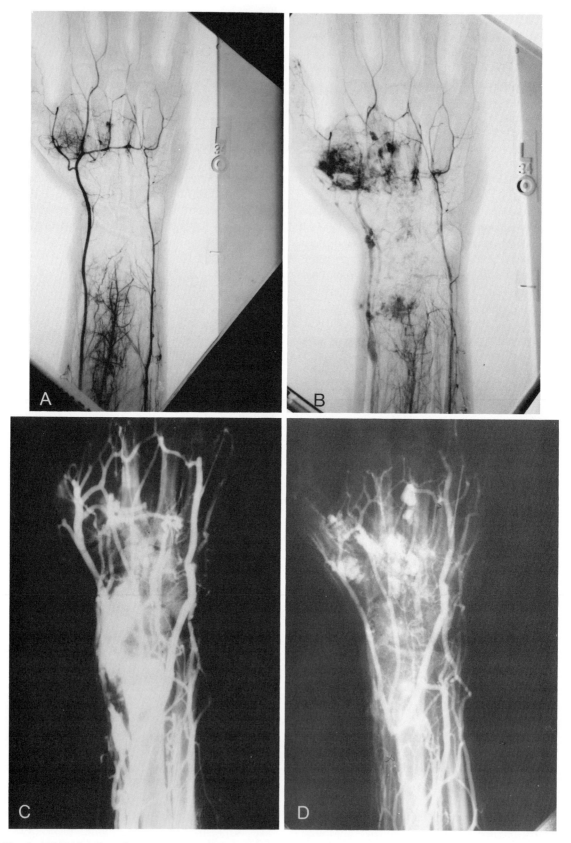

Figure 2.6.10. **A.** AP right hand arteriogram, early phase. Note normal size of inflow arteries. **B.** Same study, late venous phase. Note contrast pooling in venous malformation. **C.** AP closed system venogram, pre-therapy. Note enlarged abnormal venous vascular spaces at the wrist. **D.** AP closed system venogram, 18 months post-therapy. Note the decreased amount of abnormal venous vascular spaces. (From Yakes WF, Parker SH, Gibson MD, et al: Alcohol embolotherapy of vascular malformations. *Semin Intervent Radiol* 1989;6:146–161. Reprinted with permission.)

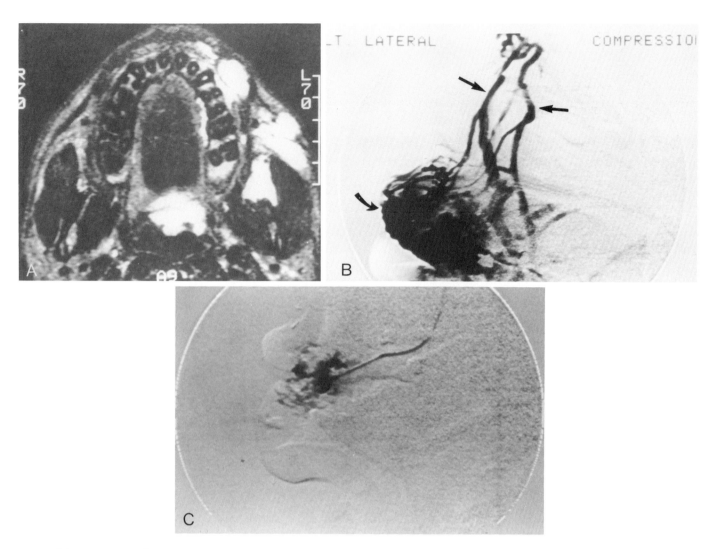

Figure 2.6.11. **A.** Axial T2 weighted MR of the face at the level of the superior alveolar area of the maxilla. Note the multifocal areas of venous malformation involvement characterized by the bright signal. **B.** Lateral direct puncture DSA of the upper lip, pre-therapy. Note the filling of abnormal vascular mass *(curved arrow)* and the draining normal angular veins *(arrows).* **C.** Lateral direct puncture DSA, post-ethanol ablation. Note misregistration artifact secondary to contrast media within areas of thrombosis. Note small area of contrast opacification due to significant thrombosis. The patient has suffered no complication.

dures and clinical applications has led to improved care and better clinical outcomes in patients with complex neurovascular problems. Broader applications of these surgical neuroangiographic techniques and the unveiling of newer procedures will undoubtedly occur in the 1990s. This process would proceed even faster if a better dialogue occurred between interventional neuroradiologists and interventional radiologists. Frequently, one group has solved a vascular problem with which the other is wrestling, and vice versa.

A thorough understanding of neurovascular anatomy and physiology of the brain, the head and neck, and the spine is crucial to minimize complications in these sensitive, high-risk neural areas and to maximize the therapeutic efficacy of interventional neuroradiologic procedures. Significant extracranial to intracranial anastomoses exist between the internal carotid artery, the external carotid artery branches, and vertebral arteries. Knowledge of these anastomoses is crucial to minimize complications that can result in cranial nerve paralysis, blindness, and infarction in the cerebral and posterior fossa vascular territories. An example is the important ascending phalangeal artery, a proximal external carotid artery branch.[81,82] The ascending pharyngeal artery supplies the pharynx, the skull base, and anastomoses to the posterior fossa. Cranial nerves supplied by the ascending pharyngeal artery include III, IV, V, VI, IX, X, XI, and XII. The ascending pharyngeal artery has anastomoses to the inferolateral trunk (or lateral mainstem artery) and meningohypophyseal trunk of the internal carotid artery, the middle meningeal artery, the distal internal maxillary artery, the occipital artery, and the vertebral artery via odontoid and spinomuscular branches. The middle meningeal artery and accessory meningeal arteries are important external carotid artery branches.

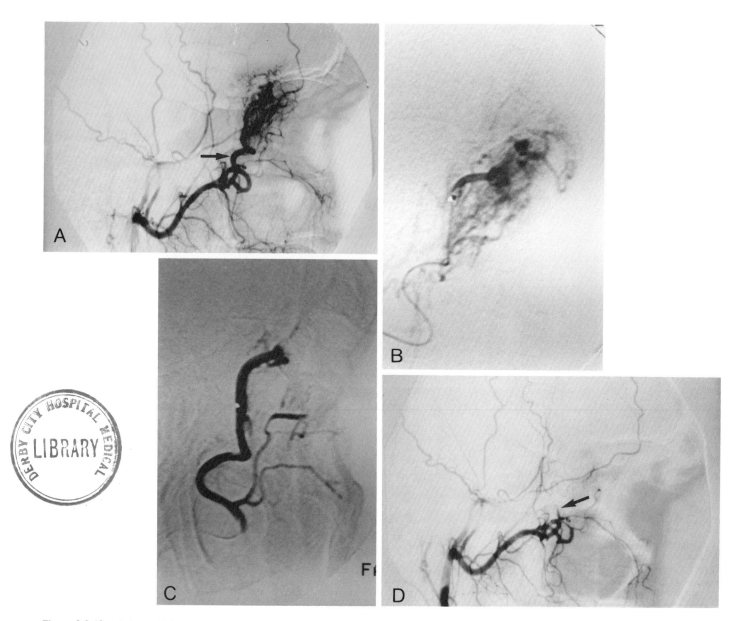

Figure 2.6.12. **A.** Lateral left internal maxillary arteriogram. Note hypertrophy of internal maxillary and deep temporal *(arrow)* arteries. Note dense contrast stain in temporalis muscle. **B.** Lateral DSA with microcath-eter in deep temporal artery prior to treatment. **C.** Lateral DSA post-PVA embolization. Compare to **B. D.** Lateral left internal maxillary arteriogram post-therapy. Note thrombosis of deep temporal artery *(arrow)*.

They supply the dura mater, the skull base, dural tumors, vascular malformations, and they supply cranial nerves III, IV, V, VI, and VII. The middle meningeal artery has normal anastomoses with the cavernous portion of the internal carotid artery and ophthalmic artery as well.

A thorough familiarity with intracranial vascular supply to eloquent areas of the brain such as the motor-sensory cortex, the visual cortex, speech areas, optic tract, internal capsule, and brain stem is essential prior to treating lesions in these vascular territories. An example is the anterior choroidal artery which arises from the internal carotid artery distal to the origin of the posterior communicating artery. If embolization of this artery is to be performed, then catheter placement should be distal to the plexal point to lessen the potential for visual field cuts (optic tract),

hemiparesis and hemianesthesia (internal capsule) and aphasia. Another example is the posterior inferior cerebellar artery which supplies the medulla, cerebellar vermis, fourth ventricle choroid, and cerebellar hemisphere. Catheter induced vascular spasm or embolization of this artery proximally can cause a lateral medullary syndrome (Wallenburg's syndrome).

Because of the need for constant neurologic monitoring during a procedure, neuroleptic analgesics are the most commonly used drugs to induce analgesia and sedation in a patient. General anesthesia is usually required in pediatric patients. The use of nalbuphine hydrochloride (Nubain; Du Pont Pharmaceuticals, Wilmington, DE) and midazolam hydrochloride (Versed; Roche Laboratories, Nutley, NJ) are particularly helpful in sedating and maintaining the

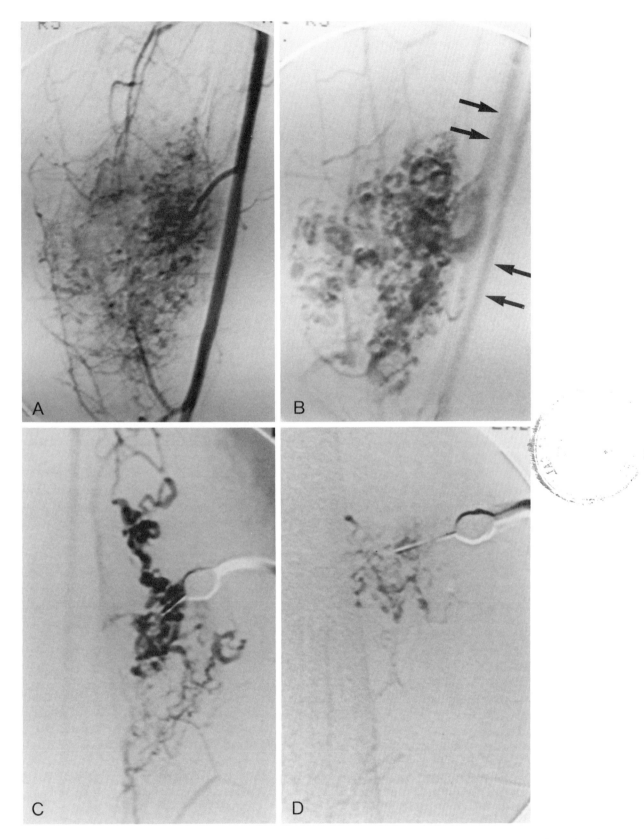

Figure 2.6.13.   A. AP posterior tibial artery DSA. Note inflow arterial hypertrophy and dense venous puddling. **B.** AP DSA, venous phase. Note abnormal venous malformation draining into posterior tibial veins *(arrows)*. **C.** AP pre-therapy direct puncture DSA. Note filling of venous malforma- tion. **D.** AP post-therapy direct puncture DSA. Note significant thrombo- sis. (From Yakes WF, Haas DK, Parker SH, et al: Symptomatic vascular malformations: ethanol embolotherapy. *Radiology* 1989;170:1059–1066. Reprinted with permission.)

ability to neurologically evaluate the patient. Physiologic monitoring by somatosensory evoked potentials (SEP) and brain stem auditory evoked potentials may be employed when a lesion near the sensory-motor cortex or brain stem is being embolized.[83] Electroencephalographic monitoring can be utilized during endovascular ablation of a brain AVM because increases in delta activity can be indicative of inadequate cerebral perfusion.[83]

Total systemic heparinization during interventional neuroradiologic procedures is an extremely controversial issue. Some authors advocate its use[84,85] and others do not.[86] The rationale for total systemic heparinization (5000-unit (ISP) bolus, then 2000 units/hr) is that heparin may decrease the risk of clot embolization from coaxillary placed seating catheters and navigational catheters. However, those who do not advocate its use counter that heparin increases the risks of significant or fatal hemorrhage while treating AVMs. The debate over this issue is ongoing.

Provocative testing has aided in the prediction of potential functional neural loss in anatomic vascular areas prior to endovascular obliteration.[87] Superselective injection of 2% lidocaine (Xylocaine 2%, Astra Pharmaceuticals, Worchester, MA) in the extracranial head and neck arterial circulation is useful as a predictor of potential neural functional loss. Superselective injection of amobarbital (Amytal, Eli Lilly, Indianapolis, IN) is useful in assessing potential neural functional loss in the intracerebral arterial circulation. Lidocaine is never used intracranially because seizures may result. It must be remembered that, throughout a procedure, provocative testing must be repeated because hemodynamic changes can occur as progressive thrombosis causes collateral vessel filling and less vascular steal from normal tissues. Provocative testing may induce deficits later in the procedure that were not present initially. Lidocaine and Amytal provocative testing are not infallible indicators of potential neural injury, just as a positive provocative test does not absolutely mean that a neural injury will always occur. Provocative testing is a useful adjunct in lessening the morbidity and mortality of interventional neuroradiologic procedures.

Normal perfusion pressure breakthrough phenomenon is an important concept in neurovascular procedures as well as peripheral vascular procedures. This phenomenon can occur after endovascular therapy of all or part of a vascular malformation or traumatic AVF.[41,88–90] Because of the chronic vascular steal from adjacent normal tissues to the high-flow lesion (AVM, AVF), chronic arteriolar dilation occurs with resultant atrophy of the muscular media. This medial muscular atrophy causes a loss of arterial contractile strength and, therefore, a loss of normal vascular autoregulation. Furthermore, the chronic arteriolar steal to the high-flow lesion results in a reactive hypotension in adjacent tissues. Once normal tissue perfusion is reestablished with thrombosis of all or part of a high-flow lesion, there is a change from tissue hypotension to increased arteriolar flow and tissue hypertension. Because of the inability

to regulate the increased flow, significant edema or even hemorrhage may occur. Organs such as the brain or spinal cord (surrounded by dura mater and bone) are particularly susceptible to injury when edema and/or hemorrhage causes expansion within an unforgiving confined space.

As with peripheral vascular malformation therapy, the team approach with close consultations between interventional neuroradiologists, neurosurgeons, neurologists, and radiation therapists is essential for the full evaluation of a particular patient's problem. Furthermore, decision making for therapeutic options is optimized by the team approach and patient care is enhanced. Frequently, procedures by several of these specialists are required to treat a particular problem. Examples of this would be the preoperative endosurgical ablation of an intracranial AVM,[91] or decreasing the vascular mass of an AVM nidus by serial endosurgical procedures to optimize the effectiveness of stereotactic radiosurgery.[92]

Arteriovenous Malformations

The embryogenesis of AVMs has already been described and is correlated to the retiform stage of vascular development. Intracranial AVMs are classified as pure pial malformations (no external carotid artery supply) and mixed pial-dural malformations (with external carotid artery supply). The vast majority of AVMs are of the pial type (85%). For unknown reasons, AVMs in the parietal area, central area, and posterior fossa have a greater potential for hemorrhage than AVMs in other areas.

As in peripheral AVMs, vascular parasitization from many vascular territories can occur. On rare occasions, arteriography performed immediately after subarachnoid hemorrhage may fail to demonstrate an AVM. Small AVMs may be a cause of hemorrhage more often than large AVMs. In exceptional cases, spontaneous decrease in size and ultimate thrombosis of AVMs has occurred. More often, if left untreated, AVMs will enlarge at follow-up. Patients with intracranial AVMs present with seizures, headaches, subarachnoid and parenchymal hemorrhage, dementia, progressive neurologic deficits, and hydrocephalus. Intracranial AVMs are particularly difficult management dilemmas. The natural history of untreated intracranial AVMs is complex. Risks of subarachnoid hemorrhage 10 years after diagnosis is 30%, and at 20 years is 42%. The rate of recurrent bleeding is 6% the first year, then a 2% chance of re-bleeding per year thereafter. The risk of developing epilepsy at 10 years is 22%, and at 20 years is 30%. Neurologic disability may occur immediately after an AVM hemorrhage or as late progressive neurologic sequelae. The risk of neurological handicap is 17% at 10 years and 27% at 20 years. The risk of death from all causes at 10 years is 18% and is 29% by 20 years.[93]

AVMs are usually treated if they are causing seizures, have previously bled, or if there is an increased chance of bleeding due to location, presence of arterial or venous aneurysms, or venous outflow stenoses. Modern management of AVMs includes preoperative ablation with PVA[91] or IBCA/NBCA,[94] serial endovascular ablation to reduce the size of the AVM nidus prior to stereotactic radiosurgery,[92,95-97] or endovascular ablative therapy alone (Fig. 2.6.2). The major drawback with radiotherapy has been the one- to two-year interval it takes to produce obliterative thrombosis in the AVM nidus, during which time the patient remains at risk for recurrent hemorrhage.

With the advent of the Tracker catheter (Target Therapeutics, Los Angeles, CA) and the Magic catheter (Ingenor Medical, Paris, France) new avenues have opened in the endovascular management of intracerebral AVMs. The ability to guide a microcatheter into superselective positioning within an AVM feeding vascular pedicle allows for the delivery of many types of endovascular ablative agents. These procedures should only be performed with DSA subtraction and road-mapping guidance. Without these imaging systems, the chance for complication is unacceptably high. Inadvertent small vessel catheterization with the injection of contrast can cause cerebral infarction. Nonionic contrast material should be used to minimize parenchymal damage if contrast extravasation occurs. After provocative testing with Amytal and clinical neurological testing, the endovascular ablative procedure can proceed if no neurologic deficits occur. It must be remembered that, during a procedure, repeat Amytal testing should be performed to evaluate for collateral flow after progressive thrombosis of a portion of the AVM being treated. Endovascular ablative therapy has proven successful as a preoperative measure, as an adjunct prior to radiotherapy, to occlude large fistulous connections, to obliterate aneurysms or pseudoaneurysms associated with increased risk of recurrent hemorrhage, and as a palliative mode of therapy.

Arteriovenous Fistulae

AVF usually occur along dural surfaces and are acquired lesions secondary to trauma, surgery, infection, or other causes of venous obstruction. Dural AVF can occur in the cavernous sinus, anterior cranial fossa, tentorium cerebelli, transverse sinus, sigmoid sinus, and torcular herophili. When these lesions are arteriographically evaluated, the routes of venous drainage must be assessed. If drainage into cortical veins is present, the patient is at a much higher risk for subarachnoid hemorrhage. AVF occurring in the anterior cranial fossa and tentorial region almost always have cortical venous drainage and are at high risk (85%) for hemorrhage (Fig. 2.6.14). AVF in the cavernous sinus area rarely have cortical venous drainage and, therefore, rarely hemorrhage. Patients with AVF may also present with headache, tinnitus, bruit, neurologic deficits, and dementia.[98-101]

Treatment of dural AVF may be performed surgically or endovascularly. Endovascular ablation is usually preferred because of C-arm road-mapping DSA capability, modern microcatheter systems, and current endovascular ablative agents. Transarterial approaches and retrograde transvenous approaches have been successful in occluding dural AVF.[98-101] Multiple endovascular ablative agents have proven successful in AVF closure, such as detachable balloons, metal coils and wires, silk suture, PVA, and IBCA/NBCA. In large dural AVF, care must be taken to neurologically monitor a patient during a procedure. Acute closure of a large AVF can lead to significant neurological complications due to normal perfusion pressure breakthrough phenomenon. Therefore, staged closure with PVA and coils, or slowly inflating a detachable balloon, and constant neurological monitoring for deficits prior to detachment, may be necessary to minimize complications.

Carotid cavernous fistulae (CCF) are complex malformations that involve the cavernous sinus. Venous drainage may be through any outflow venous channel that connects to the cavernous sinus. CCF are classified as Types A, B, C, and D. Type A CCF are direct communications between the cavernous carotid artery and the cavernous sinus that are secondary to trauma or ruptured cavernous carotid aneurysms. Type B CCF are fistulae between internal carotid branch arteries arising from the meningohypophyseal trunk and/or inferolateral trunk and the cavernous sinus. Type C CCF are fistulae arising solely from external carotid artery branches, usually middle meningeal or accessory meningeal branches (Fig. 2.6.15). Type D CCF are fistulae supplied by external carotid and internal carotid artery branches.[102,103] Type A CCF are usually best treated by detachable balloons solely or in conjunction with metal coils.[98,99,104-106] Type B, C, and D CCF are smaller, slower flow fistulae that can be treated with IBCA/NBCA, hypertonic glucose, microcoils, or PVA.[98,99] Manual carotid-jugular compression, in patients without cortical venous drainage or recent decline in visual acuity, has at times proven to be a successful noninvasive method to induce spontaneous CCF closure. Maximum effect is usually achieved in four to six weeks with this manual compression technique. Fistula thrombosis is usually associated with retroorbital pain.[107]

Angiographic findings and clinical presentations have also been evaluated to determine if patients may be at increased risk for morbidity or mortality due to their CCF. After review of 155 patients, several features were associated with a poor patient outcome: presence of pseudoaneurysm, large varix of the cavernous sinus, cortical venous drainage, and thrombosis of venous outflow distal to CCF. Cortical venous drainage is related to absence or occlusion of normal venous outflow pathways and increased venous pressure in the cortical veins resulting in an increased risk of intraparenchymal and subarachnoid hemorrhage. Cavernous sinus varices extending into the subarachnoid space are associated with an increased risk of fatal hemorrhage. Clinical signs and symptoms associated with higher morbidity and mortality include rapidly progressive proptosis,

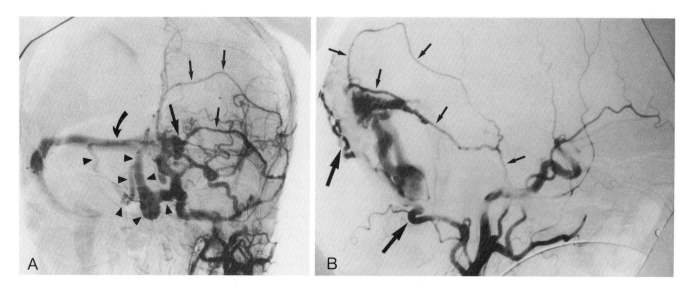

Figure 2.6.14. **A.** AP left common carotid arteriogram. Note hypertrophied meningeal arteries *(arrows)* supplying the tentorial AVF *(large arrow)*. Note prompt AV shunting into transverse sinus *(curved arrow).* Note cerebellar venous cortical drainage *(arrowheads).* **B.** Lateral left common carotid arteriogram. Note hypertrophied meningeal branches *(arrows)* and occipital artery *(large arrows)* supplying the tentorial fistula.

diminished visual activity, prior hemorrhage, increased intracranial pressure, and transient ischemic attacks.[108]

Vein of Galen malformations are AVF that drain into a dilated vein of Galen and straight sinus. Surgery has not improved survival rates (80–90% mortality).[109,110] Surgical ligation of arterial feeders in 60 neonates resulted in only six survivors, and only three neonates were neurologically intact postoperatively. The neonate usually presents with severe congestive heart failure at birth. Infants that survive this initial problem later present with hydrocephalus and seizures, or intracranial hemorrhage. Neonates that present at birth with intractable cardiac decompensation are extremely difficult to manage medically. Endosurgical vascular ablative therapy is an effective initial means to treat these fragile patients. Advances in transcatheter endovascular ablation has improved the outcome in this historically dismal disease. Arteriographic evaluation, as well as performing endosurgical procedures, are difficult in these small neonates. The usual tolerable contrast load is 10–20ml. Arteriography typically shows hypertrophied anterior and posterior choroidal arteries, pericallosal and callosomarginal arteries, thalamoperforator arteries, and, to a lesser extent, middle cerebral branches, lenticulostriate branches, and superior cerebellar artery branches. These multiple AVF may be large direct connections to the vein of Galen or smaller, more numerous fistulae. Endosurgical vascular ablative techniques include transfemoral antegrade arterial approaches, transtorcular retrograde venous approaches, and transfemoral retrograde venous approaches to the vein of Galen.[111–113] Antegrade transarterial approaches allow the use of PVA, IBCA/NBCA, metal coils, silk sutures and detachable balloons. In retrograde transvenous approaches, coils and detachable balloons may be used. Reported complication rates are in the 15–20% range, which include deep cerebral infarctions,

debilitating pulmonary embolism, and intracranial hemorrhage. Despite these potential sequelae, current techniques have successfully managed these problematic patients. Although complete cure is not the rule, by reducing the flow through the AV shunt the neonate can grow and develop to a point where other therapies may be used.

Vertebral artery fistulae are another vascular anomaly that may be congenital but usually are post-traumatic lesions whereby a connection occurs between the vertebral artery and adjacent paravertebral veins.[54,114] Neurofibromatosis, fibromuscular dysplasia, and collagen vascular diseases have been implicated as causes for vertebral AVF as well.[115,116] Patients with vertebral AVF usually present with neck pain and bruit but may also have embolic complications, neck hemorrhage and expanding hematomas, subarachnoid hemorrhage, brain or spinal cord dysfunction, and airway obstruction.[117–119] Long-standing vertebral AVF can cause progressive vascular steal from the intracranial circulation, resulting in tissue ischemia and loss of normal vascular autoregulation. If abrupt closure of the fistula occurs, normal perfusion pressure breakthrough can result in neurologic dysfunction and/or hemorrhage.[88–90,119]

Optimal treatment is with detachable balloons and/or coils placed into the drainage vein and fistula which will close the AVF and maintain patency of the vertebral artery. In some patients with severely traumatized vertebral arteries, vertebral artery closure with detachable balloons and/or coils above and below the fistula may be mandatory. It is usually well tolerated by the patient because of contralateral vertebral artery flow across the basilar artery origin to the site of vertebral artery occlusion or the last vertebral artery branch take-off. Endosurgical vascular occlusion is superior to standard surgical approaches with closure rates of 100%, low morbidity, and no mortalities reported.[54,120]

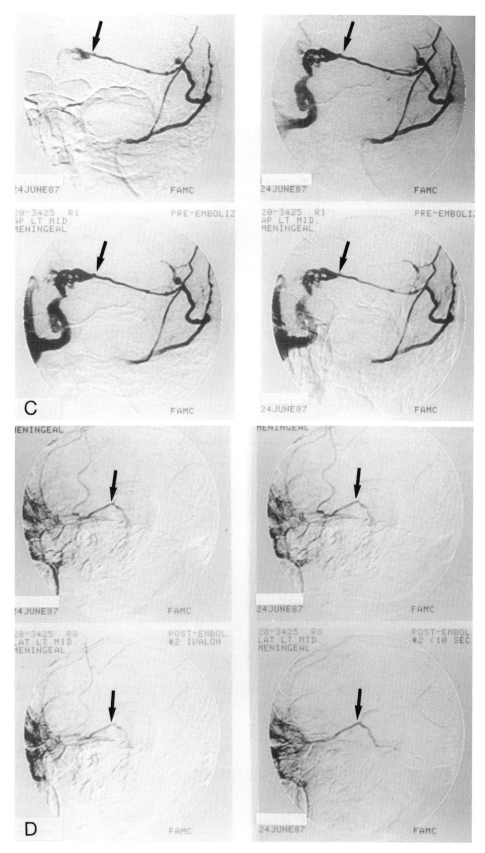

Figure 2.6.14 *(Continued).* **C.** RPO left middle meningeal DSA, pre-therapy. Note hypertrophied middle meningeal arterial branch supplying the fistula *(arrow).* **D.** Lateral left middle meningeal DSA post-PVA embo-lization. Note stasis in left middle meningeal artery branch *(arrow)* and nonfilling of AVF distally.

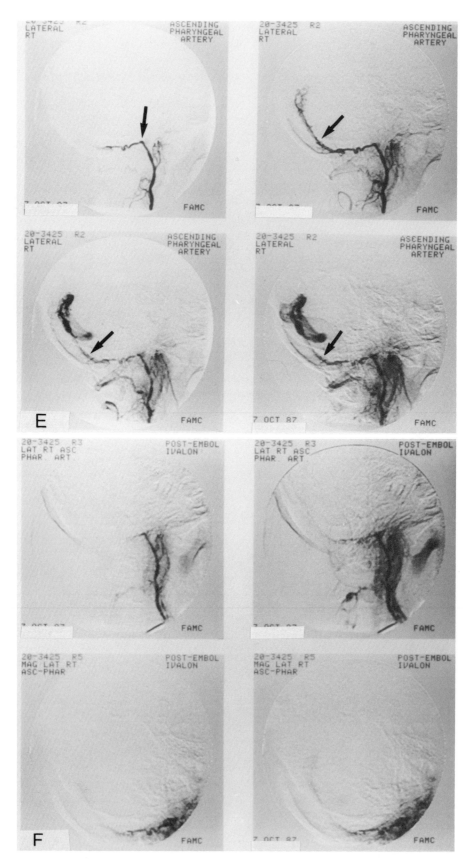

Figure 2.6.14 (Continued).   E. Lateral right ascending pharyngeal DSA, pre-therapy. Note hypertrophied tentorial feeder *(arrow).* **F.** Lateral right ascending pharyngeal DSA, post-PVA embolization. Note arterial throm-bosis and non-opacification of AVF. The patient went on to a successful surgical resection.

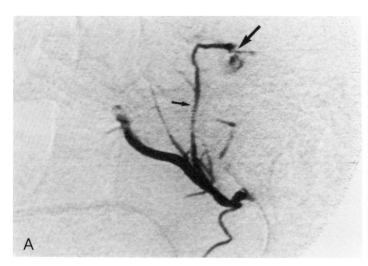 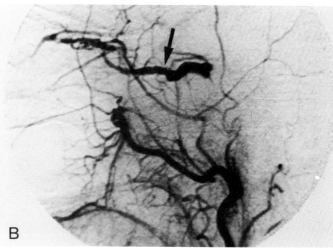

Figure 2.6.15. A. Lateral left internal maxillary DSA. Note accessory meningeal artery *(arrow)* supplying the Type C dural AVF *(large arrow).* **B.** Lateral external carotid DSA. Note accessory meningeal artery supplying dural AVF with drainage via the left superior ophthalmic vein *(arrow).*

Vertebral fistula closure should be performed in the awake patient to monitor for neurologic changes as the fistula is gradually occluded. If neurologic changes occur, the detachable balloon can be deflated immediately. Gradual closure of the AVF may be required to minimize complications arising from normal perfusion pressure breakthrough phenomenon. This technique is definitive and is the procedure of choice for treating vertebral artery fistulae.

SPINAL VASCULAR MALFORMATIONS
Vertebral Body Venous Malformations

Venous malformations of vertebral bodies may occur at any level. The typical radiographic findings are coarse, thickened trabeculae within a vertebral body. Patients may be asymptomatic and the malformation incidentally discovered on plain x-ray films. When vertebral venous malformations become neurologically symptomatic, their findings are usually related to the vertebral level involved. Pain and pathologic fractures may be other presenting complaints.

MR is the imaging modality of choice to evaluate the vertebral body itself and to determine any extraosseous extension of the venous malformation. Arteriography may be normal or show moderate arterial hypertrophy with a venous stain. Digital subtraction angiography is usually more sensitive than magnification cut-film arteriography to determine late phase venous puddling. It must be remembered that arteriography must be performed at the involved vertebral body as well as above and below the affected level to do a complete evaluation.

When patient symptoms warrant therapy, endosurgical vascular ablative therapy is an excellent treatment option. Transarterial endovascular ablation has given excellent palliation in relieving pain symptoms and in reversing neu-

rologic deficits by shrinking the vascular mass. This treatment option has also proven helpful as a preoperative measure. Retrograde injection of methyl methacrylate into a vertebral body has proven successful as a therapeutic option to stabilize the weakened vertebral body, thus obviating the need for surgery.[121-124] Other interventional procedures will most certainly come about to help manage this challenging problem.

Spinal Arteriovenous Malformations

Spinal AVMs are of several types and are classified as intradural intramedullary AVMs, intradural perimedullary AVMs, dural AVF, metameric AVMs, and paraspinal extradural AVMs.[125,126] AVMs are distinguishable from AVF in that AVMs have an intervening nidus between the inflow arteries and outflow veins and AVF are characterized by a single shunt between one or several medullary arteries to a single perimedullary vein. Another classification system of spinal cord vascular malformations is: Type I (long dorsal or dural spinal AVMs); Type II (compact or glomus lesions, usually intramedullary AVM with multiple feeders); Type III (large juvenile malformations or metameric AVM); and Type IV (direct AVF without an intervening network of small vessels).[127,128]

The spinal cord is supplied by one anterior spinal artery and two posterior spinal arteries. The anterior spinal artery traverses along the anterior median sulcus of the spinal cord. The two posterior spinal arteries lie on the dorsolateral cord surface, posterior to the dorsal nerve root on each side. These spinal arteries receive arterial supply from radicular arterial branches from the vertebral, ascending and deep cervical, intercostal, and lumbar arteries. Three of the major contributors to the anterior spinal artery circulation are radicular arteries arising from C5 or C6 (artery of the cervical enlargement), the right T6 intercostal artery, and the artery of Adamkiewicz. This artery usu-

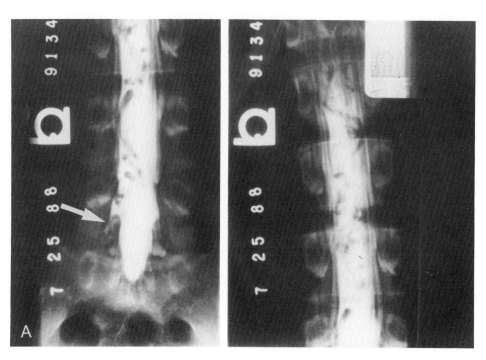

Figure 2.6.16. **A.** PA lumbar myelogram. Note multiple draining veins within the subarachnoid space causing serpiginous filling defects. Note the dilated venous varix draining through the left S-I nerve root sleeve causing the patient's pain symptoms *(arrow).*

ally arises from a lower intercostal or upper lumbar artery on the left. The anterior spinal artery supplies two-thirds to four-fifths of the cross-sectional area of the spinal cord. The paired posterior spinal arteries supply the posterior columns and a portion of the white matter anteriorly. At the tip of the conus medullaris, the two posterior spinal arteries anastomose with the anterior spinal artery forming the cruciate anastomosis. Thus, in evaluating spinal cord vascular malformations, arteriograms of both vertebral arteries, ascending and deep cervical arteries, all intercostal arteries, and all lumbar arteries are essential to determine the functional vascular anatomy of the spinal cord.

Intradural spinal cord AVMs may be located solely within the spinal cord, partially within the cord, or totally on the cord surface (Fig. 2.6.16). This group of patients usually presents between the second and third decade most commonly with subarachnoid hemorrhage or cord hemorrhage (hematomyelia). Other presenting complaints include nerve root or back pain, motor weakness, numbness, erectile dysfunction, and bowel and bladder dysfunction. Once hemorrhage occurs, the risk of a second hemorrhage in the first month is 10%, and within one year it is 40%. Hurth[129] and Djindjian[130] reported 84 intramedullary AVMs. Patients who had no therapy and were observed over time became increasingly debilitated and many progressed to complete loss of spinal cord function. Mid-thoracic AVMs were determined to have the worst prognosis with 66% of patients disabled at 20 year follow-up. Five deaths were attributable to the AVM itself. Aminoff and Logue studied 60 untreated patients and found that 36% of patients under 41 years of age and 48% of patients

between 41 and 60 years of age were confined to a bed or a wheelchair within three years from the onset of symptoms. Nine patients died from complications of chronic paraplegia.[131]

Initial therapy of spinal cord AVMs was surgical,[127,129–132] and later therapies included endosurgical vascular ablation.[132–138] Yasargil[132] reported a 48% improvement in 41 patients after surgery. An 18% recurrent subarachnoid hemorrhage rate was also seen in those patients whose AVM was incompletely resected (2 of 11 patients). Rosenblum reported a 33% improvement rate in 43 patients with intramedullary AVMs.[127] Hurth reported 56 patients treated surgically with a 60% improvement rate in those patients who had complete AVM removal.[129] In Hurth's series, only 21% of these patients were treated by particulate embolotherapy. 50% of these patients had poor long-term results. But it must be noted that these were the most difficult and complex cases which had been rejected as surgical candidates. In 33% of cases in which particulate embolization produced clinical improvement, disappearance of the AVM was noted at follow-up arteriography. Horton et al. reported three patients who had long-term benefit from particulate embolotherapy.[136] Theron et al. reported four patients who underwent particulate embolotherapy and three patients had marked clinical improvement.[137] Biondi and Merland et al. reported long-term results in 35 patients (mean follow-up six years) who underwent particulate embolotherapy and 57% of patients improved after the first therapy and 54% had persistent long-term benefit.[138] Of note in this patient series is that the authors perform annual angiographic follow-up

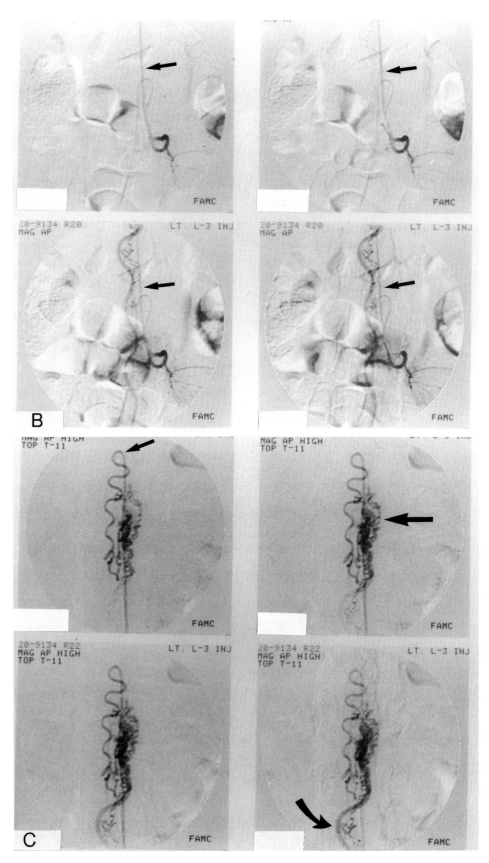

Figure 2.6.16 *(Continued).* **B.** AP left L3 lumbar DSA. Note branch coursing superiorly to supply the intradural perimedullary AVM *(arrow)*. Note the draining veins in the later phase. **C.** AP left L3 lumbar DSA cen-tered over vertebral body T11. Note the hairpin turn *(arrow)* of the feeding artery that then courses inferiorly to supply the AVM nidus *(large arrow)*. Note the inferiorly draining vein from the AVM nidus *(curved arrow)*.

whether or not the patients are symptomatic. Furthermore, repeat embolotherapy is performed if recanalizations are noted without symptom recurrence. The authors conclude that particulate embolotherapy produces better results than those of surgery. In addition, not all spinal cord AVMs are surgically accessible, thus biasing reported surgical results, whereas the most difficult and complex lesions not surgically accessible can be safely treated by particulate embolotherapy.[138]

Metameric spinal AVMs (Type II juvenile malformations) involve the paraspinal musculature, dura, and subarachnoid space. It is typically a high-flow malformation. Paraspinal AVMs involve the paraspinal musculature but not the spinal canal, dura, or subarachnoid space. Both of these rare lesions are extremely difficult management problems. Ommaya[139] and Djindjian[140] published isolated case reports of patients with metameric AVMs with symptomatic improvement following endovascular therapy. Malis reports three patients surgically treated of which one patient died, one patient became acutely paraplegic, and no change occurred in the third patient.[141,142] Spetzler reports a case that was successfully treated with endovascular ablation followed by surgery.[128] Paraspinal AVMs are rare lesions that also pose formidable management problems. We have treated two patients with paraspinal AVMs by ethanol endosurgical vascular ablation. One patient had undergone multiple surgeries which failed to control the AVM, and ultimately underwent radiation therapy which worsened her condition. After the first ethanol endosurgical procedure, the patient had a dramatic clinical improvement immediately following ablation of a portion of her AVM. After a second procedure, adjacent to the left L4 neuroforamen, the patient suffered an acute L3 and L4 neuropraxia, which significantly improved after institution of physical therapy. Follow-up arteriography at 12 months documented persistent thrombosis without evidence of recanalization or neovascular recruitment of all areas treated. A second patient underwent seven ethanol endosurgical vascular ablative procedures without complication. This patient had a midline paraspinal mass measuring 11×13cm in size. At 20 month arteriographic follow-up, the AVM is obliterated without evidence of recanalization or neovascular recruitment. The raised paraspinal mass no longer exists (the patient's back is now flat) and on physical exam the patient no longer demonstrates clonus, Babinski signs, and has recovered from bilateral leg weakness. Furthermore, the patient now successfully competes at the high school varsity level in track and field sports.[41,42]

Spinal dural AVF (Type IV malformations) and spinal AVMs have distinguishable features which suggest that spinal AVMs are congenital and spinal AVF are acquired lesions. Spinal AVMs affect children and young adults. Spinal AVF first become symptomatic in later adult life.[127] The pathophysiology of dural AVF may be related to subarachnoid hemorrhage, arterial steal, or venous hypertension.

Based on pathologic evaluation of the spinal cord, neurological deterioration in spinal AVF is attributed to increased venous pressure.[143,144] Venous hypertension occurs when arterial flow through the dural AVF into a draining medullary vein reaches the valveless coronal venous plexus and medullary veins (Fig. 2.6.17). Conversely, in spinal AVMs, increased arterial flow with vascular steal appears to be the dominant pathologic mechanism for myelopathy.

Therapy of dural AVF includes surgical ligation of the dural AVF, surgical resection of a portion of the dura involved with the AVF, or endosurgical vascular ablative therapy. Endosurgical vascular ablative therapy has emerged as the treatment modality of choice.[144] Occlusive agents used to close dural AVF are IBCA/NBCA, PVA, and microcoils. If the fistula is not completely occluded, there is the possibility of the shunt reopening necessitating further procedures. Conversely, too extensive an embolization, that is when the endovascular occlusive agents thrombose distal to the fistula into the medullary veins of the spinal cord, can lead to ascending medullary vein thrombosis. This is a lethal complication in that the medullary veins progressively thrombose cephalad and cause ascending venous infarction of the spinal cord, which is similar to the congestive venous infarction that occurs in the brain. With time and progressive ascending venous thrombosis, the spinal cord progressively infarcts cephalad until the cardiorespiratory centers in the brain stem infarct and the patient dies. Thus, only interventionalists with significant experience and/or training in managing these problems should treat these patients in which procedural morbidity is high.

SUMMARY

Vascular anomalies (hemangiomas and vascular malformations) pose some of the most significant challenges in the practice of medicine today. Peripheral and neural axis vascular anomalies cause unique clinical problems with regard to their anatomic location. Clinical manifestations of these lesions are extremely protean. Because of the rarity of these lesions, experience in diagnosis and management by most clinicians is limited, augmenting the enormity of the problem and leading to misdiagnoses and poor patient outcomes. Vascular anomalies are best treated in medical centers where patients with these maladies are seen regularly and the team approach is used. The occasional embolizer will never gain enough experience to adequately treat these problematic lesions and these patients should be referred to centers that routinely deal with vascular anomalies and the dilemmas they present. Only in this fashion can significant experience be gained, improved judgment in managing these lesions will develop, and definitive statements in the treatment of vascular anomalies can evolve.

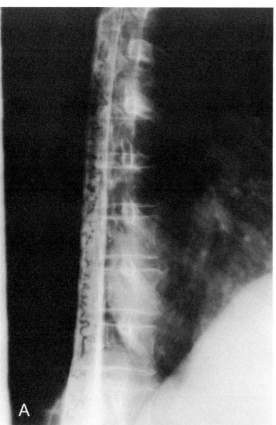

Figure 2.6.17. **A.** Left anterior oblique thoracic myelogram demonstrating the dilated dorsal medullary veins of the spinal cord as serpiginous filling defects. **B.** AP right T7 intercostal artery DSA. Note the radicular arterial feeder *(arrow)* to the AVF *(arrowhead)* and perimedullary vein (large arrow). Note prompt filling of dorsal medullary veins *(curved arrow).* **C.** Lateral right T7 intercostal DSA. Note the dorsal medullary veins *(arrows)* and ventral medullary veins *(arrow)* outlining the spinal cord. The dorsal medullary veins drain cephalad and caudad. The ventral medullary veins drain caudad. **D.** AP right T7 intercostal artery DSA through superselectively placed ''Tracker-18'' catheter. Again note the prompt opacification of the medullary veins. **E.** AP right T7 intercostal artery DSA post-NBCA embolization. Note the misregistration artifact to the NBCA ''cast'' *(arrows).* The cord medullary veins are no longer seen and only the normal arterial branches proximal to the AVF are opacified.

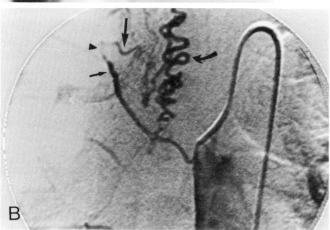

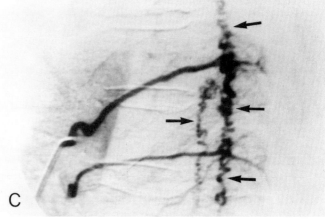

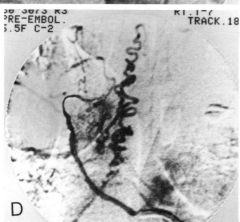

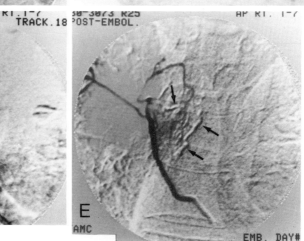

References

1. Decker DG, Fish CR, Juergens JL: Arteriovenous fistulas of the female pelvis: a diagnostic problem. *Obstet Gynecol* 1968;31:799–805

2. Szilagyi DE, Smith RF, Elliott JP, Hageman JH: Congenital arteriovenous anomalies of the limbs. *Arch Surg* 1976; 111:423–429

3. Flye MW, Jordan BP, Schwartz MZ: Management of congenital arteriovenous malformations. *Surgery* 1983;94: 740–747

4. Mulliken JB, Glowacki J: Hemangiomas and vascular malformations in infants and children: a classification based on endothelial characteristics. *Plast Reconstr Surg* 1982; 69:412–420

5. Mulliken JB, Zetter BR, Folkman J: In vitro characteristics of endothelium from hemangiomas and vascular malformations. *Surgery* 1982;92:348–353

6. Glowacki J, Mulliken JB: Mast cells in hemangiomas and vascular malformations. *Pediatrics* 1982;70:48–51

7. Finn MC, Glowacki J, Mulliken JB: Congenital vascular lesions: clinical application of a new classification. *J Pediatr Surg* 1983;18:894–900

8. Upton J, Mulliken JB, Murray JE: Classification and rationale for management of vascular anomalies in the upper extremity. *J Hand Surg* 1985;6:970–975

9. Mulliken JB, Young AE (eds): *Vascular Birthmarks: Hemangiomas and Malformations.* Philadelphia, W.B. Saunders, 1988

10. Woolard HH: The development of the principal arterial stems in the forelimb of the pig. *Contrib Embryol* 1922;14:139–154

11. Reinhoff WF: Congenital arteriovenous fistula: an embryological study with the report of a case. *Johns Hopkins Hosp Bull* 1924;35:271–284

12. Reid MR: Studies on abnormal arteriovenous communications acquired and congenital. I. Report of a series of cases. *Arch Surg* 1925;10:601–638

13. DeTakats G: Vascular anomalies of the extremities. *Surg Gynecol Obstet* 1932;55:227–237

14. Jacobs AH, Walter RG: The incidence of birthmarks in the neonate. *Pediatrics* 1976;58:218–222

15. Lowell SH, Mathog R: Head and neck manifestations of Maffuci's syndrome. *Arch Otolaryngol* 1979;105:427–430

16. Riley HD Jr, Smith WR: Macrocephaly, pseudopapilledema, and multiple hemangiomata: a previously undescribed heredofamilial syndrome. *Pediatrics* 1960;26:293–300

17. Wiedemann HR, Burgio GR, Aldenhoff P, Kunze J, Kaufmann HJ, Schirg E: The Proteus syndrome: partial gigantism of the hand and/or feet, nevi, hemihypertrophy, subcutaneous tumors, macrocephaly, or other skull anomalies and possible accelerated growth and visceral affections. *Eur J Pediatr* 1983;140:5–12

18. Bannayan GA: Lipomatosis, angiomatosis, and macrencephalia. A previously undescribed congenital syndrome. *Arch Pathol* 1971;92:1–5

19. Higginbottom MC, Schultz P: The Bannayan syndrome: an autosomal dominant disorder consisting of macrocephaly, lipomas, hemangiomas, and risk for intracranial tumors. *Pediatrics* 1982;69:632–634

20. Gorham LW, Stout AP: Massive osteolysis (acute spontaneous absorption of bone, phantom bone, disappearing bone). Its relation to hemangiomatosis. *J Bone Joint Surg* 1955;37:985–1004

21. Baskerville PA, Ackroyd JS, Browse NL: The etiology of the Klippel–Trenaunay syndrome. *Ann Surg* 1985;202:624–627

22. Gloviczki P, Hollier LH, Telander RL: Surgical implications of Klippel–Trenaunay syndrome. *Ann Surg* 1983;197:353–362

23. Phillips GN, Gordon DH, Martin EC, Haller JD, Casarella W: The Klippel–Trenaunay syndrome: clinical and radiological aspects. *Radiology* 1978;128:429–434

24. Parkes–Weber F: Haemangiectatic hypertrophy of limbs: congenital phlebarteriectasis and so called congenital varicose veins. *Br J Child Dis* 1918;15:13–17

25. Yakes WF, Stavros AT, Parker SH, Luethke JM, Rak KM, Dreisbach JN, Slater DD, Burke BJ, Chantelois AE: Color Doppler imaging of peripheral high flow vascular malformations before and after ethanol embolotherapy. Presented at the 76th Scientific Assembly and Annual Meeting of the Radiological Society of North America, Nov 25–30, 1990, Chicago, IL. *Radiology* 1990;177(P):156

26. Rak KM, Yakes WF, Ray RL, Luethke JM, Burke BJ, Dreisbach JN, Parker SH, Stavros AT, Seibert CE, Slater DD: MR imaging of symptomatic vascular malformations: diagnostic and therapeutic considerations. Presented (with concurrent scientific exhibit) at the 76th Scientific Assembly and Annual Meeting of the Radiological Society of North America; Nov 25–30, 1990, Chicago, IL. *Radiology* 1990; 177(P):204,369

27. Brooks B: The treatment of traumatic arteriovenous fistulas. *South Med J* 1930;23:100–106

28. Nakano H, Igawa M: Complication after embolization of internal iliac artery by gelatin sponge powder. *Hiroshima J Med Sci* 1986;35:21–25

29. Lee DH, Wriedt CH, Kaufman JCE, Pelz DM, Fox AJ, Vinuela F: Evaluation of three embolic agents in pig rete. *AJNR* 1989;10:773–776

30. Swarc TA, Carrasco CH, Wallace S, Richli W: Radiopaque suspension of polyvinyl alcohol foam for embolization. *AJR* 1986;146:591–592

31. Gianturco C, Anderson JH, Wallace S: Mechanical devices for arterial occlusion. *AJR* 1975;124:428–435

32. Yang PJ, Halbach VV, Higashida RT, Hieshima GB: Platinum wire: a new transvascular embolic agent. *AJNR* 1988;9:547–550

33. Vinter HV, Lundie MJ, Kaufmann JCE: Long-term pathological follow-up of cerebral arteriovenous malformations treated by embolization with Bucrylate. *N Engl J Med* 1986;314:477–483

34. Brothers MF, Kaufmann JCE, Fox AJ, Deveikis JP: N-butyl 2-cyanoacrylate-substitute for IBCA in interventional neuroradiology: histopathologic and polymerization time studies. *AJNR* 1989;10:777–786

35. Widlus DM, Murray RR, White RI Jr, et al: Congenital arteriovenous malformations: tailored embolotherapy. *Radiology* 1988;169:511–516

36. Rao VRK, Mandalam KR, Gupta AK, Kumar S, Joseph S: Dissolution of isobutyl 2-cyanoacrylate on long-term follow-up. *AJNR* 1989;10:135–141

37. Sasaki M, Tadokeoro S, Kimura S, Mori M, Kosula S, Tachibana M: Two cases of renal arteriovenous fistula treated by transcatheter embolization with absolute ethanol. *Hinyokika Kiyo* 1984;30:295–298 (Japanese)

38. Yakes WF, Pevsner PH, Reed MD, Donohue HJ, Ghaed N: Serial embolizations of an extremity arteriovenous malformation with alcohol via direct percutaneous puncture. *AJR* 1986;146:1038–1040

39. Takebayaski S, Hosaka M, Ishizuka E, Hirokawa M, Matsui K: Arteriovenous malformations of the kidneys: ablation with alcohol. *AJR* 1988;150:587–590

40. Vinson AM, Rohrer DB, Willcox CW, et al: Absolute ethanol embolization for peripheral arteriovenous malformation: report of two cures. *South Med J* 1988;81:1052–1055

41. Yakes WF, Haas DK, Parker SH, et al: Symptomatic vascular malformations: ethanol embolotherapy. *Radiology* 1989; 170:1059–1066

42. Yakes WF, Parker SH, Gibson MD, Haas DK, Pevsner PH, Carter TE: Alcohol embolotherapy of vascular malformations. *Semin Intervent Radiol* 1989;6:146–161

43. Yakes WF, Luethke JM, Parker SH, et al: Ethanol embolization of vascular malformations. *RadioGraphics* 1990; 10:787–796

44. Yakes WF, Luethke JM, Merland JJ, et al: Ethanol embolization of arteriovenous fistulas: a primary mode of therapy. *JVIR* 1990;1:89–96

45. Cho KJ, Williams DM, Brady TM, Weiss CA, Forrest ME, Oke EJ, Griffin DJ: Transcatheter embolization with sodium tetradecyl sulfate. *Radiology* 1984;153:95–99

46. Woods JE: Extended use of sodium tetradecyl sulfate in the treatment of hemangiomas and other related conditions. *Plast Reconstr Surg* 1987;79:542–549

47. Hunter DW, Moradian GP, Castañeda–Zúñiga WR, Amplatz K: Transvenous sclerotherapy of peripheral arteriovenous malformations and hemangiomas. Presented at the 75th Scientific Assembly and Annual Meeting of the Radiological Society of North America, Nov 26–Dec 1, 1989, Chicago, IL. *Radiology* 1989;173(P):179

48. Serbinenko FA: Balloon catheterization and occlusion of major cerebral vessels. *J Neurosurg* 1975;41:125–145

49. Hieshima GB, Grinnell VS, Mehringer CM: A detachable balloon for therapeutic transcatheter occlusions. *Radiology* 1981;138:227–228

50. Berenstein A, Ransohoff J, Kupersmith M, et al: Transvascular treatment of giant aneurysms of the cavernous carotid and vertebral arteries. Functional investigation and embolization. *Surg Neurol* 1984;21:3–12

51. Hieshima GB, Higashida RT, Wapenski J, Hallbach VV, Cahan L, Bentson JR: Balloon embolization of a large distal basilar artery aneurysm. *J Neurosurg* 1986;65:413–416

52. Kaufman SL, Kadir S, Barth KH, Smith JW, Walsh PC, White RI Jr: Mechanisms of recurrent varicocele after balloon occlusion or surgical ligation of the internal spermatic vein. *Radiology* 1983;147:435–440

53. White RI Jr, Lynch–Nyhan A, Terry P, et al: Pulmonary arteriovenous malformations: technique and long-term outcome of embolotherapy. *Radiology* 1988;169:663–669

54. Halbach VV, Higashida RT, Hieshima GB: Treatment of vertebral arteriovenous fistulas. *AJR* 1988;150:405–412

55. Halbach VV, Higashida RT, Hieshima GB, Hardin CW, Dowd CF, Barnwell SL: Transarterial occlusion of solitary intracerebral arteriovenous fistulas. *AJNR* 1989;10:747–752

56. Riche MC, Hadjean E, Tran–Ba–Huy P, Merland JJ: The treatment of capillary-venous malformations using a new fibrosing agent. *Plast Reconstr Surg* 1983;71:607–612

57. Stigmar G, Crawford JS, Ward CM, Thomson HG: Ophthalmic sequelae of infantile hemangiomas of the eyelids and orbit. *Am J Ophthalmol* 1978;85:806–813

58. Overcash KE, Putney FJ: Subglottic hemangioma of the larynx treated with steroid therapy. *Laryngoscope* 1973; 83:679–682

59. Larcher VF, Howard ER, Mowat AP: Hepatic hemangioma: diagnosis and management. *Arch Dis Child* 1981;56:7–14

60. Argenta LC, Bishop E, Cho KJ, Andrews AF, Coran AG: Complete resolution of life-threatening hemangioma by embolization and corticosteroids. *Plast Reconst Surg* 1982;760:739–742

61. Bowles LJ: Perinatal hemorrhage associated with the Kasabach–Merritt syndrome. *Clin Pediatr* 1981;20:428–429

62. Esterly NG: Kasabach–Merritt syndrome in infants. *J Am Acad Derm* 1983;8:504–513

63. Bartoshesky LE, Bull M, Feingold M: Corticosteroid treatment of cutaneous hemangiomas: how effective? A report on 24 children. *Clin Pediatr* 1978;17:625–638

64. Hurvitz CH, Alkalay AL, Slovinsky L, Kallus M, Pomerance JJ: Cyclophosphamide therapy in life-threatening vascular tumors. *J Pediatr* 1986;109:360–363

65. Warrell RP Jr, Kempin SJ: Treatment of severe coagulopathy in the Kasabach–Merritt syndrome with aminocaproic acid and cryoprecipitate. *N Engl J Med* 1985;313:309–312

66. Olcott C, Newton TH, Stoney RJ, Ehrenfell WK: Intraarterial embolization in the management of AVMs. *Surgery* 1976;79:3–12

67. Kaufman SL, Kumar AAJ, Roland JMA, et al: Transcatheter embolotherapy in the management of congenital arteriovenous malformations. *Radiology* 1980;137:21–29

68. Gomes AS, Busutill RW, Baker JD, et al: Congenital AVMs: the role of transcatheter arterial embolization. *Arch Surg* 1983;118:817–825

69. Clouse ME, Levin DC, Desautels RE, et al: Transcatheter embolotherapy for congenital renal AVMs. *Urology* 1983;22:360–365

70. Trout HH, Tievsky AL, Rieth KG, Druy EM, Giordano JM: Arteriovenous fistula simulating arteriovenous malformation. *Otolaryngol Head Neck Surg* 1987;97:322–325

71. Lawdahl RB, Routh WD, Vitek JJ, McDowell HA, Gross GM, Keller FS: Chronic arteriovenous fistulas masquerading as arteriovenous malformations: diagnostic considerations and therapeutic implications. *Radiology* 1989; 170:1011–1015

72. Keller FS, King CE: Delayed detachable balloon migration: a cause of recurrent arteriovenous fistula. *J Intervent Radiol* 1986;1:37–39

73. Geiser JH, Eversmann WW: Closed system venography in the evaluation of upper extremity hemangioma. *J Hand Surg* 1978;3:173–178

74. Boxt LM, Levin DC, Fellows KE: Direct puncture angiography in congenital venous malformations. *AJR* 1983;140:135–136

75. Jones KG: Cavernous hemangioma of striated muscle: a review of the literature and report of four cases. *J Bone Joint Surg* 1953;35:717–728

76. Connors JJ, Khan G: Hemangioma of striated muscle. *South Med J* 1977;70:1423–1424

77. Welsh D, Hengerer AS: The diagnosis and treatment of intramuscular hemangiomas of the masseter muscle. *Am J Otolaryng* 1980;1:186–190

78. Luessenhop AJ, Spence WT: Artificial embolization of cerebral arteries. Report of use in a case of arteriovenous malformation. *JAMA* 1960;172:1153–1155

79. Leussenhop AJ, Kachmann R, Shevlin W, et al: Clinical evaluation of artificial embolization in the management of large cerebral arteriovenous malformations. *J Neurosurg* 1965;23:400–417

80. Kricheff II, Madayag M, Braunstein P: Transfemoral catheter embolization of cerebral and posterior fossa arteriovenous malformations. *Radiology* 1972;103:107–111

81. Lasjaunias P, Moret J: The ascending pharangeal artery: normal and pathologic radioanatomy. *Neuroradiology* 1976;11:77–82

82. Lasjaunias P, Berenstein A: Functional vascular anatomy of the craniofacial arteries, in *Surgical Neuroangiography*, Vol I. Heidelberg, Springer–Verlag, 1987

83. Grundy DL: Monitoring of sensory evoked potentials during neurosurgical operations: methods and applications. *Neurosurgery* 1982;11:556–575

84. Halbach VV, Higashida RT, Hieshima GB, Hardin CW: Embolization of branches arising from the cavernous portion of the internal carotid artery. *AJNR* 1989;10:143–150

85. Eskridge JM: Interventional neuroradiology. *Radiology* 1989;172:991–1006

86. Merland JJ: Personal communication 1990. University of Paris VII, Hopital Lariboisiere, Service de Neuroradiologie et d'Angiographic Therapeutique, Paris, France

87. Horton JA, Kerber CW: Lidocaine injection into external carotid branches: provocative test to preserve cranial nerve function in therapeutic embolization. *AJNR* 1986;7:105–108

88. Spetzler RF, Wilson CB, Weinstein P, et al: Normal perfusion pressure breakthrough theory. *Clin Neurosurg* 1978;25:651–672

89. Jones FD, Boone SC, Whaley RA: Intracranial hemorrhage following attempted embolization and removal of large arteriovenous malformations. *Surg Neurol* 1982;10:278–283

90. Halbach VV, Higashida RT, Hieshima GB, Norman D: Normal perfusion pressure breakthrough occurring during treatment of carotid and vertebral fistulas. *AJNR* 1987;8:751–756

91. Purdy PD, Samson D, Batzer HH, Risser RC: Preoperative embolization of cerebral arteriovenous malformations with polyvinyl alcohol particles: experience in 51 adults. *AJNR* 1990;11:501–510

92. Dawson RC III, Tarr RW, Hecht ST, et al: Treatment of arteriovenous malformations of the brain with combined embolization and stereotactic radiosurgery: results after 1 and 2 years. *AJNR* 1990;11:857–864

93. Crawford PM, West CR, Chadwick DM, Shaw MDM: Arteriovenous malformations of the brain: natural history in unoperated patients. *J Neurol Neurosurg Psychiatry* 1986;49:1–10

94. Pelz DM, Fox AJ, Vinuela F, Drake CC, Ferguson GG: Preoperative embolization of brain AVMs with isobutyl-2-cyanoacrylate. *AJNR* 1988;9:757–764

95. Kjellberg RN, Hanamura T, Davis KR, Lyons SL, Adams RD: Bragg-peak proton beam therapy for arteriovenous malformations of the brain. *N Engl J Med* 1983;309:269–274

96. Steiner L: Radiosurgery in cerebral arteriovenous malformations, in: Flamm E, Fein J (eds): *Textbook in Cerebrovascular Surgery*. Vol 4. New York, Springer–Verlag, 1986, pp 1161–1215

97. Lunsford DL, Fleckinger J, Lindner G, Maitz A: Stereotactic radiosurgery of the brain using the first United States 201 cobalt 60 source gamma knife. *Neurosurgery* 1989;24:151–158

98. Lasjaunias P, Chiu M, Ter Brugge K, Tolia A, Hurth M, Bernstein M: Neurological manifestations of intracranial dural arteriovenous malformations. *J Neurosurg* 1986;64:724–730

99. Picard L, Bracard S, Moret J, Per A, Giacobbe HL, Roland J: Spontaneous dural arteriovenous fistulas. *Semin Intervent Radiol* 1987;4:219–241

100. Halbach VV, Higashida RT, Hieshima GB, Mehringer CM, Hardin CW: Transvenous embolization of dural fistulas involving the transverse and sigmoid sinuses. *AJNR* 1989;10:385–392

101. Barnwell SL, Halbach VV, Dowd CF, Higashida RT, Hieshima GB. Dural arteriovenous fistulas involving the inferior petrosal sinus: angiographic findings in six patients. *AJNR* 1990;11:511–516

102. Smith MD, Russell EJ, Levy R, Crowell RM: Transcatheter obliteration of a cerebellar arteriovenous fistula with platinum coils. *AJNR* 1990;11:1199–1202

103. Viñuela F, Fox AJ, Kan S, Drake CG: Balloon occlusion of a spontaneous fistula of the posterior inferior cerebellar artery. *J Neurosurg* 1983;58:287–290

104. Debrun GM: Treatment of traumatic carotid-cavernous fistulae using detachable balloon catheter. *AJNR* 1983;4:355–356

105. Hallbach VV, Higashida RT, Hieshima GB, Reicher M, Normal D, Newton TH: Dural fistulas involving the cavernous sinus: results in treatment in 30 patients. *Radiology* 1987;163:437–442

106. Wilms G: Unilateral double carotid cavernous fistula treated with detachable balloons. *AJNR* 1990;11:517

107. Higashida RT, Hieshima GB, Halbach VV, Bentson JR, Goto K: Closure of carotid cavernous fistulae by external compression of the carotid artery and jugular vein. *Acta Radiol Suppl (Stockh)* 1986;369:580–583

108. Halbach VV, Hieshima GB, Higashida RT, Reicher M: Carotid cavernous fistulae: indications for urgent treatment. *AJNR* 1987;8:627–633

109. Johnston IH, Whittle IR, Besser M, Morgan MK: Vein of Galen malformation: diagnosis and management. *Neurosurgery* 1987;20:747–758

110. Hoffman HJ, Chuang S, Hendrick EB, Humphreys RP: Aneurysms of the vein of Galen: experience at the Hospital for Sick Children, Toronto, Canada. *J Neurosurg* 1982; 57:316–322

111. Edwards MSB, Hieshima GB, Higashida R, Halbach V: Management of vein of Galen malformations in the neonate. *Int Pediatr* 1988;3:184–188

112. Mickle JP, Quisling RG: The transtorcular embolization of vein of Galen aneurysms. *J Neurosurg* 1986;64:731–735

113. Dowd CF, Halbach VV, Barnwell SL, Higashida RT, Edwards MSB, Hieshima GB: Transfemoral venous embolization of vein of Galen malformations. *AJNR* 1990;11:643–648

114. Hayes P, Gerlock AJ Jr, Cobb CA: Cervical spine trauma: a cause of vertebral artery injury. *J Trauma* 1980;20:904–905

115. Deans WR, Block S, Leibrock L, Berman BM, Skultety FM: Arteriovenous fistula in patients with neurofibromatosis. *Radiology* 1982;144:103–107

116. Reddy SV, Karnes WE, Earnest F IV, Sundt TM Jr: Spontaneous arteriovenous fistulas of cerebral vessels in association with fibromuscular dysplasia. *J Neurosurg* 1981; 54:399–402

117. Nagashima C, Iwasaki T, Kawanuma S, Sakaguchi A, Kamisas A, Suzuki K: Traumatic arteriovenous fistula of the vertebral artery with spinal cord symptoms: a case report. *J Neurosurg* 1977;46:681–687

118. Miller RE, Hieshimas GB, Giannotta SL, Grinnell VS, Mehringer CM, Kerin DS: Acute traumatic vertebral arteriovenous fistula: balloon occlusion with the use of the contralateral approach. *Neurosurgery* 1984;14:225–229

119. Kondoh T, Tamaki N, Takeda N, Suyama T, Oi SZ, Matsumoto S: Fatal intracranial hemorrhage after balloon occlusion of an extracranial vertebral arteriovenous fistula: a case report. *J Neurosurg* 1988;69:945–948

120. Higashida RT, Halbach VV, Tsai FY, et al: Interventional neurovascular treatment of traumatic carotid and vertebral artery lesions: therapeutic results in 234 cases. *AJR* 1989;153:577–582

121. Benati A, Da Pian R, Mazza C, et al: Preoperative emboli-

zation of the vertebral hemangioma compressing the spinal cord. *Neuroradiology* 1974;7:181–183

122. Gross C, Hodge C, Binet E, et al: Relief of spinal block during embolization of a vertebral body hemangioma. *J Neurosurg* 1976;45:327–330

123. Graham J, Yang W: Vertebral hemangioma with compression fracture and paraparesis treated with preoperative embolization and vertebral resection. *Spine* 1984;9:97–101

124. Nicola N, Lins E: Vertebral hemangioma: retrograde embolization-stabilization with methyl methacrylate. *Surg Neurol* 1987;27:481–486

125. Riche MC, Reizine D, Melki JP, Merland JJ: Classification of spinal cord vascular malformations. *Radiat Med* 1985;3:17–24

126. Merland JJ, Reizine D: Malformations vasculaires vertebromedullaires. *Encycl Med Chir Paris: Radiodiagnostic II-5* 1987;311671 G10

127. Rosenblum B, Oldfield EH, Doppman JL, DiChiro G: Spinal arteriovenous malformations: a comparison of dural arteriovenous fistulas and intradural AVMs in 81 patients. *J Neurosurg* 1987;67:795–802

128. Spetzler RF, Zambramski JM, Flom RA: Management of juvenile spinal AVMs by embolization and operative excision. *J Neurosurg* 1989;70:628–632

129. Hurth M, Houdart R, Djindjian R, Rey A, Djindjian M: Arteriovenous malformations of the spinal cord: clinical, anatomical, and therapeutic considerations—a series of 150 cases. *Progr Neurol Surg* 1978;9:238–266

130. Djindjian M: Les malformations arterioveneuses de la moelle epiniere. Thesis. Hôpital de la Pitie-Salpetrière, Paris, 1976

131. Aminoff MJ, Logue V: The prognosis of patients with spinal vascular malformations. *Brain* 1974;97:211–218

132. Yasargil MG, Symon L, Teddy PJ: Arteriovenous malformations of the spinal cord, in Symon L (ed): *Advances and Technical Standards in Neurosurgery.* Vol 11. Vienna, Springer–Verlag, 1984, pp 61–102

133. Doppman JL, DiChiro G, Ommaya AK: Percutaneous embolization of spinal cord arteriovenous malformations. *J Neurosurg* 1971;34:48–55

134. Djindjian R, Cophignon J, Rey A, Theron J, Merland JJ, Houdart R: Superselective arteriographic embolizations of the femoral route in neuroradiology: study of 50 cases—embolizations in vertebromedullary pathology. *Neuroradiology* 1973;6:132–142

135. Riche MC, Melki JP, Merland JJ: Embolization of spinal cord malformations via the anterior spinal artery. *AJNR* 1983;4:378–381

136. Horton JA, Latchaw RE, Gold LH, Pang D: Embolization of intramedullary arteriovenous malformations of the spinal cord. *AJNR* 1986;7:113–118

137. Theron J, Cosgrove R, Melanson D: Spinal arteriovenous malformations: advances in therapeutic embolization. *Radiology* 1986;158:163–169

138. Biondi A, Merland JJ, Reizine D, et al: Embolization with particles in thoracic intramedullary arteriovenous malformations: long-term angiographic and clinical results. *Radiology* 1990;177:651–658

139. Ommaya AK, DiChiro G, Doppman J: Ligation of arterial supply in the treatment of spinal cord arteriovenous malformations. *J Neurosurg* 1969;30:679–692

140. Djindjian R: Embolization of angiomas of the spinal cord. *Surg Neurol* 1975;4:411–420

141. Malis LI: Microsurgery for spinal cord arteriovenous malformations. *Clin Neurosurg* 1979;26:543–555

142. Malis LI: Arteriovenous malformations of the spinal cord, in Youmans JR (ed): *Neurological Surgery,* Ed 2, Vol 3, Philadelphia, WB Saunders, 1982, pp 1850–1874

143. Aminoff MJ, Barnard RO, Logue V: The pathophysiology of spinal vascular malformations. *J Neurol Sci* 1974;23:255–263

144. Merland JJ, Riche MC, Chiras J: Les fistules arterioveineuses intracanalaires extra-medullaires a drainage veineux medullaire. *J Neuroradiol* 1980;7:271–320

Part 7. Ferromagnetic Microembolization for Treatment of Hepatocellular Carcinoma

—Masao Sako, M.D., Shozo Hirota, M.D., and Masakazu Hasegawa, M.D.

Transcatheter arterial embolization is one of the most reliable adjuncts for the treatment of well localized neoplasms. Various occlusive agents have been used, most of which primarily obliterate major feeding arteries rather than small peripheral vessels. As a result, collateral circulation to the distal vascular bed subsequently develops, thus reducing the therapeutic effects of the embolization.

For optimal tumor infarction, occlusive agents must be small enough to reach the precapillary vascular bed of the tumor but too large to stray into the venous vascular bed through tumoral arteriovenous communications. To serve this purpose, the ferromagnetic effect has been investigated to try to entrap small iron particles within the target vessels.[1–4]

REAGENTS AND EQUIPMENT

Ferropolysaccharide

Ferropolysaccharide (FPS) is a dark gray, viscous, aqueous suspension of iron microspheres (Fig. 2.7.1). The particles are pure (99.99%) iron, 10–30 μm in diameter, with numerous micropores (Iron Metal Sponge; Wako Pure Chemical Industries, Ltd). The polysaccharide solution consists of 14% dextran 40, and 2% sodium carboxymethyl cellulose in saline. Dextran 40 is a popular plasma expander that can be excreted by the kidneys (mol wt: 40,000). Sodium carboxymethyl cellulose, a nontoxic polysaccharide (mol wt: 60,000–80,000), is widely used as a protective

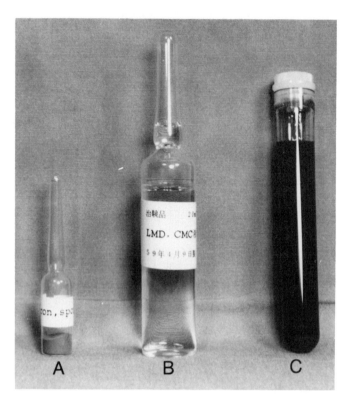

Figure 2.7.1. Ferropolysaccharide:iron sponge microspheres (30–50 μm) (**A**) and viscous polysaccharide solution (**B**) were each enclosed in glass ampules and sterilized. Prior to use, 1g of the particles was homogeneously suspended in 10ml of polysaccharide solution by thorough shaking for a few minutes in a sterilized test tube (**C**).

colloid for food, cosmetics, and medicines and is added to increase the dispersion of the iron particles. The pH of the solution is 5.1. For storage, 20ml of the polysaccharide solution and 1g of the iron sponge are sterilized in glass ampules by autoclaving. Before use, 1g of the iron sponge is suspended homogeneously in 10ml of polysaccharide solution by thorough shaking for a few minutes in a sterile test tube.

Microembolization with FPS works by macroaggregation of the iron particles: when exposed to a strong magnetic field, they become magnetized and subsequently exert a magnetic force on each other, forming larger conglomerates of particles, which grow by aggregating with fibrin in the blood until occlusion occurs.[4] The high molecular weight polysaccharide solution lowers the velocity of blood flow, allowing the viscous medium to adhere to some degree to the vascular intima, where the iron particles can be held while they aggregate progressively in the magnetic field. The iron particles can be demonstrated within the vessels by computed tomography (CT) examinations as a high-density striated pattern. The autopsy specimen of a patient who died from hepatic failure due to severe cirrhosis one year after treatment showed that small vessels around the lesion were still filled with aggregated iron particles, indicating long-term or permanent vascular occlusion.[4]

If excessive doses of FPS are injected, the aggregated iron particles will occlude, at the proximal subsegmental or segmental level, the arteries feeding not only neoplastic tissue but also normal liver tissue. However, liver infarction does not necessarily occur, as demonstrated by CT examination, if portal blood flow was normal before embolization.

The Magnetic Device

Early experimental studies have shown the optimal magnetic intensity for microembolization with FPS to be about 300 gauss; a magnetic intensity of >500 gauss causes occlusion of vessels >400 μm in diameter (Fig. 2.7.2).[5]

A box-shaped, 10 × 10 × 5cm, rare earth-cobalt magnet (Toshiba Corporation) is used. It can be placed over any part of the body surface by using an antimagnetic holder attached to the angiographic table (Fig. 2.7.3). The magnetic field intensity curves at various distances (Fig. 2.7.4) indicate that 300 gauss can be exerted at a depth of 10cm.

Care should be taken to prevent a magnetic effect on the fluoroscopic units, because use of a strong magnet close to an image intensifier temporarily or permanently distorts the image. To prevent this, before the magnet is activated, the patient is moved at least 1m away from the image intensifier. This has the disadvantage that fluoroscopic observation is not available during FPS injection. An antimagnetic fluoroscopic unit is now available commercially for observation during the injection.

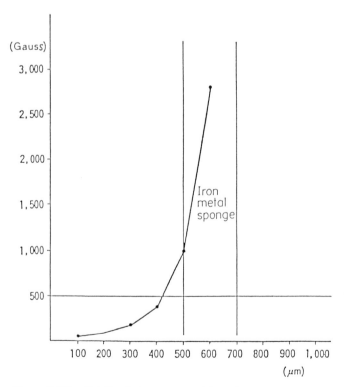

Figure 2.7.2. Relation between magnet intensity and size of vessel occluded.

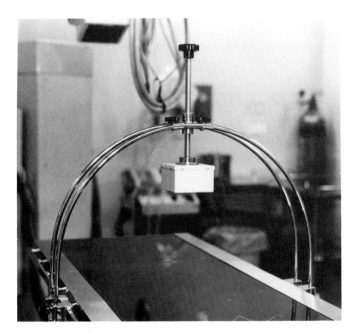

Figure 2.7.3. The magnetic device: a box-shaped, rare earth-cobalt magnet (3000 gauss) can be placed on any part of the body surface by using an antimagnetic steel holder attached to the angiographic table.

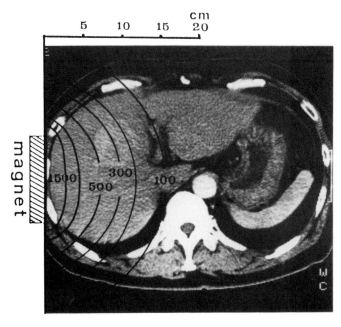

Figure 2.7.4. The magnetic field strength curves at various distances. Before embolization, the strength curves were projected on the CT image of a patient to obtain optimal positioning of the magnet.

CLINICAL APPLICATIONS OF FERROMAGNETIC MICROEMBOLIZATION TO PATIENTS WITH HEPATOCELLULAR CARCINOMA

Technique

One-hundred and forty-three ferromagnetic microembolization (FME) procedures have been performed in 48 men and 10 women aged 37 to 81 years with hepatocellular carcinoma (HCC). The diagnosis was established by biopsy, operation, autopsy, or clinical examination such as angiography and α-fetoprotein assay. In 33 patients, embolization was repeated more than two times (mean total: 2.6 treatments). In eight patients, hepatectomy was performed after the initial FME procedure.

Before the embolization, preliminary celiac and superior mesenteric arteriography is carried out to identify the feeding arteries as well as to evaluate the extent of the tumor and the presence or absence of portal vein involvement. If the portal trunk or the right or left main branches of the portal vein are occluded, embolization is contraindicated. If portal vein patency is demonstrated, superselective catheterization is done with a soft, long (3–10cm), tapered 6.5Fr catheter (inner diameter: 1.4mm). If the tumor is located in the right lobe of the liver, the catheter tip is advanced beyond the origin of the cystic artery to avoid gallbladder infarction; for lesions in the left lobe of the liver, the catheter tip is introduced into the left hepatic artery.

After selective catheterization has been achieved, the patient is moved away from the angiographic table to avoid damage to the image intensifier by the magnet. The magnet is then positioned and activated over the area of interest, and FPS is injected slowly through the catheter. After completion of the injection, the catheter is rinsed with 2–3ml of saline, and the magnet is left in place for 10 minutes.

The dose of FPS depends on the size and vascularity of the tumors; 1–2ml is routinely injected initially, and the need for additional injections is determined by fluoroscopic evaluation of hepatic blood flow or by repeat angiography. Usually, tumors of 5–6cm in diameter require 3–4ml of FPS. When necessary, FME was repeated in a subsequent session in the same manner.

Evaluation of Therapeutic Effect

The therapeutic effect of embolization of hepatic tumors is generally evaluated by tumor markers, ultrasonography, CT, and angiography. However, determination of tumor extent, including size, presence of small (<1cm) metastatic nodules, recanalization, and development of collateral circulation, can be done accurately only by angiography.

Angiograms are studied for tumor type: solitary (sharply defined lesion), multinodular (more than two sharply defined lesions), infiltrating (ill-defined lesions), and mixed; extent (number of feeding vessels, rated T1 to T4), vascularity (+ to +++), size of tumor stain (width × length), portal vein involvement (of main portal vein, right branch or left lobe branch (P3), of a first-order branch (P2), of a second-order branch (P1), or of a third-order or more peripheral branch (P0)), and presence of intrahe-

Figure 2.7.5. Angiographic classification of hepatocellular carcinoma as tumor factors.

patic metastases (number of segments, rated IM0 to IM3) (Fig. 2.7.5). For example, an ill-defined lesion with two feeding vessels, considerable vascularity, involvement of a main branch of the portal vein, and intrahepatic metastases in two segments would be classified as infiltrative T2, ++, P3, IM2 and the extent of the tumor stain in centimeters would be specified.

Regression of the primary tumor is evaluated by comparing tumor stain before and after embolization. The degree of tumor regression is divided into three categories: "marked" when there is complete disappearance or >50% decrease in tumor size, "moderate" (between 25 and 50% regression), and "poor" (<25% regression).

RESULTS

Primary Tumor Regression

A marked result was noted in 18 cases, including 9 in which there was complete disappearance of the tumor stain (Fig. 2.7.6A,B). Moderate results were seen in seven patients and poor results in eight (Table 2.7.1).

The relation between primary tumor regression and angiographic findings is shown in Table 2.7.2. In the patients with marked and moderate results (72–86% of the cases), tumors were localized within a segment (T1), and 72% had portal vein involvement limited to third-order branches (P0). The tumors in these groups were for the most part sharply demarcated, either solitary or multiple. In contrast, the group with poor results had tumors that were >T2 in 62% of cases, with portal vein involvement of >P1 in 60%. The degree of vascularity had no relation to the frequency of primary tumor regression. Intrahepatic metastases were present in 21 cases, and in 18 disappearance or marked diminution in number and size occurred (Fig. 2.7.7).

Development of collateral bypassing circulation was

Table 2.7.1. Angiographic Comparison of Tumor Size before and after Ferromagnetic Microembolization[a]

Degree of Tumor Diminution	Number of Cases	Angiographic Evaluation of Primary Effect
Disappearance	9 (27%)	Marked
More than 50%	9 (27%)	Marked
25–50%	7 (21%)	Moderate
Less than 25%	8 (24%)	Poor

[a]Angiography performed 2–5 months after ferromagnetic microembolization.

Table 2.7.2. Relation between Primary Effect and Tumor Factors

Tumor Factor	Primary Effect		
	Marked Group (18)	Moderate Group (7)	Poor Group (8)
Extent			
T1	72	86	38
T2	17	14	38
T3	11		24
Portal Involvement			
P0	72	72	50
P1	22	14	13
P3	5	14	47
Tumor Types			
Expansive	44	42	25
Multinodular	33	29	13
Infiltrative			25
Mixed	23	29	47

observed in only five patients, two with infiltrative and three with mixed-type hepatomas, in whom the extrahepatic collaterals developed from duodenal, omental, and subphrenic arteries. In these cases, the results were poor (Fig. 2.7.8).

It is difficult to compare the frequency of recanalization with the results of other vaso-occlusive agents, because FME is used with the intention of occluding peripheral intraparenchymal tumor vessels. In fact, 40% of the patients had occlusion only of the tumor vasculature. The remaining 19 patients showed occlusion of subsegmental or segmental arteries, probably because of injection of excessive amounts of FPS. Of these 19 cases, 12 showed recanalization.

Histological Examination

Histological examination was made on eight resected tumors ranging in size from 3 to 5cm. The area of necrosis on a section taken from the widest part of the tumor was calculated. In all tumors, the mean area of necrosis was more than 90% of the section taken. However, one tumor had capsular infiltration of tumor cells extending outside of the tumor capsule where the tumor cells were still viable, suggesting a certain limitation of the effect of embolization alone. On the other hand, one patient who had a FME procedure for several metastatic nodules less than 1cm in diameter in the left lobe, showed a complete necrosis of all nodules at autopsy. This patient died from cerebral hemorrhage 14 days after embolization.

Cumulative Survival Rates

Overall cumulative survival rate of 50 patients calculated by the Kaplan–Meier method was 65% at one year, 38% at two years, and 22% at three years (Fig. 2.7.9). Since survival rate is to be discussed in relationship to disease

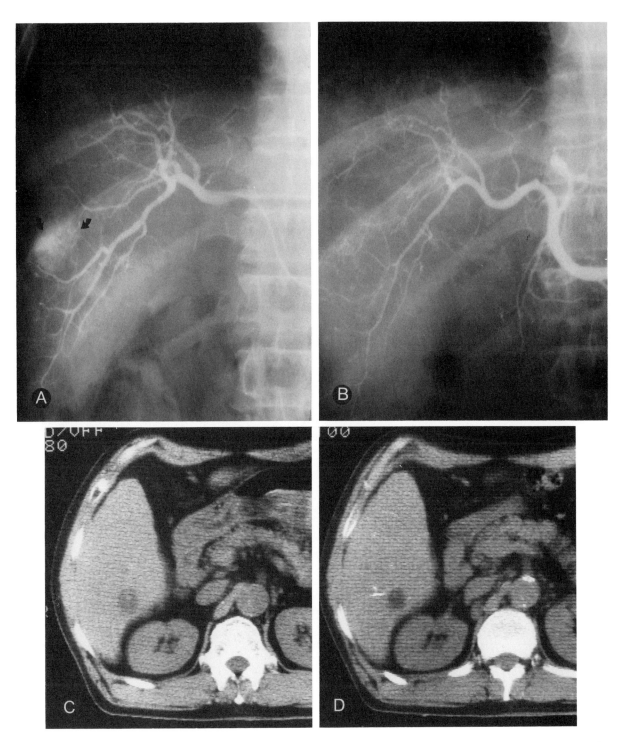

Figure 2.7.6. A 54-year-old man with hepatoma in posterior segment of the right lobe. **A.** Angiographic tumor characteristics: large vascular mass in right lobe of the liver with dense tumor stain *(arrows)*. Ferromagnetic microembolization with 3ml of FPS. **B.** Follow-up angiography performed 10 months after embolization shows no tumor stain (i.e., primary tumor regression "marked"). **C.** CT scan before embolization shows sharply defined, round, low-density area on the posterior segment of right lobe. **D.** CT scan 10 months after procedure shows diminution in both density and size of mass. Aggregated iron particles are visible as a high-density striated pattern without any abnormal density on the normal parenchyma to indicate infarction. Unfortunately, the patient died of rupture of esophageal varices 45 months after embolization.

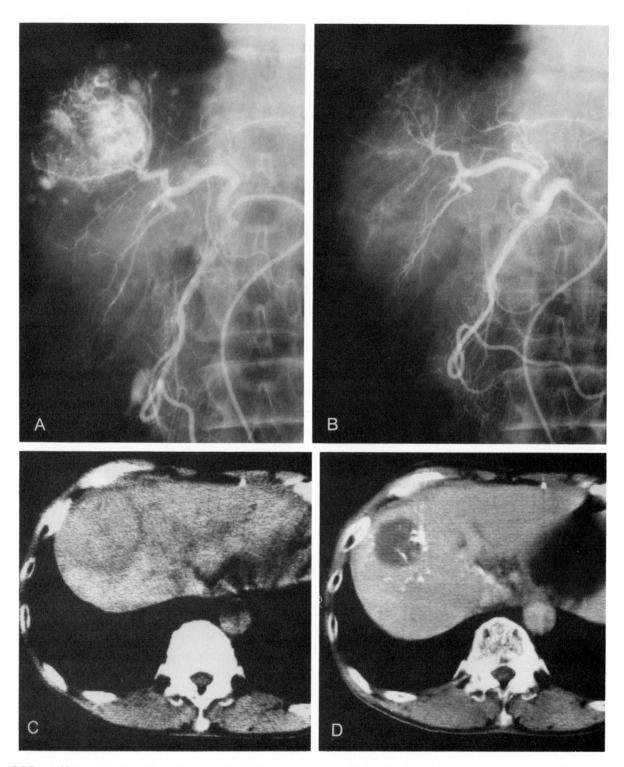

Figure 2.7.7. A 62-year-old man with hepatoma. **A.** Preliminary angiography reveals hepatoma in anterior segment of the right lobe. Angiographic tumor characteristics: expansive, T1, +++ vascularity, 6 × 6cm stain, P1, and multiple 3–20mm intrahepatic metastases. Embolization with 5ml of FPS. **B.** Follow-up angiography two months after embolization shows almost complete disappearance of tumor vessels, stain, and minute (<5mm) intrahepatic metastases, while normal hepatic arter-

ies, which had been distributed along the lesion, remain encircled. **C.** CT scan before embolization shows a round mass in the right lobe. **D.** Scan made three months after embolization reveals markedly diminished density and size of the mass, indicating widespread necrosis. Scattered, aggregated iron particles noted around and within the lesion. Patient lived for 34 months.

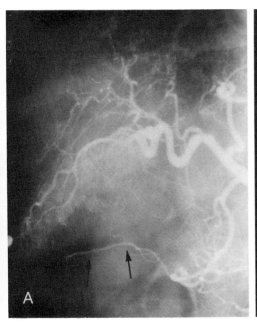
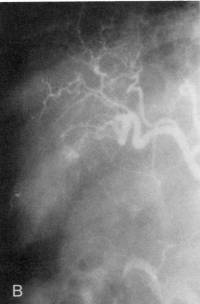
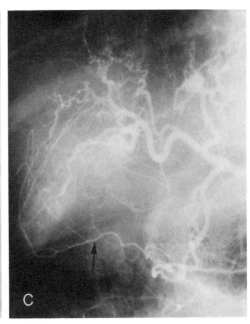

Figure 2.7.8. A 65-year-old man. **A.** Preliminary angiograms reveal hepatoma with ill-defined margin in the posterior segment of the right lobe. Extrahepatic collaterals from both omental and duodenal branches are noted *(arrows).* Superior mesenteric arteriography revealed occlusion of a first-order portal branch. Thus, tumor factors are: infiltrative, T1, + + + vascularity, 3 × 8cm stain, P2. Embolization with 5ml of FPS. **B.** Angiograms immediately after embolization reveal complete disappearance of tumor vessels and stain. **C.** Angiograms three months later show development of extrahepatic collaterals and recanalization of the posterior segmental artery feeding the tumor, which has grown slightly *(arrow).* Embolization with FPS was repeated. Patient lived seven months after repeat embolization.

stage, HCC was classified into four stages following the general rules proposed by the liver cancer study group of Japan (Table 2.7.3). Fifty patients were divided into four groups, including 1 patient in Stage I, 10 in Stage II, 22 in Stage III, and 17 in Stage IV, and each survival rate was calculated.

There was no significant difference between the survival rates of Stages I, II, and III, showing results of 78% at one year, 53% at two years, and 28% at three years. In contrast, however, the results of Stage IV were significantly poor, being 39% at one year and 8% at two and three years (Fig. 2.7.9). Concerning the relation between survival rates and angiographic tumor characteristics such as T, P, IM, and vascularity, survival rates were prone to become poor as the degree of tumor characteristics advanced. Of the tumor types, expansive and multinodular had better results in comparison to the infiltrative and mixed types.

Primary tumor regression does not necessarily correlate with the survival rates in recent data.

Postembolization Symptoms and Serologic Data

The most common postembolization symptoms were abdominal pain and abdominal distension. Pain usually subsided within 24-48 hours with the administration of sedatives and analgesics (30 mg of Pentazocine).

Fever (37–39 °C) was noted in 95% of the patients and lasted for three to seven days. Patients with fever of more than 30 °C were usually given steroids and antipyretics. Serum liver enzymes, total bilirubin, and albumin all increased transiently. However, all the concentrations returned to the pre-embolization levels within one to two weeks (Fig. 2.7.10). In addition, deterioration of the hepatic functional reserve before and after the FME pro-

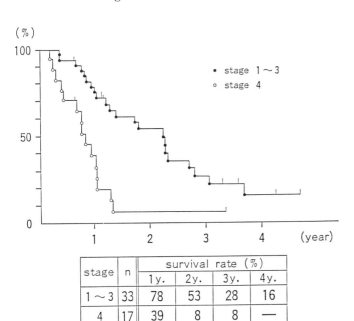

stage	n	survival rate (%)			
		1y.	2y.	3y.	4y.
1~3	33	78	53	28	16
4	17	39	8	8	—

Figure 2.7.9. Cumulative survival rate.

Table 2.7.3. Staging of Hepatocellular Carcinoma[a]

Stage	T		N	M
I	T1:single nodule (<2cm φ),	Vascular involvement (−)	N0	M0
II	T2:single nodule (<2cm φ), T2:multiple nodules (2cm φ), T2:single nodule (>2cm φ),	Vascular involvement (+) One lobe Vascular involvement (−)	N0	M0
III	T3:single nodule (>2 cm φ), T3:multiple nodules (>2cm φ), T1-3	Vascular involvement (+) One lobe	N0 N1	M0 M0
IV-A IV-B	T4:multiple nodules, >two lobes T1-4		N0-1 N0-1	M0 M1

[a]Liver Cancer Study Group of Japan, 1987.

cedure was assessed by a hepaplastin test and indocyanine green retain (ICG-R) test in 12 patients. In 2 (17%) of 12 patients, more than 20% reduction of hepatic functional reserve occurred.

DISCUSSION

HCC is one of the most common tumors in Japan. Unfortunately, it is often unresectable because of advanced cirrhosis. In such cases, hepatic embolization, usually with Gelfoam or chemo-Lipiodol with gelatin sponge cubes has been widely used. In order to improve the prognosis of this disease, correct choice of the available agents must be made for each patient on an individual basis, not only to maximize the effect on the tumor mass, but also to minimize the adverse effects on the remaining liver parenchyma.

For this purpose, a correct evaluation of therapeutic effect must be made on the basis of the degree of HCC. For this reason we attempted to classify HCC into four stages, mainly by angiographic and computed tomographic findings, following the general rules of the liver cancer study group of Japan. Interestingly enough, there was no significant difference among the survival rates of Stages I, II, and III. This may be caused by not excluding factors such as liver cirrhosis or esophageal varices in the general evaluation of results. In fact, some patients died from hepatic failure or rupture of esophageal varices, despite their good, tumor-controlled conditions. From this point of view, it could be reasonable to determine the stage of the disease, not only by using the tumor characteristics, but also the associated problems of the liver cirrhosis. This is, however, difficult to achieve since there are so many factors to evaluate that the determination of the stages will become extremely complicated; hence, in this paper, the staging was primarily attempted only based on the tumor characteristics.

Indication and Pre-embolization Assessment of the Patients

1. *Liver function*: Poor liver function with total bilirubin <3mg/dl, serum albumin <3.0g/dl, and ascites nonresponsive to diuretics was considered a contraindication because hepatic failure frequently occurs after embolization.
2. *Esophageal varices*: If the patient has esophageal varices with "red cherry sign," endoscopic sclerotherapy by injecting sclerosing agent is to be undertaken before embolization, since it is well known that portal vein pressure increases after hepatic arterial embolization.[6]
3. *Portal vein involvement*: When the portal vein or its main branches are occluded, embolization is contraindicated.
4. *Diabetes mellitus*: Diabetic patients should be well controlled before embolization, because poorly controlled patients tend to have an elevation of blood sugar after embolization.[7]

Comparison of Hepatic Embolization with FPS with Other Embolic Agents

At the beginning of application of embolotherapy for HCC, only gelatin sponge cubes were widely used, with one- and two-year survival rates of 44 and 29%, respectively.[8]

Our recent studies on a comparison of survival rates after embolization with FPS, Gelfoam, and chemo-Lipiodol have shown a one-year survival of 70, 52, and 51%, respectively, and the two-year survival was 40, 18, and 32%, respectively. FPS had greatest effect on tumor mass regression and the longest survival rate. The Gelfoam-only group had the poorest survival rate. The effect on tumor mass reduction of chemo-Lipiodol-Gelfoam was greater than Gelfoam alone. Concerning the deterioration of hepatic

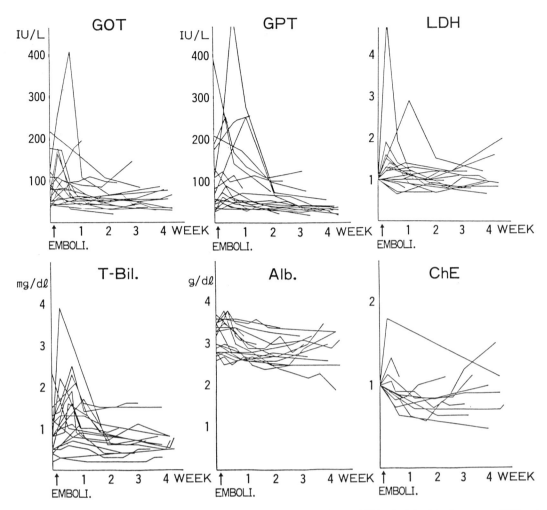

Figure 2.7.10. Serologic data after ferromagnetic microembolization. *GOT* = glutamic oxaloacetic transaminase; *GPT* = glutamic pyruvic transaminase; *LDH* = lactate dehydrogenase; *T-Bil.* = total bilirubin; *Alb.* = albumin; *ChE* = cholinesterase.

function as assessed by hepaplastin and ICG-R tests, more than 20% reduction of hepatic reserve was noted in 17% of the FPS group (12), 16% in the Gelfoam group (19), and 48% in the chemo-Lipiodol group (25). This indicated that chemo-Lipiodol-Gelfoam should be avoided in poor-risk patients. In cases where it is used, minimal doses of Lipiodol (less than 5ml) and superselective catheterization as close as possible to the tumor is advised.[9]

Advantages and Disadvantages of Ferromagnetic Microembolization

The better results obtained by FME seem to be related to several factors, including microembolization of tumor vessels with histologically proven widespread tumor necrosis (Fig. 2.7.11), long-acting or permanent occlusion, decreased incidence of collateral formation, no reflux of particles, reliable effect on small (less than 5mm) lesions, and ease of repeat embolization.

Collateral formation has been reported in 65–80% of

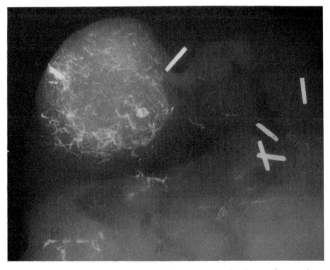

Figure 2.7.11. Low-kilovolt soft-tissue examination of specimen resected after ferromagnetic microembolization; note widespread occlusion of tumor vessels with aggregated iron particles. Histologic examination confirmed necrosis throughout the lesion.

cases after embolization with Gelfoam due to primary occlusion of major feeding arteries. This makes repeat embolization difficult and, as has been shown, this is considered essential to improve survival rates in patients with hepatocellular carcinoma. In contrast, FME has prevented the development of collaterals from both intrahepatic and extrahepatic pathways in 88% of patients. An additional procedure was easily performed when required, since major feeding arteries were commonly (76%) patent.

It is well known that distal embolization with small particles is more effective against tumors, than is occlusion of proximal vessels with other types of agents. However, small particles are more prone to reflux into proximal arteries, causing undesirable infarction of the gallbladder or pancreas, even if the injection is made at a peripheral level. An FPS embolization utilizing $30-50\mu m$ particles provides sufficient microembolization, with reflux of particles being prevented by the use of the external magnetic control.

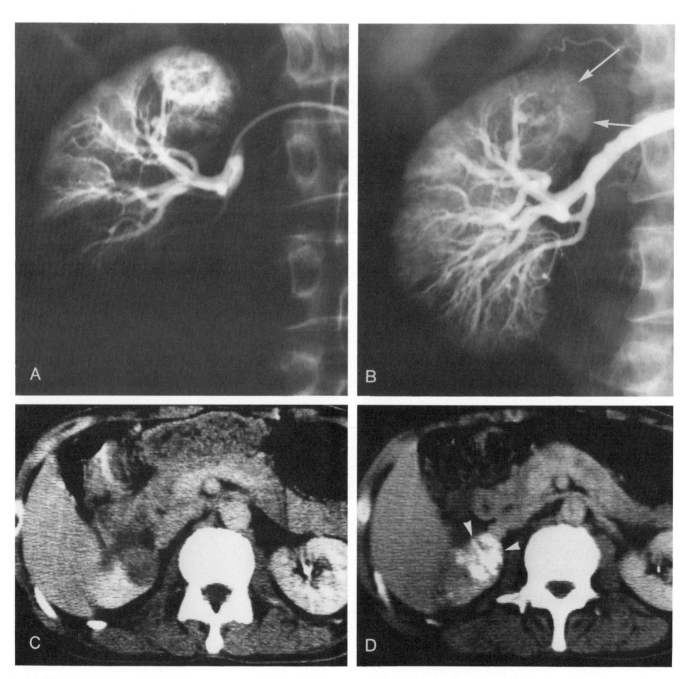

Figure 2.7.12 A 51-year-old man with renal cell carcinoma. **A.** Preliminary angiography reveals tumor in ventral segment of the right kidney. **B.** Angiograms immediately after embolization with 6ml of FPS show almost complete disappearance of tumor vessels *(arrows)*. **C.** Pre-embolization CT scan demonstrates low-density mass in upper pole of the right kidney. **D.** Plain CT film obtained ten days later shows aggregated iron particles as scattered high-density areas corresponding to the lesion *(arrowheads)*. Histologic examination confirmed widespread necrosis.

One of the disadvantages of FME is the need for a superselective catheterization to avoid gallbladder infarction. If catheterization of target vessels is not successful due to anatomic variations or to arteriosclerosis, FME must be forgone in favor of Gelfoam embolization. To extend the indications of this procedure, new devices or techniques to permit superselective catheterization will be required.

In addition to its use for hepatic embolization, FME has been applied to eight patients with renal cell carcinoma (Fig. 2.7.12) and one patient with advanced lung cancer, resulting in excellent tumor infarction.

In summary, FME provides widespread microembolization of tumors with reliable, excellent therapeutic effect and without any undesirable reactions by the normal organs. No severe complications or abnormal serologic data due to FME were observed.[10-12] In general, the therapeutic effect of FME on hepatocellular carcinoma depends on tumor characteristics: tumors of the mixed and infiltrative types are less susceptible than those of the sharply localized type.[13,14] In addition, the therapeutic effects are less prominent in the presence of portal vein involvement. To overcome this limitation, chemoembolotherapy is being tested.[15] In addition, induction heating (hyperthermia) of the magnetic particles placed in the target lesion can be used for selective heating of the lesions.[16] This induction heating is still in the experimentation stage, but recent results look promising for use in clinical practice.

In conclusion, the authors consider FME to be one of the most reliable potential methods for extending the capability of interventional radiology in oncologic patients.

References

1. Mosso JA, Rand WR: Ferromagnetic silicone vascular occlusion: a technique for selective infarction of tumors and organs. *Ann Surg* 1973;178:663
2. Albrechtsson U, Hansson GA, Olin T: Vascular occlusion with a ferromagnetic particles suspension: an experimental investigation in rabbits. *Acta Radiol [Diagn]* 1977;18:279
3. Barry JW, Bookstein JJ, Alksne JF: Ferromagnetic embolization: experimental evaluation. *Radiology* 1981;138:341
4. Sako M, Yokogawa S, Sakamoto K, et al: Transcatheter microembolization with ferropolysaccharide: a new approach to ferromagnetic embolization of tumors (preliminary report). *Invest Radiol* 1982;17:573
5. Sako M, Ohtsuki S, Arai M, et al: Cancer therapy by ferromagnetic microembolization: studies on a new electromagnetic device. *J Jpn Soc Cancer Ther* 1983;18:92
6. Okuda K, Sako M, Hirota S: Experimental and clinical studies of hemodynamic changes of the liver after hepatic arterial embolization. *J Jpn College of Angiol* 1989;29:143
7. Sakamoto K, Sako M, Nagae T, et al: Influence of hepatic arterial embolization on diabetic patients with hepatocellular carcinoma. *Nippon Acta Radiol* 1989;49:986
8. Yamada R, Sato M, Kawabata M, et al: Hepatic artery embolization in 120 patients with unresectable hepatoma. *Radiology* 1983;148:397
9. Sako M, Hasegawa M, Hirota S, et al: Comparison of hepatic arterial embolization with iron microspheres, Gelfoam, and chemo-Lipiodol-Gelfoam in 167 patients with hepatoma. *J Intervent Radiol* 1989;4:173
10. Yuri H, Sako M: Ferromagnetic microembolization in the treatment of metastatic tumors of the liver. *J Jpn Soc Cancer Ther* 1984;19:50
11. Hirota S, Sako M: Experimental and clinical study of ferromagnetic microembolization for a treatment of malignant tumors. *J Jpn Soc Cancer Ther* 1982;17:1936
12. Morita M, Sako M: Experimental and clinical studies on embolotherapy of lung cancer. *J Jpn Soc Cancer Ther* 1985;20:71
13. Sato M: Experimental and clinical studies on the hepatic artery embolization for treatment of hepatoma. *Nippon Acta Radiol* 1983;43:977
14. Nakashima T: Vascular changes and hemodynamics in hepatocellular carcinoma, in Okuda K, Peter R (eds): *Hepatocellular Carcinoma*. New York, John Wiley & Sons, 1976, p 169
15. Shimizu T, Sako M, Hirota S: Intraarterial infusion therapy with polysaccharide solution as a carrier of anticancer agents. *Nippon Acta Radiol* 1988;48:702
16. Hase M, Sako M, Hirota S: Experimental study of ferromagnetic induction heating combined with hepatic arterial embolization for treatment of liver tumor. *Nippon Acta Radiol* 1990;50:1402

3

GASTROINTESTINAL BLEEDING

Part 1. Vasoactive Drugs and Embolotherapy in the Management of Gastrointestinal Bleeding

—John F. Cardella, M.D., S. Murthy Tadavarthy, M.D., Joseph W. Yedlicka, Jr., M.D., David W. Hunter, M.D., and Wilfrido R. Castañeda–Zúñiga, M.D., M.Sc.

No aspect of angiographic and interventional radiology can be at once so frustrating and so gratifying as the diagnosis and therapy of gastrointestinal bleeding. This chapter considers the use of vasoactive drugs and embolotherapy for this purpose. The preceding chapters review embolotherapy in more detail.

The literature has an abundance of estimates of how briskly a patient must bleed for it to be detectable angiographically, ranging from 0.5 to 3.0ml/min (1.5–9 units/24 hr).[1–4] The authors' experience has shown that bleeding of 1.5–2.0ml/min (4–6 units/24 hr) is usually detectable, whereas less rapid bleeding is difficult to detect. The other component of detectability is constancy, i.e., the patient must be bleeding during the angiographic run.

NONINVASIVE DIAGNOSTIC EVALUATION

Radionuclide studies using tagged red blood cells have enhanced the ability to detect and document gastrointestinal (GI) bleeding with an image.[5–17] However, although these studies are useful for confirmation of slow oozing and widely spaced intermittent episodes by virtue of their high sensitivity, they contribute little information about etiology because of their poor specificity. Nevertheless, if properly performed with carefully timed scans, the site of bleeding can be placed at least in the proper quadrant of the abdomen and frequently in the stomach, small bowel, or colon (Fig. 3.1.1), and this information can guide the angiographer in the search for the actual site of extravasation.

OVERVIEW OF PHARMACOTHERAPY

Once a bleeding site has been identified, recent progress in occlusive therapy allows the angiographer to step from diagnostician to therapist.[18–28] Transcatheter treatment for GI bleeding includes pharmacologic agents and embolic materials. The mainstay of pharmacologic control is vasopressin (Pitressin). Epinephrine, which was used in early trials, is seldom used now.

Vasopressin can be administered intravenously without diagnostic arteriography or empirically when no bleeding site is located to produce a systemic vasoconstrictive effect to slow or arrest bleeding. Doses are 1000–2000 units/hr, with administration continued for 48 hours if the patient shows decreased melena-hematemesis, decreasing blood transfusion requirements, and stabilized hemodynamics. If 48 hours of intravenous vasopressin produces no slowing in the rate of GI blood loss, the drug should be discontinued, because further administration is unlikely to be successful.

Intra-arterial vasopressin can be used effectively immediately after arteriography when a bleeding site is identified.[26–31] Although ideally the drug is delivered selectively into the bleeding branch, when selective catheterization is not possible, delivery into the superior or inferior mesenteric artery is adequate, although less efficacious. The danger in nonselective delivery is constrictive bowel ischemia.[32,33] The currently recommended intra-arterial dose is 0.2 unit/min initially; no loading dose is given. If, after 20–30 minutes of infusion, repeat arteriography shows no vasoconstrictive effect, the dose should be doubled to 0.4 unit/min. Higher doses are seldom required. Intra-arterial infusion is continued until angiographic evidence of vasoconstriction is seen or until bleeding stops. Patients then leave the procedure room with the arterial catheter in place and the infusion running by means of a pump (Harvard pump) capable of generating suprasystemic pressure. Generally, patients undergo follow-up angiography 12–24 hours after the infusion was started. At that time, if bleeding has been arrested clinically and angiographically, the vasopressin is slowly withdrawn by tapering the dose every 6–8 hours over a 12–24-hour period. When the vasoconstrictor infusion has been discontinued, the catheter is left in place and flushed with a slow pressurized infusion of heparinized saline (3–10ml/hr flush with 5 units of heparin/ml); this allows re-infusion of vasopressin should bleeding resume. The small heparin dose (15–50 units/hr) does not cause bleeding problems and avoids pericatheter thrombosis. If all goes well and bleeding remains arrested, the catheter is removed at a convenient time. Success rates for intra-arterial vasopressin infusions are between 65 and 85%, depending on the size and location of the bleeding vessel.[31–34] Most investigators contend that intra-arterial vasopressin is more effective than intravenous systemic therapy, even with the lower doses allowed by selective delivery.

Epinephrine was also given intra-arterially for pharmacotherapy of GI bleeding in the early experience.[32,33] Its α-agonist properties caused vasoconstriction of the splanchnic bed, but its β-agonist properties caused chronotropic cardiac effects, which were a problem in some patients during long-term infusion. The reported dosages for epinephrine are:

1mg/kg/min infused into the celiac trunk in dogs[32];
8–16mg/min for the left gastric, gastroduodenal, or inferior mesenteric arteries in humans;
20–30mg/min for the celiac or superior mesenteric arteries of humans.[33]

Because of the cardiac effects of epinephrine, it has been supplanted by vasopressin in most medical centers.

OVERVIEW OF EMBOLOTHERAPY

Alternatively, GI bleeding can be arrested by embolotherapy with various temporary or permanent materials. Bleeding from transient lesions, such as ulcers, erosions, diverticula, spontaneous leaks, and traumatic tears, requires embolization with temporary materials to get the patient through the acute episode and then to permit vessel recanalization so that organ function loss in minimized. On the other hand, bleeding resulting from tumors, arteriovenous malformations (AVMs), large areas of angiodysplasia, and varices that will not heal spontaneously requires permanent embolization, both to control the immediate bleeding problems and as definitive therapy for the underlying pathologic process.

Temporary embolic agents include Gelfoam in powder and pieces[18–20] and autologous blood clot.[24,25,35,36] Gelfoam is prepared as a suspension in dilute contrast medium to facilitate viewing as the particles are deposited. The particle size is chosen on the basis of the pathology of the lesion and the size of the vessels requiring embolization; the general principle is to deposit the smallest particles that arrest bleeding and to deposit them as far peripherally as possi-

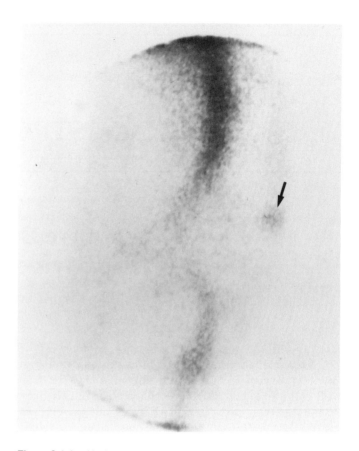

Figure 3.1.1. Nuclear medicine scan with tagged red blood cells shows accumulation of radionuclide activity in left flank *(arrow)*.

ble. The authors typically "backpack" a vessel with larger particles as the catheter is withdrawn.

Autologous blood clot is an agent mainly of historical interest[24,25]; particle (clot) size is difficult to control, the clots tend to sludge in the catheter because of their gelatinous nature, and deranged coagulation status in the patient makes clot induction difficult in some cases.

Permanent embolic agents are more numerous and include polyvinyl alcohol (Ivalon), coils, balloons, polymers and glues, alcohol, and hot contrast medium. The first two are characteristically used for bleeding in the GI tract; the last four are not used because the far distal occlusion they produce may induce wall ischemia.[37] Ivalon is prepared in a slurry with a 2:2:1 volume mixture of contrast medium:albumin:high molecular weight dextran (e.g., 20ml of contrast, 20ml of albumin, 10ml of dextran).[38] Enough Ivalon particles are then added to make a slurry that will pass through the catheter without occluding it. The small size of the Ivalon powder (0.5mm diameter) provides good end-organ embolization; injection of powder can be followed by Ivalon particles 1.0–2.0mm in diameter for occlusion of small feeding branches. For bleeding resulting from a large AVM or tumor that has caused hypertrophy of the feeding artery(ies) and large draining veins, the authors have used Ivalon particles (1.0–1.5mm diameter) followed by 3, 5, or 8mm Gianturco–Wallace–

Chuang (GWC) coils, a combination that gives excellent permanent embolization.

Whether temporary or permanent embolotherapy is chosen, a postembolization angiogram must be obtained to document cessation of bleeding, because clinical signs are not accurate. The colon, in particular, will continue to pass melanotic stool long after active bleeding has been stopped. Theoretically, the catheter could be left in place after embolization, as with infusions of vasopressin, but the authors do not do this routinely because of the thrombogenicity of that foreign body and the need for intensive care unit (ICU) monitoring of a patient with an arterial catheter in place. Furthermore, rebleeding after a successful embolization is far less likely than following a vasopressin infusion.

INDICATIONS FOR INTERVENTION

Gastrointestinal bleeding can be caused by a wide variety of lesions that may be located anywhere from the esophagus to the anus. This section of the chapter discusses specific bleeding entities from a pathophysiologic and therapeutic approach.

Mallory–Weiss Esophageal Tears

Spontaneous rupture of the esophagus is uncommon and most often is caused by severe coughing or vomiting, particularly in alcoholic patients; presumably, an existing weakness in the esophageal wall ruptures under the increased intraesophageal pressure. Typically, the lower third of the esophagus ruptures longitudinally along its posterolateral wall. The symptoms include sudden onset of excruciating epigastric and left-sided chest pain radiating to the back. Pneumothorax or hydropneumothorax, particularly on the left side, and pneumomediastinum are worrisome radiographic findings in a patient with the symptoms described. Frequently, the patients present in shock of sudden onset. Many patients have profound hematemesis. Morbidity and mortality of this entity are high, even with no associated hemorrhage. Concomitant hemorrhage worsens the prognosis even more.

The arterial blood supply of the esophagus is complex. The primary supply of the cervical portion is from the terminal branches of the inferior thyroid artery, which gives rise to multiple ascending and descending esophageal branches. The inferior thyroidal arteries, in turn, originate from the left and right subclavian arteries. There is considerable variability in the arterial supply to the esophagus, with accessory cervical esophageal arteries originating from the subclavian, carotid, and vertebral arteries as well as from the ascending pharyngeal and caudal cervical trunk.

The thoracic segment of the esophagus receives arterial blood from the bronchial arteries, the aorta, and the right intercostal arteries. Bronchial artery patterns are variable, but the most common pattern is two left and one right bronchial arteries (about 50% of individuals). Other variations include one right and one left (25% of the population), two right and two left (15% of the population), and one left and two right bronchial arteries (8% of the population). A few instances of three right and three left bronchial arteries have been described.

There are two direct aortic branches to the esophagus, which are unpaired. The superiormost branch is 3–4 cm long and usually arises from the aorta at the T6 or T7 level. The inferior aortic branch is longer, measuring 6–7 cm, and arises at the T7 to T8 level.

The abdominal portion of the esophagus receives its blood supply from branches of the left gastric, short gastric, and left inferior phrenic arteries. The complex arterial supply to the esophagus and its segmental nature make selective arterial embolization for refractory bleeding from Mallory–Weiss tears possible although complicated and technically difficult.

The angiographic evaluation of a Mallory–Weiss tear

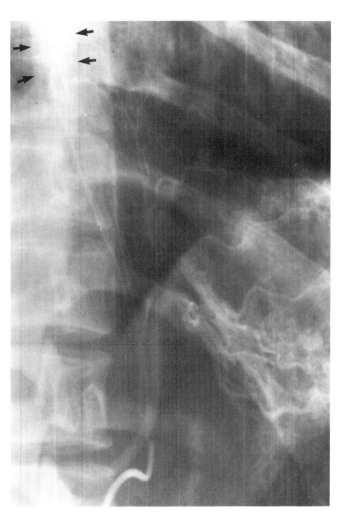

Figure 3.1.2. Patient with bleeding from Mallory–Weiss esophageal tear; selective injection into left inferior phrenic artery shows extravasation of contrast medium from lower esophagus *(arrows).*

requires a methodical search for esophageal branches, first in the brachiocephalic vessels, then progressively down the thoracic aorta, and finally into the celiac axis to locate any arterial bleeding in the distal esophagus (Fig, 3.1.2).

Variable success has been achieved with embolization of esophageal bleeding from Mallory–Weiss tears.[39–41] Because of the multiple sources of arterial bleeding, successful embolization of bleeding lesions may be difficult if collateral pathways can deliver blood to the bleeding site. If a definite site of bleeding can be identified angiographically (Fig. 3.1.2), the feeding artery should be embolized as far distally as possible with Gelfoam plugs to control the hemorrhage. Surgical repair of the tear or esophageal resection with bypass is still required but becomes more controlled if the bleeding has been stopped.

Large Mallory–Weiss tears that involve multiple arterial sites of bleeding are very difficult to embolize, and these patients are better managed surgically. Preoperative occlusion of bleeding sites makes surgery less difficult.

Successful use of intra-arterial vasopressin for Mallory–Weiss tears has not been reported.

Bleeding Esophageal Varices

Esophageal varices develop by one of two mechanisms. Varices in the lower portion develop in response to high resistance to blood flow through the liver parenchyma and may have presinusoidal or postsinusoidal causes. In each case, passage of blood from the portal venous system to the systemic venous system is impeded. As the disease worsens, the portal hypertension causes retrograde flow through the portal venous system, with reversal of blood flow through the splenic, mesenteric, and coronary veins, causing tremendous collateralization and dilatation of the esophageal venous plexus; this "uphill" flow of blood in the esophageal venous plexus permits portal venous blood to reach the systemic venous system via the azygous-hemiazygous system and the superior vena cava (Figs. 3.1.3 and 3.1.4). The other type, "downhill" esophageal varices, can develop, predominantly in the upper esophagus, in response to superior vena caval obstruction. In this case, the blood flow in the esophageal venous plexus is reversed (caudad), and portal venous blood flow is in the normal

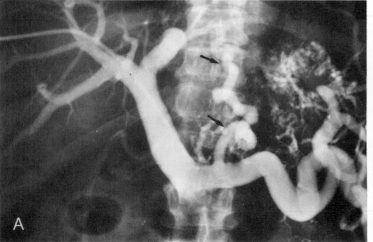

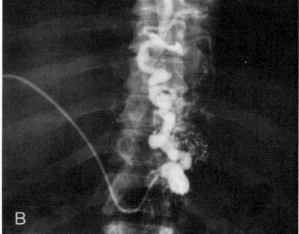

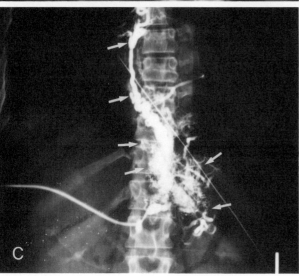

Figure 3.1.3. Forty-year-old man with alcoholic cirrhosis and esophageal varices who had several bleeding episodes. **A.** Percutaneous transhepatic portal venogram shows large coronary vein *(arrows)*. **B.** Selective coronary venogram shows large coronary vein with flow toward lower esophageal venous plexus. **C.** Selective injection into coronary vein reveals extensive esophageal and gastric varices *(arrows)*. (Reproduced from Becker GJ, Holden RW, Klatte EC: On therapeutic embolization with absolute ethanol. *Semin Intervent Radiol* 1984;1:118, with permission from Thieme–Stratton.)

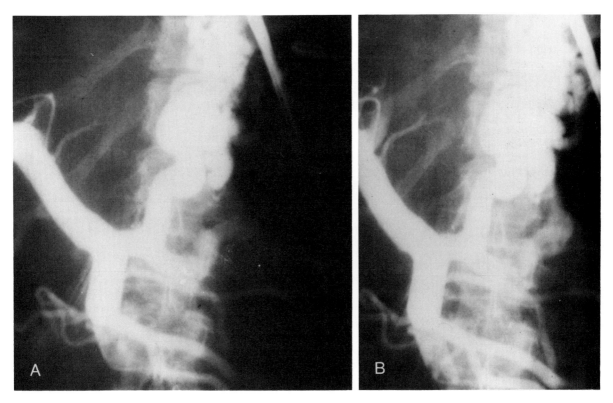

Figure 3.1.4. A,B. Transhepatic portal venogram shows markedly dilated coronary vein with large esophageal varix connecting directly to azygous vein. (Courtesy of E. Russell, M.D., University of Miami.)

direction. Thus, blood from the arm, head, and neck drains down the esophageal venous plexus into the short gastric and coronary veins, to the splenic vein, portal vein, and inferior vena cava (IVC) (through the liver).[42,43]

Historically, the diagnosis of esophageal varices has been made with an upper GI series and a barium esophagogram or esophageal endoscopy. Techniques for endoscopic sclerosis of esophageal varices with absolute ethanol or isobutyl 2-cyanoacrylate polymers are well accepted.[44] Sclerosis has been used primarily for prophylaxis, because the technique is technically more difficult and less successful in cases of bleeding esophageal varices, particularly those in which bleeding is brisk.[45-48] Intravariceal vasopressin injection was abandoned because of its ineffectiveness, but intravenous systemic vasopressin will arrest bleeding in some cases in combination with the Sengstaken balloon. This result would obviate transhepatic portal venography. A report from France studied the use of terlipressin plus nitroglycerin vs. balloon tamponade to control acute variceal bleeding.[49] The inactive vasopressin analog terlipressin is converted to active vasopressin in vivo and was equally effective in controlling variceal hemorrhage associated with balloon tamponade with fewer vasoconstrictive side effects (myocardial infarction, cerebrovascular accident, and bowel ischemia) than Pitressin.[45]

Transcatheter embolization of bleeding esophageal varices is performed using a transhepatic portal vein approach from the right midaxillary line, as first described by Wie-

chal in 1964.[50] Lunderquist et al. introduced transhepatic portal vein catheterization to the United States in 1974.[42] More recently, Widrich and others have performed more than 300 transhepatic portal venograms at the Boston Veterans Administration Medical Center.[51] The technique has been modified and improved in recent times.[44,52-58,60] Basically, a portal vein branch in the liver parenchyma is entered with the aid of a skinny (22-gauge) needle in a fashion similar to that used for percutaneous transhepatic cholangiography. Gentle aspiration of the needle is performed until blood is obtained. Small test injections are then given to distinguish portal radicles from hepatic veins and hepatic artery branches. Once the correct vessel has been entered, a guidewire is introduced and a steerable catheter is passed into the portal vein (Fig. 3.1.5A). Under fluoroscopy, the guidewire and catheter are manipulated into the splenic vein, and an angiogram is performed to demonstrate the dilated, varicose venous channels (Fig. 3.1.5B). Subsequently, the catheter is passed into the coronary vein and then into the different varices as far peripherally as possible to demonstrate anatomy, size of venous channels, and associated anomalies (Fig. 3.1.6A,B).

Various embolic materials have been used to obliterate varices.[52-58] Lunderquist and his coworkers have used a coaxial catheter system for embolization, with isobutyl 2-cyanoacrylate (Bucrylate) injected through the smaller catheter. The polymer is immediately flushed from the catheter with isotonic glucose solution and the coaxial sys-

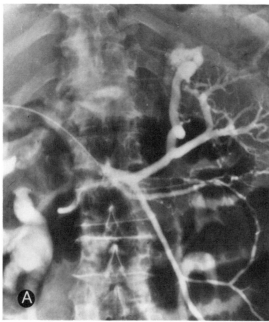
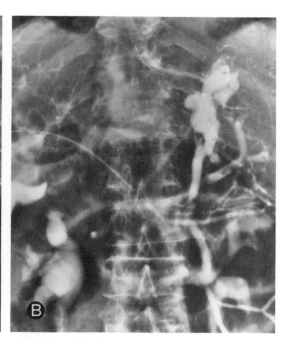

Figure 3.1.5. Patient with alcoholic cirrhosis and bleeding esophageal varices. **A,B.** Transhepatic portal venography performed with tip of catheter within splenic vein shows huge varices arising from short gastric veins.

tem is immediately withdrawn 1–2cm to prevent its adherence to the vessel wall.[44] If Bucrylate or other suitable polymers are not available, other embolic materials such as Gelfoam/Sotradecol (Fig. 3.1.7),[53,55] ethanol (Fig. 3.1.8), and GWC steel coils[51] can be used to obliterate the large feeding veins.

The present authors have used a combined technique

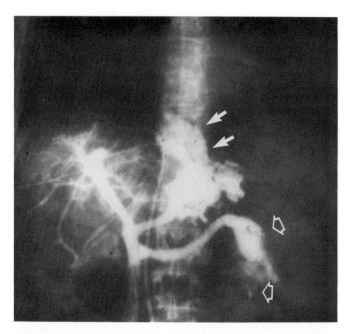

Figure 3.1.6. Transhepatic portal venogram shows spontaneous splenorenal shunt *(open arrow).* Huge gastroesophageal varices arise from coronary vein *(closed arrows).* (Courtesy of E. Russell, M.D., University of Miami.)

for embolization of esophageal varices in which a catheter is passed as far peripherally into the varix as possible. Gelfoam soaked in Sotradecol is then injected to obliterate and sclerose the venous channels. Following this, GWC coils are introduced to obliterate the large varicose channel proximally (Fig. 3.1.9*A,B*). This combined approach has arrested active bleeding, and the rebleeding rate has been low, certainly similar to that following decompressive portal-to-systemic surgical shunts and other embolic techniques. All visible varices should be embolized (Fig. 3.1.7) after which angiography is performed to demonstrate the complete obliteration of all the varicosities (Fig. 3.1.8).

Two other approaches to varices are available. An umbilical vein approach through a surgical cutdown has been advocated[58] for entering the portal system by passing through the connection of the umbilical vein with the left portal vein (Fig. 3.1.10). A recent report describes a combined surgical and radiologic approach to varices involving direct exposure and cannulation of the mesenteric vein.[59] Another approach is a transjugular route.[60] The hepatic veins are catheterized selectively, and the portal system is entered using a sharp needle passed through the guiding catheter and advanced blindly. Once the needle's position within the portal vein has been confirmed by injection of contrast medium, a guidewire is passed through the needle into the vein, and the needle and guiding catheter are replaced by an angiographic catheter that is passed over the guidewire. Catheterization and embolization of the varices are then performed. With embolization, Widrich and others report effective control of esophageal variceal bleeding at one month in 60% of 86 patients.[51] Complications of transhepatic portal vein embolization therapy

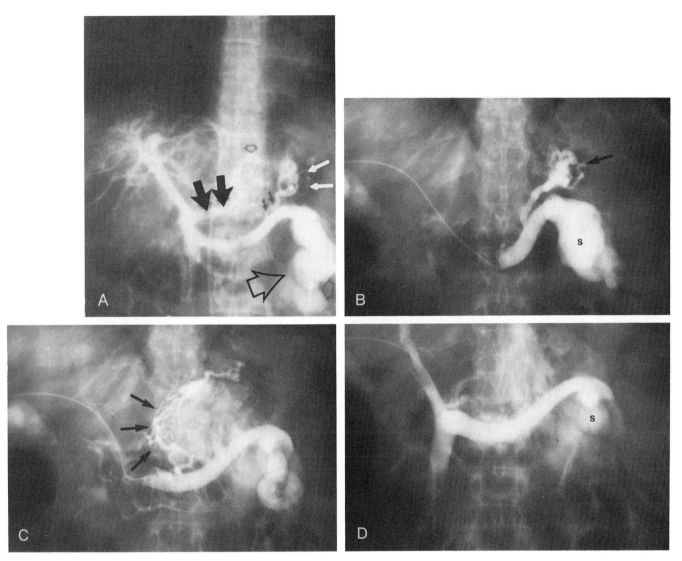

Figure 3.1.7. Patient with cirrhosis and bleeding esophageal varices. **A.** Complete thrombosis of coronary vein after embolization with Gelfoam; *large black arrows* point to left gastric vein and *small open arrow* points to distal stump. There is now opacification of a smaller short gastric vein supplying additional gastric varices *(small white arrows)*. Note increased flow across splenorenal shunt *(large open arrow)*. **B.** Bleeding recurred five years postembolization; injection into splenic vein shows enlargement of gastric varices arising from short gastric vein *(arrow)* and spontaneous splenorenal shunt *(s)*. **C.** After occlusion of short gastric veins, repeat splenic venogram shows additional varices arising from most proximal part of splenic vein *(arrows)*. **D.** Repeat portal venogram shows obliteration of all short gastric and coronary vein feeders with patent splenorenal shunt *(s)*. Patient is alive seven years after embolization. (Courtesy of E. Russell, M.D., University of Miami.)

include intra-abdominal bleeding from the transhepatic puncture, particularly in patients with coagulopathy secondary to the liver disease and with diminished platelet number or poor platelet function. The transvenous or transumbilical routes are better approaches in these patients, since they avoid extrahepatic extravasation. Intrapleural bleeding and hemothorax have been reported when the lateral costophrenic angle has been crossed during the transhepatic approach. By careful fluoroscopy monitoring during deep inhalation and exhalation by the patient, this complication should be avoidable. Portal vein thrombosis has been described related both to manipulation within the portal vein and as a response to a backflow of embolic material, such as particles (Gelfoam, Ivalon),

polymers, or alcohol. This complication should be uncommon if occlusion balloon techniques are used for fluid embolic materials and with judicious deposition of particles and coils. To avoid complications such as intraperitoneal or intrapleural bleeding, the authors have been reluctant to undertake transhepatic portal venography in patients with a platelet count <50,000/ml or in patients with prothrombin times or partial thromboplastin times >1.5 of control values. These contraindications become relative in the presence of exsanguinating esophageal bleeding, when the procedure is undertaken to save the patient's life. To help decrease bleeding from the puncture tract, a plug of Gelfoam can be inserted at the conclusion of the procedure.

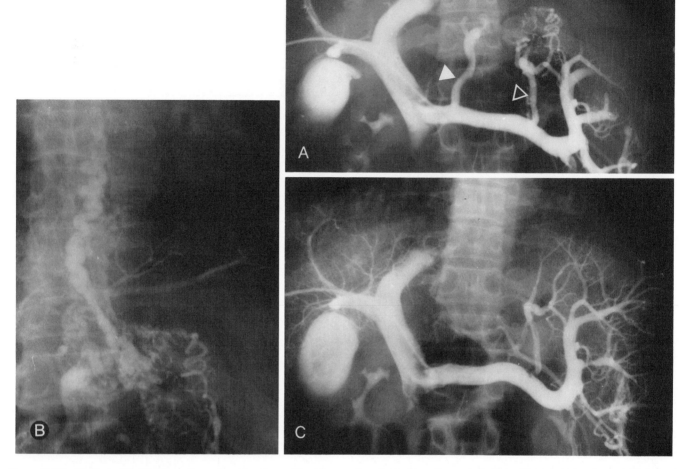

Figure 3.1.8. Patient with cirrhosis and esophageal varices with endoscopically documented variceal bleeding. **A.** Percutaneous transhepatic portal venogram shows large coronary vein *(white arrowhead)* and short gastric vein *(open arrowhead)*. **B.** Selective coronary venogram shows esophageal varices and intercommunication with short gastric veins. **C.** Portal venogram after embolization with ethanol shows obliteration of coronary vein, short gastric veins, and esophageal varices. (Reproduced from Becker GJ, Holden RW, Klatte EC: On therapeutic embolization with absolute ethanol. *Semin Intervent Radiol* 1984;1:118, with permission from Thieme-Stratton.)

Gastritis

Gastritis has two basic causes: drug- or alcohol-induced injury and idiopathic factors. Stress ulceration will be discussed under "Gastric Peptic Ulcer." In the diagnostic study of a patient presumed to have gastrointestinal bleeding from gastritis, a single focus of extravasation into the stomach is unlikely to be identified; instead, multiple sites of extravasation may be seen in the lumen of the stomach, which is diffusely hyperemic (Fig. 3.1.11).

The evaluation of these patients should include a selective left gastric artery injection if possible, because this study will often identify extravasation into the lumen and provide a more interpretable study inasmuch as there is no superimposition of splenic and pancreatic branches, as occurs with a celiac trunk injection. Depending on the size

of the patient and the aorta, selective left gastric artery catheterization can be most easily performed using a left gastric, sidewinder-1, or sidewinder-2 type of catheter in which the distal tip has been turned upward with steam. Once the sidewinder is engaged in the celiac trunk, it is pulled down slowly, with small contrast injections, until it is nearly straightened, at which point the tip will be directed superiorly and in most cases will engage the left gastric artery selectively. When gastroscopy has identified ooze or bleeding from gastritis in the distal part of the stomach, it may be necessary to perform a selective gastroduodenal artery injection with filling of the gastroepiploic arcade along the greater curvature of the stomach. Selective catheterization of the gastroduodenal artery is more difficult, especially when the vessel arises far to the right of a long common hepatic artery.

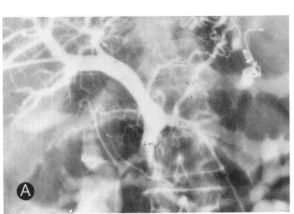

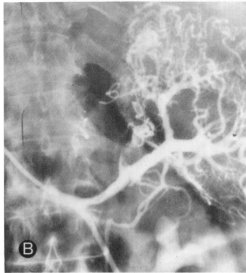

Figure 3.1.9. **A.** Portal venogram after embolization of short gastric veins with GWC spring embolus shows complete thrombosis of these vessels, but additional varices are seen arising from coronary veins. **B.** Repeat portal venography after embolization of all the short gastric and coronary vein varices shows no further opacification of varices.

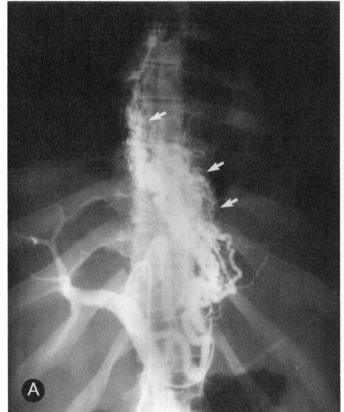

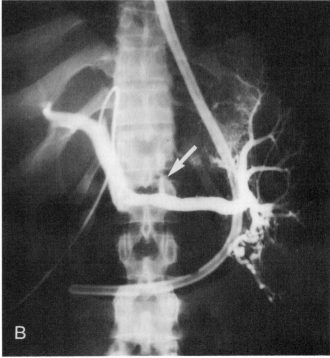

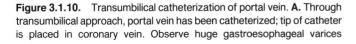

Figure 3.1.10. Transumbilical catheterization of portal vein. **A.** Through transumbilical approach, portal vein has been catheterized; tip of catheter is placed in coronary vein. Observe huge gastroesophageal varices *(arrows).* **B.** After embolization of coronary vein with Gelfoam plugs, observe complete thrombosis of esophageal varices *(arrow).* (Courtesy of Dimitri Spigos, M.D., University of Illinois.)

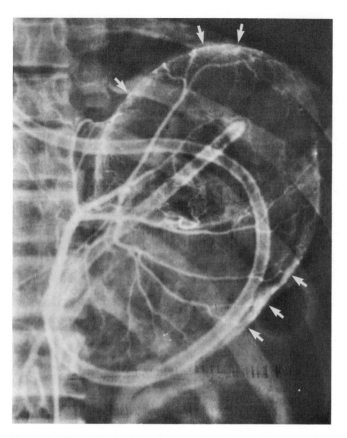

Figure 3.1.11. Selective left gastric arteriogram in patient with diffuse mucosal bleeding in erosive gastritis demonstrated by endoscopy. Note diffuse mucosal stain *(arrows)* suggestive of mucosal extravasation of contrast medium.

Once an area of extravasation has been identified along with the confirmatory hyperemic changes of gastritis, intra-arterial vasopressin should be given for the control of diffuse bleeding. In general, the bleeding from gastritis is from small (arteriolar-size) vessels, and vasoconstriction is adequate to control it. The standard infusion rate and doses outlined earlier are sufficient in most cases, although the authors recommend extending the infusion time to 24–36 hours after a response has been achieved before starting to decrease the dose; otherwise, rebleeding is more likely.[35,37,61,62] Selective infusion of vasopressin into the left gastric artery controls bleeding from gastritis in slightly more than 80% of cases[61]; in this report, approximately 16% of patients had recurrent bleeding and were judged to be suitable candidates for a repeat vasopressin infusion. Only in extremely refractory cases of gastritis bleeding, bleeding from a large hyperemic vessel, or severe coagulation abnormalities should particulate embolization for gastritis be necessary.[63,64] Because of the "four-quadrant" arterial supply to the stomach, embolization is rarely accompanied by gastric necrosis.

Gastric Peptic Ulcer

Gastric peptic ulcers occur by three mechanisms: 1) idiopathic; 2) in association with hypergastrinemia (Zollin-

ger–Ellison syndrome); and 3) stress, particularly postoperatively or following severe body burns. Regardless of the etiology of the ulceration, gastrointestinal bleeding is caused by erosion into a small artery. The angiographic evaluation of the hemorrhage is generally performed by selective injections of the left gastric artery, the gastroduodenal artery, or the superior pancreaticoduodenal arteries. In contradistinction to the arteriographic picture of gastritis, the angiographic appearance of a bleeding ulcer is one in which stomach vascularity is normal, and the bleeding is usually confined to one or two locations rather than being diffuse (Fig. 3.1.12). Occasionally, with erosions into large branch arteries, extravasation of contrast medium from the vessel can be identified.

After identification of a bleeding site, the angiographic catheter is left in place for intra-arterial vasopressin infusion. In most cases in which the bleeding originates from a small branch vessel, this treatment controls the hemorrhage. However, when the ulcer crater erodes into a larger vessel, such as the gastroduodenal or left gastric artery, vasopressin usually fails (Fig. 3.1.13A).[21,64,65] Particulate embolization of the bleeding vessel is frequently required (Fig. 3.1.13B).[21,64,66–69]

The philosophy of management of patients with gastric ulcer bleeding is evolving, especially with the advent of histamine antagonists (cimetidine) and antacid therapy.[70] In addition, gastroscopy enables peroral coagulation of bleeding points with electrocautery. Endoscopic management of GI bleeding, as well as transcatheter embolization and pharmacotherapy, has significantly reduced the frequency of surgery for bleeding ulcer disease.

Vasopressin infusion into the left gastric, gastroduodenal, or pancreaticoduodenal arteries has resulted in almost no complications.[29,32,56] Similarly, particulate embolization of these same vessels has not caused infarction of the stom-

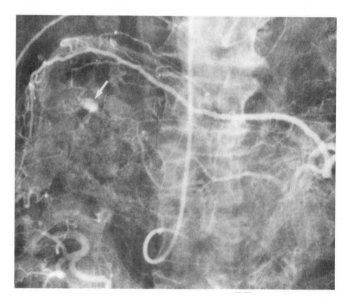

Figure 3.1.12. Stress ulceration demonstrated by a common hepatic artery injection *(arrow)* in patient with massive bleeding after major surgery for multiple trauma.

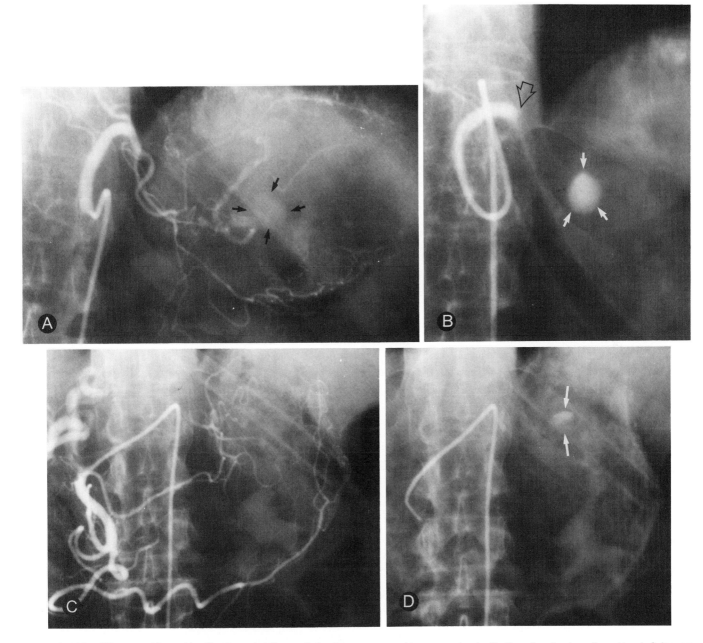

Figure 3.1.13. Fifty-year-old man bleeding from ulcer in gastric fundus. **A.** Selective left gastric arteriogram after infusion of vasopressin shows continued extravasation of contrast medium, which collects within ulcer crater *(arrows).* Observe marked decrease in caliber of left gastric artery branches due to the vasopressor effect. **B.** Selective left gastric arteriogram after embolization with Gelfoam plugs; note stump of left gastric artery *(open arrow)* and collection of contrast medium at level of ulcer crater *(small arrows).* **C.** Because of persistent bleeding, arteriography was repeated. Selective gastroduodenal arteriogram shows good opacification of right gastric and gastroepiploic arteries, with extravasation of contrast medium in area of ulcer crater in gastric fundus in late phase (**D**) *(arrows).*

ach.[71,72] The particulate material chosen for embolization should be a temporary one such as Gelfoam.[73,74] The luxurious four-quadrant blood supply of the stomach provides such excellent collateral flow that, even in the stomach that has been operated on, embolization has been almost complication free. Indeed, the dual blood supply to some areas makes control of bleeding difficult by either vasoconstrictor infusion or selective embolotherapy (Fig. 3.1.13*C,D*). Nonetheless, embolization should be approached cautiously in patients with previous gastric surgery; the extent of the surgical interruption of the vascular bed is unknown,

and embolization of an additional vessel can cause gastric infarction.[71,72]

Malignant Gastric Ulcers

Malignant gastric neoplasms are a well recognized cause of bleeding. Frequently, the site is identifiable angiographically as extravasation into the lumen of the stomach (Fig. 3.1.14) as well as by neovascularity within the tumor itself. The general principle of placing a catheter superselectively as near to the lesion as possible also applies to malignant

Figure 3.1.14. Fifty-two-year-old patient with lymphocytic leukemia presenting with gastro-intestinal bleeding from diffuse erosive gastritis during chemotherapy. **A.** Selective left gastric arteriogram shows extensive extravasation of contrast medium *(arrows)* from branch of left gastric artery. **B.** Postembolization with 2 × 2mm Gelfoam plugs; observe selective occlusion of branches in area of previous extravasation. Filling defects within proximal left gastric artery *(arrow)* represent Gelfoam plugs.

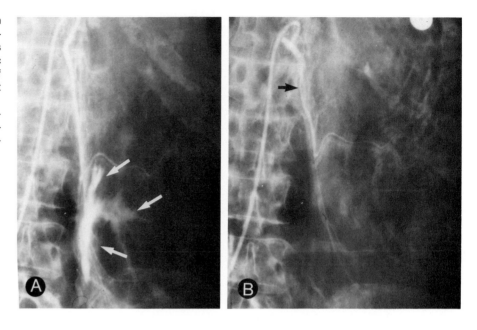

tumors. Selective infusion of tumors with drugs such as epinephrine or vasopressin has not been successful, as the abnormal tumor vessels appear unresponsive to these agents.

Goldstein et al. reported their experience with embolization of bleeding gastrointestinal tumors.[20] The preferred method of dealing with tumors in the stomach and duodenum has been embolization with permanent agents, particularly Ivalon, when superselective catheterization can be performed; not only has this been helpful in stopping the hemorrhage, but it has caused considerable tumor shrinkage prior to resection. When the tumor is larger and more

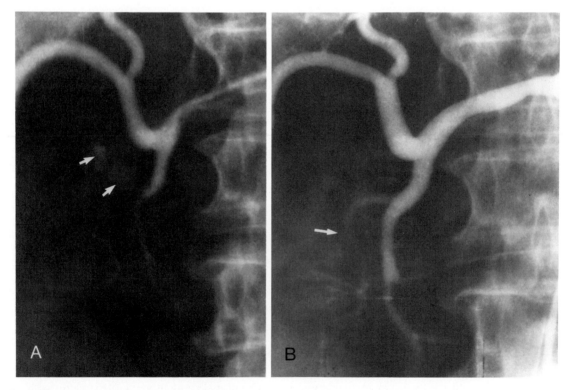

Figure 3.1.15. A 62-year-old man with metastatic renal cell carcinoma presenting with severe gastrointestinal bleeding from malignant ulcer in second portion of duodenum. **A.** Selective gastroduodenal arteriogram shows extravasation from a pancreatoduodenal arterial branch *(arrows).*

B. Common hepatic arteriogram after selective embolization of bleeding vessel shows thrombosis of this artery with no evidence of extravasation *(arrow).*

diffuse and superselective embolization is not possible, subselective embolization with a temporary particulate material such as Gelfoam can be used to control the acute hemorrhage and allow time for the patient to be stabilized and to achieve a better condition for surgical resection.[20,75]

Duodenal Peptic Ulcer Disease

Bleeding originating in the region of the pylorus or duodenum has been managed both by vasopressin infusion and by embolization, as well as by a combination of the two (Fig. 3.1.15). Vasopressin's success rate for control of bleeding in the duodenum has been only 35–45%.[64,66,70] Of those patients who underwent embolization after vasopressin failure, the procedure has been successful in 65–70%.[64,66,70,75,76] The success rate and expected outcome of vasopressin or embolization for duodenal ulcer bleeding can be predicted from the size of the vessel supplying the bleeder. A small tertiary branch of the gastroduodenal artery should respond to vasopressin, whereas more proximal large feeders from the gastroduodenal artery will require particulate embolization (Fig. 3.1.16).

The diagnosis is established by a combination of gastroscopy to identify potential ulcer bleeding sites and, if possible, by superselective arteriography into the gastroduodenal artery.

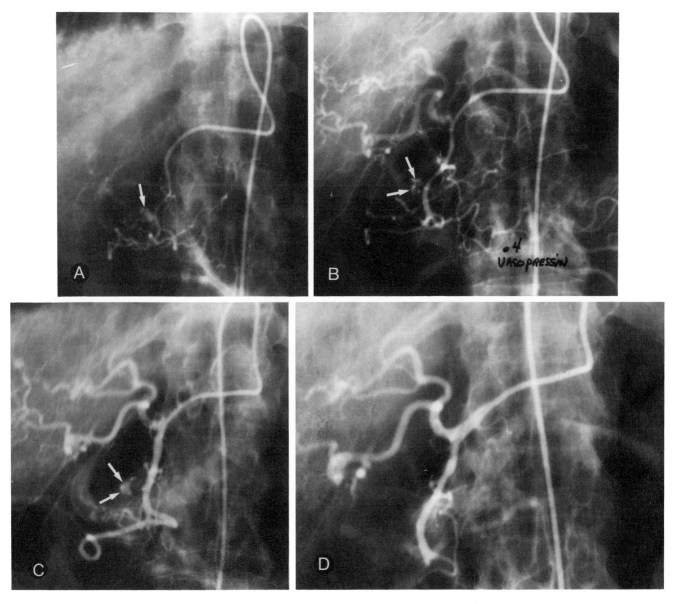

Figure 3.1.16. Patient with bleeding from duodenal ulcer. **A.** Selective infusion of vasopressin into gastroduodenal artery (0.2 unit/min) fails to halt bleeding *(arrow)*. **B.** Repeat gastroduodenal arteriogram after infusion of 0.4 unit of vasopressin/min shows continued extravasation of contrast medium *(arrows)*. **C.** Repeat gastroduodenal arteriogram after 2.5 hour of vasopressin infusion at 0.6 unit/min shows continued extravasation *(arrows)*. **D.** Repeat gastroduodenal arteriogram after embolization with Gelfoam shows adequate control of bleeding.

Postsurgical Anastomotic Bleeding

The basic principle of hemorrhage control at surgical anastomoses in the GI tract is selective injection of the appropriate vessel supplying the segment of bowel used in the anastomosis.[77,78] In cases of esophagogastrostomy, it is important to study the blood supply of the native upper esophagus and stomach used to create the anastomosis. In gastrojejunostomy anastomoses, it is important to study the blood supply of the remaining stomach and jejunum. The jejunum is supplied by the superior jejunal branches of the superior mesenteric artery. Gastroenterostomies are

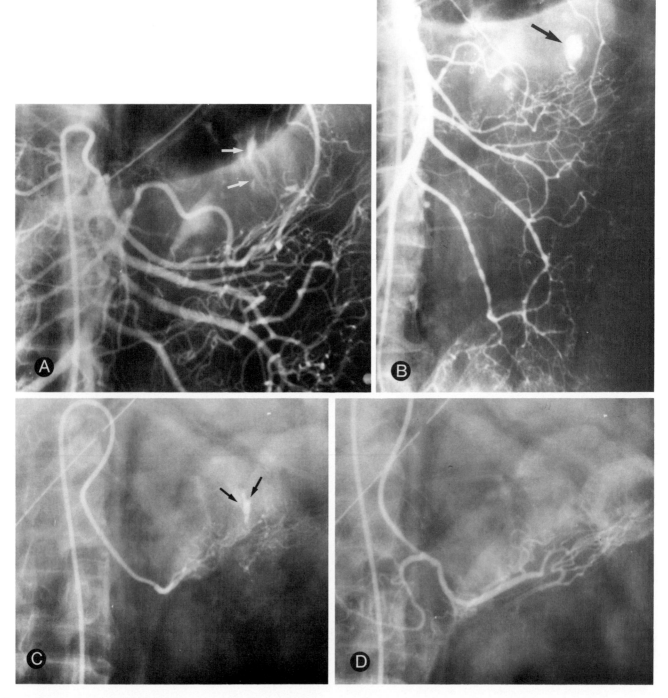

Figure 3.1.17. Gastrointestinal bleeding after Billroth I anastomosis in patient who had ingested acid. **A.** Selective superior mesenteric arteriogram shows extravasation of contrast medium from proximal jejunal branch *(arrows)*. **B.** Repeat superior mesenteric arteriogram after infusion of 0.4 unit of vasopressin/min into superior mesenteric artery shows continued extravasation of contrast medium from jejunal branch *(arrow)*. **C.** Selective catheterization of jejunal branch shows persistence of bleeding after selective infusion of 0.4 unit of vasopressin/min *(arrows)*. **D.** Repeat jejunal branch arteriogram after embolization with Gelfoam shows complete occlusion of bleeding artery with no further extravasation.

studied primarily by superior mesenteric arteriography. In these situations (Fig. 3.1.17) it is frequently necessary to perform superselective catheterization into second- and third-order branches of the superior mesenteric artery, not only to identify the bleeding site without superimposition of other vessels but also to attempt vasopressin infusion (Fig. 3.1.12). Ileocolostomies and colocolostomies require study of the appropriate superior mesenteric arterial branches, branches of the inferior mesenteric artery, or both.

The primary means of bleeding control postoperatively is vasopressin infusion, which provides good short-term cessation of bleeding and allows time for healing so that bleeding does not recur.[77]

Because GI resective surgery and bowel anastomoses frequently involve the ligation of several collateral vessels, permanent embolization is to be avoided if at all possible

because of the risk of bowel infarction, particularly after previous partial gastrectomies. Also, in cases involving resection of long segments of small bowel, many potential collateral pathways are eliminated, so, again, embolization in the small bowel is to be avoided. A similar principle applies to patients with previous colonic resections.

Bleeding in Meckel's Diverticulum

The classic picture of small bowel bleeding occurs in the young patient with a Meckel's diverticulum. The presence of Meckel's diverticulum can be established with high sensitivity and high specificity by radionuclide scanning using ^{99m}Tc-pertechnetate preparations,[12,14−16,79,80] which are avidly taken up and secreted by gastric mucosa, with which the diverticulum typically is lined (Fig. 3.1.18A). In the proper setting of GI bleeding in a young patient, in whom

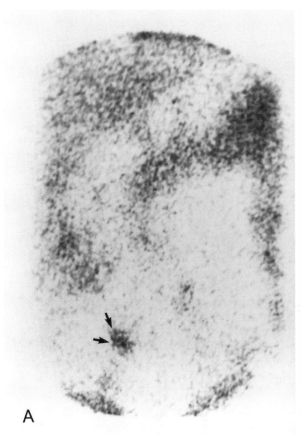
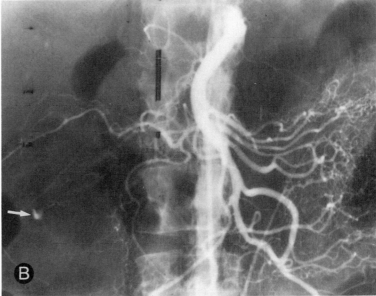
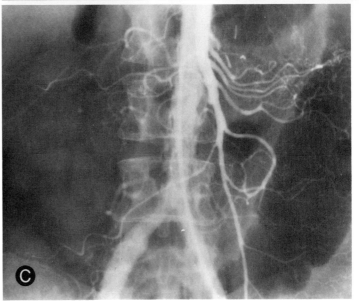

Figure 3.1.18. Control of ileocolic bleeding. **A.** Nuclear medicine scan with tagged red blood cells shows accumulation of contrast medium in right lower quadrant *(arrows)*. Observe also large amount of radionuclide activity within colon. **B.** Selective superior mesenteric arteriogram shows extravasation of contrast medium from branch of ileocolic artery *(arrow)*. **C.** Repeat superior mesenteric arteriogram after infusion of vasopressin shows adequate control of bleeding with no extravasation of contrast medium.

endoscopy is negative and who has a positive radionuclide Meckel's scan, superior mesenteric arteriography can be undertaken to identify the bleeding site. If a bleeding site is identified, superselective catheterization of the superior mesenteric artery branch supplying the region can be attempted for vasopressin infusion.[81] If superselective catheterization is difficult or impossible, infusion into the superior mesenteric artery itself is effective in stopping Meckel's diverticular bleeding, although understandably less so than direct superselective infusion.

Diverticular Disease in the Small Bowel

Occasionally, adult patients with diverticular disease in the small bowel also demonstrate gastrointestinal hemorrhage beyond the ligament of Treitz, particularly when the diverticulum is large and has been colonized by enteric organisms.[81,82] In such cases, the bleeding is of an oozing nature and is frequently difficult to identify angiographically, especially as it often is intermittent. Radionuclide scanning with ^{99m}Tc-labeled red blood cells may help confirm and, to a lesser extent, locate the region of bleeding (Fig. 3.1.18A). Again, vasopressin infusion as superselectively as possible is the mainstay of therapy (Fig. 3.1.18B,C). Antibiotics in high enteral doses should also be given to attempt to sterilize the diverticulum. Vasopressin infusion for bleeding small bowel diverticula is a temporary measure, and operation is the preferred definitive therapy.

Small Bowel Ulcerations

For the most part, ulcerations in the small bowel are ischemic, most commonly from emboli. The angiographic series may show an abruptly truncated superior mesenteric artery branch with a small embolus within the vessel, although it is rare to demonstrate the blockage. Other arteriographic signs of ischemic lesions include an intense blush of the bowel wall in the region. The mechanism by which bleeding occurs is thought to be sloughing of the bowel mucosa and erosion into small arterioles in the submucosal layers of the bowel wall. The use of vasopressin in the management of these patients may at first seem paradoxical, but bear in mind that the vessels that respond to this hormone are the medium-sized arterioles, i.e., those vessels containing smooth muscle fibers. Again, vasopressin administration is a temporizing measure and should be used only to permit stabilization of the patient in preparation for a definitive operation.

It has been helpful to leave the catheter in the superior mesenteric vessels when the patient is sent to surgery so that intraoperative injections of methylene blue can be given to assist the surgeon in locating the ulcerated, bleeding segment of the small bowel.[83,84] In this way, the extent of small bowel resection is minimized, reducing postoperative morbidity and avoiding the inconvenience to the patient of short bowel syndrome.

Tumors of the Small Bowel

Generally, small bowel tumors bleed intermittently, and because these patients are frequently studied electively between bleeding episodes, it is unusual to identify the actual site of extravasation or bleeding.[81,85,86] Tumor neovascularity itself may be seen within the small bowel. In cases of multiple small bowel tumors, the angiographic evaluation is particularly frustrating, inasmuch as any of these tumors could be the bleeding site and, in all likelihood, bleeding will be in abeyance at the time of the study.

Leiomyomas and leiomyosarcomas in the small bowel display a typical angiographic appearance, with hypervascularity and irregular corkscrew tumor vessels.[85] Intra-arterial vasopressin therapy is, again, primarily a temporizing measure while the patient is prepared for surgery. Definitive particulate embolization of these tumors is both technically difficult, because of the superselective catheterization techniques required, and fraught with complications, particularly small bowel infarction, and thus it should be undertaken reluctantly.[85,87]

A small bowel carcinoid is identifiable arteriographically by the fibroblastic reaction in the mesenteric root, which causes retraction, displacement, and occlusion of multiple superior mesenteric artery branches.[88] Vasopressin infusion is, again, a temporizing measure until definitive operation can be done when the patient is in stable condition.

Birns and coworkers reported a case of intramural small bowel hematoma presenting with severe upper GI bleeding.[89] Crawford et al. reported locating a jejunoileal arteriovenous malformation using segmental bowel staining.[90]

Granulomatous Disease of the Small Bowel (Inflammatory Bowel Disease)

Angiographically, the bowel wall involved by Crohn's disease reveals hyperemia with arteriovenous shunting and, frequently, intense venous opacification during midarterial films. The bleeding associated with inflammatory bowel disease is generally diffuse, similar to that seen with gastritis; rarely is a focal site of extravasation identified (Fig. 3.1.19A).[91,92] Gastrointestinal bleeding can be controlled acutely with intra-arterial vasopressin infusion (Fig. 3.1.19B), but the definitive therapy is surgical, particularly in Crohn's disease severe enough to cause stenosis in the terminal ileum or other segments of small bowel. Vasopressin may actually be contraindicated in these situations because of the risk of infarcting segments of bowel whose blood supply is already severely compromised by granulomatous infiltration of the wall.

Cecal Ulceration in Immunosuppressed Patients

Immunosuppressed patients can present with severe GI bleeding secondary either to steroid administration or to

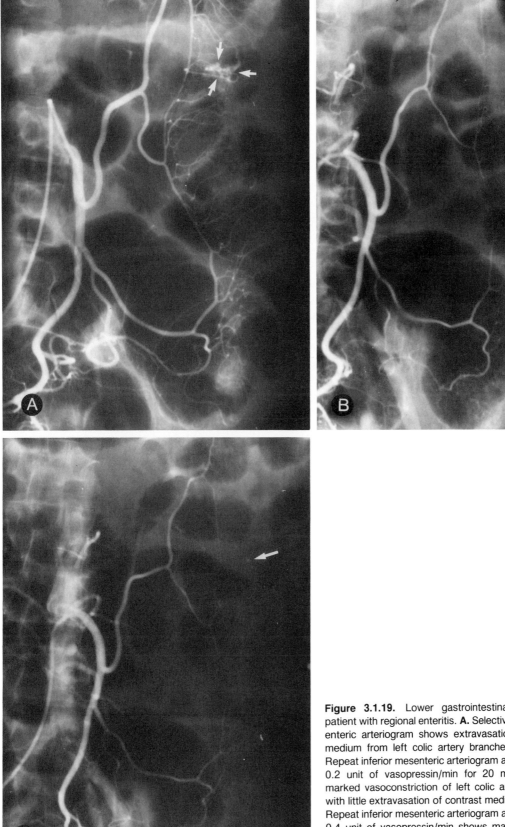

Figure 3.1.19. Lower gastrointestinal bleeding in patient with regional enteritis. **A.** Selective inferior mesenteric arteriogram shows extravasation of contrast medium from left colic artery branches *(arrows).* **B.** Repeat inferior mesenteric arteriogram after infusion of 0.2 unit of vasopressin/min for 20 minutes shows marked vasoconstriction of left colic artery branches with little extravasation of contrast medium *(arrow).* **C.** Repeat inferior mesenteric arteriogram after infusion of 0.4 unit of vasopressin/min shows marked vasoconstriction and control of extravasation. Observe residual contrast medium in ulcer *(arrow).*

overwhelming cytomegalovirus infection that can cause miliary ulcerations in the GI tract. Frequently, the latter presents as localized cecal ulcerations that respond transiently to vasopressin infusion via the superior mesenteric artery but resume bleeding as soon as the vasoconstrictor is discontinued.[87] Stopping the immunosuppressors and operation are the main avenues of therapy.[93]

Arteriovenous Malformations in the Colon

Arteriovenous malformations in the colon are congenital abnormalities, anatomically different from the acquired angiodysplastic lesions in aortic stenosis. The angiographic characteristics of both angiodysplasis and AVMs include early filling of draining veins, slow emptying of tortuous intramural venous channels, and dilatation of the feeding arteries (Fig. 3.1.20). Less commonly seen are a local stain within the colonic wall, a true vascular tuft of tangled vessels, and prolonged venous opacification (Fig. 3.1.21).[94–96] True congenital AVMs are most commonly encountered in the rectum and sigmoid colon.[97] Both angiodysplasia and AVMs of the colon tend to bleed intermittently (Fig. 3.1.22); therefore, arteriographic diagnosis is difficult, and false-negative results are frequently obtained. Identification of the nonbleeding lesions with barium enema studies

and, more commonly, by colonoscopy are important prior to angiography, especially in the patient with documented slow or intermittent colonic blood loss.[98] The abnormal vessels in both of these entities preclude success with intra-arterial vasopressin. The lesions can be managed by embolization either with Gelfoam, if temporary embolization is required, or with Ivalon particles, when permanent embolization is indicated (Fig. 3.1.22B,C).[26,99]

Embolization of the colon has a significant risk of bowel infarction, especially if small Gelfoam particles or Ivalon particles are used. These particles, if small enough, will occlude the colonic vasa rectae, end arteries, beyond the mesenteric collateral arcades, leading to segmental colonic infarcts. In a Japanese study,[100] canine intestinal embolization was universally fatal when Ivalon (polyvinyl alcohol) particles of $<250\mu m$ were used, while 9 of 11 dogs embolized with medium size $(420–590\mu m)$ and large $(590–1000\mu m)$ particles showed no ischemic gut changes.

The authors have recent experience with a bleeding AVM of the cecum. The patient, an elderly woman unsuitable for surgery, had undergone endoscopic fulguration for a bleeding cecal AVM; two days post-fulguration, she rebled and underwent arteriography. Although no bleed-

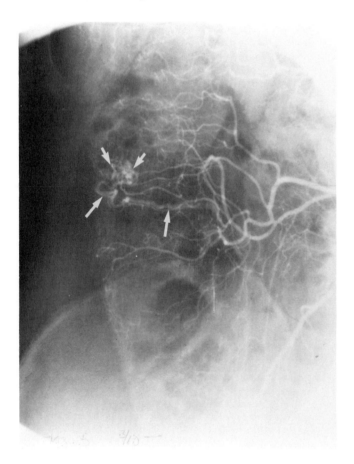

Figure 3.1.20. Abnormal cluster of vessels in cecal area, with early venous opacification *(arrows)*.

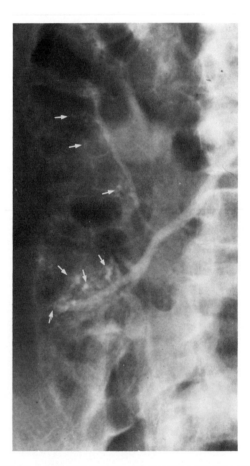

Figure 3.1.21. A 56-year-old man with repeated episodes of lower gastrointestinal bleeding. Selective superior mesenteric arteriogram reveals a localized area of dense vascular stain *(arrows)* and early venous opacification.

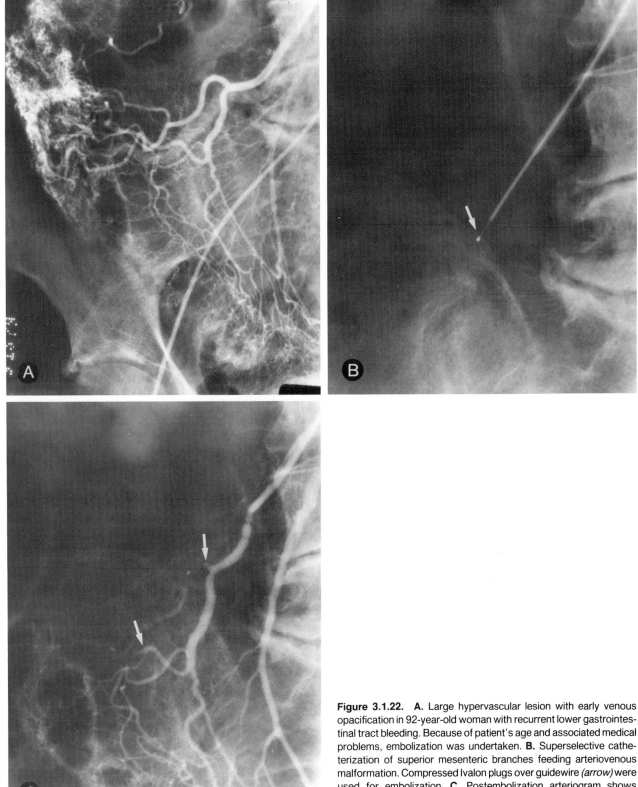

Figure 3.1.22. **A.** Large hypervascular lesion with early venous opacification in 92-year-old woman with recurrent lower gastrointestinal tract bleeding. Because of patient's age and associated medical problems, embolization was undertaken. **B.** Superselective catheterization of superior mesenteric branches feeding arteriovenous malformation. Compressed Ivalon plugs over guidewire *(arrow)* were used for embolization. **C.** Postembolization arteriogram shows occlusion of main feeders *(arrows)*; lesion is significantly devascularized.

ing site was seen angiographically, an empiric Gelfoam embolization of the ileocolic artery was performed. Her GI bleeding stopped and transfusions were no longer needed. Unfortunately, four days postembolization, she required laparotomy for a necrotic cecum and terminal ileum.

Grossly visible AVMs do not present a difficult surgical problem and can be resected easily. On the other hand, small angiodysplastic lesions are nearly invisible intraoperatively, and empiric colon resection frequently is necessary when bleeding is a problem. The specimen must be sent for high-resolution magnification angiography, if possible using a small focal spot unit. In addition, the predominant feeding arteries of the colon should be injected with a silicone preparation when the specimen is sectioned by the pathologist in the hope of locating AVMs.

Diverticulitis of the Colon

Diverticulosis is the most common cause of bleeding in the large intestine and generally occurs in patients older than 60 years.[101] Although diverticula are more common in the left side of the colon, bleeding from diverticula occurs three times more often from the right side. The primary origin of diverticular bleeding is thought to be erosion into a peridiverticular artery by fecal material or bacterial overgrowth. The only definite angiographic criterion for diverticular bleeding is extravasation into the precise diverticular site (Fig. 3.1.23A). Intra-arterial vasopressin is

reportedly the more successful way to control diverticular bleeding (Fig. 3.1.23B).[99,101] Those cases in which vasopressin infusion fails are thought to be the result of the age of the patient and the atherosclerotic changes in the vessels involved. In this situation, the arterioles may not be capable of constricting in response to the infusion of vasopressin.

Inflammatory Bowel Disease (Granulomatous and Ulcerative Colitis)

Boijsen and Reuter have shown that in granulomatous enterocolitis, the arteries and veins fill more rapidly than in the surrounding normal bowel, with increased vascularity, and that there is a slight dilatation of the feeding arteries, with dilatation and tortuosity of the draining veins.[91] Those authors also showed that during the capillary phase of the arteriogram, thickened, edematous bowel wall can be detected in the presence of active ulcerative or granulomatous colitis.

The bleeding from inflammatory bowel disease of the colon, whether it be granulomatous or ulcerative, is generally diffuse oozing from the involved segment.[27,28] Correspondingly, the bleeding from inflammatory bowel disease is perhaps amenable to vasopressin infusion but certainly is not an appropriate indication for embolization. Again, the bleeding is intermittent and oozing, and frequently no evidence of the bleeding site will be visible on

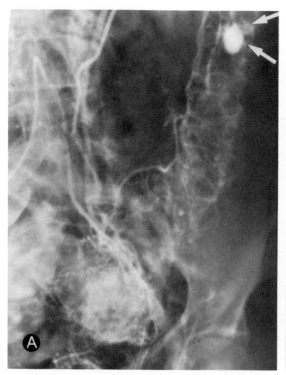

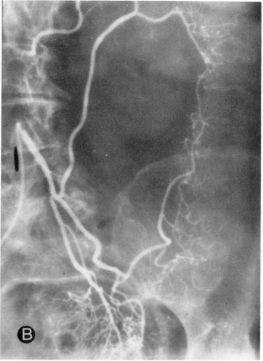

Figure 3.1.23. A 76-year-old woman with bright red hemorrhage through rectum. **A.** Selective inferior mesenteric arteriogram shows extensive extravasation of contrast medium from diverticulum in descending colon *(arrows)*. **B.** Repeat inferior mesenteric arteriogram after vasopressin infusion for 24 hours shows thrombosis of bleeding vessel with no further extravasation of contrast medium.

arteriography. Several publications discuss in detail the angiographic findings in both ulcerative and granulomatous colitis and the differentiation of the two.[27,28,91]

Tumors of the Colon

More than 75% of all polyps and cancers in the colon occur in the tissue served by the inferior mesenteric artery.[102–104] Several reports have suggested a role for arteriography in the diagnosis of carcinoma of the colon, but more recently, these techniques have been abandoned as insufficiently sensitive and certainly not cost effective in screening for this common cancer.[91,105–107] When changes are visible, the angiographic appearance is one of tortuous vessels that are randomly distributed, have irregular walls, and taper more rapidly than adjacent normal vessels. Many colon carcinomas accumulate contrast medium with some puddling in the capillary and early venous phase, and many also demonstrate premature venous filling.[108]

The role of vasopressin infusion for bleeding carcinomas has not been established, but this method is generally ineffective because of the nonresponsiveness of the tumor vessels. Particulate embolization with permanent agents such as Ivalon is a theoretical, although not widely accepted, method of dealing with the bleeding carcinoma of the colon. However, embolization for tumor control is difficult in the inferior mesenteric arterial circulation because of the frequent inability to pass catheters superselectively into this vessel. In addition, operation remains the definitive treatment for the disease because problems of obstruction, tumor bulk, and detection of metastases cannot be managed percutaneously at this time. The primary tumors in the colon that are most likely to contribute to lower GI bleeding are villous adenomas, adenocarcinomas, and, less frequently, carcinoids in the region of the cecum.

COMPLICATIONS

The complications of the percutaneous management of gastrointestinal bleeding can be divided into three categories. The first group of complications is related to the catheter, which, with modern equipment and technology, should be uncommon. Thrombosis at the arterial puncture site probably occurs most frequently (about 0.1% of the studies performed in the United States[109,110]).

With long-term vasopressin infusion, the catheter is frequently left in place for several days, during which time it accumulates a fibrin sheath. However, this sheath appears to be well tolerated by the patient if care is exercised during catheter removal. The present authors remove the catheter in the following way. First, peripheral pulses in the leg are checked. Then the physician's assistant applies gentle continuous suction to a large syringe attached to the catheter as it is slowly withdrawn. The artery is compressed below the puncture site, and the catheter is removed under continuous suction. After the catheter leaves the artery, the vessel is allowed to bleed for several seconds to expel any thrombus or fibrin sheath that has been stripped off the catheter at the puncture site. After several seconds of bleeding, the vessel is controlled from above and the artery compressed in the standard fashion. Using this pull-out technique, the authors have had no distal embolization from long-term indwelling catheters left in place up to 96 hours. Two cases of distal embolization of thrombus have occurred despite this technique (one in a patient on intra-arterial chemotherapy (7 days) and the second in a patient receiving urokinase therapy (48 hours) without concomitant heparin).

The second category of complications is attributable to vasopressin. Most patients complain initially of some abdominal cramping, which is thought to be related to the direct effect of the hormone on the smooth muscle of the gut, with increased peristalsis. This cramping persists for as long as 0.5 hour and is unlikely to recur. The physicians performing this study and the staff caring for the patient should be alert for abrupt changes in the patient's comfort level, with particular attention to complaints of severe localized pain. This frequently indicates a shift in catheter position to a more supraselective location, causing vasopressin to be delivered into a smaller blood vessel, producing intense vasospasm and local ischemia. Although the intra-arterial vasopressin dose is low in comparison to the systemic dose, during long-term infusion, the antidiuretic effect appears, usually after 6–8 hours. Therefore, the patient's urinary output and electrolyte status must be monitored. Diuretic therapy or electrolyte replacement must be started if urinary output falls or electrolyte imbalances develop. Some patients experience profound peripheral vasoconstriction, which is believed to be an idiosyncratic reaction to vasopressin. The extremities can become mottled and painful to the point of necessitating discontinuation of the drug. At the recommended local doses, reduction in cardiac output should not be a problem, but this is almost certainly dependent on the individual patient's cardiac status.

The third category of complications involves improper deposition of embolic material. Generally, once embolic particles or devices are released from the catheter, they cannot be retrieved, so it is incumbent upon the physician performing the procedure to be absolutely meticulous in positioning the catheter tip so that the embolic material is deposited as close to the bleeding site as possible and so that there is no backflow of material into blood vessels supplying normal tissue. The complications resulting from embolic particulate matter include end-organ necrosis and reflux of embolic material. As mentioned earlier in this chapter, embolic reflux should be avoidable with the use of occlusion balloon techniques, especially when fluid embolic material, such as absolute alcohol or cyanoacrylate, is used. Necrosis of normal tissue has been described to occur even after seemingly properly placed embolic material.[111]

After embolizations, particularly extensive ones, the patients may have fever as high as 102 °F. Local areas of ischemic pain and pain from necrotic tissue may also be experienced.

PERIPROCEDURAL CARE

Patient Preparation

Close cooperation between the interventional radiologist and the referring clinician is mandatory in the management of these patients. Adequate preangiographic workup is also necessary to facilitate a tailored examination in which selected high-suspicion areas within the GI tract can be examined. "Search and destroy" arteriographic procedures are to be avoided, because they require large contrast volumes and are frequently nonrewarding diagnostically. Collection of all available data, including barium GI studies and radionuclide bleeding studies, should be the responsibility of the interventional radiologist before diagnostic or therapeutic angiography.

Patients should be in as good a coagulation status as possible, which is usually not a problem in cases of GI bleeding. Exceptions are the patient with bleeding esophageal varices secondary to cirrhosis, patients receiving chemotherapy, and recipients of bone marrow transplants, in whom coagulation studies are likely to be significantly abnormal. If the hemorrhage is not life-threatening, the authors prefer to correct the coagulation factors with fresh-frozen plasma, cryoprecipitate, vitamin K, and platelet transfusions as appropriate. An additional consideration is the frequent coagulation abnormality in patients who have received several transfusions before angiography. Although these patients may have coagulation studies within the normal range, they frequently bleed extensively at the time of catheter removal.

It is imperative that the interventional radiologist discuss the diagnosis and treatment plan with the patient. At the authors' institutions, the patient's permission is obtained for both diagnostic angiography and therapeutic embolization as indicated before preprocedure drugs are given.

Sedative medication that will transiently lower blood pressure is to be avoided in the preangiographic period, because a decrease in blood pressure in response to narcotic medications can transiently stop or slow the bleeding, thereby masking the bleeding site. The GI bleeding evaluation, particularly if embolization is being considered, should be performed in a fully equipped angiographic suite, with ready access to anesthesia and patient monitoring services.

Postprocedure Care

Patients receiving a vasopressin infusion will of necessity return from the special procedure room with an arterial catheter in place. This is best monitored in an ICU setting where the patient has a primary, one-to-one nurse. Frequent catheter checks and groin observation for hematoma are essential. The authors deliver 0.2–0.4 unit of vasopressin/min using an autosyringe or Harvard pump mechanism, both of which are capable of generating suprasystemic pressures and of precisely controlling the delivery rate. Generally, using a 5Fr to 7Fr catheter, flow rates of 50–75ml/hr are required to keep the catheter open, and the concentration of vasopressin is formulated by the pharmacy to fulfill this requirement.

The typical GI bleeding case is referred late in the afternoon or in the early evening. Assuming the bleeding site is identified and vasopressin is begun, an angiogram is performed after 20–30 minutes of infusion. If bleeding is still identified, the dose is doubled to 0.4 unit/min. In another 20–30 minutes, angiography is repeated to see if bleeding has been controlled, and the patient is sent to the ICU with the infusion running. Generally, the patient is returned for the first follow-up angiogram 12–24 hours after the infusion was started. If bleeding has subsided clinically and angiographically, the infusion is continued at an effective rate for another 12 hours and then slowly reduced, as described earlier. If bleeding does not resume, the vasopressin infusion is stopped and the patient is sent to the ward with flush solution infusing through the catheter. If there are no clinical signs of bleeding over the next 8–12 hours the catheter is removed.

References

1. Baum S, Nusbaum M, Blakemore A, Finkelstein K: The preoperative radiographic demonstration of intra-abdominal bleeding from undetermined sites by percutaneous selective celiac and superior mesenteric arteriography. *Surgery* 1965;58:797
2. Margulis AR, Heinbecker P, Bernard HR: Operative mesenteric arteriography in the search for the site of bleeding in unexplained gastrointestinal hemorrhage. *Surgery* 1960;48:534
3. Nusbaum M, Baum S: Radiographic demonstration of unknown sites of GI bleeding. *Surg Forum* 1963;14:374
4. Rahn NH III, Tishler JMA, Han SY, Russinovich NAE: Diagnostic and interventional angiography in acute gastrointestinal hemorrhage. *Radiology* 1982;143:361
5. Kalff V, Kelly MJ, Dudley F, et al: Management of acute intermittent gastrointestinal bleeding. *Radiology* 1984;152:270
6. Smith RK, Arterburn JG: Advantages of delayed imaging and radiographic correlation in scintigraphic localization of gastrointestinal bleeding. *Radiology* 1981;136:707
7. Smith RK, Arterburn JG: Detection and localization of gastrointestinal bleeding using Tc-99m-pyrophosphate in vivo labeled red blood cells. *Radiology* 1980;136:287
8. Bunker SR, Brown JM, McAuley RJ, et al: Detection of gastrointestinal bleeding sites: use of in vitro technetium Tc 99m-labeled RBCs. *Radiology* 1982;145:286
9. Winzelberg GG, McKusnick KA, Froelich JW, et al: Detection of gastrointestinal bleeding with 99m-Tc-labeled red blood cells. *Radiology* 1982;142:139
10. Alavi A: Detection of gastrointestinal bleeding with 99m-Tc-sulfur colloid. *Radiology* 1982;12:126
11. Som P, Oster ZH, Atkins HL, et al: Detection of gastroin-

testinal blood loss with 99m-Tc-labeled, heat-treated red blood cells. *Radiology* 1981;138:207

12. Markisz JA, Front D, Royal HD, et al: Evaluation of Tc-99m labeled red blood cell scintigraphy for the detection and localization of gastrointestinal bleeding sites. *Radiology* 1983;147:316

13. Winn M, Weissmann HS, Sprayregen S, et al: Radionuclide detection of lower gastrointestinal bleeding sites. *Radiology* 1984;151:835

14. Alavi A: Radionuclide localization of gastrointestinal hemorrhage. *Radiology* 1982;142:801

15. Miskowiak J, Nielsen SL, Munck O: Scintigraphic diagnosis of gastrointestinal bleeding with 99m-Tc-labeled blood-pool agents. *Radiology* 1981;141:499

16. Bunker SR, Lull RJ, Tanasescu DE, et al: Scintigraphy of gastrointestinal hemorrhage: superiority of 99m-Tc red blood cells over 99m-Tc sulfur colloid. *Radiology* 1984;143:543

17. Ferrant A, Dehasque N, Leners N, et al: Scintigraphy with In-111-labeled red cells in intermittent gastrointestinal bleeding. *Radiology* 1981;139:270

18. Rösch J, Antonovic R, Dotter CT: Current angiographic approach to diagnosis and therapy of acute gastrointestinal bleeding. *Fortschr Röntgenstr* 1976;125:301

19. Goldman ML, Land WC, Bradley EL III, Anderson J: Transcatheter therapeutic embolization in the management of massive upper gastrointestinal bleeding. *Radiology* 1976;120:513

20. Goldstein HM, Medellin H, Ben-Menachem Y, Wallace S: Transcatheter arterial embolization in the management of bleeding in the cancer patient. *Radiology* 1975;115:603

21. Rösch J, Dotter CT, Brown MJ: Selective arterial embolization. *Radiology* 1972;102:303

22. Ring EJ, Oleaga JA, Freiman D, Husted JW, Waltman AC, Baum S: Pitfalls in the angiographic management of hemorrhage: hemodynamic considerations. *AJR* 1977;129:1007

23. Higgins CB, Bookstein JJ, Davis GB, Galloway DC, Barr JW: Therapeutic embolization for intractable chronic bleeding. *Radiology* 1977;122:473

24. Reuter SR, Chuang VP, Bell RL: Selective arterial embolization for control of massive upper gastrointestinal bleeding. *AJR* 1975;125:119

25. Reuter SR, Chuang VP: Control of abdominal bleeding with autologous embolized material. *Radiology* 1974;114:86

26. Kaufman SL, Kumar AAJ, Harrington DP, et al: Transcatheter embolization in the management of congenital arteriovenous malformations. *Radiology* 1980;137:21

27. Lunderquist A: Angiography and ulcerative colitis. *AJR* 1967;99:18

28. Tsuchiaya M, Miura S, Asakura H, et al: Angiographic evaluation of vascular changes in ulcerative colitis. *Angiology* 1980;31:147

29. Clark RA, Colley DP, Eggers FM: Acute arterial gastrointestinal hemorrhage: efficacy of transcatheter control. *Radiology* 1981;136:1185

30. Jander HP, Russinovich NAE: Transcatheter Gelfoam embolization in abdominal, retroperitoneal, and pelvic hemorrhage. *Radiology* 1980;136:337

31. Feldman L, Greenfield AJ, Waltman AC, et al: Transcatheter vessel occlusion: angiographic results versus clinical success. *Radiology* 1983;147:1

32. Baum S, Nusbaum M: The control of gastrointestinal hemorrhage by selective mesenteric arterial infusion of vasopressin. *Radiology* 1971;98:497

33. Nusbaum M, Baum S, Blakemore WS, Tumen H: Clinical experience with selective intra-arterial infusion of vasopressin in the control of gastrointestinal bleeding from arterial sources. *Am J Surg* 1972;123:165

34. Gomes AS, Lois JF, McCoy RD: Angiographic treatment of gastrointestinal hemorrhage: comparison of vasopressin infusion and embolization. *AJR* 1986;146:1031

35. Baum S, Athanasoulis CA, Waltman AC, Ring EJ: Angiographic diagnosis and control. *Adv Surg* 1973;7:49

36. Bookstein JJ, Chlosta EM, Foley D, Walter JF: Transcatheter hemostasis of gastrointestinal bleeding using modified autogenous clot. *Radiology* 1974;113:227

37. White RI, Harrington DP, Novak G, Miller FJ, Giargiana FA, Sheff RN: Pharmacologic control of hemorrhagic gastritis: clinical and experimental results. *Radiology* 1974;111:549

38. Herrera M, Castañeda WR, Kotula F, Rysavy J, Rusnak B, Amplatz K: Ivalon shavings, a new embolic agent: technical considerations. *Radiology* 1982;144:683

39. Carsen GM, Casarella WJ, Spiegel RM: Transcatheter embolization for treatment of Mallory–Weiss tears of the esophagogastric junction. *Radiology* 1978;128:309

40. Fisher RG, Schwartz JT, Graham DY: Angiotherapy with Mallory–Weiss tear. *Radiology* 1980;134:679

41. Eisenberg H, Steer ML: The nonoperative treatment of massive pyloroduodenal hemorrhage by retracted autologous clot embolization. *Surgery* 1976;79:414

42. Lunderquist A, Hoevels J, Owman T: Transhepatic portal venography, in Abrams HL (ed): *Abrams' Angiography: Vascular and Interventional Radiology*, Ed 3. Boston, Little, Brown, and Company, 1983, p 1505

43. Fleig WE, Stange EF, Ditschuneit H: Upper gastrointestinal hemorrhage from downhill esophageal varices. *Radiology* 1982;144:699

44. Lunderquist A, Borjesson B, Owman T, Bengmark S: Isobutyl II cyanocrylate (Bucrylate) in obliteration of gastric coronary vein in esophageal varices. *AJR* 1978;130:1

45. Hanna SS, Warren WD, Galambos JT: Bleeding varices: emergency management. *Radiology* 1981;140:583

46. Hanna SS, Warren WD, Galambos JT: Bleeding varices: elective management. *Radiology* 1981;140:585

47. Agha FP: Esophagus after endoscopic injection sclerotherapy: acute and chronic changes. *Radiology* 1984;153:37

48. Tihansky DP, Reilly JJ, Schade RR, Van Thiel DH: Esophagus after injection sclerotherapy of varices: immediate postoperative changes. *Radiology* 1984;153:43

49. Fort E, Sautereau D, Silvain C, et al: A randomized trial of terlipressin plus nitroglycerine vs. balloon tamponade in the control of acute variceal hemorrhage. *Hepatology* 1990;11:678

50. Wiechal KL: Tekniken vid perkutan transhepatisk portapunktion (PTP). *Nord Med* 1971;86:912

51. Widrich WC: Embolization therapy of esophageal varices. Presented at the Eighth Annual Course on Diagnostic and Therapeutic Angiography and Interventional Radiology, Society of Cardiovascular Radiology, San Francisco, February 1983

52. Widrich WC, Robbins AH, Nabseth DC, Johnson WC, Goldstein SA: Pitfalls of transhepatic portal venography and therapeutic coronary vein occlusion. *AJR* 1978;131:637

53. Pereiras R, Viamonte M Jr, Russel E, LaPage J, White P, Hutson D: New technique for interruption of gastroesophageal venous blood flow. *Radiology* 1977;124:313

54. Mendez G Jr, Russell E: Gastrointestinal varices: percutaneous transhepatic therapeutic embolization in 54 patients. *Radiology* 1980;135:1045

55. Funaro AH, Ring EJ, Freiman DB, Oleaga JA, Gordon RL:

Transhepatic obliteration of esophageal varices using the stainless steel coil. *AJR* 1979;133:1123

56. Viamonte M Jr, Pereiras R, Russel R, LaPage J, Hutson D: Transhepatic obliteration of gastro-esophageal varices: results in acute and nonacute bleeders. *AJR* 1977;129: 237

57. L'Hermine CL, Chastanet P, Delemazure O, et al: Percutaneous transhepatic embolization of gastroesophageal varices: results in 400 patients. *AJR* 1989;152:755

58. Spigos DG, Tauber JW, Tau WS, Mulligan BD, Espinoza GL: Umbilical venous cannulation: a new approach for embolization of esophageal varices. *Radiology* 1983; 146:53

59. Durham JD, Kumpe DA, VanStiegmann G, et al: Direct catheterization of the mesenteric vein: combined surgical and radiologic approach to the treatment of variceal hemorrhage. *Radiology* 1990;177:229

60. Goldman ML, Fajman W, Galambos J: Transjugular obliteration of the gastric coronary vein. *Radiology* 1976;118:453

61. Athanasoulis CA, Baum S, Waltman AC, Ring EJ, Imbembo A, Vander Salm TJ: Control of acute gastric mucosal hemorrhage: intra-arterial infusion of posterior pituitary extract. *N Engl J Med* 1974;290:597

62. Rösch J, Dotter CT, Antonovic R: Selective vasoconstrictor infusion in the management of arterio-capillary gastrointestinal hemorrhage. *AJR* 1972;116:279

63. Rösch J, Keller FS, Kozak B, Niles N, Dotter CT: Gelfoam powder embolization of the left gastric artery in treatment of massive small-vessel gastric bleeding. *Radiology* 1984;151:365

64. Reuter ST, Chuang VP, Bree RL: Selective arterial embolization for control of massive upper gastrointestinal bleeding. *AJR* 1975;125:119

65. Dempsey DT, Burke DR, Reilly RS, et al: Angiography in poor-risk patients with massive nonvariceal gastrointestinal bleeding. *Surgery* 1990;159:282

66. Katzen BT, McSweeney J: Therapeutic transluminal arterial embolization for bleeding in the upper part of the gastrointestinal tract. *Surg Gynecol Obstet* 1975;141:523

67. White RI Jr, Giargiana FA Jr, Bell W: Bleeding duodenal ulcer control: selective arterial embolization with autologous blood clot. *JAMA* 1974;229:546

68. Bookstein JJ, Chlosta EM, Foley D, et al: The transcatheter hemostasis of gastrointestinal bleeding using modified autologous clot. *Radiology* 1974;113:277

69. Lang EV, Picus D, Marx MV, Hicks ME: Massive arterial hemorrhage from the stomach and lower esophagus: impact of embolotherapy on survival. *Radiology* 1990;177:249

70. Collen MJ, Hanan MR, Maher JA, et al: Cimetidine vs. placebo in duodenal ulcer therapy. *Radiology* 1981;139:524

71. Bradley EL, Goldman M: Gastric infarction after therapeutic embolization. *Surgery* 1976;79:421

72. Prochaska JM, Flye MW, Johnsrude IS: Left gastric artery embolization for central gastric bleeding: a complication. *Radiology* 1973;107:521

73. Castañeda–Zúñiga WR, Jauregui H, Rysavy J, Amplatz K: Selective transcatheter embolization of the upper gastrointestinal tract: an experimental study. *Radiology* 1978;127:81

74. Gold RE, Grace M: Gelfoam embolization of the left gastric artery for bleeding ulcer. *Radiology* 1975;116:575

75. Waltman AC, Greenfield AJ, Novelline RA, Athanasoulis CA: Pyloroduodenal bleeding and intra-arterial vasopressin: clinical results. *AJR* 1979;133:643

76. Athanasoulis CA: Therapeutic applications of angiography. *N Engl J Med* 1980;302:1117 and 1174

77. Athanasoulis CA, Waltman AC, Ring EJ, Smith JC, Baum S: Angiographic management of postoperative bleeding. *Radiology* 1974;113:37

78. Rosenbaum A, Siegelman S, Sprayregen S: The bleeding marginal ulcer: catheterization, diagnosis and therapy. *AJR* 1975;125:812

79. Sfakianakis GN, Conway JJ: Detection of ectopic gastric mucosa in Meckel's diverticulum and in other aberrations by scintigraphy: indications and methods—a 10 year experience. *Radiology* 1982;143:299

80. Gordon I: Gastro-intestinal hemorrhage unrelated to gastric mucosa diagnosed on 99m-Tc pertechnetate scans. *Radiology* 1980;136:821

81. Briley CA Jr, Jackson DC, Johnsrude IS, Mills SR: Acute gastrointestinal hemorrhage of small-bowel origin. *Radiology* 1980;136:317

82. Spiegel RM, Schultz RW, Casarella WJ, Wolff M: Massive hemorrhage from jejunal diverticula. *Radiology* 1982;143:367

83. Fazio VW, Zelas P, Weakley FL: Intraoperative angiography and the localization of bleeding from the small intestine. *Radiology* 1980;139:524

84. Athanasoulis CA, Moncure AC, Greenfield AJ, et al: Intraoperative localization of small bowel bleeding sites with combined use of angiographic methods and methylene blue injection. *Surgery* 1980;87:77

85. Uflacker R, Amaral NM, Lima S, et al: Angiography in primary myomas of the alimentary tract. *Radiology* 1981;139:361

86. Zornoza J, Dodd GD Jr: Lymphoma of the gastrointestinal tract. *Semin Roentgenol* 1980;15:272

87. Palmaz JC, Walter JF, Cho KJ: Therapeutic embolization of the small-bowel arteries. *Radiology* 1984;152:377

88. Song-Nian L, Wan-Zhong Z, Xie Jing-Xia, et al: Gastrointestinal tract carcinoid: radiologic and pathologic morphology. *Chin Med J* 1982;95:136

89. Birns MT, Katon RM, Keller F: Intramural hematoma of small intestine presenting with major upper gastrointestinal hemorrhage: case report and review of literature. *Radiology* 1980;134:816

90. Crawford ES, Roehm JOF Jr, McGavren MH: Jejunoileal arteriovenous malformation: localization for resection by segmental bowel staining techniques. *Radiology* 1980; 137:880

91. Boijsen E, Reuter SR: Mesenteric arteriography in the evaluation of inflammatory and neoplastic disease of the intestine. *Radiology* 1966;87:1028

92. Brahme F: Mesenteric angiography in regional enterocolitis. *Radiology* 1966;87:1037

93. Castañeda–Zúñiga WR, Jauregui J, Garera Reyes R, Amplatz K: Bleeding from cecal ulcers in renal transplant patients. *Rev Interam Radiol* 1978;3:27

94. Boley SJ, Sprayregen S, Sammartanor J, Adams A, Kleinhaus S: The patho-physiologic basis for the angiographic signs of vascular ectasias of the colon. *Radiology* 1977;125:615

95. Nyman U, Boijsen E, Lindstrom C, et al: Angiography in angiomatous lesions of the gastrointestinal tract. *Radiology* 1981;138:521

96. Lewis HJE, Gledhill T, Gilmour HM, et al: Arteriovenous malformation of intestine. *Radiology* 1980;135: 264

97. Talman EA, Dixon DS, Gutierrez FE: Role of arteriography in rectal hemorrhage due to arteriovenous malformations and diverticulosis. *Radiology* 1980;134:816

98. Max MH, Richardson JD, Flint LM Jr, et al: Colonoscopic diagnosis of angiodysplasias of the gastrointestinal tract. *Radiology* 1981;140:855

99. Walker WJ, Goldin AR, Shaff MI, Allibone GW: Per catheter control of hemorrhage from the superior and inferior mesenteric arteries. *Clin Radiol* 1980;31:71

100. Kusano S, Murata K, Ohuchi H, et al: Low-dose particulate polyvinyl-alcohol embolization in massive small artery intestinal hemorrhage; experimental and clinical results. *Invest Radiol* 1987;22:388

101. Shaff ME, Becker H: Diagnosis and control of diverticular bleeding by arteriography and vasopressin infusion. *S Afr Med J* 1979;56:72

102. Maglinte DDT, Keller KJ, Miller RE, Chernish SM: Colon and rectal carcinoma: spatial distribution and detection. *Radiology* 1983;147:669

103. Johnson CD, Carlson JC, Taylor WF, et al: Barium enemas of carcinoma of the colon: sensitivity of double- and single-contrast studies. *Radiology* 1983;140:1143

104. Thoemi RF, Petras AF: Detection of rectal and rectosigmoid lesions by double-contrast barium enema examination and sigmoidoscopy: accuracy of technique and efficacy of standard overhead views. *Radiology* 1982;142:59

105. Halpern N: Selective inferior mesenteric arteriography. *Vasc Dis* 1964;1:294

106. Strom BG, Winberg T: Percutaneous selective arteriography of the inferior mesenteric artery. *Acta Radiol (Stockh)* 1962;57:401

107. Wholey NH, Bron KM, Haller JB: Selective angiography of the colon. *Surg Clin North Am* 1965;45:1283

108. Stromb G, Winberg T: Percutaneous selective arteriography of the inferior mesenteric artery. *Acta Radiol (Stockh)* 1962;57:401

109. Hessel SJ, Adams DF, Abrams HL: Complications of angiography. *Radiology* 1981;138:273

110. Jacobson B, Curtin H, Rubenson A, et al: Complications of angiography in children and means of prevention. *Radiology* 1981;138:273

111. Brow KT, Friedman WN, Marks RA, Saddekni S: Gastric and hepatic infarction following embolization of the left gastric artery: case report. *Radiology* 1989;172:731

Part 2. Site and Etiology of Hemobilia

—Ivan Vujic, M.D.

In 50% of cases of hemobilia, bleeding originates from the liver parenchyma, whereas the biliary ducts and the gallbladder are the source in approximately 45% of the cases. Hemobilia due to pancreatic disease is rare (see Chapter 3, Part 3).

CAUSES

Trauma is by far the most common cause of hemobilia, accounting for 50% of the cases (Fig. 3.2.1). Approximately one-third are iatrogenic. With the many traffic accidents and the recent introduction of invasive percutaneous radiographic procedures, one should expect to see an increasing percentage of cases of hemobilia of traumatic origin.[1]

Although hemobilia is present in only 2.5% of cases of accidental liver trauma,[2] the incidence following diagnostic biopsy is 3–7%[3] and that following percutaneous transhepatic cholangiography (Fig. 3.2.2) with an 18-gauge needle is 4%.[4] An incidence of 14% after percutaneous transhepatic biliary drainage was reported by Monden et al.[5] Similarly, late angiography in 83 patients who had undergone percutaneous transhepatic biliary drainage revealed a substantial number of vascular complications, with four patients presenting with severe hemobilia due to a pseudoaneurysm adjacent to the drainage catheter.[6] More recently, sporadic cases of hemobilia following endobiliary prosthesis placement and the use of an infusion pump for intra-arterial delivery of chemotherapy have been described.[1] Hemobilia is usually of no clinical significance and subsides spontaneously, although occasionally, signif-

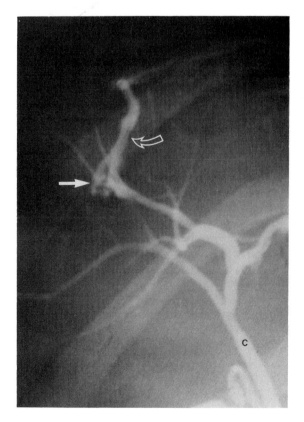

Figure 3.2.1. Endoscopic retrograde cholangiogram with bile ducts injected via catheter positioned in common bile ducts *(c)* opacifies fistula *(white arrow)* and segmental branch of right hepatic vein *(open arrow).*

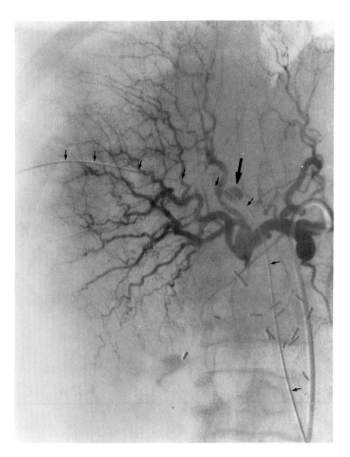

Figure 3.2.2. Common hepatic arteriography reveals false aneurysm arising from right hepatic artery *(large arrow)* in patient following percutaneous biliary drainage. *Small arrows* show position of drainage catheter.

icant bleeding follows diagnostic percutaneous procedures.[7]

Another form of iatrogenic hemobilia is caused by cholecystectomy and surgical manipulations in the biliary tree.[8] The extraction of stones in conjunction with the exploration of biliary ducts can result in bleeding secondary to mucosal laceration by the instruments. Occasionally, bleeding can be due to a pseudoaneurysm following surgical exploration.[1]

Gallstones and stones in the common bile duct are associated with hemobilia in 25 and 37% of cases, respectively.[9] In most of these cases, the bleeding is caused by mucosal irritation during stone passage. This type of bleeding is minor and ceases spontaneously. Pressure necrosis of the wall, however, allows the stone to migrate to adjacent hollow structures and can cause severe hemobilia if vascular erosion occurs (Fig. 3.2.3).[10]

Hemobilia can also be caused by inflammatory lesions, the most common of which has been coexisting gallstones and cholecystocholangitis.[1,8,11] On the other hand, in the Far East, "tropical hemobilia" caused by *Ascaris* is by far the most common form.[12]

Extensive necrosis of the liver due to drug-induced hepatitis[13] and halothane anesthesia[14] has been blamed for

severe hemobilia. Similarly, on very rare occasions, hemobilia has been associated with abscess (Fig. 3.2.4),[15] hydatid cyst,[16] and amebic infection.[17]

Primary or metastatic malignancy of the liver, gallbladder, or bile ducts may result in severe hemobilia. Single adenomatous polyps, diffuse biliary papillomatosis, aberrant pancreatic tissue in the wall of the gallbladder,[10] and other benign tumors[18–22] have been occasional sources of profuse hemorrhage. Coagulopathy is a rare cause.[1]

Only 7% of cases of hemobilia are caused by vascular abnormalities.[10] The passage of blood into the biliary tree is the result of arteriobiliary (Fig. 3.2.5A,B) or, rarely, of venobiliary (Fig. 3.2.6) fistulae. An arteriobiliary fistula is usually the consequence of penetrating trauma but may result from spontaneous rupture of hematomas, necrotic liver tissue (Fig. 3.2.4), or aneurysms into the bile ducts (Figs. 3.2.5 and 3.2.6). Venobiliary fistulae may occur between the portal or hepatic vein and the biliary radicles and may be associated with hemobilia (Fig. 3.2.7).[23,24] Aneurysms or pseudoaneurysms involving the hepatic artery have a great tendency to rupture, and, if this happens, free communication with the biliary tree is not uncommon.[25] Hemobilia due to ruptured gastroduodenal and cystic arteries has been recorded in a number of patients.[26]

Arteriovenous fistulae are often present in association with hemobilia. The most common fistula is one between the hepatic artery and the portal vein.[27] If the fistula is large, it may lead to severe portal hypertension.[28,29]

Portal hypertension may cause hemobilia, most often when large varices along the biliary ducts or gallbladder wall rupture. Varices of this type have been reported accompanying severe portal hypertension due to a primary hepatic malignancy invading the portal system or to cirrhosis.[30,31] The varices can enlarge, compress nearby tissues, and subsequently cause obstructive jaundice. It is essential to realize that these patients are prone to bleed spontaneously or following any invasive radiologic or surgical procedure.[32]

CLINICAL PRESENTATION AND DIAGNOSIS

Hemobilia remains difficult to diagnose even with the newer imaging modalities. The combination of gastrointestinal bleeding and biliary colic resembling gallstone disease should raise the suspicion of hemobilia. A classic triad of gastrointestinal bleeding, biliary colic, and obstructive jaundice is present in about one-third of patients.[27] Gastrointestinal bleeding occurs as melena or hematemesis. Additional symptoms include anemia in 70% of cases, fever, a palpable mass in the right upper quadrant, and dull pain (Fig. 3.2.3).[10] Shock due to significant blood loss is not uncommon. When blood seeps into the duodenum slowly, the cardinal symptoms are not present, and the only manifestation may be chronic anemia. Another important feature is the time lag between the initial injury and the evi-

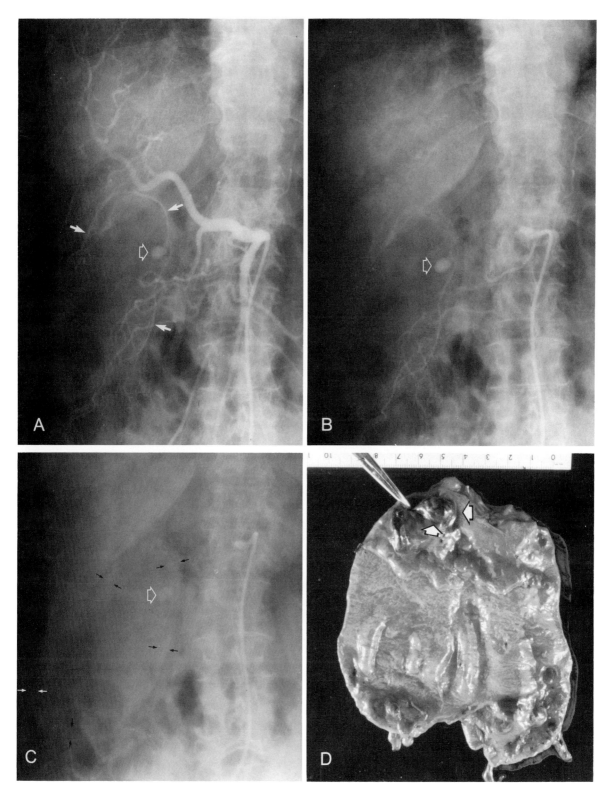

Figure 3.2.3. **A.** Early arterial phase of hepatic injection demonstrates branches of cystic artery *(white arrows)* outlining gallbladder and pool of contrast medium *(open arrow)* in region of gallbladder neck. **B.** Late arterial phase shows persistent collection of contrast medium *(open arrow)* within dilated gallbladder. **C.** Venous phase demonstrating a thickened and irregular gallbladder wall *(small arrows)*. Collection of contrast medium persists *(open arrow)*. **D.** Approximately 1cm below the gallbladder neck, note partially organized thrombus *(arrows)* adherent to area of ulceration, corresponding to angiographically demonstrated bleeding site. (Reproduced from Ryvecher MY, Schatz SL, Deutch AM, Cohen HR: Angiographic demonstration of bleeding into the gallbladder. *Radiology* 1980;136:326.)

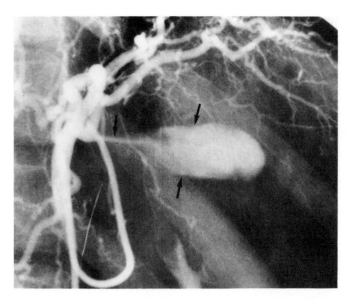

Figure 3.2.4. Patient with bacterial liver abscess presenting with severe gastrointestinal bleeding. Selective left hepatic arteriography reveals extensive extravasation of contrast medium *(arrows)* in area of hepatic abscess.

dence of subtle bleeding and recurrence of hemorrhage, which may be present for weeks, months, or years.

The diagnosis of hemobilia is difficult unless the condition is suspected. Percutaneous transhepatic cholangiography (Fig. 3.2.1) or endoscopic retrograde cholangiopancreatography may show filling defects, but they are not pathognomonic for hemobilia. Ultrasonic examination may identify a hypoechogenic hematoma within the liver[23] or a dense echogenic intraluminal mass within the gallbladder without acoustic shadowing.[33,34]

A preliminary report suggests that computed tomography (CT) can reveal the presence of blood clots in the gallbladder[35] and therefore may serve as the initial screening procedure if hemobilia is suspected. The normal gallbladder density measures from 0–20 Hounsfield units (HU). In experimental work on monkeys, it was shown that hemobilia homogeneously or nonhomogeneously increases the attenuation coefficient of bile to >50–60 HU (Fig. 3.2.8). Follow-up CT scans show a gradual increase in the attenuation coefficient of retracted blood clots over time, a feature that makes CT an attractive screening modality. On endoscopy and angiography one can miss the diagnosis because of the intermittent character of the bleeding episodes. An additional important advantage of CT is its ability to identify cholelithiasis, milk of calcium, tumors, and liver trauma as possible causes of hemobilia.

The observation of a dense accumulation of contrast medium in the biliary tree after selective hepatic angiography (Figs. 3.2.6A and 3.2.7) is another finding that suggests hemobilia.[36] However, this finding should be interpreted cautiously, because use of cholecystographic agents, vicarious excretion of urographic water-soluble

contrast media, and reflux of orally administered contrast medium through the papilla of Vater due to a malfunctioning sphincter all may increase the attenuation value of bile.[35] Strax et al. demonstrated that the usual increase in the density of bile follows the use of contrast medium with >37g of iodine.[37] Therefore, the identification of contrast medium in the biliary system after angiographic examination occurs normally by itself and should be diagnostic of hemobilia only if it is associated with endoscopic proof.

A definitive diagnosis of hemobilia is made by direct observation of blood coming through the ampulla of Vater. Unfortunately, because of the intermittent character of the bleeding, endoscopic diagnosis is made in only approximately 50% of patients.[27,38] Because the principal reason for failure in diagnosis is this intermittent type of bleeding, extended endoscopic observation of the papilla is recommended.[39] With minor bleeding, a hemoglobin-positive duodenal content, in the presence of otherwise normal endoscopic findings, may be the only positive test.

The most rewarding evaluation is obtained by selective celiomesenteric angiography. The angiographic feature most frequently associated with hemobilia originating in the liver and bile ducts is a pseudoaneurysm (Figs. 3.2.2, 3.2.4, and 3.2.6A). Hepatic artery-portal vein fistulae are also common, whereas communication between the hepatic artery and the hepatic veins is rare. Only a few cases of direct venobiliary fistulae have been reported (Fig. 3.2.7).[24] In spite of the proximity of the hepatic artery, portal vein, and bile ducts, extravasation of contrast medium into the biliary tree is seen in only 25% of patients.

TREATMENT

Significant hemobilia seldom ceases spontaneously and thus usually necessitates surgical or, more recently, angiographic intervention. Surgical treatment consists of either liver suturing or partial hepatic resection for peripheral lesions and ligation of the hepatic artery for more central injuries. Early recognition and prompt intervention seem to be the reasons for the gradual decrease in the mortality rate.[1] Cholecystectomy is the procedure of choice for every case in which the gallbladder is a source of bleeding (Fig. 3.2.3).

In recent years, since Walter et al. described a case of hemobilia controlled by angiographic techniques, there has been wide acceptance of this method as the first choice for the treatment of relatively stable patients.[40] Vaughan et al., in a review of 34 published cases, found that vascular embolization controlled hemobilia in every case.[38] In most cases, Gelfoam particles were successful (Fig. 3.2.6B), although for larger hepatoportal or hepatobiliary fistulae, the use of GWC spring coils or detachable balloons is indicated (Fig. 3.2.9).[41–43] The primary goal of embolic therapy should be to reduce the pulsatile blood pressure distal to the artificial occlusion rather than to devascularize the hepatic parenchyma. Peripheral placement of the catheter

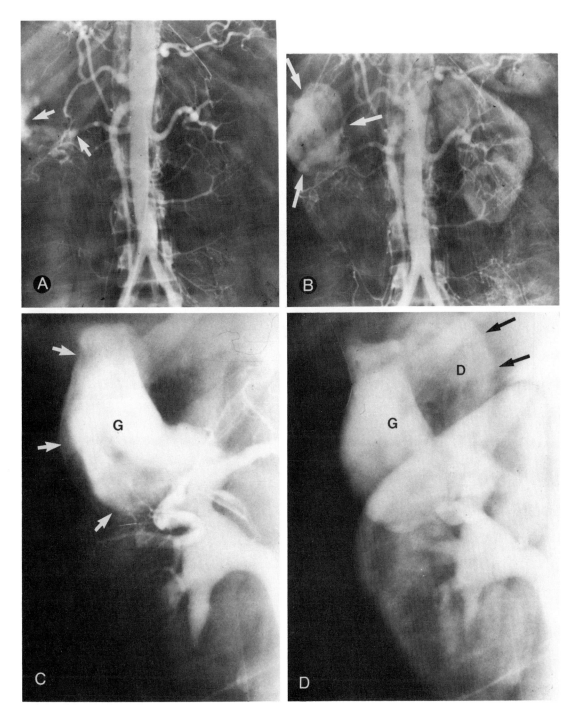

Figure 3.2.5 A,B. Patient with profuse upper gastrointestinal bleeding. Abdominal aortogram reveals massive extravasation from the right renal artery *(A, arrows)* with a localized collection in the right upper quadrant *(B, arrows)*. **C.** Selective right renal arteriogram shows massive extravasation of contrast medium into the gallbladder *(G, arrows)*. **D.** Late phase of arte-

riogram reveals passage of contrast medium from the gallbladder *(G)* into the duodenum *(D) (arrows)*. Surgery demonstrated a communication between the gallbladder and a patch that was performed to correct severe fibromuscular dysplasia of the renal artery 10 years previously.

in the vessel feeding the abnormality and embolization with absorbable particulate material seems to be most effective. Central embolization of the main hepatic artery or one of its principal branches is indicated whenever a peripheral branch cannot be catheterized or if the patient's deteriorating condition mandates prompt intervention. Spring coils or detachable balloon catheters can be used for these

occlusions. Infarctions and necrosis of liver parenchyma usually do not occur with central embolization because of the enormous potential for collateral circulation distal to the site of interruption of the blood flow.

The low rate of complications of embolic therapy in the liver is the result of the dual hepatic vascular supply. The portal vein contributes 75–80% of the oxygen and meta-

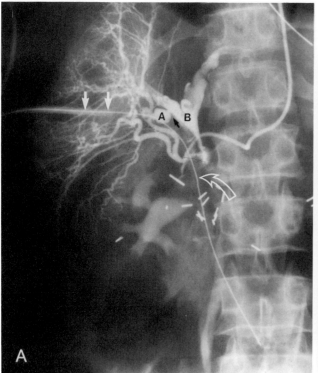

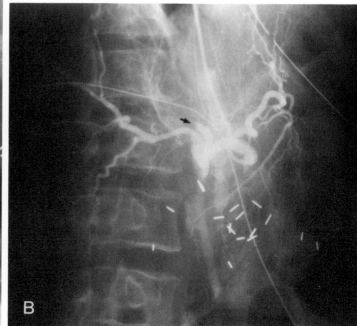

Figure 3.2.6. False aneurysm. **A.** Selective right hepatic arteriogram confirms to better advantage the presence of a false aneurysm *(A)*. Note also opacification of biliary radicle *(B)* from false aneurysm *(black arrow)* after partial pull-back of tamponading drainage catheter *(white arrows)* over a guidewire *(curved open arrow)*. Same patient as in Figure 3.2.2. **B.** Repeat right hepatic arteriogram after embolization reveals occlusion of hepatic artery branch feeding false aneurysm *(arrow)*.

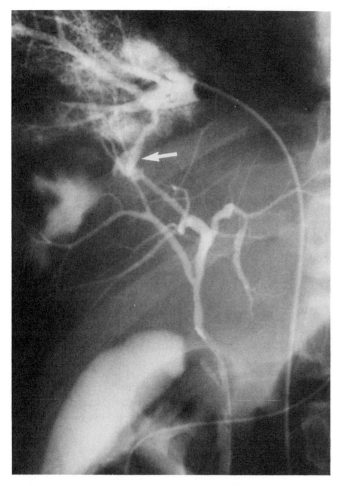

Figure 3.2.7. Wedge hepatic venogram in patient with severe hemobilia following blunt abdominal trauma shows opacification of biliary radicles from hepatic veins *(arrow)*.

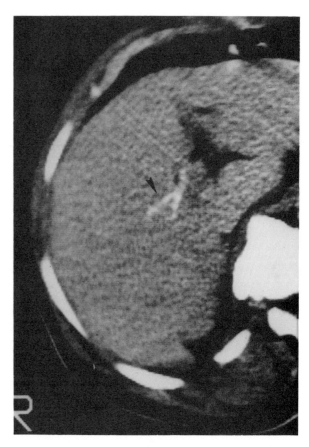

Figure 3.2.8. CT obtained after hepatic arteriography in patient with known hemobilia shows dense opacification of biliary radicles *(arrowhead)*.

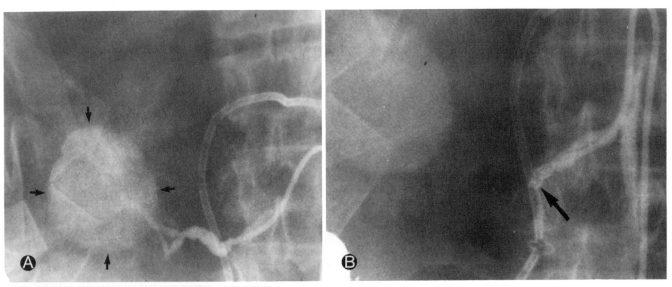

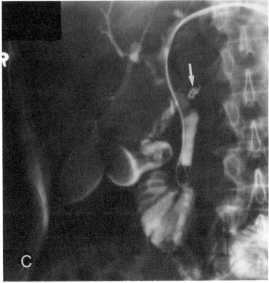

Figure 3.2.9. Patient with severe bleeding after partial hepatic resection. **A.** Selective common hepatic arteriogram shows extravasation into large false aneurysm *(arrows)*. **B.** Angiogram after embolization with GWC coils shows complete occlusion of hepatic artery branches supplying false aneurysm *(arrow)*. **C.** Cholangiogram through drainage catheter shows large amount of blood clots in bile ducts and gallbladder. *Arrow* points to coils in hepatic artery.

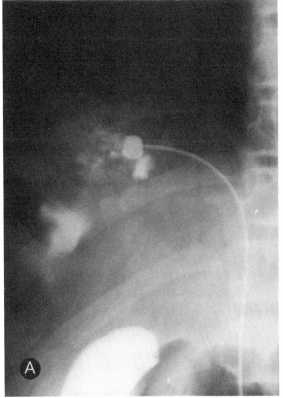

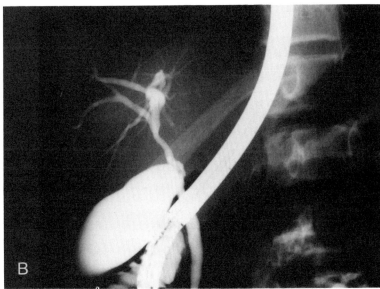

Figure 3.2.10. Venobiliary fistula. **A.** Balloon in wedge position to occlude fistula. Same patient as in Figure 3.2.6. **B.** Endoscopic retrograde cholangiogram 3.5 weeks later. Normal biliary pattern. (Reproduced from Struyven J, Cremer M, Pirson P, Jennty P, Jeanmart Y: Posttraumatic bilhemia: diagnosis and catheter therapy. *AJR* 1982;138:746.)

bolic needs, so prior to any interventional occlusive therapy, one should cautiously evaluate the portal anatomy and hemodynamics and avoid embolization procedures in patients with severely compromised portal flow. Minor liver damage manifested as a transient elevation of serum liver enzyme concentrations is present in approximately 20% of patients. Major complications are rare and associated with obstructive jaundice.[6] It is believed that decreased portal perfusion of the liver is associated with obstruction of bile ducts. As a result of this hemodynamic change, the liver parenchyma becomes more and more dependent on the arterial blood flow and consequently very sensitive to the ischemic conditions created by embolization of hepatic arteries.[44]

Venobiliary fistulae with clinical evidence of bilemia may be treated by temporary occlusion of the venous end of the fistula with a balloon catheter (Fig. 3.2.10A,B). This results in thrombosis and permanent occlusion of the abnormal channel.[24]

References

1. Sanblom P, Saegesser F, Mirkovitch V: Hepatic hemobilia: hemorrhage from the intrahepatic biliary tract: a review. *World J Surg* 1984;8:41

2. Fekete F, Guillet R, Giuli R, Goyer S: Hemobilies traumatiques. *Ann Chir* 1969;23:1199

3. Raines DR, VanHeertum RL, Johnson LF: Intrahepatic hematoma: a complication of percutaneous liver biopsy. *Gastroenterology* 1979;67:284

4. Cahow CE, Burell M, Greco R: Hemobilia following percutaneous cholangiography. *Ann Surg* 1977;185:235

5. Monden M, Okamura J, Kobayashi N, et al.: Hemobilia after percutaneous transhepatic biliary drainage. *Arch Surg* 1980;115:161

6. Hoevees J, Nilsson U: Intrahepatic vascular lesions following nonsurgical percutaneous transhepatic bile duct intubation. *Gastrointest Radiol* 1980;5:127

7. Merion de Villasante JRE, Alvarez–Rodriquez J, Hernandez–Ortiz J: Management of post-biopsy hemobilia with selective arterial embolization. *AJR* 1977;128:668

8. Larmi TK: Hemobilia associated with cholecystitis, post cholecystectomy conditions and trauma. *Ann Surg* 1966;163:373

9. Gad P: Okkult blodning ved galdesten. *Nord Med* 1962; 68:1069

10. Ryvicker MY, Schatz SL, Deutch AM, Cohen HR: Angiographic demonstration of bleeding into the gallbladder. *Radiology* 1980;136:326

11. Salem R, Boesby S, Bowley N, Blumgart LH: Haemobilia and haemoperitoneum. *J R Coll Surg Edinb* 1984;29:262

12. Chen S: On the etiology, pathogenesis, diagnosis and treatment of massive hemorrhage from the intrahepatic bile duct (abstract), in *Proceedings of the VIII National Congress of Surgery*, Peking, 1963, p 28

13. Lichtman SS: Gastrointestinal bleeding in disease of the liver and biliary tract. *Am J Dig Dis* 1936;3:439

14. Makela V, Landesmaki M: Hemobilia associated with hepatic necrosis after halothane anesthesia: a case report. *Ann Chir Gynecol Tenn* 1969;58:183

15. Karam JH, Jacobs T: Hemobilia: report of a case of massive gastrointestinal bleeding originating from a hepatic abscess. *Ann Intern Med* 1961;54:319

16. Goulston E: Massive hemobilia from an hydatid cyst of the liver. *Aust NZ J Surg* 1963;105:662

17. Forestier M: Un cas d'hemobilie après un absces amibien du foie. *Mem Acad Chir* 1963;34:83

18. Fisher ER, Creed DL: Clot formation in common duct: unusual manifestation of primary hepatic carcinoma. *Arch Surg* 1956;73:261

19. Rudstom P: Hemobilia in malignant tumours of the liver. *Acta Chir Scand* 1951;101:243

20. Bismuth H, Hernandez C, Hepp J: Les hemobilies d'origine vestibulaire. *Ann Chir* 1976;30:376

21. Hudson PB, Johnson PP: Hemorrhage from gallbladder. *N Engl J Med* 1946;234:438

22. Goldner F: Hemobilia secondary to metastatic liver disease. *Gastroenterology* 1979;76:595

23. Curet P, Baumer R, Roche A, Grellet Y, Mercadier M: Hepatic hemobilia of traumatic or iatrogenic origin: recent advances in diagnosis and therapy. Review of the literature from 1976 to 1981. *World J Surg* 1984;8:2

24. Struyven J, Cremer M, Pirson P, Jeanty P, Jeanmart Y: Post-traumatic bilhemia: diagnosis and catheter therapy. *AJR* 1982;138:746

25. Guida PM, Moore SW: Aneurysm of the hepatic artery: report of five cases with a brief review of the previously reported cases. *Surgery* 1966;60:299

26. Warmath MA, Usselman JA: Hemobilia developing from aneurysm of the left gastric artery. *Gastrointest Radiol* 1980;5:21

27. Foley WJ, Turcotte JG, Hoshins PA, Brant RL, Ause RG: Intrahepatic arteriovenous fistulae between the hepatic artery and portal vein. *Ann Surg* 1971;174:849

28. Cleveland RJ, Jackson BM, Newman PH, Nelson R: Traumatic intrahepatic artery–portal vein fistula with associated hemobilia. *Ann Surg* 1970;171:451

29. Markgraf WH: Traumatic hemobilia associated with hepato-portal biliary fistula. *Arch Surg* 1960;81:860

30. Barzilia R, Kleckner MS Jr: Hemocholecyst following ruptured aneurysm of portal vein. *Arch Surg* 1956;72:725

31. Martelli CF: Contributo allo studio delle emorragie colecistiche. *Arch Osp Mare* 1958;10:259

32. Meredith HC, Vujic I, Schabel SI, O'Brien PH: Obstructive jaundice caused by cavernous transformation of portal vein. *Br J Radiol* 1978;51:1011

33. Ruiz R, Teyssou H, Tessier JP: Apport de l'echographie dans le diagnostic des hemobilies: a propos d'un cas après ponction biopsie hepatique transparietale. *Ann Radiol* 1980; 22:52

34. Grant EG, Smirniotopoulos JG: Intraluminal gallbladder hematoma: sonographic evidence of hemobilia. *J Clin Ultrasound* 1983;11:507

35. Krudy AG, Doppman JL, Bissonette MB, Girton M: Hemobilia: computed tomographic diagnosis. *Radiology* 1983; 148:785

36. Vujic I, Stanley JH, Tyminski L, Cunningham JT, Adams K: Computed tomographic demonstration of hemobilia. *J Comput Assist Tomogr* 1983;7:219

37. Strax R, Toombs BD, Kam J, Rauschkolb EN, Patel S, Sandler CM: Gallbladder enhancement following angiography: a normal CT finding. *J Comput Assist Tomogr* 1982;6:766

38. Vaughan R, Rösch J, Keller FS, Antonovic R: Treatment of hemobilia by transcatheter vascular occlusion. *Eur J Radiol* 1984;4:183

39. Lehman GA, Bash D: Endoscopic observations of hemobilia. *Gastrointest Endosc* 1979;25:110

40. Walter JF, Paaso BT, Cannon BW: Successful transcatheter embolic control of massive hematobilia secondary to liver biopsy. *AJR* 1976;127:847

‌

41. Clark RA, Frey RT, Colley DP, Eiseman WS: Transcatheter embolization of hepatic arteriovenous fistula for control of hemobilia. *Gastrointest Radiol* 1981;6:353

42. Tegtmeyer CJ, Besirdjian DR, Fergerson WW, Hess CE: Transcatheter embolic control of iatrogenic hemobilia. *Cardiovasc Intervent Radiol* 1981;4:88

43. Dunnick NR, Doppman JL, Brereton HD: Balloon occlusion of segmental hepatic arteries: control of biopsy induced hemobilia. *JAMA* 1977;238:2524

44. Doppman JL, Girton M, Vermess M: The risk of hepatic artery embolization in the presence of obstructive jaundice. *Radiology* 1982;143:37

Part 3. Bleeding as a Complication of Pancreatic Disease

—Ivan Vujic, M.D.

Bleeding in association with pancreatic disease is not uncommon, but most of these patients bleed from peptic ulcer disease, hemorrhagic gastritis, or, rarely, Mallory–Weiss syndrome.[1] Far fewer bleed from the direct sequelae of pancreatic disease. Such bleeding is caused either by direct erosion of pancreatic or peripancreatic vessels or by thrombosis, usually involving portal vein tributaries.

MECHANISMS OF BLEEDING

Erosion of vascular structures is caused by the proteolytic activity of pancreatic enzymes, which are released during subacute or recurrent chronic pancreatitis after severe trauma. The result is acute pancreatitis, often leading to formation of a pseudoaneurysm, which has been reported by White et al. in 10% of cases of pancreatitis.[2] The process is usually also associated with formation of pancreatic pseudocysts. Once formed, the pseudoaneurysm has a tendency to enlarge[3] and ultimately ruptures into the gastrointestinal tract, the abdominal cavity, or, rarely, the pancreatic ductal system. In some cases, the hemorrhage will be confined to the pseudocyst cavity; but on rare occasions, the pseudocyst erodes the large vessels such as the aorta[4] and portal vein.[5,6] The vessels most commonly involved are, in descending order of frequency, the splenic (Fig. 3.3.1), gastroduodenal, and pancreaticoduodenal arteries, although virtually every peripancreatic vessel may be involved (Fig. 3.3.2).[7] This type of hemorrhage is severe and, until recently, had a high mortality rate,[8,9] principally because of inadequate preoperative workup and too conservative treatment.

Hemorrhage may take place prior to, during, or after operation (Fig. 3.3.3). Frey[10] and Sankaran and Walt[11]

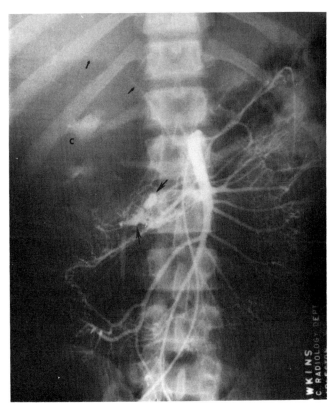

Figure 3.3.2. Enlarging hemorrhagic cyst *(c)* with two pseudoaneurysms originating from small colic branches *(large arrows)*. Note the displacement of vessels by enlarging hemorrhagic pseudocysts in the head of the pancreas *(small arrows)*.

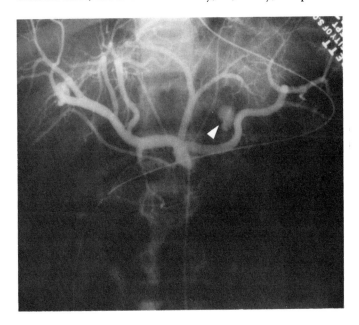

Figure 3.3.1. Post-traumatic pancreatitis with pseudoaneurysm *(arrowhead)* originating in the region of the small pancreatic branches of the splenic artery.

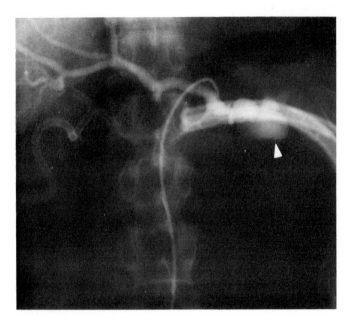

Figure 3.3.3.   Active bleeding from the stump of the splenic artery *(arrowhead)* into the pseudocyst and abdominal cavity following splenectomy and distal pancreatotomy.

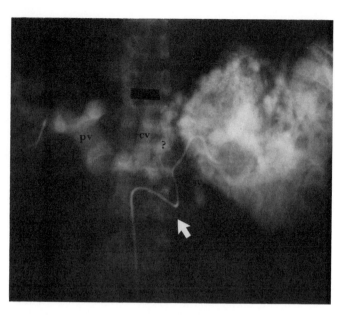

Figure 3.3.4.   Left-sided portal hypertension caused by splenic vein *(sv)* thrombosis *(arrow)* due to chronic pancreatitis. Collateral hepatopetal flow through gastric varices, coronary vein *(cv)*, and additional vein paralleling the coronary vein serves as the predominant route for decompression. *pv* = portal vein.

reported severe preoperative and postoperative bleeding in 7.6–9.8, 6.0–7.6, and 7.6–10% of patients with pancreatic pseudocysts. Similarly, Nielsen reported an 18% postoperative incidence of bleeding following internal drainage of pancreatic pseudocysts.[12] Recently, with more liberal use of angiography and earlier and more aggressive operation, the mortality rate has been reduced considerably.[8]

Although encasement of major arteries is frequently seen in disease of the pancreas, thrombosis of these arteries is not a prominent feature. Occasionally, smaller arteries may thrombose in the course of fatty necrosis in hemorrhagic pancreatitis, leading to bowel infarction.[13,14] On the other hand, thrombotic processes frequently involve the peripancreatic tributaries of the portal vein. Splenic vein thrombosis is by far the most common, being reported in 8.5–45% of patients with pancreatitis.[15–18]

The next most common causes of bleeding are tumors of the pancreas, usually carcinomas but occasionally islet cell tumors and cystadenomas.[19] The iatrogenic causes include thrombosis following splenectomy,[20] distal splenorenal shunt,[21] and umbilical vein catheterization.[22] The result of splenic vein thrombosis is gastric varices, which usually develop from the abundant collateral flow through the short gastric veins, which drain into the right and left gastric veins and finally the portal vein (Fig. 3.3.4). Another major collateral pathway consists of the left gastroepiploic vein, which drains through the omentum into the right gastroepiploic and superior mesenteric to the portal vein (Fig. 3.3.5). Occasionally, however, the left gastroepiploic vein drains through the omental branches of the left colic vein into the inferior mesenteric vein, resulting in colonic varices[23] that are highly suggestive of splenic

vein thrombosis, although in a review of the cases reported in the English language literature, Moosa and Gadd noticed that esophageal varices were present in almost 50% of cases.[19] Such varices develop when the short gastric veins are inadequate to decompress left-sided portal hypertension,[19] which is likely when the coronary vein drains into

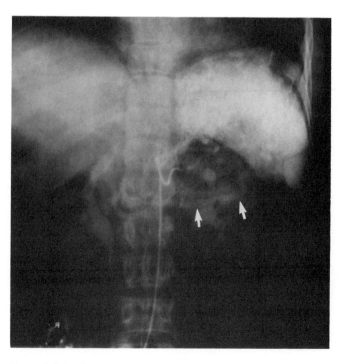

Figure 3.3.5.   Splenic vein thrombosis at the level of the splenic hilum with collateral circulation predominantly through the gastroepiploic veins *(arrows)*.

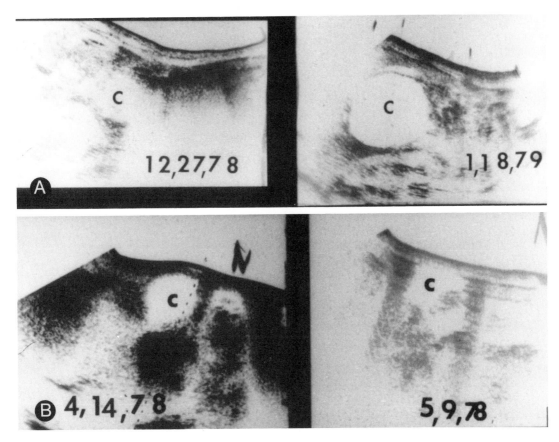

Figure 3.3.6.   Hemorrhagic pseudocysts. **A.** Bleeding is manifested by the rapid enlargement of the pseudocyst *(C)* over a period of three weeks; compare with Figure 3.3.2. **B.** Small pseudoaneurysm in the tail region of

the pancreas bleeding into the pseudocyst. Mild to moderate enlargement of the cavity with change in internal echogenicity indicating bleeding.

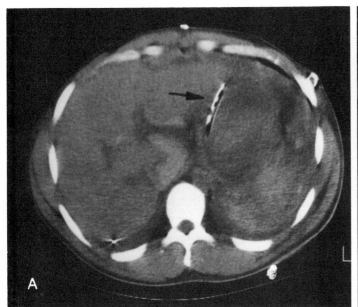
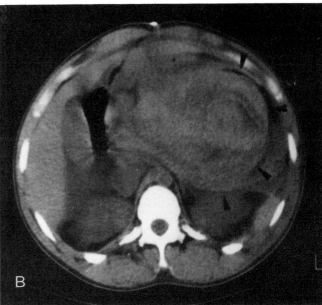

Figure 3.3.7.   Sudden drop in the hematocrit in a patient with known pancreatic disease and retrograde cystic mass. **A.** Acute formation of a pseudocyst displacing the stomach anteriorly and medially *(arrow).* **B.**

Lower level, high-density number within the pseudocyst *(arrowheads),* indicative of extensive bleeding.

the splenic rather than the portal vein, an anatomic arrangement present in 70% of persons.[18,24]

Thrombosis involving the portal and superior mesenteric veins is rare and is associated with either a septic stage of severe necrotizing pancreatitis or with carcinoma of the pancreatic head causing pancreatitis.[13,19,25]

CLINICAL PRESENTATION AND DIAGNOSIS

Early recognition of bleeding in patients with known pancreatitis is essential for appropriate successful management. The chief presenting complaints are gastrointestinal bleeding in one-half the patients and vague recurrent abdominal pain in one-fourth. Splenomegaly is present in approximately one-third of patients. The combination of a palpable abdominal mass, particularly if it is pulsatile, an audible bruit in the vicinity of the mass, abdominal pain, and clinical evidence of bleeding into the gastrointestinal tract or abdominal cavity in association with hyperamylasemia should alert the clinician.

Endoscopy may rule out bleeding from peptic ulcer disease, gastritis, Mallory–Weiss tears, and varices and occasionally may permit diagnosis of pancreatic hemobilia.[26] On rare occasions, it will reveal the site of the erosion of the pseudocyst directly into the gastrointestinal tract.

Ultrasonic patterns associated with a bleeding pancre-

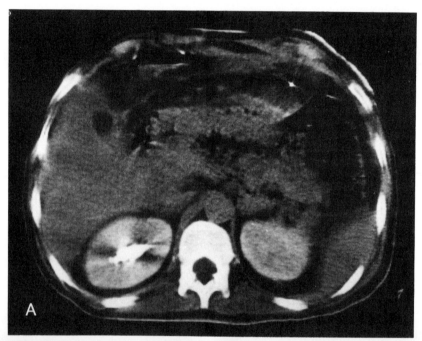

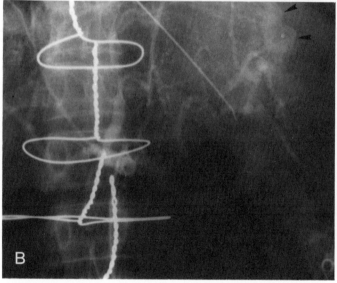

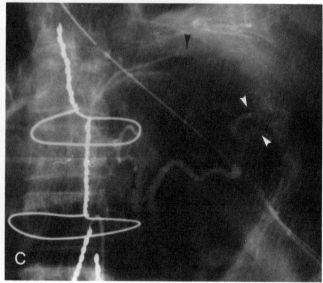

Figure 3.3.8. Phlegmon. **A.** CT scan; pancreas and peripancreatic tissues are not recognizable. **B.** Celiac angiogram demonstrates severe encasement of splenic and left gastric arteries and area of extravasation in left upper quadrant *(black arrowheads).* **C.** Hemostasis was established by limited embolization of the branches of the splenic and left gastric arteries *(white arrowheads).*

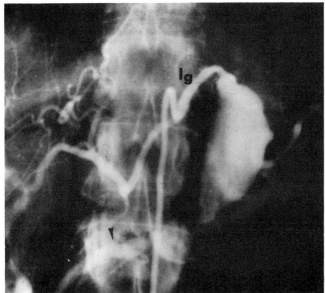

Figure 3.3.9. Left gastric angiogram after Billroth gastrectomy reveals extensive extravasation from the stump of the left gastric artery *(lg)* into a pancreatic pseudocyst and drainage via the pancreatic duct into the duodenum *(arrowhead)*.

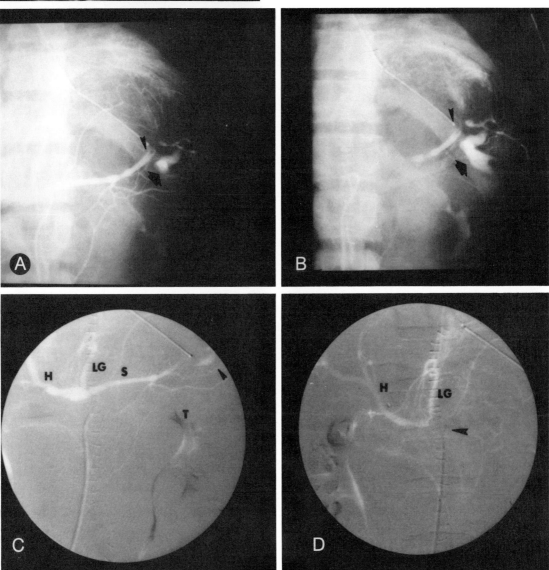

Figure 3.3.10. Trauma case. **A,B.** Injury to distal pancreas and distal portion of splenic artery *(small arrowhead)* with active extravasation in the same area *(large arrow)*. **C.** Digital subtraction angiography also demonstrates bleeding from the distal portion of the splenic artery *(arrowhead)*.

D. An occlusion balloon has been placed in the origin of the splenic artery for temporary control of bleeding, which was followed by definitive surgical procedure. *H* = hepatic artery; *LG* = left gastric artery; *S* = splenic artery; *T* = upper pole of left kidney.

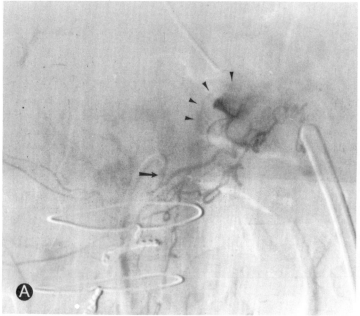

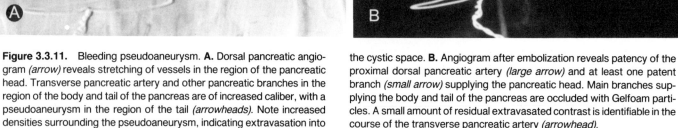

Figure 3.3.11. Bleeding pseudoaneurysm. **A.** Dorsal pancreatic angiogram *(arrow)* reveals stretching of vessels in the region of the pancreatic head. Transverse pancreatic artery and other pancreatic branches in the region of the body and tail of the pancreas are of increased caliber, with a pseudoaneurysm in the region of the tail *(arrowheads)*. Note increased densities surrounding the pseudoaneurysm, indicating extravasation into the cystic space. **B.** Angiogram after embolization reveals patency of the proximal dorsal pancreatic artery *(large arrow)* and at least one patent branch *(small arrow)* supplying the pancreatic head. Main branches supplying the body and tail of the pancreas are occluded with Gelfoam particles. A small amount of residual extravasated contrast is identifiable in the course of the transverse pancreatic artery *(arrowhead)*.

atic pseudocyst consist of rapid enlargement of a cystic mass and a sudden change in the echogenicity of the inner structures of the cystic space (Fig. 3.3.6).[27] Recent work suggests that an acute hemorrhagic pancreatic fluid collection presents as a well defined mass with homogeneous echogenicity. Remote hemorrhagic collections of more than several weeks' duration present as simple appearing cysts. Hemorrhagic collections studied one week after a bleeding episode appear as a cystic mass containing solid tissue or septa.[28] It should be remembered, however, that occasionally it is impossible to distinguish between pseudoaneurysms and pseudocysts.[29]

Computed tomography (CT) is an excellent way to demonstrate an acute hemorrhage in or around the pancreas. The finding of increased density numbers (>30 Hounsfield units) is diagnostic of acute bleeding (Fig. 3.3.7).[30] Occasionally, CT will identify the aneurysm within the pseudocyst.[31] In addition, CT is the appropriate modality for identification of abnormalities following pancreatic trauma.[32]

Angiography is the procedure of choice for identification of the site and source of bleeding. Its widespread and prompt use in the past decade has led to earlier and more accurate diagnosis, which resulted in more aggressive surgical treatment and a considerable decrease in the mortality rate.[7] Thus, the angiographic distinction of acute bleeding due to peptic ulcer disease, hemorrhagic gastritis, or the Mallory–Weiss syndrome from bleeding due to pancre-

atitis and its sequelae has had a tremendous impact on clinical management. Angiography is indispensable in the evaluation of the portal system, which should be part of a standard evaluation of bleeding patients with pancreatic disease. Identification of splenic vein thrombosis as the sole abnormality or confirmation of associated generalized portal hypertension due to liver disease is important, because the surgical treatment of these two entities is completely different.

The source and site of bleeding are usually diagnosed by identification of the erosive arterial changes or pseudoaneurysm formation. If the pseudoaneurysm is huge, angiography usually confirms its nature and distinguishes it from the pseudocyst. Occasionally, however, the angiogram identifies multiple small pseudoaneurysms that cannot be diagnosed by any other means.[33] These abnormalities are usually associated with encasement of the intrapancreatic arteries and, occasionally, with active bleeding (Fig. 3.3.8).[34] Rarely, frank extravasation of contrast medium from the pseudoaneurysm is seen. This occurs more frequently when the pseudoaneurysm ruptures into the abdominal cavity into or around the pancreatic bed. The next most common rupture is into the gastrointestinal tract, usually the duodenum.[11] Extravasation into the pseudocyst with drainage via the pancreatic ductal system is rare.[35] In a few cases, bleeding into the pancreatic duct has been demonstrated by angiography (Fig. 3.3.9).[36–38]

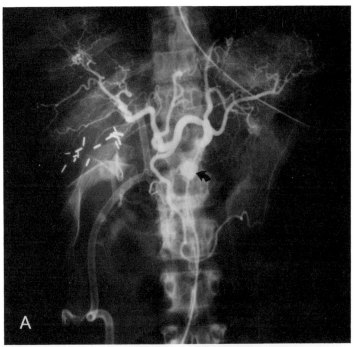

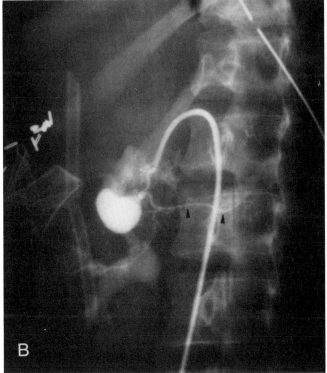

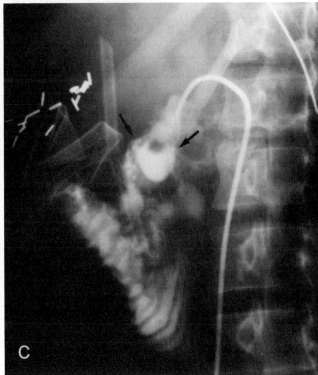

Figure 3.3.12. Patient with hemobilia. **A.** Celiac angiogram demonstrates a large pseudoaneurysm in the region of the pancreas *(arrow)*. **B.** Subselective angiogram demonstrates the dorsal pancreatic artery to be the feeding artery *(arrowheads)*. **C.** During embolization with Gelfoam particles the pseudoaneurysm ruptured, with extravasation of contrast medium *(arrows)* into the common bile duct and duodenum.

MANAGEMENT

As a rule, bleeding complications of pancreatic disease require prompt diagnosis and an aggressive surgical approach. Preoperative angiography is one of the most important steps in patient management.

Once the source of bleeding has been identified, surgical celiotomy is indicated. The operative technique remains somewhat controversial, although recent data suggest that arterial ligation or intracystic suture ligation in conjunction with drainage procedures, splenectomy, and gastrectomy, rather than partial or total pancreatectomy,

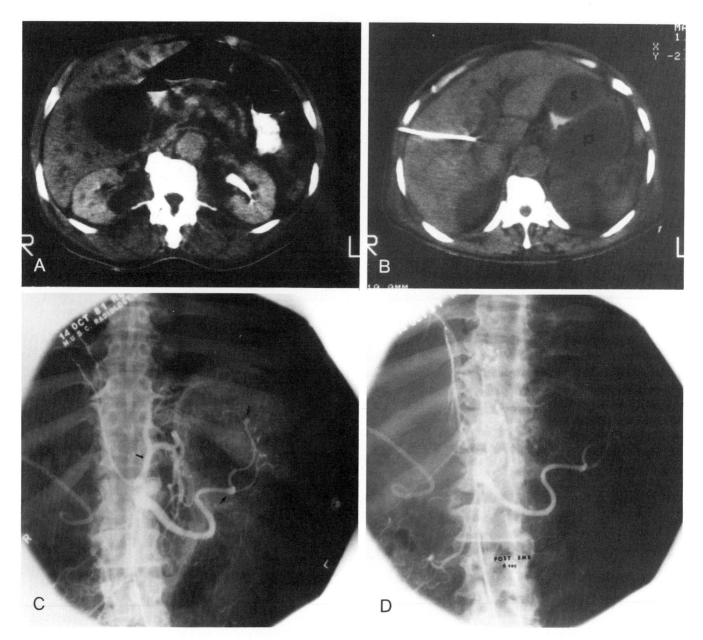

Figure 3.3.13. Appearance of bleeding during percutaneous drainage. **A.** CT scan demonstrates dilated biliary ducts, gallbladder, and main pancreatic duct. **B.** After successful percutaneous external drainage of the biliary tree, there was a drop in the hematocrit associated with the sudden appearance of a pancreatic pseudocyst in the retrogastric area. *s* = stomach; *p* = pancreatic pseudocyst. **C.** An angiogram done because of clin-ical evidence of continued bleeding demonstrates encasement of left gastric *(small arrow)* and splenic arteries with small pseudoaneurysms identified in the distribution of the splenic artery *(large black arrows)*. Note the common trunk of the left hepatic and left gastric arteries. **D.** After embolization with small particles of Gelfoam, smaller branches of splenic and left gastric arteries do not opacify.

is effective. In patients with ductal pancreatic bleeding or with bleeding as a result of pancreatitis triggered by a mass lesion in the head of the pancreas, partial or total pancre-atectomy is required for definitive control of bleeding.[7]

There are several situations, however, in which angio-graphic management of hemorrhage is appropriate. First, in unstable patients with a severely bleeding pseudoaneu-rysm, temporary hemostasis can be obtained by occlusion with mechanical devices (Fig. 3.3.10).[7,37] Occlusion balloon catheters, detachable balloons, and GWC coils are ideal for the occlusion of large arteries. However, because the

bleeding vessel may be supplied by collateral pathways, which form rapidly after embolotherapy, a definitive oper-ation should be done as soon as possible after angiographic occlusion and restoration of blood volume.

Second, if the patient bleeds from a small pseudoaneu-rysm involving the intrapancreatic branches, embolization with Gelfoam particles may control a bleeding episode and obviate operation (Fig. 3.3.11).[39–41] These small pseudo-aneurysms have extremely fragile walls that are prone to rupture during the delivery of particulate embolic mate-rial, so use of the minimal volume of carrier fluid and min-

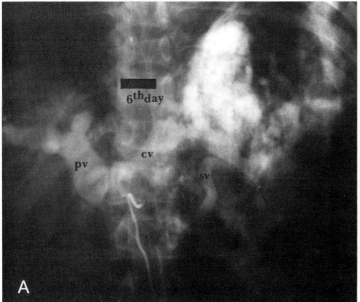 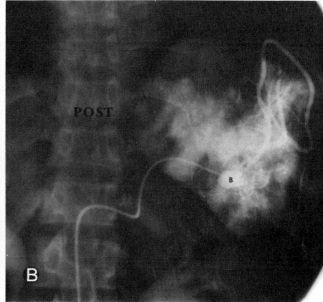

Figure 3.3.14. Left-sided portal hypertension after embolization of spleen with Gelfoam particles in the patient in Figure 3.3.4. **A.** Despite extensive embolization, flow to the spleen is preserved. Thrombosis of the splenic vein *(sv)* is demonstrated, with collateral circulation through gastric varices into the portal vein *(pv)* through the dilated coronary vein *(cv)*. **B.**

To decrease flow to the spleen and varices, a balloon catheter was placed in splenic hilum and inflated. The inflated balloon completely blocks circulation in the splenic bed. The patient was immediately sent to the operating room for surgical splenectomy.

imal injection pressure during delivery of the emboli is appropriate (Fig. 3.3.12).[39]

Third, angiographic management may be indicated in patients with obvious bleeding in or around the pancreas and convincing findings on ultrasound and CT examinations who have unimpressive findings on angiography. This happens mostly in cases of encasement of small arterial branches and pseudoaneurysms. Occasionally, bleeding is demonstrated, but its source is not identified. In such cases, limited embolization of branches of the splenic and left gastric arteries with Gelfoam particles immediately stops the bleeding (Fig. 3.3.13). A semipermanent resorbable material rather than a permanent material is recommended in these patients, because the resorbable material occludes the vessels over a crucial period of several weeks, allowing conservative treatment of the underlying disease, yet permits restoration of flow to the diseased region as the clinical condition improves.

Finally, the angiographer may assist the surgeon in the preoperative management of patients with left-sided portal hypertension due to splenic vein thrombosis. A simple splenectomy cures this condition, but the operation is not easy because considerable venous engorgement and inflammatory reaction due to pancreatitis extend the operating time, and the procedure is often complicated by extensive bleeding during dissection of the numerous adhesions. In such cases, the relatively easy placement of an occlusion balloon catheter in the splenic artery and its inflation during the crucial stage of the operative procedure reduce the need for blood transfusion (Fig. 3.3.14). In addition, the

catheter can be left in place with the balloon deflated for 24–48 hours postoperatively to permit control of bleeding by inflation of the balloon. Leaving the balloon catheter in place seems particularly justifiable in those patients in whom partial or total pancreatectomy or internal pseudocyst-drainage procedures are done in addition to splenectomy (I. Vujic, unpublished data). Published data suggest that the mortality rate from hemorrhage following surgical ligation of a bleeding vessel or pancreatic resection is almost twice that in patients with spontaneous hemorrhage due to pancreatic disease. Therefore, angiographic workup and management of postoperative bleeding in patients with pancreatic disease seems to be justified in every patient who is hemodynamically stable. Even in those patients who are hypotensive, a quick insertion of an occlusive balloon into the bleeding vessel may considerably reduce both morbidity and mortality.

References

1. Gadacz TR, Trunkey D, Kieffer RF Jr: Visceral vessel erosion associated with pancreatitis. *Arch Surg* 1978;113:1438
2. White AF, Baum S, Buranasiri S: Aneurysm secondary to pancreatitis. *AJR* 1976;127:393
3. Boisen E, Tylen U: Vascular changes in chronic pancreatitis. *Acta Radiol [Diagn]* 1972;12:35
4. Sindelar WF, Mason GR: Aortocystoduodenal fistula: rare complication of pancreatic pseudocyst. *Arch Surg* 1979;114:953
5. Zeller M, Hetz HH: Rupture of pancreatic pseudocyst into the portal vein. *JAMA* 1966;196:869
6. Takayama T, Kato K, Katada N, et al: Radiological demon-

stration of spontaneous rupture of a pancreatic pseudocyst into the portal system. *Am J Gastroenterol* 1982;76:55

7. Stabile BE, Wilson SE, Debas HT: Reduced mortality from bleeding pseudocysts and pseudoaneurysms caused by pancreatitis. *Arch Surg* 1983;118:45

8. Cogbill CL: Hemorrhage in pancreatic pseudocysts: review of literature and report of two cases. *Ann Surg* 1968;167:112

9. Stanley JC, Frey CF, Miller TA, et al: Major arterial hemorrhage: complication of pancreatic pseudocysts and chronic pancreatitis. *Arch Surg* 1976;111:435

10. Frey CF: Pancreatic pseudocyst: operative strategy. *Ann Surg* 1978;188:652

11. Sankaran S, Walt AJ: The natural and unnatural history of pancreatic pseudocysts. *Br J Surg* 1975;62:37

12. Nielsen OS: Bleeding after pancreatic cystogastrostomy. *Acta Chir Scand* 1979;145:247

13. Collins JJ, Peterson LY, Wilson RE: Small interstitial infarction as a complication of pancreatitis. *Ann Surg* 1968; 167:433

14. Hunt DR, Mildenhall P: Etiology of strictures of the colon associated with pancreatitis. *Am J Dig Dis* 1975;20:941

15. Leger L, Lenroit J, Lamaitre G: Hypertension portale segmentaire des pancreatities: aspects angiographiques. *J Chir (Paris)* 1968;95:599

16. Rignault D, Mine J, Moire D: Splenoportographic changes in chronic pancreatitis. *Surgery* 1968;63:571

17. LeMaitre G, L'Hermine C, Maillard JP, Toison FL: Hypertension portale segmentaire des pancreatities: aspects angiographiques. *Lille Med* 1971;16:928

18. Little AG, Moossa AR: Gastrointestinal hemorrhage from left sided portal hypertension. *Am J Surg* 1981;141:153

19. Moossa AR, Gadd MA: Isolated splenic vein thrombosis. *World J Surg* 1985;9:284

20. Zannini G, Musciariello S, Pagano G, et al: Prehepatic portal hypertension: experience with eighty-eight cases. *Int Surg* 1982;67:311

21. Nordlinger BM, Fulenwider JT, Millikan WJ, Warren WD: Splenic artery ligation in distal splenorenal shunt. *Am J Surg* 1978;136:561

22. Vos LJM, Potocky V, Broker FHL, et al: Splenic vein thrombosis with esophageal varices: a late complication of umbilical vein catheterization. *Ann Surg* 1974;180:52

23. Burbige EJ, Tarder G, Carson S, et al: Colonic varices: a complication of pancreatitis with splenic vein thrombosis. *Am J Dig Dis* 1978;23:752

24. Stone RT, Wilson SE, Passaro E Jr: Gastric portal hypertension. *Am J Surg* 1978;136:73

25. Case records of Massachusetts General Hospital. *N Engl J Med* 1945;233:443

26. Brintall BB, Laidlaw WW, Papp JP: Hemobilia: pancreatic pseudocyst hemorrhage demonstrated by endoscopy and arteriography. *Am J Dig Dis* 1974;19:186

27. Vujic I, Seymour EQ, Meredith HC: Vascular complications associated with sonographically demonstrated cystic epigastric lesions: an important indication for angiography. *Cardiovasc Intervent Radiol* 1980;3:75

28. Hashimoto BE, Laing FC, Jeffrey RB Jr, Federle MP: Hemorrhagic pancreatic fluid collections examined by ultrasound. *Radiology* 1984;150:803

29. Jhaveri HS, Gerlock AJ Jr, Smith CW, Goncharenko V: Value of arteriography in the evaluation of a sonolucent pancreatic mass. *Cardiovasc Intervent Radiol* 1979;2:55

30. Isikoff MB, Hill MC, Silverstein W, Barkin J: The clinical significance of acute pancreatic hemorrhage. *AJR* 1981; 136:679

31. Borlaza GS, Kuhns LR, Seigel R, Posderac R, Eckhauser F: Computed tomographic and angiographic demonstration of gastroduodenal artery pseudoaneurysm in a pancreatic pseudocyst. *J Comput Assist Tomogr* 1979;3:612

32. Jeffrey RB Jr, Federle MP, Crass RA: Computed tomography of pancreatic trauma. *Radiology* 1983;147:491

33. Harris RD, Anderson JE, Coel MN: Aneurysms of small pancreatic arteries: a cause of upper abdominal pain and intestinal bleeding. *Radiology* 1975;115:17

34. Vujic I, Anderson BL, Stanley JH, Gobien RP: Pancreatic and peripancreatic vessels: embolization for control of bleeding in pancreatitis. *Radiology* 1984;150:51

35. Bivins BA, Sachatello CR, Chuang VP, Brody P: Hemosuccus pancreaticus (hemiductal pancreatitis). *Arch Surg* 1978; 113:751

36. Koehler PR, Nelson JR, Berenson MM: Massive extra-enteric gastrointestinal bleeding: angiographic diagnosis. *Radiology* 1976;119:41

37. Walter YE, Chuang VP, Bookstein JJ, et al: Arteriography of massive hemorrhage secondary to pancreatic disease. *Radiology* 1977;124:337

38. Vujic I, Jones WN, Bradham GB, Meredith HC: Angiographic demonstration of gastrointestinal bleeding through the pancreatic duct. *Gastrointest Radiol* 1980;5:43

39. Lina JR, Jaques P, Mandell V: Aneurysm rupture secondary to transcatheter embolization. *AJR* 1979;132:553

40. Vujic I, Anderson MC, Meredith HC, Cullom JW: Successful embolization of dorsal pancreatic artery to control massive upper gastrointestinal bleeding. *Am Surg* 1980;46: 184

41. Knight RW, Kadir S, White RI Jr: Embolization of bleeding transverse pancreatic artery. *Cardiovasc Intervent Radiol* 1982;5:37

4

PERCUTANEOUS TRANSLUMINAL ANGIOPLASTY

Part 1. Pathology of Atherosclerotic Vascular Disease

—Danna E. Johnson, M.D.

INTRODUCTION

The vasculature serves a much more complex function than simple conduction of blood throughout the body. Vessels also regulate distribution of blood flow and selective exchange of molecules and cells between the blood and interstitial spaces and produce factors crucial for thrombosis and thrombolysis. Dynamic adaptation to stress and injury is characteristic of blood vessels, and plays a role in the pathogenesis of arteriosclerosis, stenosis of vein and synthetic grafts, and restenosis after therapeutic vascular interventions.

STRUCTURE AND FUNCTION OF NORMAL ARTERIES

All arteries, regardless of size, are composed of three concentric layers, or tunics: the tunica intima, tunica media, and tunica adventitia.[1] The innermost tunic is the intima, consisting of a monolayer of endothelial cells overlying a thin subendothelium and the internal elastic lamina. Endothelial cells are modified epithelial cells and have a multitude of functions. These include control of inter- and transcellular transport, procoagulant and anticoagulant activities, regulation of inflammatory and immune responses, synthesis of growth factors and connective tissue components, modulation of vascular tone, and formation of new vessels (angiogenesis).[2] The subendothelium consists only of collagen, ground substance, and a few myointimal cells which have some properties of smooth muscle cells. This layer can become greatly thickened in response to aging and injury and in atherosclerosis.[3-5]

Normally, the thickest layer, the tunica media, is particularly prominent in muscular medium-size and small arteries and in arterioles. Smooth muscle cells aligned in a heli-cal array form the bulk of the media of muscular arteries. Contraction and relaxation of these cells causes rapid changes in lumen size which regulate the distribution of blood flow by muscular arteries and vascular tone by arterioles. The larger elastic arteries, including the aorta, aortic arch branches, and common iliac arteries, have abundant elastic tissue in the media. Elastic fibers form parallel and interconnecting networks that assist in conversion of systolic pressure to arterial wall tension.[1] Dissipation of this wall tension during diastole helps maintain hydrostatic blood pressure.

The tunica adventitia is separated from the media by the external elastic lamina; veins and arterioles do not possess this outer elastica. The adventitia is composed of loose connective tissue, nerves, lymphatics, and small blood vessels. Some of these vessels, known as the vasa vasorum, penetrate and provide circulation to the outer media of larger arteries.

PATHOLOGY OF ATHEROSCLEROSIS

Atherosclerosis and its complications have long been recognized as major causes of morbidity and mortality. The pathology of atherosclerotic lesions is variable, and probably plays a major role in determining the success or failure of therapeutic vascular interventions.

Fatty Streaks and Intimal Thickenings

Fatty streaks are small, slightly raised, yellow intimal lesions initially seen during the first decade of life with a peak prevalence during the third decade.[6,7] They consist of intimal aggregates of lipid-rich cells known as "foam cells," most of which are macrophages.[8] The relationship between fatty streaks and atherosclerotic plaques is controversial.[9]

On the one hand, coronary artery fatty streaks may occur in the same proximal regions favored by atherosclerotic plaques.[6] Yet, aortic fatty streaks are most heavily concentrated in the proximal aorta, whereas atherosclerosis preferentially involves the distal abdominal aorta.[10] Also, the prevalence of fatty streaks during childhood is the same for human populations at low and high risk for atherosclerosis during adulthood.[11] Most likely some fatty streaks do evolve to plaques whereas others regress or persist unchanged.

"Branch pads" and "cushions" are areas of slight fibrous intimal thickening located at ostia of arterial branches which are evident in early childhood.[7] So-called "intimal thickenings" are histologically similar to branch pads, but they occur in proximal to middle segments of medium-sized muscular arteries. In a detailed autopsy study, Velican and Velican were able to document histologic evidence for progression of coronary branch pads and intimal thickenings to atherosclerotic plaques.[7]

Distribution of Atherosclerotic Plaques

Atherosclerotic plaques are localized or diffuse intimal growths which may impede or block blood flow to organs and tissues. Plaques develop mainly at sites of altered shear stress and flow velocity, including bifurcations, curves, and branch points.[12] In decreasing order of frequency, plaques involve the abdominal aorta below the renal arteries, proximal coronary arteries, popliteal arteries, descending thoracic aorta, internal carotid arteries, and arteries of the circle of Willis.[10] The pulmonary, upper extremity, mesenteric, and renal arteries are generally relatively free of disease, except at their ostia.

Uncomplicated Atherosclerotic Plaques

The primary pathologic manifestation of atherosclerosis is the "atherosclerotic plaque." Atherosclerotic plaques consist of variable quantities of 1) mesenchymal cells, 2) collagen and other connective tissue elements, 3) lipids, and 4) calcium salts.[10]

The simplest lesion is the "fibrous plaque" which has a matrix of predominantly Types I and III collagen,[13] basement membrane material,[13] elastin, and proteoglycans[14] (Fig. 4.1.1). Also present are smooth muscle cells that contain numerous synthetic organelles including rough endoplasmic reticulum, mitochondria and Golgi apparatus.[15] These smooth muscle cells are known as "synthetic" type cells and they synthesize and release the connective tissue components that make up the bulk of atherosclerotic plaques.[15]

"Atheromatous plaques," named after the Greek word "atheroma" for gruel, contain a large central pool of lipids and cellular debris. Grossly, this lipid core is soft and yellow and exudes from the cut surface of an artery with slight pressure (Fig. 4.1.2). The lipid-rich zone appears microscopically as amorphous material or as crystalline structures known as "cholesterol clefts" (Fig. 4.1.3). The lipid core has a complex composition of free cholesterol, cholesterol esters,[16] apolipoproteins,[17,18] and foam cells. It develops through progressive binding of plasma-derived lipids and apolipoproteins to the collagen and elastic fibers in the plaque and rupture of foam cells. The "fibrous cap" overlying the lipid core may be quite thin and is susceptible to fissuring and ulceration. Finally, the basal regions of plaques are often neovascularized by ingrowth of proliferated capillary buds from the vasa vasorum.[19]

Figure 4.1.1. A concentric fibrous atherosclerotic plaque composed of dense collagen and virtually no lipid. (H & E, original magnification × 50).

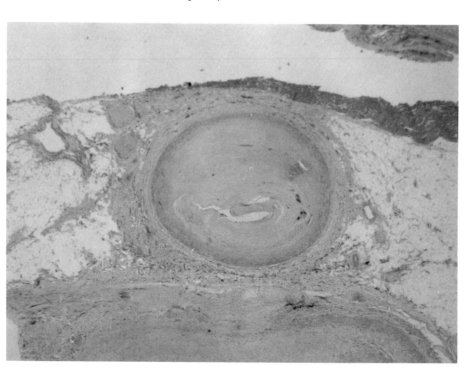

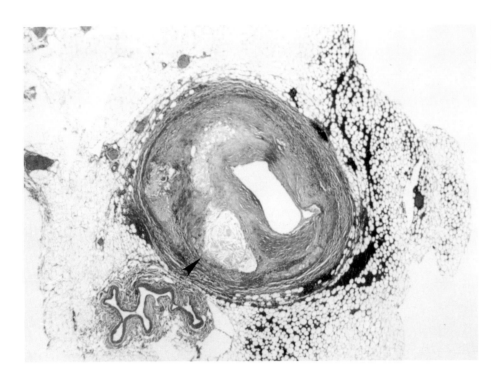

Figure 4.1.2. Atheromatous coronary artery plaque with fibrous tissue overlying a core rich in lipids *(arrowhead)*. (H & E, original magnification × 50).

Complicated Atherosclerotic Plaques

Most advanced, high-grade, and clinically significant atherosclerotic stenoses have undergone one or more "complications." These complications include: 1) calcification, 2) plaque surface ulceration, 3) thrombosis, 4) intraplaque hemorrhage, and 5) aneurysmal dilatation.[10]

CALCIFICATION

Dystrophic calcification of atherosclerotic plaques is common and, when severe, produces rigid, noncompliant vessels. Calcification of the lipid core, surrounding fibrous tissues and occasionally overlying surface thrombus may be seen to varying degrees (Fig. 4.1.4). Plaque mineralization occurs through a vesicle matrix mechanism and involves

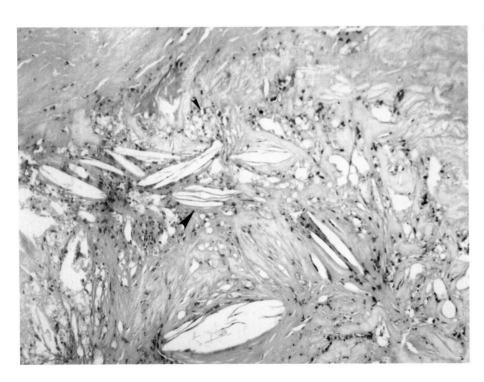

Figure 4.1.3. Numerous cholesterol clefts *(large arrowhead)* and clusters of foam cells *(small arrowhead)* comprise the lipid core of this plaque. (H & E, original magnification × 300).

Fig. 4.1.4. Dark, irregular calcium deposits *(arrowhead)* are evident in and surrounding the atheromatous core. (H & E, original magnification × 230).

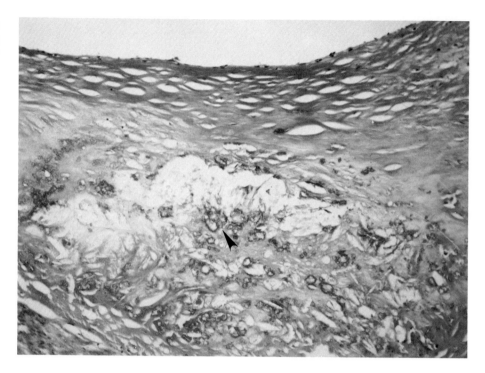

progressive deposition of calcium carbonate apatites with significant amounts of sodium and magnesium.[20]

Plaque Surface Ulceration

The fibrous cap overlying atheromatous lesions may undergo fissuring, erosion, or frank ulceration probably precipitated by hemodynamic stresses or arterial spasm.[21-23] Ulceration may, in turn, lead to serious consequences such as thrombosis, hemorrhage into a plaque, or peripheral embolization of fatty debris (cholesterol emboli).[21]

Thrombosis

Acute arterial thrombosis is the most significant plaque complication. Up to 90% of patients who die of acute transmural myocardial infarcts are found at autopsy to have recent thrombotic occlusions of one or more coronary arteries.[22,24] Recent reviews have emphasized that plaque fissuring or ulceration is the precipitating cause of most thrombotic occlusions.[25,26] Plaque surface ulceration presumably exposes thrombogenic substances such as collagens and lipids to the flowing blood, with resultant platelet adhesion, aggregation, release reaction and activation of the clotting cascade. The head of a thrombus, which overlies the ulcerated plaque, consists largely of platelets whereas the propagating distal tail is composed of enmeshed fibrin and erythrocytes with few platelets. In addition to blocking perfusion through an artery, the distal thrombus tail may fragment to form thromboemboli.

Arterial thrombosis is a dynamic process. As soon as thrombus formation is initiated, thrombolytic processes are also activated. Indeed, most small thrombi are probably completely and spontaneously lysed with few or no clin-

ical consequences. Larger, occlusive thrombi may not be entirely lysed. Over several weeks to months, these thrombi undergo a process known as "organization." Organization of thrombi occurs through infiltration by inflammatory cells, enzymatic degradation of blood products within the thrombus, thrombus replacement by collagen synthesized by infiltrating fibroblasts, and ingrowth of capillary buds (neovascularization)[10] (Fig. 4.1.5). Sometimes these vascular channels completely traverse an occlusive, organized thrombus (recanalization). However, the size of these recanalizing vessels is usually inadequate to restore sufficient blood flow. Most chronic, total occlusions of arteries represent thrombi in various stages of organization.

Intraplaque Hemorrhage

Hemorrhage into plaques usually occurs through erosion of the plaque fibrous cap with entry of plasma and blood cells. This may cause increased intraplaque pressure followed by plaque rupture and thrombosis.[26] A second potential source of bleeding is the small capillary branches of the vasa vasorum which penetrate the basal regions of plaques.[19] Leakage from these capillaries is less significant than hemorrhage from the arterial lumen.

Aneurysmal Dilatation

Aneurysms are localized dilatations of vessels, the most common cause of which is atherosclerosis.[10] In decreasing order of frequency, atherosclerotic aneurysms involve the lower abdominal aorta, iliac arteries, ascending aorta and descending thoracic aorta. However, any atherosclerotic artery may be affected.

Aneurysms occur because the tunica media underlying plaques becomes progressively thinned and atrophic and

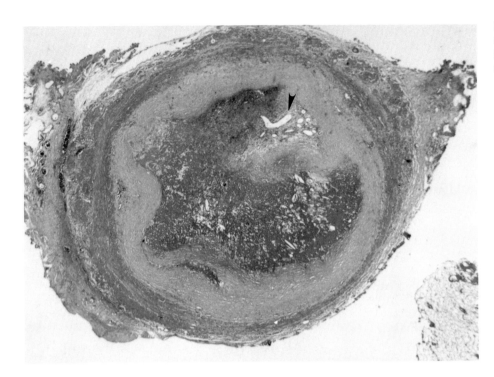

Figure 4.1.5. An organizing thrombus with early recanalization (*arrowhead*) occludes this coronary artery. (H & E, original magnification × 60).

may even be replaced by fibrous tissue.[27] This weakens the arterial wall which may, particularly in the setting of hypertension, become stretched to form a saccular or fusiform aneurysm. Aneurysm sacs almost always contain laminated thrombus. Surface thrombus may be fresh and friable and is prone to embolization. Other complications of atherosclerotic aneurysms include rupture, compression of adjacent structures such as vertebral bodies and branch arteries, and secondary infection by blood-borne organisms.[10]

PATHOGENESIS OF ATHEROSCLEROSIS

Numerous hypotheses to explain the pathogenesis of atherosclerosis have been put forth. The "lipid insudation" theory, which proposed increased seepage of plasma lipids into the intima, and the "thrombogenic" theory, which suggested that plaques develop through fibrous organization of thrombi, have been popular. These hypotheses are incomplete, however, in that they can only account for relatively late phenomena in the evolution of atherosclerotic plaques. They do not adequately explain the initiation of early lesions.

A third proposal, the "response to injury" theory, has attracted renewed attention in recent years. This hypothesis maintains that atherosclerotic lesions represent a reparative reaction to some form of vascular insult.[4,5,28] In 1976, Ross and Glomset suggested that the inciting injury may be endothelial cell denudation,[4] based upon observations from experimental balloon catheter injury.[29] Loss of the endothelium would promote: 1) adherence of platelets to denuded sites, 2) monocyte attachment to exposed areas and migration into the subendothelium to become macrophages, 3) local release of potent mitogens such as plate-let-derived growth factor (PDGF) from degranulated platelets, 4) mitogen stimulation of media smooth muscle cells, causing them to undergo ultrastructural changes, proliferation and migration into the intima, 5) synthesis and release of collagen and other connective tissue elements by these modified smooth muscle cells, and 6) accumulation of lipids and lipoproteins from the plasma within intimal macrophages and smooth muscle cells.

One problem with this theory is that frank endothelial denudation is observed only rarely, even overlying atherosclerotic plaques.[30] Subsequently, it has been suggested that nondenuding endothelial injuries such as those caused by hypercholesterolemia,[30-32] endotoxin,[33] hemodynamic stresses,[34] components of cigarette smoke,[35] and viruses[36] may alter the vessel wall in such a way as to induce early plaque formation. These insults may alter endothelial cell structure, metabolism, permeability, and turnover rates and thereby affect normal vessel wall homeostasis.

It is also now clear that inflammatory cells, mainly monocytes/macrophages and lymphocytes, play an important role in atherogenesis. Blood monocytes adherent to endothelium may pass into the subendothelium through spaces between endothelial cells; hypercholesterolemia enhances monocyte adherence.[30,31] Once within the intima, these cells can take up oxidized low density lipoproteins to become foam cells,[37] release chemoattractant substances such as interleukin-1 (IL-1),[38] and secrete growth factors with mitogenic properties. The growth factors released by macrophages which may have relevance in atherosclerosis include PDGF-like substances, fibroblast growth factor (FGF), transforming growth factor-α (TGF-α) and transforming growth factor-β (TGF-β).[28] T-lymphocytes are also found in atherosclerotic plaques[39] perhaps having been recruited by IL-1 released from macrophages or through as yet unknown cell-mediated immune reactions. The significance of these cells is likewise unclear, but they might represent a delayed type hypersensitivity immune response.

Finally, in addition to platelets and macrophages, smooth muscle cells themselves have been found to release a variety of growth factors, including PDGF[40] and FGF,[41] raising the possibility that autocrine, or self-stimulatory, effects may promote and maintain smooth muscle cell proliferation in plaques. Autonomous growth may partially explain the observation of clonal proliferations of smooth muscle cells in plaques by Benditt.[42]

CONCLUSION

As can be seen from this brief review, the pathology of atherosclerosis is complicated and variable. The composition of atherosclerotic plaques no doubt impacts upon the success or failure of vascular interventions. With so many new interventional techniques becoming available, it will be possible to select therapy on the basis of plaque morphology and configuration. Also, the pathogenetic mechanisms of atherosclerosis are extremely complex and encompass a number of forms of vascular injury and response to injury.

References

1. Simionescu N, Simionescu M: The cardiovascular system, in Weiss L (ed): *Histology. Cell and Tissue Biology.* New York, Elsevier Biomedical, 1983, pp 372–423
2. Fajardo LF: The complexity of endothelial cells: a review. *Am J Clin Pathol* 1989; 92:241–250
3. Velican C, Velican D: Study of coronary intimal thickening. *Atherosclerosis* 1985;56:331–344
4. Ross R, Glomset JA: The pathogenesis of atherosclerosis. *N Engl J Med* 1976;295:369–377, 420–425
5. Ross R: The pathogenesis of atherosclerosis—An update. *N Engl J Med* 1986;314:488–500
6. McGill HC Jr: Fatty streaks in the coronary arteries and aorta. *Lab Invest* 1968;18:560–564
7. Velican C, Velican D: The precursors of coronary atherosclerotic plaques in subjects up to 40 years old. *Atherosclerosis* 1980;37:33–46
8. Munro JM, Van Der Walt JD, Munro CS, Chalmers JAC, Cox EL: An immunohistochemical analysis of human aortic fatty streaks. *Hum Pathol* 1987;18:375–380
9. McGill HC Jr: Persistent problems in the pathogenesis of atherosclerosis. *Arteriosclerosis* 1984;4:443–451
10. Cotran RS: Blood vessels, in Cotran RS, Kumar V, Robbins SL (eds): *Robbins Pathologic Basis of Disease.* 4th Ed. Philadelphia, WB Saunders, 1989, pp 553–595
11. McGill HC Jr, Arias–Stella J, Carbonell LM, Correa P, de Veyra EA Jr, Donoso S, Eggen DA, Galindo L, Guzman MA, Lichtenberger E, Loken AC, McGarry PA, McMahaon CA, Montenegro MR, Mossy J, Perez–Tamayo R, Restrepo C, Robertson WB, Salas J, Solberg LA, Strong JP, Tejada C, Wainwright J: General findings of the International Atherosclerosis Project. *Lab Invest* 1968;18:498–502

12. Glagov S, Zarins C, Giddens DP, Ku DN: Hemodynamics and atherosclerosis. *Arch Pathol Lab Med* 1988;112:1018–1031
13. Barnes MJ: Collagens in atherosclerosis. *Collagen Relat Res* 1985;5:65–97
14. Berenson GS, Radhakrishnamurthy B, Srinivasan SR, Vijayagopol P, Dalferes ER: Arterial wall injury and proteoglycan changes in atherosclerosis. *Arch Pathol Lab Med* 1988; 112:1002–1010
15. Mosse PRL, Campbell GR, Wang ZL, Campbell JH: Smooth muscle phenotypic expression in human carotid arteries: I. Comparison of cells from diffuse intimal thickenings adjacent to atheromatous plaques with those of the media. *Lab Invest* 1985;53:556–562
16. Smith EB, Slater RS: The microdissection of large atherosclerotic plaques to give morphologically and topographically defined fractions for analysis: The lipids in isolated fractions of plaques. *Atherosclerosis* 1972;15:37–56
17. Yomantas S, Elner VM, Schaffner T, Wissler RW: Immunohistochemical localization of apolipoprotein B in human atherosclerotic lesions. *Arch Pathol Lab Med* 1984;108:374–378
18. Bedossa P, Poynard T, Abella A, Paraf F, Lemaigre G, Martin E: Localization of apolipoprotein A-I and apolipoprotein A-II in human atherosclerotic arteries. *Arch Pathol Lab Med* 1989;113:777–780
19. Zamir M, Silver MD: Vasculature in the walls of human coronary arteries. *Arch Pathol Lab Med* 1985;109:659–662
20. Tomazic BB, Brown WE, Queral LA, Sadovnik M: Physiochemical characterization of cardiovascular calcified deposits. I. Isolation, purification, and instrumental analysis. *Atherosclerosis* 1988;69:5–19
21. Falk E: Plaque rupture with severe pre-existing stenosis and precipitating coronary thrombosis. Characteristics of coronary atherosclerotic plaques underlying fatal occlusive thrombi. *Br Heart J* 1983;50:127–134
22. Ridolfi R, Hutchins GM: The relationship between coronary artery lesions and myocardial infarcts: ulcerations of atherosclerotic plaques precipitating coronary thrombosis. *Am Heart J* 1977;93:468–486
23. Hellstrom HR: Evidence in favor of the vasospastic cause of coronary artery thrombosis. *Am Heart J* 1979;97:449–452
24. Davies MJ, Woolf N, Robertson WB: Pathology of acute myocardial infarction with particular reference to occlusive coronary thrombi. *Br Heart J* 1976;38:659–669
25. Davies MJ, Thomas AC: Plaque fissuring—the cause of acute myocardial infarction, sudden ischemic death, and crescendo angina. *Br Heart J* 1985;53:363–373
26. Buja LM, Willerson JT: The role of coronary artery lesions in ischemic heart disease: insights from recent clinicopathologic, coronary arteriographic, and experimental studies. *Hum Pathol* 1987;18:451–460
27. Isner JM, Donaldson RF, Fortin AH, Tischler A, Clarke RH: Attenuation of the media of coronary arteries in advanced atherosclerosis. *Am J Cardiol* 1986;58:937–939
28. Munro JM, Cotran RS: Pathogenesis of atherosclerosis: atherogenesis and inflammation. *Lab Invest* 1988;58:249–261
29. Stemerman MB, Ross R: Experimental arteriosclerosis. I. Fibrous plaque formation in primates, an electron microscope study. *J Exp Med* 1972;136:769–789
30. Hansson GK, Bondjers G: Endothelial proliferation and atherogenesis in rabbits with moderate hypercholesterolemia. *Artery* 1980;7:316–329
31. Faggiotto A, Ross R, Harker L: Studies of hypercholesterolemia in the nonhuman primate. I. Changes that lead to fatty streak formation. *Arteriosclerosis* 1984;4:323–340
32. Faggiotto A, Ross R: Studies of hypercholesterolemia in the nonhuman primate. II. Fatty streak conversion to fibrous plaque. *Arteriosclerosis* 1984;4:341–356

33. Hansson GK, Chao S, Schwartz SM, Reidy MA: Aortic endothelial cell death and replication in normal and lipopolysaccharide-treated rats. *Am J Pathol* 1985;121:123–127

34. Davies PF, Remuzzi A, Gordon EJ, Dewey CF Jr, Gimbrone MA Jr: Turbulent shear stress induces vascular endothelial cell turnover in vitro. *Proc Natl Acad Sci USA* 1986;83:2114–2117

35. Sieffert GF, Keown K, Moore SW: Pathologic effect of tobacco smoke inhalation on arterial intima. *Surg Forum* 1981;32:333–335

36. Petrie BL, Adam E, Melnick JL: Association of herpesvirus/cytomegalovirus infections with human atherosclerosis. *Prog Med Virol* 1988;35:21–42

37. Quinn MT, Parthasarathy S, Fong LG, Steinberg D: Oxidatively modified low density lipoproteins: A potential role in recruitment and retention of monocyte/macrophages during atherogenesis. *Proc Natl Acad Sci USA* 1987;84:2995–2998

38. Luger TA, Charon JA, Colot M, Micksche M, Oppenheim JJ: Chemotactic properties of partially purified human epidermal cell-derived thymocyte-activating factor for polymorphonuclear and mononuclear cells. *J Immunol* 1983;131:816–820

39. Jonasson L, Holm J, Skalli O, Bondjers G, Hansson GK: Regional accumulation of T cells, macrophages and smooth muscle cells in the human atherosclerotic plaque. *Arteriosclerosis* 1986;6:131–138

40. Walker LN, Bowen-Pope DF, Ross R, Reidy MA: Production of PDGF-like molecules by cultured arterial smooth muscle cells accompanies proliferation after arterial injury. *Proc Natl Acad Sci USA* 1988;85:2810–2814

41. Winkles JA, Friesel R, Burgess WH, et al: Human vascular smooth muscle cells both express and respond to heparin-binding growth factor 1 (endothelial cell growth factor). *Proc Natl Acad Sci USA* 1987;84:7124–7128

42. Benditt EP, Benditt JM: Evidence for a monoclonal origin of human atherosclerotic plaques. *Proc Natl Acad Sci USA* 1973;70:1753–1756.

Part 2. Mechanism of Transluminal Angioplasty

—Christoph L. Zollikofer, M.D., Andrew H. Cragg, M.D., David W. Hunter, M.D., Joseph W. Yedlicka, Jr., M.D., Wilfrido R. Castañeda–Zúñiga, M.D., M.Sc., and Kurt Amplatz, M.D.

Percutaneous transluminal angioplasty (PTA) was introduced by Dotter and Judkins in 1964.[1,2] After a rather slow start, it has gained wide acceptance during the past 10 years for the treatment of both atherosclerotic and nonatherosclerotic vascular disease, even though its mechanism has not been well understood until recently. This review presents the authors' experimental work on human cadavers and living animals to explain the morphologic changes seen after angioplasty. The changes in arachidonic acid metabolism induced by the dilation of arterial segments are also described. A special section deals with the theoretical consequences of drug administration for the prevention of stenosis recurrence and of thrombosis. Finally, the effects of compliance and bursting characteristics of the various balloon materials on the results of angioplasty are stressed.

HISTORICAL DEVELOPMENT OF TRANSLUMINAL ANGIOPLASTY

Early Equipment

On January 16, 1964, the first PTA, of a popliteal artery, was performed in an elderly woman with gangrene, and by November of that year Dotter and Judkins could describe their experience with the new technique in 11 patients.[2] Over the next few years, Dotter and Judkins further documented the value of their nonsurgical technique.[3-6] The dilation system they used consisted of coaxial Teflon dilators, which were introduced over a guidewire after antegrade puncture of the femoral artery (Fig. 4.2.1). The technique was subsequently modified by Staple and Van Andel.[7,8] The latter investigator designed a series of tapered catheters of increasing size that are introduced one after another, a system with the theoretical advantage of avoiding the "snowplow effect" of the relatively blunt Dotter system. With the gradually tapered dilators, more radial than axial or longitudinal force was applied to the atheromatous vessel wall (Fig. 4.2.2).

In spite of the reported success in Europe,[9-15] particularly from the groups headed by Andreas Grüntzig[12] and Eberhart Zeitler,[13] minimal acceptance was given the new method in the United States. Furthermore, the Dotter procedure was limited to the femoral and popliteal arteries because larger diameter dilators were needed for the iliac arteries.[16-19] Latex balloons proved unsatisfactory because of the large compliance and stretching deformity of the latex.[20,21] Then, in 1973, Porstmann described a "caged" or "corset" balloon catheter (Fig. 4.2.3), further modified by Dotter et al., which could be used in iliac arteries.[22] The corset or cage formed by the struts of Teflon prevented undesirable deformation of the latex balloon. However, because of fear of excessive damage to the vessel wall and because of its higher thrombogenicity, the caged balloon catheter was never widely accepted. It was not until Andreas Grüntzig reported successful transluminal angioplasty in peripheral as well as renal and coronary arteries using a new double-lumen polyvinyl chloride (PVC) balloon catheter that transluminal angioplasty finally became popular in the United States.[23-25]

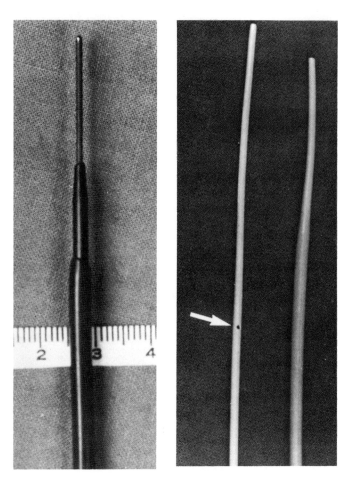

Figure 4.2.1. *(left)* Dotter coaxial Teflon catheter system with 1.12mm guidewire and 8Fr inner and 12Fr outer catheter.

Figure 4.2.2. *(right)* Van Andel catheters with long tapered tips. Proximal sidehole *(arrow)* was added later by E. Zeitler for injection of contrast medium.

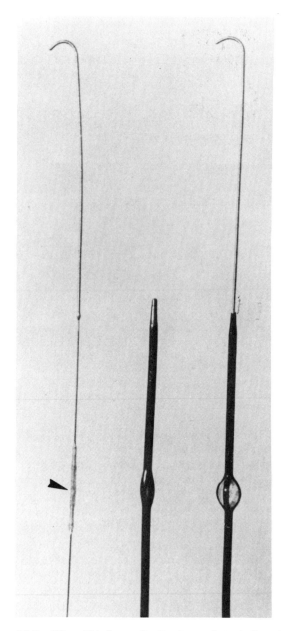

Figure 4.2.3. ''Corset'' balloon, after Portsmann. Latex balloon *(arrowhead)* mounted on guidewire is inflated within Teflon catheter with three longitudinal struts. The Teflon catheter prevents overstretching of the balloon.

Grüntzig Balloon Catheter

After his original report of a single-lumen balloon catheter,[21] Grüntzig introduced a double-lumen, single end hole balloon catheter in 1976.[23] Over an inner catheter, a PVC coaxial catheter was mounted that had an inflatable distal balloon (Fig. 4.2.4). This balloon could be filled via a side channel at the proximal end of the catheter, which connected to a longitudinal groove cut along the outer surface of the inner catheter. With this new design, pressures of 3–5 atm could be applied to the stenosis with balloons as large as 10mm in diameter. This permitted dilation of iliac artery stenoses using a catheter with a maximum outer diameter of 3.0mm. Also, with a balloon, radial rather than axial forces were applied to the atherosclerotic lesions, thereby minimizing the risk of embolization.[21]

Thanks to the ingenious Grüntzig balloon catheter, angioplasty, or the Dotter procedure, was rediscovered in the United States and spread rapidly. Continued modifications and improvements, especially in the compliance of

the balloons, made it possible to treat increasingly difficult cases. Also, strictures and stenoses outside the vascular system, such as those in the gastrointestinal and genitourinary tracts, could be treated successfully.

By 1981, about 100,000 Grüntzig balloon catheters were being sold yearly in the United States.[26] A study by Doubilet and Abrams pointed out that, as a consequence of the use of PTA in the treatment of iliac and femoral lesions, more than 300 patients' lives and $100,000,000 in health expenses could be saved annually in the United States.[27] The numbers for coronary artery disease are even more impressive: according to Hall and Grüntzig, 15–20%

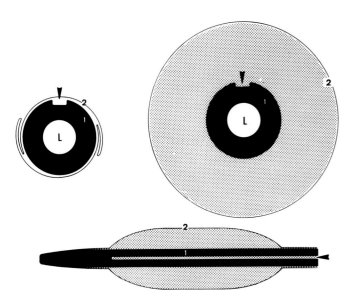

Figure 4.2.4. Diagram of the Grüntzig balloon dilatation catheter in cross- and longitudinal sections. *1* = inner catheter with side channel *(arrowhead); L* = lumen of the inner catheter; *2* = balloon and coaxial outer catheter made of PVC. In the deflated state, the balloon folds around the inner catheter in an umbrella-like fashion *(top left). Top right and bottom,* balloon inflated. (After A. Grüntzig, 1977.)

of patients requiring coronary bypass surgery are candidates for PTA,[28] with annual savings in health expenses of $170,000,000.[29] The percentage of patients with coronary artery disease who are candidates for PTA has climbed in an accelerated fashion over the last few years.

THEORIES OF THE MECHANISM OF TRANSLUMINAL ANGIOPLASTY

Original Theories Offered by Dotter and Other Pioneers of Transluminal Angioplasty

According to Dotter,[5,6,20,30,31] the principal mechanism of angioplasty is compression and remodeling of the atheromatous plaque. In other words, it was believed that the dilating catheter or balloon causes a cold flow that remodels the atheromatous material, much as if a balloon were being inflated in soft cheese. By this inelastic compression-remodeling of the atheromatous core—possibly with release of fluid contents—a stable autogenous tube would be formed, with maximum preservation of the existing vessel lining (Fig. 4.2.5).[20,30,31] This theory was largely accepted by the two other pioneers of transluminal angioplasty, Grüntzig[12,21] and Zeitler.[13] Grüntzig also mentioned a role for stretching of the media, with an increase in the outer

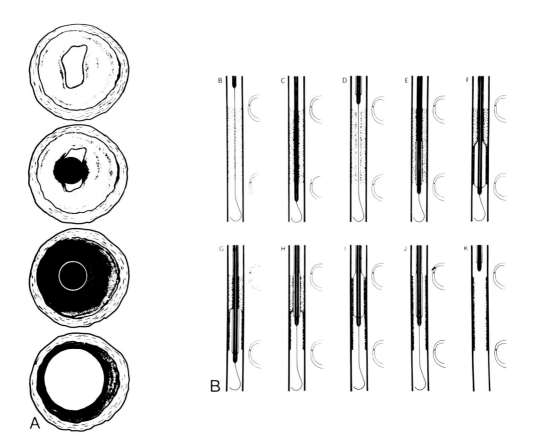

Figure 4.2.5. Original theory of the mechanism of angioplasty as described by Dotter (**A**) and Grüntzig (**B**). Widening of lumen (**A**) or recanalization of atherosclerotic obstruction (**B**) occurs with no evidence of increase in the caliber of the artery or change in the length of the lesion.

arterial diameter, which was suggested by the work of Jester et al.[32]

Challenging the Old Theory

With the more frequent use of PTA, it became clear that the original theory was not tenable. Atheromatous plaques, being semiliquid or solid without true empty spaces, are virtually incompressible unless liquid is extruded. Therefore, if the balloon causes cold flow inside a relatively rigid tube, the plaque, like soft cheese, should spread, i.e., the stenosis should elongate (Fig. 4.2.6). However, this effect has almost never been seen during balloon dilatation, although with Dotter's original coaxial dilator system some pushing of lesion material (snowplow effect) can occur.[8,13] Furthermore, fibrotic or calcified lesions also can be dilated by balloon angioplasty, yet, in these lesions, remodeling by cold flow can be excluded. Significant extrusion of liquid is highly unlikely in such cases, which eliminates significant compression of the plaque as a mechanism. In addition, the radiolucent lines so frequently seen in arteriograms after successful angioplasty could not be explained on the basis of the original theory. There was a clear need for experimental data on which to base a better theory, but before 1979 there were few experimental data on the mechanism of angioplasty,[24,32-36] and all of these papers, with the exception of that by Leu and Grüntzig,[36] described experiments with coaxial dilators.

Four papers presented at the American Heart Association's 1978 annual meeting dealt with histologic changes after balloon angioplasty of coronary arteries.[37-40] How-

ever, the results were contradictory. Whereas Jester et al. described extensive dissections and tears in the intima with stretching of the media during successful angioplasty,[32] Baughman et al.[37] and Freudenberg et al.[38] called dissection and rupture of the intima a complication. In other words, successful dilatation of an atherosclerotic stenosis was thought to be possible while leaving the intima intact and without stretching of the media and adventitia.

These contradictory findings and conclusions, together with the physical fact that solid or semisolid substances are noncompressible in the absence of extrusion of liquids, prompted the present authors to begin an extensive experimental study of the mechanism of angioplasty in 1978. Their research was conducted in three principal directions: the morphologic changes that follow PTA, the changes in vessel wall metabolism after PTA, and the physical properties of the balloon catheters and their influence on PTA results.

Experimental Data

INTRODUCTORY REMARKS ON BLOOD VESSEL ANATOMY AND PHYSIOLOGY

Anatomy of the Arterial Wall

The arterial wall consists of three layers, the tunica intima, the tunica media, and the tunica adventitia. This three-layer design is found in all mammalian arteries (Fig. 4.2.7), although the individual components differ with the function and size of the vessel. Accordingly, the authors distinguish between the large central or elastic arteries, the distributing or muscular arteries, and the arterioles.

Tunica Intima

The inner surface of the artery, toward the blood stream, is sealed by a flat endothelium that covers a layer of amorphous ground substance and longitudinal elastic fibers (Fig. 4.2.8). Occasionally, smooth muscle cells are present. The intima is separated from the media by a strong, fenestrated tube of elastic fibers, the internal elastic lamina (IEL), which limits the compliance of arteries and helps to reconstitute the original lumen after limited stretching of the wall.

Tunica Media

The media is the thickest of the three layers of the arterial wall. It consists of principally concentric, fenestrated elastic laminae and circumferentially oriented smooth muscle fibers (Fig. 4.2.8). Between layers of elastic and muscle fibers, collagen fibers and an amorphous intercellular substance are found. According to the numbers of smooth muscle cells and elastic fibers, arteries of the elastic or muscular type are distinguished. Smooth muscle cells are pluripotent and probably produce not only elastin and collagen but also the intercellular substance. The outer border of the media is formed by the external elastic lam-

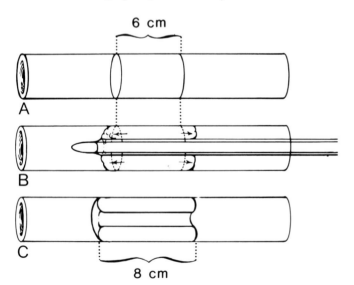

Figure 4.2.6. Diagram of a 6cm-long localized obstruction (**A**), through which a 12Fr Dotter dilator is introduced (**B**). If no material is removed or compressed, the atheroma will have to be redistributed proximally and distally to make room for the dilator. The calculated volume of the cylinder that has been displaced would lead to elongation of the atheromatous lesion to 8cm (**C**). (Reproduced from Castañeda–Zúñiga WR, Amplatz K, Laerum F, et al: Mechanics of angioplasty: an experimental approach. *Radiographics* 1981;1:1–14.)

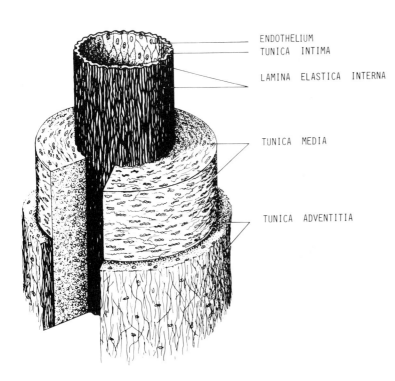

Figure 4.2.7. Schematic drawing of a medium-sized muscular artery showing its three distinct layers.

Labels in figure: ENDOTHELIUM, TUNICA INTIMA, LAMINA ELASTICA INTERNA, TUNICA MEDIA, TUNICA ADVENTITIA

ina, which is usually developed to a lesser degree than is the IEL.

Tunica Adventitia

The adventitia consists of fibrous connective tissue with collagen and elastic fibers oriented in a longitudinal or spiral fashion. In this layer, also, the vasa vasorum are found (more pronounced in the elastic and large muscular arteries), as are lymph vessels and nerves. Peripherally, the adventitia merges with the loose surrounding connective tissue.

Oxygenation of the Arterial Wall (Vasa Vasorum)

Oxygenation of the arterial wall is accomplished in two ways: first, by direct diffusion through the endothelium from the bloodstream and, second, through the vasa vasorum, which are found in the elastic and the larger muscular arteries. The vasa vasorum are tiny vessels—about the size of arterioles or capillaries—that originate from the mother artery or its branches or from neighboring arteries.[41] In the aorta, the vasa vasorum originate mainly from intercostal and lumbar arteries. Newer studies using various methods to demonstrate the vasa vasorum[42-45] or to measure the blood flow in the arterial wall of humans and several animal species[46] have shown the intima and inner media to be without any vasa vasorum. That is, only the outer media and adventitia contain vasa vasorum in the normal animal, whereas the inner layers of the artery are oxygenated by diffusion from the bloodstream.

MORPHOLOGIC CHANGES AFTER ANGIOPLASTY

In order to prove the hypothesis that transluminal angioplasty is effective primarily because of stretching of and controlled damage to the arterial layers, with subsequent healing, a series of experiments was performed on human cadaver arteries and on normal and atherosclerotic dog and rabbit arteries in vivo. On the basis of the radiologic, macroscopic, histologic, and ultrastructural changes seen in the dilated arteries, a new theory of the mechanism of PTA was proposed.

Experiments on Human Cadaver Arteries[47-50]

Materials and Methods

Fifty-six coronary, renal, mesenteric, and iliac arteries and abdominal aortas were removed at autopsy and dilated within 24 hours of death. Spot films in two projections of the arteries filled with a suspension of barium served to demonstrate the location and degree of stenoses. Because postmortem arteries have a tendency to shrink considerably due to the absence of blood pressure,[51-54] the arteries were dilated using a system that provided physiologic pressure (100mm Hg) (Fig. 4.2.9). Under the same pressure, the dilated vessels were afterward fixed in formalin. One group of arteries was dilated three times for 1 min each time using Grüntzig balloons 4–12mm in diameter at 4–5 atm of pressure. A second group of 19 arteries was dilated using PVC balloons 12–21mm in diameter (Fig. 4.2.10) at pressures of 2.5–11 atm. A third group was dilated using Foley catheters at 3 atm of pressure. The morphologic effects were assessed by the radiographic appearance, macroscopic alterations, including changes in outer diameter of the artery and histologic changes.

Results

Histologic changes. In the first group of arteries, dilatation caused intimal rupture, fragmentation, and partial

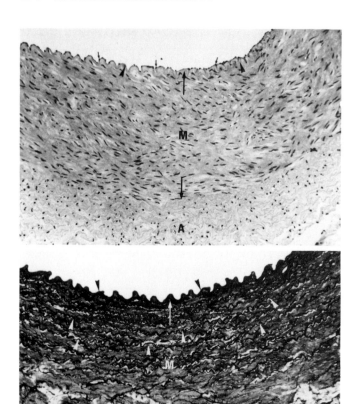

Figure 4.2.8. Cross-section of a normal canine carotid artery (× 100). Hematoxylin and eosin *(top)* and Verhoeff–van Gieson (VVG) *(bottom)*. Endothelium *(small arrows)* seals intima toward the vessel lumen. Wavy IEL *(black arrowheads)* divides intima from media *(M)*, which consists of predominantly circumferentially oriented smooth muscle fibers alternating with layers of elastic laminae. Elastic laminae are nearly continuous in spite of small fenestrations and ramifications *(white arrowheads)*. Adventitia *(A)* forms outer layer of the arterial wall toward the loose surrounding connective tissue.

dehiscence from the media. These changes generally were found at zones of transition from marked intimal thickening to areas with less plaque. In high-grade stenoses, additional rupture of the media was found (Fig. 4.2.11).

In the other two groups of arteries, analogous changes were seen in those vessels that had not completely ruptured. In addition, some areas of the media showed signs of compression, and other areas demonstrated partial or complete rupture of the media. Tears in the media were frequently combined with stretching of the adventitia (Fig. 4.2.12).

Changes of vessel diameter. The changes in external arterial diameter in response to polyethylene and PVC catheters are shown in Tables 4.2.1 and 4.2.2. The increase in diameter in the first group was only 0.8mm, and three arteries could not be dilated at all because of circumferential calcification. In the second group, which was dilated

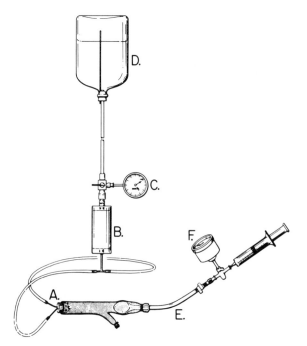

Figure 4.2.9. Diagram of system for angioplasty under physiologic pressure. Stopper to seal vessel *(A)*, with two small tubes that connect vessel to infusion system consisting of a small reservoir *(B)*, manometer *(C)*, and main reservoir *(D)*. E, F, balloon catheter with manometer for dilatation. (Reproduced from Laerum F, Vlodaver Z, Castañeda–Zúñiga WR, Edwards JE, Amplatz K: The mechanism of angioplasty: dilatation of iliac cadaver arteries with intravascular pressure control. *RöFo* 1982; 136:573–576.)

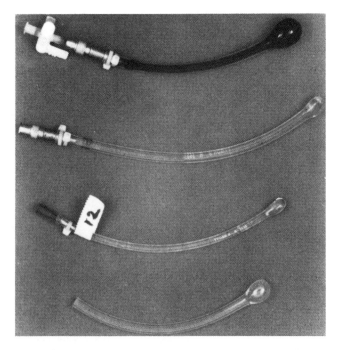

Figure 4.2.10. PVC balloons with diameters of 12–21mm. (Reproduced from Laerum F, Vlodaver Z, Castañeda–Zúñiga WR, Edwards JE, Amplatz K: The mechanism of angioplasty: dilatation of iliac cadaver arteries with intravascular pressure control. *RöFo* 1982;136:573–576.)

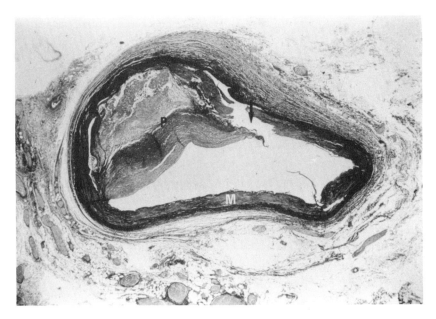

Figure 4.2.11. Superior mesenteric artery after dilatation with 9mm balloon for 3 min; there is a tear *(arrow)* at the edge of the plaque *(P)*. Media *(M)* shows marked degenerative changes, mainly where it is covered by plaque. The tear also involves degenerative parts of the media. Verhoeff–van Gieson; original magnification × 8. (Reproduced from Castañeda–Zúñiga WR, Formanek A, Tadavarthy M, et al: The mechanism of balloon angioplasty. *Radiology* 1980;135:565–571.)

Table 4.2.1. Angioplasty of 10 Distal Abdominal Aortas and Iliac Arteries with PE Balloons of 8–12mm Diameter (Inflation Pressure: 5 atm)

	No. of Dilatations		
	1	2	3
Increase of outer diameter (mm)	0.5 (0–1.0)	0.6 (0–1.3)	0.7 (0–2.0)

Table 4.2.2. Angioplasty of 19 Iliac Arteries with PVC Balloons of 12–21mm Diameter (Inflation Pressure: 5.5 atm (1.5–11))

	No. of Dilatations			
	1	2	3	4
Increase of outer diameter (mm)	0.7 (0–2.5)	1.0 (0–2.5)	1.0 (0–2.5)	1.2 (0.5–3)
Number of arterial ruptures	5	1	3	1
Inflation pressure (atm) at arterial rupture	5.8 (2.5–11)	3.5	5.2 (2.5–8)	7.5

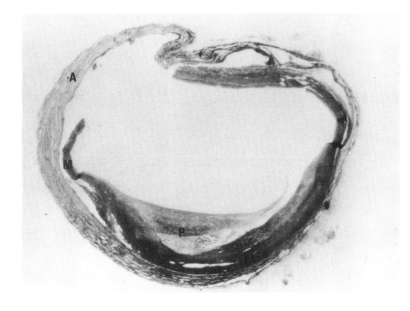

Figure 4.2.12. Iliac artery after dilatation with PVC balloon; rupture of intima and media where intima is only slightly thickened. Adventitia *(A)* has been stretched in this area. Media is partially detached from adventitia. *P* = plaque. Elastic stain; original magnification × 6.

Table 4.2.3. Angioplasty of Six Iliac Arteries with Foley Catheters (Inflation Pressure: 3 atm)

	No. of Dilatations			
	1	2	3	4
Increase in outer diameter (mm)	0.7 (0.5–1.0)	0.8 (0.5–1.2)	1.2 (0.7–2.0)	1.4 (1.0–2.0)
Number of arterial ruptures	0	0	0	2

with large PVC balloons, several arteries could be dilated only by using increased pressures. The vessels that did not rupture completely showed an average increase in outer diameter of only 1.25mm (12%). In the third group, the maximum average increase in diameter was 1.4mm (Table 4.2.3). In all groups, the largest increase in diameter was achieved with the last or fourth dilatation. All arteries showed an inverse correlation between the amount of calcification and the increase in diameter—i.e., vessels with marked circumferential calcification could not be dilated measurably.

Radiographic changes. The increase in inner luminal diameter, as measured on x-ray films of the barium-filled arteries, was similar to the changes in the outer diameter. Again, heavily calcified arteries did not show a measurable increase in lumen (Fig. 4.2.13). All increases in lumen in the dilatable vessels resulted from rupture or tears in the

plaques, with intimal dehiscence from the media, changes visible radiographically as radiolucent linear defects (Fig. 4.2.14*A,B*) that closely resembled those seen after clinical PTA (Fig. 4.2.14*C*). Histologically, these lucent lines matched the areas of intimal dehiscence or flaps. They were always oriented longitudinally. No signs of plaque redistribution could be found.

Discussion

The results of these first experiments confirmed the hypothesis that balloon dilatation does not compress atheromatous plaque but rather works by intimal rupture and partial dehiscence of this layer from the media, thus producing large clefts. These longitudinal clefts corresponded well with the radiolucent linear defects seen on postangioplasty arteriograms in clinical PTA. Noteworthy was the small increase in outside, and often also in luminal, diameter of the dilated arteries, a fact that was confirmed by LeVeen et al.[55] Circumferential plaque thickening resulted in especially limited luminal widening. On the other hand, asymmetric intimal thickening led to marked stretching and localized rupture of the media. Also, aneurysmal dilatation of the adventitia on the side opposite the plaque was found in these cases. Heavily calcified arteries could not be dilated at all unless the intimal plaque ruptured. This fact was again proved when dilating an atherosclerotic vessel within a test tube (Fig. 4.2.15), which prevents increase of the outer diameter and thereby plaque rupture. Arteries

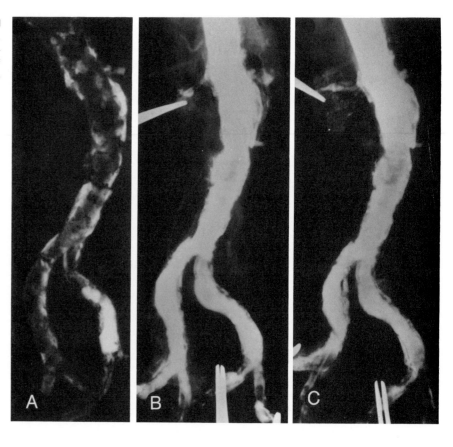

Figure 4.2.13. Specimen of heavily calcified abdominal aorta including proximal pelvic arteries. **A.** Severe calcification. **B.** Specimen filled with suspension of barium; before dilatation. **C.** After dilatation of aortic bifurcation and common iliac arteries; no measurable dilatation because of the circumferential calcification.

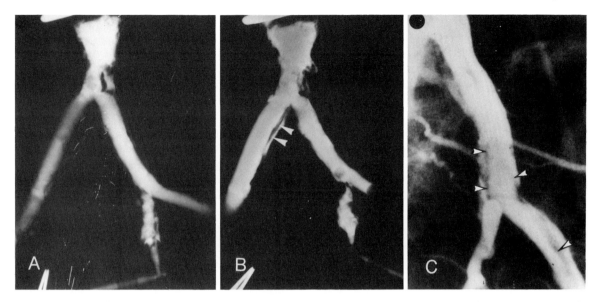

Figure 4.2.14. Specimen (filled with barium suspension) of distal abdominal aorta with proximal pelvic arteries (**A,B**). Iliac angiogram of a patient after PTA of left pelvic axis (**C**). **A.** Before dilatation. **B.** After dilatation of bifurcation and right iliac artery; definite luminal widening, with a longitudinal lucent defect due to plaque dehiscence *(arrowheads)*. **C.** Analogous findings in vivo, with linear contrast defects after dilatation *(arrowheads)*.

with comparatively mild atheromatous disease often ruptured completely even when dilated with Foley catheters and pressures of only 3 atm (group 3; Table 4.2.3). Chin et al. demonstrated that plaque dehiscence is already apparent at dilating pressures of 1–1.5 atm.[56]

Cadaver arteries obviously have a markedly reduced range of mechanical stretch as compared with living vessels, probably because of the lack of muscle tone and of autolytic changes that hasten rupture of the arterial wall. Nonetheless, even if experiments on cadaver arteries have limited value in defining optimal pressures and duration of balloon inflation for dilating atherosclerotic vessels, the authors were able to draw some important conclusions from studying these specimens to confirm their hypothesis:

1. No significant compression or redistribution of the plaque takes place.
2. The mechanism for widening of the arterial lumen consists of a combination of rupture and tears in the intima, with consequent dehiscence of this layer from the media. Another important factor is stretching of the media and adventitia, which had already been mentioned by Hempel in 1969[34] and by Jester et al. in 1976.[32] Thus, successful dilatation that leaves the endothelium and intima intact, as proposed by Baughman et al.[37] and Simpson et al.,[40] seems unlikely.
3. The longitudinal radiolucent defects in angiograms made after PTA and the transient intramural accumulations of contrast medium originally thought to represent complicating dissections[37,38] are a consequence of this rupture and the dehiscence of the intima. This phenomenon is common, especially with fibrous, calcified lesions, and should be interpreted as a normal finding as long as there is no obstruction of flow or embolization.[57]

Animal Experiments

The authors further hypothesized that the extent of damage to the arterial wall depends on balloon size, the pressure applied, and the duration of balloon inflation. The time factor, especially, can be investigated appropriately only in living arteries. Therefore, a series of experiments was designed using normal canine and atherosclerotic rabbit arteries.

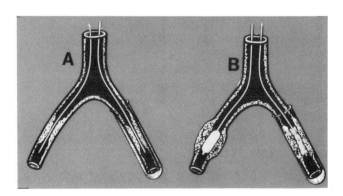

Figure 4.2.15. Drawing of cadaver aortic-iliac specimen with severe bilateral iliac atherosclerosis. Left iliac artery has been placed in a glass test tube *(A)*. With dilatation *(B)*, right iliac artery expands at dilatation site, while the segment of left common iliac artery being dilated is restrained by a test tube. (Reproduced from Wolinsky H, Glagov S: Nature of species differences in the medial distribution of aortic vasa vasorum in mammals. *Circ Res* 1967;20:409–421.)

Angioplasty in Normal Canine Arteries Using Inflation Pressures of 4–5 Atmospheres[47,48,58,59]

Materials and methods. As a pilot study, the infrarenal aorta and iliac arteries of three anesthetized mongrel dogs were dilated with 9mm balloons (approximately 25% greater than the normal size for the abdominal aorta and more than 100% for the iliac arteries). In another dog, the aorta was dilated using a 15mm balloon, and, in a fifth dog, two 9mm balloons were used simultaneously to dilate the aorta more than 100% oversize. Follow-up angiograms were taken immediately after and at intervals of 1 week to 4 months following PTA. The animals were euthanized 4 weeks to 4 months postangioplasty, and the dilated vessels, including normal control segments, were processed for histologic study.

Forty carotid and femoral arterial segments were dilated using 25 and 60–80% oversized balloons, which were inflated for 1 min to 4.5 atm three times. Animals were euthanized for examination at 30 min; at 6, 18, 24, 48, and 72 hours; at 1 and 2 weeks; and at 1–6 months after angioplasty. Follow-up angiograms were taken immediately after dilatation and before sacrificing the animals. Dilated and normal control segments were excised and prepared for histologic and electron microscopic examination. The arterial lumen was measured on the angiograms before and after dilatation.

Results. Already in the pilot study, a correlation between the histologic changes in the abdominal aorta and iliac arteries and the balloon size or duration of inflation was suggested. With 25% overdilatation at 5 atm for three min, histologic changes remained limited to the intima and endothelium, whereas with 100% or more overdilatation, the abdominal aortas showed extensive changes, with locally complete disruption of the media. At three to four months after angioplasty, the medial tears had been

bridged by scar (neomedia) and there was extensive intimal hyperplasia (Fig. 4.2.16). The adventitia was hyperplastic and intact, and there were no signs of local aneurysmal dilatation. In spite of this, after four months the aortas showed, both in situ and after excision, definite widening of the outer circumference (Fig. 4.2.17). The iliac arteries overdilated by more than 100% showed analogous changes, although the intimal hyperplasia tended to be localized rather than circumferential (Fig. 4.2.18).

Angiographically, 25% overdilatation of the aorta or iliac arteries did not cause any measurable widening of the lumen. Dilation of 100% or more resulted in marked widening of the arterial lumen lasting about one month and then slowly decreasing over the following two to three months (Fig. 4.2.19).

Histologic and electron microscopic examination of the carotid and femoral arteries revealed two important new observations: that significant stretching of normal arteries leads to intimal hyperplasia, which persists for at least six months, and that stretching causes irreversible changes in the medial architecture. These findings are in contrast to the results of studies on the significance of endothelial damage in the pathogenesis of atherosclerosis, the hallmark of which is intimal hyperplasia or "fibrous plaque formation" and the re-endothelialization of the luminal surface secondary to trauma to the endothelium but not to the underlying media.[60] These changes are limited to the intima and result from migration and proliferation of smooth muscle cells along with production of collagen and elastin.[61–64] In these studies, intimal hyperplasia was transient, with complete regression over three to six months.

The authors' light and electron microscopic studies showed endothelial abrasion with various degrees of medial damage in the acute stage, followed by intimal hyperplasia and medial fibrosis. Slight differences were noted according to balloon size. That is, balloons of 25%

Figure 4.2.16. Abdominal aorta four months after >100% overdilatation. Elastic stain; original magnification × 7. Media *(M)* is missing over a considerable area; thick neointima *(I)* composed of laminated fibrous tissue covers the entire internal surface of the vessel. Adventitia *(A)* appears intact. (Reproduced from Castañeda–Zúñiga WR, Formanek A, Tadavarthy M, et al: The mechanism of balloon angioplasty. *Radiology* 1980; 135:565–571.)

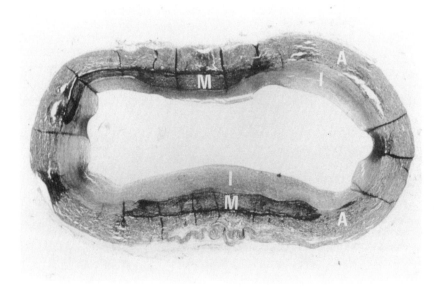

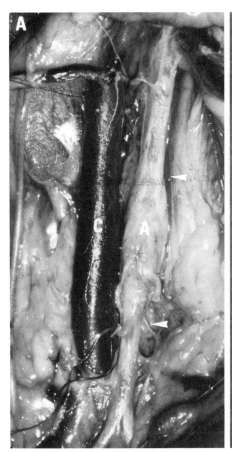
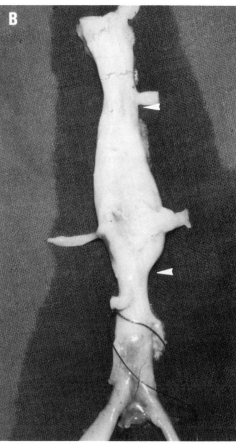

Figure 4.2.17. Abdominal aorta four months after >100% overdilatation. **A.** *In situ.* **B.** After excision. Marked widening of outer aortic contour (A) at the area of previous dilatation *(between arrowheads). C =* vena cava.

oversize caused focal fractures and stretching of the IEL, and damage to the media was limited to the inner third of this layer; whereas dilation with 60–80% oversized balloons caused extensive destruction of the IEL and penetrating damage through more than half of the medial thickness (Figs. 4.2.20 and 4.2.21). After use of large balloons, separation of collagen and elastic fibers from the myocytes

was common (Fig. 4.2.21). Within 18–48 hours, the damaged media had "empty" spaces filled with edema and debris but lacking any intact cellular elements (Fig. 4.2.22). It remains unclear how the cellular debris was removed, inasmuch as leukocytes and macrophages were present in large numbers only in those areas where blood had access to the interior of the arterial wall, i.e., in medial dissections.

Figure 4.2.18. Iliac artery from same animal four months after 100% overdilatation; media *(M)* and IEL show focal rupture *(arrowheads).* Defect is covered by neointima *(I).* Note irregular distribution of intimal hyperplasia. Adventitia shows proliferation particularly at area of medial rupture. Elastic stain; original magnification × 16.

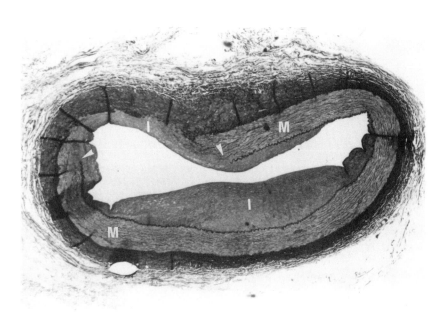

Figure 4.2.19. Abdominal aortic angiograms of same animal after overdilatation with two 9mm balloons. **A.** Before dilatation. **B.** After dilatation. **C.** Four weeks after dilatation; persistent luminal widening is apparent. **D.** At 3.5 months after dilatation, luminal widening has regressed.

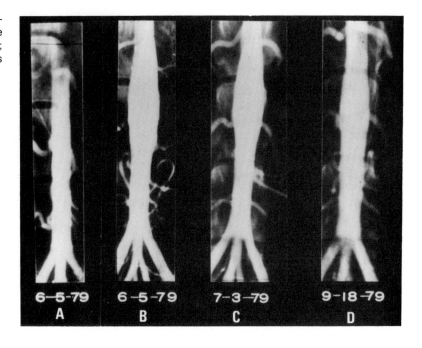

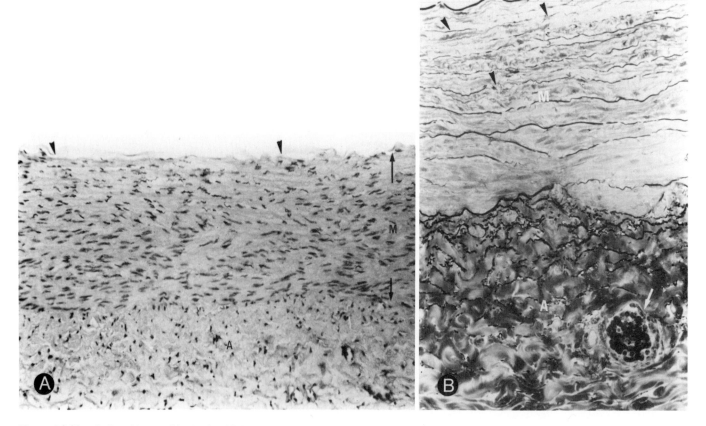

Figure 4.2.20. **A.** Carotid artery 20 min after 80% overdilatation. Hematoxylin and eosin; original magnification × 120. Endothelium is completely erased, and IEL *(arrowheads)* is partially detached. Inner media shows corkscrew-like deformation and pyknoses of smooth muscle nuclei. Inner media is edematous with multiple acellular areas. *M* = media, *A* = adventitia. **B.** Same vessel; note stretched elastic laminae *(arrowheads)* with increased fragmentation and thinning. There is a dilated vasa vasorum in adventitia containing several polymorphonuclear leukocytes *(arrows).* Toluidine blue; original magnification × 200.

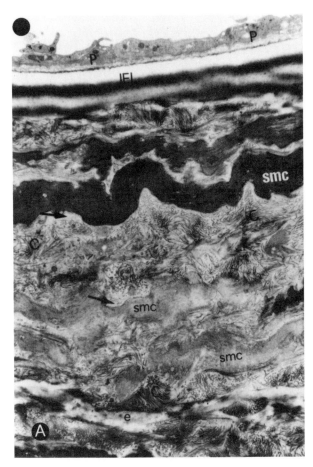
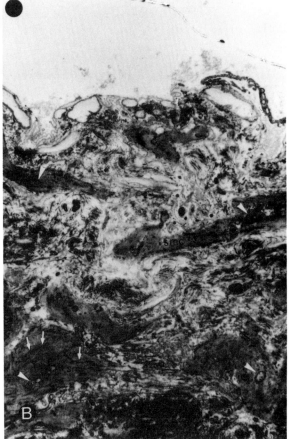

Figure 4.2.21. Electron micrographs of carotid artery 30 min after dilatation. Original magnification × 5300. **A.** 25% dilatation; platelets *(P)* adhere to denuded and stretched IEL; note degenerating myocytes *(smc)* with corkscrew formation, loss of dense bodies, and loss of stainability. Collagen *(C)* and elastic fibers *(e)* have lost their close relation to smc *(arrow)*. Edematous intercellular spaces are seen. **B.** 60% dilatation; complete destruction of IEL. Note chaotic structure and interstitial edema. Changes are much more severe than in **A.** Myocytes show myofilaments *(arrows)* and swollen mitochondria *(arrowheads)*.

Very soon after the dilatation injury, platelets could be observed attached to the denuded surface. These findings correspond closely to those reported after endothelial abrasion using the Baumgartner method[60,62-64] as well as to the studies of PTA in normal canine coronary arteries reported by Pasternak et al.[65] and O'Gara et al.[66] These aggregated platelets could be followed for up to three days, at which time modified smooth muscle cells were seen invading the neointima, and re-endothelialization could be observed, which was complete at one to three weeks (Fig. 4.2.23). Intense proliferation and migration of smooth muscle cells and increased production of elastin and, especially, collagen caused marked intimal thickening at one month (Fig. 4.2.24). A similar repair process, with proliferation of smooth muscle cells and fibrosis secondary to irregular deposition of collagen and elastic fibers, was seen in the media. Reconstitution of the fractured or destroyed IEL was not seen (Fig. 4.2.24).

After three to six months, no significant regression of the irregular cushion-like intimal hyperplasia was noted.

The fibrotic changes of the media with proliferation of collagen also persisted, and thus the irregular medial architecture correlated well with the degree of initial overdistension (Fig. 4.2.25).

The increase in the arterial lumen as measured on angiograms immediately after angioplasty was 0–7% (average 2.6 ± 3.3) with overdilation of 25% and 8–30% (average 17.4 ± 7.1) with overdilation of 60–80% (Fig. 4.2.26). Two-thirds of the dilated arteries exhibited short, spasm-like luminal narrowings adjacent to the site of dilatation (Figs. 4.2.26 and 4.2.27). Occasionally, these spasms extended over several centimeters (Fig. 4.2.27), and they appeared to have no correlation with the extent of arterial dilatation. They persisted for as long as 48 hours.

By 18–48 hours after 80% overdilation, the luminal widening had diminished to 10–12% (Fig. 4.2.28), and one to two weeks later no increase in luminal diameter could be measured. Angiograms four weeks or more after angioplasty revealed no significant changes from the control films made before angioplasty. In cases of 25% over-

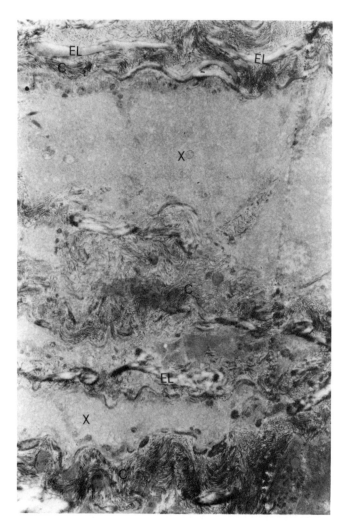

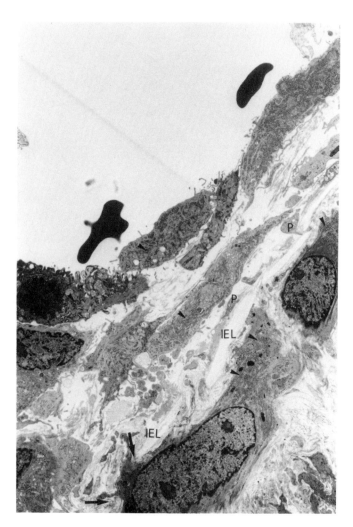

Figure 4.2.22. Carotid artery 18 hours after 80% dilatation. Approximate original magnification × 5300. Transition of outer to middle third of media shows ''empty'' spaces *(X)* filled with edema and debris between original layers of collagen and elastic laminae *(EL)*. Many EL are fragmented. Collagen fibers *(C)* remain in contact with EL. There are no cellular blood elements within the damaged wall. (Reproduced from Zollikofer CL, Salomonowitz E, Sibley R, et al: Transluminal angioplasty evaluated by electron microscopy. *Radiology* 1984;153:369–374.)

Figure 4.2.23. Carotid artery one week after dilatation (75%). Original magnification × 4500. Electron micrograph shows intima and inner media. Two or three layers of modified smooth muscle cells (fibromyoblasts) with prominent endoplasmic reticulum *(arrowheads)* are seen on luminal side of IEL. Some platelets *(P)* are still visible close to IEL. A fibromyoblast seems to be migrating into intima through gap in IEL *(between arrows)*.

dilation, luminal widening persisted no longer than 18 hours.

Discussion. These results proved that even dilatation of the normal vessel cannot be achieved without damage to the arterial wall structures. This damage is clearly dependent on the amount of wall stretching. The chronologic steps of platelet aggregation on the denuded inner vascular surface, followed by proliferation and invasion of smooth muscle cells that results in a hypertrophied neointima covered by a neoendothelium, support the theory that platelets play a major role in stimulating migration and proliferation of smooth muscle cells by releasing mitogenic factors leading to intimal hyperplasia.[62–64,67] In contrast to the results of Ross and Glomset,[62,68] Stemerman and colleagues,[64,69] and others,[61,63,70] the present authors did not

find regression of this intimal hyperplasia. Also, Leu and Grüntzig, in their study of canine arteries, found persistent intimal thickening after a seven-month period.[36]

An 80% overdilation of nonaortic canine vessels caused widespread changes in the intima and media without definitely traumatizing the adventitia. Only dilated vasa vasorum were noted in the adventitia immediately after angioplasty. Complete medial destruction in excessively dilated (>100%) aortic and proximal iliac vessels resulted in healing with marked intimal hyperplasia. However, again, no signs of adventitial tears or localized, saccular aneurysm formation could be detected in areas of formerly complete medial rupture. The latter healed by scar formation resulting in a neomedia and proliferation of the adventitia which obviously compensate for the missing media after excessive

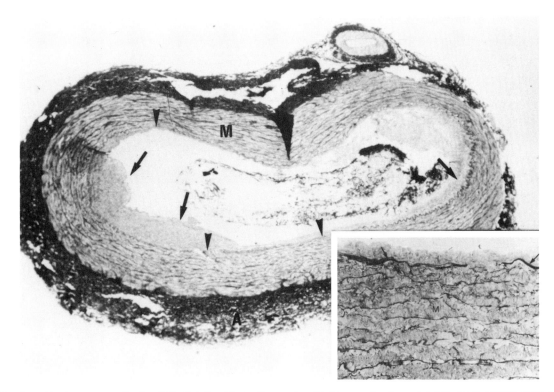

Figure 4.2.24. Carotid artery one month after 60% dilatation. Verhoeff–van Gieson; original magnification × 20. Irregular intimal hyperplasia *(arrows)*. Internal elastic lamina is interrupted in several areas *(arrowheads)*. M = media, A = adventitia. *Inset,* carotid artery one month after 60% dilatation. Toluidine blue; original magnification × 200. Intimal hyperplasia *(I)*; IEL *(arrows)* is not reconstituted.

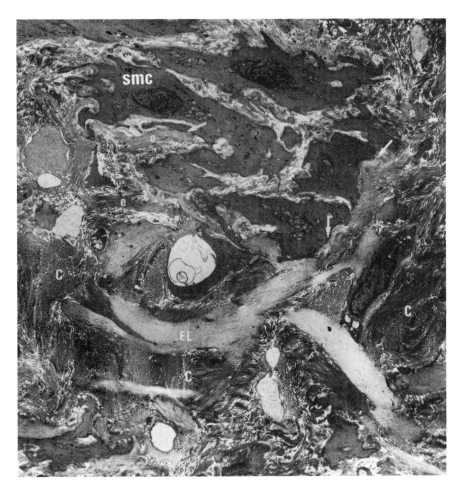

Figure 4.2.25. Electron micrograph of carotid artery three months after 80% dilatation. Original magnification × 3700. Media exhibits irregular pattern with increased collagen *(C)*. Elastic laminae *(EL)* are irregular and fragmented. Smooth muscle cells *(smc)* show prominence of mitochondria but no increase in rough endoplasmic reticulum. Note that close relation of collagen and elastin with smc has been re-established *(arrows)*. Overall, there is fibrosis from increase in collagen and irregular elastin. (Reproduced from Zollikofer CL, Salomonowitz E, Sibley R, et al: Transluminal angioplasty evaluated by electron microscopy. *Radiology* 1984; 153:369–374.)

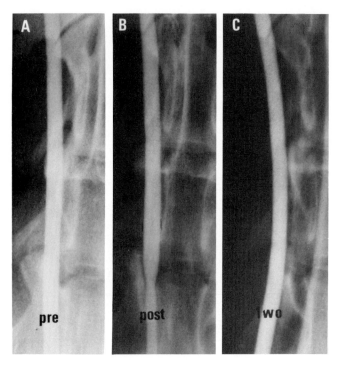

Figure 4.2.26. Carotid artery angiogram before (**A**), immediately after (**B**), and one week after (**C**) 25% dilatation. Lumen increase in **B** amounts to 6%. Note local spasm at the proximal end of the dilated segment. One week after dilatation, there is no appreciable luminal widening.

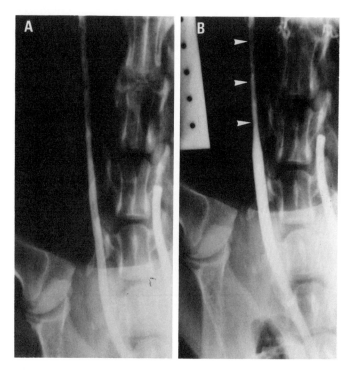

Figure 4.2.27. Carotid artery angiogram before (**A**) and after (**B**) 80% dilatation. Note extensive spasm distal to the dilatation (*arrowheads*). Luminal widening of dilated segment is 23%.

dilation. A compensatory mechanism may also explain the persistence of intimal thickening as opposed to the findings of experiments where the arterial lesion was limited to the endothelium. Unlike the fibrosis in the media, the amount of intimal hyperplasia was not definitely dependent on the degree of overdilation and medial damage. This phenomenon may have some importance in the etiology of recurrent stenosis following balloon dilatation; i.e., angioplasty with insufficient luminal widening may cause rapid recurrence of stenoses due to intimal hyperplasia, especially in nonatherosclerotic disease. Therefore, it seems noteworthy that experimentally, intimal hyperplasia may be reduced by antiplatelet therapy.[71]

Whether intimal hyperplasia occurs to the same degree in atherosclerotic vessels is not certain. Faxon et al. have shown in atherosclerotic rabbits that restenosis occurs four weeks after angioplasty as a result of extensive intimal thickening.[72,73] Thrombotic occlusions also were found, suggesting that the intimal thickening may have been due to organization of thrombotic material rather than to genuine intimal hyperplasia.

Obviously, these findings in animals cannot simply be transferred to human atherosclerotic disease. The more complex condition of human atherosclerosis, with frequent necrosis and calcification, may respond differently to, and progress more slowly after, angioplasty. On the other hand, Waller et al. found severe restenosis at areas of previous PTA at autopsy two to five months after successful clinical coronary angioplasty.[74,75] Possibly, the intimal pro-

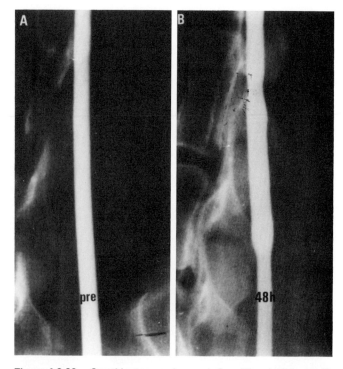

Figure 4.2.28. Carotid artery angiogram before (**A**) and 48 hours after (**B**) 70% dilatation. Luminal widening in **B** is 10%; immediately after dilatation, the lumen increase had been 14%. Again, note spasm proximal and distal to dilatation.

liferation stimulated after PTA in arteries of relatively small diameter is of greater importance and may explain the higher recurrence rate (approximately 30%) in coronary compared with peripheral PTA. Furthermore, in the presence of hyperlipidemia, atherosclerosis may be accelerated by simple mechanical damage to the endothelium,[62,76–79] a fact also noted after the use of arterial clamps. Therefore, it is theoretically advisable to put patients on a low-cholesterol diet after PTA until re-endothelialization has occurred and to prescribe antiplatelet drugs. Indeed, Faxon et al. showed in the atherosclerotic animal model that aspirin and dipyridamole or sulfinpyrazone significantly reduce intimal thickening and restenosis, as well as the rate of thrombotic occlusions, after PTA.[72]

In excessively dilated abdominal aortas, a long-lasting increase in arterial diameter could be demonstrated angiographically after angioplasty. The luminal widening tended to decrease simultaneously with the increasing intimal hyperplasia and scar formation. Nonetheless, the outer circumference was still definitely enlarged even after four months. To explain such an aneurysmal widening of the outer contour, adventitial stretching must take place in addition to medial damage.

The cause and significance of local spasm adjacent to the dilated arterial segments are discussed below under "Pharmacologic Phenomena and Metabolic Changes of the Arterial Wall after PTA."

In summary, these studies led to the following conclusions:

A long-lasting dilatation of the normal vessel can be achieved only by means of marked damage to the intima and media and stretching of the media and, to some degree, of the adventitia. As long as the adventitia is not severely damaged, healing without aneurysm formation can be expected. Intimal hyperplasia may compensate for medial destruction and therefore probably is irreversible. Intimal thickening may also be important in the atherosclerotic vessel after PTA.

How antiplatelet drugs affect healing of the vessel wall, intimal thickening, and early reocclusion needs further investigation, if possible in primates.

Angioplasty in Normal Canine Arteries Using Higher Inflation Pressures (8–12.5 atm)[50,80]

In the previous studies of normal canine arteries, the authors noticed that balloons 50–100% oversized compared with the arterial lumen did not reach their full diameter at the usual inflation pressures of 4–5 atm (Fig. 4.2.29). They therefore studied the behavior of the balloons in situ and the histologic changes caused by higher inflation pressures. Of special interest were potential differences between balloons of differing compliances.[80]

Materials and methods. Twenty-five carotid and femoral arteries were dilated with balloon catheters with a diameter equal to that of the vessel, 30% larger, and 80–100% larger than the original vessel diameter as measured on the angiogram (groups A, B, and C, respectively). The two brands of balloon catheters used were made from PVC or polyethylene. Spot films and cinefluorography (cine)

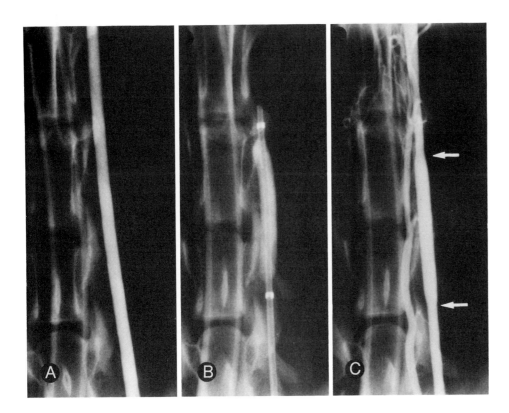

Figure 4.2.29. Effect of 80% dilatation of left carotid artery. **A.** Angiogram before dilatation; arterial diameter measures 4.5mm. **B.** An 8mm balloon catheter in situ; diameter is 5.7mm at 4.5 atm. **C.** Angiogram postdilatation; dilated segment measures 5mm (+12%). Note spasms proximal and distal to dilated segment *(arrows)*.

films were taken of the balloon catheters filled with diluted contrast medium within the vessel at 4.5 atm as well as at inflation pressures of 6, 8, 10, and 12.5 atm. In this way, the diameters of the arterial lumen on the angiogram as well as the diameters of the balloons in situ could be compared with the aid of a micrometer caliper. After the animals were killed, the dilated arterial and normal vessel segments were excised and stained for histologic examination.

Results. Table 4.2.4 shows the diameters the balloons reached intravascularly, given as a percentage of their requested (inflated) diameter as stated by the manufacturer, at 4.5 and 8–12.5 atm (before possible rupture of the artery). At pressures of 4.5 atm, the diameters of the PVC balloons were less than those of the polyethylene bal-

Table 4.2.4. Diameters of Balloons Attained Intravascularly (in % of Their Requested Diameter) at 4.5 and 8–12.5 atm: Comparison of PVC and PE Balloons

	4.5atm		8–10atm	
	PVC	PE	PVC	PE
A. Dilation 80–100% (balloon diameter 8–9mm)				
% of requested diameter	68 (67–70)	82 (81–84)	80 (70–96)	95 (83–100)
B. Dilation 30% (balloon diameter 6mm)				
% of requested diameter	85 (78–96)	87 (77–92)	95 (85–114)	101 (100–101)
C. Dilation 0% (balloon diameter 4mm):				
% of requested diameter	131 (120–145)	110 (107–112)	150 (145–158)	121 (110–142)

Figure 4.2.30. Iliac artery 30 min after 80% dilatation at 10 atm. **A.** PE balloon. At two places, media *(M)* has completely ruptured *(arrows);* adventitia *(A)* bulges slightly in these areas. There is marked stretching of elastic lamina, and there are ruptures of the IEL *(arrowheads).* Adventitia prevents complete rupture of the artery. Thrombus is seen in lumen. Verhoeff–van Gieson; original magnification × 25. **B.** PVC balloon. Close-up view of area with medial rupture that reaches down to adventitia *(arrows).* There is severe damage to myocytes and elastic lamina of the media bordering the rupture, which is covered by thrombus. Hematoxylin and eosin; original magnification × 50. (Reproduced from Zollikofer CL, Salomonowitz E, Brühlmann WF, Castañeda–Zúñiga WR, Amplatz K: Dehnungs-, Verformungs und Berstungs-Charakteristika haufig verwendeter Balloon-Dilatationskatheter: in vivo Untersuchungen an Hundegefassen (Teil 2). *RöFo* 1986; 144:189–195.)

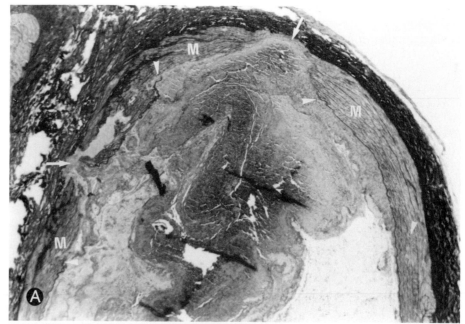

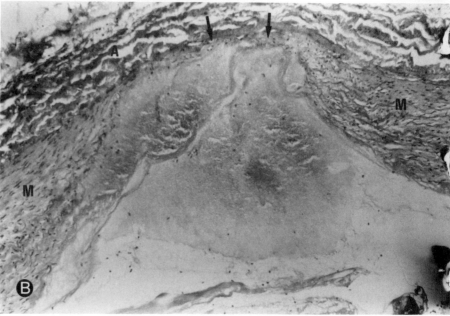

loons in the nine specimens overdilated by 80–100%. Accordingly, the histologic changes were less penetrating with PVC balloons. At pressures of 8–10 atm, the differences in the diameters of the two types of balloons were again noted, although the differences in the histologic changes were less obvious (Fig. 4.2.30). With both balloons, extensive damage to the intima and media was noted, with focal stretching of the latter (Fig. 4.2.30). In addition, local thrombosis occurred, particularly in areas of complete medial rupture. Only one artery showed less penetrating lesions, and here the balloon catheter reached

barely 70% of its requested diameter because of its relatively high compliance and elongation. In three cases (two polyethylene and one PVC balloon), complete rupture of the artery resulted at pressures of 10 atm. All three balloons reached 100% of their requested diameter after rupture of the vessel.

At 4.5 atm, neither the balloon diameters nor the histologic changes differed significantly for the two balloon materials in the eight cases of 30% overdilation (Table 4.2.4). At high pressures (10–12.5 atm), all of the polyethylene balloons reached their requested diameter (Fig.

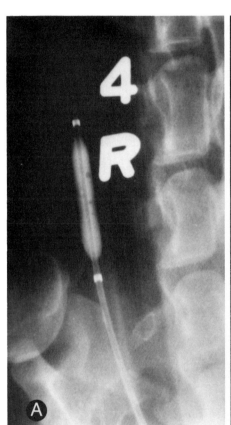
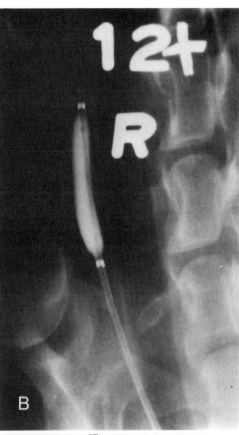
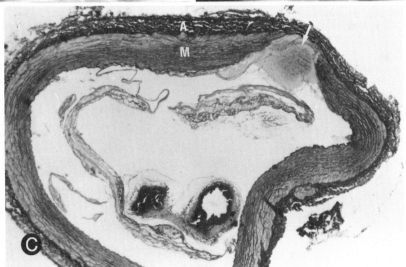

Figure 4.2.31. Carotid artery, 30% dilatation to maximum of 12.5 atm with 6mm PE balloon. **A.** Balloon in situ at 4.5 atm attains 77% of full diameter. **B.** Balloon in situ at 12.5 atm is 100% inflated, to 6mm. **C.** Histologic section (Verhoeff–van Gieson stain) of artery shows local rupture of media *(M) (arrow)* with slight bulging of adventitia *(A)*. Nonruptured parts of media (elastic laminae) seem less stretched and less compressed than in **A.**

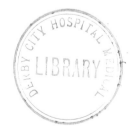

4.2.31), whereas the PVC balloons showed a wide range in attained diameters, with two balloons not reaching their requested diameters while exhibiting severe deformation and elongation (Fig. 4.2.32). Compared to group A, the arterial wall damage was less distinct in the areas of dilatation: only focal medial disruptions in two cases and no complete ruptures of the vessel (Fig. 4.2.31C). However, elongation and deformation of the PVC balloons, as shown in Figure 4.2.32, damaged the vessel wall far beyond the original balloon length.

As shown in Table 4.2.4, the range of attained diameters was much wider for PVC balloons at 4.5 atm as well as at 10–12.5 atm in the cases that were not overdilated. In addition, due to their greater compliance, the PVC balloons enlarged above the requested diameter more readily than did the polyethylene balloons (Figs. 4.2.33 and 4.2.34). Accordingly, the histologic changes were more penetrating with the PVC balloons (Fig. 4.2.35). Five of the eight balloons ruptured in situ at 10–12.5 atm. However, there were no local histologic changes attributable to a jet of saline from the rupturing balloon.

Discussion. This study definitely demonstrated progressive histologic changes in the arterial wall with increasing balloon diameter as well as with increasing inflation pressure. Balloons oversized 30% and more do not reach their requested diameters at normal working pressures as suggested by the manufacturer; to achieve the requested diameter, the inflation pressure must be substantially increased. The study also showed that the result of angio-

plasty depends on the compliance of the balloon material. An oversized balloon of low compliance has more dilating strength and may even cause vessel rupture, whereas a balloon of the same size but with a comparatively large compliance may cause less local damage. However, because of the deformation and elongation of the balloon, the arterial wall may undergo changes far beyond the actual dilated segment, and this can lead to extensive vascular spasm and difficulties in retracting the balloon catheter. Balloons the diameter of the lumen or slightly larger that have large compliance, on the other hand, can cause more histologic damage than noncompliant balloons because of their considerable tendency to overinflate and "grow" at high pressures.

In addition, this study demonstrated that with high balloon pressures, rupture of the media may lead to focal stretching of the adventitia. Such aneurysmal outpouchings were also seen in the present authors' study on cadaver arteries (Fig. 4.2.12) and were described after PTA in atherosclerotic rabbits by Sanborn et al.[81]

A further important observation concerns the tendency to extensive local thrombus formation in areas of severe medial damage with complete rupture. Organization of such thrombi may play an important role in healing and in preventing aneurysm formation as a delayed complication. If the media was not completely destroyed and torn through to the adventitial layer (as shown in the previous study with inflation pressures limited to 4.5 atm), thrombus formation was much less prominent.

Figure 4.2.32. Carotid artery, 30% dilatation to maximum of 10 atm with 6mm PVC balloon. **A.** Angiogram before dilatation (arterial lumen = 5.1mm). **B.** Balloon in situ at 4.5 atm attains 78% of its full diameter. **C.** Balloon in situ at 10 atm attains 85% of its full diameter. Severe elongation and deformation of balloon with marked dilatation of catheter shaft *(arrowheads)* are caused by spreading of injected fluid between inner and outer catheter sleeve (dissection between the two coaxial catheters). A further increase in the balloon pressure could not be achieved.

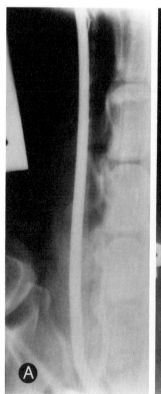
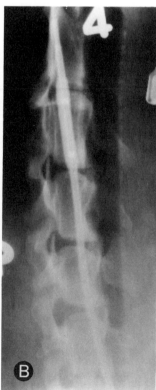
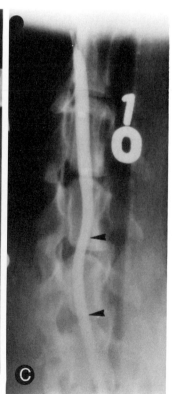

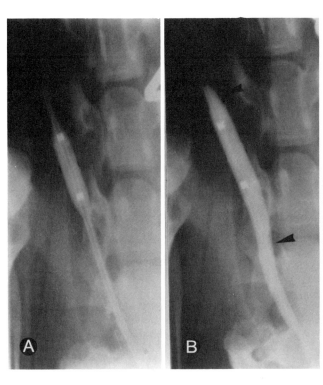
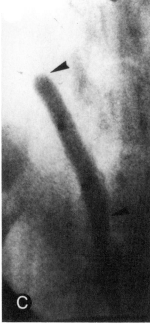

Figure 4.2.33. Carotid artery (4.8mm diameter) with 4mm PVC balloon in situ. **A.** 4.5 atm; balloon diameter 5.8mm. **B.** 8 atm; balloon diameter 6.3mm (=157%). There is severe deformation and elongation of balloon *(arrowheads)* and dissection of injected fluid between the inner and outer catheter sleeve at region of catheter shaft. **C.** 10 atm; no further increase in diameter. Balloon has extended toward tip of catheter and catheter shaft *(arrowheads),* causing enormous increase in diameter of shaft.

Angioplasty in Atherosclerotic Rabbits[82]

For clinical PTA, the often strictly followed rule of three dilations for 30–60 seconds each with a balloon approximately equal in diameter to the original (nondiseased) lumen has been advocated without a solid scientific basis.[48,83,84] According to the authors' studies on canine arteries, a close correlation exists between the histologic alterations of the vessel wall and the diameter and inflation pressures of the balloon catheter. Healthy arteries were able to withstand >100% overdilation as long as inflation

pressures were not above 4–5 atm. On the other hand, studies of atherosclerotic cadaver arteries have revealed differences in behavior during angioplasty depending on the configuration and the amount of calcification of the atherosclerotic plaque.[47–50,85] However, the effects of various balloon sizes and inflation times had not been investigated in experimental animals by Block, Faxon, Sanborn, and their colleagues.[81,85–87] To gain better insight into the influence of balloon size and time of inflation on atherosclerotic arteries, the present authors studied normal and atherosclerotic rabbits.

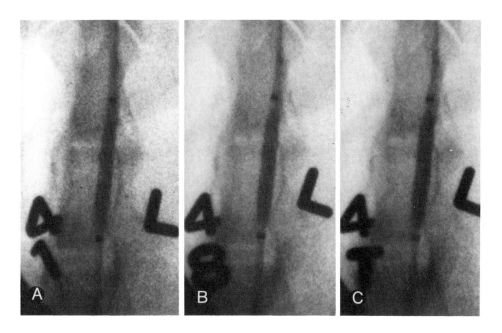

Figure 4.2.34. Carotid artery (diameter = 4.6mm) with 4mm PE balloon in situ. **A.** 4.5 atm; balloon diameter = 4.3mm. **B.** 8 atm; balloon diameter = 4.4mm. **C.** 10 atm; balloon diameter = 4.6mm (=115%). No significant deformation or elongation of balloon is noted.

Figure 4.2.35. Carotid artery after dilatation with 4mm balloons (0% group). H & E; original magnification × 32. **A.** Dilatation with PVC balloon; dissection into media *(M)*, with rupture and partial destruction of IEL *(arrowheads)*. There is significant stretching of elastic laminae and pyknotic nuclei are seen within media. *A* = adventitia. **B.** Dilatation with PE balloon; changes in media are significantly less penetrating than in **A**. There are no dissections, only interruptions, of IEL *(arrowheads)*. (Reproduced from Zollikofer CL, Salomonowitz E, Brühlmann WF, Castañeda–Zúñiga WR, Amplatz K: Dehnungs-, Verformungs und Berstungs-Charakteristika haufig verwendeter Balloon-Dilatationskatheter: in vivo Untersuchungen an Hundegefassen (Teil 2). *RöFo* 1986;144:189–195.)

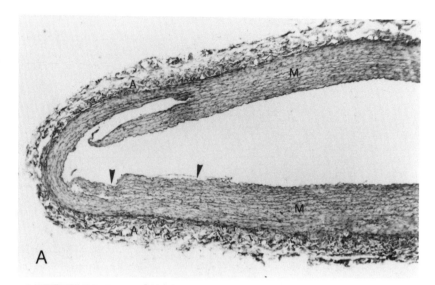

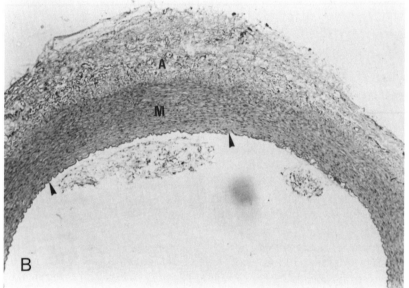

Materials and methods. Two groups of eight 3.6kg New Zealand rabbits were studied. The rabbits in group I served as controls and were fed standard rabbit chow, whereas those in group II were fed a 2% cholesterol-enriched diet. The thoracic and abdominal aortas were dilated with Grüntzig-type balloon catheters of 25 and 50% oversize, respectively, compared with the original lumen of the aorta measured on the angiogram. The inflation time ranged from 15–60 seconds. The animals were then killed, and dilated and nondilated aortic segments were prepared for histologic and electron microscopic examination.

Results. In nonatherosclerotic rabbits, there was a progressive increase in wall changes with time and balloon diameter (Table 4.2.5 and Fig. 4.2.36).

In the atherosclerotic rabbits, the atheromatous plaques were primarily fibrous and associated with both circumferential and focal plaques (Fig. 4.2.37). The histologic and electron microscopic studies revealed no linear correlation either with balloon size or with time of inflation (Table 4.2.6). Instead, the histologic changes were governed by the thickness and location of the plaques. Fracture of plaque or dissection into the media, mainly at the edges of plaques or at sites of fracture, were seen with as little as 50% dilation for 15 seconds and were accompanied by extensive damage to the smooth muscle cells (Fig. 4.2.38). These findings were even more pronounced and accompanied by local hematoma formation when multiple plaques were present (Fig. 4.2.37). The extent of dissection did not correlate linearly with either balloon size or inflation time. Segments with minor plaque formation exhibited more stretching and compression but less medial dissection. These changes were seen best with light microscopy, since the large field facilitated comparison of various areas. Even with prolonged inflation, no plaque compression was seen; however, electron microscopy revealed superficial abrasion with production of plaque debris (Fig. 4.2.39).

Table 4.2.5. Changes in Normal Rabbits after Vessel Dilatation[a]

	15 sec		30 sec		45 sec		60 sec	
	+25%	+50%	+25%	+50%	+25%	+50%	+25%	+50%
Intima								
Focal denudation	+	+	+	+	+	+	+	+
Complete denudation	−	−	−	−	−	+	−	+
IEL								
Stretching	+	+	+	+	+	++	++	++
Fractures	−	+	−	+	+	++	+	++
Dehiscence	−	−	−	+	−	+	++	++
Abrasion	−	−	−	−	−	+	+	++
Media								
Damage to smooth muscle cells	+1	+1	+1	+3	+3	++3	+3	++3
Intercellular edema	+1	+1	+1	+1	+3	++3	+3	++3
Destruction of the elastic lamina	−	−	−	+1	−	+1	−	+2
Separation of myocytes	−	−	−	−	−	+1	−	++2
Dissection	−	−	−	−	−	−	−	−

[a]Key: + = present but limited; ++ = present and extensive; − = absent. 1 = inner one-third of media; 2 = inner two-thirds of media; 3 = entire media.

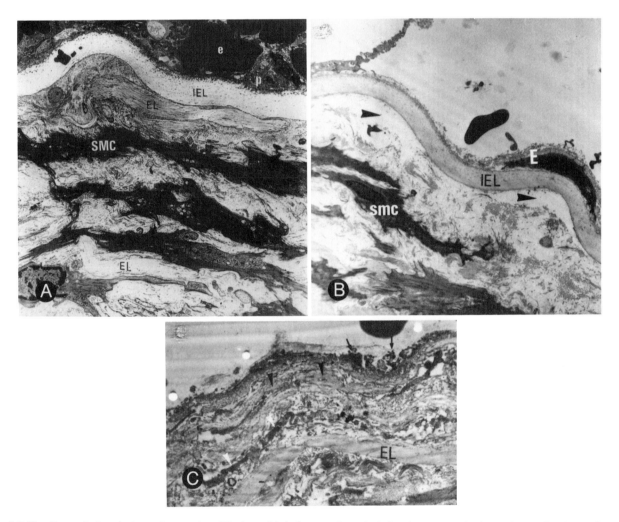

Figure 4.2.36. Transmission electron micrographs of the inner third of nonatherosclerotic, dilated aorta. Original magnification × 3000. **A.** +50%, 15 seconds; denuded endothelium is covered with thrombus. Smooth muscle cells *(SMC)* show hydropic changes, including swollen mitochondria. Otherwise, there are no definite changes in IEL and media. *EL* = elastic lamina; *P* = platelets; *e* = erythrocyte. **B.** +50%, 30 seconds; endothelium *(E)* is partially missing, and IEL has separated from media *(arrowheads)*. Note marked interstitial edema. **C.** +50%, 45 seconds; endothelium is now completely missing, and luminal surface is covered by platelets *(arrows)*. Media shows marked compression as well as fragmentation of elastic fibers *(black arrows)*. Note various grades of disintegration and other severe changes of smooth muscle cells *(white arrowheads)*. (Reproduced from Zollikofer CL, Chain J, Salomonowitz E, et al: Percutaneous transluminal angioplasty of the aorta. *Radiology* 1984;151:355–363.)

271

Figure 4.2.37. Dilated atherosclerotic aorta. H & E; original magnification × 20. **A.** +50%, 45 seconds; several focal plaques *(P)* show dehiscence at edges *(arrowheads). LA* = lumbar artery. **B.** +50%, 30 seconds; semicircular plaque with dissections at edges. Plaque-free wall shows marked stretching and thinning. Compression and stretching of plaque-free media *(M)* seems greater than in **A.** In both sections, there are no signs of plaque compression. (Reproduced from Zollikofer CL, Chain J, Salomonowitz E, et al: Percutaneous transluminal angioplasty of the aorta. *Radiology* 1984; 151:355–363.)

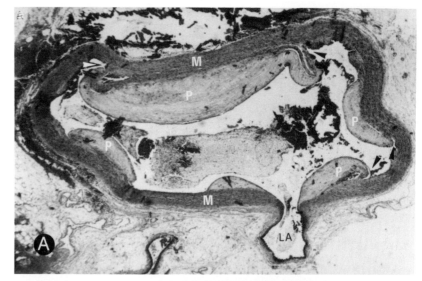

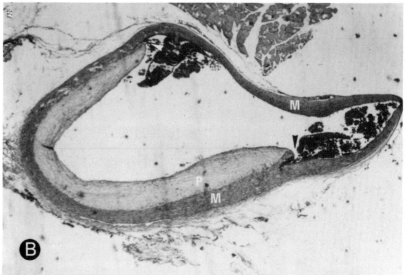

Table 4.2.6. Changes in Atherosclerotic Rabbits after Vessel Dilatation[a]

	15 sec		30 sec		45 sec		60 sec	
	+25%	+50%	+25%	+50%	+25%	+50%	+25%	+50%
Intima								
Focal denudation	+	−	−	−	−	−	−	−
Complete denudation	−	+	+	+	+	+	+	+
Plaque configuration	Circumferential	Circumferential	Circumferential	Semicircular ("horseshoe")	Semicircular ("horseshoe")	Multiple focal plaques	Multiple focal plaques	Multiple focal plaques
Plaque compression	−	−	−	−	−	−	−	−
Plaque fracture or splitting	−	+	−	−	−	−	−	−
Plaque dehiscence	−	+	+ +	+	−	+[c]	+[c]	+[c]
IEL								
Stretching	−	+	+ +	+ +	+ +	+[c]	+[c]	+[c]
Fractures	−	+	+ +	+ +	+	+[c]	+[c]	+[c]
Dehiscence	−	−	+ +	+ +	+	+[c]	+[c]	+[c]
Media[b]								
Damage to smooth muscle cells	−	+ +	+ +	+ +	+	+[c]	+ +[c]	+ +[c]
Compression	−	+	+ +	+ +	+ +	+[c]	+[c]	+[c]
Dissection	−	+ +	+ +	+	+	+ +[c]	+ +[c]	+ +[c]

[a]Key: + = present but limited; + + = present and extensive; − = absent.
[b]Multiple plaques.
[c]Changes seen only in areas of plaque and dehiscence or dissection or plaque-free areas.

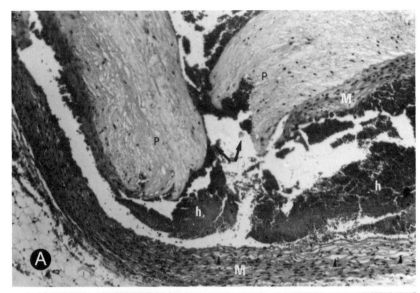

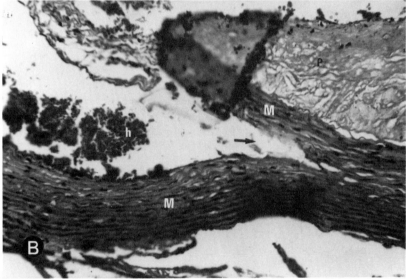

Figure 4.2.38. Dilated atherosclerotic aorta. **A.** + 50%, 15 seconds; rupture of plaque *(P; arrows)*, with dissection and compression of media *(M)*. Note pyknosis of nuclei of smooth muscle cells and increased space between elastic laminae that is filled with edema fluid *(arrowheads)*. There is a hematoma *(h)* within dissection. H & E; original magnification × 80. **B.** +25%, 30 seconds; dissection into media *(M)* at edge of plaque *(P, arrow)*. There are corkscrew nuclei in damaged smooth muscle cells and edema in medial layers. *H* = hematoma. H & E; original magnification × 150. (Reproduced from Zollikofer CL, Chain J, Salomonowitz E, et al: Percutaneous transluminal angioplasty of the aorta. *Radiology* 1984;151:355–363.)

Discussion. The current study again revealed that histologic changes in the nonatherosclerotic arterial wall after balloon dilatation are related to the size of the balloon and the duration of inflation, progressing in an approximately linear fashion as these factors increase. In contrast, histologic changes in atherosclerotic vessels are governed by the thickness and location of the plaques. That is, with a thick plaque, the underlying media remains unchanged. However, the wall is stretched in plaque-free areas and sites of dehiscence or rupture, and there is a tendency toward medial dissection, the extent of which correlates to only a limited degree with balloon size or length of inflation. This dissection is usually seen at the edges of the plaque or sites of rupture. Most likely, the force the dilating balloon exerts on the edge of the plaque causes dehiscence followed by rupture of the underlying tissues into the media. The wall of the atherosclerotic artery becomes stretched between the individual plaques, unlike normal arteries, in which the entire wall is stretched uniformly. This means that, in a way, the plaque protects the underlying media. Similar findings were described by Faxon et al. in a study of three rabbit models of atherosclerosis.[87] The results of the current study also confirm the observations made in cadaver arteries, that in atherosclerotic disease with circumferential plaque, luminal widening can be accomplished only by cracking or rupture of the plaque. This study also clearly demonstrated that the wall of an atherosclerotic artery is more vulnerable than that of a normal vessel, as shown by the fact that changes penetrating into the media occur even with small balloons and short inflation times.

Although with extensive atherosclerosis, increased stretching results in greater plaque dehiscence and rupture accompanied by more pronounced medial dissection, which is in accord with observations in clinical PTA,[88–90] the current study showed that neither the amount nor the

Figure 4.2.39. Transmission electron micrograph of dilated atherosclerotic aorta (+50%; 30 seconds). Original magnification × 8000. Luminal surfaces of plaques show abrasion of superficial elements *(arrowheads)* and denudation of endothelium. No definite signs of compression. *e* = erythrocytes. (Reproduced from Zollikofer CL, Chain J, Salomonowitz E, et al: Percutaneous transluminal angioplasty of the aorta. *Radiology* 1984; 151:355–363.)

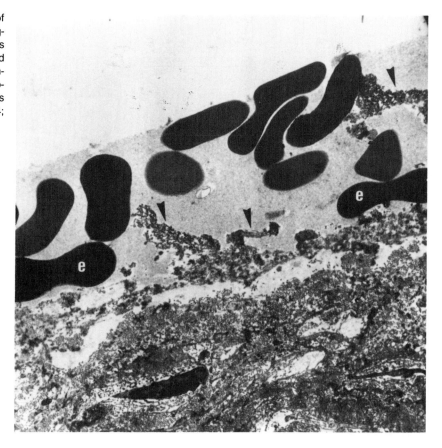

duration of the balloon dilatation necessarily correlated with the nature and extent of histologically visible damage to the wall of atherosclerotic arteries. In spite of the increased overall vulnerability of the atherosclerotic vessel, intimal and medial dissections remained limited to the dilated region; they measured 2–8mm and were always oriented parallel to the long axis of the vessel. Occluding intimal flaps were not observed, and intramural hematomas remained localized, without formation of dissecting aneurysms. In accord with the authors' findings in atherosclerotic cadaver arteries, and also with the findings of other investigators,[85–87,91] no signs of plaque compression could be detected. However, the observation of endothelial abrasion and desquamation of superficial plaque elements is important because of the possibility of distal embolization, which is probably common, although silent. The incidence of embolization in peripheral angioplasty is only 3–5%.[92,93] When clinically evident, it is probably the result of complete plaque dehiscence rather than of atherosclerotic debris.[94] Although marked intimal and medial splitting and partial plaque dehiscence were observed, neither peripheral embolization of the plaques nor true dissection producing an intimal hematoma large enough to obstruct the lumen was seen.

Because of the more complex conditions in human atherosclerosis, extrapolation of the findings in this animal model may legitimately be criticized. Human atherosclerotic lesions have significantly greater amounts of necrosis and calcifications. Also, the media often is involved to an extensive degree, with substantial alteration and thinning of this layer. No calcified lesions could be provoked in this model; the atheromas were mainly fibrous, similar to the models described by Faxon et al.[72,73] and LeVeen et al.[95] In addition, the present authors were able to initiate focal, cushion-like atheromas by mechanically damaging the endothelium prior to feeding the cholesterol diet. With this technique, the results of their animal experiments have closely paralleled the histologic findings after clinical angioplasty.

In summary, the following conclusions can be drawn from this study:

The mechanism of PTA is multifactorial, the result of a combination of rupture and dissection of the atheromatous plaque together with stretching of the plaque-free arterial wall segments. There is some desquamation of superficial plaque elements.

The wall of the atherosclerotic vessel is much more vulnerable than that of the normal artery.

Because of the limited correlation of balloon size and duration of inflation with the arterial wall damage in atherosclerosis and the difference in the tissue quality of the arterial wall in the animal model and human atherosclerosis, this study does not allow a definite recommendation on optimal balloon size and duration of inflation in clinical PTA.

Morphology of the Vasa Vasorum after PTA[50,96–98]

As stated earlier, the vasa vasorum are responsible for oxygenation of the outer layers of the media and adventitia in the central, elastic, and larger muscular arteries, whereas the intima and inner media are oxygenated by direct diffusion from the blood stream. This fact renders the middle media a critical area with regard to oxygenation, because thickening of the intima, as in atherosclerosis, must reduce this diffusion capacity. Geiringer found the maximum thickness of the intima at which the inner media is still adequately oxygenated by diffusion to be 0.5mm.[99] Thereafter, further thickening leads to proliferation of the vasa vasorum into the intima, thus increasing the blood flow in the vessel wall.[99,100] This phenomenon of vascularization of the intima and media was confirmed in animal studies by Heistad et al.[101] The importance of the vasa vasorum was further substantiated by Wilens et al., who were able to induce medial necrosis of the aorta by blocking the blood supply to the vasa vasorum.[43] Possibly, atherosclerotic changes in the vasa vasorum are a causative factor in the pathogenesis of atherosclerotic aneurysm formation.[102] Because angioplasty induces severe changes in the intima and media, it is conceivable that the blood supply to the arterial wall could be jeopardized by this procedure. Therefore, theoretically, PTA-induced injury of the vasa vasorum could provoke late complications such as aneurysms or medial necrosis. To investigate the impact of PTA on the microcirculation of the blood vessel wall, the authors studied the morphology of the vasa vasorum using a latex infusion technique before and after angioplasty in normal canine arteries as well as in human cadaver arteries.

Materials and Methods

Thoracic and abdominal aortic segments in three anesthetized dogs were dilated with 50–100% oversized Grüntzig balloons at 4 atm of inflation pressure. An additional three dogs underwent dilatation of aortic segments to >100% oversize.

Three specimens of human cadaver abdominal aorta including the iliofemoral arteries were excised at autopsy. After roentgenologic location of the stenotic areas in the barium-filled specimens, the vessels were flushed clear with saline. The stenotic segments were then dilated using two 9mm balloons for the aorta and a 12- or 8mm balloon for the iliac vessels (>100%).

After death, the dilated vessels of the dogs were clamped proximally and distally, and large visceral branches of the aorta were ligated in situ. In the cadaver specimens, all visceral branches and lumbar arteries were ligated after angioplasty. A latex solution (Campton Biomedical Products, Inc.; Boulder, CO) was infused into the canine vessels in situ and into the cadaver specimens at 120mm Hg during 10 minutes. After preparation, the latex-filled canine vessels were excised. Together with the cadaver arteries, the specimens were processed by the clearing technique of Spalteholz (alcohol dehydration and methylsalicylate) for macroscopic and microscopic examination.

Results

Canine arteries. The morphology of the vasa vasorum of a nondilated aorta is shown in Figure 4.2.40A. Most of the vasa vasorum originate from the lumbar arteries, close to the aorta. In cross-section, the vasa vasorum can be seen to run from the surface of the adventitia toward the outer third of the media, at which site they end in several ramifications (Fig. 4.2.40B).

In the specimens dilated to no more than 80% oversize, no definite alteration in the morphology or penetration of the vasa vasorum was noted. No tears were detectable in

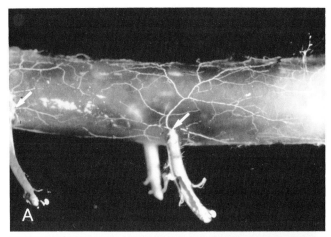

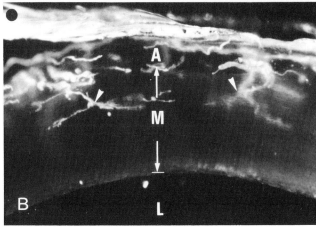

Figure 4.2.40. Nondilated canine thoracic aorta after latex infusion. **A.** Extensive network of vasa vasorum arising from intercostal arteries *(arrows)*. **B.** Cross-section shows adventitial vasa vasorum reaching and branching into outer media *(arrowheads)*. A = adventitia; M = media; L = lumen. (Reproduced from Cragg AH, Einzig S, Rysavy JA, Castañeda-Zúñiga WR, Borgwardt B, Amplatz K: The vasa vasorum and angioplasty. *Radiology* 1983;148:75–80.)

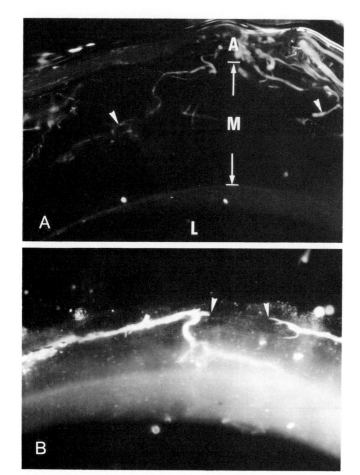

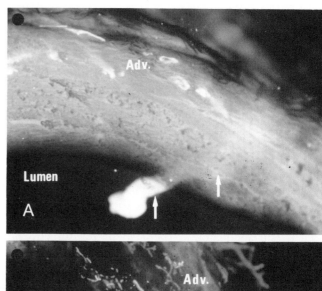

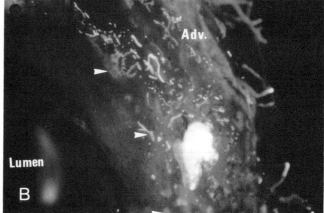

Figure 4.2.41. Canine aorta after latex infusion. **A.** Cross-section after 80% dilatation shows adventitial vasa vasorum running into outer media. Branching and structure of vasa vasorum in outer media appear intact *(arrowheads).* A = adventitia; M = media; L = lumen. **B.** Thinning of wall and severe stretching of vasa vasorum with rupture *(arrowheads)* after >100% dilatation.

Figure 4.2.42. Nondilated human abdominal aorta after latex infusion. **A.** Cross-section shows vasa vasorum penetrating from adventitia through to lumen *(arrows).* **B.** Cross-section shows bush-like ramifications and proliferation of vasa vasorum *(arrowheads),* which show marked caliber changes. P3 = calcified plaque; Adv. = adventitia.

the small peripheral branches of the vasa vasorum (Fig. 4.2.41A). In contrast, overdilatation by 100% or more produced definite changes, with marked stretching or rupture of the vasa vasorum in areas of significant thinning of the aortic wall (Fig. 4.2.41B).

Human cadaver arteries. Nondilated segments with pronounced intimal plaques showed abundant proliferation of the vasa vasorum, some of which penetrated through the intima into the lumen (Fig. 4.2.42A). The bush-like ramifications of the vasa vasorum were of irregular caliber with multiple ectasias (Fig. 4.2.42B). In the dilated segments, the findings were practically identical; but in addition, the vasa vasorum had been severed at sites where the intimal plaques had been ruptured by angioplasty (Fig. 4.2.43).

Discussion

Significant overdilatation of a nonatherosclerotic aortic wall may severely damage the integrity of the vasa vaso-

rum. Nevertheless, follow-up angiograms as much as six weeks later did not show any evidence of aneurysm formation.

Despite the lack of morphologic changes in the vasa vasorum in canine arteries dilated <100%, Cragg and coworkers found a significant change in vessel wall perfusion after PTA, with a striking increase in blood flow over more than four hours.[96-98] Similarly Train et al. described three cases of fine perivascular networks visible on angiography after clinical PTA, which they interpret as the vasa vasorum.[103] However, these minute vessels run at some distance along the mother artery and therefore may also represent adventitial collaterals. The present authors were never able, either in living canine or in human cadaver arteries, to demonstrate the intramural vasa vasorum angiographically after PTA. Indeed, the vasa vasorum of the inner adventitia and the media are below the limit of angiographic resolution. Nevertheless, it can be argued that through the same mediators that cause hyperemia of

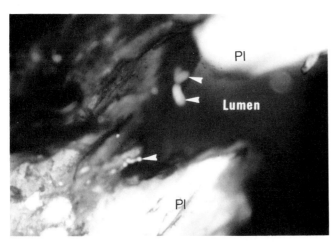

Figure 4.2.43. Dilated human iliac artery after latex infusion. Cross-section shows area with rupture of plaque *(Pl)*. Multiple vasa vasorum *(arrowheads)* end in lumen where plaque has been ruptured.

the vasa vasorum, dilatation of the adventitial collaterals also may be provoked.

The effects on the atherosclerotic cadaver vessels were difficult to distinguish. The nondilated atherosclerotic artery showed a very irregular pattern of the vasa vasorum, with vessel cut-offs, so only severance of the vasa vasorum at sites of plaque rupture could be definitely attributed to the dilating trauma. However, it is conceivable that advanced atherosclerosis with extensive proliferation of vasa vasorum throughout the arterial wall layers has a propensity for intramural hematoma formation after PTA. This, again, may be a cause of early reocclusion in clinical angioplasty.

Summary and Conclusions

The permanent widening of the arterial lumen by PTA could be the result of one or more of the following[104]:

1. Compression of the atherosclerotic plaque;
2. Redistribution of the plaque;
3. Embolization of the plaque;
4. Regression of plaque secondary to phagocytosis or metabolic changes; and
5. Stretching of the arterial wall.

In the authors' studies on cadaver arteries and atherosclerotic animals, no significant compression or redistribution was found. This has been confirmed by other investigators.[56,81,85–87] Compression of an atherosclerotic plaque is not possible without simultaneous extrusion of liquid constituents. This may be possible with "soft" edematous atheromas or relatively fresh thrombi[36,105,106]; however, according to the experimental results of Chin et al. in atherosclerotic cadaver arteries, the expressible liquid contents of the plaque amount to no more than 12% of the total lumen increase, and the portion of the lumen increase attributable to plaque compression is <2%.[56] Hence, 87–

93% of the total lumen increase results from rupture of the plaque and stretching and tearing of the media and adventitia. This rule does not apply to fibrinous thrombotic deposits with little cellular attachment to the intima; such deposits are pulverized by balloon compression and carried downstream by the blood without sequelae.[106] According to the current experiments, redistribution of plaque occurs only with the use of dilating Teflon catheters according to the original Dotter method, but not when using balloon catheters. With the former, the axial (forward) force of the dilating catheter may displace atheromatous material by a snowplow effect.[8,13]

Peripheral embolization is encountered in 3–5% of clinical PTA procedures and is often asymptomatic.[92,93,107] According to the authors' experimental studies, only superficial plaque elements are loosened, so their loss does not significantly increase the arterial lumen.[82,108] Clinically significant embolization, therefore, is the result of a completely detached atheromatous plaque or of dislocation of relatively fresh thrombi.

After dilatation of normal arteries, only occasional macrophages were encountered, and no significant phagocytosis of necrotic wall material could be detected.[59] Also, in long-term studies in atherosclerotic animals, there were no signs of significant phagocytosis of atherosclerotic wall constituents after PTA.[72,73,86]

Hence, stretching of the arterial wall is the principal mechanism for permanent widening of the arterial lumen after PTA. Since atheromatous plaques are essentially noncompressible and nonelastic, this stretching is possible only after rupture and partial detachment of the plaque. The increasing balloon diameter leads to tears and crevices in the plaque at its weakest point. Once the cuirass-like plaque has been torn, the freed parts of the media and adventitia are stretched by the further increase in the balloon diameter. This mechanism has been proved by the present authors' studies on cadavers and atherosclerotic animal arteries[47,49,82] and has been confirmed several times by other authors.[72,73,81,87,88] In addition, histologic findings in human arteries after successful clinical angioplasty parallel the findings in experimental angioplasty (Figs. 4.2.44 through 4.2.46). However, in severe atherosclerosis involving the entire wall with thinning of the media, it is not always possible to recognize wall changes after clinical PTA.[75,109]

The dilating effect (wall stretching) in normal canine or rabbit artery is directly proportional to the size of the balloon as well as to the duration and pressure of balloon inflation. Unfortunately, this is not true in the atherosclerotic vessel. Although the authors found a general tendency toward progressive wall damage with increasing balloon diameter and inflation time, there was no predictable correlation due to the greater vulnerability and the heterogeneous behavior of the atherosclerotic vessel. They therefore can give no definite recommendation on the ideal bal-

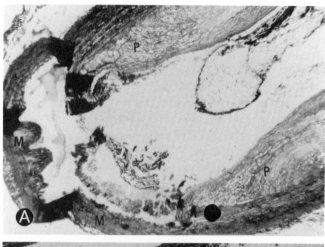

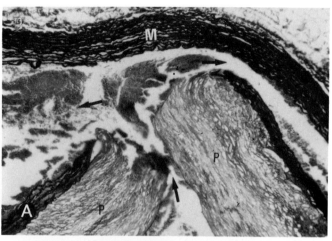

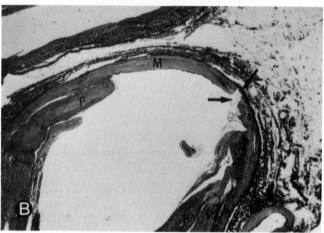

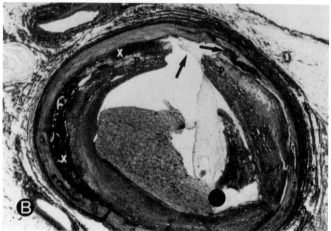

Figure 4.2.44. Atherosclerotic rabbit aorta after 50% overdilatation for 60 seconds (**A**) and human femoral artery 5 days after transluminal angioplasty (**B**). In both instances, there is stretching, with rupture of media at places where it is free of plaque *(arrows)*. M = media, P = plaque. (Courtesy of PD. Dr. J. Schneider, Department of Pathology, University Hospital, Zurich.)

Figure 4.2.45. Atherosclerotic rabbit aorta after 50% overdilatation for 15 seconds (**A**) and human femoral artery 5 days after transluminal angioplasty (**B**). In both cases, there is rupture of plaque *(P)* and dissection into media *(M) (arrows)*. In addition, the case of clinical PTA shows marked dehiscence of plaque from media. Spaces of dehiscence are filled with thrombi *(x)*. (Courtesy of PD. Dr. J. Schneider, Department of Pathology, University Hospital, Zurich.)

loon size and duration of inflation for clinical PTA, although there is a difference between treating circumferential and asymmetric, cushion-like atheromas (Fig. 4.2.47). That is, with an asymmetric, localized plaque, a comparatively low balloon pressure may significantly stretch those parts of the arterial wall with little atheromatous involvement, whereas in a severe circumferential stenosis, the plaque must be torn by the dilating balloon before the arterial wall can stretch (Fig. 4.2.47*B,C*). The smaller the plaque-free area of the arterial wall, the greater the local wall-stretching at this site needed to enlarge the arterial lumen to a given degree (Fig. 4.2.47*B, C*). Simultaneously, the danger of wall rupture increases. Therefore, careful analysis of the angiogram is important to avoid overstretching the artery.

As demonstrated in the authors' experiments in normal canine arteries,[47,59] postangioplasty healing of the arterial wall occurs with fibrotic scar formation in the media and

hyperplasia in the intima secondary to widespread stimulation and migration of smooth muscle cells. Even severe stretching of the arterial wall with complete disruption of the medial layers does not result in significant localized aneurysm formation in the patent lumen, and healing without aneurysm formation can be expected as long as the adventitia is not too severely damaged.

The process of healing in the atherosclerotic vessel cannot be followed as easily, although it is apparent that scar formation and intimal hyperplasia are not of the same nature as in normal vessels. Faxon et al. found the atherosclerotic process to be accelerated following angioplasty of rabbit arteries[72,73]; restenoses and thrombotic occlusion in various stages of organization were apparent four weeks after angioplasty. The thickened neointima was of a more complex nature than the intimal hyperplasia found in nonatherosclerotic vessels. The study also suggested that intraluminal thrombosis plays a significant role in reocclusion

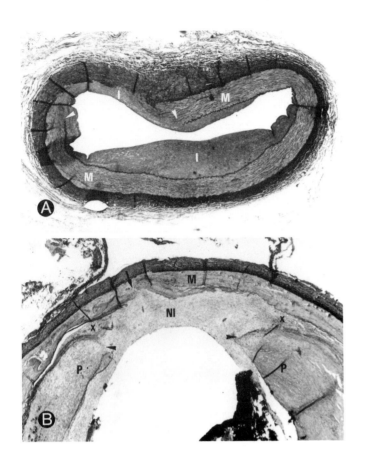

Figure 4.2.46. Canine iliac artery 4 months after >100% overdilatation (**A**) and human superficial femoral artery 44 days after transluminal angioplasty (**B**). In the canine artery, there is focal rupture of media *(M)* and IEL *(arrowheads)*. Defect is covered by neointima and medial scar *(I)*, which merges with nonruptured medial areas. In the human artery, plaque rupture is clearly noticeable *(arrowheads)*. Focally ossified media is partially torn *(arrow)*. Rupture has been covered by thick neointima *(NI)*, which has also filled spaces and crevices of original plaque *(P)* dehiscence *(x)*, thereby smoothing luminal surface. Much as in the animal experiment, the new intima may serve as a compensatory layer where arterial wall had been partially ruptured. (Courtesy of PD. Dr. J. Schneider, Department of Pathology, University Hospital, Zurich.)

after angioplasty, because administration of antiplatelet drugs significantly reduced restenoses and reocclusions.[72] In clinical PTA, also, antiplatelet drugs and anticoagulants significantly improved the patency rate.[110–116]

In clinical practice, the higher stenosis recurrence rate after dilatation of smaller (e.g., coronary) arteries may be due to thrombosis or to an accelerated atherosclerotic process secondary to release of platelet factors. According to the authors' experimental findings, recurrence of stenosis may also be due to intimal hyperplasia; and this seems especially likely if a nonatherosclerotic stenosis has not been dilated sufficiently. Intimal hyperplasia causing restenosis after PTA of an atherosclerotic stenosis has not been definitely shown. However, occasionally, uncommonly long and rapidly occurring restenoses are found at the site of previous angioplasty. Such recurrences are attributed to a reaction of the intima and media.[117]

Extrapolation of the results of experimental atherosclerosis in rabbits to human atherosclerosis may be criticized because of the differences in the nature and complexity of the human disease. Therefore, in spite of the many animal experiments, the exact mechanism of healing and smoothing of the arterial wall after clinical PTA has not been clarified. The few examinations of human arteries following clinical PTA have revealed bridging of the plaque ruptures and medial tears by a neointima that probably represents organized thrombus (Fig. 4.2.46*B*).

The radiolucent linear filling defects seen in postdilatation angiograms could also be demonstrated in vitro after angioplasty of cadaver arteries. These radiolucent lines correspond to the crevices in the atherosclerotic plaque and sites of dehiscence of the thickened intima from the media. In advanced atherosclerosis, intima and media both may be partly dehisced from the adventitia. Similar filling defects were found in the animal experiments. In the atherosclerotic rabbits, a widening of the lumen was regularly accompanied by dehiscence or rupture of the plaque, proving that such dehiscence and rupture are integral parts of successful dilatation. Angiographically and histologically, these phenomena differ from true intraluminal dissections, because they are confined to the dilatation site and do not have a tendency to propagate. Therefore, rupture and dehiscence of plaques should not be interpreted as complications of PTA as long as there is no obstruction to flow or detachment of the plaque.[57] According to the histologic findings in the animal experiments, the degree of dehiscence of atherosclerotic plaques that is seen angiographically probably depends on both the amount of dilatation (balloon size, pressure, duration of inflation) and the nature and configuration of the atherosclerotic plaques. However, the present authors do not agree with Roth et al.[117] that a rupture or dehiscence limited to the intimal plaque can be differentiated angiographically from a penetrating dehiscence that includes the media. In advanced atherosclerosis, the media is usually markedly thinned and involved in the pathologic process, so it is likely that this layer frequently is included to some extent in the rupture and dehiscence (Figs. 4.2.44 through 4.2.46).

Simultaneously with the healing process, at which time the crevices and clefts in the plaque are covered by a neointima (organized thrombi), smoothing of the contours is visible angiographically. Additional widening of the artery visible on follow-up angiograms over several months is probably caused by adaptation to blood flow. That is, once the media and adventitia are freed from the encasing atherosclerotic plaque (as after endarterectomy), the stretched arterial wall may dilate further as a response to the demand for increased blood flow. Enlargement of the lumen because of shrinkage (fibrosis) and metabolic degradation of atheromatous material are additional possible mechanisms for long-term patency.[36,106,118]

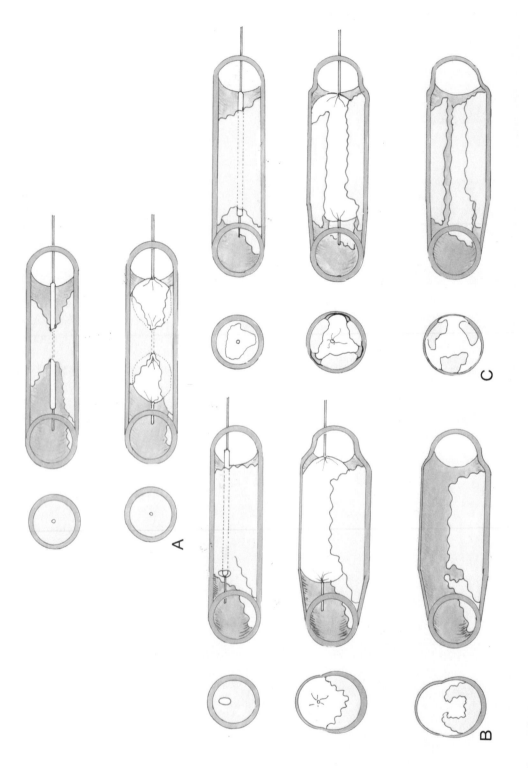

Figure 4.2.47. Mechanisms of PTA. **A.** Schematic drawing of mechanism with high-grade circular stenosis. *Above,* high-grade circumferential stenosis has been crossed with dilating balloon. *Below,* inflation of balloon. As long as atheromatous plaque cannot be torn, the lumen cannot widen; the balloon merely expands proximal and distal to stenosis, forming a waistline. **B.** Schematic drawing of mechanism with high-grade eccentric stenosis. *Above,* stenosis has been crossed by dilatation catheter. *Center,* inflated balloon has ruptured plaque at its weakest area; freed media and adventitia can now be stretched. *Below,* after dilatation, the widened lumen stays open. Plaque shows longitudinal dehiscence at edges where plaque has been ruptured. **C.** Schematic drawing of mechanism with irregular stenosis. *Above,* stenosis has been crossed by balloon catheter. *Center,* with inflation of the balloon, there is rupture of plaque in several places, with local wall stretching. *Below,* lumen increase after rupture and local dehiscence of plaque with stretching of the wall in plaque-free areas.

Pharmacologic Phenomena and Metabolic Changes of the Arterial Wall after PTA

It was the authors' hypothesis that the response of dilated arteries to vasoactive substances is altered by the destruction of contractile elements and by the scar formation and medial fibrosis seen in their animal experiments. To verify this hypothesis, vasoconstriction of dilated and nondilated canine arteries in response to vasopressin was tested. According to the studies of Cragg and coworkers, which showed significant hyperemia of the arterial wall after PTA,[96] they further postulated that metabolic changes as well as the direct mechanical trauma were responsible for paralysis of the arterial wall after angioplasty. Therefore, they investigated potential alterations in arachidonic acid metabolism in normal canine arteries.

Paralysis of the Arterial Wall after PTA[119]

Materials and Methods

In this pilot study, carotid and iliac arteries in anesthetized dogs were dilated with Grüntzig balloons 80–100% larger than the original lumen as measured on the angiogram. Dilatations were performed twice for 1 minute at an inflation pressure of 4 atm. The arterial lumen was again measured, and 0.2–0.4 unit of vasopressin (Pitressin; Parke–Davis) was infused per minute until the mean arterial pressure had risen by 10mm Hg. At this time, the angiogram was repeated, and the dilated lumen was compared with that on the postdilatation angiogram. In two dogs, angiography was repeated before and after administration of vasopressin two months after PTA.

Results

As in the previously described studies, luminal widening was frequently accompanied by spasms adjacent to the dilated segments (Fig. 4.2.48A,B). After vasopressin administration, the dilated segments remained unchanged. However, the tendency toward proximal and distal constriction increased, and these areas now covered several centimeters (Fig. 4.2.48C). At follow-up, the wall paralysis persisted after administration of vasopressin (Fig. 4.2.49). Again, definite constriction of the nondilated areas was apparent.

Discussion

As discussed earlier, the mechanism of luminal widening in PTA consists of a controlled injury to the arterial wall. The immediate trauma to the media obviously prevents vasoconstriction of the dilated segments. This condition may persist for months if there has been sufficient damage to the media, with fibrous scarring and permanent loss of elastic elements. The authors' results were recently confirmed by Wolf and coworkers,[120] who found that in rabbit

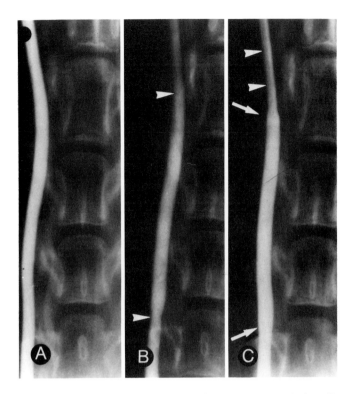

Figure 4.2.48. Paralysis after PTA. **A.** Carotid arteriogram before dilatation. **B.** Angiogram immediately after dilatation; luminal widening is 22%. Note local vasoconstriction proximal and distal to dilated segment *(arrowheads)*. **C.** Angiogram after dilatation and administration of vasopressin. No change in widening of dilated segment *(between arrows)*; contraction in the adjacent segments, especially distally, has progressed *(arrowheads)*. (Reproduced from Castañeda–Zúñiga WR, Laerum F, Rysavy J, Rusnak B, Amplatz K: Paralysis of arteries by intraluminal balloon dilatation. *Radiology* 1982;144:75–76.)

aortas, wall paralysis depends on the extent of dilatation, with 50% overdilation abolishing vasoconstriction. However, these findings in normal animal vessels are difficult to confirm in human arteries.

The spontaneous spasm-like contractions proximal and distal to the dilated segments seen in this and earlier studies were unexpected. Histologically, these areas were damaged to a significantly lesser degree than the dilated segment itself and responded to vasoactive drugs. The phenomenon may be explained by the work of Price et al.[121] and Tallaride et al.,[122] who showed a direct correlation between the state of stretch of the arterial wall and the vasoconstrictor response. The studies of Wolf et al. further showed that slight stretching in vitro enhances the vasoconstrictor response, whereas great stretching attenuates the vasoconstriction response to both depolarizing agents (potassium) and receptor-mediated agonists (norepinephrine).[123] It is therefore conceivable that with only limited stretching of the media in the areas adjacent to the dilated arterial segments, such a mechanism causes spontaneous vasoconstriction. These observations are also important with regard to clinical PTA, where spasms are not uncommon in spite of advanced atherosclerosis with calcification and may lead to early thrombotic reocclu-

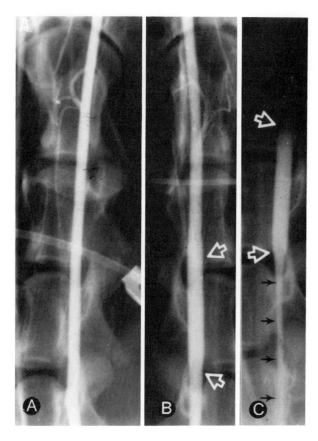

Figure 4.2.49. Persisting paralysis after PTA. **A.** Carotid artery angiogram before dilatation. **B.** Angiogram immediately after dilatation shows widening of dilated segment *(between arrows).* **C.** Follow-up angiogram after two months shows persisting paralysis of dilated segment *(between open arrows)* during infusion of vasopressin. Note severe contraction of adjacent proximal nondilated segment *(small arrows).* (Reproduced from Castañeda–Zúñiga WR, Laerum F, Rysavy J, Rusnak B, Amplatz K: Paralysis of arteries by intraluminal balloon dilatation. *Radiology* 1982; 144:75–76.)

sion.[24,83,107,112,124–126] For this reason, especially in renal and coronary angioplasty, prophylactic administration of vasodilating drugs (i.e., nifedipine, nitroglycerin) is recommended.[83,125,127] Furthermore, on the basis of the authors' experimental findings and the study by Wolf and Lentini,[123] vasodilating drugs seem especially indicated in PTA of nonatherosclerotic disease.

Because the reduction of the vasoconstrictor response is roughly proportional to the effectiveness of the stretch, Wolf et al. discuss the possibility that this response might be used to determine the endpoint of clinical PTA.[120] However, on the basis of the present authors' observations of frequent spontaneous spasms adjacent to sites of dilation, they consider this maneuver dangerous and contraindicated, especially for nonatherosclerotic vessels, where contractability is not compromised by atherosclerotic plaque.

Role of Prostaglandins after PTA[128]

In the animal studies by Cragg et al., an increase in vessel wall blood flow after PTA was demonstrated (Fig. 4.2.50).[97,98] The segments directly adjacent to the dilated areas also showed increasing flow although to a lesser degree and for a shorter time (Fig. 4.2.50). When acetylsalicylic acid (ASA) was given intravenously before angioplasty, vessel wall hyperemia was significantly attenuated when compared to the controls (283 vs. 2356%) (Fig. 4.2.51). On the basis of these studies, it was concluded that vessel wall hyperemia was caused by release of vasoactive compounds as well as by the effects of mechanical damage. Because post-PTA hyperemia could be influenced by ASA, which is a cyclooxygenase blocker, it was further hypothesized that prostaglandins play a key role in changing the vasoactive response. Such an effect is of particular clinical

Figure 4.2.50. Sequential vessel wall blood flow (VWBF) measurements up to four hours using radioactive microspheres (group 1). Dramatic increase (+ 1200%) in blood flow in dilated carotid artery persisted throughout experiment. Briefer rise in VWBF is also found in segments directly adjacent to dilatation site. No elevation of blood flow in the thoracic aorta. (Reproduced from Cragg AH, Einzig S, Rysavy JA, Castañeda–Zúñiga WR, Borwardt B, Amplatz K: The vasa vasorum and angioplasty. *Radiology* 1983;148:75–80.)

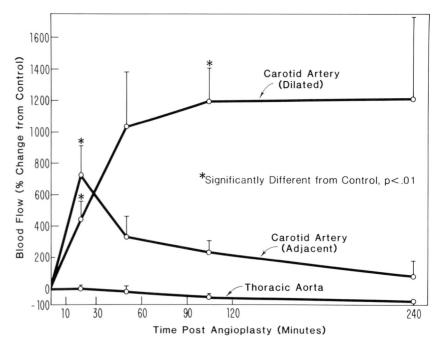

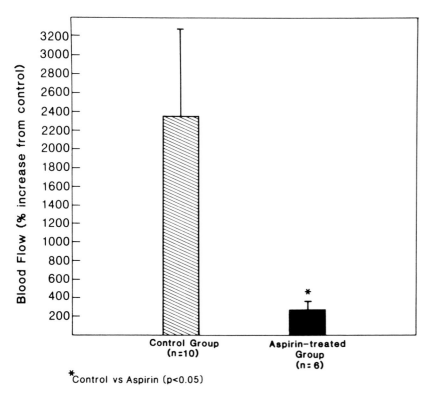

Figure 4.2.51. Vessel wall blood flow measurement using radioactive microspheres 60 minutes after angioplasty. ASA significantly attenuates increase produced by angioplasty (2356 vs. 283%). (Reproduced from Cragg A, Einzig S, Rysavy J, Castañeda–Zúñiga WR, Borwardt B, Amplatz K: Effect of aspirin on angioplasty-induced vessel wall hyperemia. *AJR* 1983;140:1233–1238.)

interest, because cyclooxygenase inhibitors such as ASA are recommended to prevent platelet aggregation after PTA.[23,28,116,127,129] Cyclooxygenase inhibitors prevent synthesis of the proaggregating thromboxane A_2 (TXA_2) in platelets by blocking the conversion of arachidonic acid into the unstable intermediate endoperoxide (PG) H_2. Likewise, PGI_2, which is formed in the blood vessels, is also synthesized from PGH_2.[130,131] Therefore, ASA blocks not only the formation of TXA_2, but also the antiaggregating and vasodilating effects of PGI_2 (Fig. 4.2.52). It may be postulated then, that the attenuation of post-PTA vessel wall hyperemia by ASA reflects a direct influence of this drug on PGI_2 production in the arterial wall. If indeed PGI_2 is produced and released by the damaged vessel wall after PTA, this would be beneficial and so should not be blocked. The following experiments were performed to investigate this hypothesis.

MATERIALS AND METHODS

Carotid arteries in anesthetized dogs were dilated with Grüntzig-type polyethylene balloon catheters three times for one minute each time at 4.5 atm of inflation pressure. The balloon diameters were 25–100% larger than the arterial lumen, as measured on a baseline angiogram. The dilated segments were divided into three groups:

Group A: Six arteries dilated to 50–100% above normal size and studied within six hours;
Group B: Three arteries dilated to 25–30% above normal size, of which two were studied 24 hours after dilation and one after 1 week;

Group C: Four arteries dilated to 70–100% above normal size, of which two were studied at 24 hours, one after 1 week, and one after 3 months.

Eight nondilated arteries served as controls (group D). Dilated and control segments were carefully excised and cut into rings 3mm wide. These were attached to a transducer, which measures isometric contractile force (ICF) in grams, and then suspended in an organ bath containing

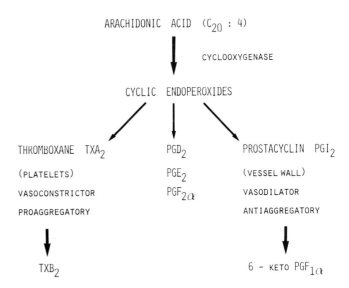

Figure 4.2.52. Metabolism of arachidonic acid, showing synthesis of prostacyclin (*PGI₂*) and thomboxane (*TXA₂*) and their stable derivatives. (Reproduced from Zollikofer C, Cragg A, Einzig S, et al: Prostaglandins and angioplasty. *Radiology* 1983;149:681–685.)

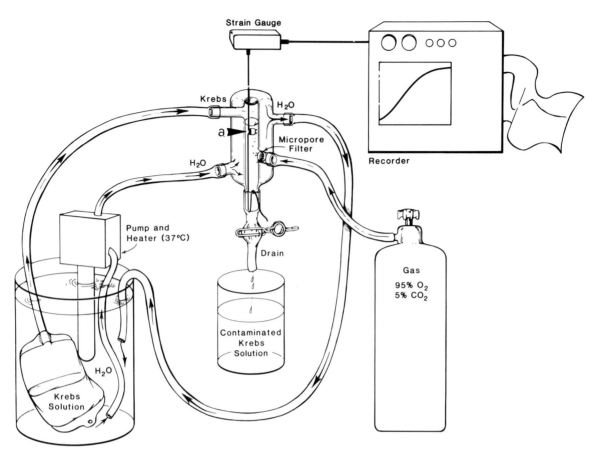

Figure 4.2.53. System used to measure isometric contractile force of carotid arterial rings. Ring *(a)* is suspended in organ bath. Oxygenated Krebs' solution is kept at constant temperature of 7 °C by perfusion pump. Contractions measured by strain gauge are displayed on fiberoptic strip-chart recorder. (Reproduced from Zollikofer C, Cragg A, Einzig S, et al: Prostaglandins and angioplasty. *Radiology* 1983;149:681–685.)

buffered Krebs' solution (Fig. 4.2.53). After sequential administration of 30ng, 100ng, and 1 μg of norepinephrine/ml to the bath, the ICF was measured. The bath was then changed, 3 μg of indomethacin was added per ml, and contraction was again measured after administration of the same norepinephrine doses. Any increased contraction following indomethacin administration was compared with short- and long-term studies and analyzed using Student's paired and unpaired t tests.

RESULTS

As expected, the normal arterial rings exhibited progressive increases in ICF with increasing doses of norepinephrine. Contraction increased significantly when indomethacin was added (Fig. 4.2.54*A*), with the maximum ICF rising from a mean ($\pm$ SE) of 3.71 ± 0.29 to 4.63 ± 0.37g ($p < 0.02$) (Table 4.2.7). Of the dilated arteries, those in group A showed significantly decreased contraction compared with the controls (0.95 ± 0.11 vs. 3.71 ± 0.29g; $p < 0.01$). In the presence of indomethacin, contraction rose to 2.84 ± 0.25g ($p < 0.001$) (Fig. 4.2.54*B* and Table 4.2.7). Although the absolute contraction with indometh-

acin was lower than in the controls, the average percentage increase was 10 times greater in the dilated arteries (468 vs. 42%; $p < 0.01$).

The percentage increase in contraction due to indomethacin in all groups is shown in Table 4.2.8 and Figure 4.2.55. In group B, there was no significant difference from the controls before or after indomethicin administration (Tables 4.2.7 and 4.2.8). Although not quite statisti-

Table 4.2.7.   Total Mean Concentration ($\pm$ SE) before and after Indomethacin

	Contraction (g)	
	Without Indomethacin	With Indomethacin
Normal ($n = 8$)	3.71 ± 0.29	4.63 ± 0.37^a
Short-term ($>50\%$) ($n = 6$)	0.95 ± 0.22^b	2.84 ± 0.25^c
Long-term		
$\leq 30\%$ ($n = 3$)	3.83 ± 0.60	4.51 ± 0.40
$\geq 70\%$ ($n = 4$)	2.88 ± 0.49	3.89 ± 0.27

[a] $p < 0.02$ for normal (with vs. without).
[b] $p < 0.01$ for with (normal vs. short-term).
[c] $p < 0.001$ for short-term (with vs. without).

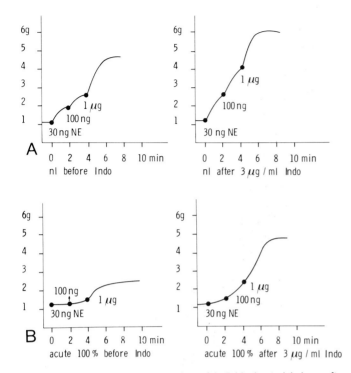

Figure 4.2.54. Isometric contraction of individual arterial rings after sequential administration of 30ng, 100ng, and 1 μg of norepinephrine *(NE)* (indomethacin *(Indo)*) per ml. **A.** Normal nondilated artery; indomethacin moderately enhances contraction *(right)*. **B.** Carotid artery overdilated by 100% in short-term study; contraction is decreased compared to control *(A)* and increases markedly after addition of indomethacin *(right)*. (Reproduced from Zollikofer C, Cragg A, Einzig S, et al: Prostaglandins and angioplasty. *Radiology* 1983;149:681–685.)

Discussion

These findings indicate that mechanical damage to carotid arteries dilated for a short time in situ reduces the responsiveness to exogenous norepinephrine in vitro. Treatment of damaged arterial rings with the cyclooxygenase inhibitor indomethacin significantly increased responsiveness to norepinephrine, although contraction was never completely restored. These results suggest that synthesis of PGI_2 by the damaged arterial wall is responsible for the decreased response to norepinephrine before cyclooxygenase blockade, because the local vasodilating effect of PGI_2 may have been sufficient to override the constrictor effect of norepinephrine. These effects lasted for at least 6 but less than 24 hours after dilatation, in accord with earlier flow studies of the vasa vasorum.[97]

Although PGI_2 synthesis may certainly be a favorable side effect of PTA, preventing early reocclusion, these data indicate that this is an acute event. They are in general agreement with the fact that tissue damage may increase prostaglandin synthesis over the short term, whereas in the long term, synthesis at the site may actually be reduced. This is especially true of blood vessels, because cyclooxygenase is produced principally in the endothelium, with production gradually declining toward the peripheral media.[132,133] Damage to these layers by PTA may cause immediate local release of PGI_2, as suggested by these findings. Inasmuch as PGI_2 is a potent antiaggregatory and vasodilating drug and its release seems limited to a short time (at least 6 but less than 24 hours) ASA treatment may be delayed for 12–24 hours, in order not to affect PGI_2 synthesis. Nevertheless, it should be noted that platelets form aggregates in vitro in two distinct phases. The primary phase is initiated by adenosine diphosphate (ADP) or epinephrine; the second phase is due to TXA_2 synthesis, which initiates further release of ADP. Only the second phase is prevented by drugs such as ASA or indomethacin, which inhibit formation of TXA_2.[134] In contrast, substances such as adenosine and PGI_2, which elevate platelet levels of cyclic adenosine monophosphate (cAMP), block primary as well as secondary aggregation.[135] Therefore, treatment with ASA alone will not eliminate all the factors responsible for platelet aggregation.

cally significant, there was a distinct trend toward reduced contraction for arteries dilated 70–100% and studied after one week to three months (Table 4.2.7 and Fig. 4.2.56). Similarly, ICF in group C tended to be lower than in group B. Arteries dilated to no more than 30% and studied 24 hours or more after angioplasty did not show a significant difference from the controls before and after indomethacin administration (Tables 4.2.7 and 4.2.8). The overall percentage increase in ICF after indomethacin was greater at lower doses of norepinephrine in all groups studied (Fig. 4.2.56).

Table 4.2.8. Percent Increase in Contraction with Indomethacin (Mean ± SE)

	Short-term		Long-term	
	Normal (n = 8)	>50% (n = 6)	≤30% (n = 3)	≥70% (n = 4)
Norepinephrine				
30 ng	54.0 ± 27.0	699.0 ± 254.3	32.5 ± 42.5	81.4 ± 47.6
100 ng	43.6 ± 16.4	489.4 ± 108.9	44.2 ± 35.5	86.3 ± 33.1
1 μg	26.9 ± 10.1	216.6 ± 38.7	21.6 ± 13.8	41.1 ± 13.2
Average	42.0 ± 10.8	468.3 ± 99.7[a]	32.8 ± 16.8	69.6 ± 18.9

[a]$p < 0.01$ (normal vs. short-term).

Figure 4.2.55. Relative mean percentage increase in contractile force after indomethacin (norepinephrine (*NE*)) in the normal controls and the three groups of dilated arteries. (Reproduced from Zollikofer C, Cragg A, Einzig S, et al: Prostaglandins and angioplasty. *Radiology* 1983;149:681–685.)

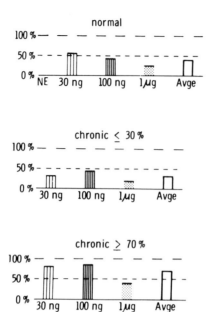

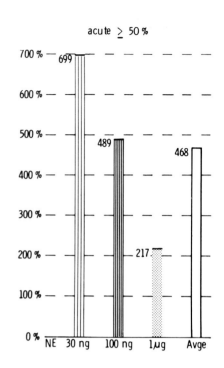

This experiment was performed in nonatherosclerotic canine carotid arteries, which may behave much differently from atherosclerotic human vessels. Whereas in normal vessels, synthesis of PGI_2 is greatest in the endothelium and gradually decreases toward the adventitia,[132] in atherosclerosis there is evidence that, in vitro, PGI synthesis is generally reduced.[136,137] Therefore, the release of prostacyclin might also be reduced after PTA of atherosclerotic vessels. However, these results have been challenged. Probst et al. demonstrated release of prostacyclin soon after coronary angioplasty,[138] and in vivo studies measuring excretion of urinary prostacyclin metabolites in patients with severe atherosclerosis showed a significant increase in endogenous biosynthesis of prostacyclin compared with healthy subjects.[139] Furthermore, the vessel wall may synthesize prostacyclin not only from its endogenous endoperoxides, but also from exogenous endoperoxides released from platelets.[132] Consequently, platelet aggregation on the denuded surface of the dilated segment may lead to increased prostacyclin synthesis in the arterial wall. Therefore, one must not rely on the ability of the blood vessels to produce prostacyclin, but rather on the ability of the platelets to adhere to the damaged surface.

This raises the question of whether a selective inhibitor of TXA_2 synthesis should be used instead of a cyclooxygenase inhibitor for PTA. Aiken et al.[140] and Yarger et al.[141] have shown that selective thromboxane synthetase inhibitors have a greater antiaggregating efficacy than do cyclooxygenase inhibitors due to the enhanced responsiveness of the platelets to endogenous PGI_2. Probably even more important is the fact that the antithrombotic action of these compounds can be blocked by previous treatment with ASA. Therefore, a selective thromboxane inhibitor may be preferable to ASA for preventing early reocclusion

after PTA, because local PGI_2 synthesis would be unaffected and platelet aggregation at the damaged site would be impaired. On the other hand, it has recently been reported that the TXA_2 produced by platelets is more sensitive to ASA than to PGI_2 produced by the vessel wall, so that low-dose ASA has been advocated as having a lesser effect on PGI_2 synthesis.[142–146] Some authors have recommended giving one ASA tablet per day on the grounds that prostacyclin synthesis returns to normal within 24–36 hours after a single dose, whereas blockade of TXA_2 in the platelets is irreversible.[142,144] Weksler et al. recently demonstrated differential inhibition of vascular and platelet prostaglandin synthesis by ASA in atherosclerotic patients undergoing aortocoronary bypass.[147] With low-dose (80 mg/day) ASA, a reliable blockade of TXA_2 was achieved, with only minor effects on prostacyclin synthesis. However, other investigators could not entirely confirm such beneficial differential effects of low-dose ASA on prostaglandin synthesis. Consequently, the response of PGI_2 synthesis to ASA and the appropriate dosage remain controversial, since there are wide in vivo differences in ASA sensitivity.[147–153]

Although the percentage of contraction increased 10-fold after indomethacin administration in the short-term study (Fig. 4.2.54), the arterial rings showed a decreased absolute response (Fig. 4.2.55). Therefore, in addition to the prostaglandin effect hypothesized above, there must be direct mechanical damage to the media that reduces responsiveness even after several weeks if the arterial wall has been stretched far enough. Such damage is obviously related to the amount of stretching by the balloon, as shown by the authors' long-term studies (groups B and C) as well as by the histomorphologic investigations.[47,59,82]

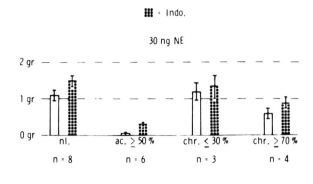

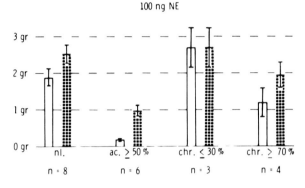

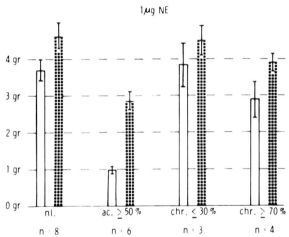

Figure 4.2.56. Absolute mean increase ($\pm$ SE) in contractile force (g) after indomethacin (norephinephrine (*NE*)) administration in the controls and the three groups of dilated arteries. (Reproduced from Zollikofer C, Cragg A, Einzig S, et al: Prostaglandins and angioplasty. *Radiology* 1983;149:681–685.)

Summary and Conclusions

Local paralysis and hyperemia of the arterial wall after PTA can now be explained by some combination of mechanical damage and release of vasoactive substances. These studies strongly suggest that prostaglandins are responsible for the pharmacologically induced vasodilation. Acetylcholine, ATP and ADP, histamines, and bradykinins are not active without an intact endothelium,[154] so one can logically conclude that cyclooxygenase inhibitors reduce vessel wall hyperemia by direct action on prostacy-

clin synthesis. Partial restitution of arterial contractibility following administration of cyclooxygenase inhibitors can be similarly explained. Furthermore, it is tempting to speculate that cyclooxygenase inhibition with ASA or indomethacin might predispose a recently dilated vessel to spasm or amplify its response to circulating norepinephrine. It is known that inhibition of the cyclooxygenase pathway can shunt arachidonic acid metabolism into the lipoxygenase pathway (Fig. 4.2.57),[155] increasing the production of hydroxyeicosatetraenoic acid (HPETE), a potent vasoconstrictor.

The local spasms proximal and distal to the dilated segments as seen on angiograms after experimental PTA can be explained by two mechanisms: increased release of HPETE in the dilated arterial segments and an enhanced vasoconstrictor response of those segments immediately adjacent to the dilation site that have been stretched only slightly.[123] Increased synthesis of HPETE after PTA of canine carotid arteries has recently been reported by Cragg et al.[156] Hence, the administration of ASA could, theoretically, cause vasospasm leading to early thrombotic occlusion by shunting arachidonic acid pathway metabolites into the lipoxygenase pathway. In addition, animal experiments have shown an ASA dosage of >10mg/kg to enhance platelet deposition on the de-endothelialized vascular surface.[157,158]

In short, the problem of prophylactic ASA remains unsolved and controversial (at least for the common dose of 0.5–1.0 g/day).[142,147,151–153,159,160] Other means of preventing thrombosis after PTA must therefore be considered. Selective thromboxane inhibitors, stimulation of prostacyclin production by the vessel wall, development of inhibitors of phosphodiesterase (which might be potentiating endogenous prostacyclin production), and administration of synthetic prostacyclin offer new possibilities.[132] Because prostacyclin is the most powerful substance currently known for preventing platelet aggregation and simultaneously increasing cAMP production, it or a stable synthetic analog, alone or in combination with a phosphodiesterase inhibitor, should provide better prophylaxis against platelet aggregation.

However, one must be cautious in extrapolating these conclusions, derived from studies on normal canine arteries in vitro and in vivo, to the clinical situation in human atherosclerosis. Only detailed experiments on diseased vessels of primates and clinical trials with prostacyclin and TXA_2 inhibitors can validate these first experimental data.

Significance of Balloon Pressure Recording and Relation between Arterial and Balloon Rupture in Experimental Angioplasty[161,162]

In clinical PTA, the number of repetitions of balloon inflation and the duration for a given lesion are still arbitrary.[84,163] Commonly, the balloon is inflated to an arbitrar-

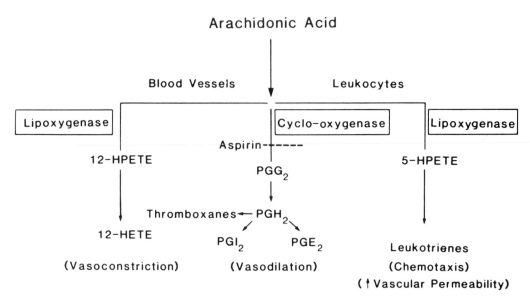

Figure 4.2.57. Arachidonic acid metabolism and cyclooxygenase metabolites. Cyclooxygenase is blocked by ASA. Several other vasoactive substances are produced by the separate lipoxygenase pathway, including the potent vasoconstricting hydroxymetabolite hydroxyeicosa- tetraenoic acid *(HPETE)*. (Reproduced from Cragg A, Einzig S, Rysavy J, Castañeda–Zúñiga WR, Borgwardt B, Amplatz K: Effect of aspirin on angioplasty-induced vessel wall hyperemia. *AJR* 1983;140:1233–1238.)

ily selected diameter for 15 seconds to 1 minute when treating renal or peripheral arteries; indeed, this "recipe" is often followed religiously despite the absence of scientific validation. Normal and atherosclerotic arteries differ considerably in their compliance and response to PTA, and this fact is of great importance in clinical practice, where careful fluoroscopic monitoring provides the only means of assessing the yielding of a lesion and where the impending rupture of the artery cannot be detected directly. In order to define the moment of optimal dilation, and because the causal and temporal relations between vascular and balloon rupture were open to controversy,[84,164,165,166] an experiment was designed to characterize the compliance of a vascular lesion during dilatation.

MATERIALS AND METHODS

Three experiments were performed in atherosclerotic cadaver arteries and normal canine arteries. Volumes and pressures of the dilation balloons were monitored in digital and analog form using the special apparatus shown in Figure 4.2.58. In the experiments on cadaver vessels, atherosclerotic, stenotic lesions in iliac arteries were dilated. In addition to monitoring pressure-volume curves, volume was plotted against pressure during balloon inflation and deflation and the hysteresis cycle (difference in the pathways of the pressure-volume curves during inflation and deflation[53,167]) was recorded on an oscilloscope.

In the second series of experiments, normal carotid arteries of anesthetized dogs were dilated to 80% oversize, and the pressure and volume in the balloon were recorded. For assessment of possible stress effects on the arterial wall (changes in the viscoelastic property), dilations and recordings, including hysteresis cycles, were performed three or

four times for each vessel at intervals of five minutes to permit stress relaxation in the artery.[167]

In the third series of experiments, carotid, iliac, and femoral arteries were dilated using PE balloon catheters with inflation pressures of 4.5 atm. Inflation pressures were then increased in 2-atm increments to a maximum pressure of 12.5 atm or until the balloon burst. Pressure and volume tracings of the balloons were recorded throughout. Deformation and bursting of the balloon during pressure increases were simultaneously recorded by cinefluorography at 30 frames/sec. The balloon sizes were selected according to the vessel diameters: equal to the arterial size (0 group), 50% larger, and 100% larger than the artery. Burst balloons remained in situ until after sacrifice of the dog and dissection of the artery. After the animals had been killed, the dilated vascular segments were examined macroscopically and by light microscopy.

RESULTS

Partial or total disruption of human atherosclerotic plaques could be clearly appreciated on the pressure recordings (Fig. 4.2.59). Partial intimal and medial tears, as well as rupture of intimal plaques, were seen better on the pressure curves than on the volume curves. Hysteresis cycles did not add any information but rather obscured significant pressure changes (Fig. 4.2.60).

Figure 4.2.61*A* shows a typical volume and pressure recording during dilatation of a normal canine carotid artery at a pressure of 4.5 atm. Repeated dilation of the same arterial segment did not alter the pattern of the curves (Fig. 4.2.61*B*), and the configuration of the hysteresis cycle did not change. The findings of increasing volume of the balloons with repeated dilations were incon-

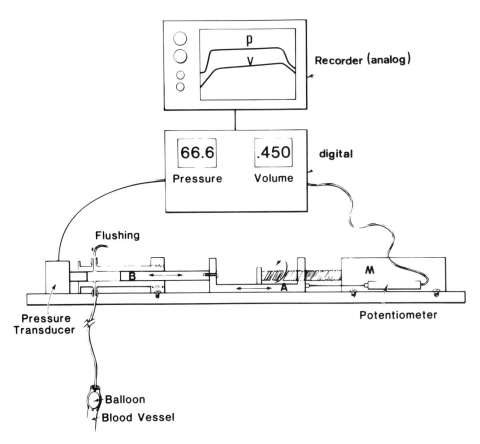

Figure 4.2.58. Medi–tech apparatus for recording balloon pressure to 12.5 atm and measuring volume and flow of saline into and out of balloon (potentiometer). Motor *(M)* turns lead screw *(A)* coupled to metal piston *(B)* of a noncompliant syringe. The syringe has two outlets, one for the balloon catheter and one to allow flushing and refilling of the syringe. For a given pressure setting, the saline volume in the balloon is adjusted automatically by the motor, which is controlled by an electronic feedback mechanism. Pressure *(p)* and volume *(v)* changes are recorded digitally on a fiberoptic strip-chart recorder. (Reproduced from Zollikofer CL, Salomonowitz E, Castañeda–Zúñiga WR, Brühlmann WF, Amplatz K: The relationship between arterial rupture and balloon bursting in experimental angioplasty. *AJR* 1985;144:777–779.)

sistent and could not be differentiated from the balloon's own compliance.

In a variation of the experimental set-up, using a noncompliant inflation system without the pressure-volume apparatus, a sudden yielding of human cadaver or normal canine arteries could be recorded faithfully simply by monitoring the pressure of the balloon with a high-pressure Statham transducer (Fig. 4.2.62).

In the dogs, with increasing pressures, arterial rupture

with complete transmural tears could be demonstrated with 100% overdilation (Table 4.2.9). Rupture of the vessel preceded bursting of the balloon in every case, as shown on the pressure-volume tracings (Fig. 4.2.63). Arterial rupture allowed the balloon to expand suddenly, which caused a sharp pressure drop that activated the electronic servo-loop feedback system to compensate for the pressure loss in the balloon; fluid was automatically injected until the original pressure was restored. Bursting of the balloon was

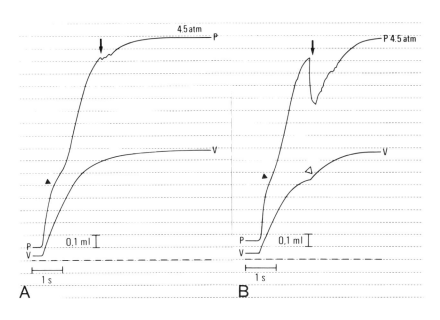

Figure 4.2.59. Pressure *(P)* and volume *(V)* curves of angioplasty in cadaver iliac artery with 8mm PE balloon at 4.5 atm. **A.** Discrete tear in atherosclerotic intimal plaque is shown as slight pressure drop *(arrow)* but cannot be appreciated on volume curve. *Arrowhead* indicates delay in pressure buildup due to unfolding of balloon. **B.** With rupture of plaque, there is a marked pressure drop *(arrow)*. Note gradual change in slope of volume curve *(open arrowhead)* secondary to balloon expansion with injection of more fluid. (Reproduced from Zollikofer CL, Salomonowitz E, Brühlmann WF, Frick MP, Castañeda–Zúñiga WR, Amplatz K: Significance of balloon pressure recording during angioplasty. *RöFo* 1985;142:526–530.)

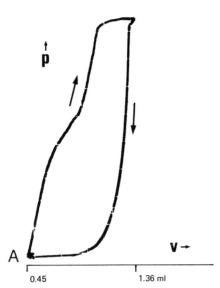

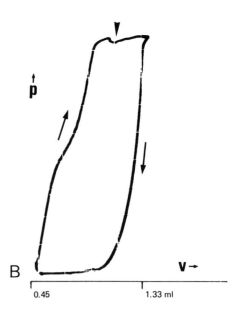

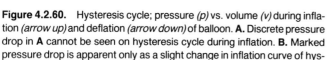

Figure 4.2.60. Hysteresis cycle; pressure *(p)* vs. volume *(v)* during inflation *(arrow up)* and deflation *(arrow down)* of balloon. **A.** Discrete pressure drop in **A** cannot be seen on hysteresis cycle during inflation. **B.** Marked pressure drop is apparent only as a slight change in inflation curve of hysteresis cycle *(arrowhead).* (Reproduced from Zollikofer CL, Salomonowitz E, Brühlmann WF, Frick MP, Castañeda–Zúñiga WR, Amplatz K: Significance of balloon pressure recording during angioplasty. *RöFo* 1985; 142:526–530.)

Figure 4.2.61. Pressure *(P)*-volume *(V)* curves and corresponding hysteresis cycles at first (**A**) and third (**B**) dilatation of canine carotid artery at 4.5 atm; pressure-volume curves during inflation and deflation are practically identical. Arterial wall creep during progressive dilation from the first to the third inflation cannot be detected. *Arrowhead* indicates pressure curve "shoulder" due to unfolding of balloon. *Broken vertical line* indicates point at which paper speed changed from 25 to 2.5mm/sec. (Reproduced from Zollikofer CL, Salomonowitz E, Brühlmann WF, Frick MP, Castañeda–Zúñiga WR, Amplatz K: Significance of balloon pressure recording during angioplasty. *RöFo* 1985;142:526–530.)

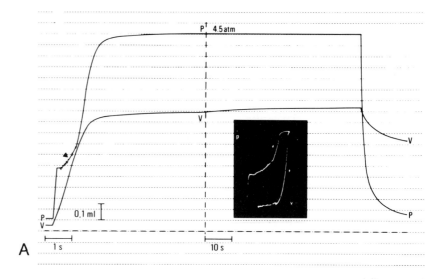

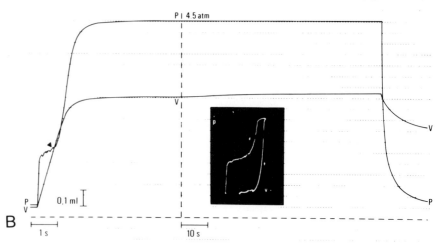

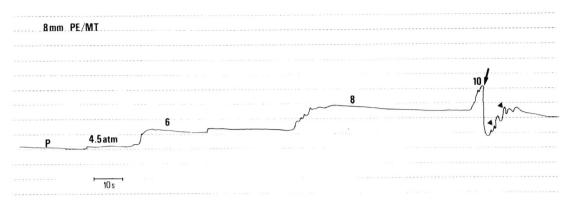

Figure 4.2.62. Pressure curve during dilation of cadaver iliac artery with 8mm PE balloon using a noncompliant injection system (noncompliant syringe, tubing, and high-pressure Statham transducer). Balloon inflation to 4.5 atm with sequential pressure increases up to 10 atm. The slight slope after each fractional pressure increase at 6 and 8 atm corresponds to compliance of balloon and artery. A sudden pressure drop at 10 atm *(arrow)* signals rupture of plaque. Under continuous balloon inflation, pressure buildup is irregular *(arrowheads)* due to stretching of arterial wall, which has been freed from the plaque.

then signified by a complete pressure loss that could not be reversed by injection of saline (Fig. 4.2.63).

In both the 50% and the 0 groups, rupture of the balloon did not cause transmural rupture of the artery (Table 4.2.9). In the 50% group, intimal abrasion, medial stretching, and medial tears were seen, but the adventitia remained intact. In the 0 group, arterial wall damage was limited to intimal abrasion and stretch effects, which were restricted to the inner one-third to one-half of the media.

Balloon bursting pressures ranged from 8–12.5 atm (Table 4.2.10). Examination of burst balloons revealed longitudinal tears with smooth margins. The time between arterial rupture and balloon bursting ranged from 3–4 to 45 seconds.

DISCUSSION

The author's experiments in atherosclerotic cadaver and normal canine arteries indicate that progress of angioplasty can be monitored by following pressure and volume changes in the balloon. With a sophisticated noncompliant system, a sudden yielding of the arterial wall can be recorded exactly. Sudden tears of the media and splitting or rupture of intimal plaques also are demonstrated on the pressure-volume curves of the dilating balloons.

In contrast, the assessment of viscoelastic properties of the dilated artery or the changing compliance of the slowly stretching arterial wall during repeated dilations could not

be picked up by the pressure-volume curves; and the configurations of the curves could not be correlated with the nature of a lesion, as suggested by Abele.[163] Furthermore, the present authors were not able to demonstrate alterations in the hysteresis loops after repeated angioplasty,

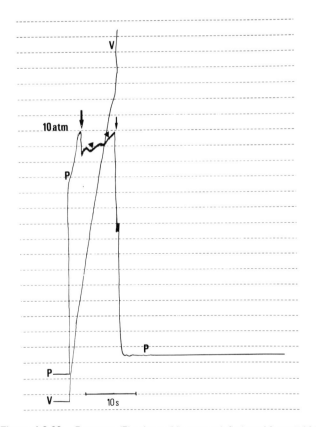

Figure 4.2.63. Pressure *(P)*-volume *(V)* curve at inflation of 9mm (100% oversized) PE balloon in canine iliac artery from 0 to 10 atm. A sudden pressure drop *(large arrow)* marks rupture of the artery. With subsequent automatic injection of fluid, pressure in the balloon is restored *(arrowheads)*. Irregular pressure buildup *(wavy line)* represents gradually increasing tear in the artery (see Fig. 4.2.64). With rupture of balloon *(small arrow)*, there is complete pressure loss, and volume increases to infinity.

Table 4.2.9. Number and Sequence of Arterial and Balloon Ruptures

	Rupture of:				
Overdilation	Artery Followed by Balloon	Balloon Followed by Artery	Balloon Only	Artery Only	No Rupture
0% (*n* = 8)	0	0	5	0	3
50% (*n* = 8)	0	0	3	0	5
100% (*n* = 10)	6	0	2	0	2

Table 4.2.10.   Balloon Bursting Pressures

Overdilation	Balloon Pressure		
	≤8 atm	≤10 atm	≤12.5 atm
0% (*n* = 5)	0	1	4
50% (*n* = 3)	0	2	1
100% (*n* = 8)	1	5	2

although they had expected that the changing compliance of the vessel wall would change the loop configuration.[167,168] Finally, the complicated recording of hysteresis loops proved unrewarding in detecting the sudden yielding of a lesion.

In this study, volume recordings were relatively insensitive when compared with the pressure curves. Hence, recording of the balloon pressure alone seems adequate. For clinical use, a noncompliant inflation system (syringe, connecting tubes, and balloon catheter) is necessary. Under laboratory conditions, such a system proved practical in picking up a sudden yielding of the vessel wall, such as a disruption of an atherosclerotic plaque. This system is more sensitive than looking for the famous "pop" of the lesion, as demonstrated by a sudden change of the balloon's shape on fluoroscopy. Therefore, a pressure-recording system should be valuable in determining when a procedure must be terminated to avoid overdistension of the vessel wall. This seems particularly important during use of high-pressure balloons.

With the advent of recording of balloon pressure and volume during PTA, the authors were able to demonstrate that balloon rupture occurs secondary to overdistension of the vessel and not vice versa.[169,170] With vascular rupture, the external restraint on the balloon is lost, allowing a sudden increase in the balloon diameter. Because of the lack of a retaining arterial sheath, the tensile strength of the balloon material is exceeded within seconds, and the balloon bursts even without a further pressure increase.

The authors did not observe a single case of arterial rupture caused by a bursting balloon. Furthermore, the histologic changes could not be definitely attributed to a jet phenomenon caused by a rupturing balloon[164]; rather, diffuse changes of general overdistension were found. Localized ruptures in the medial layer were found irrespective of whether the balloon had ruptured in situ. If vascular ruptures were indeed caused by the jet from a rupturing balloon, the pressure curves should have dropped to zero and remained at this level. However, with activation of the pump and saline injection by the electronic feedback mechanism, balloon pressure was reconstituted, indicating an intact balloon.

During fluoroscopic observation, rupture of the nonopaque arterial wall cannot be seen, although cine recording may reveal an eccentric deformation of the balloon preceding extravasation of contrast medium at rupture (Fig. 4.2.64). However, the entire series of events, with the sequence and causal relations of arterial rupture and balloon bursting, was best displayed on the pressure-volume curves, with which the sequence was convincingly clarified.

An exception to these findings may occur with equatorial balloon ruptures, as described by Yune and Klatte[171] and Waltman et al.[84] Such ruptures produce irregular, sometimes sharp, edges that could harm the stretched arterial wall, especially when the balloon catheter is withdrawn. With today's improved balloon materials, however, such unusual and irregular ruptures should not occur.

SUMMARY AND CONCLUSIONS

The results of these tests of the various balloon dilation catheters support the use of the true double-lumen catheter or the Olbert system. The latter offers the potential advantage of high working pressures (10–12 atm). However, with these balloons, the operator should be reluctant to exceed the manufacturer's suggested pressures, especially with the larger (≥6mm) balloons, because the outer nylon mesh may rupture, leading to significant expansion of the inner PU component. By contrast, in all the other balloons tested, the suggested working pressures are much lower, 4–6 atm. The PVC/S and PE/MT balloons, owing to their low compliance (an increase in diameter of no more than 1mm), can exceed the manufacturer's suggested pressures by several atmospheres without the risk of untoward effects. Furthermore, these tests demonstrated that PE has no definite advantages over modern PVC materials with respect to compliance and tensile strength, as was formerly the case. Conventional PVC/C and PE/C balloons of the coaxial type should not be inflated above their suggested pressures, however, because of their considerable compliance. It should be stressed that there is a new balloon catheter, manufactured by Cook, Inc., that has a true double-lumen system that considerably improves the balloon's compliance.

In general, the results of angioplasty depend much less on the number of balloon inflations than on the inflation pressure and duration. Therefore, as a general rule (always bearing in mind that balloon characteristics and configuration must also be appropriate for the anatomic site and the nature of the vascular lesion), balloons with the lowest possible compliance should be used. In this way, maximum dilation force with exact definition of the balloon diameter should be achieved even with high inflation pressures.

As demonstrated, oversized balloons attained their full diameter in healthy arteries only at considerably increased inflation pressures. Accordingly, histologic changes increase and eventually culminate in rupture of the artery in parallel with increasing balloon diameter and inflation pressure. Applying high pressures in clinical PTA thus increases the risk of vascular rupture; sufficient attention must therefore be given to the selection of balloon diameter. Normally, balloon size is chosen according to the estimated diameter of the nondiseased vessel. As noted earlier, however, some experienced investigators always use

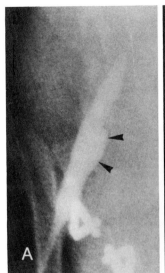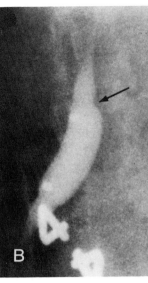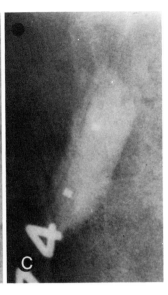

Figure 4.2.64. Cine film recording of rupture of canine iliac artery followed by balloon rupture at 10 atm (30 frames/sec; same experiment as in Fig. 4.2.63). **A.** Asymmetric bulging of balloon *(arrowheads)* caused by rupture of artery at dilation site. Distal half of balloon is still contained by intact part of arterial wall. **B.** 500 milliseconds later, the bulge is more prominent and has increased in length because of progressing arterial rupture. Note transition between balloon segments contained by the artery and unsupported expanded portion *(arrow).* **C.** Another five seconds later, balloon has ruptured, with extravasation of contrast medium. (Reproduced from Zollikofer CL, Salomonowitz E, Castañeda–Zúñiga WR, Brühlmann WF, Amplatz K: The relationship between arterial rupture and balloon bursting in experimental angioplasty. *AJR* 1985;144:777–779.)

slightly oversized (1- or 2mm) balloons, whereas others oppose this tactic. In the present authors' opinion, use of a slightly oversized balloon seems justified as long as inflation pressures do not exceed 4–6 atm; but when high pressures (10–12 atm or more) are used, it is prudent not to use oversized balloons.

Despite the authors' extensive attempts to characterize the nature of stenotic lesions, they cannot give definite recommendations on optimal dilation because of the wide variation in compliance of atherosclerotic lesions. Generally, it seems that nonatherosclerotic disease, especially of the inflammatory and fibrous type, requires longer inflation times and higher pressures. Continuous monitoring of balloon pressure may demonstrate a gradual or abrupt yielding of a lesion to a much better degree than does fluoroscopic observation of the balloon shape, so pressure monitoring can help improve PTA results, particularly when using high inflation pressures. Furthermore, if one uses only state-of-the-art balloon dilatation catheters, arterial rupture secondary to a bursting balloon should not occur. Finally, the initial result of transluminal angioplasty still must be evaluated by follow-up angiograms, recording of pressure gradients, or both.

References

1. Dotter CT, Judkins MP: Transluminal treatment of arteriosclerotic obstruction. *Circulation* 1964;30:654
2. Dotter CT, Judkins MP: Percutaneous transluminal treatment of arteriosclerotic obstruction. *Radiology* 1965; 84:631
3. Dotter CT, Judkins MP, Frische LH, Mueller R: The "nonsurgical" treatment of ilio-femoral arteriosclerotic obstruction. *Radiology* 1966;86:871
4. Dotter CT, Judkins MP, Frische LH, Rosch J: Nonoperative treatment of arterial occlusive disease: a radiologically facilitated technique. *Radiol Clin North Am* 1967;5:531
5. Dotter CT, Judkins MP, Rosch J: Nichtoperative transluminale Behandlung der arteriosklerotischen Verschlussaffektionen. *RöFo* 1968;109:125
6. Dotter CT, Rosch J, Judkins MP: Transluminal dilatation of atherosclerotic stenosis. *Surg Gynecol Obstet* 1968; 127:794
7. Staple TW: Modified catheter for percutaneous transluminal treatment of atherosclerotic obstructions. *Radiology* 1968;91:1041
8. Van Andel GJ: *Percutaneous Transluminal Angioplasty: The Dotter Procedure.* Amsterdam, Excerpta Medica, 1976
9. Brahme F, Swedenborg J, Tibel B: Evaluation of transluminal recanalization of the femoral artery. *Acta Chir Scand* 1969;135:697
10. Berglund G, Bodvall B, Eldh J, Yden S: Nytt Behandlingsalternative vid Artiell insufficiens i benen. *Lakartidningen* 1969;66:129
11. Dow J, Hardwick C: Transluminal arterial recanalization. *Lancet* 1966;1:73
12. Grüntzig A, Bollinger A, Brunner U, Schlumpf M, Wellauer J: Perkutane rekanalisation chronischer arterieller Verschlusse nach Dotter: eine nicht-operative Kathetertechnik. *Schweiz Med Wochenschr* 1973;103:825
13. Zeitler E, Schoop W, Zahnow W: The treatment of occlusive arterial disease by transluminal catheter angioplasty. *Radiology* 1971;99:19
14. Brunner U, Grüntzig A: Das Dilatationsverfahren nach Dotter in gefässchirurgischer Sicht. *Vasa* 1975;4:334
15. Brunner U, Schneider E, Gygax P: Kombination der PTA mit chirurgischen Eingriffen im femoropoplitealen Bereich. *Vasa* 1982;11:278
16. Abbot WM: Percutaneous transluminal angioplasty: surgeon's view. *AJR* 1980;135:917
17. Alpert J: Grüntzig's plaque pressing: "verbum sapienti." *J Med Soc N Jersey* 1981;78:87
18. Vetto RM: Further comment (editorial). *JAMA* 1974; 230:92
19. Vollmar J, Trede M, Laubach K, Forrest M: Principles of reconstructive procedures for chronic femoro-popliteal occlusion: report on 546 operations. *Ann Surg* 1968; 168:215
20. Dotter CT, Rosch J, Anderson JM, Antonovic R, Robinson M: Transluminal iliac artery dilatation: nonsurgical

catheter treatment of atheromatous narrowing. *JAMA* 1974;230:117

21. Grüntzig A, Hopff H: Perkutane rekanalisation chronischer arterieller Verschlusse mit einem neuen Dilatationskatheter. *Dtsch Med Wochenschr* 1974;99:2502

22. Porstmann W: Ein neuer Korsett-Balloonkatheter zur transluminalen Rekanalization nach Dotter unter besonderer Berücksichtigung von Obliterationen an den Beckenarterien. *Radiol Diagn (Berl)* 1973;2:239

23. Grüntzig A: Die perkutane Rekanalisation chronischer arterieller Verschlusse (Dotter–Prinzip) mit einem neuen doppellumigen Dilatationskatheter. *RöFo* 1976;124:80

24. Grüntzig A: *Die Perkutane Transluminale Rekanalisation Chronischer Arterienverschlusse mit einer Neuen Dilatationstechnik.* Baden–Baden, Witzstrock, 1977

25. Grüntzig A, Kuhlmann U, Vetter W, Lutolf U, Meier B, Siegenthaler W: Treatment of renovascular hypertension with percutaneous transluminal dilatation of a renal-artery stenosis. *Lancet* 1978;1:801

26. Dotter CT: Transluminal angioplasty: results and future outlook, in Dotter CT, Grüntzig A, Schoop W, Zeitler E (eds): *Percutaneous Transluminal Angioplasty.* Berlin, Springer–Verlag, 1983, p 337

27. Doubilet P, Abrams HL: The cost of underutilization: percutaneous transluminal angioplasty for peripheral vascular disease. *N Engl J Med* 1984;310:95

28. Hall D, Grüntzig A: Percutaneous transluminal coronary angioplasty: current procedure and future direction. *AJR* 1984;142:13

29. Jang GC, Block PC, Cowley MJ, et al: Comparative cost analysis of coronary angioplasty and coronary bypass surgery: results from a national cooperative study. *Circulation* 1982;66(Suppl 2):123

30. Dotter CT: Clinical indications for transluminal dilatation in the management of atheromatous leg ischemia. *Cardiovasc Clin* 1971;3:104

31. Dotter CT: Transluminal angioplasty: pathologic basis, in Zeitler E, Grüntzig A, Schoop W (eds): *Percutaneous Vascular Recanalization.* Berlin, Springer–Verlag, 1978, p 3

32. Jester HG, Sinapius D, Alexander K, Leitz KH: Morphologische Veranderungen nach transluminaler Rekanalisation chronischer arterieller Verschlusse, in Zeitler E (ed): *Hypertonie-Risikofaktor in der Angiologie.* Baden–Baden, Witzstrock, 1976

33. Jester HG, Sinapius D: Morphologic alterations after percutaneous transluminal recanalization of chronic femoral atherosclerosis, in Zeitler E, Grüntzig A, Schoop W (eds): *Percutaneous Vascular Recanalization.* Berlin, Springer–Verlag, 1978, p 51

34. Hempel KJ: Morphologische Befunde zur Kompressibilität atheromatoser und thrombotischer Intimaveranderungen, in 2. *Angiologisches Symposiom.* Frankfurt, Aggertalklinik Engelskirchen, 1969

35. Hohn P, Wagner R, Zeitler E: Histologische Befunde nach der Katheterbehandlung arterieller Obliterationen nach Dotter und ihre Bedeutung. *Herz/Kreislaufforsch* 1975; 7:13

36. Leu HJ, Grüntzig A: Histopathologic aspects of transluminal recanalization, in Zeitler E, Grüntzig A, Schoop W (eds): *Percutaneous Vascular Recanalization.* Berlin, Springer–Verlag, 1978, pp 39

37. Baughman KL, Pasternak RC, Fallon JT, Block PC: Coronary transluminal angioplasty in autopsied human hearts (abstract). *Circulation* 1978;57/58(Suppl 2):II-80

38. Freudenberg H, Wefing H, Lichtlen PR: Risks of transluminal coronary angioplasty: a postmortal study (abstract). *Circulation* 1978;57/58(Suppl 2):II-80

39. Lee G, Ikeda R, Mason DT, et al: Effective dilatation of human coronary artery obstruction due to atherosclerosis utilizing a balloon-tip catheter. *Circulation* 1978;57/58 (Suppl 2):II-80

40. Simpson JB, Robert EW, Billingham ME, Myler RK, Harrison DC: Coronary transluminal angioplasty in human cadaver hearts (abstract). *Circulation* 1978;57/58(Suppl 2):II-80

41. Ramsey MR: Nutrition of the blood vessel wall: review of the literature. *Yale J Biol Med* 1936/37;9:14

42. Clarke JA: The vasa vasorum of normal human lower limb arteries. *Acta Anat* 1965;61:481

43. Wilens SL, Malcolm JA, Vazquez JM: Experimental infarction (medial necrosis) of the dog's aorta. *Am J Pathol* 1965;47:695

44. Woerner CA: Vasa vasorum of arteries: their demonstration and distribution, in Lansing AJ (ed): *The Arterial Wall.* Baltimore, Williams & Wilkins, 1959

45. Wolinsky H, Glagov S: Nature of species differences in the medial distribution of aortic vasa vasorum in mammals. *Circ Res* 1967;20:409

46. Heistad DD, Marcus ML, Law EG, Armstrong ML, Ehrhardt JC, Abboud FM: Regulation of blood flow to the aortic media in dogs. *J Clin Invest* 1978;62:133

47. Castañeda–Zúñiga WR, Formanek A, Tadavarthy M, et al: The mechanism of balloon angioplasty. *Radiology* 1980; 135:565

48. Castañeda–Zúñiga WR, Amplatz K, Laerum F, et al: Mechanics of angioplasty: an experimental approach. *RadioGraphics* 1981;1:1

49. Laerum F, Vlodaver Z, Castañeda–Zúñiga WR, Edwards JE, Amplatz K: The mechanism of angioplasty: dilatation of iliac cadaver arteries with intravascular pressure control. *RöFo* 1982;136:573

50. Zollikofer CL: Experimentelle Grundlagen der perkutanen transluminalen Angioplastie. *Habilitationsschrift,* 1985

51. Bunce DF: Structural differences between distended and collapsed arteries, in *Atlas of Arterial Histology.* St. Louis, Green, 1974

52. Cook TA, Yates PO: A critical survey of techniques for arterial mensuration. *J Pathol* 1972;108:119

53. Dobrin PB: Mechanical properties of arteries. *Physiol Rev* 1978;58:397

54. Pesonen E, Martimo P, Rapola J: Histometry of the arterial wall. *Lab Invest* 1974;31:550

55. LeVeen RF, Wolf GL, Turco MA: Morphometric changes in normal arteries and those undergoing transluminal angioplasty. *Invest Radiol* 1983;18:63

56. Chin AK, Kinney TB, Rurik GW, Shoor PM, Fogarty TJ: A physical measurement of the mechanisms of transluminal angioplasty. *Surgery* 1984;95:196

57. Castañeda–Zúñiga WR, Tadavarthy SM, Laerum F, Amplatz K: "Pseudo" intramural injection following percutaneous transluminal angioplasty. *Cardiovasc Intervent Radiol* 1984;7:104

58. Zollikofer CL, Castañeda–Zúñiga WR, Amplatz K: Results of animal experiments with balloon dilatation, in Dotter CT, Grüntzig A, Schoop W, Zeitler E (eds): *Percutaneous Transluminal Angioplasty.* Berlin, Springer–Verlag, 1983, p 60

59. Zollikofer CL, Salomonowitz E, Sibley R, et al: Transluminal angioplasty evaluated by electron microscopy. *Radiology* 1984;153:369

60. Baumgarter HR: Eine neue Methode zur Erzeugung von Thromben durch gezielte Überdehnung der Gefasswand. *Arch Ges Exp Med* 1963;137:227

61. Chidi CC, DePalma RG: Collagen formation by trans-

formed smooth muscle cells after arterial injury. *Surg Gynecol Obstet* 1981;152:8

62. Ross R, Glomset JA: Atherosclerosis and the arterial smooth muscle cell. *Science* 1973;180:1332

63. Spaet TH, Stemerman MB, Veith FJ, Lejnieks I: Intimal injury and regrowth in the aorta: medial smooth muscle cells as a source of neointima. *Circ Res* 1975;36:58

64. Stemerman MB, Ross R: Experimental arteriosclerosis: fibrous plaque formation in primates: an electron microscopic study. *J Exp Med* 1972;136:769

65. Pasternak RC, Baughman KL, Fallon JT, Block PC: Scanning electron microscopy after coronary transluminal angioplasty of normal canine coronary arteries. *Am J Cardiol* 1980;45:592

66. O'Gara PT, Guerrero JL, Feldman B, Fallon JT, Block PC: Effect of dextran and aspirin on platelet adherence after transluminal angioplasty of normal canine coronary arteries. *Am J Cardiol* 1984;53:1695

67. Fishman JA, Ryan GB, Karnovsky MJ: Endothelial regeneration in the rat carotid artery and the significance of endothelial denudation in the pathogenesis of neointimal thickening. *Lab Invest* 1975;32:339

68. Ross R, Glomset JA: The pathogenesis of atherosclerosis. *N Engl J Med* 1976;295:369

69. Stermerman MB, Spaet TH, Pitlick F, Clintron J, Lejnieks I, Tiell ML: Intimal healing: the pattern of reendothelialization and intimal thickening. *Am J Pathol* 1977;87:125

70. Nam SC, Lee WM, Jarmolych J, Lee KT, Thomas WA: Rapid production of advanced atherosclerosis in swine by a combination of endothelial injury and cholesterol feeding. *Exp Mol Pathol* 1973;18:369

71. Hagen P, Wang Z, Mikat EM, Hackel DB: Antiplatelet therapy reduces aortic intimal hyperplasia distal to small diameter vascular prostheses (PTFE) in non-human primates. *Ann Surg* 1981;195:328

72. Faxon DP, Sanborn TA, Haudenschild CC, Ryan TJ: Effect of antiplatelet therapy on restenosis after experimental angioplasty. *Am J Cardiol* 1984;53:72C

73. Faxon DP, Sanborn TA, Weber JV, et al: Restenosis following transluminal angioplasty in experimental atherosclerosis. *Arteriosclerosis* 1984;4:189

74. Waller BF: Early and later morphologic changes in human coronary arteries after percutaneous transluminal coronary angioplasty. *Clin Cardiol* 1983;6:363

75. Waller BF, Gorfinkel HJ, Rogers FJ, Kent KM, Roberts WC: Early and late morphologic changes in major epicardial coronary arteries after percutaneous transluminal coronary angioplasty. *Am J Cardiol* 1984;53:42C

76. DePalma RG: Atherosclerosis in vascular grafts. *Atheroscleros Rev* 1979;5:147

77. Lee WM, Lee KT: Advanced coronary atherosclerosis in swine produced by combination of balloon catheter injury and cholesterol feeding. *Exp Mol Pathol* 1975;23:492

78. Ross R, Harker L: Hyperlipidemia and atherosclerosis: chronic hyperlipidemia initiates and maintains lesions by endothelial cell desquamation and lipid accumulation. *Science* 1976;193:1094

79. Scott RF, Imai H, Makita T, Thomas WA, Reiner JM: Lining cell and intimal smooth muscle cell response and Evans blue staining in abdominal aorta of young swine after denudation by balloon catheter. *Exp Mol Pathol* 1980;33:185

80. Zollikofer CL, Salomonowitz E, Brühlmann WF, Castañeda–Zúñiga WR, Amplatz K: Dehnungs-, Verformungs, und Berstungs-Charakteristika haufig verwendeter Balloon-Dilatations- katheter: in vivo Untersuchungen an Hundegefassen (Teil 2). *RöFo* 1986;144:189

81. Sanborn TA, Faxon DP, Haudenschild C, Gottsman SB, Ryan TJ: The mechanism of intraluminal angioplasty: evidence for formation of aneurysms in experimental atherosclerosis. *Circulation* 1983;68:1136

82. Zollikofer CL, Chain J, Salomonowitz E, et al: Percutaneous transluminal angioplasty of the aorta. *Radiology* 1984;151:355

83. Levin DC, Harrington DP, Bettmann MA, et al: Equipment choices, technical aspects and pitfalls of percutaneous transluminal angioplasty. *Cardiovasc Intervent Radiol* 1984;7:1

84. Waltman AC, Greenfield AJ, Athanasoulis CA: Transluminal angioplasty: general rules and basic considerations, in Athanasoulis CA, Pfister RC, Greene RE, Roberson GH (eds): *Interventional Radiology*. Philadelphia, WB Saunders, 1982, p 253

85. Block PC, Fallon JT, Elmer D: Experimental angioplasty: lessons from the laboratory. *AJR* 1980;135:907

86. Block PC, Baughman KL, Pasternak RC, Fallon JT: Transluminal angioplasty: correlation of morphologic and angiographic findings in an experimental model. *Circulation* 1980;61:778

87. Faxon DP, Weber VJ, Haudenschild C, Gottsman SB, McGovern WZ, Ryan TJ: Acute effects of transluminal angioplasty in three experimental models of atherosclerosis. *Arteriosclerosis* 1982;2:125

88. Block PC, Myler RK, Stertzer S, Fallon JT: Morphology after transluminal angioplasty in human beings. *N Engl J Med* 1981;305:382

89. Clouse ME, Tomashefski JF Jr, Reinhold RE, Costello P: Mechanical effect of balloon angioplasty: case report with histology. *AJR* 1981;137:869

90. Hoffman MA, Fallon JT, Greenfield AJ, Waltman AC, Athanasoulis CA, Block PC: Arterial pathology after percutaneous transluminal angioplasty. *AJR* 1981;137:147

91. Saffitz JE, Totty WG, McClennan BL, Gilula LA: Percutaneous transluminal angioplasty: radiological-pathologic correlation. *Radiology* 1981;141:651

92. Grüntzig A, Kumpe DA: Technique of percutaneous transluminal angioplasty with the Grüntzig balloon catheter. *AJR* 1979;132:547

93. Zeitler E, Ernsting M, Richter EI, Seyferth W: Komplikationen nach PTA femoraler und iliakaler Obstruktionen. *Vasa* 1982;11:270

94. Katzen BT, Chang J, Knox WG: Percutaneous transluminal angioplasty with the Grüntzig balloon catheter: a review of 70 cases. *Arch Surg* 1979;114:1389

95. LeVeen RF, Wolf GL, Villanueva TG: New rabbit atherosclerosis model for the investigation of transluminal angioplasty. *Invest Radiol* 1982;17:470

96. Cragg A, Einzig S, Rysavy J, Borgwardt B, Castañeda W, Amplatz K: Arterial wall hyperemia following transluminal angioplasty (abstract). *Am J Cardiol* 1982;49

97. Cragg AH, Einzig S, Rysavy JA, Castañeda–Zúñiga WR, Borgwardt B, Amplatz K: The vasa vasorum and angioplasty. *Radiology* 1983;148:75

98. Cragg A, Einzig S, Rysavy J, Castañeda–Zúñiga W, Borgwardt B, Amplatz K: Effect of aspirin on angioplasty-induced vessel wall hyperemia. *AJR* 1983;140:1233

99. Geiringer E: Intimal vascularization and atherosclerosis. *J Pathol Bacteriol* 1951;63:201

100. Schutte HE: Plaque localization and distribution of vasa vasorum. *Angiologica* 1966;3:21

101. Heistad DD, Armstrong ML, Marcus ML: Hyperemia of the aortic wall in atherosclerotic monkeys. *Circ Res* 1981;48:669

102. Schutte HE: Changes in the vasa vasorum of the atherosclerotic aortic wall. *Angiologica* 1968;5:210

103. Train JS, Mitty HA, Efremidis SC, Rabinowitz JG: Visualization of a fine periluminal vascular network following transluminal angioplasty: possible demonstration of the vasa vasorum. *Radiology* 1982;143:399

104. Wolf GL, LeVeen RF, Ring EJ: Potential mechanism of angioplasty. *Cardiovasc Intervent Radiol* 1984;7:11

105. Leu HJ: Morphologie der Arterienwand nach perkutaner transluminaler Dilatation. *Vasa* 1982;11:265

106. Leu HJ: The morphological concept of percutaneous transluminal angioplasty, in Dotter CT, Grüntzig A, Schoop W, Zeitler E (eds): *Percutaneous Transluminal Angioplasty.* Berlin, Springer–Verlag, 1983, p 46

107. Seyfert W, Ernsting M, Grosse–Vorholt R, Zeitler E: Complications during and after percutaneous transluminal angioplasty, in Dotter CT, Grüntzig A, Schoop W, Zeitler E (eds): *Percutaneous Transluminal Angioplasty.* Berlin, Springer–Verlag, 1983, p 161

108. Block PC, Elmer D, Fallon JT: Release of atherosclerotic debris after transluminal angioplasty. *Circulation* 1982; 65:950

109. Sinapius D: Pathological basis for percutaneous catheter balloon revascularization, in Dotter CT, Grüntzig A, Schoop W, Zeitler E (eds): *Percutaneous Transluminal Angioplasty.* Berlin, Springer–Verlag, 1983, p 56

110. Hess H, Muller–Fassbender H, Ingrisch H, Mietaschk A: Verhutung von Wiederverschlussen nach Rekanalisation obliterierter Arterien mit der Kathetermethode. *Dtsch Med Wochenschr* 1978;103:1994

111. Hess H, Mietaschk A: Rezidivprophylaxe nach PTA: Antikoagulatien oder Aggregationshemmer. *Vasa* 1982; 11:344

112. Horvath L, Illes I, Fendler K: Prevention of complications in percutaneous transluminal angioplasty, in Dotter CT, Grüntzig A, Schoop W, Zeitler E (eds): *Percutaneous Transluminal Angioplasty.* Berlin, Springer–Verlag, 1983, p 170

113. Schneider E, Grüntzig A, Bollinger A: Langzeitergebnisse nach perkutaner transluminaler Angioplastie (PTA) bei 882 konsekutiven Patienten mit iliakalen und femoropoplitealen Obstruktionen. *Vasa* 1982;11:322

114. Schneider E, Grüntzig A, Bollinger A: Long-term patency rates after percutaneous transluminal angioplasty for iliac and femoropopliteal obstructions, in Dotter CT, Grüntzig A, Schoop W, Zeitler E (eds): *Percutaneous Transluminal Angioplasty.* Berlin, Springer–Verlag, 1983, p 175

115. Zeitler E, Reichold J, Schoop W, Loew D: Einfluss von Acetylesalicylsaure auf das Fruhergebnis nach perkutaner Rekanalization arterieller Obliterationen nach Dotter. *Dtsch Med Wochenschr* 1973;98:1285

116. Zeitler E: Percutaneous dilatation and recanalization of iliac and femoral arteries, in Athanasoulis CA, Abrams HL, Zeitler E (eds): *Therapeutic Angiography.* New York, Springer–Verlag, 1981, p 11

117. Roth FJ, Cappius G, Fingerhut E: Radiological pattern at and after angioplasty, in Dotter CT, Grüntzig A, Schoop W, Zeitler E (eds): *Percutaneous Transluminal Angioplasty.* Berlin, Springer–Verlag, 1983, p 73

118. Block PC: Mechanism of transluminal angioplasty. *Am J Cardiol* 1984;53:69C

119. Castañeda–Zúñiga WR, Laerum F, Rysavy J, Rusnak B, Amplatz K: Paralysis of arteries by intraluminal balloon dilatation. *Radiology* 1982;144:75

120. Wolf GL, Lentini EA, LeVeen RF: Reduced vasoconstrictor response after angioplasty in normal rabbit aortas. *AJR* 1984;141:1023

121. Price JM, Davis DL, Knauss EB: Length-dependent sensitivity in vascular smooth muscle. *Am J Physiol* 1981; 241:H557

122. Tallaride RJ, Sevy RW, Harakal C, Bendrick J, Faust R: The effect of preload on the dissociation constant of norepinephrine in isolated strips of rabbit thoracic aorta. *Arch Int Pharmacodyn Ther* 1974;210:67

123. Wolf GL, Lentini EA: The influence of short duration stretch on vasoconstrictor response in rabbit aortas. *Invest Radiol* 1984;19:269

124. Cowley M, Bentivoglio L, Block P, et al: Emergency coronary artery bypass surgery for complications of coronary angioplasty: NHLBI PTCA Registry experience (abstract). *Circulation* 1981;64(Suppl 4):IV-193

125. Holmes DR, Vliestra RE, Mock MB, et al: Angiographic changes produced by percutaneous transluminal coronary angioplasty. *Am J Cardiol* 1983;51:676

126. Sos TA, Sniderman KW: Percutaneous transluminal angioplasty. *Semin Roentgenol* 1981;16:26

127. Sos TA, Pickering TG, Sniderman KW, et al: Percutaneous transluminal renal angioplasty in renovascular hypertension due to atheroma or fibromuscular dysplasia. *Semin Intervent Radiol* 1984;1:237

128. Zollikofer C, Cragg A, Einzig S, et al: Prostaglandins and angioplasty. *Radiology* 1983;149:681

129. Richter EI, Zeitler E: Percutaneous transluminal angioplasty: adjunct drug therapy, in Dotter CT, Grüntzig A, Schoop W, Zeitler E (eds): *Percutaneous Transluminal Angioplasty.* Berlin, Springer–Verlag, 1983, p 84

130. Moncada S, Higgs EA, Vane JR: Human arterial and venous tissues generate prostacyclin (prostaglandin x), a potent inhibitor of platelet aggregation. *Lancet* 1977;1:18

131. Weksler BB, Marcus AJ, Jaffe EA: Synthesis of prostaglandin I$_2$ (prostacyclin) by cultured human and bovine endothelial cells. *Proc Natl Acad Sci USA* 1977;74:3922

132. Moncada S: Prostacyclin and arterial wall biology. *Arteriosclerosis* 1982;2:193

133. Smith WL, Bell TG: Immunohistochemical localization of the prostaglandin forming cyclooxygenase in renal cortex. *Am J Physiol* 1978;235:F451

134. Gorman RR, Bundy GL, Peterson DC, Sun FF, Miller OV, Fitzpatrick FA: Inhibition of human platelet thromboxane synthetase by 9,11-azoprosta-5,13-dienoic acid. *Proc Natl Acad Sci USA* 1977;74:4007

135. Gorman RR: Modulation of human platelet function by prostacyclin and thromboxane A$_2$. *Fed Proc* 1979;38:83

136. Dembinskia–Kiec A, Gryglewska T, Zmuda A, Gryglewski RJ: The generation of prostacyclin by arteries and the coronary vascular beds is reduced in experimental atherosclerosis in rabbits. *Prostaglandins* 1977;14:1025

137. Sinzinger H, Feigl W, Silberbauer K: Prostacyclin generation in atherosclerotic arteries. *Lancet* 1979;2:469

138. Probst P, Pachinger O, Sinzinger H, Kaliman J: Release of prostaglandins after percutaneous transluminal coronary angioplasty. *Circulation* 1983;68(Suppl 3):144

139. Fitzgerald GA, Smith B, Pedersen AK, Brash AR: Increased prostacyclin biosynthesis in patients with severe atherosclerosis and platelet activation. *N Engl J Med* 1984;310:1065

140. Aiken JW, Shebuski RJ, Miller OV, Gorman RR: Endogenous prostacyclin contributes to the efficacy of a thromboxane synthetase inhibitor for preventing coronary artery thrombosis. *J Pharmacol Exp Ther* 1981;219:299

141. Yarger WE, Schocken DD, Harris RH, et al: Obstructive nephropathy in the rat: possible roles for the renin-angiotensin system, prostaglandins, and thromboxanes in postobstructive renal function. *J Clin Invest* 1980;65:400

142. Harter HR, Burch JW, Majerus PW, et al: Prevention of

thrombosis in patients on hemodialysis by low-dose aspirin. *N Engl J Med* 1979;301:577

143. Lorenz R, Siess W, Weber PC: Effects of very low versus standard dose acetyl salicylic acid, dipyridamole and sulfinpyrazone on platelet function and thromboxane formation in man. *Eur J Pharmacol* 1981;70:511

144. Masotti G, Galanti G, Poggesi L, Abbate R, Neri Serneri GG: Differential inhibition of prostacyclin production and platelet aggregation by aspirin. *Lancet* 1979;2:1213

145. Shaikh BS, Bott SJ, Demers LM: The differential inhibition of prostaglandin synthesis in platelets and vascular tissue in response to aspirin. *Prostagland Med* 1980;4:439

146. Jaffe EA, Weksler BB: Recovery of endothelial cell prostacyclin production after inhibition by low doses of aspirin. *J Clin Invest* 1979;63:532

147. Weksler BB, Pett SB, Alonso D, et al: Differential inhibition by aspirin of vascular and platelet prostaglandin synthesis in atherosclerotic patients. *N Engl J Med* 1983; 308:800

148. Burch JW, Stanford N, Majerus PW: Inhibition of platelet prostaglandin synthetase by oral aspirin. *J Clin Invest* 1978;61:314

149. Kelton JG: Antiplatelet agents: rationale and results. *Clin Hematol* 1983;12:311

150. Killackey JJ, Killackey BA, Philp RB: Structure–activity studies of aspirin and related compounds on platelet aggregation, arachidonic acid metabolism in platelets and artery, and arterial prostacyclin activity. *Prostagland Leukotrienes Med* 1982;9:9

151. Marcus AJ: Aspirin as an antithrombotic medication. *N Engl J Med* 1983;24:1515

152. O'Brien JR: Platelets and the vessel wall: how much aspirin? (letter). *Lancet* 1980;1:372

153. Preston FE, Whipps S, Jackson CA, French AJ, Wyld PJ, Stoddard CJ: Inhibition of prostacyclin and platelet thromboxane A_2 after low dose aspirin. *N Engl J Med* 1981;304:76

154. Furchgott RF: Role of endothelium in responses of vascular smooth muscle. *Circ Res* 1983;53:558

155. Hamberg M, Svensson J, Samuelsson B: Prostaglandin endoperoxides: a new concept concerning the mode of action and release of prostaglandins. *Proc Natl Acad Sci USA* 1974;71:3824

156. Cragg A, Einzig S, Castañeda–Zúñiga WR, Amplatz K, White JG, Rao GHR: Vessel wall arachidonate metabolism after angioplasty: possible mediators of postangioplasty vasospasm. *Am J Cardiol* 1983;51:1441

157. Buchanan MR, Dejana E, Gent M, Mustard JF, Hirsh J: Enhanced platelet accumulation onto injured carotid arteries in rabbits after aspirin treatment. *J Clin Invest* 1981;67:503

158. Buchanan MR, Hirsch J: Effect of aspirin and salicylate on platelet–vessel wall interactions in rabbits. *Arteriosclerosis* 1984;4:403

159. Lewis HD, Davis JW, Archibald DG, et al: Protective effect of aspirin against acute myocardial infarction and death in men with unstable angina. *N Engl J Med* 1983;309:396

160. Lorenz RL, Weber M, Kotzur J, et al: Improved aortocoronary bypass patency by low-dose aspirin (100mg daily). *Lancet* 1984;1:1261

161. Zollikofer CL, Salomonowitz E, Castañeda–Zúñiga WR, Brühlmann WF, Amplatz K: The relationship between arterial rupture and balloon bursting in experimental angioplasty. *AJR* 1985;144:777

162. Zollikofer CL, Salomonowitz E, Brühlmann WF, Frick MP, Castañeda–Zúñiga WR, Amplatz K: Significance of balloon pressure recording during angioplasty. *RöFo* 1985;142:526

163. Abele JE: Balloon catheters and transluminal dilatation. *AJR* 1980;135:901

164. Athanasoulis CA, Abbott WM, Fidrych AM, et al: Balloon catheters for transluminal angioplasty: balloon bursting characteristics and clinical significance (abstract). Presented at 66th Scientific Meeting of the Radiological Society of North America, Dallas, TX, 1980

165. Waltman AC: Percutaneous transluminal angioplasty: iliac and deep femoral arteries. *AJR* 1980;135:921

166. Simonetti G, Rossi P, Passariello R, et al: Iliac artery rupture: a complication of transluminal angioplasty. *AJR* 1983;140:989

167. McDonald DA: *Blood Flow in Arteries*. Baltimore, Williams & Wilkins, 1960, p 153

168. Altose MD: Pulmonary mechanics, in Fishman AP (ed): *Pulmonary Diseases and Disorders*. New York, McGraw–Hill, 1980, p 359

169. Burton AC: *Physiology and Biophysics of the Circulation*. Chicago, Year Book Medical Publishers, 1972, p 67

170. Olbert F, Kasparzak Muzika N, Schlegl A: Percutaneous transluminal dilatation and recanalization: long-term results and report on experience with a new catheter system. *Ann Radiol* 1984;27:349

171. Yune HY, Klatte EC:. Circumferential tear of percutaneous transluminal angioplasty catheter balloon. *AJR* 1980;135:395

Part 3. Noninvasive Evaluation of Peripheral Vascular Disease

Introduction to Doppler Physics

—Keith M. Horton, M.D.

GENERAL PRINCIPLES

Ultrasound utilizes high frequency sound waves in order to noninvasively image and characterize motion within tissues. Audible waves lie within the 20–20,000Hz (cycles/sec) range. Commonly used ultrasound frequencies are in the 2–20mHz (million cycles/sec) range.

By using a piezoelectric crystal commonly referred to as a transducer (a device which converts electrical energy into sound energy and vice versa), a brief burst of sound is sent into the soft tissues. This is followed by analysis of the echoes reflected from structures within the tissues. This information can then be used to determine depth, composition, and relative motion of the tissues studied.

Depth can be judged by the time it takes for the reflected echo to return to the transducer face. By knowing that sound travels approximately 1540m/sec, distance that the echo traveled can be calculated using the equation:

$$D = \frac{\nu T}{2}$$

where D = distance from transducer to object; ν = velocity of sound in tissue (1540m/sec); and T = time it takes for the echo to return to the probe face. (Since time is a measure of a round trip for the echo, it must be divided by 2 for one trip.)

Sound emitted from the transducer undergoes many interactions within the tissues before it returns. Most of the sound beam is absorbed or scattered as it travels through the body. Some of the beam is reflected back to the transducer. The amount and type of interaction is dependent upon the tissue characteristics. Adjacent tissues with large differences in density or "acoustic impedance" will generate large signals at their interfaces. Tissues which are reflectors of sound and are perpendicular to the beam reflect the most sound and, therefore, generate the largest signal.

Images are thus obtained by sending multiple thin parallel sound waves into tissues and analyzing the returning echoes. The strength of the signal is determined by the amount of tissue interaction.

The location or depth of the signal is determined by the amount of time it took for the signal to return to the transducer. If one were to send out one sound burst and analyze

the returning signal, one still frame image would be obtained. By repeating this process multiple times per second, the illusion of motion, "real-time" images, are obtained, much like motion pictures. The number of images displayed per second is referred to as the "frame rate." Frame rates of greater than 30 are commonly used to produce flicker-free B-mode real-time images.

DOPPLER SONOGRAPHY

The Doppler principle was first described by the 19th century Austrian physicist, Christian Johann Doppler. He showed that the frequency of light or sound emitted by a source traveling toward the observer is perceived as higher than its transmitted frequency, and vice versa.[1]

This is well illustrated in common practice by the increasing pitch of approaching trains, sirens, or race car engines on a track. The faster the object moves toward or away from the detector, in our case the ear, the more pronounced the perceived change in pitch (Fig. 4.3.1). This change in pitch is known to the Doppler physicist as frequency shift. By using red blood cells as the moving object and a Doppler probe as the detector, these principles can be applied to flowing blood. By analyzing these perceived changes in frequency shifts, certain features such as the direction and speed of the red blood cells can be determined.

Two basic types of Doppler probes, continuous wave and pulsed wave, can be used to assess blood flow. Bidirectional continuous wave Doppler probes have been available since the early 1970s and until the mid-1980s were the predominant means of evaluation of vascular disease. They are often still used to evaluate faint or nonpalpable peripheral pulses. Because of the continuous nature of these instruments, these probes contain two slightly offset ultrasound piezoelectric crystals. One crystal continuously emits an ultrasound wave, and the other constantly monitors returning signals. The two crystals are minimally offset, creating a zone where the Doppler shift frequency can be detected (Fig. 4.3.2). This information can be analyzed and output as either an audible signal or a display on a television monitor. If output as an audible signal, it can be transmitted through a loud speaker. Blood flow moving toward the transducer results in a higher pitched signal. If processed by a fast Fourier transform calculation, the signal could also be displayed on a television monitor. The horizontal axis reflects time and the vertical axis displays the Doppler frequency shift, which is proportional to the velocity of blood flow. The brightness or amplitude of the

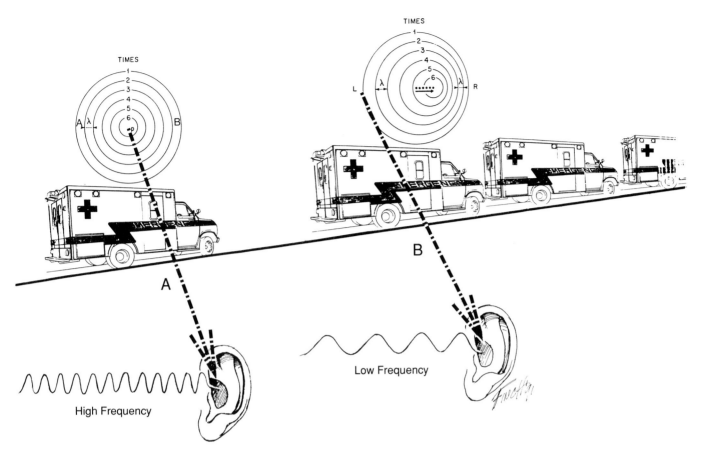

Figure 4.3.1. **A.** When stationary, sound emitted from a source travels at the same speed in all directions. Therefore, to an observer, sound is perceived at the same frequency as it is emitted at any point. Therefore, sound emitted from *Point P* will be perceived as the same frequency by Observer A or B. **B.** When sound is emitted from a moving source, those waves moving in the same direction as the object are traveling at a slightly higher speed than those on the trailing edge. Because of this, the waves on the leading edge are closer in time, or have a higher frequency than those on the trailing edge, and those on the trailing edge are slightly lower in frequency. To an observer, this is detected by the ear as a change in frequency or pitch and is proportional to the speed of the moving object. Therefore, the observer at *Point L* will hear a slightly lower frequency than the observer at *Point R*. (Adapted with permission from Curry TS III, Dowdey JE, Murry RC Jr (eds): *Christensen's Introduction to the Physics of Diagnostic Radiology.* ed 3. Philadelphia, Lea & Febiger, 1984.)

signal reflects, in part, the number of red blood cells at that particular point within the vessel.

Because of the continuous output of the emitting crystal and the inability to image vessels, it is not possible to know the precise origin of a Doppler shift signal. Therefore, Doppler signals generated from anywhere within the region of emitting and receiving transducer overlap are detected.

In the early 1980s pulsed Doppler ultrasound was developed which, when combined with B-mode real-time images, permits accurate localization of the source of a Doppler signal. As with routine B-mode imaging, the transducer acts as both the transmitter and receiver but cannot act as both simultaneously. The probe must take turns in its duty by emitting a pulse of sound and then for a fraction of a second listening for the returning echo. The amplitude of the reflected echo is dependent upon the tissue composition and the amount of acoustical interfaces encountered. Using these data, an image can thus be produced.

Pulsed Doppler allows one to localize the source of the signal by only accepting and decoding echoes from a set window of time which corresponds to the depth of the returning echo. This combination of B-mode imaging with pulsed Doppler is what is commonly known today as duplex ultrasound. In practice, the B-mode image is frozen and range-gated with a cursor to define the area for pulsed-Doppler interrogation. Such range-gating allows precise placement of the sampling volume, assisting in determination of the angle between the probe face and the blood vessel, an important parameter in the calculation of the Doppler frequency shift or blood flow velocity.

To measure the Doppler shift, pulses must be repeated at a constant rate (Fig. 4.3.3). The frequency at which these pulses, or echoes, are sent out is known as the pulse repetition frequency (PRF). Knowing that sound travels at approximately 154,000cm/sec, it can be easily calculated that sound travels 1cm in 6.5 microseconds, or a round trip of 13 microseconds.[2] For most applications the depth of sampling is usually less than 5cm, which means that it would take 68 microseconds for a round-trip pulse. Utiliz-

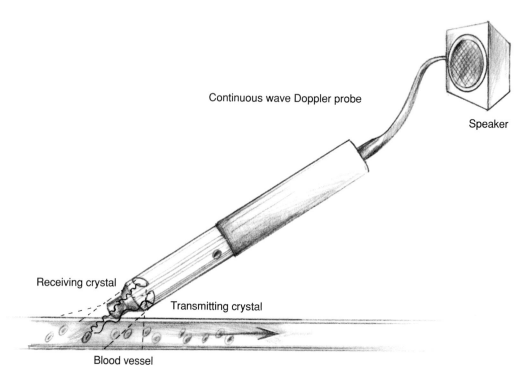

Figure 4.3.2. Continuous wave Doppler probe. The transmitting crystal sends out continuous waves of sound. The receiving crystal constantly monitors the returning echoes for changes in frequency. Increased changes in frequency mean that the RBCs are reflecting sound toward the transducer and this is represented as an increase in frequency of the sound or pitch.

ing this, it is easily calculated that up to 14,700 (14.7kHz) pulses can be generated per second. Typically, pulse repetition frequencies used for arterial flow analysis are between 7 and 15,000Hz. The closer the target area is, the faster the echo returns. It is, therefore, easy to see that sampling at lesser depths allows for faster pulse repetition frequencies. This becomes important because improper setting of the pulse repetition frequency can lead to the generation of falsely low and apparently misleading Doppler frequency shifts. When this occurs it is known as aliasing, and it occurs when the pulse repetition frequency is less than twice the Doppler shift frequency (Fig. 4.3.4). This is the same phenomenon that causes the illusion of backward spinning wagon wheels in old Western movies. This maximal Doppler shift frequency is known as the Nyquist frequency. Aliasing can be eliminated first by simply increasing the pulse repetition frequency. Other methods include ways to decrease the apparent Doppler shift frequency which can be done by examining the Doppler equation

$$f = \frac{2\nu f_0}{c} \cos \theta.$$

For practical purposes, f_0 and θ are the only nonconstants in the equation. By lowering f_0 or the transducer frequency or increasing θ (increasing θ causes the cosine of θ to decrease toward zero when approaching 90°), frequency shift can be decreased.

Doppler measurements are less reliable when the sampling angle is greater than 60° or less than 30°; therefore, for accurate representation of flow velocity θ should be kept between 30°–60°. Doppler shift frequency is directly proportional to red blood cell velocity. If the probe angle and the transmitted frequency are known, then flow velocity can also be determined. Flow velocity data, rather than frequency shift, are more often displayed on the y-axis of a time graph because they are a more easily standardized from machine to machine and often simpler to understand.

SPECTRAL ANALYSIS

Spectral analysis is the key to objective and reproducible interpretation of Doppler examinations. When displayed graphically with time on the x-axis and velocity on the y-axis, speed and direction of flow can instantly be evaluated. Positive deflections represent flow towards the transducer (or acceleration) while the negative deflections depict flow traveling away from the transducer (or deceleration) (Fig. 4.3.5).

When displayed as such, arterial and venous waveforms possess distinguishing characteristics. Most normal arterial waveforms demonstrate an early positive deflection depicting accelerating flow during systole. This is followed by a negative deflection representing deceleration of flow during early diastole, followed by another positive deflection representing antegrade flow during diastole. The height or velocity of flow during diastole is a measure of the relative vascular resistance (the more flow, the less the vascular resistance) in the system that that particular vessel supplies.

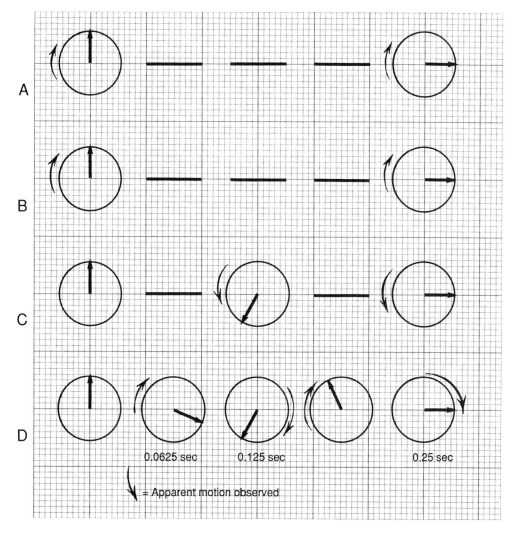

Figure 4.3.3. We will observe two clockwise spinning discs by taking pictures of the two discs at a set rate (analogous to pulse repetition frequency) over 0.25 sec. **A.** Disc A spins at 1 rev/sec (analogous to Doppler shift frequency). **B.** Disc B spins at 5 rev/sec (analogous to Doppler shift frequency). However, if pictures of the spinning disc are taken at 4 pictures/sec (pulse repetition frequency), then both appear to spin at the same rate. **C.** If the pictures are taken of Disc B at a faster rate (8 pictures/

sec) (increased pulse repetition frequency), then the disc appears to spin backward (or counterclockwise) instead of 5 rev/sec forward (clockwise). **D.** If the rate of the pictures is increased to 16 pictures/sec, then the true rate for Disc B can be determined ($16 > 2 \times 5$). Thus the pulse repetition frequency now exceeds the Nyquist limit where 16 = pulse repetition frequency and 5 is the Doppler shift frequency.

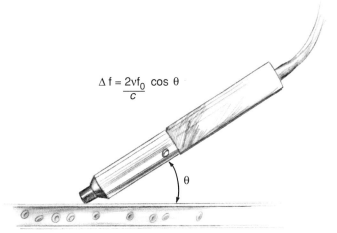

$$\Delta f = \frac{2vf_0}{c} \cos \theta$$

Figure 4.3.4. $\Delta f = \dfrac{2vf_0}{c} \cos \theta$, where f_0 = frequency of the transmitting transducer; θ = angle between the transducer and vessel; v = velocity of the flowing RBCs; c = speed of sound in soft tissues (1540m/sec); Δf = Doppler frequency shift.

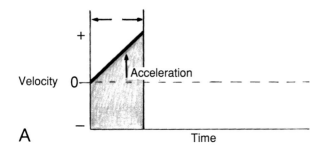

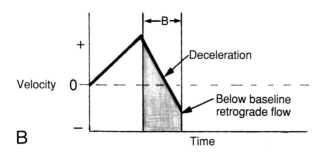

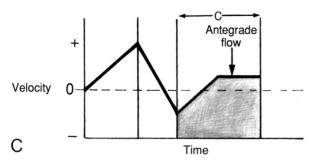

Figure 4.3.5. Typical arterial waveform. Positive deflections represent flow toward the transducer (or acceleration) while the negative deflections depict flow traveling away from the transducer (or deceleration). **A.** Early positive deflection depicts accelerating flow during systole. **B.** Negative deflection represents decelerating flow during early diastole. Flow below baseline represents retrograde flow (seen only in higher resistance arteries). **C.** Late diastole flow again assumes antegrade direction.

As will be discussed later, each vascular system has its own characteristics which determine its typical waveform.

Venous Doppler tracings demonstrate several differences from their arterial counterpart. First, venous flow is typically nonpulsatile unless one is examining abnormal veins or those close to the heart demonstrating reflected atrial pulsations.

Venous flow is phasic, meaning that the velocity varies with respiration. Flow is normally spontaneous in the medium to large veins and can be abruptly increased or augmented by compression of the extremity distal to the site of examination. Flow can also be halted, often by performing the Valsalva maneuver. The loss of any of these basic findings makes one suspicious of pathology in the venous system being examined.

Therefore, by examining the spectral characteristics of

flow, whether arterial or venous, inferences about abnormalities can be confidently and reproducibly made. Using the above techniques, noninvasive duplex examination of most vascular systems can be obtained.

COLOR FLOW DOPPLER

Color flow Doppler (CFD) takes the data acquired from the duplex signal and assigns color to objects moving within a designated area. Ideally, CFD detects only the signals from flowing blood, not other signals generated from "stationary" tissues. Various filters and discriminators have been designed to optimize color imaging of blood flow. Wall filters are used to eliminate low frequency shifts, such as patient or transducer movement, from the higher frequency shifts caused by flowing blood. Other data manipulation includes color thresholding which assigns color only to anechoic regions. Both of these parameters can be varied during an examination.

By convention, blood flow toward the transducer is assigned a red color, and that flowing away blue. This can easily be adjusted by the operator. In addition, color hue varies according to the mean flow velocity within the vessel. However, because the probe angle to blood flow is not consistently known, quantitative data are difficult to generate with CFD. However, there are studies at this time describing the value of color imaging alone in determining the significance of stenoses.[3-6]

CFD offers several advantages over conventional duplex imaging in the evaluation of vascular disease. Because of color, indicating the presence of flow, ability to select and follow the course of vessels is greatly enhanced. As the course of a vessel can be defined more accurately, the Doppler angle for velocity measurements can be determined more precisely. Using the change in color intensity, the ability to select areas of abnormal blood flow, velocity and turbulence is greatly facilitated. Consequently, the area within a vessel with the most abnormal flow characteristics can be rapidly selected for conventional pulsed Doppler interrogation. In general the use of CFD has decreased scanning time for the experienced vascular sonographer and shortened the learning curve for the novice examiner.

Extracranial Carotid Artery Disease

INTRODUCTION

Stroke is the third leading cause of death in the United States today. Each year 400,000 Americans suffer strokes. Nearly two-thirds of survivors may be handicapped, with an estimated two million people in the United States currently disabled by stroke. When direct medical expenses are combined with lost income and productivity, the total cost of stroke in the United States is estimated to be 14 bil-

lion dollars annually, impacting significantly on the American health care system.[7] Most strokes are caused by atherosclerotic disease involving the extracranial carotid near the bifurcation.[8] Transient ischemic attacks can also be linked to atherosclerotic disease and the risk for strokes in a patient so affected approaches 10% per year.[9] It is felt that, with adequate screening, carotid artery disease could be detected and, therefore, many strokes prevented. Over the years, this hypothesis has sparked several technologic developments for the evaluation of extracranial carotid artery disease, including oculoplethysmography, continuous wave Doppler, and duplex sonography. Currently, the most accurate, noninvasive method of evaluating carotid vascular disease is conventional duplex or color flow Doppler (CFD) ultrasound.

The management of patients with carotid artery disease remains very controversial; consequently, the indications for imaging are clouded as well. This is largely because of the lack of significant data documenting the natural progression of carotid artery disease. Most of this controversy centers on the management of asymptomatic patients with carotid artery bruits and/or stenosis, and patients with nonlocalizing symptoms and carotid stenosis.[10]

Patients have been traditionally screened for the presence of stenosis demonstrating at least a 50% transluminal diameter reduction or a 70% cross-sectional area of stenosis. Patients that are judged to have so-called critical stenosis, or greater than 80% decrease in diameter, are generally felt to have an increased risk of cerebral infarction and are generally considered surgical candidates.

One of the major indications for duplex examination is the presence of a carotid bruit. In a study done on 1,000 normal patients, there was a 31% incidence of carotid bruits. In this same survey, 12% of patients greater than 60 years of age had a carotid bruit.[11] Cervical bruits can originate from the external carotid artery, subclavian and even transmitted superior mediastinal murmurs.

Other studies show that 30–50% of patients with asymptomatic bruits have significant carotid stenosis by duplex scanning.[9,12,13] Classically, a carotid bruit can be detected on physical exam at approximately a 50% diameter stenosis and paradoxically will often disappear with stenosis greater than 85%, making the patients in whom detection of asymptomatic stenosis is the most desirable, the most difficult to identify. However, at least 50% of patients with hemispheric symptoms have less than a 50% diameter stenosis. Some studies suggest that plaque characterization may some day help in defining therapy in these patients.

Another often cited indication is a history of transient ischemic attacks (TIA). Patients with TIAs have a 2.5- to 5-fold increased risk per year of having a stroke when compared with normal patients. Ninety percent of the spontaneous symptoms of TIAs were associated with an 80% or greater stenosis at the time of occurrence. Progression of a lesion to more than an 80% stenosis is a warning observation since it reportedly carries a 35% risk of ischemic symptoms or ipsilateral occlusion within 6 months and a 46% risk at 12 months.[9,14]

Patients with known atherosclerotic disease involving either the peripheral vascular tree or coronary arteries have an increased risk of carotid disease. In one study of patients undergoing coronary artery bypass grafting, 18% were shown to have significant stenosis of the carotid artery.[15] A significant portion of the morbidity and mortality resulting from coronary artery surgery emanates from carotid artery disease, making screening prudent in these patients.

Other indications include: 1) nonhemispheric symptoms; 2) to follow-up endarterectomy; 3) high-risk patients with diabetes or strong family history of cardiovascular disease; 4) patients with amaurosis fugax; 5) patients with known carotid plaque receiving medical therapy for atherosclerotic disease; and 6) patients with a pulsatile neck mass.

EXAMINATION

Examination is performed with the patient in the supine position and the examiner at the patient's head. The patient's head is turned toward the contralateral side to facilitate access to the region of interest. We currently utilize a 5mHz linear transducer for examination of the carotid arteries.

We first obtain longitudinal images of the proximal carotid artery. This allows us to identify sites of atherosclerotic disease and assess its severity. Then, utilizing pulsed Doppler, we obtain a representative velocity spectrum of the common carotid artery. Following the common carotid artery to the bifurcation, examination of the branch vessels is then performed. Views of the bifurcation and branch vessels can sometimes be obtained on the same image when scanning from the posterolateral position. With the addition of color flow Doppler, sites of significant stenosis can usually be easily identified and sampled to obtain flow velocities in these regions. If no stenoses are detected, representative Doppler waveforms are obtained of the proximal internal carotid arteries (ICA) and external carotid arteries (ECA).

Identification of the internal and external carotid can be performed in several ways. Visually, when scanning posterolateral, the ICA is usually the artery closer to the transducer (greater than 90% of patients)[16] (Fig. 4.3.6). It is often the larger of the two branches. In addition, one can often see branches originating from the ECA. Using Doppler waveform analysis, the classic differentiating point is that the ICA waveform remains above baseline during diastole because of the decreased vascular resistance within the cerebral bed (Fig. 4.3.7). Using color, one should see continuous color in the ICA. The ECA can be identified easily by using a maneuver in which the superficial temporal

Figure 4.3.6. Drawing of neck. Patient is scanned from posterior lateral position. In this position, the ICA is more often the closer of the bifurcation vessels to the transducer.

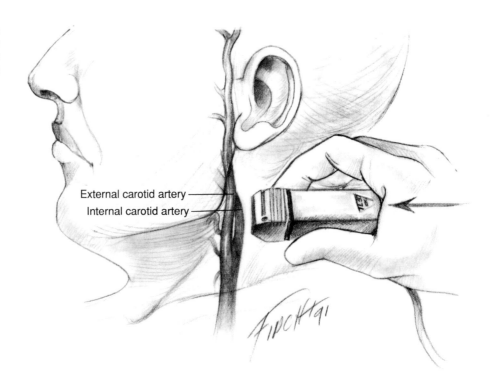

External carotid artery
Internal carotid artery

artery is tapped and a corresponding deflection can be traced on the Doppler waveform. These maneuvers are often useful when scanning tortuous carotid vessels.

Transverse scans of the carotid and branch vessels are also obtained and can be very helpful in locating plaque and grading stenoses. Lastly, the vertebral artery is imaged by locating a pulsatile signal between the transverse processes of the cervical vertebra. A Doppler waveform tracing is obtained at this level in order to document antegrade flow to rule out subclavian steal (Fig. 4.3.8).

INTERPRETATION

Interpretation of duplex Doppler carotid examinations utilizes the Gray scale images and Doppler data measurements. When taken separately, these individual components have a 70–80% rate of accuracy in assessing the degree of carotid stenosis.[9,17–20] Combined reported sensitivities range from 91 to 99% with specificities and accuracies ranging from 84 to 97% and 92 to 96%, respectively.[4,21–23]

Gray scale images permit direct imaging of the arterial lumen and wall, allowing an estimation of the degree of relative diameter or area stenosis. The diameter of areas in question can be compared with more normal areas and an estimate of luminal narrowing can be obtained. Because most plaques are eccentric, careful transverse imaging of the vessel must be done, as well as longitudinal imaging for correlation. Also, because of the sometimes similar sonographic characteristics of the arterial lumen and echolucent plaque along the vessel wall, the exact margins of the artery may be difficult to determine (Fig. 4.3.9A,B).

With the increased use of high resolution imaging, some researchers have found a correlation between plaque echogenicity and its histology.[24–28] This suggests that there may be some prognostic information obtainable from analysis of plaque composition. The echogenicity of plaque tends to correlate best with collagen content. Simply, the more echogenic the plaque, the higher its collagen content.[17–20] Hyperechoic plaques with acoustic shadowing tend to represent calcified regions (Fig. 4.3.10). These plaques tend to be more stable and are not usually linked to significant symptoms. A notable pitfall is that calcified plaques can often block the ultrasound beam and hamper Doppler investigation deep to the plaque.

Fibrofatty plaque, often quite homogeneous, is felt to be the least echogenic type of plaque. It may be difficult to detect sonographically, as it may be isoechoic to flowing blood (Fig. 4.3.9A). These plaques tend to be more symptomatic than calcified plaque. Some researchers have found that plaque with fatty components predominates in tissue removed from symptomatic endarterectomy patients when compared with that from asymptomatic patients.[28] Additionally, Bluth has suggested that hypoechoic plaques with areas of increased echogenicity have sustained intraplaque hemorrhage[24]; it is also felt that these lesions occur more commonly in symptomatic than in asymptomatic patients.[25,26,28] Lusby has associated intraplaque hemorrhages with plaque surface ischemia and intimal tears, stimulating thrombus formation and peripheral emboli. These lesions are associated with rapid progression of symptomatology and luminal stenosis.[9] Accuracy rates for the detection of these types of lesions, as quoted by Lusby and Bluth, range from 82 to 90% with sensitivities ranging from 91 to 94%.[29,30]

Ulceration remains one of the most difficult lesions to

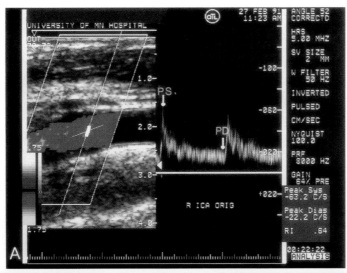

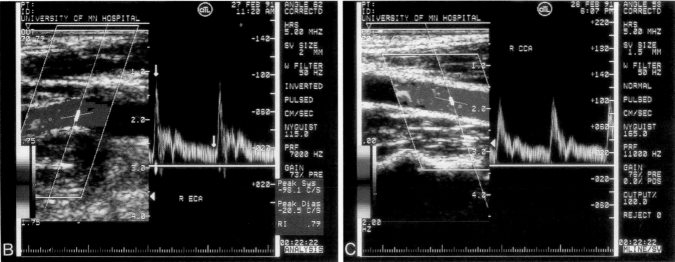

Figure 4.3.7. **A.** ICA waveform. Sharp upstroke. *Arrows* measuring peak systole and end diastolic velocities. Note diastolic flow remains above baseline (*PS* = peak systolic; *PD* = peak diastolic). **B.** ECA wave-form. Sharper upstroke with diastolic flow less than ICA flow. **C.** CCA. Hybrid of the above waveforms. However, since the ICA carries 80% of the CCA flow, the waveform resembles the ICA more than the ECA.

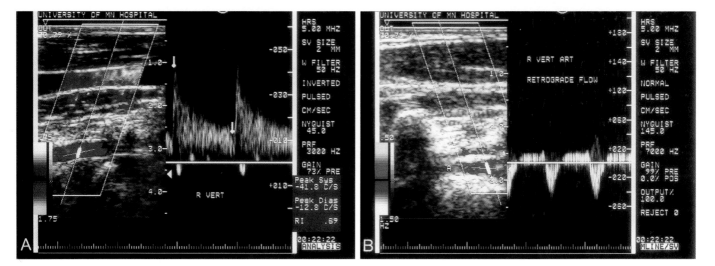

Figure 4.3.8. **A.** Normal antegrade flow vertebral artery depicted as *red*. Jugular vein in the near field is *blue*. **B.** Retrograde flow in vertebral artery with accompanying vertebral vein. Both *blue*. Flow is in the same direction.

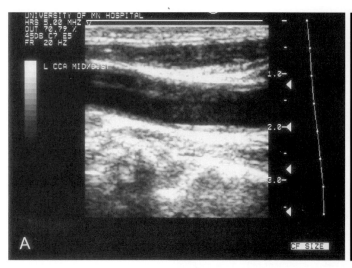

Figure 4.3.9. **A.** Longitudinal image of CCA partially echogenic lumen. However, margins are difficult to determine. **B.** Using color, margin of hypoechoic plaque and lumen easily differentiated demonstrating the value of color.

detect. Ulcers also tend to have a high correlation with symptoms. Studies suggest that the significance and ease of detection of ulcers varies with the degree of luminal stenosis. Comerota found that in his series of symptomatic patients, 100% of plaques with less than or equal to 50% stenosis contained ulcers, whereas 63% of plaques with greater than 50% stenosis were ulcerated.[31] This suggests that it is easier to detect ulcerations in patients with less than 50% stenosis. Studies have shown that the sensitivity for detection of ulcers approaches 77% for B-mode images when there is less than 50% stenosis. This compares with a 41% detection rate for lesions of greater than 50% steno-

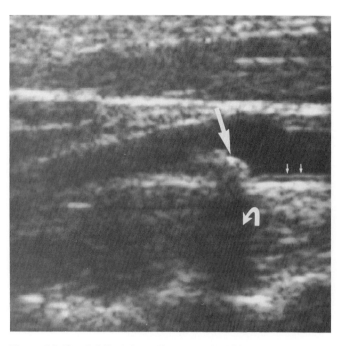

Figure 4.3.10. Calcified plaque (*large arrow*) in ICA with acoustic shadowing (*curved arrow*) and thickening of arterial wall (*small arrows*).

sis, which correlates reasonably well to arteriography, which has a 77 and 48% rate, respectively.[31]

Doppler criteria for relative stenoses were developed based on the premise that flow velocity is proportional to the cross-sectional area of the arterial lumen. In areas where there is greater than 50% cross-sectional diameter narrowing, there is a significant increase in blood flow velocity. It has also been noted that peak flow velocities are more reliable criteria for stenosis than are mean flow velocities.[22,32–34] Various criteria have been established to determine the significance of these stenoses. A commonly used set of criteria was developed by Bluth[34] (Table 4.3.1); it relies on peak systolic, as well as peak diastolic, flow velocities. This system also relies on the fact that both parameters are elevated once stenosis exceeds 55% (Fig. 4.3.11*A*). For stenoses within the range of 55–70% the peak systolic velocities correlate best with luminal diameters. Above 75% stenosis peak diastolic velocities seem to correlate better with vessel stenosis. Peak diastolic velocity ratios are also very effective for assessing 75–95% diameter stenoses; these values rely less on cardiac output, peripheral vascular resistance, or tandem lesions in either the ipsilateral and contralateral carotid systems (Fig. 4.3.11*B*). In practice, these ratio criteria are less often utilized than are absolute velocity measurements (Fig. 4.3.12).

Spectral broadening, which is a measure of turbulence produced in the lumen, has also been used to evaluate the degree of luminal stenosis. "Filling-in" of the spectral window, manifested by increased echoes within the normal echolucent area under the systolic peak, is the most reliable quantitative measure of turbulence and suggests that at least a 50% diameter stenosis is present (Fig. 4.3.13).

As the severity of the stenosis increases, so does the velocity of flow. When internal carotid artery stenosis approaches near occlusion, the vascular resistance increases and slows blood flow. More blood is shifted

Table 4.3.1. **Criteria for Grading Disease Severity**

Category	Diameter Stenosis (Category)	Peak Systolic Velocity (cm/sec)	Peak Diastolic Velocity (cm/sec)	Systolic Velocity Ratio (VICA/VCCA)[a]	Diastolic Velocity Ratio (VICA/VCCA)
Normal–mild	0–39	<110	<40	<1.8	<2.4
Moderate	40–59	110–130	40	<1.8	<2.4
Severe	60–79	130–250	40–100	1.8–3.7	2.4–5.5
Critical	80–99	>250	>100	>3.7	>5.5
Occlusion	100	0	0	NA[b]	NA

[a]VICA = velocity of internal carotid artery; VCCA = velocity of common carotid artery.
[b]NA = not applicable.
(From Bluth EI, Wetzner SM, Stavros AT, et al: Carotid duplex sonography: a multicenter recommendation for standardized imaging and Doppler criteria. *RadioGraphics* 1988;8:487–506.)

toward the higher resistance of the ICA. The Doppler tracing obtained proximal to an obstruction demonstrates a dampened or "water-hammer pulse" waveform. Also, the normal high diastolic flow seen in lower resistance vessels is often lost, and flow approaches that normally seen in the external carotid artery. However, if the ipsilateral ECA is supplying collateral flow to the carotid artery, this will often decrease the resistance and often result in a nearly normal ICA flow pattern in the ECA. Maneuvers discussed before may be of help in this situation to differentiate the ECA from the ICA. Also, an asymmetric ICA waveform, when compared with the contralateral ICA, may reveal an unsuspected occlusion.

The most difficult area for interpretation of duplex examinations is in the evaluation of at least 95% luminal stenosis of the ICA. Because the high velocity of flow within the stenotic segment requires the use of relatively high pulse repetition rates and high wall filters, it may be difficult to detect slow flow in the segment of the vessel distal to the stenosis. This can be overcome by lowering the pulse repetition frequency when a high-grade stenosis or total occlusion is suspected. This is a critical differentiation to

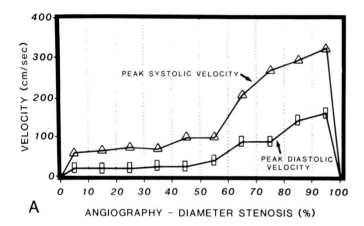

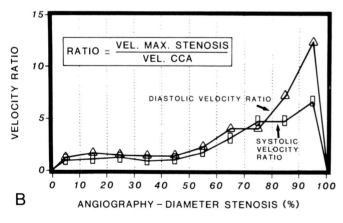

Figure 4.3.11. Velocity/velocity ratios. **A.** Graph compares diameter stenosis with velocity. There is no significant increase in peak velocity until patient has a 55% or greater diameter stenosis. There is a more linear relationship between peak systolic velocity (PSV) and percent diameter stenosis, until one reaches a 75% diameter stenosis where peak diastolic velocities correlate better. Once stenosis exceeds 95%, flow rapidly decreases. **B.** Peak diastolic velocity ratios have a much more linear relationship with diameter stenosis than systolic velocity ratios at all points. (Reproduced with permission from Bluth EI, Wetzner SM, Stavros AT, et al: Carotid duplex sonography: a multicenter recommendation for standardized imaging and Doppler criteria. *RadioGraphics* 1988;8:487–506.)

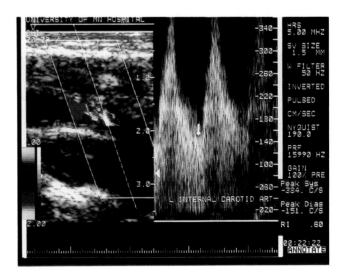

Figure 4.3.12. Critical carotid artery stenosis. Peak systolic velocity > 340cm/sec. End diastolic velocity 151cm/sec.

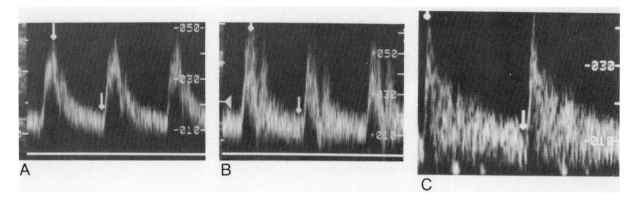

Figure 4.3.13. **A.** Mild turbulence. However, spectral window remains open. **B.** Moderate turbulence demonstrates increased echoes within spectral window. **C.** Severe turbulence with filling-in of spectral window.

make because a total occlusion is usually deemed inoperable, whereas a critical stenosis can be treated with endarterectomy. Angiography is indicated for definitive diagnosis in most of these cases.

CONCLUSION

Duplex sonography of the extracranial carotid system is a reliable diagnostic method for accessing and grading stenotic lesions. Its ability to characterize plaque morphology may be promising in the future. Although angiography has been the gold standard for many years, CFD has proved to be as reliable, if not better, in detecting stenoses and ulcerations in the extracranial carotids.

References

1. Gerlock AJ, Giyanani VL, Krebs C: *Applications of Noninvasive Vascular Techniques.* Philadelphia, W.B. Saunders, 1988, p 4
2. Curry TS III, Dowdey JE, Murry RC Jr (eds): *Christensen's Introduction to the Physics of Diagnostic Radiology.* ed 3. Philadelphia, Lea & Febiger, 1984
3. Erickson SJ, Mewissen MW, Foley WD, et al: Stenosis of the internal carotid artery: assessment using color Doppler imaging compared with angiography. *AJR* 1989;152:1299–1305
4. Jacobs NM, Grant EG, Schellinger D, Byrd MC, Richardson JD, Cohan SL: Duplex carotid sonography: criteria for stenosis, accuracy, and pitfalls. *Radiology* 1985;154:385–391
5. Hallem MJ, Reid JM, Cooperberg PL: Color-flow Doppler and conventional duplex scanning of the carotid bifurcation: prospective, double-blind correlative study. *AJR* 1989;152:1101–1105
6. Steinke W, Kloetzsch C, Hennerici M: Carotid artery disease assessed by color Doppler flow imaging: correlation with standard Doppler sonography and angiography. *AJR* 1990;154(5):1061–1068
7. *Stroke: Hope Through Research.* U.S. Department of Health and Human Services. NIH Publication No. 83-2222. August 1983:1
8. Hass WK, Fields WS, North RR, Kricheff II, Chase NE, Bauer RB: Joint study of extracranial arterial occlusion II: arteriography techniques, sites, and complications. *JAMA* 1968;203:961–968
9. Wong WS: *The Art of Carotid Duplex Scan.* Acuson, p 2
10. Gosink BB: *Carotid Duplex Evaluation: A Practical Approach.* Presented at the 76th Scientific Assembly of the Radiological Society of North America; Chicago, November, 1990
11. Hammon JH, Eisinger RP. Carotid bruits in 1000 normal subjects. *Arch Intern Med* 1962;109:563
12. Breslau PJ, Phillips DJ, Greep JM, Strandness E: The impact of duplex scanning on the evaluation of patients of asymptomatic bruits in the region of the carotid arteries. *Netherlands J Surg* 1983;35(4):134–138
13. David THE, Humphries AW, Younger TR, et al: A correlation of neck bruits and arteriosclerotic carotid arteries. *Arch Surg* 1973;107:729
14. Check WA: Ultrasound shows carotid stenosis in just half of cervical bruit cases. *JAMA* 1984;252:593–594
15. Lusiani L, Visona A, Castellani V, Ronsisvalle G, Pagnan A, et al: Prospective evaluation of combined carotid and coronary surgery. *Eur J Cardiothoracic Surg* 1987;111:16–19
16. Trigaux JP, Delchambre F, van Beers B: Anatomical variations of the carotid bifurcation: implications for digital subtraction angiography and ultrasonography. *Br J Radiol* 1990;63:181–185
17. Zweibel WJ, Knighton R: Duplex examination of the carotid arteries. *Semin Ultrasound CT MR* 1990;11(2):97–135
18. Chambers BR, Norris JW: Outcome in patients with asymptomatic neck bruits. *N Engl J Med* 1986;315:860–865
19. Caplan LR. Carotid artery disease. N Engl J Med 1986;315:886–888
20. Moneta GL, Taylor DC, Nicholls L, et al: Operative versus nonoperative management of asymptomatic high-grade internal carotid artery stenosis: improved results with endarterectomy. *Stroke* 1987;18:1005–1010
21. Cardoso TJ, Middleton WD: Duplex and color Doppler ultrasound of the carotid arteries. *Semin Intervent Radiol* 1990;7(1):1–8
22. Langlois Y, Roederer GO, Chan A, et al: Evaluating carotid artery disease: the concordance between pulsed Doppler/spectrum analysis and angiography. *Ultrasound Med Biol* 1983;9:51–63
23. Taylor DC, Strandness DE: Carotid artery duplex scanning. *J Clin Ultrasound* 1987;15:635–644
24. Lusby RJ, Ferrell LD, Ehrenfeld WK, et al: Carotid plaque hemorrhage. *Arch Surg* 1981;117:1479–1487
25. Imparato AM, Riles TS, Gorstein F: The carotid bifurcation plaque: pathologic findings associated with cerebral ischemia. *Stroke* 1979;3:238–245
26. Weinberger J, Marks SJ, Gaul JJ, et al: Atherosclerotic

plaque at the carotid artery bifurcation: correlation of ultrasonographic imaging with morphology. *J Ultrasound Med* 1987;6:363–366

27. Bluth EI, McVay LV, Merritt CRB, et al: The identification of ulcerative plaque with high resolution duplex carotid scanning. *J Ultrasound Med* 1988;7:73–76

28. Seeger JM, Klingman N: The relationship between carotid plaque composition and neurologic symptoms. *J Surg Res* 1987;43:78–85

29. Reilly L, Lusby R, Hughes L, Ferrell L, Stoney R, Ehrenfeld W: Carotid plaque history using real-time ultrasonography. *Am J Surg* 1983;146:188–193

30. Bluth EI, Kay D, Merritt CRB, et al: Sonographic characterization of carotid plaque: detection of hemorrhage. *AJNR* 1986;7:311–315

31. Comerota AJ, Katz ML, White JV, Grosh JD: The preoperative diagnosis of the ulcerated carotid atheroma. *J Vasc Surg* 1990;11(4):505–510

32. Blackshear WM, Phillips DJ, Chikos PM, Harley JD, Thiele BL, Strandness DE: Carotid artery velocity patterns in normal and stenotic vessels

33. Garth KE, Carroll BA, Sommer FG, Oppenheimer DA: Duplex ultrasound scanning of the carotid arteries with velocity spectrum analysis. *Radiology* 1983;147:823–827

34. Bluth EI, Wetzner SM, Stavros AT, Aufrichtig D, Marich KW, Baker JD: Carotid duplex sonography: a multicenter recommendation for standardized imaging and Doppler criteria. *RadioGraphics* 1988;8:487–506

35. Towne JB, Weiss DG, Hobson RW: First phase report of cooperative VA asymptomatic carotid stenosis study—operative morbidity and mortality. *J Vasc Surg* 1990;11(2):252–258

36. Brown PB, Zwiebel WJ, Call GK: Degree of cervical carotid artery stenosis and hemispheric stroke: duplex US findings. *Radiology* 1989;170:541–543

37. Carroll BA: Duplex sonography in patients with hemispheric symptoms. *J Ultrasound Med* 1989;8:535–540

Noninvasive Assessment of Lower Extremity Arterial Disease

—Sandra J. Althaus, M.D., Deborah G. Longley, M.D., and Janis Gissel Letourneau, M.D.

Introduction

Angiography is accepted as the "gold standard" for demonstrating the presence of arterial occlusive disease; however, it provides anatomic rather than hemodynamic information, is subject to significant variability at the time of interpretation, is relatively invasive, exposes the patient to contrast media, and is costly. Arteriography is not a test that can be used easily to evaluate the effects of therapy or for interval evaluation of the natural progression of underlying arterial disease.

Currently, numerous noninvasive methods of evaluating lower extremity arterial perfusion are in use. These include duplex sonography, color Doppler sonography, ankle-brachial indices, segmental limb pressures, and $tcPO_2$ measurements. More recently, magnetic resonance imaging angiography is being investigated as a noninvasive method for vascular imaging. Although many of these techniques rely on different physiologic principles and utilize a variety of instrumentation, they all indirectly assess arterial perfusion.

Noninvasive tests can, to a variable extent, locate and objectively quantify the severity of hemodynamic abnormalities. This information is useful for preprocedural tailoring of an angiographic study, pre- and postprocedural evaluation of revascularization with angioplasty, atherectomy, or surgical bypass grafting; therefore, they provide valuable physiologic information to the interventional radiologist and vascular surgeon. The purpose of this section is to discuss the noninvasive evaluation of the lower extremity arterial system.

Hemodynamics of the Lower Extremity Arterial System

A complete but succinct review of the hemodynamic principles of blood flow has been published recently.[1]

A summary description of the hemodynamic theory of blood flow follows.

Poiseuille's law describes the relationship between pressure and flow in an idealized fluid system. It states that fluid of a viscosity (η) flowing through a tube with a length (l) and a radius (r), the pressure difference (P1 − P2) at two points in the system is:

$$P1 - P2 = \frac{q8l\eta}{\pi r^4}$$

Poiseuille's law indicates that the pressure change across an arterial stenosis is directly proportional to the length (l), inversely proportional to the radius (r) to the fourth power, and proportional to the volume of flow (q). The equation applies to a rigid tube and, therefore, only predicts the theoretical minimum pressure gradient of an arterial system.[1] Disturbances of flow produced from arterial stenoses can be described in terms of energy losses as well as pressure changes. The radius of a stenosis is the predominant factor in determining viscous energy loss. Inertial energy losses are related to the kinetic energy of the blood and are proportional to the square of the blood velocity as follows: $^E(k) = \frac{1}{2}pv^2$, where k = kinetic energy, p = specific gravity, and v = velocity. The viscous losses originate within the stenotic segment and inertial losses occur at the entrance (contraction effects) and exit (expansion effects) of a stenosis. Poststenotic turbulence is an expansion effect that can result in considerable energy loss. Even mild stenoses can become significant when arranged in a series. Multiple short segmental stenoses of equal diameter are more clinically significant than a single long stenosis of equal diameter because of multiple sites of inertial energy loss.

A hemodynamically significant stenosis is defined as one

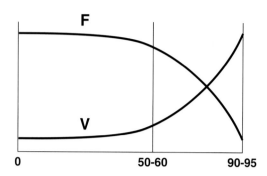

Figure 4.3.14. Increase in percent diameter stenosis causes the blood flow volume rate (*F*) to decrease and the blood flow velocity (*V*) to increase.

with a diameter reduction of 50% or greater; this corresponds to a 75% or greater cross-sectional area reduction. As the degree of stenosis increases, the blood flow volume rate decreases and the blood flow velocity increases (Fig. 4.3.14). Lesions that narrow the artery by less than 50% can become hemodynamically significant when exercise is performed or when a vasodilating drug such as papaverine is administered. This dilatation decreases the resistance in the peripheral vascular bed and increases the blood flow across a stenosis.

A laminar blood flow pattern exists only in an idealized vessel; in such a condition all motion is parallel to the vessel walls. The velocity is lowest adjacent to the tube wall and increases toward the center of the tube to create a parabolic flow profile. The transition from laminar to turbulent flow, for example at a stenosis, depends on Reynold's number,[2] a scaling factor that takes into account flow velocity and vessel size so that blood vessels with similar Reynold's numbers have similar flow characteristics. Reynold's number is determined by the equation

$$\mathrm{Re} = \frac{p\mathrm{d}\nu}{\eta}$$

where p is the fluid density (grams/cm to the second power), d is the vessel diameter in centimeters, ν is the flow velocity in centimeters/sec, and η is the fluid viscosity in Newton's seconds/M[2]. Turbulence occurs at Reynold's numbers greater than 2000. Reynold's numbers are usually less than 2000 in normal arterial flow; however, they may exceed this value in the ascending aorta or distal to a hemodynamically significant stenosis.

ANATOMY AND DISEASE

Atherosclerotic disease may affect any or all of the vessels from the aorta to the toes, including the aorta-iliac system, the femoropopliteal system, and the tibial-peroneal peripheral run-off. An obstructive lesion anywhere within these systems may cause symptomatology in the lower extremities.

The aortoiliac inflow system extends from the level of the renal arteries to that of the inguinal ligaments. This is the second most common site of arteriosclerotic obstruction affecting the extremities. Lesions at this level will limit blood inflow into one or both of the lower extremities.

The femoropopliteal outflow system begins at the level of the inguinal ligament with the common femoral artery (CFA) and ends at the bifurcation of the popliteal artery into the anterior tibial artery and posterior tibial peroneal trunk. The common femoral artery is below the inguinal ligament and is a continuation of the internal iliac artery. There is a high incidence of simultaneous involvement in the aortic inflow and common femoral arteries.

The superficial femoral artery (SFA) descends along the anteromedial aspect of the thigh, whereas the profunda femoral artery (PFA) penetrates deeply into the thigh lateral to the SFA. The SFA is the most common site of atherosclerotic obstructive disease in the lower extremity. Obstructions in the SFA generally occur at its origin from the CFA or at the level of the adductor canal. The PFA and its branches act as a collateral pathway into the popliteal artery. The popliteal artery begins at the termination of the adductor canal; anatomically this correlates with the tendinous insertion of the adductor magnus thigh muscle on the medial aspect of the femur.

The tibioperoneal run-off system begins at the popliteal artery in the popliteal fossa posterior to the knee and terminates at the ankle. Sites of obstruction commonly involve the proximal segments. The first branch from the popliteal artery is the anterior tibial artery, which passes forward between the interosseous membrane of the tibia and fibula and ultimately forms the dorsalis pedis artery in the dorsum of the foot. In 5% of the population the dorsalis pedis pulse is unobtainable; in this situation, large plantar branches usually arise from an enlarged posterior tibial artery.[3] The posterior tibial and peroneal arteries arise as terminal branches of the popliteal artery from a common trunk (the posterior tibial peroneal trunk). The posterior tibial artery ends at the ankle to form the plantar arteries of the foot. Doppler examination of this vessel is best obtained behind the medial malleolus at the ankle. The peroneal artery descends in the deep muscles located between the tibia and fibula and terminates at the ankle; the communicating branches of this vessel can act as a source of collateral blood flow to the anterior and posterior tibial arteries.

CONVENTIONAL DUPLEX AND COLOR DOPPLER ULTRASOUND

Doppler sonography is a valuable noninvasive test for obtaining anatomic and physiologic information concerning arterial flow. As flow disturbances are manifested at sites of arterial narrowing, duplex scanning can be used to assess the relative significance of stenoses in patients with suspected peripheral vascular disease. Duplex scanning and color Doppler sonography are well established methods for assessing the carotid bifurcation and are now being utilized more commonly for lower extremity arterial disease. In 1959, Satomura examined the blood flow and its patterns from specific vessels and was the first to use Doppler technology to assess human blood flow.[4]

The highest frequency scanning transducer that provides adequate depth penetration should be utilized for lower extremity evaluation. Transducer frequencies of approximately 3mHz are most suitable for evaluating the abdominal vessels in the average sized adult. The arteries of the lower extremity can be examined with a 5, 7.5, or 10mHz transducer. Generally, the Doppler probe is positioned to create an angle 30–60° between the ultrasound beam and the presumed direction of blood flow along the longitudinal axis of the artery.

The normal arterial Doppler waveform of a peripheral artery has three main components[5] (Fig. 4.3.15): 1) prominent forward flow during systole; 2) a small but distinct flow reversal in early diastole (dicrotic notch); and 3) forward flow in late diastole. During systole each left ventricular contraction ejects blood into the aortic root; at this point in time a Doppler probe over an artery in the lower extremity will detect a positive deflective velocity wave which reaches a peak at the end of systole. The elasticity of the arterial walls limits luminal distension as this increased blood volume enters the peripheral arterial system. Because of peripheral arterial resistance, blood cannot easily pass out into the venous circulation.

In early diastole the arteries begin to contract and recoil; this causes a reversal of flow toward the lower resistance, larger diameter aorta. This negative wave deflector is termed the dicrotic notch. The magnitude of flow reversal is proportional to the amount of resistance caused by arterioles in the peripheral vascular bed. A larger artery leading to a constricted peripheral vascular bed will have marked reversal of flow in diastolic forward flow, whereas a dilated hyperemic arteriole system will cause the feeding vessel Doppler waveform to have little or no flow reversal or even antegrade diastolic flow.

An additional notch in the peripheral waveform is the incisura, which begins to form before the aortic valve closes at the end of systole or in early diastole as the aortic valve closes. When the left ventricle relaxes at the end of systole the decreased intraventricular pressure allows blood to flow backward through the open aortic valve cusps, which is transmitted through the peripheral arteries.

The third arterial waveform component, late diastolic forward flow, is often absent in the distal vessels if the examination is performed when the leg is cold because of increased peripheral resistance; this should not be confused with occlusive arterial disease. A repeat examination after warming the patient could show late antegrade diastolic flow.

The dicrotic notch and incisura are most pronounced in the larger peripheral arteries of the leg such as the common femoral, superficial femoral, and popliteal arteries, rather than in the tibial arteries and small peripheral arteries of the foot. Correlative Doppler studies are shown (Figs. 4.3.16 and 4.3.17).

The criteria for grading the severity of a stenosis have been established and are based on changes in the normal triphasic waveform with a narrow spectral band width. In a prospective clinical study by Kohler et al.,[6] duplex scanning had a sensitivity of 82% and a specificity of 92% in identifying significant arterial stenoses with a positive and negative predictive value of 80 and 93%, respectively. Duplex scanning in the iliac region had an 89% sensitivity and 90% specificity with 75 and 96% positive and negative predictive values, when compared to angiography. In a 1985 article by Jager,[7] the grading of peripheral arterial stenoses is summarized (Table 4.3.2) (Fig. 4.3.18). Stenoses in the 1–19% range show normal waveform contours and peak systolic frequency but are associated with mild spectral broadening. Lesions causing 20–49% stenosis are characterized by spectral broadening, filling in the clear window under the systolic peak, and a peak systemic velocity over but less than double that of the proximal prestenotic area. Severe stenoses in the 50–99% range cause complete loss of reversal flow, extensive spectral broadening and more than a doubling in the peak systolic velocity. Relative measurements are usually used in the peripheral system, as increased age is associated with decreased aortic peak systolic velocity. Totally arterial occlusion is diagnosed when no flow can be detected from within the vessel and when monophasic flow is seen distally due to collateral blood flow. Kohler[8] concluded that clinical decisions made using duplex sonography are very similar to those made using arteriography and the duplex criteria established by Jager.[7] Nicholls[9] found that the direction and magnitude of velocity of diastolic flow correlated best with the degree of stenosis. There have not been additional supporting articles regarding diastolic flow correlating with the degree of stenosis and presently it is not routinely relied on in the peripheral circulation. At the University of

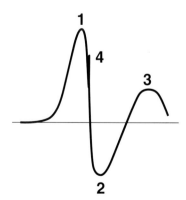

Figure 4.3.15. Normal peripheral artery triphasic waveform. *1*, positive wave peak of systolic segment; *2*, negative wave of early diastolic segment (dicrotic notch); *3*, positive wave of late diastolic segment; *4*, incisura.

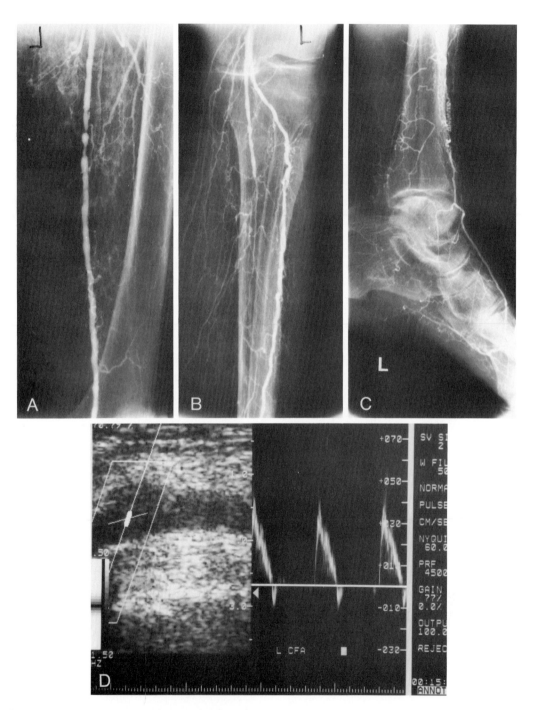

Figure 4.3.16. Doppler waveform study of the lower extremities with correlative unilateral angiography of arterial stenosis. **A–H.** Critical stenosis of the mid-left superficial femoral artery with increased velocity and loss of the triphasic waveform. Biphasic anterior tibial artery and posterior tibial artery waveforms suggest stenosis or occlusion with reconstitution.

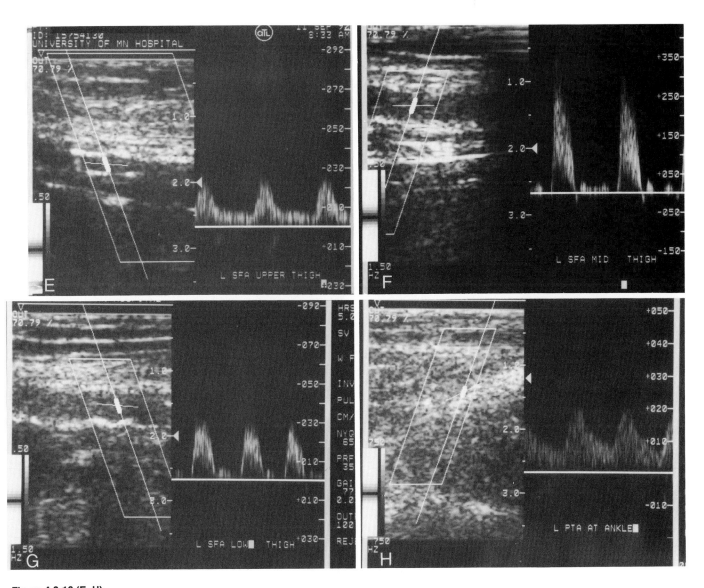

Figure 4.3.16 (E–H).

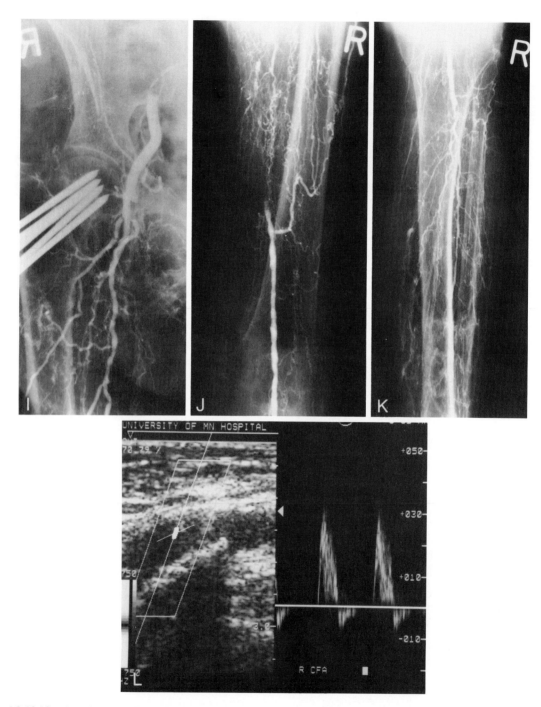

Figure 4.3.16 (*Continued*). I+N. Occlusion of right superficial femoral artery with reconstitution in the mid-superficial femoral artery.

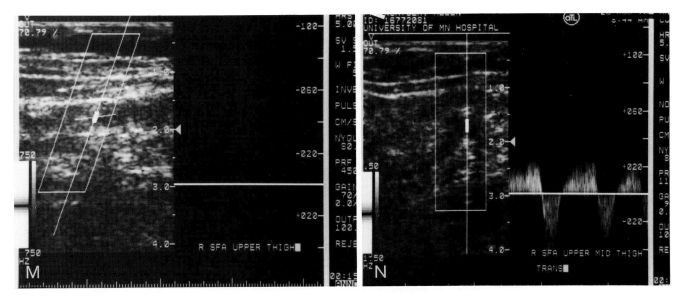

Figure 4.3.16 (M–N).

Minnesota[10] preliminary laboratory results show that the systolic component correlated very well with the degree of stenosis and that the ratio of the proximal velocity to the maximum velocity, the velocity index, yielded the best correlation. Consequently, conventional and color flow Doppler appear to have promise in the assessment of suspected peripheral arterial disease affecting the native lower extremity vessels.

Duplex or color Doppler sonography of lower extremity arterial bypass grafts is useful for early detection of failing grafts and possible limb salvage. Ankle-brachial pressure indices frequently confirm a deterioration of distal extremity perfusion but do not differentiate between an occluded graft and a hemodynamically compromised, yet patent, graft. A prospective study by Bartlett and associates[11] concluded that duplex sonography was a superior method for postoperative in situ saphenous vein bypass surveillance. Duplex sonography can accurately identify incompletely lysed valves restricting flow, patent arteriovenous fistulae, and areas of graft or anastomotic stenoses. Bandyk et al.[12] maintained that graft failure can be predicted on the basis of peak systolic velocities in the graft and the distal anastomosis; velocities less than 40–45cm/sec associated with a monophasic Doppler waveform predict impending graft failure. A retrospective review at the University of Minnesota[13] revealed that 20% of the patients with in situ bypass grafts had a significant alteration in their clinical diagnosis and management based on data from the duplex examination that could not be determined by physical examination.

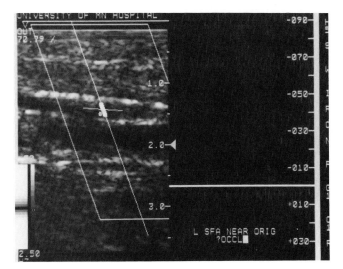

Figure 4.3.17. Duplex examination of heavily calcified vessel can obscure intraluminal thrombus and is technically difficult to detect blood flow within the vessel lumen. Lack of Doppler waveform does not necessarily indicate occlusion of the vessel in this instance.

Table 4.3.2. Classification Criteria for Estimating Severity of Stenosis in Peripheral Arteries

Normal
  Triphasic waveform, no appreciable spectral broadening.
1–19% Diameter Reduction
  Normal waveform with slight spectral broadening and peak velocities increased no more than 30% greater than in the proximal adjacent segment.
20–49% Diameter Reduction
  Spectral broadening filling in the clear window under the systolic peak, peak velocity less than 100% greater than that of the next most proximal segment.
50–99% Diameter Reduction
  Peak systolic velocity 100% greater than proximal adjacent segment and reverse velocity component usually absent in the stenosis. Monophasic velocity waveform beyond the stenosis with reduced systolic velocity.
Occlusion
  No flow in the imaged artery. Monophasic, preocclusive "thump" heart proximal to the occlusion; velocities markedly diminished and waveforms monophasic beyond the stenosis.

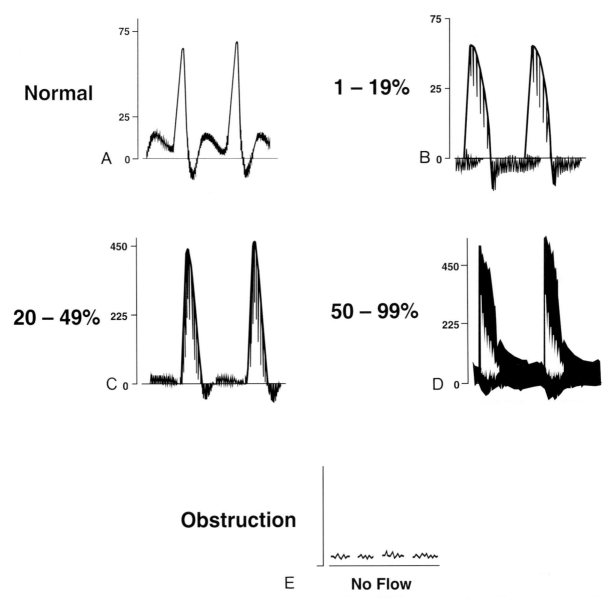

Figure 4.3.18.   Representative velocity waveforms from lower extremity arteries. **A.** Normal. **B.** 0–19% diameter reduction. **C.** 20–49% diameter reduction. **D.** 50–99% diameter reduction. **E.** Obstruction.

Noninvasive techniques may be used to assess the intraprocedural or immediate postprocedural results of angioplasty or atherectomy. When multiple stenoses are present it is important to determine which stenoses are hemodynamically significant and after dilatation which stenoses continue to be hemodynamically significant. Sacks[14] noted that it is important to have a follow-up study at six weeks after percutaneous transluminal angioplasty because immediate post-PTA velocities may be elevated secondary to the expected associated intimal dissections.

The recent development of color flow Doppler systems has allowed the superimposition of duplex sonography with color flow documentation of blood flow. Color Doppler decreases scan time, facilitates localization of stenoses and facilitates visualization of these above-mentioned areas (Fig. 4.3.19A,B). It allows better visualization of the

small arteries in the calf and permits imaging of the superficial arteries of the ankle and foot. Further research will determine if color flow sonography can selectively replace diagnostic angiography for the lower extremity.

ANKLE-BRACHIAL PRESSURE MEASUREMENT

The ankle-brachial index (ABI) is one of the simplest and most useful parameters to objectively assess lower extremity arterial perfusion. This study helps to define the severity of the disease and successfully screens for hemodynamically significant disease. The patient is placed in a supine position. The brachial and ankle systolic pressure measurements are obtained. Each ankle pressure measurement is divided by the highest brachial systolic pressure in order to obtain an ankle-brachial pressure ratio. There

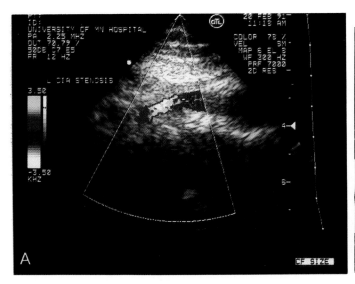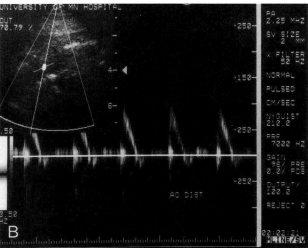

Figure 4.3.19. Internal iliac artery stenosis. **A.** Color flow Doppler of the left common iliac artery. **B.** The color saturation is consistent with the increased velocity.

should be less than 10mm Hg difference between each brachial pressure measurement (Fig. 4.3.20). Ankle-brachial indices between 0.92 and 1.10 are normal; abnormal values are less than 1.0. The majority of the patients with claudication have ABIs ranging from 0.30 to 0.92.[3] Rest pain or severe occlusive disease typically occurs with an ABI less than 0.50. Indices less than 0.20 are associated with ischemic or gangrenous extremities. In diabetic patients with heavily calcified vessels, the arteries are frequently incom-

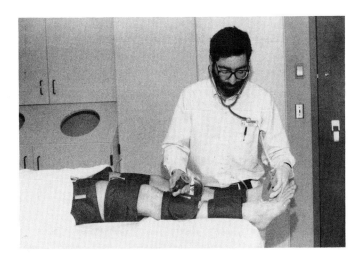

Figure 4.3.20. Ankle-brachial index measurement. A Doppler probe is positioned over the posterior tibial artery at the ankle; a pressure cuff is inflated, then slowly deflated and the pressure at which the pulse reappears is registered. Note only the ankle cuff is inflated for this procedure. Procedure is repeated over the dorsalis pedis artery. The higher of the two values is taken as a reference for ankle pressure. Not shown, the procedure is repeated in both the arms with the cuff above the elbow and the probe over the radial artery. The higher value registered is taken as the brachial pressure. Ankle-brachial index is given by the ratio of the two values.

pressible. This results in an artifactually elevated ankle pressure which can underestimate disease severity. In these patients toe pressure determinations, discussed later, more accurately reflect perfusion. Berkowitz and colleagues[15,16] concluded that 77% of vein graft stenoses can be detected within the first postoperative year based on the ABI values. A decrease of greater than 0.20 in ABI is consistent with a hemodynamically significant stenosis due to inflow disease, stenosis in the graft itself, or pressure of outflow disease.

Stress testing is particularly helpful in patients with borderline ABI values at rest but who present with claudication symptoms. During exercise, increased resistance within the diseased segment will become the limiting factor for arterial flow and downstream pressure will decrease. Normally there is no change in extremity pressure with exercise. Any drop in pressure ABIs is abnormal and can be graded by recording the recovery time. Single level disease returns to baseline within 2–6 minutes, multiple level disease returns to baseline in 12 minutes, and occlusive disease returns to baseline in as much as 30 minutes. Hyperemic testing may be performed in patients unable to exercise. A wide thigh cuff is inflated for three minutes 20mm above systolic blood pressure. Postocclusion ankle pressures are obtained for three minutes; in severe disease states there is greater than a 50% pressure drop.

TOE PRESSURE

Like ankle pressures, toe pressure measurements are typically obtained with a pneumatic cuff, also known as a photoplethysmography, or less frequently a Doppler probe or strain gauge plethysmography (plethysmos, in Greek, means "increase"; graphein means "to write"). In photoplethysmography a photoelectric cell measures changes in cutaneous blood content. A small occlusion cuff is placed around the proximal phalanx of the great toe. The cuff is inflated to a pressure which obliterates digital perfusion and then is slowly deflated. The toe pressure is recorded when pulsations return.

In all plethysmographic systems a waveform is obtained. In normal conditions, the pulse contour is characterized by a sharp systolic upstroke with a narrow peak followed by slow drop-off toward the baseline interrupted by a dicrotic notch. The pathologic findings distal to occlusion are easily recognized: the wave becomes rounded, the amplitude is reduced, and the upswing is more gradual. In total occlusion the waveform is flat. From the analysis of the waveform, the hemodynamic significance of an obstruction and its approximate site can be detected. These results are easily obtained with low cost equipment. Normal values are 5–10mm Hg less than the brachial pressure. A normal toe pressure should be 60% of the ankle pressure or greater and, therefore, the toe-ankle index should be 0.60 or greater.[17] Toe pressure measurements less than 30mm Hg correlate with the threshold value for rest pain and portend a poor prognosis for healing of toe ulcers.[18] As previously mentioned, medial arterial wall calcifications typically seen in diabetic patients may affect ankle pressures; however, they seldom affect toe pressure measurements and, thus, toe pressure measurements may be of particular value in this set of patients. Atherosclerotic disease significantly lowers toe pressures to a degree proportional to the extent of proximal hemodynamic obstruction. Toe pressure measurements also aid in the identification of pedal arch disease, an important factor in healing of ischemic foot ulcers.

SEGMENTAL LIMB PRESSURE RECORDINGS

Segmental limb pressure examination is a noninvasive tool which can locate the level of a peripheral arterial stenosis. This method was first introduced by Winsor in 1950.[19] A pneumatic cuff is inflated above systolic pressure and deflated until the Doppler signal reappears. Measurements are obtained at four levels: high thigh, above the knee, below the knee, and ankle. Typical ratios of measured pressure to brachial pressure are high thigh 1.35, above the knee 1.25, calf 1.18, and ankle 1.10. Between any level, an absolute pressure decrease of greater than 30mm Hg is indicative of a hemodynamically significant stenosis. The high thigh pressure determination is typically 20–30mm Hg higher than the brachial pressure due to the discrepancy in measurements from narrower and wider blood pressure cuffs.

A limitation of the technique is that it can be difficult to differentiate aortoiliac inflow disease from concomitant profunda and femoral artery disease (Fig. 4.3.21). Rutherford used angiography as a gold standard and obtained an accuracy for segmental pressures of 97% in normal limbs, 75% in isolated aortoiliac disease, 78% for combined

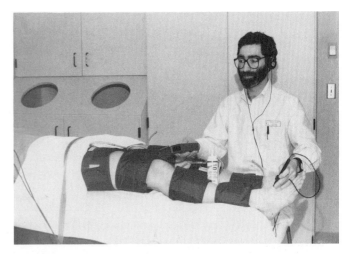

Figure 4.3.21. Segmental pressure measurement. This full procedure is performed when the ankle-brachial index is abnormal. In each leg four pressure cuffs are placed, two above the knee and two below. The pressure measurement is begun at the ankle. A Doppler probe is positioned over the posterior tibial artery or the dorsalis pedis artery (where the pressure is higher). Each cuff is inflated separately and the pressure at which the pulse is heard during deflation is recorded. The four cuff method is generally performed because it aids in differentiation of aortoiliac disease from superficial femoral artery disease. However, the three-cuff method is more accurate due to wider cuffs. This latter method does not provide as extensive information and is generally only used on patients with short legs.

aortoiliac and superficial femoral artery disease, 55% for superficial femoral artery disease, 60% for superficial femoral artery and popliteal disease, and 36% for popliteal-tibial disease.[20]

Typical artifacts which may give erroneous measurements include[3]: 1) pulsatile venous signals in patients with congestive heart failure which can be confused with arterial signals; 2) occlusive disease with collateral flow that might yield inadequate measurements for the native vessel; 3) incompressible calcified vessels producing artifactually high pressure values; 4) low flow or occlusion preventing measurements at certain levels; or 5) obesity or large thighs distorting pressure values.

tcPO$_2$ MEASUREMENT

Transcutaneous oxygen pressure measurements (tcPO$_2$) assess tissue metabolism as a function of perfusion and, therefore, can be used to measure the degree of extremity ischemia. Such tcPO$_2$ measurements are particularly helpful in detecting the severity of arterial occlusive disease and assessing the likelihood that pedal ulcers or amputations will heal. The basis of transcutaneous oxygen tension measurements is detection of oxygen that has diffused through the skin. To facilitate this process local hyperthermia is produced by heating the sensing electrode to 44°C. This produces maximal vasodilatation. In addition, there is increased skin oxygen consumption and enhanced oxyhemoglobin dissociation. Normal patients have no gradient in tcPO$_2$ values from proximal to distal in the lower extremity.

tcPO$_2$ levels greater than 38mm Hg are uniformly associated with extremity healing, while values less than 38mm Hg are associated with nonhealing or delayed healing.[21] tcPO$_2$ values normally increase if the patient moves to an erect from a supine position. A failure to increase the absolute tcPO$_2$ foot reading by 15mm Hg with standing has a poor prognosis for arterial reconstruction. tcPO$_2$ values are dependent on cardiac output and arterial oxygen content; both vary with each patient. Some authors[22] recommend calculating a regional perfusion index (RPI) by dividing the tcPO$_2$ of the extremity by that of a well perfused region, such as the anterior chest wall. This would reflect the severity of obstructive disease rather than tissue ischemia per se.

MAGNETIC RESONANCE ANGIOGRAPHY

Flowing blood may produce complex signal patterns, depending on the flow velocity, direction, and profile. Vascular magnetic resonance imaging utilizes one of two fundamental approaches: time of flight (TOF) or phase contrast (PC) angiograms. Each method has specific applications and various methods for data acquisition.[2] The most widely used approach is the time-of-flight angiography, which relies on the inflow of fully magnetized blood into the imaging plane, also known as flow-related enhancement. This phenomenon occurs in gradient echo images obtained perpendicular to the axis of the vessel. In these images flow compensation is usually used to reduce flow-related signal roll. The information can be obtained in two- or three-dimensional data bases. PC angiography generates vascular images by detecting changes in the phase of the blood's transverse magnetization as it moves along a time-varying magnetic field gradient whose net effect on stationary tissue is negligible. It is dependent on alterations of spin phase for image contrast. A brief outline of the history of magnetic resonance angiography (MRA) follows.

Macovski, in 1982, postulated the use of motion-induced phase contrast and subtraction as a method for producing projective MR angiograms.[23] Dixon et al.[24] was the first to be successful in utilizing the time-of-flight effects for providing vascular contrast to create angiographic images. Their work involved tagging incoming carotid blood flow with a special radiofrequency coil located at the base of the neck. Dixon also introduced a twister pulse to improve vascular contrast. By saturating spins and taking advantage of paradoxical enhancement of inflowing spins in transverse slices, a vascular image was obtained without subtraction. Nishimura and colleagues[25] were successful with a time-of-flight technique that utilizes thick slab images generated with use of a locally placed coil at the carotid bifurcation. In 1986 and 1987 Wehrli and colleagues[26] suggested that a blood vessel could be imaged

with two-dimensional Fourier transform gradient echo images oriented perpendicular to the direction of flow on the basis of flow-related enhancement. Subsequent to this, Ruggieri and colleagues utilized time-of-flight angiography techniques performed with three-dimensional Fourier transform sequences. Edelman et al.[27] used sequential two-dimensional Fourier transform images with selectively applied saturation pulses to produce arteriograms and venograms in the abdomen.

Since there is no nonvascular physiologic motion in the extremities they are ideal areas for vascular studies. Wedeen[28] described an initial large field of view study that is sensitive to disease. It can act as a screening examination, although eddy currents may degrade subtracted images. A subsequent high-resolution scan may be obtained for suspicious areas of vascular disease using the gradient rephase/dephase sequence described. This technique can consistently detect normal and occluded popliteal trifurcation. The difficulty is that stenotic segments cannot be portrayed consistently and are frequently overestimated. The less pronounced effects of turbulence and motion are also present.

Many problems need to be solved in order for magnetic resonance angiography to achieve full clinical utility. However, perhaps in as little as five years a diagnostic peripheral angiogram will be a study of the past, replaced with noninvasive magnetic resonance angiography and duplex sonography, which could depict vascular anatomy and function.

CONCLUSION

Numerous noninvasive methods for evaluating the lower extremities are available and continue to be developed. A thorough understanding of the capabilities and limitations of the methods employed is essential for the interventional radiologist. Although the information obtained from many tests may appear redundant, the diagnostic accuracy and the therapeutic decision-making process may be facilitated.

References

1. Zierler RE: Hemodynamic considerations in evaluation of arterial disease by Doppler ultrasound. *Clin Diagn Ultrasound* 1990;26:13–22
2. Turski P, Bernstein M, Boyko O: Vascular magnetic resonance imaging. *Signa Applications Guide,* Volume III, 1st Ed, August 1990
3. Huber JF: The arterial network supplying the dorsum of the foot. *Anat Rev* 1941;80:373–376
4. Strandness DE Jr: Clinical applications of Doppler ultrasound in the assessment of arterial disease. *Clin Diagn Ultrasound* 1990;26:5–8
5. Gerlock AJ, Giyananoi VL, Krebs C: *Applications of Noninvasive Vascular Techniques.* Philadelphia, WB Saunders, 1988, pp 292–380
6. Kohler TR, Nance DR, Cramer MM, Vandenburghe N,

Strandness DE Jr: Duplex scanning for diagnosis of turbulence and femoropopliteal disease: a prospective study. *Circulation* 1987;76:1074–1080

7. Jager KA, Ricketts HF, Strandness DE Jr: Duplex scanning for evaluation of lower limb arterial disease, in Bernstein EF (ed). *Noninvasive Diagnostic Techniques in Vascular Disease*. St. Louis, CV Mosby, 1985, p 619

8. Kohler TR, Andrews G, Porter J, Clowes A, Goldstone J, Johansen K, Nance D, Strandness DE Jr: Can duplex scanning replace arteriography for lower extremity arterial disease? *Ann Vasc Surg* 1990;4:280–287

9. Nicholls SC, Kohler TR, Martin R, et al: Diastolic flow as prediction of arterial stenosis. *J Vasc Surg* 1986;3:498

10. Althaus SJ, Yedlicka JW Jr, Aeppli D, Hunter DW: Comparison of duplex sonography and arteriography for lower extremity stenoses in a dog model. Presented at the Sixteenth Annual Meeting of the Society of Cardiovascular and Interventional Radiology, San Francisco, CA, February 16–21, 1991

11. Bartlett ST, Killewich LA, Fischer C, Ward RE: Duplex imaging if in situ saphenous vein bypass grafts and late failure reduction. *Am J Surg* 1988;136:484–487

12. Bandyk DF, Cato RF, Towne JB: A low flow velocity predicts failure of femoropopliteal and femorotibial grafts. *Surgery* 1985;98:799–809

13. Althaus SJ, Rolfs A, Hunter DW: Duplex evaluation following in-situ saphenous vein bypass grafts. Presented at the 1991 Annual Meeting of the American Roentgen Ray Society, Boston, MA, May 5–10, 1991

14. Sacks D, Robinson M, Marinelli D, Perlmutter G: Evaluation of the peripheral arteries with duplex ultrasound after angioplasty. *Radiology* 1990;176:39–44

15. Berkowitz HD, Hobbs CL, Roberts B, Freiman D, Oleaga J, Ring E: Value of routine vascular laboratory studies to identify graft stenoses. *Surgery* 1981;90:971–979

16. Berkowitz HD, Greenstein SM: Improved patency in reversed femoral-infrapopliteal autogenous vein grafts by early detection and treatment of the failing graft. *J Vasc Surg* 1987;5:755–761

17. Kempczinski R, Yas J: *Practical Noninvasive Vascular Diagnosis*. Chicago, Year Book Medical Publishers, 1983, p 90

18. Ramsey DE, Manke DA, Sumner DS: Toe blood pressures—a valuable adjunct to ankle pressure measurement for assessing peripheral arterial disease. *J Cardiovasc Surg* 1983;24:43–48

19. Winsor T: Influence of arterial disease in the systolic blood pressure gradient of the extremity. *Am J Med Sci* 1950;220:117

20. Rutherford RB, Lowenstein DH, Klein MF: Combining segmental systolic pressures and plethysmography to diagnose arterial occlusive disease of the legs. *Am J Surg* 1979;138:211–218

21. Byrne P, Prarnan JL, Ameli FM, Jones DP: The use of transcutaneous oxygen tension measurements in the diagnosis of peripheral vascular insufficiency. *Ann Surg* 1984;200:159–165

22. Ana C, Katsamouris A, Meyerman J, Brewster DC, Strayhorn EC, Robeson JG, Abbott WM: Utility of transcutaneous oxygen tension measurements in peripheral arterial occlusive disease. *J Vasc Surg* 1984;1:362–371

23. Macovski A: Selective projection imaging: applications to radiography and NMR. *IEEE Trans Med Imaging* 1982;1:42–47

24. Dixon WT, Du LN, Faul DD, Gado M, Rosnick S: Projection angiograms of blood labeled by adiabatic fast passage. *Magn Reson Med* 1986;3:454–462

25. Nishimura DG, Macovski A, Pauly JM, Conolly SM: MR angiography by selective inversion recording. *Magn Reson Med* 1987;4:193–202

26. Wehrli FW, Shimakawa A, Gullberg GT, MacFall JR: Time-of-flight MR flow imaging: selective saturation recovery with gradient refocusing. *Radiology* 1986;160:781–785

27. Edelman RR, Wentz KA, Mattle H, et al: Projection arteriography and venography: initial clinical results with MR. *Radiology* 1989;173:527–532

28. Wedeen VJ, Meuli RA, Edelman RR, et al: Projective imaging of pulsatile flow with magnetic resonance imaging. *Science* 1985;230:946–948

Diagnosis of Deep Vein Thrombosis with Ultrasound Technique

—Haraldur Bjarnason, M.D., Deborah G. Longley, M.D., and Janis Gissel Letourneau, M.D.

LOWER EXTREMITY

Introduction

Acute deep venous thrombosis (DVT) of the lower extremity is the most common disease of the vascular system; as many as 20,000,000 new cases occur annually in the United States.[1,2] Autopsy findings have shown that the incidence of DVT in hospitalized patients ranges from 27 to 80%.[3] It has been estimated that, without adequate treatment, one patient in three with DVT will have a pulmonary embolus.[4] Moreover, up to 50% of patients eventually develop post-thrombotic syndrome.[5] Deep venous thrombosis is, therefore, a very important disease and is responsible for morbidity and mortality that can partly be avoided by early and accurate diagnosis.

The pathogenesis of DVT was described by Virchow as a triad of slow flow, intimal lesion, and/or coagulopathy. First, slow blood flow or stagnation of blood flow occurs in patients with heart failure or with immobilization, as is the case with hospitalization or long journeys. Second, intimal injury in the vein occurs with trauma, irritating infusion fluids, or catheter manipulations, for example. Third, coagulopathies can be seen with increased coagulability secondary to malignant disease or estrogen therapy.

The clinical diagnosis is, as has repeatedly been demonstrated, very difficult and only approximately 50% of patients clinically believed to have DVT appear to have proved DVT. Conversely, up to two-thirds of DVTs are silent and are never detected clinically.[6]

The major clinical features are swelling of the affected extremity with tenderness on palpation and increased temperature of the skin. All these signs are nonspecific and "Homan's sign" appears to be of little diagnostic value.[7]

Almost all lower extremity deep venous thromboses begin in the calf; some thromboses migrate to the popliteal and femoral veins and even up to the iliac veins and inferior vena cava. It is rare to have de novo formation of DVT in the proximal leg or pelvis. It has been estimated that approximately 40% of calf DVTs resolve spontaneously without any therapy and another 40% become organized, retract, or recanalize without any extension, leaving locally abnormal veins. Approximately 20% of calf clots propagate into the popliteal vein, superficial femoral vein, iliac vein, or inferior vena cava, and those are responsible for 90% of pulmonary emboli.[8,9] De novo thrombosis within the above-the-knee or pelvic veins and the inferior vena cava are responsible for a minority of pulmonary emboli. These cases are generally associated with abdominal or pelvic masses, trauma to the pelvis, hip, or femur, venous instrumentation, and, occasionally, long-term immobilization as in patients with neurologic impairment.[10]

Until relatively recently, the goal for treatment of DVT has been to stop further progression of thrombosis with anticoagulation, first using intravenous heparin and then treatment with oral anticoagulation for three to six months. This course of therapy requires that the patient stay in bed for several days while the greatest risk for pulmonary embolism exists. In more recent years, the development of thrombolytic therapy has changed the therapeutic approach to DVT. Thrombosis in the large proximal veins is especially well suited for thrombolytic treatment. Consequently, it has become even more important to make an early and accurate diagnosis and have a single, repeatable diagnostic tool that can be used to follow the effect of treatment.

Inferior vena cava (IVC) filters are an effective therapy in preventing pulmonary embolism in cases of DVT with a contraindication for anticoagulation or in cases of recurrent pulmonary embolism in patients adequately treated with anticoagulation. IVC filters are usually inserted via the common femoral vein or internal jugular vein and are placed within the IVC just below the renal veins. To do this, large-bore introducer sheaths are used, risking the development of thrombosis at the introducer site. With IVC filters, one has also to be aware of the risks of cava thrombosis (2–7%) and filter migration. Duplex and color flow Doppler studies are excellent means of following up the puncture site after filter placement. The position of the filter and flow in the IVC are readily examined. The study is noninvasive and usually easy to perform; usually one is able to visualize the IVC and the filter (Fig. 4.3.22). If so, establishing patency of flow is possible, and by so doing, thrombosis of the IVC is excluded.

Another field where duplex and color flow Doppler sonography are ideal methods for follow-up is in the situation of venous stent placement. Venous stents are often used in patients when the iliac veins have been closed or severely stenosed for longer periods and a good collateral system has developed around the occlusion, yet symptoms persist. The stents are usually visualized within the iliac veins and conventional or color flow Doppler technologies can be used to verify flow and define flow characteristics inside, proximal to, and distal to the stents (Fig. 4.3.23).

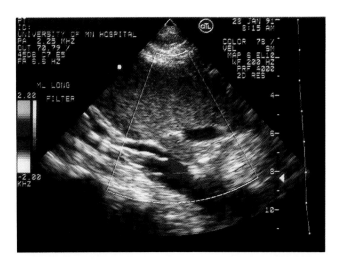

Figure 4.3.22. Titanium Greenfield filter in inferior vena cava (IVC). IVC is patent as seen by *red* color flow. The filter is seen as high echogenic threads within the IVC.

There are, however, cases where abdominal gas obscures the iliacs and renders the study nondiagnostic. A preprocedural duplex study distal to the stent insertion site provides valuable data on the flow and waveform characteristics for follow-up.

Anatomy

The veins of the lower extremity can be divided into deep and superficial venous systems (Fig. 4.3.24). The deep veins accompany the principal arteries and have the same names. There is usually a single iliac vein, common, superficial, and deep femoral veins, and popliteal vein.

Below the knee the veins are usually paired and lie on

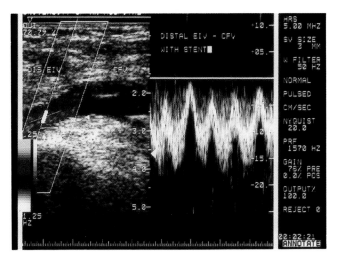

Figure 4.3.23. Longitudinal view of distal external iliac vein (EIV) and common femoral vein (CFV) showing distal end of vascular stent in the EIV *(three arrows)*. Patency of the vessel is shown by color flow filling the lumen. Doppler waveform reflects atrial contractions and respiratory phasicity, with some spectral broadening.

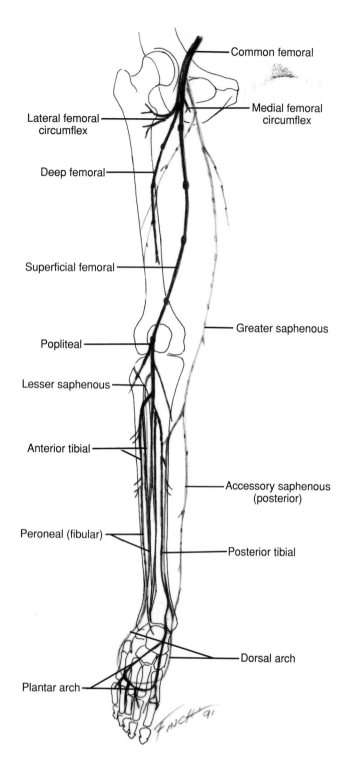

Figure 4.3.24. The anatomy of the venous system in the lower extremity.

each side of the arteries. The paired calf veins are the posterior tibial vein which drains the deep plantar part of the foot, the anterior tibial vein which drains the dorsum of the foot, and the peroneal (fibular) vein which drains the foot and the ankle region. Those veins drain then into the popliteal vein, usually as a single but, occasionally, as paired veins. The superficial femoral vein can also be paired,

although the deep femoral and common femoral veins are usually single. It is important to be familiar with variants in the popliteal and superficial femoral vein because, although one vein of the pair may be patent, the other can be thrombosed.

The superficial venous system is composed roughly of two major veins. The short saphenous vein drains the lateral and the posterior part of the calf; this vein courses into the popliteal region to join the popliteal vein. The other major superficial vein is the greater saphenous vein draining the medial and posterior part of the calf and thigh and coursing anteriorly and medially joining the common femoral vein.

There are several communicating veins between the deep and the superficial systems, with one-way valves that direct the flow from the superficial system into the deep system under normal circumstances. In the deep system there are several valves directing the flow toward the heart. Those valves are numerous in the calf region but more sparse proximal to the calf. The superficial venous system is considered in the diagnosis of DVT when the clot extends into the proximal saphenous vein.

Diagnostic Methods

The ideal diagnostic evaluation for DVT would be noninvasive, repeatable, painless, and easy to perform and would have a sensitivity and specificity of 100%. Ideally, such studies would use instruments used for other purposes also. The common venogram has been regarded as 100% sensitive and 100% specific; however, some reports indicate that venography does not have perfect sensitivity or specificity, due to problems with execution of the studies and interpretation errors.[11] Venography is considered the "gold standard" for the diagnosis of DVT because of the extensive experience that exists with this examination and because it does have a high, albeit imperfect, sensitivity and specificity. Nonetheless, the venogram is invasive and uncomfortable for the patient. It requires a special laboratory and injection of potentially thrombogenic contrast material.[12,13] With the use of newer nonionic contrast materials, injection complications are minimized, but these compounds may be allergenic and nephrotoxic and are expensive for routine use.

Many other diagnostic methods have been utilized in the setting of suspected DVT. Most have been noninvasive, such as impedance plethysmography, fibrinogen labeled with iodine-125, duplex sonography, and, most recently, color flow Doppler sonography. All of these techniques have a role in the diagnosis of DVT.

IMPEDANCE PLETHYSMOGRAPHY

With impedance plethysmography one measures the rate of emptying of the venous system in the lower extremity after placement and release of a tourniquet on the proximal thigh. Impedance plethysmography records variation in the electrical resistance of the leg to pulses of weak alternating electrical current. Under normal circumstances, venous emptying should be abrupt, but if there is thrombosis proximally in the venous system, emptying will be slowed. This test is quite sensitive in detecting thrombosis within the veins in the knee region and those more proximally situated, but is very insensitive in detecting thrombosis in the calf region. It is also rather nonspecific, as one can have slow flow from other causes, such as with narrowing of the veins by external compression with increased central venous pressure, with cardiac failure, and increased intra-abdominal pressure from ascites. False-negative results may also occur with nonocclusive thrombosis. Plethysmography is rather simple to perform, but requires expertise for interpretation. It can be repeated without risk to the patient.[9]

125I MARKED FIBRINOGEN TEST

The principle behind this study is that fibrinogen labeled with ^{125}I accumulates in progressing thromboses and can be detected with a γ camera. This test is as sensitive for calf vein thromboses as venography. The study generally requires 24–48 hours to complete and it can be carried out for as long as seven days to follow-up progression. Because ^{125}I is a low energy emitter, this test is not well suited for diagnosis of DVT in the proximal veins or pelvis. False-positive results can occur if inflammatory conditions exist in the area being monitored. Such false-positive results could be expected when a surgical wound, trauma, fractures, cellulitis, hematoma, edema, and arthritis are in the region being examined.

Because this examination requires the use of blood products, there is a risk of acquiring hepatitis. This risk is very small as the donors are screened. Additionally, this test cannot be performed in pregnant or lactating women, as fibrinogen crosses the placenta and is excreted in breast milk.[9]

ULTRASOUND: CONVENTIONAL DUPLEX AND COLOR FLOW DOPPLER

Compression ultrasound with or without Doppler technology has become one of the most widely used and readily accepted of the noninvasive techniques for the diagnosis of DVT. In many institutions, it has replaced venography as the first diagnostic study for suspected DVT. Because of the high sensitivity and specificity of conventional duplex and color flow Doppler sonography, venography can be reserved for cases with high proximal extension or for instances fraught with technical difficulties. Ultrasound has many advantages over venography, the most apparent being its noninvasiveness. It is also relatively painless and is easily repeatable to assess potential progression or response to treatment. As duplex equipment is usually portable, the study can be done at the bedside. In 8% of cases other clinically unsuspected abnormalities, including hematomas, aneurysms, Baker cysts, lymph nodes, and

superficial phlebitis have been identified that explain the presenting symptomatology.[2] Additionally, ultrasound is a safe method of detecting DVT, with no significant complications reported except in one presumptive case of dislodgment of a floating thrombus resulting in pulmonary embolism.[14]

Instrumentation and Examination Technique

The most commonly used transducers for the compression ultrasound in diagnosis of DVT vary from 5 to 7.5mHz. Linear array transducers are commonly used because the "footprint" of the transducer face is well suited for compression, but sector transducers can also be used. When the patient is thin and the vessels are superficial, a high frequency transducer can easily be used to optimize accuracy of the study. In the pelvis and inner thigh, especially in the adductor channel, a 5mHz or even a 3.5mHz transducer may be needed.

The proximal part of the venous system of the legs is usually examined with the patient in the supine position and the head of the examination table tilted up approximately 20° to optimize filling and distension of the veins. The iliac vessels are examined as proximally as possible, most preferably up to the IVC. At these levels it is important to interrogate with Doppler during attempted augmentation and with the Valsalva maneuver to verify patency and phasicity of flow. This portion of the study is often difficult because of the deep location of the veins and the presence of intervening bowel. (Venography may be required to determine the proximal extent of thrombosis in the iliac veins or inferior vena cava and to provide anatomic data for therapeutic caval filter placement.) The femoral vein should be examined transversely and followed distally without and with compression at 2cm intervals. One should also note dynamics of the vessel, changes in size of the vessel, and flow with respiration. The drainage of the saphenous vein into the femoral vein should also be noted (Fig. 4.3.25). Special attention should be paid to the bifurcation of the common femoral vein (Fig. 4.3.26) and to the proximal part of the deep femoral vein because thrombosis can occur in this deep branch. One has also to be aware of possible duplication of the superficial femoral vein, a common congenital variant. The examination often becomes difficult at the adductor canal and color flow Doppler will facilitate tracing the veins in this area. Although the patient can remain supine for this portion of the study, bending the knee laterally, it may be necessary to place the patient in a prone position for examination of the popliteal vein. The popliteal vein is usually superficial to the artery in the popliteal fossa distal to the adductor canal.

The calf veins are most successfully examined from the medial aspect of the calf just behind the tibia. The Gray scale imaging of these veins is often difficult and one often has to rely on color flow Doppler for the entire examination. No spontaneous flow may be identified within the calf with flow only detectable with an augmentation maneuver.

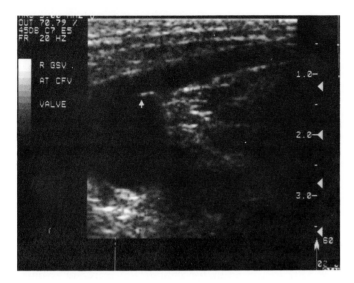

Figure 4.3.25. The draining of the great saphenous vein (GSV) into the common femoral vein. Notice a valve at the ostium of the GSV *(arrow).*

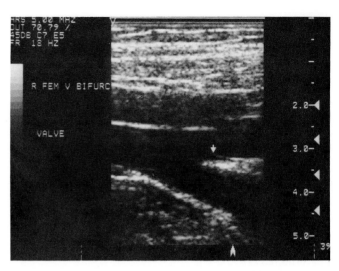

Figure 4.3.26. The common femoral vein bifurcating into the superficial femoral vein (SFV) above and the deep profunda femoral vein below. A valve is seen proximally in the SFV *(arrow).*

Calf veins should be examined in the longitudinal and transverse plane. Important landmarks are the arteries following pairs of veins. The examination can be done scanning from the knee or from the ankle; it is often easier to start at the ankle and follow the veins proximally to the knee. One should be aware that the anterior tibial veins are probably of little clinical importance in the diagnosis of deep venous thrombosis.[15] The best approach for examination of the anterior tibial veins is just lateral to the tibia. The peroneal vein can often be better visualized by a posterior approach instead of a medial approach.

Normal Vein in Duplex and Color Flow Doppler Sonography

A normal lower extremity vein is similar in size or slightly larger than the adjacent artery. The vessel wall is

thin and almost imperceptible (Fig. 4.3.27A). Thickening of the vessel wall is abnormal and suggests previous or even fresh thrombosis. The lumen of the vessel is usually echo-free, but with newer high-resolution instruments the lumen can be minimally echogenic because of the movement of blood cells.[2] With high resolution imaging, valves and their movement can often be seen (Figs. 4.3.25 and 4.3.26). The size of the vein may change slightly with respiration and increase with the Valsalva maneuver.

Normally the vein is completely compressible when compared with the incompressible artery. Compression is best tested with the probe in a transverse orientation so that the vein is fixed beneath the transducer and so that the vein and the artery can be seen simultaneously. The vein should be totally compressible, meaning the opposing walls should touch each other. When thrombosis is present the

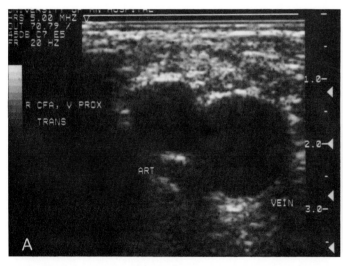

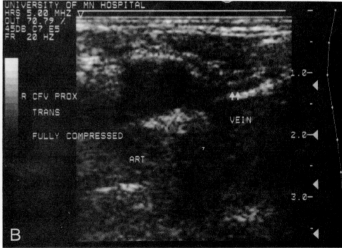

Figure 4.3.27. The normal sonographic appearance of the common femoral vein (CFV). **A.** The common femoral artery is seen to the *left* of the CFV which is slightly larger than the artery. The CFV walls are thin and

barely seen. The lumen is anechogenic. **B.** The vein is completely compressed by the transducer *(two arrows).* The artery is just slightly compressed.

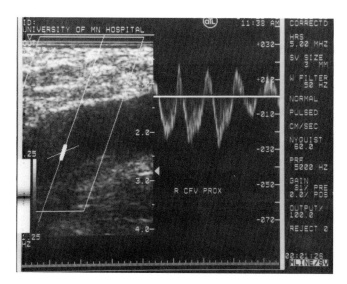

Figure 4.3.28. Normal Doppler waveform of the common femoral vein showing atrial contraction waves and respiration changes (phasicity).

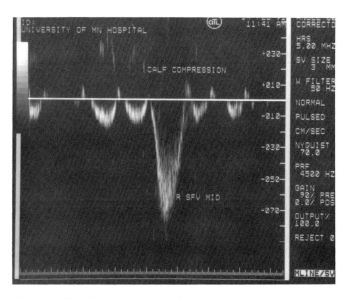

Figure 4.3.29. Normal response of superficial femoral vein to distal compression. There is a sharp increase in flow (augmentation) seen with calf compression.

vein may be partly or totally incompressible; incompressibility has been shown to be extremely reliable in the diagnosis of DVT (Fig. 4.3.27*B*).

The presence of valves in the venous system causes the flow to be unidirectional toward the heart. The flow is continuous in most of the large and medium-sized vessels, even at rest, but can be stagnant in smaller vessels. The normal flow pattern is phasic, meaning that it varies with respiration (Fig. 4.3.28). Nonphasic flow or continuous flow without any variation with respiration should arouse suspicion of occlusion or narrowing of the vessel proximal to the region examined. Alternatively, blood may be traversing a recanalized vein or collateral vessels. Although loss of phasicity indicates partial or total obstruction to flow, flow can be phasic in nonocclusive thromboses.

Squeezing of the leg or foot distal to the region examined increases venous flow proximally (augmentation) (Fig. 4.3.29). This is a reliable sign of patency of the vein between the region of Doppler integration and the site of distal pressure. A similar test is the Valsalva maneuver, where the patient bears down; spontaneous flow within the vein should stop abruptly, indicating patency of venous flow between the thorax and the region of examination (Fig. 4.3.30).

Incompetent valves can most easily be diagnosed by the color flow Doppler. This is best done by asking the patient to bear down with a Valsalva maneuver. The color flow Doppler demonstrates the reversed flow by a change in the luminal color. Normally there is a small amount of reversed flow with Valsalva, but there is much more flow reversed with incompetent valves. This is also easily seen with Doppler waveform analysis.

The color should fill the vein completely in transverse and longitudinal planes. This is not always possible and often one has to compress the calf or foot to get this effect (called augmentation). This should be a reliable sign but needs further evaluation (Fig. 4.3.31).

DVT as Seen by Duplex and Color Flow Doppler Sonography

The diagnostic features of DVT by compression ultrasound, conventional duplex and color flow Doppler have been briefly mentioned earlier. The main criteria are:

1. Compressibility. A vein with thrombosis is partially or totally noncompressible. This is the most commonly used and most reliable sonographic feature of DVT (Figs. 4.3.27*A*, 4.3.27*B*, 4.3.32*A*, and 4.3.32*B*). Occasionally complete compression of a normal vein is not possible because of the tissues surrounding the vein, as in a muscular region; for example, the adductor channel is routinely a difficult area to examine. In such

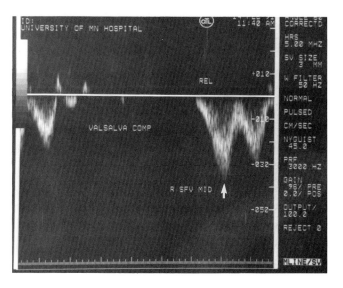

Figure 4.3.30. Normal response to Valsalva maneuver in superficial femoral vein. The forward flow ceases as the patient bears down. The flow is augmented upon exhalation *(white arrow).*

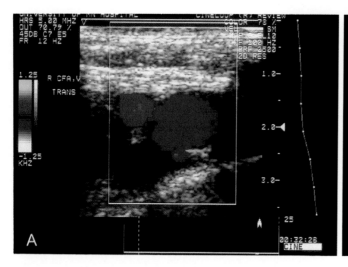

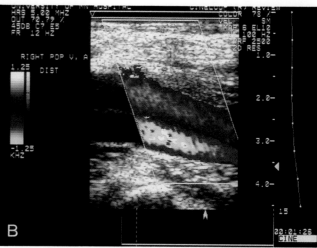

Figure 4.3.31. Normal color flow. **A.** Normal color flow Doppler appearance of popliteal artery and vein seen in longitudinal section. The vein is *blue* and the artery *red* in this instance. **B.** Normal transverse view of femoral vessels.

instances duplex and color flow Doppler examinations are helpful in verifying normalcy of the vein.

2. Direct visualization of the thrombus inside the vessel lumen (Fig. 4.3.33). Acute thrombus, hours to days old, can be almost anechoic (Fig. 4.3.32A). In such cases, it is important to have Doppler interrogation to verify the absence of flow and, with color flow Doppler, one may see flow between the recent thrombus and the vein wall. Typically, with increasing age, echogenicity of the thrombus increases.

3. Distension of the vein with acute and subacute thrombosis. This can be used to differentiate between an acute event and chronic or long-standing thrombosis (months to years).

4. Absence of phasic flow. This indicates thrombosis or partial obstruction in the vein proximally (Fig. 4.3.34). The same is the case with an abnormal response to a Valsalva maneuver.

5. If compression of the tissues distal to the region of Doppler interrogation does not result in increased flow, this suggests thrombosis in the intervening region.

6. Abnormal color flow pattern. The color flow Doppler is probably of most value where there is fresh anechoic thrombus in a vein and continuous flow around the thrombus as a color signal (Fig. 4.3.35). Such color flow can often be augmented by squeezing the extremity distal to the thrombus.

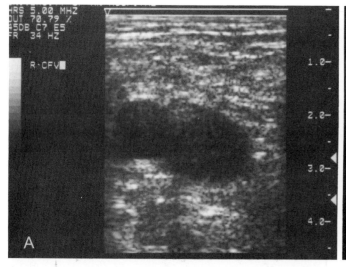

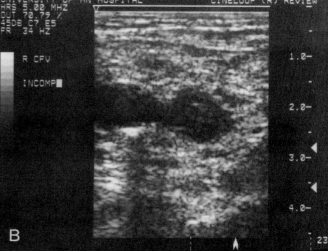

Figure 4.3.32. Transverse view of right common femoral artery and vein. **A.** The vein to the *right* appears anechogenic. **B.** Anechogenic thrombus in the common femoral vein. When the artery and vein are compressed by the ultrasound transducer, the vein does not compress due to thrombus.

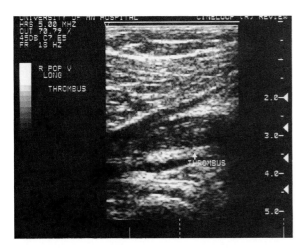

Figure 4.3.33. Direct visualization of thrombus in popliteal vein. Thrombus is echogenic, as opposed to anechoic thrombus seen in Figure 4.3.11*A*.

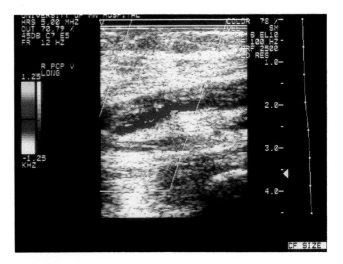

Figure 4.3.35. Popliteal vein with thrombus seen in longitudinal view. The color around the thrombus is clearly seen. This is the same picture as Figure 4.3.10*A* but with color flow imaging.

Acute thrombus is hypoechoic or is anechoic. The vein is usually distended and flow around the thrombus may be seen. Free-floating thrombus is relatively common acutely. Such terminology describes acute thrombus that is not totally adherent to the wall; this is most commonly seen at the proximal aspect of the clot. Typically over a period of several weeks, the echogenicity of the thrombus increases. The thrombus will shrink and the vessel will become more normal in size. Resumption of flow may be seen by conventional color flow Doppler, but this is variable. Months to years after thrombosis, the vessel is characterized by thick and irregular walls. The flow within such vessels is often continuous because of associated vascular abnormalities. Valvular incompetence may develop (Fig. 4.3.36).

Accuracy of Ultrasound

Above the Popliteal Trifurcation

Most of the studies assessing the accuracy of diagnosis of DVT have used comparisons with venography. Until recently, the results of ultrasound in diagnosing DVT below the trifurcation of the popliteal vein have been discouraging; color flow Doppler technology may improve the capability. However, there have been many reports citing high accuracy for the diagnosis of DVT above the level of the trifurcation. Dorfman and Cronan compared six almost identical studies comparing compression ultrasound and venography in 602 patients. The mean sensitivity was 93% (ranging from 89 to 100%) and the mean specificity was 99% (ranging from 97 to 100%). Zwiebel and Priest compared 10 series done from 1984 to 1989, comparing duplex sonography with venography in DVT within

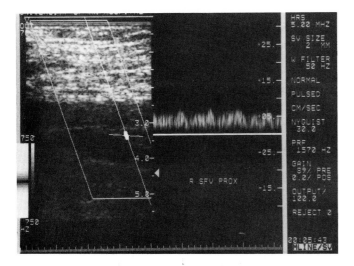

Figure 4.3.34. Nonphasic flow in superficial femoral vein. Flat waveform indicates flow in a collateral vessel or incomplete occlusion more proximally.

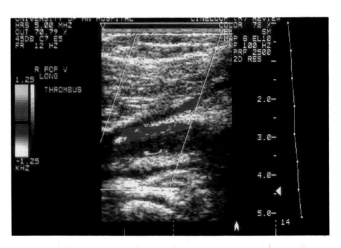

Figure 4.3.36. Old thrombus detected in the popliteal vein. High echogenic material is seen within a partially compressible vein with recanalization seen by color flow Doppler sonography.

the femoropopliteal region. Those studies demonstrated sensitivities from 88 to 100% and specificities from 92 to 100%.

Color flow Doppler is a relatively new technique applied to the diagnosis of DVT. Bjarnason and Sandbaek undertook a prospective study comparing compression ultrasound with color flow Doppler (using a defect in color filling of the veins as the main criterion for DVT) to venography in 72 patients in the femoropopliteal region. A sensitivity of 100% and specificity of 98% were found for DVT in the femoroiliac region and a sensitivity of 95% and specificity of 98% were found for DVT in the popliteal region (unpublished data). The time necessary to complete a color flow Doppler study was 13 minutes compared to 16 minutes for venography. It has been postulated that color flow Doppler permits a faster study, vessels can be located more easily, and flow within the lumen can be identified immediately. Color flow Doppler is also helpful in the examination of the iliac vessels, where compression techniques cannot be used, but the presence of flow may be verified.

Diagnosis of Deep Vein Thrombosis in the Calf Region

The calf is difficult to examine by compression ultrasound alone and studies citing accuracy of diagnosis of DVT in this area are inconsistent. However, Semrow et al. have reported a sensitivity of 98% and specificity of 94% for compression ultrasound using venography as the standard. Color flow Doppler sonography facilitates the identification of calf veins. Early reports on the accuracy of color flow Doppler in DVT of calf veins are promising[17,18]; Zwiebel and Priest reported a sensitivity of 95% and specificity of 100% in 45 examinations.[19]

Difficulties and Pitfalls in Diagnosis of DVT

The diagnosis of DVT by ultrasound is somewhat subjective and examiner-dependent. In particular, examination and interpretation of studies of the obese patient and patients with previous DVT can be difficult. The sonographer must, therefore, be aware of the limitation of ultrasound and recommend venography when the study is indeterminate. Areas consistently difficult to examine are the iliac veins, calf veins, and femoropopliteal veins at the adductor canal. In these areas the use of color flow Doppler facilitates the identification of patency of flow.

Another potential pitfall is the common variations of duplication of femoral and popliteal veins. Systematic examination of duplications with compression is necessary as the presence of peripheral vascular disease, particularly with occlusion, may make a venous examination difficult as arterial landmarks cannot be used. As a general rule, a collateral or superficial vein is likely being examined if an artery is not seen in the immediate vicinity.

Ease and accuracy of diagnosing acute DVT in the patient with a history of previous DVT is compromised; these veins are often tortuous and thick-walled. Conse-quently, it can be difficult to differentiate between acute DVT with clot characterized by low echogenicity and a recanalized thick-walled post-thrombotic vessel. Such chronically diseased vessels are usually not completely compressible and feature abnormal contours with inadequate responses to augmentation and Valsalva maneuvers.

UPPER EXTREMITY

Introduction

The incidence of DVT of the upper extremity has been recognized as being higher in recent years than previously reported. Horattas et al. made a literature review in 1988 in addition to reporting a retrospective review of patients with subclavian and axillary DVTs.[20] They found that 28% of patients with subclavian catheters developed DVTs of the subclavian vein and that approximately 12% of patients with thrombosis of the upper extremity got pulmonary embolism. This was a much higher number than previously anticipated. Of all subclavian vein thrombosis, catheters are the major cause, particularly large-bore catheters.

The main complications of upper extremity DVTs are swelling of the arm and major long-term disability of the upper arm, pulmonary embolism (approximately 12%), septic thrombophlebitis, and superior vena cava syndrome. The subclavian, internal jugular, and innominate veins are the major central venous access routes and in cases of thrombosis of those veins, such an access is often impossible. Patients with dialysis fistulas in the arm need good venous return for proper fistula function and it is, therefore, important to have a good and easily repeatable method to evaluate the status of the proximal outflow veins as well as the more distal veins.

Several diagnostic methods have been tried for evaluation of the upper extremity. As in the lower extremity, a venogram is the most reliable study and the gold standard. Plethysmography is relatively unreliable and the ^{125}I marked fibrinogen test is also unreliable. There has, therefore, been increasing interest in using duplex and color flow Doppler sonography. This is now a relatively accepted way of ruling out stenosis or thrombosis of the upper extremity central veins but is still not fully evaluated.

Anatomy

The anatomy of the upper extremity is, in many ways, analogous to the lower extremity (Fig. 4.3.37). The deep veins follow the arteries and are duplicated distal to the elbow. There are two major superficial veins: the basilic and the cephalic veins. The first one drains into the proximal brachial vein and the latter one drains into the axillary vein. The proximal innominate vein and the superior vena cava cannot usually be easily seen with ultrasound; therefore, careful examination of the more distal veins with duplex sonography and comparative analysis of the Dopp-

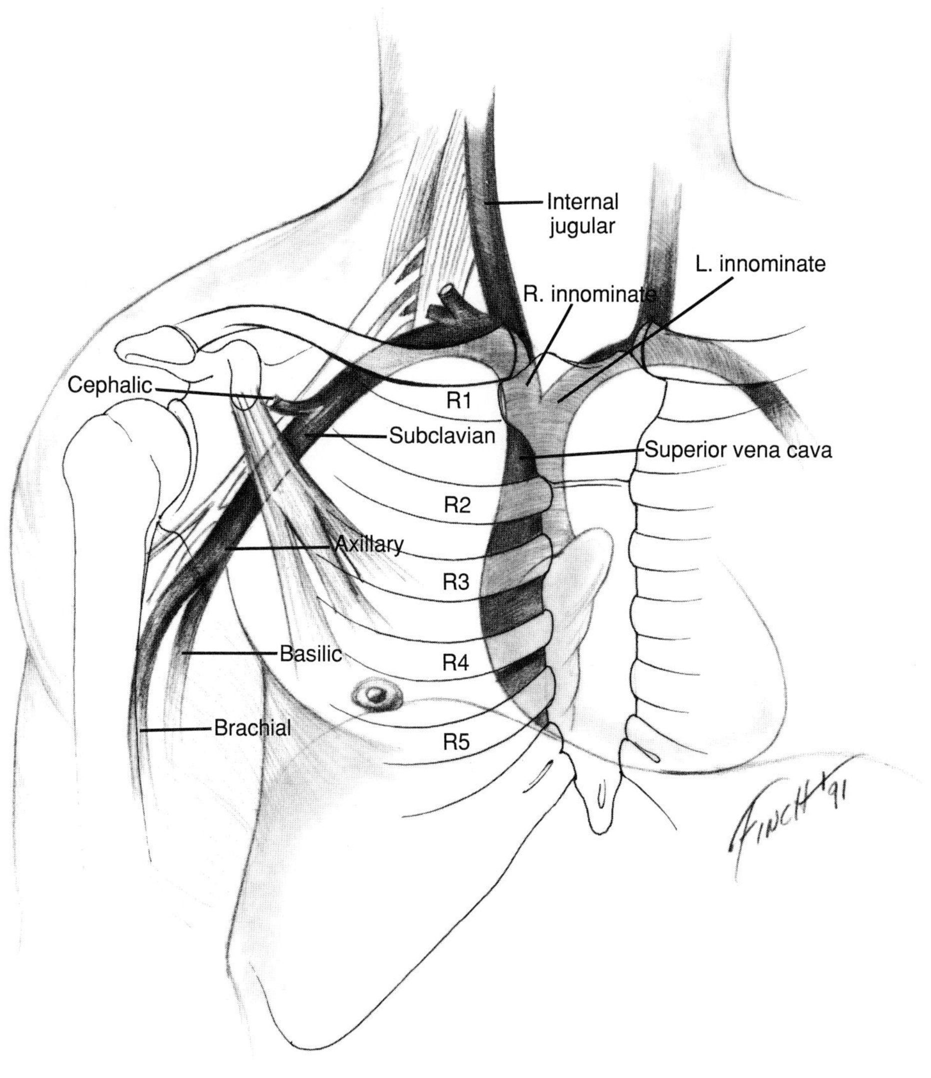

Figure 4.3.37. The anatomy of the proximal veins of the upper extremity and neck.

ler waveforms must be used to indirectly rule out thrombosis of the large proximal veins.[19]

Ultrasound: Doppler and Color Flow Doppler

INSTRUMENTS AND EXAMINATION TECHNIQUE

The patient is examined in the prone position with the arm in resting position beside the body. Usually a 5mHz sector array transducer is used. The internal jugular vein is identified from the lateral aspect of the neck and followed inferiorly in transverse section with light pressure without compressing the vein. The vein is followed at the junction to the subclavian vein. The subclavian vein is examined in longitudinal and transverse view and color flow Doppler or conventional Doppler is used to differentiate between artery and vein. Doppler tracing is obtained from the internal jugular vein from the junction of the internal jugular vein and the subclavian vein and also deep into the innominate vein if possible. The medial part of the subclavian vein

is examined transversely from the supraclavicular aspect in transverse and longitudinal view. The Doppler signal is obtained from the medial part of the subclavian vein as well. The lateral part of the subclavian vein and the axillary vein are examined from below the clavicle. Here, as well, a Doppler tracing is obtained from the whole length of the vessel[21,22] if color flow Doppler is not available.

It is very important to localize the vein in the immediate neighborhood of the artery to ensure that one is not observing a collateral vein, such as the cephalic vein, for example. Collaterals can be very large in this region but they do not follow arteries. The compression technique described for lower extremity studies can be used in the internal jugular vein and in most of the subclavian vein. The analysis of Doppler waveforms rather than relying on venous compression or color flow visualization is very important in the upper extremity examination because the innominate vein is not well seen; especially in the proximal part the superior vena cava (SVC) is not visualized and stenosis (or thrombus) can also be overlooked in the part of

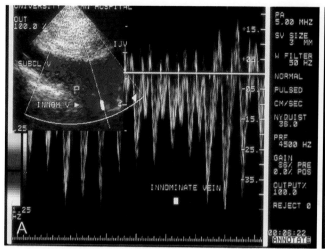

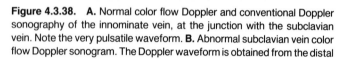

Figure 4.3.38. **A.** Normal color flow Doppler and conventional Doppler sonography of the innominate vein, at the junction with the subclavian vein. Note the very pulsatile waveform. **B.** Abnormal subclavian vein color flow Doppler sonogram. The Doppler waveform is obtained from the distal subclavian vein. The flow is nonphasic with spectral broadening. This waveform is suggestive of more central stenosis or occlusion in innominate vein or superior vena cava.

the subclavian vein where it goes beneath the clavicle, with flow maintained. The waveform is examined by looking at respiratory and atrial pulsatility components.

The reflected atrial contraction and the respiratory variations are very prominent in the upper extremity veins and the waveforms are normally very sharp and pulsatile. The spectral band width is normally narrow (Fig. 4.3.38A). In case of central stenosis or occlusion, the atrial contraction waveform and the respiration waveform diminish or disappear and the spectral bands broaden (Fig. 4.3.38B). However, large collateral veins may be effective enough to maintain a pulsatile venous waveform laterally in the subclavian vein, so waveform analysis must be combined with attention to the course of the normal subclavian vein. Comparison of waveforms obtained bilaterally is often helpful.

The cephalic vein is often prominent if there is stenosis or occlusion of the subclavian or innominate veins.

In cases where there is an arteriovenous dialysis fistula in the arm, the flow velocity increases and the spectral band gets broader and the waveform somewhat more irregular. It is important to be aware of this.

Conclusion

There has been a rapid evolution in the use of ultrasound in the diagnosis of human disease. Conventional Doppler and color flow Doppler technologies have also rapidly evolved and we continue to grow in our understanding of applications for those techniques. Venography has been, and still is, considered to be the definitive radiographic study of the deep veins of the legs.

Nonetheless, compression ultrasound and, more recently, conventional duplex and color flow Doppler, have attained important positions in the diagnosis of DVT.

These examinations are highly accurate, in the face of their ease, portability, and relative inexpense. Although such studies will likely replace venography for many routine cases, contrast studies will continue to be done for patients with high proximal venous extension, candidates for filter placement, and patients with suspected superimposed acute and chronic thrombotic processes.

Duplex and color flow Doppler studies of the central veins in the upper extremity are a promising method of studying those vessels, but more experience and clinical data must be collected.

References

1. Killewich LA, Bedford GR, Beach KW, Strandness DE: Diagnosis of deep venous thrombosis. *Circulation* 1989; 79(1):810–814
2. Dorfman GS, Cronan JJ: Sonographic diagnosis of thrombosis of the lower extremity veins. *Semin Intervent Radiol* 1990;7(1):9–19
3. Langsfeld M, Hershey FB, Thorpe L, Auer AI, Binnington HB, Hurley JJ, Woods JJ: Duplex B-mode imaging for the diagnosis of deep venous thrombosis. *Arch Surg* 1987; 122:587–591
4. Coon WW, Willis PW: Deep venous thrombosis and pulmonary embolism—prediction, prevention and treatment. *Am J Cardiol* 1959;4:611–621
5. Strandness DE, Langlois Y, Cramer M, Randlett A, Thiele BL: Long-term sequelae of acute venous thrombosis. *JAMA* 1983;250(10):1289–1292
6. Salzman EW: Venous thrombosis made easy. *New Engl J Med* 1986;314(13):847–848
7. Cranley JJ, Canos AJ, Sull WJ: The diagnosis of deep venous thrombosis. *Arch Surg* 1986;111:34–36
8. Kakkar VV, Flanc C, Howe CT, Clarke MB: Natural history of postoperative deep-vein thrombosis. *Lancet* 1969;2:230–232
9. Kakkar VV: Deep vein thrombosis. *Circulation* 1975;51:8–19
10. Dorfman GS, Froehlich JA, Cronan JJ, Urbanek PJ, Hern-

don JH: Lower-extremity venous thrombosis in patients with acute hip fractures: determination of anatomic location and time of onset with compression sonography. *AJR* 1990; 154:851–855

11. Lund F, Diener L, Ericsson JLE: Postmortem intraosseous phlebography as an aid in studies of venous thromboembolism. *Angiology* 1969;20:155–176

12. Bettmann MA, Paulin S: Leg phlebography: the incidence, nature and modification of undesirable side effects. *Radiology* 1977;122:101–104

13. Laerum F, Holm HA: Postphlebographic thrombosis - a double-blind study with methylglucamine metrizoate and metrizamide. *Radiology* 1981;140:651–654

14. Yedlicka JW, Hunter DW, Letourneau JG: Pulmonary embolism after femoral vein compression during sonography: case report. *Semin Intervent Radiol* 1990;7(1):24–26

15. van Bemmelen PS, Bedford G, Strandness DE: Visualization of calf veins by color flow imaging. *Ultrasound Med Biol* 1990;16(1):15–17

16. Cronan JJ, Dorfman GS, Grusmark J: Lower-extremity deep venous thrombosis: further experience with and refinements of US assessment. *Radiology* 1988;168:101–107

17. Polak JF, Culter SS, O'Leary DH: Deep veins of the calf: assessment with color Doppler flow imaging. *Radiology* 1989;171:481–485

18. Foley WD, Middleton WD, Lawson TL, Erickson S, Quiroz FA, Macrander S: Color Doppler ultrasound imaging of lower-extremity venous disease. *AJR* 1989;152:371–376

19. Zweibel WJ, Priest DL: Color duplex sonography of extremity veins. *Semin Ultrasound CT MR* 1990;11(2):136–167

20. Horattas MC, Wright DJ, Fenton AH, Evans DM, Oddi MA, Kamienski RW, Shields EF: Changing concepts of deep vein thrombosis of the upper extremity—report of a series and review of the literature. *Surgery* 1988;104(3):561–567

21. Falk RL, Smith DF: Thrombosis of upper extremity thoracic inlet veins: diagnosis with duplex Doppler sonography. *AJR* 1987;149:677–682

22. Longley D, Yedlicka JW Jr, Molina E, Schwabacher S, Letourneau JG: Color Doppler ultrasound of thoracic outlet syndrome. *Semin Intervent Radiol* 1990;7(3–4):230–235

An Overview of the Role of Duplex and Color Doppler Sonography in the Evaluation of the Hepatic and Portal Vasculature and Solid Organ Transplants (Renal, Hepatic, and Pancreatic)

—Richard N. Aizpuru, M.D. Deborah G. Longley, M.D., Janis Gissel Letourneau, M.D., David W. Hunter, M.D., and Joseph W. Yedlicka, Jr., M.D.

The purpose of this section is to give a brief overview of the salient duplex color Doppler sonographic findings in evaluating disorders involving the hepatic and portal vasculature and organ transplants. Duplex sonography and color Doppler sonography are useful in the diagnosis of portal hypertension and in following the progression of portal hypertension. Doppler sonography also provides a noninvasive screening test to direct subsequent angiographic diagnosis and intervention. Finally, Doppler

sonography is routine at major transplant centers, essential for expedient diagnoses of peritransplant vascular complications.

TECHNIQUE AND INSTRUMENTATION

The basic principles of abdominal Doppler sonography are derived from peripheral Doppler evaluation.[1] However, since the hepatic and splanchnic vessels are both tortuous and deep structures, low wall filters (<50Hz), low transducer frequencies (2–3mHz), and low pulse repetition frequency are used to detect blood flow.

To evaluate the main portal vein and its right tributaries, the right intercostal approach is used. The left portal vein, its branches, and the hepatic veins are best studied via an oblique subcostal approach. The splenic vein is seen in a midline transverse orientation while the superior mesenteric vein can best be evaluated from a sagittal anterior abdominal approach.

NORMAL FLOW PATTERNS IN THE HEPATIC AND SPLANCHNIC VASCULATURES

The portal vein and its branches, the superior mesenteric vein, and the splenic vein have flow patterns characterized by steady flow directed to the liver (hepatopedal)[2] (Figs. 4.3.39, 4.3.40, and 4.3.41). Small pulsations reflecting the cardiac cycle are present in the waveforms. Postprandial increases in the flow in these vessels have been reported.[3,4]

The inferior vena cava and the hepatic veins have triphasic flow. The first two phases reflect right atrial and right ventricular diastole. The third phase of reversed flow reflects atrial systole (Figs. 4.3.42 and 4.3.43).[1] Flow within the inferior vena cava increases with expiration. Hepatic artery flow is biphasic, reflecting the low resistance of the liver (pattern of flow can be similar to the internal carotid and renal arteries) (Fig. 4.3.44).

Flow patterns within the portal vein and hepatic artery are intimately related. When flow within the portal vein is high, flow within the hepatic artery is low and vice versa. In patients who are fasting, hepatic artery flow usually is high, whereas portal vein flow is low. Alcoholic patients often demonstrate increased hepatic artery flow with decreased portal venous flow (seen best in the periphery of the liver); these changes likely represent a state of diminished portal venous flow in patients developing portal hypertension.

FLOW PATTERNS IN THE HEPATIC AND PORTAL VASCULATURE IN DISEASE STATES

Portal hypertension can be diagnosed based on a number of flow patterns. Reversed flow in the intrahepatic portal vein or splenic vein is the most reliable sign of portal hypertension.[1] "To-and-fro flow" (i.e., inspiration draws

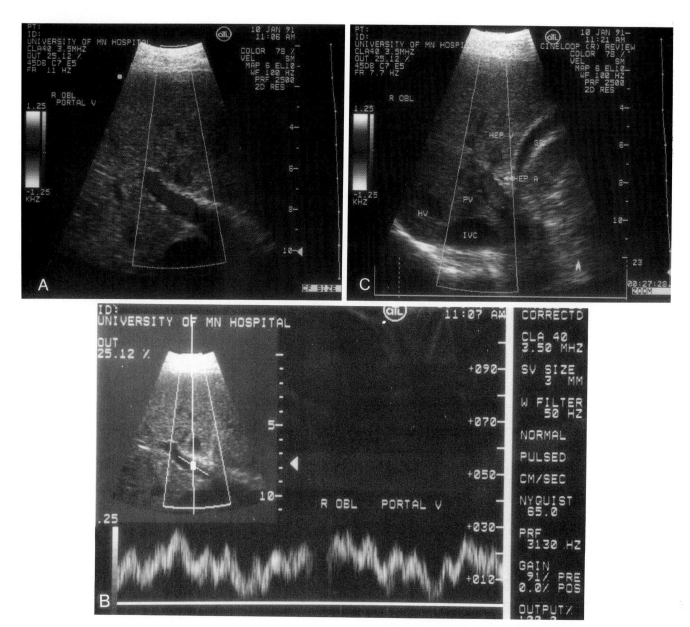

Figure 4.3.39. Portal vein. **A.** Right oblique view from a color Doppler study shows normal hepatopedal flow. **B.** Doppler wave form shows hepatopedal flow and slight pulsatility reflecting cardiac cycle. **C.** Color Doppler demonstrates the relationship of the portal vein (*PV*), hepatic artery (*HEP A*), and inferior vena cava (*IVC*) as labeled in the diagram.

blood toward the liver (hepatopedal) and expiration reverses flow (hepatofugal)) is a less reliable sign of portal hypertension since this can be seen in right-sided heart failure.[1]

Currently, the use of Doppler sonography in the abdomen is confined to qualitative analysis of blood flow and direction of flow. Clinical use for more quantitative flow measurements is not routine. Diagnostic goals in evaluating hepatic and portal vasculature should include the presence and direction of flow in the splenic veins, portal veins, hepatic veins, and the inferior vena cava.[5-7] Detection of portosystemic collaterals is also important if portal hypertension is suspected.[8]

Certain pitfalls when evaluating the direction of portal

vein flow should be avoided. Portal vein flow reversal is a sign of portal hypertension. The direction of flow in the portal vein, whether it is hepatofugal (reversed flow) or hepatopedal (normal flow direction) should be demonstrated; if using color Doppler equipment, the orientation of the color display should be known. Also, the angle of the Doppler beam to the vessel is usually less than 60°, and the relationship of the transducer to the expected direction of flow must be known. If confusion about the direction of flow is encountered, comparison to a control vessel with known flow direction (i.e., celiac, hepatic, or splenic artery) may be helpful.

Absence of flow in the portal vein can be difficult to establish because often the portal vein becomes very small

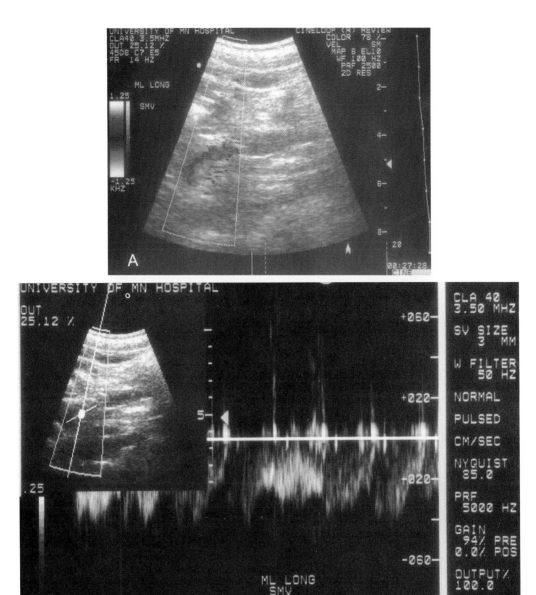

Figure 4.3.40. Superior mesenteric vein. **A.** Color Doppler shows normal flow in the superior mesenteric vein distal to the portal confluence. **B.** Doppler waveform shows hepatopedal flow and cardiac cycle reflections.

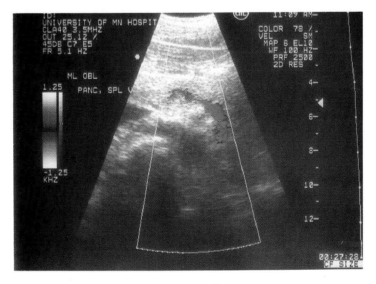

Figure 4.3.41. Splenic vein. Color Doppler shows normal splenic vein.

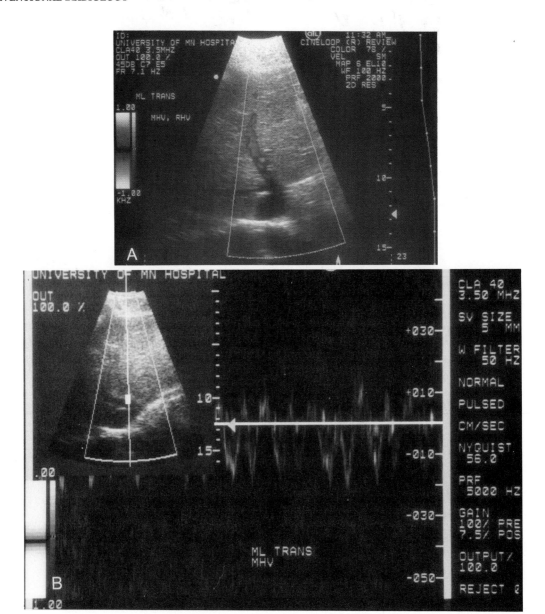

Figure 4.3.42. Hepatic veins. **A.** Normal color Doppler of middle hepatic vein. **B.** Doppler waveform demonstrates triphasic flow.

and low flow can mimic no flow. Generally, if one is using a 3mHz transducer, full Doppler gain, low pulse repetition frequency, and a 50Hz wall filter, and no Doppler signal is obtained, then blood is flowing with a velocity less than 2.5cm/sec.[1] A flow velocity of 2.5cm/sec is extremely slow and may be reflective of either portal vein thrombosis or a prethrombotic state (Fig. 4.3.45). Portal vein thrombosis is followed by the formation of a system of collateral veins known as cavernous transformation of the portal vein.[9]

Arterial-portal fistulae are rare and characterized by a portal vein flow pattern with systolic peaks and high diastolic Doppler shifts.[10]

In addition to these Doppler flow patterns in patients with portal hypertension and cirrhosis, a careful search for portosystemic collaterals is routine (Fig. 4.3.46). A predisposition to esophageal bleeding exists when distension of periesophageal veins via the left gastric veins is present. If one images a left gastric vein greater than 5.0mm, portal hypertension is most likely present.[1] Another common portosystemic route is the paraumbilical vein (this represents hepatofugal flow from the left portal vein to the periumbilical venous plexus). Hepatofugal flow in this vein suggests thrombosis of the portal vein.

In addition to the above Doppler and collateral findings in portal hypertension, morphologic signs include splenomegaly, changes in liver architecture, and ascites.[11–17]

Ultrasound findings of Budd–Chiari syndrome include an enlarged caudate lobe, ascites, and an unusual course of the hepatic veins.[18,19] Doppler sonography evidence of Budd–Chiari syndrome includes absence of flow in the hepatic veins and an association with portal vein thrombosis which reaches nearly 20%.[18,19]

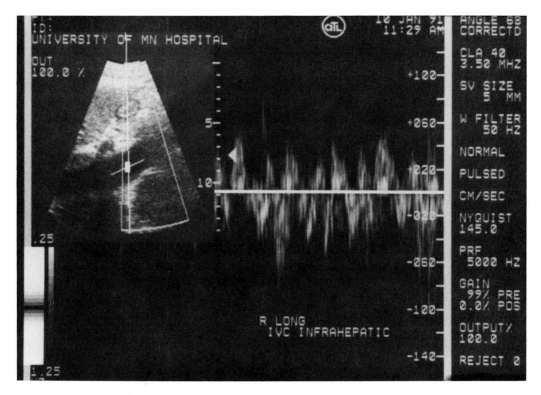

Figure 4.3.43. Inferior vena cava. Doppler waveform demonstrates triphasic flow.

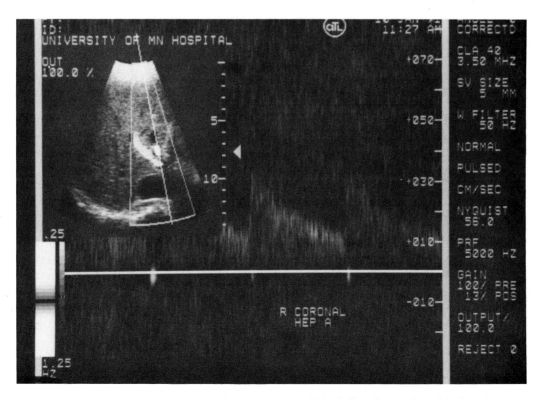

Figure 4.3.44. Hepatic artery. Doppler waveform demonstrates biphasic flow characteristic of the hepatic artery.

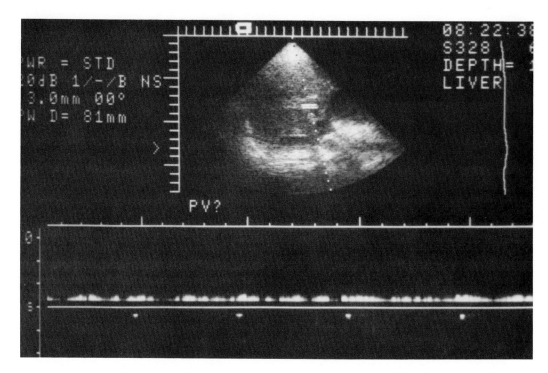

Figure 4.3.45. Portal vein thrombosis. Doppler waveform shows that there is virtually no flow in the portal vein in this patient with a liver allograft.

Doppler evaluation of surgical portosystemic shunts is reliable in establishing their patency. There are two broad categories of surgical portosystemic shunts: total and partial. An example of a total shunt is a portocaval shunt in which a communication (side-to-side) between the portal vein and the inferior vena cava directs high-pressure flow into the systemic circulation. Partial shunts allow diversion of high-pressure splanchnic venous flow with preservation of portal venous perfusion of the liver and thereby decrease the risk of hepatic encephalopathy; the Warren–Zeppa distal splenorenal shunt selectively shunts blood from the splenic vein to the inferior vena cava via the left renal vein. When the shunt is patent, blood flow is easily discovered at the shunt site (Fig. 4.3.47). Increased velocity at an anastomotic site may indicate stenosis.[20] Evaluation of a shunt site and hepatic and portal vasculature should be included in the evaluation of portosystemic shunts.

DUPLEX AND COLOR DOPPLER SONOGRAPHIC EVALUATION OF SOLID ORGAN TRANSPLANTS

An understanding of the techniques and methods required for the duplex and color Doppler sonographic evaluation of the hepatic and portal vasculature is most helpful in evaluating renal, hepatic, and pancreatic allografts. Renal transplantation is very common and represents a therapeutic alternative to peritoneal dialysis or hemodialysis. Although less frequent, hepatic and pancreatic transplantations are performed at a number of institutions around the world.

Real-time ultrasound examination is used to exclude complications of transplantation such as fluid collection, hematoma, abscess, malignancy, or other fluid collections specific to the transplanted organ, including lymphocele, bilomas, or pseudocysts. Biliary obstruction and hydronephrosis are also common complications after liver or kidney transplantation, respectively. Duplex and color Doppler sonography are used to screen for vasculature complications of transplant revascularization. Since the development of these techniques, the number of diagnostic invasive tests performed has decreased, avoiding unnecessary complications.

Renal Transplants

The reported incidence of allograft renal artery stenosis ranges from 1 to 12%.[21–25] Factors that predispose to renal artery stenosis are atherosclerosis in the native or transplanted vessel, injury during graft harvesting, allograft rejection, and technical problems such as kinking,[23] or difficult surgical anastomosis of the blood vessels. Since allograft renal artery stenosis is treated by angioplasty or surgery if the patient has uncontrolled hypertension or graft ischemia, it is important to recognize its presence. A number of other causes of hypertension after renal transplantation are recognized, such as allograft rejection and hydronephrosis. Screening patients with Doppler ultrasound can narrow the differential diagnosis.

A number of studies have shown that a peak systolic frequency shift of 7.5kHz and distal turbulence are sensitive (94.1%) and specific (86.7%) criteria for the accurate diag-

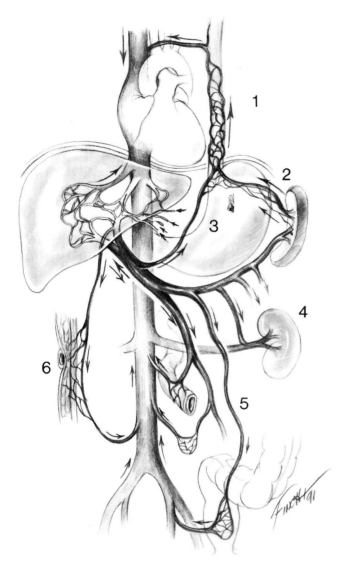

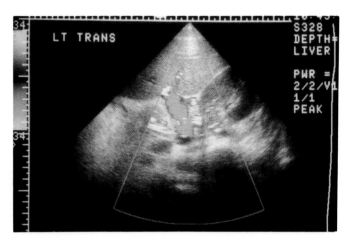

Figure 4.3.47. Distal spleno-renal shunt. Color Doppler shows patent spleno-renal shunt with flow away from the transducer *(blue)*.

Figure 4.3.46. Portal systemic collaterals. Major routes of portosystemic collaterals are demonstrated in this diagram. *1,* Esophageal veins (varices) seen in 82% of patients with portal hypertension.[56] *2,* Short gastric veins seen in 54% of patients with portal hypertension.[56] *3,* Abnormally enlarged left gastric vein seen in 80% of patients with portal hypertension.[56] *4,* Lower splenic hilus veins seen in 24% of patients with portal hypertension.[56] *5,* Inferior mesenteric vein varices seen in less than 15% of patients with portal hypertension.[56] *6,* Periumbilical vein collaterals seen in less than 15% of patients with portal hypertension.[56]

nosis of allograft renal artery stenosis.[26] The frequency shift corresponds to a peak systolic velocity of 1.7m/sec using a 3mHz Doppler transducer.[13] Angiography with a plan for angioplasty is recommended with a renal artery anastomotic velocity over l.7m/sec. Often, angiography reveals that a tortuous vessel is the cause for an evaluated renal artery anastomotic velocity (Fig. 4.3.48), rather than a significant stenosis.

In the immediate postoperative stage, color Doppler analysis of renal artery waveforms can be helpful to differentiate acute renal artery thrombosis from hyperacute or accelerated acute rejection.[27] The absence of arterial flow is compatible with renal artery thrombosis although not always diagnostic since elevated end-organ impedance of any cause can significantly decrease arterial flow.[26] More commonly, absence of arterial signal is secondary to severe vascular rejection, the main renal artery remains patent, but severe occlusive changes are found in the smaller intrarenal vessels.

Renal vein thrombosis is more common than renal artery thrombosis.[23,24] This complication typically occurs in the early postoperative period, and it causes renal allograft failure since the renal transplant does not have available native venous collateral blood supply.[27] Characteristic duplex findings include absent venous Doppler signal and an altered arterial waveform with an abruptly peaked systolic shift followed by a retrograde plateau-like diastolic shift[28] (Fig. 4.3.49). Normally, one sees slowly falling systolic peak and abundant antegrade diastolic flow in the main renal artery and its proximal branches. Hyperacute rejection also can produce loss of detectable main renal vein flow.

Pseudoaneurysms and arteriovenous fistulae are uncommon vascular complications that are detected with Doppler ultrasound. These are found in renal, hepatic, and pancreatic transplants. Pseudoaneurysms and arteriovenous fistulae are often complications of biopsy or vascular reconstructions. Accurate diagnosis is important because of their associated life-threatening complications such as rupture, hemorrhage, and infection. Pseudoaneurysms are characterized by a variably sized, well circumscribed hypoechoic or complex mass with a pulsatile Doppler waveform and a high velocity jet at the neck of the pseudoaneurysm.[29] Color Doppler examination of the pseudoaneurysm reveals multidirectional, whirling flow (Fig. 4.3.50). Arteriovenous fistulae are characterized by decreased resistive indices in the supplying arteries which also have increased flow (Fig. 4.3.51). The draining vein also has an arterialized pattern. Color Doppler evaluation reveals increased color saturation.

The real-time sonographic criteria for acute allograft rejection include changes in graft size, changes in the

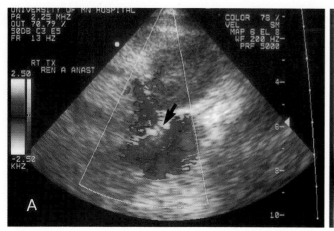

Figure 4.3.48. Renal artery. **A.** Color Doppler shows a focal area of increased velocity with color saturation *(arrow)*. **B.** Doppler waveform at the renal artery anastomosis shows increased systolic velocity (1.8 m/sec) with an interrogation angle corrected for the course of the renal artery. However, at angiography the anastomosis was normal.

appearance of the renal sinus fat and renal pyramids, and the thickening of the wall of the renal collecting system.[30,31] Quantification of arterial inflow within the graft as a means of predicting acute rejection has received a lot of attention.[32–40] Calculation of a pulsatility or resistive index as a measure of impedance to arterial inflow within the graft is no longer accepted as an accurate means to diagnose allograft rejection since it is nonspecific and reflects only an increase in vascular impedance.[32–36,37–40] Vascular impedance can increase in a number of situations including acute tubular necrosis, renal vein thrombosis, graft infection, extrarenal compression of the graft, obstructive hydronephrosis, and acute and chronic rejection.[27]

Doppler sonography is very useful in differentiating mild hydronephrosis, creating a dilated renal pelvis, from a prominent central venous structure.[41]

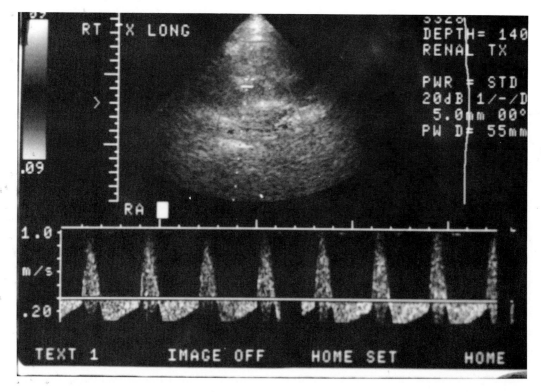

Figure 4.3.49. Renal vein thrombosis. Duplex sonogram of renal transplant artery shows complete reversal of diastolic flow with a spike of systolic flow, indicating severely increased resistance to flow. Renal vein flow was not identified. Graft nephrectomy showed renal vein thrombosis.

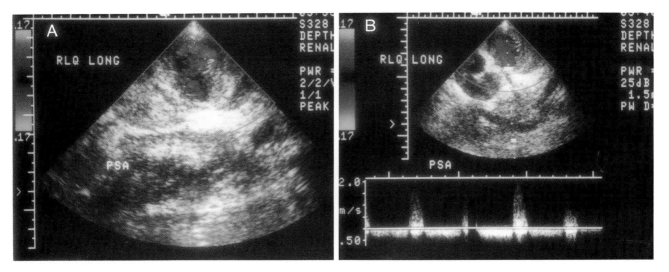

Figure 4.3.50. Postbiopsy pseudoaneurysm. **A.** Color sonography depicts an intrarenal pseudoaneurysm after biopsy. Note characteristic whirling blood flow. **B.** Doppler waveform shows typical "to-and-fro" waveform with antegrade systolic and retrograde diastolic flow.

Liver Transplants

Duplex and color Doppler sonography play an important role in evaluating liver transplant recipients both before and after surgery. Preoperative studies focus on evaluating extrahepatic portal vein patency, as has been discussed earlier in this section. Preoperative evaluation can be difficult and may require angiographic evaluation; particularly when the portal vein has been thrombosed and partially recanalized or collaterals or cavernous transformation of the portal vein is present.[42] Systemic venous drainage of the liver is also evaluated preoperatively since this is critical to operative planning. In approximately 10% of cases of extrahepatic biliary atresia, there is anomalous venous drainage of the liver; usually this is azygous continuation of an interrupted inferior vena cava.[43]

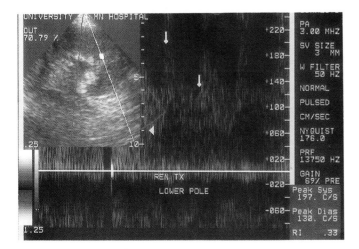

Figure 4.3.51. Renal arteriovenous fistula. Postbiopsy arteriovenous fistulas demonstrated with high flow as well as increased diastolic flow as seen by Doppler waveform.

Hepatic artery thrombosis and portal venous thrombosis are seen in approximately 10% of liver transplant recipients.[44,45] Inferior vena cava thrombosis occurs in approximately 5% of cases.[44,45] Hepatic artery thrombosis is characterized by the abrupt onset of fever, septicemia, elevated liver function tests, and deteriorated coagulation parameters.[46] Portal vein thrombosis and inferior vena cava thrombosis are characterized by nonspecific clinical findings such as impaired hepatic function, gastrointestinal bleeding, ascites, peripheral edema, fever, and sepsis.[47] Doppler sonography allows the noninvasive preliminary diagnosis of hepatic artery thrombosis, portal venous thrombosis, or inferior vena cava thrombosis.[44,48–50] The Doppler findings of absent flow should be corroborated by the presence of echogenic thrombus in cases of suspected portal venous or inferior vena caval thrombosis; relying solely on Doppler findings of absent flow can be problematic in these two instances (Fig. 4.3.45). Hepatic artery thrombosis seen by Doppler evaluation requires angiographic confirmation if intervention is planned, as false-positive examinations can occur.

Hepatic artery, portal venous, and inferior vena caval stenosis have all been reported after liver transplantation, but the true incidence is not known.[45,49,51] Narrowing of the portal vein and inferior vena caval anastomosis is seen frequently, but the hemodynamic significance is not always clear. Anastomotic stricture should be considered in the face of increased velocities; angiographic confirmation followed by angioplasty or vascular stenting may be required.

The presence of portal venous gas produces high acoustic impedance foci within the portal vein, detected as "blips" on the Doppler signal.[52] Studies have shown that portal venous gas may not portend the same grave prognosis after transplant as it does in other clinical settings.[52]

Studies from the University of Pittsburgh show a lack of correlation of the loss of hepatic artery diastolic flow with

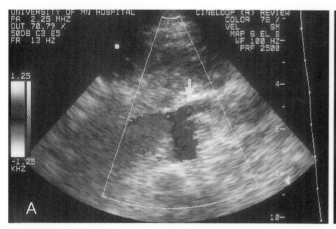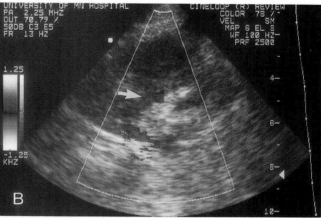

Figure 4.3.52. Pancreatic artery transplant thrombosis. **A.** Transverse color Doppler sonogram shows flow only in the very most proximal portion of the artery *(white arrow)*. The remainder of the artery is thrombosed. Thrombosis occurred secondary to acute severe rejection. Iliac vein and artery flow is normal. **B.** Color sonography shows minimal flow in a pancreatic vein *(white arrow)*.

histopathologic evidence of acute rejection.[53,54] Therefore, as in renal transplants, hepatic arterial resistive indices have no value in evaluating acute liver transplant rejection.

Color Doppler sonography is helpful in differentiating dilated intrahepatic biliary ducts from small vascular structures; consequently, the diagnosis of biliary obstruction in hepatic recipients with graft dysfunction can be greatly facilitated.

Pancreatic Transplants

Approximately 10% of pancreatic transplants are complicated by graft thrombosis. Since the signs and symptoms are nonspecific, imaging is important in identifying this complication. Allograft thrombosis can occur acutely or later, usually secondary to infection or rejection. Presently scintigraphy is the mainstay of diagnosis of graft thrombosis; however, duplex sonography is also sensitive and specific in the diagnosis.[55] The definitive diagnosis with duplex technology alone is problematic as thrombosis is characterized by a lack of arterial and/or venous signal; more certainty of diagnosis is possible when progressive changes in the arterial waveform are seen (Fig. 4.3.52).

The precise role of duplex sonography in the setting of pancreatic transplant rejection has not been defined. Real-time examination shows graft inhomogenicity, although this finding is nonspecific.

References

1. Lafortune M, Patriquin H: Doppler sonography of the liver and splanchnic veins. *Semin Intervent Radiol* 1990;7(1):27-38
2. Burns P, Taylor KJW, Blei AT: Doppler flowmetry and portal hypertension. *Gastroenterology* 1987;92:824–826
3. Pugliese D, Ohnishi K, Tsunoda T, Sabba C, Albano O: Portal hemodynamics after meal in normal subjects and in patients with chronic liver disease studied by echo Doppler flowmeter. *Am J Gastroenterol* 1987;82:1052–1056
4. Lee SS, Hadengue A, Moreau R, Sayegh R, Hilton P, Lebrec

D: Postprandial hemodynamic responses in patients with cirrhosis. *Hepatology* 1988;8:647–651
5. Patriquin H, Lafortune M, Burns PN, et al: Duplex Doppler evaluation in portal hypertension: technique and anatomy. *AJR* 1987;149:71–76
6. Patriquin HB, Babcock D, Paltiel H: Color Doppler: applications in children. *Ultrasound Q* 1989;7:243–269
7. Vanleeuwen MS: Doppler ultrasound in the evaluation of portal hypertension. *Clin Diagn Ultrasound* 1989;26:53–76
8. Subramanyam BR, Balthazar EJ, Madamba MR, et al: Sonography of portosystemic venous collaterals in portal hypertension. *Radiology* 1983;146:161–166
9. Weltin G, Taylor KJW, Carter AR, et al: Duplex Doppler: identification of cavernous transformation of the portal vein. *AJR* 1985;144:999–1001
10. Burns PN, Jaffe CC: Quantitative measurements with a Doppler ultrasound: techniques, accuracy and limitations. *Radiol Clin North Am* 1985;23:641–657
11. Lafortune M, Constantin A, Bregon G, et al: The recanalized umbilical vein in portal hypertension: a myth. *AJR* 1985;144:549–553
12. Kauzlaric D, Petrovic M, Barmeir E: Sonography of cavernous transformation of the portal vein. *AJR* 1984;142:383–384
13. Kane RA, Katz SG: The spectrum of sonography findings in portal hypertension: a subject review and new observations. *Radiology* 1982;142:453–458
14. Marchal GJF, Van Holsbeeck M, Tshibwabwa-Ntumba E, et al: Dilatation of the cystic vein in portal hypertension: sonographic demonstration. *Radiology* 1985;154:187–189
15. Von Koischwitz D, Paquet K, Schulz D: Sonographische Beurteiling des portalen Gefassystems bei der portalen Hypertension. *Fortschr Röntgenstr* 1982;137:509–517
16. Juttner HV, Jenny JM, Ralls PW, et al: Ultrasound demonstration of portosystemic collaterals in cirrhosis and portal hypertension. *Radiology* 1982;142:459–463
17. Waller RM, Oliver TW, McCain AH, et al: Computed tomography and sonography of hepatic cirrhosis and portal hypertension. *RadioGraphics* 1984;4:677–715
18. Menu Y, Alison D, Lorphelin JM, et al: Budd-Chiari syndrome: US evaluation. *Radiology* 1985;157:761–764
19. Baert AL, Fevery J, Marchal G, et al: Early diagnosis of Budd-Chiari syndrome by computed tomography and ultrasonography: report of five cases. *Gastroenterology* 1983;84:587–595
20. Lafortune M, Patriquin H, Pomier G, et al: Hemodynamic

changes of portal circulation following porto-systemic shunts: a study of 45 patients using duplex ultrasonography. *AJR* 1987;149:71–76

21. Smellie WAB, Vinik M, Hume DM: Angiographic investigation of hypertension complicating renal transplantation. *Surg Gynecol Obstet* 1969;128:963–969

22. Margules RM, Belzer FO, Kountz SL: Surgical correction of renovascular hypertension following renal allotransplantation. *Arch Surg* 1973;106:13–16

23. Belzer FO: Technical complications after renal transplantation, in Morris PJ (ed): *Kidney Transplantation*. New York, Grune & Stratton, 1979, pp 267–284

24. McGrath BP, Ledingham JGG: Cardiovascular complications after renal transplantation, in Morris PJ (ed): *Kidney Transplantation*. New York, Grune & Stratton, 1979, pp 282–325

25. Tilney NL, Kirkman RL: Surgical aspects of kidney transplantation, in Garovoy MR, Guttmann RD (eds): *Renal Transplantation*. New York, Churchill Livingstone, 1986, p 93

26. Snider JF, Hunter DW, Moradian GP, et al: Transplant renal artery stenosis: evaluation with duplex sonography. *Radiology* 1989;172:1027–1030

27. Letourneau JG, Day DL: Vascular evaluation of renal, hepatic, and pancreatic allografts with duplex sonography and color Doppler scanning. *Semin Intervent Radiol* 1990; 7(1):44–56

28. Reuther G, Wanjura D, Bauer H: Acute renal vein thrombosis in renal allografts: detection with duplex Doppler US. *Radiology* 1989;170:557–558

29. Abu-Yousef MM, Wiese JA, Shamma AR: The "to-and-fro" sign: duplex Doppler evidence of femoral artery pseudoaneurysm. *AJR* 1988;150:632–634

30. Hoddick W, Filly RA, Backman U, et al: Renal allograft rejection: US evaluation. *Radiology* 1986;161:469–473

31. Hricak H, Terrier F, Marotti M, et al: Post transplant renal rejection: comparison of quantitative scintigraphy, US, and MR imaging. *Radiology* 1987;162:685–688

32. Rigsby CM, Taylor KJW, Weltin G, et al: Renal allografts in acute rejection: evaluation using duplex sonography. *Radiology* 1986;158:375–378

33. Rigsby CM, Burns PN, Weltin GG, et al: Doppler signal quantitation in renal allografts: comparison in normal and rejecting transplants, with pathologic correlation. *Radiology* 1987;162:39–42

34. Rifkin MD, Needleman L, Pasto M, et al: Evaluation of renal transplant rejection by duplex Doppler examination: value of the resistive index. *AJR* 1987;148:759–762

35. Buckley AR, Cooperberg PL, Reeve CE, et al: The distinction between acute renal transplant rejection and cyclosporine nephrotoxicity: value of duplex sonography. *AJR* 1987; 149:521–525

36. Steinberg HV, Nelson RC, Murphy FB, et al: Renal allograft rejection: evaluation by Doppler US and MR imaging. *Radiology* 1987;162:337–342

37. Warshauer DM, Taylor KJB, Bia MJ, et al: Unusual causes of increased vascular impedance in renal transplants: duplex Doppler evaluation. *Radiology* 1988;169:367–370

38. Don S, Kopecky KK, Filo RS, et al: Duplex Doppler US of renal allografts: causes of elevated resistive index. *Radiology* 1989;171:709–712

39. Allen KS, Jorkasky DK, Arger PH, et al: Renal allografts: prospective analysis of Doppler sonography. *Radiology* 1988; 169:371–376:

40. Genkins SM, Sanfilippo FP, Carroll BA: Duplex Doppler sonography of renal transplants: lack of sensitivity and specificity in establishing pathologic diagnosis. *AJR* 1989;152:525–529

41. Platt JF, Rubin JM, Ellis JH, et al: Duplex Doppler US of the kidney: differentiation of obstructive from nonobstructive dilation. *Radiology* 1989;171:515–517

42. Nelson RC, Lovett KE, Chezmar JL, et al: Comparison of pulsed Doppler sonography and angiography in patients with portal hypertension. *AJR* 1987;149:77–81

43. Abramson SJ, Berden WE, Altman RP, et al: Biliary atresia and non-cardiac polysplenic syndrome: US and surgical considerations. *Radiology* 1987;163:377–379

44. Dalen K, Day DL, Ascher NL, et al: Imaging of vascular complications after hepatic transplantation. *AJR* 1988; 150:1285–1290

45. Wozney P, Zajko AB, Bron KM, et al: Vascular complications after liver transplantation: a 5 year experience. *AJR* 1986; 147:657–663

46. Tzakis AG, Gordon GD, Shaw BW Jr, et al: Clinical presentation of hepatic artery thrombosis after liver transplantation in the cyclosporine era. *Transplantation* 1985;40:667–671

47. Webb LJ, Sherlock S: The etiology, presentation and natural history of extra-hepatic portal venous obstruction. *Q J Med* 1979;48:627–639

48. Longley DG, Skolnick ML, Zajko AB, et al: Duplex Doppler sonography in the evaluation of adult patients before and after liver transplantation. *AJR* 1988;151:687–696

49. Taylor JKW, Morse SS, Weltin GG, et al: Liver transplant recipients: portable duplex US with correlative angioplasty. *Radiology* 1986;159:357–363

50. Letourneau JG, Day DL, Ascher NL, et al: Abdominal sonography after liver transplantation: results in 36 patients. *AJR* 1987;149:299–303

51. Abad J, Hildago EG, Cantarero JM, et al: Hepatic artery anastomotic stenosis after transplantation: treatment with percutaneous transluminal angioplasty. *Radiology* 1989; 171:661–662

52. Chezmar JL, Nelson RC, Bernadino ME: Portal venous gas after hepatic transplantation: sonographic detection and clinical significance. *AJR* 1989;153:1203–1205

53. Longley DG, Skolnick ML, Sheahan DG: Acute allograft rejection in liver transplant recipients: lack of correlation with loss of hepatic artery diastolic flow. *Radiology* 1988;169:417–420

54. Harder DM, DeMarino GB, Sumkin JH, et al: Liver transplant rejection: value of the resistive index in Doppler US of hepatic arteries. *Radiology* 1989;173:127–129

55. Snider JF, Hunter DW, Kuni CC, et al: Pancreas transplantation: radiographic evaluation of vascular complications. *Radiology* 1991;178:749–753

56. Hoevels J, Lunderquist A, Ihse I: Portosystemic collaterals in cirrhosis of the liver: selective percutaneous transhepatic catheterization of the portal venous system and portal hypertension. *Acta Radiol (Stockh)* 1979;20:865

Part 4. Intravascular Ultrasound

—Christopher E. Engeler, M.D., and Joseph W. Yedlicka, Jr., M.D.

EQUIPMENT AND METHODS

Instrumentation

Miniaturization of ultrasonic transducers has recently been achieved with crystal thicknesses under 0.1mm. Accordingly, feasible transducer frequencies are in the range of 15–25mHz. Axial resolution can be expected to be very high. Lateral resolution will depend on focusing of the ultrasonic beam. However, depth of field is limited as tissue penetration decreases with higher frequency.

Such high-frequency ultrasound transducers have been mounted on catheters for intraluminal imaging and are now commercially available. Either a linear array arrangement or mechanical scanning is possible.[1] In the linear array transducer, there are no moving parts. However, the volume of the transducer increases with the number of crystals mounted at the catheter tip. With mechanical scanning, the crystal is rotated 360° to accumulate B-mode data for axial display. Both types of transducers have been introduced.

The illustrations in this chapter are from a rotating type transducer with a crystal frequency of 20mHz. Mounted on a long flexible shaft, the transducer is rotated at 900 rpm within a catheter. Real-time images are thus obtained.

INTRODUCTION AND GUIDANCE

The shaft with the transducer tip is introduced into a sterile catheter filled with water which provides internal acoustical coupling. This assembly can then be advanced through any vascular sheath of at least 7Fr diameter. A monorail guidewire has been added to improve the safety of transducer positioning, particularly after interventional procedures. As is well known, intimal dissections are common after angioplasty. Blind advancement of a transducer through an area of recently performed angioplasty can result in an extension of the intimal dissection and/or peripheral embolization of detached segments. Current limitations include catheter stiffness, poor torque control, and a relatively short catheter length (100cm). Access to most major arterial or venous systems is possible by using directional sheaths or guidewire systems. Even transvenous advancement through the right heart chambers into pulmonary artery branches has been accomplished.

DISPLAY AND IMAGING RECORDING

Real-time images are projected on the monitor of the ultrasound machine at a rate of 15 frames/sec. The time gain compensation setting is critical to proper image interpretation. Due to the high frequency of the ultrasound beam, significant scattering from cellular blood compo-nents is observed.[2] It is important to reduce these echoes as much as possible. Once the appropriate settings have been selected, the images may then be displayed on video-tape or on film.

ENDOSONOGRAPHY OF VASCULAR DISEASE

Pathological Overview

Figure 4.4.1 summarizes the spectrum of arteriosclerosis. The normal arterial wall consists of three layers: intima, media, and adventitia. Intimal edema, thickening, and proliferation are early responses to endothelial injury. Atherosclerosis is characterized by the accumulation of lipids in the intima. Atheromatous disease may progress to fibrous plaques, cholesterol deposition, and calcification. Complications include hemorrhage and ulceration. Specific degeneration of the tunica media is known as Möncke-berg's sclerosis. In large and medium-sized muscular arteries, characteristic calcification of the media is seen in some of these patients; these vessels are radiographically visible and may be clinically palpable.

Sonography of Intimal Hyperplasia

It is possible with high-resolution ultrasonography to differentiate the layers of the arterial wall as they demonstrate characteristic morphologic changes. Intimal hyperplasia is particularly evident in vascular grafts when veins have been employed as arterial conduits for long periods of time. In the lower extremities, in situ grafts utilizing the saphenous vein are common surgical procedures. Progressive luminal narrowing leads to recurrent arterial insufficiency. Intimal hyperplasia in a 15-year-old saphenous vein graft is demonstrated sonographically in Figure 4.4.2.

Sonography of Atheromatous Lesions

Simple atheromas are echogenic due to the deposition of lipids in the tunica intima. The size of atheromatous lesions and the degree of echogenicity vary considerably. An increased fibrous component is expected to decrease echogenicity while cholesterol deposits likely increase echogenicity. Previous investigators have correlated histologic and magnetic resonance findings with images from a prototype high-resolution intravascular ultrasound unit in vitro.[3,4] Calcification of an atheroma is obvious when there is reflection of the ultrasound beam with distal acoustic shadowing. Figures 4.4.3 and 4.4.4 show variations of atheromatous disease.

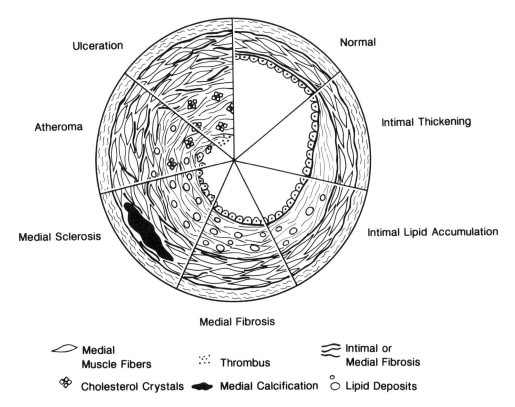

Figure 4.4.1. Diagrammatic representation of arterial wall changes related to arteriosclerosis.

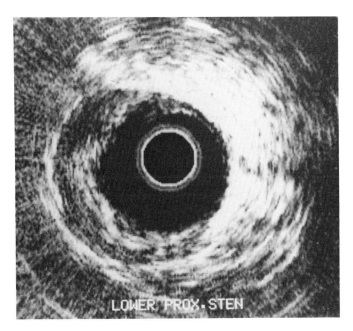

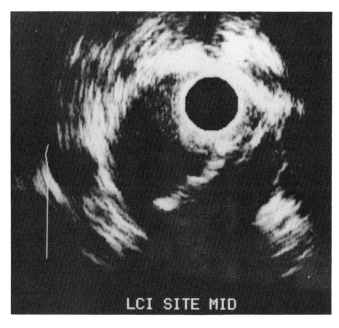

Figure 4.4.2. Intravascular ultrasound of a patient with a high-grade stenosis of the left common iliac shows a densely fibrotic lesion with heavy calcifications.

Figure 4.4.3. Intravascular ultrasound following dilation of left common iliac artery stenosis with an 8mm balloon shows a large intimal flap floating free within the vascular lumen. Note shadowing behind the calcified fibrotic plaque.

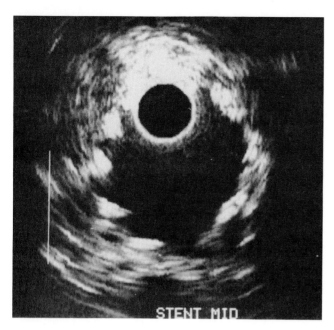

Figure 4.4.4. Following placement of a Palmaz intravascular stent, the lumen has been restored. Dense white dots represent the struts of the stent. The transducer is lying against the densely fibrotic calcified plaque.

Sonography of Medial Sclerosis

Atheromatous disease and medial sclerosis may overlap in many patients. With advanced disease, there is circumferential involvement of the affected artery. Ultrasound waves are then unable to pass beyond the tunica media. The calcifications of medial sclerosis and other arteriosclerotic pathology can be differentiated sonographically. Figure 4.4.5 demonstrates a case of severe medial sclerosis in a popliteal artery.

INTRAVASCULAR ULTRASOUND OF REVASCULARIZATION PROCEDURES

Methods

Adequate access to the diseased vessel is established for both the introduction of interventional catheters and the ultrasound probe. For the latter, a 7Fr or greater sheath size is required. Characterization of the general degree of arteriosclerosis and the specific local vascular disease is accomplished angiographically and sonographically. The locations of the stenotic areas are marked on the drape covering the patient for future reference. The progress of the revascularization procedure can be intermittently monitored without contrast by using intravascular ultrasound to assess the degree of any residual stenosis. Further technical advances may lead to coaxial procedures where the ultrasound probe is used to directly monitor the effects of intervention. This could be achieved when, for example, the balloon is mounted around the probe itself.

Assessment by Intravascular Ultrasound

ANGIOPLASTY

Various success rates for immediate and long-term results of angioplasty have been reported. Obviously, the nature of the lesion and the immediate effect of dilatation are both critical variables in the eventual result. Intravascular ultrasound can both characterize the diseased vessel as well as confirm the effect of angioplasty.[5]

The cross-sectional image furnished by intravascular ultrasound can be used to calculate the area and flow through a vessel. This information is similar to that obtained by measuring pressure gradients and is probably more accurate in situations with impaired runoff or distal occlusions. Breaks in the vessel wall, either in the intima or media, may be visualized, particularly if this occurs in a calcified lesion. Intimal flaps are commonly encountered after angioplasty, but may not be evident angiographically. Such flaps increase the risk of restenosis at the site of angioplasty. Intravascular ultrasound has proved to be of great value in recognizing these complications,[6] thus allowing for treatment of these complications and hopefully improving the long-term outcome (Figs. 4.4.3 and 4.4.5).

ATHERECTOMY

The goal of atherectomy is to remove pathologic deposits or accumulations that are obstructing vessels. A cutting device such as the Simpson atherectomy catheter is used. Large amounts of material can be extracted. Atherectomy can be used to supplement angioplasty and vice versa. As a secondary procedure, the atherectomy device is capable of removing intimal flaps after angioplasty. Its role as a pri-

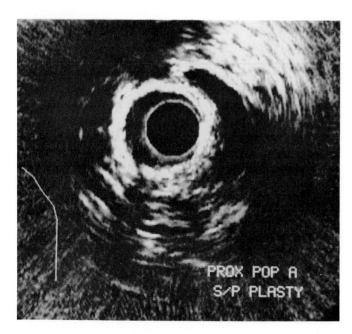

Figure 4.4.5. Intravascular ultrasound in a patient with medial sclerosis. Following angioplasty, minimal increase in diameter of the lumen at the site of severe narrowing of the popliteal artery was seen.

mary procedure is currently under long-term evaluation. Intravascular ultrasound characterizes arterial disease by demonstrating the thickness and composition of the wall. Although further experience is necessary, it is becoming evident that the larger the pathologic deposit, the greater the relative merits of atherectomy over angioplasty (i.e., severe intimal hyperplasia and large intimal flaps). Figure 4.4.2 illustrates such a case in a diseased saphenous in situ graft. In some cases of severe calcific arterial disease, atherectomy was able to remove enough material to allow for successful angioplasty.

STENTS

Both arterial and venous stents are coming into widespread clinical use. They are designed to overcome the inherent elasticity of vessels which causes them to collapse.[7] The true lumen of a stent cannot be established on a conventional basis without multiple radiographic projections. With intravascular ultrasound, it is possible to measure directly the cross-sectional area of a stented vessel as well as to establish the relationship of the stent to adjacent structures including normal and abnormal vessels as well as masses (Fig. 4.4.4).[8]

Intravascular Lasers: Role of Intravascular Ultrasound

Vascular recanalization with lasers is a potential alternative to other techniques described previously. At the present time, the risk of perforation and lack of guidance limit its clinical applications severely. Intravascular ultrasound delivers essential information on the exact location of the native vessel wall and may serve as a guide to the laser beam.[9] The technical challenge lies in mounting the ultrasound transducer near the tip of the laser catheter. Longitudinal as well as radial imaging capabilities are necessary prerequisites.[10]

CONCLUSIONS

Intravascular ultrasound provides interesting new insights into vascular disease and interventional radio-graphic procedures. The information it gives to the interventionalist has greatly increased with the availability of the new catheter-based units. With further experience, it is hoped that the relative indications and results of different revascularization procedures may be better defined by intravascular ultrasound. Direct guidance and real-time monitoring of interventional procedures will become possible with further technical advances. With the use of smaller sonographic (e.g., 4.8Fr) catheters designed for intracoronary imaging, access to vessels below the knee is possible.

References

1. Bom N, ten Hoff H, Lancee CT, Gussenhoven WJ, Bosch JG: Early and recent intraluminal ultrasound devices. *Int J Card Imaging* 1989;4(2–4):79–88
2. Zagzebski JA: Physics and instrumentation in Doppler and B-mode ultrasonography, in Zwiebel WJ (ed): *Vascular Ultrasonography.* Orlando, Grune and Stratton, 1986, pp 21–51
3. Meyer CR, Chiang EH, Fechner KP, Fitting DW, Williams DM, Buda AJ: Feasibility of high-resolution, intravascular ultrasonic imaging catheters. *Radiology* 1988;168:113–116
4. Gussenhoven WJ, Essed CE, Lancee CT, et al: Arterial wall characteristics determined by intravascular ultrasound imaging: an in vitro study. *J Am Coll Cardiol* 1989;14:947–952
5. Tobis J, Mallery J, Gessert J, et al: Intravascular ultrasound cross-sectional arterial imaging before and after balloon angioplasty in vitro. *Circulation* 1989;80:873–882
6. Isner JM, Rosenfield K, Losordo DW, et al: Percutaneous intravascular US as adjunct to catheter-based interventions: preliminary experience in patients with peripheral vascular disease. *Radiology* 1990;175:61–70
7. Palmaz JC, Richter GM, Noeldge G, et al: Intraluminal stents in atherosclerotic iliac artery stenosis: preliminary report of a multicenter study. *Radiology* 1988;168:727–731
8. Losordo DW, Chokshi SK, Harding M, et al: Three dimensional intravascular ultrasound images of intraarterial stents: validation of technique by histologic morphometry. *Circulation* 1990;82(4):Suppl.III-103 (abstr)
9. Borst C, Rienks R, Mali WPTM, van Erven L: Laser ablation and the need for intra-arterial imaging. *Int J Card Imaging* 1989;4(2–4):127–133
10. Gregory KW, Martinelli MA, Aretz TH, et al: Intravascular ultrasound guided Holmium laser atherectomy. *Circulation* 1990;82(4):Suppl.III-677 (abstr)

Part 5. Balloon Catheter Technology

—John E. Abele

As balloon angioplasty has matured since its "official" introduction in 1973,[1] improvements in materials, design, and technique have dramatically expanded the indications and success rates.[2] Despite large investments and optimism for "next generation" devices,[3,4] "POBA" (plain old balloon angioplasty) remains the mainstay for interventional therapy of stenosed and occluded vessels.

A review of principles and performance criteria as well as remaining issues and developments is helpful in being able to continue to improve these results as well as improve assessment of newer technologies. Although balloon dilatation of blood vessels is relatively new, catgut balloons were used to dilate urethral strictures over one and a half centuries ago[5] and wire-guided balloons were used for dila-

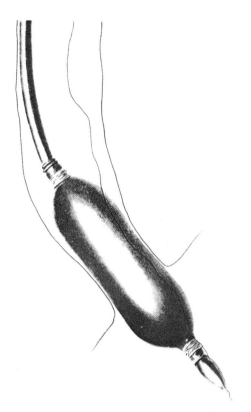

Figure 4.5.1. Esophageal balloon dilator, 1919.

tation of esophageal narrowings by Plummer and Vinson in 1919[6] (Fig. 4.5.1). The smaller size of arteries as well as the complications of introduction, tortuosity, debris, and thrombosis made the development of PTA catheters considerably more difficult. Differences in anatomy, lesion type, size, and location have necessitated the development of a number of balloon catheter variations specifically tailored to the individual situation. Only recently have standardized descriptions been developed for commonly found lesions.[7] In addition, driven by coronary angioplasty applications where small variations in catheter design result in a big difference in performance, a series of catheter performance criteria has been developed which improves the ability to compare different designs and better understand the trade-offs of one attribute versus another.[8,9]

TRACKABILITY

Trackability refers to the characteristics of a catheter which allow it to follow over a guidewire through tortuous paths to its ultimate destination. It is a collection of "subcharacteristics" that include lateral flexibility of the shaft, lumen friction with the guidewire, and column strength. Catheters with varying degrees of stiffness must have very smooth and gradual transitions from one segment to another. Balloon catheters tend to have stiff segments where the balloon joins the shaft, which can make tracking difficult. Although smaller catheters tend to have greater

flexibility, they tend to have lower column strength. Since users want to have smaller outer diameters without losing the inner lumen size, it has been necessary to reduce wall thickness resulting in an increased tendency for the catheter to kink as well as a reduced column strength. This has led to the development of higher strength shaft materials as well as shafts reinforced with braiding, coils, or stylets. Most percutaneous transluminal angioplasty (PTA) catheter shafts are 5Fr for balloon sizes from 4 to 8mm. Percutaneous transluminal coronary angioplasty (PTCA) catheters and peripheral small vessel catheters are now available with shafts of 3Fr and smaller.

CROSSABILITY

The key subcharacteristics of crossability are profile of the tip and deflated balloon segment as well as frictional properties of the surfaces. Profile refers not only to the deflated diameter of the balloon, but the tip taper and abruptness of the change in diameter underneath the radiopaque marker and the beginning of the balloon taper. A test protocol has been developed to characterize this attribute.[8]

PUSHABILITY

This refers to the ability to transfer axial force applied at the proximal end of the catheter to the tip. When there is tortuosity involved, as in a contralateral femoral or an ostial renal, the pushability characteristic is tested to its utmost. Catheters with good flexibility are more prone to be compressed when pushed, or to kink. Therefore, the most important subcharacteristic of pushability is "column strength." Different materials, reinforced materials, laminated materials, lumen geometry, and gradually increased flexibility toward the tip tend to enhance this characteristic.

DILATING FORCE

One of the most misunderstood performance attributes of balloon catheters, dilatation force refers to the radial force applied to the lesion in order to enlarge its inner diameter.[10] Pressure applied inside the balloon not only pushes outward against the membrane but also forces the membrane to become taut. This circumferential force is known as "hoop stress." Larger diameter balloons have a larger inside surface area over which pressure is applied and, since Force = Pressure × Area, they experience more hoop stress at a given pressure than do smaller balloons. This relation is expressed by LaPlace's law, $HS = P \times D$, where HS is the hoop stress, P is the pressure in the balloon, and D is the inside diameter of the balloon.

Dilating force is the sum of the hydrostatic force plus a mechanical vector force which occurs when the circumference of the balloon, in the process of straightening out, exerts a radial component. As the depression in the circumference is straightened with increasing tension, force vectors are created, resulting in an outward or radial force on the lesion. This latter force vector is greatest when the balloon is more "hourglassed." The radial force vector diminishes as the line straightens (Fig. 4.5.2). It is like trying to lift a weight in the center of a sagging clothesline by pulling on one end. The lifting force is greatest when the depression is deepest, since the vector forces are more perpendicular. The dilatation balloon can be visualized as a collection of clotheslines because, as pressure is applied, the surface becomes taut in many directions simultaneously. To the person doing angioplasty, this has several important implications. First, applying more pressure to eliminate a small dent in the balloon produces little dilating force, and it is more likely to break the balloon. Second, for the same lesion at the same pressure, more force will be applied by a larger balloon because it will be "hourglassed" more and, thus, the radial force vector will be greater. Third, larger balloons will require much less pressure to exert substantial dilating force than small balloons because their large diameters generate more hoop stress. Conversely, small balloons require much more pressure to produce adequate force for dilatation. Fourth, hoop stress

occurs in vessels as well as in balloons. Larger vessels require less pressure to dilate . . . and to rupture.

The amount of force applied to a lesion also depends on the resistance of that lesion. In a heterogeneous lesion with soft and hard segments as well as an elastic component, the balloon will push in the direction of least resistance. This can result in a distorted lumen or, in the case of an elastic segment, an unsuccessful dilatation. The use of a longer balloon in these situations enlarges the "platform" from which the balloon "pushes off," resulting in a greater force on the lesion.

DILATING FORCE VERSUS BALLOON PRESSURE

For the same size balloon, an increase in pressure increases the dilating force in a linear fashion provided there is no change in the diameter of either the lesion or the balloon.

DILATING FORCE VERSUS STENOSIS AREA

A dilating balloon produces more force on a lesion with a large surface area. The significance of this observation is

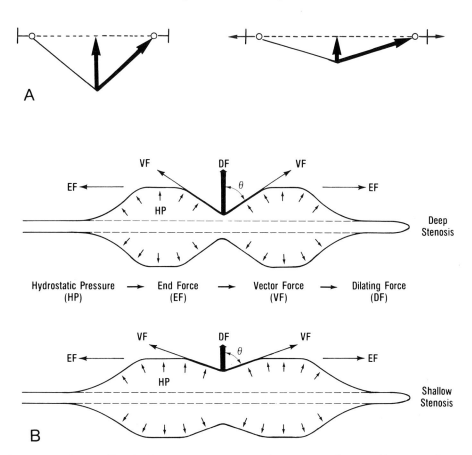

Figure 4.5.2. Dilating force and clothesline effect. **A.** When weight hanging in center of clothesline is lifted by pulling on each end of the line, force vector pushing upward decreases as line straightens. **B.** Same principle applied to balloon dilatation. If balloon surface is indented by localized stenosis, component force pushing outward corresponds to dilating force. With progressive expansion of balloon or dilatation of stenosis, dilating force decreases.

that short and shallow focal lesions are frequently more difficult to dilate because they have less area and receive less total dilating force.

DILATING FORCE VERSUS DEGREE OF STENOSIS

At the same pressure, a dilating balloon will produce more force in a tight or narrow stenosis than in a shallow or open one because the radial force vector decreases as the circumference of the balloon straightens out.

DILATING FORCE AND BALLOON COMPLIANCE

Compliance is a measure of how much the balloon surface stretches when force is applied to it. Because all balloon materials stretch slightly and to varying degrees, the balloon diameter will increase with pressure. These diameter-vs.-pressure curves vary for different materials and also with temperature and sometimes with degree of use. If the "yield strength" (the force that causes permanent deformation of the material) approximates the "ultimate tensile strength" (the force required to break the material), then the diameter will change very little with pressure. A low compliant (non-stretch) balloon will have:

A. *More dilating force.* Balloons with the same dimensions will produce considerably greater dilating force at the same pressure if the material does not stretch. If the balloon stretches or deforms under pressure, this prevents a concentration of force at the stenosis; the balloon stretches around the lesion rather than exerting force on it.
B. *Predictable diameter.* What you see is what you get. Repeat inflations produce the same results.
C. *Better "feel" of the lesion.* The feel at the syringe barrel is a result of changes in the lesion, not in the balloon.
D. *Retention of profile.* A non-stretch balloon will retain its sausage shape rather than expand to dilate normal vessels on either side of the lesion or expand in the aorta, as in the case of an ostial renal stenosis.
E. *Safer failure mode.* The balloon will not stretch before rupture. An expanded balloon is difficult to remove without entry-site trauma.

Most manufacturers today have relatively low compliant balloons. The challenge is to produce a low compliant balloon that is smooth, flexible, has a low profile on deflation, and is reasonably scratch-resistant (an important concern when extremely thin wall materials are inserted through abrasive calcified lesions).

Present catheter designs have achieved many of the original objectives of the ideal balloon catheter.

1. *Balloon-on-a-wire.* Originally developed for coronary purposes,[11] the balloon-on-a-wire for peripheral

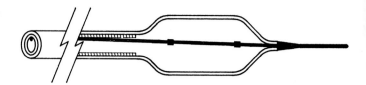

Figure 4.5.3. Balloon-on-a-wire.

applications[12] is particularly useful for renal applications and distal peripheral stenosis. The through-lumen is sacrificed in order to reduce both the shaft diameter and deflated diameter. The objective is to have a dilatation catheter that behaves like a guidewire. The shaft may be part hypodermic tubing, part guidewire encased in a low friction sleeve. Large balloon sizes require a special guiding catheter. The low profile of the balloon-on-a-wire allows it to be used coaxially through small diameter introducer sheaths or guiding catheters (Fig. 4.5.3).

2. *Low profile.* Great progress has been made in this area. High-strength, ultra-thin wall polymers (PET, nylon, polyamide, new composites) allow most catheters up to 8mm in diameter to be introduced through a 5Fr shaft and do not rely on folding to produce low profile; instead, the fabric-reinforced balloon is stretched using the coaxial design originally described in 1978.[13]

3. *High pressure.* High-pressure balloons (up to 20 atmospheres) have been available for a number of years in 7Fr sizes and are now becoming available in 5Fr as well. The same polymers developed for the low profile applications have been thickened slightly to provide this greater strength. New processing techniques allow "molecular braiding" within the polymer to produce a film with extremely low compliance and high burst strength.

4. *Short tip and "no tip."* Blunt tip balloon catheters have always been technically difficult because of the need to have adequate surface area to bond the balloon to the shaft and to provide "folding space" for the balloon material at the front end. Although there are still some trade-offs in tip profile, these designs get better and better and will see an increasing role in specialized applications (Fig. 4.5.4).

5. *Monorail.* This catheter, originally developed for coronary use,[14] primarily because of the ability to rapidly exchange one catheter for another without the need for an extended length guidewire, is now being made available for peripheral use (Schneider USA, Inc., Minneapolis, MN). The rapid exchange feature is balanced by a decrease in trackability and pushability, lack of ability to inject contrast, and a slightly increased trauma from having a wire and catheter side by side in the vessel. It is not clear whether it will have wide application (Fig. 4.5.5).

6. *Tapered balloons, pre-curved balloons, balloons with proximal side holes or distal side holes* were previously

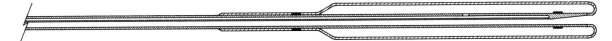

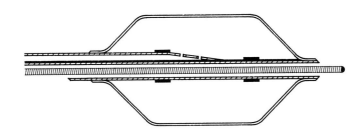

Figure 4.5.4. "No-tip" dilatation balloon.

Figure 4.5.5. "Monorail" balloon catheter.

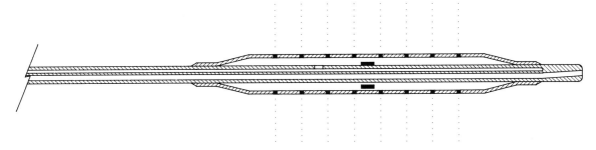

Figure 4.5.6. "Walinsky" catheter for drug delivery.

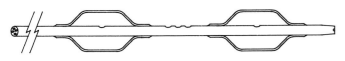

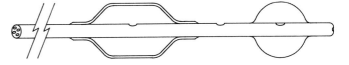

Figure 4.5.7. "Tonnesen" catheter for drug delivery.

Figure 4.5.8. Carotid angioplasty catheter with reverse flush capabilities for protecting against distal debris.

developed for improved lesion access, tight lesion crossing, improved opacification, etc. With the advent of the "super thin" balloon materials and low profile designs, as well as the practice of introducing balloon catheters through sheaths and improvements in imaging technology, the demand for these earlier styles has been reduced.

New catheter designs and trends for the future continue to extend applications of PTA to more distal lesions, total occlusions and complex lesions.

1. *Continued improvements in low profile and improved guideability.* Just when it seems that no further improvements can be made, another design is introduced. Coated balloons for improved slipperiness, composites for improving scratch resistance, flexibility, and foldability extend the ability to guide these catheters to more distal lesions as well as to cross total occlusions.

2. *Drug delivery balloons* which purport to address the problem of restenosis by delivering antiproliferative drugs at the site of dilatation[15-17] (Figs. 4.5.6 and 4.5.7).

3. *Catheters with debris protection* for use in cerebral vessels which employ distal filters, backward flushing mechanisms, etc.[18] (Fig. 4.5.8).

4. *Laser and thermal balloons.* The "laser balloon" has been developed for tacking flaps after a failed angioplasty.[19] Although the early experience with this device in the coronaries has been mixed, improvements are being made and alternative designs are being explored which hopefully will reduce the early complications of this technique (primarily thrombosis). A different approach, called percutaneous low-stress angioplasty (PLOSA),[20] involves using low-temperature thermal mediation to soften plaque so that dilatation can be accomplished at very low pressures (1 atmosphere or less) resulting in far fewer tears, dissections, etc. This approach, in addition to reducing procedural compli-

cations, may reduce restenosis by avoiding the peripheral response associated with traditional angioplasty injury.

Conclusion

The attraction of balloon dilatation in the treatment of obstructive lesions has been in its elegant simplicity. Grüntzig's treatment philosophy was to do the least amount necessary to help the body heal itself. Improvements in balloon technology have continued to reduce their invasiveness and expand their application. As imaging and sensing technologies continue to improve, including on-site through-the-balloon modalities and with adjunctive treatments such as thermal, chemical, or other approaches, improved success rates and expanded indications should be expected.

REFERENCES

1. Portsmann W: Ein neuer Korsett-Ballonkatheter zur transluminalen Rekanalisation nach Dotter unter besonderer Berucksichtigung von Obliterationen an der Beckenarterien. *Radiol Diagn (Berl)* 1973;14:239–244
2. Grüntzig A, Hopff H: Perkutane Rekanalisation chronischer arterieller Verschlusse mit einem neuen Dilatationskatheter. Modifikation der Dotter-Technik. *Dtsch Med Wochenschr* 1974;99:2502–2505
3. Waller B: Crackers, breakers, stretchers, drillers, scrapers, shavers, burners, welders and melters. The future treatment of atherosclerotic coronary artery disease? A clinical-morphologic assessment. *J Am Coll Cardiol* 1989;13:5
4. Abele J: New tools extend value of intravascular therapy. *Diagn Imaging* Sept 1990
5. Guthrie GJ: *On the Anatomy and Diseases of the Neck of the Bladder and of the Urethra.* London, Burgess & Hill, 1834
6. Vinson EP: A case of cardiospasm with dilatation and angulation of the esophagus. *Med Clin North Am* 1919;3:623–627
7. Spies J, Bakal C, Burke D, et al: Guidelines for percutaneous transluminal angioplasty. *J Vasc Intervent Radiol* 1990;1:5–15
8. Chang M, Plant M, Moon P, Vetrovec G: In vitro analysis of angioplasty balloons: characteristics affecting functional profile. *J Am Coll Cardiol* 1990;15(2):105A
9. Roubin GS, Robinson KA, Brown JE, King SB, Yognathan A, McMillan S: Proposal—evaluation of balloon catheters. Andreas R. Grüntzig Cardiovascular Center, Emory University Hospital and School of Chemical Engineering, Georgia Institute of Technology, March 1987
10. Abele J: Balloon catheters and transluminal dilatation: technical considerations. *AJR* 1980;135:901–906
11. Myler RK, Mooney MR, Stertzer SH, Clark DA, Hidalgo BO, Fishman J: The balloon on a wire device: a new ultra-low-profile coronary angioplasty system/concept. *Cathet Cardiovasc Diagn* 1988;14:135–140
12. Tegtmeyer CJ: Guidewire angioplasty balloon catheter: preliminary report. *Radiology* 1988;159:253–254
13. Olbert F, Hanecka L: Transluminal vascular dilatation with a modified dilatation catheter, in Zietler E, Grüntzig A, Schoop W (eds): *Percutaneous Vascular Recanalization.* Berlin, Springer–Verlag, 1978, pp 32–38
14. Finci L, Meier B, Roy P, Steffenino G, Rutishauser W: Clinical experience with the Monorail balloon catheter for coronary angioplasty. *Cathet Cardiovasc Diagn* 1988;14:206–212
15. Wolinsky H, Thung SN: Local introduction of drugs into the arterial wall: a percutaneous catheter technique. *J Intervent Cardiol* 1989;2:4
16. McGrath LP, Kundu SK, Spears R: Experimental application of bioprotective materials to injured arterial surfaces with laser balloon angioplasty. *Circulation* 1990;82(4):Abstr 282, Suppl. III
17. Jorgensen B, Tonnesen KH, Bulow J, Jorgensn M, Nielsen JD, Holstein P, Andersen E: Femoral artery recanalization with percutaneous angioplasty and segmentally enclosed plasminogen activator. *Lancet* May, 1989
18. Medi-Tech "Special Product," 1982
19. Spears JR: Percutaneous transluminal coronary angioplasty restenosis: potential prevention with laser balloon angioplasty. *Am J Cardiol* 1987;60:61B–64B
20. Kuhn FP: Percutaneous low stress angioplasty (PLOSA). Abstract: Third Annual International Symposium on Peripheral Vascular Intervention Meeting, Miami, FL, January 21–24, 1991

Part 6. Angioplasty of Supra-aortic Vessels

—S. Murthy Tadavarthy, M.D.

Percutaneous angioplasty has been performed extensively in the peripheral vessels, renal, and coronary arteries since the original description by Dotter and Judkins in 1964.[1] Recently, angioplasty has been performed in the brachiocephalic arteries: subclavian, innominate, vertebral, common carotid, external carotid, and internal carotid arteries. Angioplasty of the supra-aortic arteries is not commonly done because of the fear of cerebral embolization. A limited number of cases have been reported in patients who were high risk candidates for the conventional carotid endarterectomy and general anesthesia.

Preliminary Investigations Prior to Angioplasty of Supra-aortic Branches

Only interventionalists with experience in both angioplasty and cerebral catheterization should attempt supra-aortic vessel dilatation, since inexperience of the operator may lead to severe, permanent neurologic deficits.[1] Angioplasty in the brachiocephalic vessels should be limited to lesions that are clinically symptomatic. Borderline indications should be left alone. In addition, close cooperation between interventional radiologist, neurologist, and vascular surgeon is mandatory. A uniform opinion should be sought prior to transluminal angioplasty and the patient should be warned of the potential risks and complications and should be told of other therapeutic alternatives. Preliminary investigations should include arch aortography and selective catheterization of the supra-aortic branches with intracranial vascular studies to determine the hemodynamic significance of the vascular lesions. Preliminary evaluation should also include duplex ultrasound studies. Other sophisticated investigational tests include:

A. Echotomography of the carotid bifurcation;
B. Computed tomography of neck vessels;
C. Cerebral blood flow and blood volume studies;
D. Position emission tomography (PET) studies, with the determination of cerebral blood flow and volume and oxygen use.[2]

ANGIOPLASTY OF THE SUBCLAVIAN ARTERY

The subclavian steal syndrome was initially described in 1961 and much has been written about its diagnosis and its relationship to the presence or absence of clinical symptoms.[3,4] In a study of 1114 patients with extracranial arterial occlusions of the innominate and subclavian arteries, only 168 patients demonstrated signs and symptoms of the subclavian steal syndrome, and 9 of these were asymptomatic.[5,6]

A diagnosis of subclavian steal syndrome should only be made after thoracic aortography (Fig. 4.6.1), as selective injections into the subclavian vessels can produce artificial steals.[6] Stenosis of the left subclavian artery at its origin is more frequently observed than on the right side. The clinical symptoms include vertigo, ataxia, diplopia, paresis,

numbness, and arm claudication. Physical examination reveals reduction of blood pressure in one arm along with a supraclavicular bruit.[4] The authors have also seen cases of recurrent angina secondary to subclavian artery stenosis in patients who have undergone internal mammary artery bypass to the left anterior descending artery.

In the presence of associated carotid artery stenotic lesions, the precise cause of cerebral symptoms is obscure.[6] Relief of the obstruction at the carotid artery level by surgery might alleviate the symptoms of vertebrobasilar insufficiency, by improving the intracranial collateral circulation.

In the past, many patients underwent endarterectomy and bypass procedures, with complication rates as high as 23%.[7,8] The recently introduced extrathoracic surgical interventions are more appealing and include the carotid-subclavian, axillo-axillary, and femoral-axillary bypasses. The surgical procedures are associated with complications such as pneumothorax, chylothorax, thrombosis of the graft, phrenic nerve palsy, lymphatic fistulas, and Horner's syndrome.[9] Angioplasty of the subclavian arteries is an attractive alternative. In the reported data from more than 400 subclavian and innominate angioplasty procedures, a 92% technical success rate was achieved,[8] with an overall 6% complication rate, including central nervous system complications.

Methodology

One to two days prior to the angioplasty, aspirin (325mg daily) is administered orally. In the majority of cases, the subclavian angioplasty can be easily accomplished from the transfemoral route. Occasionally, the transaxillary approach has been suggested in difficult cases because of

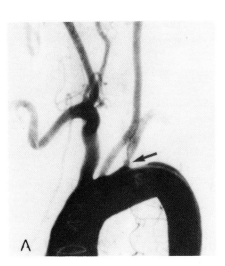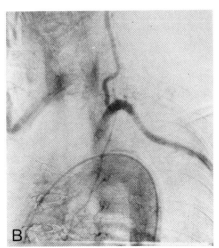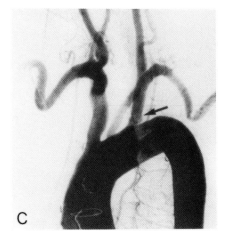

Figure 4.6.1. Atherosclerotic stenosis of left subclavian artery with steal syndrome. **A.** Early arterial phase of aortic arch angiogram, left anterior oblique projection; narrow stenosis of left subclavian artery *(arrow)*. Vertebral artery is not opacified. Poor opacification of distal left subclavian artery. **B.** Same procedure, late phase; retrograde filling of left vertebral artery. **C.** Aortic arch angiogram performed after angioplasty; early filling of left vertebral artery and enlargement of origin of left subclavian artery *(arrow)*. (Reproduced with permission from Theron JG: Angioplasty of supra-aortic arteries. *Semin Intervent Radiol* 1987;4:331–342.)

tortuosity and dilatation of the aorta. Complications such as axillary hematoma, brachial plexus trauma, and distal embolization of atherosclerotic plaques to the fingers are known sequelae of this approach.

The stenotic subclavian artery is catheterized with a 5.0Fr headhunter catheter. The roadmapping capabilities of the presently available digital subtraction angiography units greatly facilitate crossing of the stenosis. The stenotic lesions are easily crossed with soft-tip Bentson or torque-controlled guidewires.

Heparin is administered as soon as the lesion is crossed. Occasionally, spasm of the subclavian and axillary arteries is encountered. This can be promptly relieved with the administration of intra-arterial nitroglycerin in bolus of 100–200μg. The size of the balloon to be used is determined by the measurement of the normal-sized vessel both proximal and/or distal to the area of the stenosis. The balloons we frequently use are 8–10mm in diameter, occasionally 6mm balloons are used in small-sized vessels. The length of the balloons is usually between 2 and 4mm, since they have a tendency to slide away from the area of the stenosis during inflation of the balloon. The larger balloons have a propensity to a more stable position. The angioplasty balloon catheters are advanced over an exchange guidewire. We prefer for the exchange stronger guidewires such as the Rosen wire. A tightly curved tip is advantageous over straight wires since it minimizes the spasm and the risk of dissection of the subclavian artery. Balloons are usually inflated up to 4–5 atmospheres for 15–30 seconds. The end point of the dilation is indicated by the full inflation of the balloon at the site of the stenosis, this usually requires two to three inflations.

After the angioplasty, the results are documented by arch aortography, utilizing pigtail catheters and digital subtraction technique. Selective injections are not advised since the jet of the contrast medium can easily dissect the recently dilated segments. In doubtful angiographic appearances, the results can be verified by pullback pressure measurements across the area of dilatation. Following catheter removal, the residual heparin is neutralized with the administration of intravenous protamine sulfate, to minimize the formation of groin or axillary hematomas. The patients are maintained indefinitely on oral aspirin at a dose of 325mg/day.

Discussion

Out of all the supra-aortic arteries, angioplasty of the subclavian artery is the most commonly carried out procedure. The feasibility of a successful angioplasty in over 90% of the cases has been well established, both in short and large series.[2,6–19]

On the other hand, the results of angioplasty in cases of subclavian artery occlusion are poor, therefore, the treatment of choice in these cases is a surgical bypass procedure.[9] The potential for vertebral artery embolization dur-

ing the subclavian angioplasty is minimal, based on the findings of Ringelstein and Zumer.[16] They monitored the homolateral vertebral flow before, during, and after angioplasty of the subclavian artery proximal to the vertebral artery. Despite a successful recanalization, the direction of blood flow within the vertebral artery did not change immediately to antegrade, but did so over a period of 27 seconds to several minutes.[16] This observation diminished the fear of cerebral embolization, and, if it occurs, the debris would be directed across the dilated segment toward the axillary artery. Also, Block and Elmer reported that release of atherosclerotic debris with distal embolization is a rare occurrence.[20] This event does occur, and when it does it is frequently fatal.

Balloon dilatation of a stenotic subclavian artery either proximal or distal to the vertebral artery origin does not cause occlusion of the vertebral artery, in spite of the balloon being inflated across the origin of the vertebral artery.[17] Vertebral artery occlusion can occur if the stenotic plaque is adjacent to the origin of the vertebral artery.[2,17] Occasionally, even if the vertebral artery is occluded, the symptoms may not be aggravated, but may be ablated.[2] In case of proximal subclavian artery stenosis on the right side, the balloon position might compromise flow to the carotid artery. The carotid artery circulation can be protected by placing an angiographic catheter from the contralateral femoral approach.[8]

The simplicity of subclavian angioplasty along with the low complication rate, fewer hospitalization days and its low cost, are appealing in comparison to the surgical alternative.

INNOMINATE AND CAROTID ARTERY ANGIOPLASTY

Angioplasty of the carotid arteries is controversial due to the low morbidity and mortality of surgical carotid endarterectomy. Furthermore the experience with carotid angioplasty is limited and the follow-up is short, making a good comparison of results with surgical endarterectomy almost impossible. Surgical endarterectomy has a morbidity of 1–4% and a mortality of 1–8%.[21,22]

Carotid endarterectomy has been recommended in patients with transient ischemic attacks (TIAs) who have no permanent damage to the cortical tissue. In these patients, the chances of stroke are higher in the first two to three months. Surgical endarterectomy is recommended soon after the onset of TIAs since, in about 25% of patients, a stroke will develop within a period of five years.[8]

The indications for angioplasty of the carotid arteries gathered from the few reports in the literature[2,8,23–30] include:

1. Smooth stenotic lesions at the origin of the innominate and carotid arteries either from atherosclerotic or

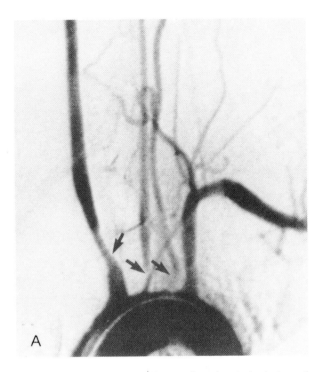
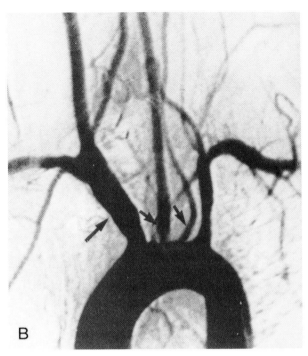

Figure 4.6.2. Takayasu's arteritis with stenotic and occlusive lesions of aortic arch vessels. Patient suffered a right hemispheric cerebral infarction a few months before. **A.** Aortic arch angiogram before angioplasty; narrow stenoses of left vertebral, left common carotid, and right common carotid arteries *(arrows)* and occlusion of origin of right subclavian artery with steal syndrome on late phase. **B.** Aortic arch angiogram after angio- plasty; enlargement of stenosed vessels *(arrows).* Origin of right subclavian artery is no longer occluded; good filling of artery is demonstrated without steal syndrome on late phase. (Reproduced with permission from Theron JG: Angioplasty of supra-aortic arteries. *Semin Intervent Radiol* 1987;4(4):331–342.)

inflammatory processes such as Takayasu's disease (Fig. 4.6.2);

2. Fibromuscular dysplasia of the internal carotid artery (Fig. 4.6.3);
3. Stenotic external carotid artery in patients with an occluded internal carotid artery (Fig. 4.6.4). Dilatation might improve the collateral circulation between the external and internal carotid artery branches;
4. Web-like stenosis of the common carotid artery;
5. Recurrent stenosis from myointimal hyperplasia following carotid endarterectomy (Fig. 4.6.5);
6. Common and internal carotid artery stenosis in patients with concomitant coronary artery disease. These are high-risk patients for carotid endarterectomy and general anesthesia.

Methodology

Carotid artery angioplasty can be performed either from the femoral or axillary approach. Two to five days prior to angioplasty, aspirin (325mg/day) is administered orally. In older patients, tortuosity of the aorta and iliac vessels can hinder the advancement of catheters across the stenotic innominate or carotid artery. In these patients, an axillary approach may be beneficial as it is easier to catheterize the acutely angled innominate and carotid arteries.[2] The origin of the aortic branches usually requires 10mm balloons for effective dilatation. The common and external carotid arteries require 8mm balloons. The internal carotid artery is dilated either with a 5 or a 6mm balloon. The tip of the balloon catheter should be 5mm in length or less. This avoids complications such as spasm in the external carotid artery.[27]

Cerebral embolic events during or after carotid angioplasty can lead to permanent neurologic deficits. This fear has stimulated various innovative ideas. These methods have been tried in a handful of cases. Therefore, their real value cannot be established at this time.

Hodgins described dilatation of a stenosis at the origin of the left common carotid artery in a patient with Takayasu's arteritis intraoperatively using a wash-out technique.[25]

Internal carotid artery stenosis from fibromuscular dysplasia was effectively treated by Smith in five patients by balloon dilatation. An arteriotomy incision was made, the balloon catheter was inserted via the incision and hemostasis was achieved with vascular loops. Following the angioplasty, the balloon catheter was removed, and the blood was allowed to egress through the arteriotomy by releasing the vascular loop. In this fashion, the potential for thrombi or debris reaching the brain was minimized or eliminated.[31]

In Derauf's report, the vessel was exposed in the neck and an arteriotomy was created on the common carotid artery. The arteriotomy was secured with proximal and dis-

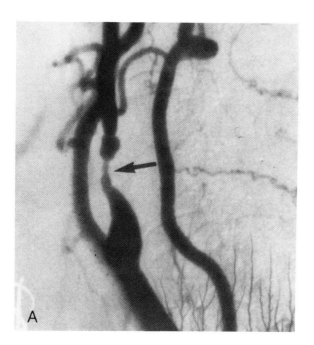

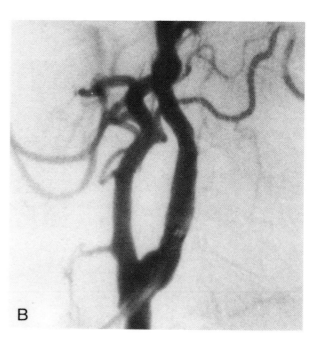

Figure 4.6.3. Fibromuscular dysplasia of internal carotid artery in a 78 year-old patient presenting with clinical signs of cerebrovascular insufficiency. **A.** Right brachial angiogram; narrow stenosis of internal carotid artery with characteristic pattern of fibromuscular dysplasia *(arrow)*. **B.** Postangioplasty angiogram of common carotid artery. Angioplasty was performed from a direct neck approach. (Reproduced with permission from Theron JG: Angioplasty of supra-aortic arteries. *Semin Intervent Radiol* 1987;4(4):331–342.)

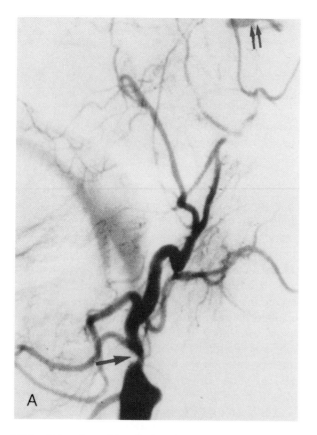

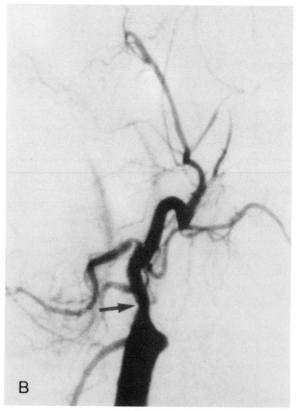

Figure 4.6.4. External carotid angioplasty in a patient presenting with thrombosis of the internal carotid artery; angioplasty was intended to improve collateral flow from external carotid toward carotid siphon via ophthalmic artery. **A.** Common carotid angiogram before angioplasty; narrow stenosis of external carotid *(arrow)*. Carotid siphon *(double arrow)* is opacified via ophthalmic artery. **B.** Postangioplasty angiogram; enlargement of external carotid artery *(arrow)*. (Reproduced with permission from Theron JG: Angioplasty of supra-aortic arteries. *Semin Intervent Radiol* 1987;4:331–342.)

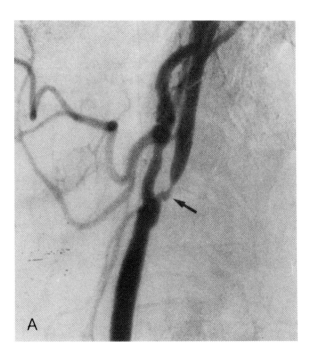
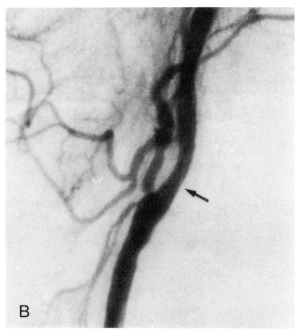

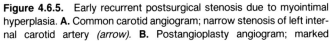

Figure 4.6.5. Early recurrent postsurgical stenosis due to myointimal hyperplasia. **A.** Common carotid angiogram; narrow stenosis of left internal carotid artery *(arrow)*. **B.** Postangioplasty angiogram; marked improvement in diameter of internal carotid *(arrow)*. (Reproduced with permission from Theron JG: Angioplasty of supra-aortic arteries. *Semin Intervent Radiol* 1987;4(4):331–342.)

tal vascular loops and the balloon was then inserted through the arteriotomy. During the angioplasty, the carotid artery was temporarily occluded. Following the dilatation, the blood and possible embolic debris from the angioplasty were allowed to egress through the arteriotomy by releasing the proximal loop. Finally, the arteriotomy incision was closed.[32]

Balloon occlusion of the common carotid artery prior to angioplasty of the innominate artery was proposed and successfully performed by Vitek.[24] The occlusion balloon catheter was continuously infused with heparinized saline and inflation was carried out for 15 minutes prior and during the angioplasty of the innominate artery. No untoward sequelae were noted in the patient. A cerebral protection technique was proposed by Theron.[2] In this technique, through a guiding catheter positioned in the common carotid artery, a thin polyethylene balloon is floated beyond the stenosis and the internal carotid artery is occluded. If the patient can tolerate the occlusion, angioplasty is performed (Fig. 4.6.6). The blood that might potentially contain the debris is aspirated through the balloon catheter and flushed into the external carotid artery system. This system is in development.[2]

Systemic heparinization is achieved during angioplasty by using 5,000 to 10,000 units of heparin. Successive rapid inflations and deflations of the balloon at the level of the stenotic lesions are recommended by Theron. The method seems to be as effective as leaving the balloon inflated for longer periods of time.[2]

Tsai infused through the balloon catheter with the patients' own heparinized blood during the angioplasty to minimize the ischemic events.[27] All patients are maintained indefinitely on aspirin (325mg daily).

Discussion

Angioplasty of the carotid arteries is controversial and at the present time is not recommended for patients who can undergo conventional surgical endarterectomy. It is an excellent nonsurgical alternative to be considered in patients with a prohibitively high surgical risk. Angioplasty has been recommended for stenotic lesions of the innominate or carotid artery origins. The lesions are usually smooth and nonulcerated.[27] Surgical endarterectomy in these patients requires a thoracotomy. The surgical bypass procedures can be associated with complication rates as high as 23%, including chylothorax, wound infection, phrenic nerve palsy, and lymphatic fistulae.[33,34]

A careful angiographic analysis of the morphologic appearance of the carotid artery stenosis is recommended.[28] Most authors have limited carotid artery dilatation to smooth, concentric, short stenotic lesions. Kachel et al. recommended scintigraphic studies of the shoulder and neck with indium-111 labeled platelets to detect thrombi at the site of stenosis. Only the patients with negative studies should undergo angioplasty, and positive studies are contraindications for dilatation.[23]

Theron stated that angioplasty of the internal carotid artery is a very effective technique from a hemodynamic point of view and can and should be used to manage cerebral vascular insufficiency. He stated, however, that the decision to perform angioplasty should be based on cere-

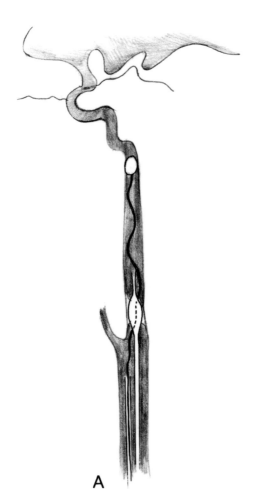

A

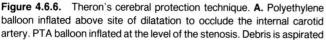

B

Figure 4.6.6. Theron's cerebral protection technique. **A.** Polyethylene balloon inflated above site of dilatation to occlude the internal carotid artery. PTA balloon inflated at the level of the stenosis. Debris is aspirated through PTA catheter lumen. **B.** If the lesion is below the bifurcation, the polyethylene balloon is kept inflated while the debris is flushed into the external carotid artery.

bral hemodynamic data. As long as the cerebral protection technique is used, even ulcerated lesions are not an absolute contraindication.[2]

Brachycephalic trunk origin stenosis secondary to Takayasu's, arteritis, fibromuscular dysplasia of the internal carotid arteries, and recurrent stenosis of the internal carotid artery from myointimal hyperplasia following surgical endarterectomy are favorable lesions for angioplasty. They are less likely to release embolic debris to the intracranial circulation. Another good procedure is angioplasty of the external carotid artery, which increases collateral circulation to branches of an occluded internal carotid artery.[2]

Carotid angioplasty in patients with coexistent coronary artery disease has been recommended. The mortality in these patients is as high as 14% following carotid endarterectomy and the incidence of stroke is 17%.[27] Combined carotid endarterectomy and coronary bypass procedure is recommended in these patients to reduce complications.[27] The indications for transluminal angioplasty in this clinical setup are controversial.

In performing these procedures, a close cooperation between the interventionalist, surgeon, and neurologist should exist. This will allow appropriate patient selection and minimize the complications.

Transluminal angioplasty of the carotid arteries at the present time cannot be proposed as a routine method of revascularization of the cerebral arteries. Furthermore, its precise role is uncertain, since its surgical counterpart, carotid endarterectomy, is under close scrutiny in the United States and Europe.

PERCUTANEOUS TRANSLUMINAL ANGIOPLASTY (PTA) OF VERTEBRAL ARTERY

The indications for angioplasty of the vertebral arteries are poorly defined mostly because the symptomatology is nonspecific. The symptomatology includes dizziness, diplopia, nystagmus, ataxia, cortical blindness, weakness, and memory disturbances.[35]

Angioplasty of the vertebral artery is an attractive non-surgical alternative, and its advantages include:

—Recanalization accomplished under local anesthesia;
—Low cost, fewer hospital days;
—Repeat angioplasty if restenosis occurs;
—Avoidance of surgical complications;
—An easier approach to the dilatation of ostial stenosis of the vertebral artery by balloon methods.[23]

In an uncertain situation, when the physician is confronted with symptoms of vertebral insufficiency and is not certain of its etiology in a patient with a proven stenosis of the proximal vertebral artery, angioplasty can be attempted as a therapeutic trial because of its low morbidity and mortality.[36]

Ostial stenosis of the vertebral artery accounts for 90% of vertebral artery lesions and 40% of all vertebral basilar insufficiency cases.[8]

The natural history of vertebral basilar insufficiency indicates that 30% of patients remain asymptomatic after one or two episodes, 50% evolve, and 18% suffer a stroke.[37] The ostial stenosis of the vertebral artery is a very smooth lesion, unlike that of the carotid arteries which is frequently ulcerated[38] (Fig. 4.6.7). These anatomical features are conducive to angioplasty and the risk seems to be small.[2,8,36]

Prior to angioplasty, Doppler examination of the carotid-vertebral system is highly recommended for the following reasons:

A. To establish a diagnosis of ostial stenosis of the vertebral artery;
B. To determine the dominant vertebral artery;
C. To identify the abnormal flow pattern in the vertebral circulation;
D. To evaluate the presence or absence of associated carotid artery stenosis;
E. Manual compression of the internal carotid arteries during the Doppler study will identify the presence or absence of effective collateral circulation through the circle of Willis.[2]

When there are associated hemodynamically significant carotid lesions present, surgical correction of the carotid lesion is recommended prior to attempting vertebral angioplasty. Improvement of collateral circulation might alleviate the symptoms of vertebral-basilar artery disease.[39]

Methodology

The angioplasty is performed under local rather than general anesthesia either from the femoral or the axillary approach. If during the procedure there is an embolic event that might evolve into a stroke, the neurologic changes are easily diagnosed if the patient is awake. One of the disadvantages of using the femoral approach is the distance between the point of entry and the target site. In older people, tortuosity and ectasia might hinder the selective placement of balloon catheters from the femoral approach. When such anatomical problems exist, an axillary artery approach is recommended.[36] The shorter and relatively straighter course between the entry point in the brachial and/or axillary artery and the vertebral artery ostium makes for an easier procedure. Prior to angioplasty, aspirin (325mg) is administered for two to five days to inhibit the platelet activity. Intra-arterial administration of

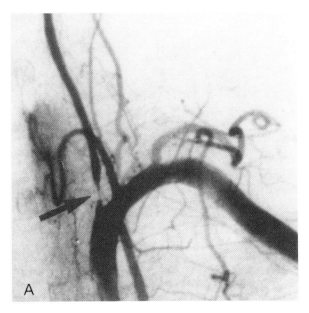

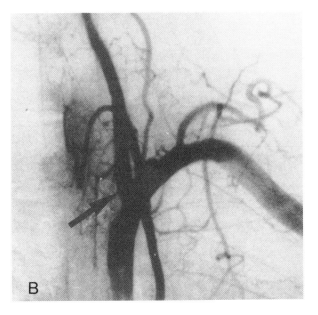

Figure 4.6.7. A 38-year-old man who presented three months before with infarction of left cerebellar hemisphere. **A.** Left subclavian artery angiogram; narrow stenosis of origin of vertebral artery *(arrow)*. **B.** Post- angioplasty angiogram; enlargement of origin of left vertebral artery *(arrow)*. (Reproduced with permission from Theron JG: Angioplasty of supra-aortic arteries. *Semin Intervent Radiol* 1987;4(4):331–342.)

5000 units of heparin is done as soon as the vertebral artery is catheterized.

When the lesion is crossed with a 5Fr catheter, an exchange wire is advanced beyond the stenoses. The balloon size used commonly varies from 4 to 7mm and the length from 2.0 to 2.5cm. The size is predetermined from the measurement of the normal vessel adjacent to the stenosis on the cut films. Rapid inflation and deflation for 10–15 seconds until the "waist" on the balloon disappears is recommended. Usually this requires two to three inflations to effectively dilate the stenosis.

In the event of complications, such as occlusion of the vertebral artery, the symptoms may not be aggravated, and in one case they were cured.[2]

Aspirin (325mg once a day) is administered indefinitely. The post-angioplasty Doppler examinations serve as a baseline for comparison with future examinations in case of recurrent stenosis.

Results

So far, 66 vertebral artery dilatations have been attempted with technical success in all but 3 cases.[8] In the series published by Courtheoux,[36] 21 of 24 patients have shown improvement. There is relative lack of data on long-term clinical follow-up. The role of vertebral angioplasty in the treatment of vertebral basilar insufficiency is not well established and is still evolving due to the lack of sufficient data.[8]

References

1. Dotter ET, Judkins MR: Transluminal treatment of arteriosclerotic obstructions: description of new technique and preliminary report of its application. *Circulation* 1964; 30:654–670
2. Theron J: Angioplasty of supra-aortic arteries. *Semin Intervent Radiol* 1987;4:331–342
3. Reivich M, Holling H, Roberts B, Toole JF: Reversal of blood flow through vertebral artery and its effect on cerebral circulation. *N Engl J Med* 1961;265:878–885
4. Editorial: New vascular syndrome: "the subclavian steal." *N Engl J Med* 1961;265:912–913
5. Fields WS, Lemak NA: Joint study of extracranial arterial occlusion. VII. Subclavian steal: a review of 168 cases. *JAMA* 1972;222:1139–1143
6. Burke DR, Gordon RL, Mishkin JD, McLean GK, Meranze SG: Percutaneous transluminal angioplasty of subclavian arteries. *Radiology* 1987;164:699–704
7. Beebe HG, Stark R, Johnson ML, Jolly PC, Hill LD: Choices of operation for subclavian-vertebral arterial disease. *Am J Surg* 1980;139:616–623
8. Becker GJ: Non coronary angioplasty. *Radiology* 1989; 170:921–940
9. Motarjeme A, Keifer JW, Zuska AJ, Nabawi P: Percutaneous transluminal angioplasty for treatment for subclavian steal. *Radiology* 1985;155:611–613
10. Erbstein RA, Wholey MH, Smoot S: Subclavian artery steal syndrome: treatment by percutaneous transluminal angioplasty. *AJR* 1988;151:291–294
11. Moore TS, Russell WF, Parent AD, Parker JL, Smith RR: Percutaneous transluminal angioplasty in subclavian steal syndrome: recurrent stenosis and retreatment in two patients. *Neurosurgery* 1982;11:512–516
12. Galichia JP, Bajaj AK, Vine DL, Roberts RW: Subclavian artery stenosis treated by transluminal angioplasty: six cases. *Cardiovasc Intervent Radiol* 1983;6:78–81
13. Wilms G, Baert A, Dewaele D, Vermylen J, Nevelsteen A, Suy R: Percutaneous transluminal angioplasty of the subclavian artery: early and late results. *Cardiovasc Intervent Radiol* 1987;10:123–128
14. Cook AM, Dyet JF: Six cases of subclavian stenosis treated by percutaneous angioplasty. *Clin Radiol* 1989;40:352
15. Theron J, Melancon D, Ethier R: "Pre" subclavian steal syndromes and their treatment by angioplasty: hemodynamic classification of subclavian artery stenoses. *Neuroradiology* 1985;27:265–270
16. Ringelstein EB, Zeumer H: Delayed reversal of vertebral artery blood flow following percutaneous transluminal angioplasty for subclavian steal syndrome. *Neuroradiology* 1984;26:189–198
17. Vitek JJ, Keller FS, Duvall ER, Gupta KI, Chandra–Sekar B: Brachycephalic artery dilation by percutaneous transluminal angioplasty. *Radiology* 1986;158:779–785
18. Damuth HD Jr, Diamond AB, Rappoport AS, Renner JW: Angioplasty of subclavian artery stenosis proximal to the vertebral origin. *AJNR* 1983;4:1239–1242.
19. Bachman DM, Kim RM: Transluminal dilatation for subclavian steal syndrome. *AJR* 1980;135:995–996
20. Block PC, Elmer D: Release of atherosclerotic debris after transluminal angioplasty. *Circulation* 1982;65:950–952
21. Imparato AM, Riles T, Ecorstein F: The carotid bifurcation plaque: pathologic finding associated with cerebral ischemia. *Stoke* 1979;10:238–245
22. Loftus CM, Quest DO: Current status of carotid endarterectomy for atheromatous disease. *Neurosurgery* 1983; 12:718–723
23. Kachel R, Endert G, Basche S, et al: Percutaneous transluminal angioplasty (dilatation) of carotid, vertebral and innominate artery stenosis. *Cardiovasc Intervent Radiol* 1987;10:142–146
24. Vitek JJ, Raymon BC, Oh SJ: Innominate artery angioplasty. *AJNR* 1984;5:113–114
25. Hodgins GW, Dutton JW: Subclavian and carotid angioplasties for Takayasu's arteritis. *J Can Assoc Radiol* 1982;33:205–207
26. Kobinia GS, Bergmann H Jr:. Angioplasty in stenosis of the innominate artery. *Cardiovasc Intervent Radiol* 1983;6:82–85
27. Tsai FY, Matovich V, Hieschima G, et al: Percutaneous transluminal angioplasty of the carotid artery. *AJNR* 1986;7:349–358
28. Wiggli U, Gratzi O: Transluminal angioplasty of stenotic carotid arteries: case reports and protocol. *AJNR* 1983; 4:793–795
29. Bockenhemer SAM, Mathias K: Percutaneous transluminal angioplasty in arteriosclerotic internal carotid artery stenosis. *AJNR* 1983;4:791–792
30. Tievsky AL, Druy EM, Mardiat JG: Transluminal angioplasty in post-surgical stenosis of the extracranial carotid artery. *AJNR* 1983;4:800–802
31. Smith DC, Smith LL, Hasso AN: Fibromuscular dysplasia of the internal carotid artery treated by operative transluminal balloon angioplasty. *Radiology* 1985;155:645–648
32. Derauf BJ, Hunter DW, Erickson DL, Castañeda–Zúñiga WR, Cardella JF, Amplatz K: "Wash-out" technique for brachycephalic angioplasty. *AJR* 1986;146:849–851

33. DeBakey ME, Crawford ES, Cooley DA, Morris GC Jr, Garrett E, Fields WS: Cerebral arterial insufficiency. One to 11 years results following arterial reconstructive operation. *Am J Surg* 1965;161:921–945

34. Diethrick EB, Garrett H, Ameriso J, Crawford ES, El-Bayer M, DeBakey ME: Occlusive disease of the common carotid and subclavian arteries treated by carotid subclavian bypass. *Am J Surg* 1967;114:800–808

35. Higashida RT, Hulbach VV, Hieshima G: Transluminal angioplasty of the vertebral and basilar artery. *AJNR* 1987;8:745–749

36. Courtheoux P, Tournade A, Theron J, et al: Transcutaneous angioplasty of vertebral artery atheromatous ostial stricture. *Neuroradiology* 1985;27:259–264

37. Baker RN, Carroll RJ, Schwartz WS: Prognosis in patients with transient cerebral ischemic attacks. *Neurology* 1968;18:1157–1165

38. Fischer CM, Gore I, Okabe N, White P: Atherosclerosis of the carotid and vertebral arteries: extracranial and intracranial. *J Neuropathol Exp Neurol* 1963;24:455–476

39. Humphries AW, Young YR, Bevan GG, Lefevre FA, DeWolfe VG: Relief of vertebrobasilar symptoms by carotid endarterectomy. *Surgery* 1965;57:48–52.

Part 7. Celiac and Superior Mesenteric Artery Angioplasty

—Wilfrido R. Castañeda–Zúñiga, M.D., M.Sc., David W. Hunter, M.D., S. Murthy Tadavarthy, M.D., Joseph W. Yedlicka, Jr., M.D., and Kurt Amplatz, M.D.

Intestinal angina is an uncommon entity that has been recognized for more than a century. The association of abdominal pain with arterial disease was initially reported by Schnitzler in 1901.[1] In 1936 Dunphy reviewed autopsy cases of intestinal infarction, and found that 7 of 12 cases had abdominal angina symptoms.[2] In 1958, Mikkelson suggested a surgical approach for correction of superior mesenteric vascular obstructions.[3]

The clinical manifestations of abdominal angina are postprandial pain and substantial weight loss. The weight loss is attributed to the fear of eating because of the anticipated abdominal pain. Nausea, vomiting, and diarrhea may be encountered but are not frequent. The disease is more common in women in a ratio of 2:1 to 4:1.[4]

The majority of the patients undergo multiple diagnostic studies including upper and lower gastrointestinal tract endoscopy, barium contrast studies, and computed tomography. The negative work-up usually prompts clinicians to obtain biplane abdominal aortography for diagnosis of visceral artery stenosis. More than two-thirds of the patients have peripheral vascular disease and aneurysmal dilatation of the abdominal aorta.[5] Coronary artery disease is a frequently associated problem and up to 33% of the patients are symptomatic.[5] Angioplasty of the iliac and superior mesenteric artery (SMA) has been recommended for chronic abdominal angina as a nonsurgical alternative.[6–17]

Pathophysiology of Abdominal Angina

It has been said that at least two of the three visceral branches (celiac, superior mesenteric, and inferior mesenteric arteries) have to be either stenosed by 50% or occluded for manifestations of abdominal angina to occur. In spite of the presence of stenosis or occlusions, most patients do not manifest intestinal angina because of the existence of significant collateral circulation.[18] Intestinal angina is uncommon, even in the presence of widespread disease in the visceral vessels, to the extent of 35–70% in autopsy series.[14]

The celiac and superior mesenteric artery narrowing can be secondary to atherosclerosis, fibromuscular dysplasia, or the median cruciate ligament.[3–5] The median cruciate ligament crosses the origin of the celiac axis and by extrinsic compression can compromise the blood flow. Obviously, this lesion cannot be effectively managed by balloon dilation, since the compression is extrinsic. If the stenosis does not improve after balloon dilatation, strong consideration should be given to the surgical division of the ligament.[3–5] Invariably, inferior mesenteric artery stenosis is related to atherosclerosis.[3–5]

It is difficult to comprehend why isolated celiac artery stenosis should produce intestinal angina.[16] In 68% of cases, relief has, however, been obtained by revascularizing the celiac artery, either by excising the diaphragmatic ligament or by surgical arterial reconstruction.[19]

Angioplasty Methodology

One to two days prior to the angioplasty procedure aspirin (325mg/day) is administered to minimize platelet activity. A lateral abdominal aortogram is obtained in inspiration and expiration. If angioplasty is indicated, the visceral branches (iliac, SMA, and inferior mesenteric artery) are catheterized either from the femoral or axillary artery approach (Fig. 4.7.1). If the origin of the vessel is acutely angled downward, it is preferable to catheterize these vessels from the axillary route, since it is easier to advance the balloon catheter over the guidewire from above (Fig. 4.7.2). From the femoral approach the celiac and superior mesenteric arteries are easily catheterized with a 5.0Fr cobra or Simmons catheter, utilizing a soft Bentson guidewire, the stenosis is easily crossed and the catheter is advanced over the wire. An exchange Rosen guidewire is then passed through the catheter to facilitate advancement of the balloon catheter. Alternatively, a Simmons balloon angioplasty catheter can be used to catheterize the artery. Once the ostium is engaged, a Bentson guidewire is passed across the stenosis and the Simmons balloon is then pulled over the wire until it bridges the area of narrowing. Another alternative is the use of a coaxial system, first catheterizing the artery with the guiding catheter, crossing the obstruction with an 0.018-inch guidewire and then advancing the balloon through the guiding catheter to the level of the obstruction over the 0.018-inch guidewire (Fig. 4.7.3).

A systemic anticoagulation effect is achieved by the administration of 5000 units of heparin either intravenously or by intra-arterial injection. The size of the balloon is predetermined from the measurement of the iliac or superior mesenteric artery adjacent to the stenosis. Usually, it requires either a 6 or an 8mm balloon. The stenosis

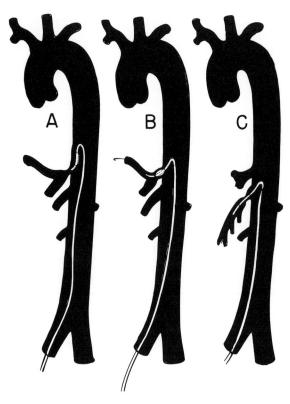

Figure 4.7.1. Diagrammatic representation of catheterization of celiac and SMA using a Simmons catheter from the femoral approach.

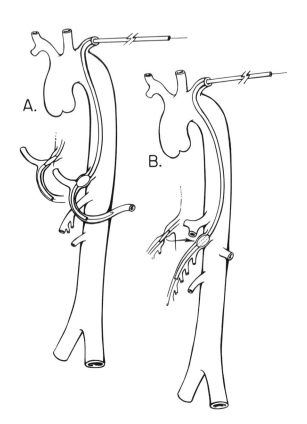

Figure 4.7.2. Diagrammatic representation of catheterization of celiac (**A**) and SMA (**B**) using a transaxillary approach.

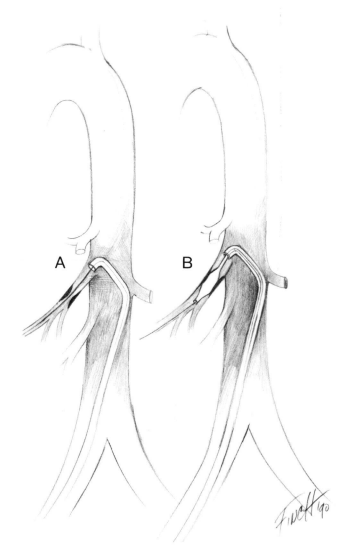

Figure 4.7.3. Coaxial technique used to catheterize the SMA.

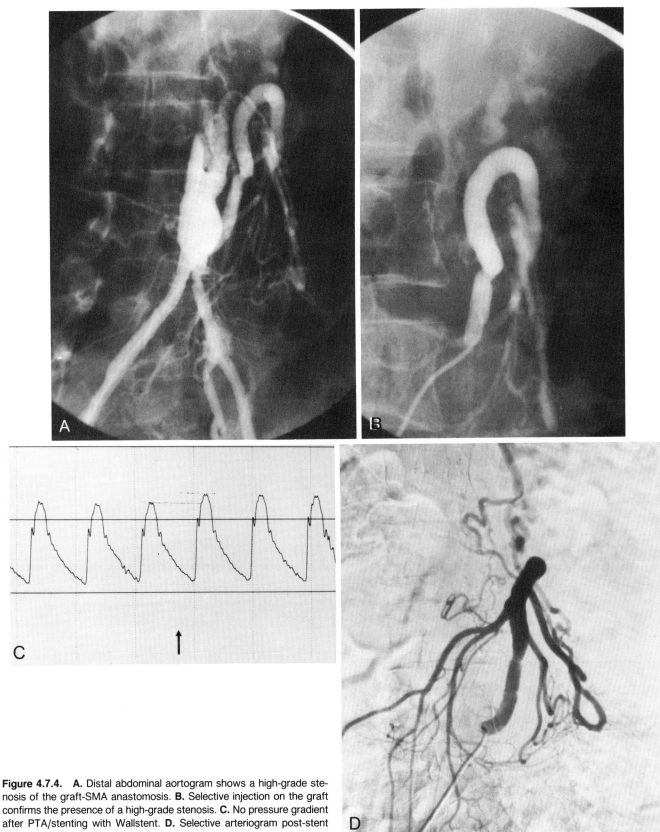

Figure 4.7.4. **A.** Distal abdominal aortogram shows a high-grade stenosis of the graft-SMA anastomosis. **B.** Selective injection on the graft confirms the presence of a high-grade stenosis. **C.** No pressure gradient after PTA/stenting with Wallstent. **D.** Selective arteriogram post-stent placement shows a widely patent lumen.

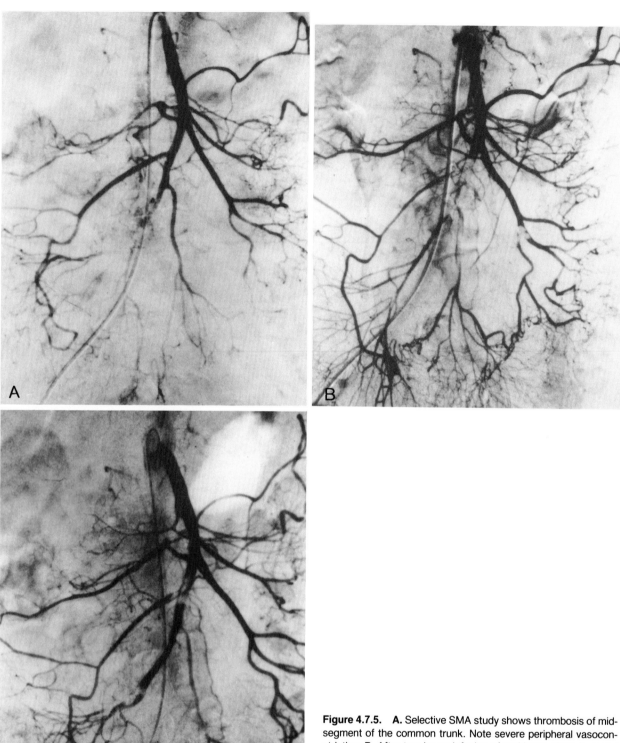

Figure 4.7.5.   A. Selective SMA study shows thrombosis of mid-segment of the common trunk. Note severe peripheral vasoconstriction. **B.** After two hours infusion of urokinase, there is partial lysis of thrombus with improved distal flow. **C.** After continued lysis with urokinase a high-grade stenosis was found. This was dilated and infusion was continued. Note thrombus present after PTA.

is dilated in the usual fashion until the "waist" in the balloon disappears. Pressure measurements and angiographic studies are taken before and after angioplasty to evaluate the results of angioplasty and the status of the vascular bed. If necessary a second balloon dilatation can be performed with a slightly larger balloon. In patients where angioplasty has failed and in whom surgery is contraindicated for medical reasons, the placement of an intravascular stent should be considered (Fig. 4.7.4).

DISCUSSION

The diagnosis of abdominal angina is a challenge since the diagnosis does not exclude or preclude the coexistence of nonvascular disorders than can account for the pain.[4] Therefore, whether to revascularize or not is a difficult decision. Prior to the advent of angioplasty, revascularization was achieved by thromboendarterectomy, vessel reimplantation, and retrograde aortovisceral bypass (prosthetic or autogenous vein). Recently, antegrade suprailiac aortic mesenteric grafts have been introduced.[5,20] The antegrade bypass provides nonturbulent flow and avoids the inherent technical pitfalls of retrograde bypasses.[21]

The mortality rate following surgery varies from 3 to 20%.[5,20-23] The majority of the patients have coexistent coronary artery disease, and the immediate operative mortality is attributed to myocardial infarction.[18] Short-term patency rates have been reported to be around 70–90%.[19,20] In the series described by McCollum, the 5-year survival was 83% and the 10-year survival rate was 62%.[20]

Many interventionalists recommend angioplasty as an excellent nonsurgical alternative because of its simplicity and repeatability.[18] In the recent series published by Odurny et al., 10 patients underwent dilatation in 19 arteries on 14 occasions.[16] Initial technical success was achieved in 17 of 19 arteries (90%), with relief of symptoms that lasted from 6 to 24 months. In 50% of the patients (5 of 10 cases), the symptoms recurred and redilatation in three of them relieved the symptoms again. They have attributed their incidence of restenosis to a slight underdilatation of visceral arteries for the fear of catastrophic rupture. The vessels were not overdilated as is commonly done in peripheral dilatation.[16] No significant complications have been reported associated with the procedure.

Angioplasty should be the initial choice of treatment for intestinal angina, as it avoids the perioperative mortality and morbidity related to the coexistent coronary artery disease. If angioplasty fails, patients can be subjected to the more invasive surgical revascularization procedures, which may involve either a thromboendarterectomy or aortovisceral bypass grafting.

The use of angioplasty in the management of acute mesenteric ischemia was initially reported by Van Denise in a patient presenting with acute onset of abdominal pain, signs of peritoneal irritation, and guaiac positive stools.[13] Classic teaching says that these symptoms are associated with a high likelihood of transmural intestinal infarction and should therefore be addressed by surgical intervention. In Boley's series, however, two patients responded to the intravenous administration of vasodilators.[24] We have treated a patient presenting with the classical symptoms and in whom a laparotomy showed no evidence of transmural infarction. On angiography the patient had thrombosis of the SMA with significant impairment of antegrade blood flow (Fig. 4.7.5*A*). After lysis of the thrombus with urokinase, a high grade stenosis of the SMA distal to the ostium was found (Fig. 4.7.5*B*). This was successfully dilated (Fig. 4.7.5*C*) and the patient recuperated uneventfully.

As stated by Van Denise there seems to be a group of patients with acute occlusive or nonocclusive intestinal ischemia, who do not have transmural necrosis of bowel and thus may respond to balloon dilatation.[13] The problem lies in identifying these patients who, if presenting with classic symptomatology, will be taken to surgery. The more expeditious way to identify them would be to perform angiography on those patients in whom the presenting signs are not classic.

References

1. Bergan JJ, Yao JST: Chronic intestinal ischemia, in Rutherford RB (ed): *Vascular Surgery*, Ed 2. Philadelphia, WB Saunders, 1984, pp 964–972
2. Dunphy JE: Abdominal pain of vascular origin. *Am J Med Sci* 1936;192:109–113
3. Mikkelson WP: Intestinal angina: its surgical significance. *Am J Surg* 1957;94:262–269
4. Stanton PE Jr, Hollier PA, Seidel TW, Rosenthal D, Clark M, Lamis PA: Chronic intestinal ischemia: diagnosis and therapy. *J Vasc Surg* 1986;4:338–344
5. Rapp JH, Reilly LM, Qvarfordt PG, et al: Durability of endarterectomy and antegrade grafts in the treatment of chronic visceral ischemia. *J Vasc Surg* 1986;3:799–806
6. Saddenkni S, Sniderman KW, Hilton S, Sos TA: Percutaneous transluminal angioplasty of nonatherosclerotic lesions. *AJR* 1980;135:975–182
7. Uflacker R, Goldany MA, Constant S: Resolution of mesenteric angina with percutaneous transluminal angioplasty of a superior mesenteric artery stenosis using a balloon catheter. *Gastrointest Radiol* 1980;5:367–369
8. Golden DA, Ring EJ, McLean GK, Freiman DB: Percutaneous transluminal angioplasty in the treatment of abdominal angina. *AJR* 1982;139:247–249
9. Van Denise WH, Zawacki JK, Phillips D: Treatment of acute mesenteric ischemia by percutaneous transluminal angioplasty. *Gastroenterology* 1986;91:475–478
10. Roberts L Jr, Wertman DA Jr, Mills SR, Moore AV Jr, Heaston DK: Transluminal angioplasty of the superior mesenteric artery: an alternative to surgical revascularization. *AJR* 1983;141:1039–1042
11. Wertman RL Jr, Mills SR, Moore AV, Heaston DK: Transluminal angioplasty of the superior mesenteric artery: an alternative to surgical revascularization. *AJR* 1983;141:1039–1042
12. Furrer J, Gruentzig A, Kugelmeier J, Goebel N: Treatment of abdominal angina with percutaneous dilatation of an arteriamesenteric superior stenosis. *Cardiovasc Intervent Radiol* 1980;5:367–369

13. Van Denise WH, Zawacki JK, Phillips D: Treatment of acute mesenteric ischemia by percutaneous transluminal angioplasty. *Gastroenterology* 1986;91:475–478
14. Beebe HG, MacFarlane S, Raker IJ: Supraceliac aortomesenteric bypass for intestinal ischemia. *J Vasc Surg* 1987;5:749–754
15. Becker GJ, Stewart J, Holden RW, Yune HY, Mail JT, Klatte EC: Abdominal angina: clinical presentation, angiography, and PTA (abstr). Program of the 13th Annual Meeting of the Society of Cardiovascular and Interventional Radiology. Reston, VA, Society of Cardiovascular and Interventional Radiology, 1988, pp 165–167
16. Odurny A, Sniderman KW, Colapinto RF: Intestinal angina: percutaneous transluminal angioplasty of the celiac and superior mesenteric arteries. *Radiology* 1988;167:59
17. Castañeda–Zúñiga WR, Gomes A, Weens C, Ketchum D, Amplatz K: Transluminal angioplasty in the treatment of abdominal angina. *Röfo* 1982;137:330–332
18. Becker GJ, Katzen BT, Dake MD: Noncoronary angioplasty. *Radiology* 1989;170:921–940
19. Reilly LM, Ammar AD, Stoney RJ, Ehrenfield WK: Late results following operative repair for celiac artery compression syndrome. *J Vasc Surg* 1985;2:79–91
20. McCollum CH, Graham JM, DeBakey ME: Chronic mesenteric arterial insufficiency: results of revascularization in 33 cases. *South Med J* 1976;69:1266–1268
21. Beebe HG, MacFarlane S, Raker EJ: Supraceliac aortomesenteric bypass for intestinal ischemia. *J Vasc Surg* 1987; 5:749–754
22. Stoney RJ, Wylie EJ: Recognition and surgical management of visceral ischemic syndromes. *Ann Surg* 1966;164:714–721
23. Reul GJ Jr, Wukash DC, Dandiford EM, Chiarillo L, Hallman GL, Cooley DA: Surgical treatment of abdominal angina. Review of 25 patients. *Surgery* 1974;75:682–689
24. Boley SJ, Spraygen S, Siegelman SS, Veith FJ: Initial results from an aggressive roentgenological and surgical approach to acute mesenteric ischemia. *Surgery* 1977;82:848–855

Part 8. Percutaneous Transluminal Angioplasty of the Renal Arteries

—Charles J. Tegtmeyer, M.D., and J. Bayne Selby, Jr., M.D.

RENAL ANGIOPLASTY

Data from the United States National Health Examination Survey indicate that hypertension (blood pressure ≥ 160/95mm Hg) occurs in 10–15% of the adult population in this country.[1] Of this group of approximately 23 million persons, 1 million (≈4%) have potentially correctable renovascular hypertension.[2] Coronary artery disease, stroke, and renal failure have all been unequivocally related to uncontrolled hypertension,[3,4] and hypertension of the renovascular type poses the additional threat of progressive renal insufficiency.

Pharmacotherapy and surgical revascularization, the traditional modes of treatment for renovascular hypertension, have significant shortcomings. For example, in many cases, drugs only partially control blood pressure; and, when several drugs are combined, side effects and poor patient compliance can become a problem.[5–7] Also, if the renal artery is severely stenotic, lowering the blood pressure with drugs further reduces renal blood flow, sometimes leading to ischemic atrophy or even renal infarction. Hunt et al. proved that surgical correction of renovascular hypertension was superior to medical therapy.[8] With 7–14 years of follow-up, 84% of their surgically treated patients were alive, in contrast to only 60% of those treated medically. Therefore, whenever possible, the treatment of choice for renovascular hypertension is correction of the renal artery stenosis. However, the operation requires general anesthesia, and many patients are poor risks because of severe diffuse atherosclerotic disease, renal insufficiency, or both. Moreover, surgical results vary, there is considerable morbidity, and the mortality rate can be as high as 5.9%.[9] Therefore, although surgery and medical therapy have significant benefits in spite of these shortcomings,[10,11] there is no question that alternative treatments are desirable.

Grüntzig reported the first successful balloon dilatation of renal artery stenosis in 1978.[12] In the relatively short period since then, several articles detailing the results of percutaneous transluminal angioplasty (PTA) in large series have been published.[13–21] The preliminary data suggest that PTA is highly successful in correcting renal artery stenoses. Only a few series have described the long-term results of renal angioplasty,[22–25] but more definitive analyses of the long-term results are now emerging.[26–29]

RENAL ARTERY STENOSES

Etiology

There are many causes of stenoses in the renal arteries, but the majority of the lesions are atherosclerotic in origin, and most of the remainder are due to fibromuscular dysplasia. For example, in the 884 hypertensive patients with renal artery lesions among the 2442 patients in the Cooperative Study on Hypertension, atherosclerosis was the cause in 557 (63.0%), fibromuscular hyperplasia in 286 (32.4%), and miscellaneous disease in 41 (4.6%).[10] In the University of Virginia series, atherosclerosis was the cause of the stenosis or occlusion in 75 patients, who had 93 lesions dilated, and fibromuscular dysplasia was the cause of 85 stenoses in 66 patients. Seven patients had stenoses in the arteries to renal allografts. One patient had his native artery dilated after his saphenous bypass graft occluded, and one patient had three stenoses due to previous irradiation.[26,29]

Significance

Renovascular hypertension can be defined as hypertension caused by obstruction of the main renal artery or one of its branches. The difficulty in making the diagnosis of true renovascular hypertension only begins after identification of an anatomic obstruction, however. The temptation to dilate a renal artery stenosis once discovered is great, especially because the absence of lateralization of renin production does not preclude a response to correction of the stenosis in 21% of patients.[30] However, in 1956, Homer Smith pointed out that only 26% of patients undergoing a nephrectomy for apparent unilateral renovascular hypertension were normotensive at the end of one year.[31] Eyler et al. studied the arteriograms of normotensive and hypertensive adults and found significant renal artery stenoses in both groups,[32] and Holley and associates found renal artery stenosis at autopsy in 49% of patients who had been normotensive during life.[33] Therefore, once a renal artery stenosis is identified in a hypertensive patient, the physiologic importance of the lesion should be assessed. If the physiologic significance of this lesion is not ascertained, optimal angioplasty results will not be achieved.

INDICATIONS FOR RENOVASCULAR EVALUATION

It is not feasible or cost effective to completely evaluate all hypertensive patients for renovascular disease. The criteria for work-up vary from one medical center to another; however, certain patients have an increased risk of renovascular hypertension and should be evaluated.

1. Patients with a documented sudden onset of hypertension;
2. Those without a family history of hypertension or other identifiable secondary causes of hypertension;
3. Young women who develop hypertension and are not taking oral contraceptives;
4. Patients, especially whites, who develop malignant hypertension;
5. Those with longstanding hypertension who suddenly develop accelerated hypertension;
6. Those who are refractory, or who become refractory, to hypertensive drugs other than blockers of the renin-angiotensin system;
7. Those with a flank bruit;
8. Those who suffer renal insufficiency while taking captopril.

The evaluation protocol also varies with the institution. Initially, peripheral blood may be assayed for renin; if the concentration is elevated, selective samples are obtained from both renal veins and the inferior vena cava. This can be performed on an outpatient basis, and an intravenous digital subtraction angiography (DSA) study can be obtained at the same time. However, intravenous radiologic studies may miss subtle lesions caused by fibromuscular dysplasia or branch stenoses. Therefore, if the renin concentrations are elevated and the DSA is negative, an arteriogram should be obtained.

Alternatively, in patients strongly suspected of having angiotensinogenic hypertension, renal vein renin sampling and an arteriogram can be performed on the same day. If the patient has impaired renal function, an intra-arterial digital study can be performed. Intra-arterial digital studies are far superior to intravenous ones, as they have better solution and require less contrast material.

INDICATIONS FOR RENAL ANGIOPLASTY

The indications for renal angioplasty include the relief of proved renovascular hypertension or of the angiotensinogenic component in patients with both essential hypertension and renovascular hypertension. Many of the patients in the University of Virginia series have a long history of hypertension with recent acceleration due to superimposed renal disease. In patients with deteriorating renal function, renal angioplasty may be indicated, because if there are underlying renal artery stenoses, correction of these lesions may preserve or improve renal function.

Techniques

Since the introduction of renal angioplasty by Grüntzig et al. in 1978, the technique has been refined and simplified.[19] Nonetheless, renal angioplasty remains more complex than peripheral angioplasty. It is far from innocuous and should be performed only by angiographers who have had considerable experience dilating peripheral vessels. Inflating one balloon is simple, but crossing a tight renal stenosis with a balloon catheter requires great skill, and selection of the proper size balloon requires experience.

A high-quality preliminary midstream arteriogram is necessary to determine the approach. Unless an abdominal arteriogram has been obtained within the previous month, this study should always be obtained before catheterizing the renal arteries, because profound changes may occur in a short time in the presence of a tight renal artery stenosis.

There are five percutaneous angiographic approaches to the treatment of stenoses in the renal arteries with Grüntzig-type balloons:

1. Guided coaxial balloon catheter system;
2. Femoral balloon catheter system via a femoral approach;

Figure 4.8.1. Technique of renal dilatation with the coaxial balloon catheter system. *A,* stenosis in left renal artery. *B,* orifice of the renal artery is selected with the guiding catheter. *C,* the 4.5Fr dilatation catheter is directed through the stenosis by the guiding catheter and is inflated, dilating the stenosis. *D,* intima is split, and a portion of media is stretched or split, relieving the obstruction in the renal artery. (Reproduced from Tegtmeyer CJ, Dyer R, Teates CD, et al: Percutaneous transluminal dilatation of the renal arteries: techniques and results. *Radiology* 1980;135:589–599.)

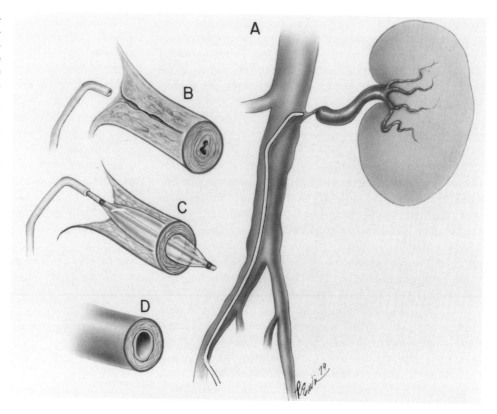

3. Femoral balloon catheter system via an axillary approach;
4. Femoral balloon catheter system with the sidewinder approach;
5. "Kissing balloon" technique

Each will be discussed.

GUIDED COAXIAL BALLOON CATHETER SYSTEM

The Grüntzig-type guided coaxial balloon catheter system utilizes an 8Fr or 9Fr renal guiding catheter and a 4.3Fr or 4.5Fr coaxial balloon catheter (Fig. 4.8.1). The renal guiding catheter is available in three configurations (Fig. 4.8.2). It is inserted by a femoral approach, and the orifice of the renal artery is carefully selected. The small coaxial catheter is then passed through the guiding catheter across the stenosis. The balloon catheter will accept a 0.014- or 0.016-inch guidewire which can be passed across the stenosis before advancing the coaxial catheter to facilitate traversing a tight stenosis. With the advent of the new platinum wires, which are highly visible radiologically, this is a very effective technique. In the presence of a tortuous renal vessel, a tight stenosis, or a stenosis in a branch, the fine guidewire greatly facilitates passage of the balloon

Figure 4.8.2. The renal guiding catheter is available in three basic configurations; the choice for a particular procedure depends on the size of the aorta and the angle that the renal artery takes as it branches from the aorta.

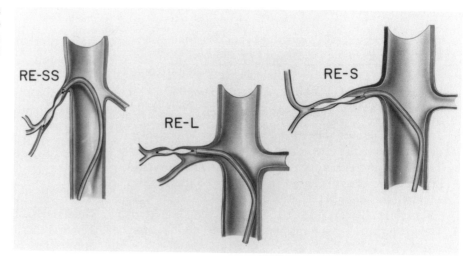

catheter. If the stenosis is not too tight, the coaxial catheter can be advanced across it without the guidewire while injecting a small amount of contrast medium.

The advantage of this coaxial technique is that the small catheter passes through the tight stenosis more readily than the 7Fr balloon catheter. It is also easy to steer this catheter out into the branches of the renal artery. Therefore, this catheter system is usually used for a tight stenosis that cannot be passed by other techniques or in the treatment of distal or branch stenoses. There are several disadvantages to the technique, however. For example, the catheters are expensive, and it is necessary to make an 8Fr or 9Fr puncture wound in the femoral artery. Also, the guiding catheter is stiff and may damage the aortic wall. It is inserted over a 0.063-inch guidewire which is also quite stiff and thus potentially traumatic. Balloons are available from 2 to 5mm, but if an 8Fr guiding system is used the balloon catheter can be no larger than 3mm.

The technique is more complex than the standard femoral balloon catheter technique. The common femoral artery is punctured, and a two-part sheath is introduced over a 0.038-inch guidewire. The sheath is advanced into the distal abdominal aorta, its inner cannula is removed, and the 0.063-inch guidewire is advanced into the abdominal aorta as far as the diaphragm. The guiding catheter is then advanced over the guidewire through the sheath and into the abdominal aorta. The guidewire is removed, and the guiding catheter is used to select the renal artery orifice. The balloon catheter is then advanced through the guiding catheter and across the stenosis. The small diameter of the balloon makes it possible to measure pressures across the stenosis. The balloon is inflated with a 1:1 mixture of contrast medium and 0.9% saline. Balloon inflation and the progress of the angioplasty can be monitored by injecting contrast medium through either the balloon catheter or the guiding catheter, which is a definite advantage. However, because of the dilatation injury to the intima, caution should be exercised when injecting contrast medium near the dilatation site.

The recent development of an angioplasty balloon on a guidewire has allowed a modification of the conventional coaxial technique.[34] This system uses a 7Fr or 8Fr renal guiding catheter and a Tegwire (Medi-Tech) angioplasty catheter. The guiding catheters come in a variety of preformed shapes specifically designed for use with the Tegwire. The angioplasty balloon is mounted on a 0.035-inch guidewire with a short floppy tip distal to the balloon. It is available in 3–6mm diameters.

A sheath is placed in the groin and an appropriately shaped guiding catheter is placed adjacent to the orifice of the renal artery. The Tegwire is then passed through a Tuohy–Borst connector on the end of the guiding catheter. While the guiding catheter is held stationary, the Tegwire is gently advanced across the stenosis. Slight clockwise or counterclockwise rotation of the guiding catheter may be necessary.

If the lesion cannot be easily crossed, the most likely cause of the problem is the guiding catheter and a new shape should be tried. Once the lesion is crossed, it is dilated in the standard manner. The result can then be checked by the injection of contrast material through the Tuohy–Borst adapter.

This technique combines the advantages of crossing a lesion with a coaxial system while using smaller size guiding catheters and larger balloon sizes. It should be noted that changing to a larger balloon size requires recrossing the lesions, but we have not found this to be a problem.

FEMORAL BALLOON CATHETER SYSTEM

Femoral Approach

This technique involves a modification of the double lumen balloon catheter designed by Grüntzig for angioplasty of superficial arteries (Fig. 4.8.3). Only catheters with a low-profile balloon located close to the catheter tip should be utilized in the renal arteries. In tight stenoses, it is important not to prepare the balloon before inserting it, because this may interfere with passage through the stenosis.

Originally the Grüntzig-type balloon catheters were only available on a 7Fr shaft. Recently, smaller 5Fr shaft

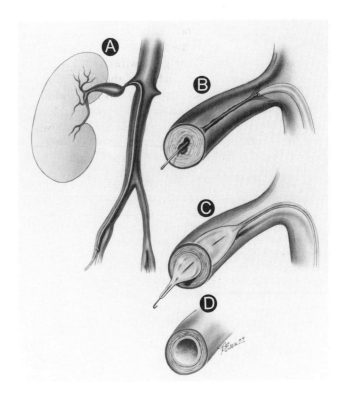

Figure 4.8.3. Technique of renal dilatation with a femoral balloon catheter system via the femoral approach. *A,* stenotic right renal artery is catheterized selectively with a cobra catheter. *B,* the guidewire is passed through the stenosis. *C,* a selective catheter is exchanged for a dilation catheter, and the balloon is inflated, compressing the stenosis. *D,* obstruction is now relieved. (Reproduced from Tegtmeyer CJ, Dyer R, Teates CD, et al: Percutaneous transluminal dilatation of the renal arteries: techniques and results. *Radiology* 1980;135:589–599.)

balloon catheters have become available with balloon diameters ranging from 4 to 7mm. Eight millimeter or larger balloons still require the larger size catheter. A 2cm long balloon is usually employed for renal angioplasty.

The femoral artery is punctured and the appropriate 5Fr diagnostic catheter is advanced into the abdominal aorta using the Seldinger technique. The orifice of the renal artery is carefully selected, and contrast medium is injected to locate the lesion. Under fluoroscopic guidance, a 0.035-inch tight J or a 0.035-inch Bentson guidewire is advanced beyond the stenosis. If these guidewires will not pass, the lesion can often be traversed with a 15mm J guidewire. It is imperative to avoid subintimal passage of the guidewire. Once the stenosis has been crossed, the 5Fr selective catheter should be passed across it because this facilitates the subsequent passage of the balloon catheter. A small amount of contrast medium is injected to confirm the intraluminal position of the catheter, and 2000–5000 IU of heparin is injected through the catheter. A movable core type J or Rosen wire is then inserted through the catheter beyond the stenosis, and the diagnostic catheter is replaced with the appropriate size renal balloon catheter, chosen by measuring the renal artery proximal and distal to the stenosis (Fig. 4.8.4) and estimating the original size of the renal artery. If the artery is estimated to have been 5mm in diameter, this is the balloon size that should be used. Because this method does not take radiographic magnification into account, the renal arteries are being slightly (~1mm) overdilated. The guidewire must not be moved back and forth in the branches of the renal artery when exchanging the catheters, because this may induce spasm or cause occlusion of the segmental branches.

If the balloon catheter will not cross the stenosis, a 5Fr catheter with a 3mm balloon is passed across the lesion and inflated, partially dilating the stenosis. The proper size balloon catheter can then be advanced easily across the stenosis.

The balloon catheter is positioned across the stenosis under fluoroscopic control, and the balloon is inflated either with a USCI inflation device or with a syringe. If a syringe is used, a 10ml size is probably ideal, because it is capable of generating approximately 9.4 atm of pressure during inflation and sufficient negative pressure to deflate the balloon rapidly. A pressure gauge should always be used. The balloon is first inflated to 2 atm of pressure to determine its position in relation to the stenosis. When it is properly positioned, it is inflated to 4–6 atm and left inflated for 30–40 seconds. It may be necessary to repeat this several times. The progress can be monitored by watching the configuration of the balloon as it is inflated.

The 0.035-inch wire is then replaced with a smaller wire and a Tuohy–Borst connector is attached. A 0.025-inch wire is used with the 7Fr catheters while a 0.021-inch wire is used with 5Fr balloon catheters. The balloon is carefully pulled back and contrast medium is injected to assess the results. The balloon catheter can be readvanced if the lesion requires further dilatation. Immediately after angioplasty, an arteriogram is performed to assess the results. Before removing the balloon catheter, it is important to completely deflate the balloon and apply suction as it is being removed from the femoral artery.

The primary advantage of this technique is that only a 5Fr or 7Fr puncture wound is needed in the femoral artery. If the stenosis permits easy passage of the balloon, this is the simplest approach. However, if the stenosis is tight or the renal artery branches from the aorta at an acute angle, the balloon catheter may be reluctant to follow the guidewire across the lesion, because it has a tendency to buckle in the aorta when pressure has to be applied. This difficulty may often be overcome by advancing, first, the

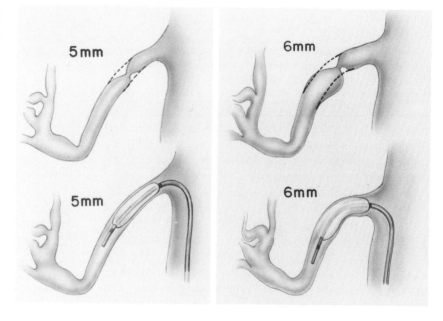

Figure 4.8.4. A balloon catheter is selected to correspond to the original diameter of the stenotic renal artery; post-stenotic dilatation must be taken into account. Because renal arteries are magnified by 15–20% on standard angiograms, arteries will be overdilated by approximately 1mm. (Reproduced from Tegtmeyer CJ, Kellum CD, Ayers C: Percutaneous transluminal angioplasty of the renal arteries. *Radiology* 1984;153:77–84.)

5Fr diagnostic catheter, and then either a 7Fr tapered Van Andel or the 3mm balloon catheter as described and then reinserting the balloon catheter.

Axillary Approach

The axillary approach may also be used to dilate the renal arteries (Fig. 4.8.5).[35] This approach greatly simplifies the procedure when the renal arteries originate from the aorta at a sharp angle, because the stenotic artery is easily selected. Once the guidewire is in place across the lesion, the dilatation catheter has a natural tendency to follow its gentle downward curve. Passage of the guidewire and then the catheter through the stenosis is often facilitated by having the patient take a deep breath. The axillary approach is also useful when severe atherosclerotic disease or a bypass graft is present in the pelvic or abdominal vessels.

The technique also uses the double lumen balloon catheter designed by Grüntzig for superficial femoral artery angioplasty. The balloon is available for renal angioplasty in 4mm through 8mm sizes and in several lengths. The 2cm-long balloon is the most popular. A left axillary approach is usually taken because it offers the straightest

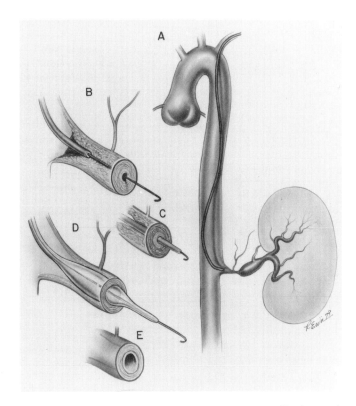

Figure 4.8.5. Technique of renal dilatation through the axilla. *A*, stenotic left renal artery is selected with diagnostic cobra catheter. *B*, the guidewire is passed through stenosis. *C*, a cobra catheter is advanced through stenosis. *D*, a selective catheter is replaced with a dilatation catheter, which is inflated. *E*, stenosis is now relieved. (Reproduced from Tegtmeyer CJ, Dyer R, Teates CD, et al: Percutaneous transluminal dilatation of the renal arteries: techniques and results. *Radiology* 1980;135:589–599.)

approach to the descending aorta and because the catheter has a tendency to buckle in the ascending aorta when the right axillary approach is attempted. The technique is otherwise similar to that of the femoral approach.

Theoretically, there is an increased risk of damage to the smaller axillary artery; however, this can be minimized by using 5Fr angioplasty balloons, deflating the balloon carefully, and rotating it as it is being inserted and removed. There is also the possibility of brachial plexus injury, the chances of which can be minimized by using the high brachial approach, in which the artery is entered just distal to the axillary crease. The artery is easier to control in this area because it can be compressed against the humerus.

Sidewinder Approach

The sidewinder approach combines the advantages of the femoral and axillary approaches (Fig. 4.8.6). The same Grüntzig-type double lumen balloon catheter used in the femoral approach is used. The femoral artery is punctured, but the renal artery is approached from above to take advantage of the natural curve of the renal artery, and it is selected with a 5Fr "shepherd's crook" or "sidewinder" catheter which is advanced across the lesion under fluoroscopic control as contrast medium is injected, with care taken to keep the tip within the lumen of the artery. Alternatively, a flexible-tip guidewire is advanced across the stenosis followed by the catheter. Once the catheter is across the lesion, 2000–3000 IU of heparin is injected through it. The guidewire is replaced with a movable-core J guidewire or a Rosen wire. The diagnostic catheter is then exchanged for the appropriate size renal balloon catheter. After the sidewinder catheter has crossed the lesion, the balloon catheter will usually cross the stenosis with ease. After dilatation, a midstream arteriogram is obtained to document the results.

The principal advantage of this technique is that withdrawing the sidewinder catheter advances the diagnostic catheter across a tight stenosis because the configuration of the catheter exerts considerable downward force as it is withdrawn over the guidewire. This technique is very helpful in traversing tight stenoses.

"Kissing Balloon" Technique

This technique, originally described for dilating lesions at the bifurcation of the abdominal aorta,[36,37] has application in selected cases in the renal arteries.[38] If two renal arteries originate from the aorta in proximity, or if the lesion involves a major bifurcation in the renal artery (Fig. 4.8.7*A*), dilating the lesion may occlude the adjacent vessel. In this situation, catheters are inserted through both femoral arteries, and a catheter is passed across the lesion in the involved branch (Fig. 4.8.7*B*). The origin of the uninvolved branch is usually protected by the diagnostic catheter (Fig. 4.8.7*C*). If the origin of the vessel is involved by the lesion or compromised by the procedure, the catheter

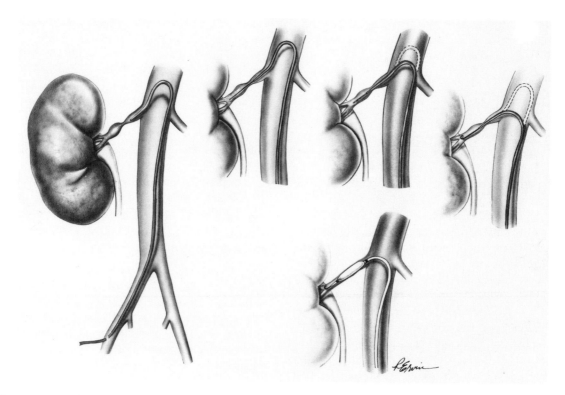

Figure 4.8.6. Technique of renal angioplasty using shepherd's crook catheter. After selection of an appropriate renal artery, a flexible-tip guidewire is advanced through the lesion under fluoroscopic control. The cath- eter is advanced across the stenosis by withdrawing the catheter at the puncture site. The guidewire is then exchanged for a heavy-duty tight J wire, and appropriate balloon catheter is inserted to dilate lesion.

is exchanged for a second balloon catheter, and the lesion is dilated.

Periprocedural Management

Proper management of candidates for renal angioplasty requires a team approach. The proper selection of patients and the management of blood pressure requires the close cooperation of a hypertension specialist. Also, inadvertent occlusion of the renal artery may create a surgical emergency so the procedure should be performed only when a skilled vascular surgeon is available.

The blood pressure must be monitored especially carefully during the first 24–48 hours after angioplasty because profound changes may occur. It is important to discontinue antihypertensive drugs before angioplasty, thereby helping to prevent a precipitous drop in the blood pressure. If the diastolic pressure rises above 110mm Hg, the blood pressure should be controlled by captopril or short-acting intravenous infusion of saline. Therefore, all patients undergoing renal angioplasty should have an intravenous line in place.

If not contraindicated, patients receive 2000 IU of heparin subcutaneously every six hours beginning eight hours after the procedure and continuing for two days. The patients also receive 75 mg of dipyridamole (Persantine) orally twice a day for at least six months and 325 mg of acetylsalicylic acid once a day beginning the day before angio- plasty and continuing for life. The patients are strongly encouraged to stop smoking. After angioplasty, the patients should be monitored by a cardiologist or a nephrologist, who specializes in the control of high blood pressures. The patient's need for antihypertensive drugs changes after a successful procedure, so blood pressure must be monitored closely. If the blood pressure rises in the ensuing months, arteriography or DSA should be repeated.

Complications

Because renal angioplasty is more complex than peripheral angioplasty, and because the potential complications are serious, the procedure should be performed only in hospitals where a skilled vascular surgeon is immediately available.

The complication rate of renal angioplasty ranges from 5 to 10%, with most complications being minor. The most frequent major complication is transient renal insufficiency, which clearly is related to the contrast medium. The frequency can be reduced by performing the diagnostic arteriogram several days before the therapeutic procedure in patients with renal insufficiency. Subintimal dissection with the guidewire or the diagnostic catheter may result when attempting to cross the stenosis. A small intimal flap will usually heal, but angioplasty should be postponed for four to six weeks. Thrombosis of the renal artery infre-

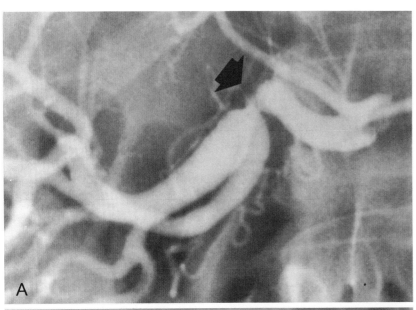

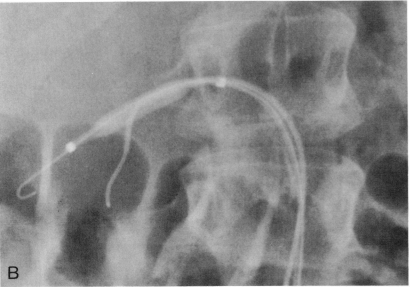

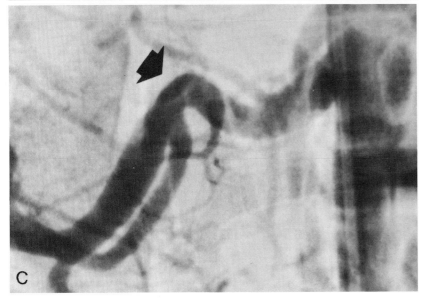

Figure 4.8.7.   A 28-year-old woman presented with a two-year history of hypertension. **A.** Midstream arteriogram demonstrates a tight stenosis *(arrow)* at the junction of the dorsal and ventral branches of the renal artery. **B.** A 100mm spot radiograph shows the balloon inflated in the upper branch, dilating the lesion, and a catheter in the lower artery, protecting the orifice of the artery. **C.** Immediately following PTA, the renal artery and both branches are widely patent *(arrow)*. (Reproduced from Tegtmeyer CJ, Sos TA: Techniques of renal angioplasty. *Radiology* 1986;161:577–586.)

quently follows balloon dilatation. This complication is sometimes treated by infusing a thrombolytic agent into the renal artery, but it is vital that sufficient collateral vessels be present if this approach is selected so that renal ischemia does not develop while waiting for the enzyme to work. Urokinase is currently the most widely accepted thrombolytic agent in this setting. Another rare major complication is rupture of the renal artery, which may result from weakening of the wall or from subintimal placement of the balloon catheter. If rupture is noted immediately after deflation of the balloon, the balloon should be re-inflated to occlude the proximal renal artery, and the patient should be operated on immediately. Distal embolization is an infrequent complication, but a recently occluded renal artery should be approached with caution, because thrombi may be dislodged by the catheter to occlude segmental branches.

The most frequent minor complication is spasm or occlusion of a renal arterial branch (Fig. 4.8.8), usually caused by movement of the tip of the guidewire back and forth within the vessel. If possible, the guidewire should not be placed within the segmental branches. Focal spasm may also be produced in the area immediately adjacent to the angioplasty site. Calcium channel blockers prevent and reverse spasm in the renal arteries. Nifedipine is the most potent vasodilator among the calcium antagonist drugs and can be given in a dose of 20 mg sublingually at the outset of procedure. If spasm occurs, verapamil may be given through the arterial catheter in a dose of 2.5–5 mg. Also, because the mechanism of action of nitroglycerin differs from that of the calcium antagonists, and since it has an additive effect with the calcium channel blockers, it may be useful against spasm in the renal arteries. It is either injected directly into the affected renal artery (50–200μg) or given sublingually (0.4–0.6mg). Calcium channel blockers may induce hypotension and should be used with caution in patients with known cardiac conduction defects.

In addition to these complications unique to renal angioplasty, there may be complications at the puncture site. The principal complication is formation of a large hematoma. Because the patient is receiving anticoagulants and there are frequent catheter exchanges when using the axillary approach, the operator should be careful to puncture high in the brachial artery and not in the axilla itself to avoid devastating effects, including brachial plexus injury, of a large hematoma in the axilla.

RESULTS

In experienced hands, renal angioplasty is a highly effective method for correcting renal artery lesions. An initial success rate greater than 90% should be achieved when dilating renal artery stenoses. Technical failures usually result from an inability to cross the lesion or from insufficient dilatation.

The long-term results of renal angioplasty can be assessed in three ways: the effects on vessel patency, on blood pressure, and on renal function. The effect of the procedure on vessel patency is related to the cause and characteristic of the lesion. The patients can be divided into five distinct groups:

1. Those with atherosclerotic renal artery stenoses or occlusions;

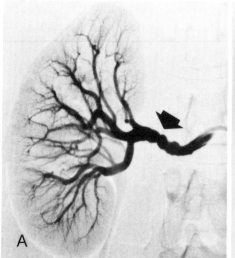
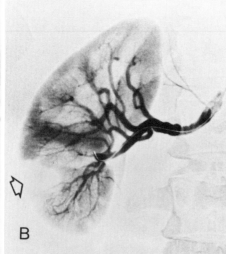
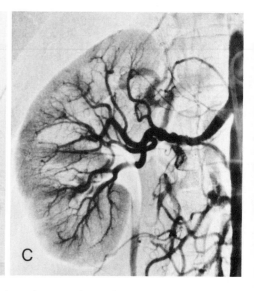

Figure 4.8.8. Renal parenchymal defect caused by guidewire during angioplasty procedure. **A.** Selective renal arteriogram reveals changes consistent with fibromuscular dysplasia *(arrow)*. **B.** Immediately after dilatation, angiogram demonstrates defect in lower pole of kidney *(arrow),* apparently caused by guidewire, which is still in place. **C.** Arteriogram obtained three months later shows resolution of the defect. Renal arteries are widely patent. (Reproduced from Tegtmeyer CJ, Kellum CD, Ayers C: Percutaneous transluminal angioplasty of the renal arteries. *Radiology* 1984;153:77–84.)

2. Those with fibromuscular dysplasia;
3. Those with renal allografts;
4. Those with saphenous bypass grafts;
5. Those treated primarily for renal insufficiency.

Atherosclerotic Lesions

Atherosclerotic disease is the most frequent cause of the stenosis subjected to renal dilatation. In the University of Virginia series, 94% of the 65 hypertensive patients with atherosclerotic lesions were helped by the procedure: 15 were cured and 46 improved. Analysis of the results in these patients revealed some factors that are important to the success of renal angioplasty. First, better results are achieved with unilateral renal artery stenoses than with bilateral stenoses, because the restenosis rate is higher in patients with severe bilateral renal artery disease than in patients with unilateral renal artery stenosis.[26] Sos et al.[25] and Martin and associates[27] also showed that success was more frequent in patients with unilateral lesions. Second, it is becoming increasingly clear that certain lesions are more amenable to balloon dilatation than are others. For example, a good result can be expected in short isolated lesions (Fig. 4.8.9), whereas when the stenosis is caused by a large plaque in the abdominal aorta that engulfs the origin of the renal artery (Fig. 4.8.10), the chances of success are diminished. Figure 4.8.11 illustrates the type of lesion in which this diminished response is often obtained. Cicuto et al.,[39] Sos et al.,[25] and Schwarten[40] all reported similar results. In the University series, the lesions requiring redilation were caused by aortic plaques that engulfed the ori-

gin of the renal artery. Finally, complete blocks are more difficult to dilate than are stenoses, and one should not try to dilate complete blocks that are not perfectly straight.

Fibromuscular Dysplasia

The best results in renal angioplasty are achieved in patients with fibromuscular lesions (Fig. 4.8.12), which respond well to balloon dilatation, usually at pressures of 4 atmospheres or less. Thus, if the lesion can be crossed, a good result can be expected. There were 66 hypertensive patients with 85 lesions caused by fibromuscular dysplasia in the authors' series and all but one of the patients benefited from renal angioplasty, with seven patients requiring a second dilatation.[29] Similar results have been achieved by several other authors. Geyskes et al. performed PTA in 21 patients with fibromuscular dysplasia, and all but one were either cured or improved.[24] Sos et al. achieved technical success in 27 of their 31 patients.[25]

Stenoses in Renal Allografts

Seven patients with stenoses in the arteries of renal allografts underwent dilation (Fig. 4.8.13). Five patients improved, and there were two failures, one of which was caused by inability to dilate the lesion, probably because of the use of a polyvinyl chloride balloon. With the polyethylene balloons now available, a better result probably would have been achieved in this patient. In another patient, a tight stenosis at the anastomosis of the allograft vessel with the hypogastric artery recurred after seven

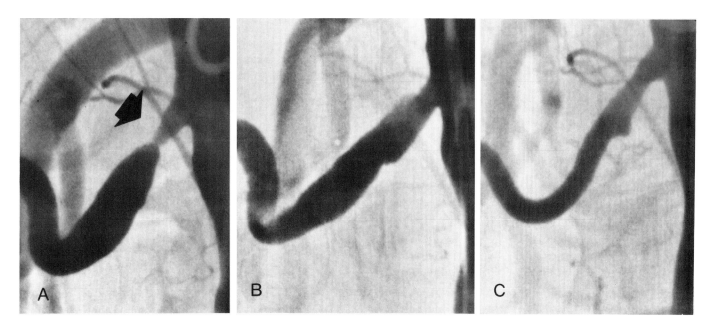

Figure 4.8.9. **A.** Abdominal aortogram shows a high-grade stenosis of the right renal artery *(arrow)*. **B.** An aortogram following transluminal angioplasty of the right renal artery shows increase in diameter at the site of balloon dilatation with no residual narrowing. **C.** A six-month follow-up aortogram shows a widely patent lumen with no evidence of recurrence of stenosis.

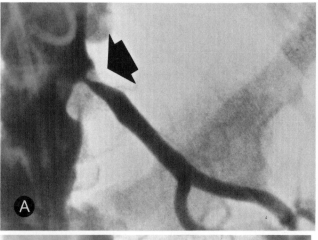

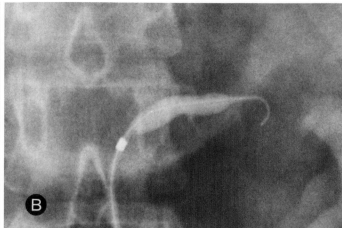

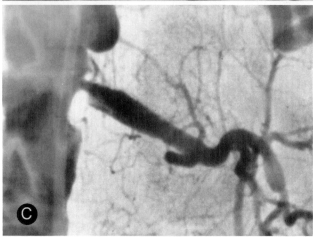

Figure 4.8.10.   Diminished response typical of renal artery orifice lesions caused by plaques in abdominal aorta, illustrated in 68-year-old woman with long-standing hypertension, tight stenosis at the origin of the left renal artery, and 60% stenosis in the right renal artery. **A.** Predilatation arteriogram reveals tight stenosis at the origin of the left renal artery *(arrow)*. **B.** The 100mm spot radiograph with 6mm balloon in place; note that the balloon is not completely expanded. **C.** Immediately after PTA, the artery is improved but stenosis remains. (Reproduced, with permission, from Tegtmeyer CJ, Kofler TJ, Ayers CA: Renal angioplasty: current status. *AJR* 1984;142:20.)

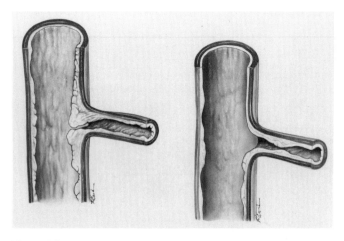

Figure 4.8.11.   This is the type of atherosclerotic lesion in which diminished response to balloon dilatation can be expected. Lesion on *left* is caused by atherosclerotic plaque in the abdominal aorta which engulfs the orifice of the renal artery. Occasionally, a good result is obtained, but usually results are poor when compared with other types of lesions. A good response can be expected in short stenoses within the renal artery *(right)*. (Reproduced, with permission, from Tegtmeyer CJ, Kofler TJ, Ayers CA: Renal angioplasty: current status. *AJR* 1984;142:20.)

months despite three dilatations with pressures as high as 14 atm. Sniderman et al. attempted to dilate stenoses in the arteries of renal allografts in 15 patients, 3 of whom underwent repeat dilatations. The procedure was technically successful in 15 of the 18 attempts in 13 of the 15 patients.[41] Gerlock et al. were successful in all seven patients in their series with allograft stenoses.[42]

Caution should be exercised when dilating lesions of renal allografts, because there are no collateral vessels to the kidney. Therefore, if the vessel is occluded, operation must be undertaken immediately. If follows that wherever allograft dilatation is done, a surgeon should be readily available.

Stenoses in Saphenous Bypass Grafts

In the University of Virginia series, three patients had PTA of stenoses in their renal saphenous bypass grafts dilated. The procedure was successful in all cases.

Renal Insufficiency

Under certain circumstances, alleviation of renal artery stenosis is important to preserve renal function. Correc-

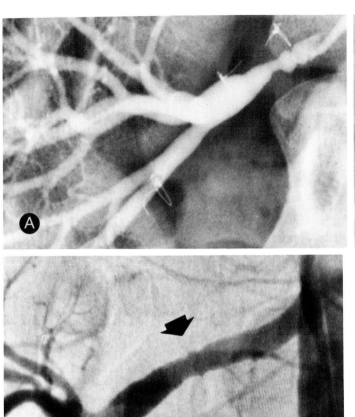

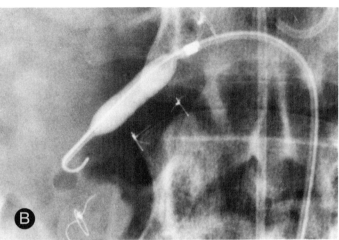

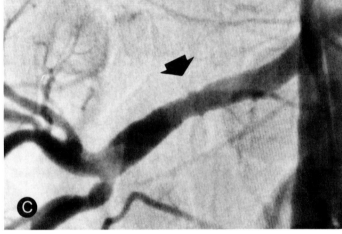

Figure 4.8.12. Balloon dilatation of lesions caused by fibromuscular dysplasia in a 24-year-old hypertensive woman. **A.** Selective right renal arteriogram reveals stenosis in the artery. **B.** Fibromuscular dysplasia is usually easy to dilate; 5mm balloon expands easily, dilating the lesion. **C.** Immediately after dilatation, the lesion has disappeared *(arrow)*.

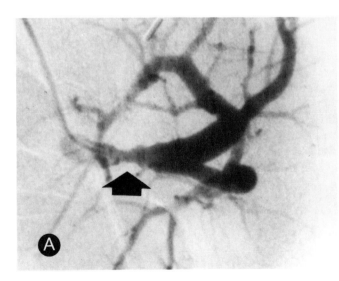

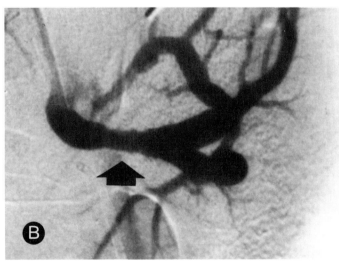

Figure 4.8.13. Percutaneous transluminal angioplasty in a 23-year-old woman with a renal allograft. **A.** Selective renal arteriogram demonstrates tight stenosis *(arrow)* at the anastomosis between the renal and hypogastric arteries. **B.** Lumen of vessel is much improved *(arrow)* after balloon angioplasty via axillary approach. (Reproduced from Tegtmeyer CJ, Brown J, Ayers CA, Wellons HA, Stanton LW: Percutaneous transluminal angioplasty for the treatment of renovascular hypertension. *JAMA* 1981;246:2068–2070.)

tion of stenosis is probably worthwhile in unilateral disease if kidney size indicates potentially significant preservation of functional tissue or if bilateral renal artery stenoses are present. In the latter case, an attempt to alleviate obstruction for the larger kidney should be given priority even if the smaller kidney is secreting all the renin.

The results of angioplasty are not as dramatic in patients treated primarily for renal insufficiency as in patients treated primarily for hypertension, but they are nonetheless encouraging. In the present authors' series, 10 patients were treated primarily for renal insufficiency, all with atherosclerotic lesions, the mean serum creatinine being 5.2 mg/dl before dilation. After angioplasty, this average decreased to 2.3 mg/dl,[26] with five of the patients having a positive response to PTA. Five of the patients have not been helped. Fourteen of the patients with fibromuscular dysplasia treated primarily for hypertension[29] also had renal insufficiency, and 12 of these patients now have better renal function, with three having normal blood urea nitrogen (BUN) and creatinine values. In the two patients who did not exhibit a decrease, their renal function stabilized and did not continue to deteriorate. In some patients, the improvement was gradual, so that the full benefit of the procedure was not apparent for several months.

SUMMARY OF RESULTS

Renal angioplasty is a clinically effective means of treating renovascular hypertension. In the present authors' series, the blood pressure response was analyzed in the 92 hypertensive patients whose initial dilatation was successful, who have been followed from 1 to 60 months (mean, 23.7 months). The mean systolic pressure was 199.74mm Hg before renal angioplasty and 140.34mm Hg afterward; the mean diastolic pressure was 117.05mm Hg before angioplasty and 83.74mm Hg afterward. Analysis of the long-term clinical results in the 98 hypertensive patients who underwent renal angioplasty to control their blood pressure reveals that 26% were cured (defined by the Cooperative Study of Renovascular Hypertension[43] as having an average diastolic pressure of less than or equal to 90mm Hg with at least a 10mm Hg decrease from the pre-dilatation level). Sixty-seven percent were improved, in that their blood pressure was easier to control with drugs as a result of the angioplasty, and 7% were nonresponders, although one of these was helped for several months. A review of the large series in the world literature shows that if the initial dilatation is successful, the vessels can be expected to remain patent in 70–90% of the patients and that if the vessel remains patent for at least eight months, it is likely to remain patent for at least five years. The recurrence rate has been variously reported as 12.9%[26] and 22.5%.[40] The rate is clearly higher in atherosclerotic stenoses than for other types. A significant factor is the success of the initial dilatation: lesions with a ≥30% residual stenosis on the immediate post dilatation films are more likely to recur than lesions in which a better result has been

obtained.[20,26] Therefore, it is essential that a good result be obtained initially. However, restenosis can usually be redilated, and the procedure is often easier than the initial one.

CONCLUSIONS

The results of the University of Virginia series and published series show that PTA of the renal arteries is a versatile and reliable procedure. Excellent results can be obtained in the control of hypertension if the patients are carefully selected. It is encouraging to note that the procedure also has the potential for stabilizing or reversing renal insufficiently. In the University of Virginia series, of the 39 patients who had high BUN and creatinine levels before PTA, 18 currently have better renal function, and 4 of these have normal BUN and creatinine values.

In experienced hands, the results of renal angioplasty compare favorably with surgical results in the treatment of renovascular hypertension. The success so far has changed the original skepticism to tempered enthusiasm. If the renal artery remains patent for at least eight months after PTA, a good long-term result can be expected. Renal angioplasty should be considered the treatment of choice in patients with hypertension and renal artery stenoses caused by fibromuscular dysplasia or short isolated atherosclerotic lesions. Good results can also be obtained in patients with stenoses in the arteries of renal allografts and in patients with stenoses in bypass grafts.

The procedure is enticing because it offers many advantages. It is relatively simple compared with surgery, and it preserves renal tissue. It avoids general anesthesia and intra-abdominal surgery, and the patient experiences less pain. The procedure is relatively inexpensive and reduces the hospital stay.[44] Recent refinements in balloon technology and manufacturing, including development of 5Fr balloon catheters and the balloon on a guidewire, have further decreased trauma to the groin.

Studies are currently underway involving new adjunctive technologies to angioplasty such as atherectomy and intravascular stents. While no conclusive results are available yet, continued investigation of new innovations can only lead to further improvement in the treatment of this disease. For the more than one million Americans who suffer from renovascular hypertension, renal angioplasty has become the initial treatment of choice.

References

1. Stokes JB III, Payne GH, Cooper T: Hypertension control: the challenge of patient education (editorial). *N Engl J Med* 1973;289:1369
2. Gifford RW Jr: Evaluation of the hypertensive patient with emphasis on detecting curable causes. *Milbank Mem Fund Q* 1969;47:170
3. Kaplan NM: *Clinical Hypertension*. New York, Medcom, 1973, pp 1–45,173–242
4. Janeway TC: A clinical study of hypertensive cardiovascular disease. *Arch Intern Med* 1913;12:755–798
5. Genest J, Boucher R, Rojo-Ortega JM, et al: Renovascular

hypertension, in Genest J, Koiw E, Kuchel O (eds): *Hypertension: Physiopathology and Treatment.* New York, McGraw-Hill, 1977, pp 815–840

6. Youngberg SP, Sheps SG, Strong CG: Fibromuscular disease of the renal arteries. *Med Clin North Am* 1977;61:623
7. Dollery CT, Bulpitt CJ: Management of hypertension, in Genest J, Koiw E, Kuchel O (eds): *Hypertension: Physiopathology and Treatment.* New York, McGraw-Hill, 1977, pp 1038–1068
8. Hunt JC, Sheps SG, Harrison EG Jr, Strong CG, Bernatiz PE: Renal and renovascular hypertension: a reasoned approach to diagnosis and management. *Arch Intern Med* 1974;133:988–999
9. Foster JH, Maxwell MH, Franklin SS, et al: Renovascular occlusive disease: results of operative treatment. *JAMA* 1975;231:1043
10. Veterans Administration Cooperative Study Group on Antihypertensive Agents: Effects of treatment of morbidity in hypertension: results in patients with diastolic blood pressures averaging 115 through 129 mm Hg. *JAMA* 1967;202:1028
11. Veterans Administrative Cooperative Study Group on Antihypertensive Agents: Effects of treatment on morbidity in hypertension: results in patients with diastolic blood pressure averaging 90 through 114 mm Hg. *JAMA* 1970;213:1143
12. Grüntzig A, Kuhlmann U, Vetter W, Lutolf U, Meier B, Siegenthaler W: Treatment of renovascular hypertension with percutaneous transluminal dilation of a renal artery stenosis. *Lancet* 1978;1:801–802
13. Boomsma JHB: *Percutaneous Transluminal Dilatation of Stenotic Renal Arteries in Hypertension.* Groningen, The Netherlands, Drukkerijvan Denderen B.V., 1982, pp 103–128
14. Katzen BT, Chang J, Knox WG: Percutaneous transluminal angioplasty with the Grüntzig balloon catheter: a review of 70 cases. *Arch Surg* 1979;114:1389–1397
15. Martin EC, Mattern RF, Baer L, Frankuchen EL, Casarella WJ: Renal angioplasty for hypertension: predictive factors for long-term success. *AJR* 1981;137:921–924
16. Puijlaert CBAJ, Boomsma JHB, Ruijs JHJ, et al: Transluminal renal artery dilatation in hypertension: technique, results and complications in 60 cases. *Urol Radiol* 1981;2:201–210
17. Schwarten DE: Percutaneous transluminal renal angioplasty. *Urol Radiol* 1981;2:193–200
18. Sos TA, Saddekni S, Sniderman KW, et al: Renal artery angioplasty: techniques and early results. *Urol Radiol* 1982;3:223–231
19. Tegtmeyer CJ, Dyer R, Teates CD, et al: Percutaneous transluminal dilatation of the renal arteries: techniques and results. *Radiology* 1980;135:589–599
20. Tegtmeyer CJ, Teates CD, Crigler N, Gandee RW, Ayers CR, Stoddard M, Wellons HA Jr: Percutaneous transluminal angioplasty in patients with renal artery stenosis. Follow-up studies. *Radiology* 1981;140:323–330
21. Tegtmeyer CJ, Brown J, Ayers CA, Wellons HA, Stanton LW: Percutaneous transluminal angioplasty for the treatment of renovascular hypertension. *JAMA* 1981;246:2068–2070
22. Tegtmeyer CJ, Elson J, Glass TA, Ayers CR, Chevalier RL, Wellons HA Jr, Studdard WE Jr: Percutaneous transluminal angioplasty: the treatment of choice for renovascular hypertension due to fibromuscular dysplasia. *Radiology* 1982;143:631–637
23. Colapinto RF, Stronell RD, Harries-Jones EP, et al: Percutaneous transluminal dilatation of the renal artery: follow-up studies on renovascular hypertension. *AJR* 1982;139:727–732
24. Geyskes GG, Puijlaert CBAJ, Oei HY, Mees EJD: Follow-up study of 70 patients with renal artery stenosis treated by percutaneous transluminal dilatation. *Br Med J (Clin Res)* 1983;287:333–336
25. Sos TA, Pickering TG, Sniderman K, et al: Percutaneous transluminal renal angioplasty in renovascular hypertension due to atheroma or fibromuscular dysplasia. *N Engl J Med* 1983;309:274–279
26. Tegtmeyer CJ, Kellum CD, Ayers C: Percutaneous transluminal angiplasty of the renal arteries. *Radiology* 1984;153:77–84
27. Martin LG, Price RB, Casarella WJ, et al: Percutaneous angioplasty in clinical management of renovascular hypertension: initial and long-term results. *Radiology* 1985;155:629–633
28. Martin LG, Casarella WJ, Alspaugh JP, et al: Renal artery angioplasty: increased technical success and decreased complications in the second 100 patients. *Radiology* 1986;159:631–634
29. Tegtmeyer CJ, Selby JB, Hartwell GD, Ayers C, Tegtmeyer V: Results and complications of fibromuscular disease. *Circulation* 1991;83(Suppl I):I-155–I-161
30. Bourgoignie J, Jurz S, Catanzaro FJ, Serirat P, Perry HM: Renal venous renin in hypertension. *Am J Med* 1970;48:332–342
31. Smith HW: Unilateral nephrectomy in hypertensive disease. *J Urol* 1956;76:685–701
32. Eyler WR, Clark MD, Garman JE, et al: Angiography of the renal areas including comparative study of renal artery stenoses in patients with and without hypertension. *Radiology* 1962;78:879–892
33. Holley KE, Hunt JC, Brown AL Jr, et al: Renal artery stenosis: a clinical pathologic study in normotensive and hypertensive patients. *Am J Med* 1964;37:14–22
34. Tegtmeyer CJ: Guidewire angioplasty balloon catheter: preliminary report. *Radiology* 1988;169:253–254
35. Tegtmeyer CJ, Ayers CA, Wellons HA: The axillary approach to percutaneous renal artery dilatation. *Radiology* 1980;135:775–776
36. Tegtmeyer CJ, Wellons HA, Thompson RN: Balloon dilatation of the abdominal aorta. *JAMA* 1980;244:2636–2637
37. Tegtmeyer CJ, Kellum CD, Kron IL, et al: Percutaneous transluminal angioplasty in the region of the aortic bifurcation: the two-balloon technique with results and long-term follow-up study. *Radiology* 1985;157:661–665
38. Baker KS, Sawyer RW, Tisnado J, et al: Percutaneous transluminal angioplasty of the renal arteries: double-catheter technique. *Radiology* 1986;159:554–555
39. Cicuto KP, McLean GK, Oleaga JA, Freiman DB, Grossman RA, Ring EJ: Renal artery stenosis: anatomic classification for percutaneous transluminal angioplasty. *AJR* 1981;137:599–601
40. Schwarten DE: Percutaneous transluminal angioplasty of the renal arteries: intravenous digital subtraction angiography for follow-up. *Radiology* 1984;150:369
41. Sniderman KW, Sos TA, Sprayregen S: Postrenal transplantation, in Castañeda–Zúñiga WR (ed): *Transluminal Angioplasty.* New York, Thieme–Stratton, 1983, p 80
42. Gerlock AJ Jr, MacDonnell RC Jr, Smith CW, et al: Renal transplant arterial stenosis: percutaneous transluminal angioplasty. *AJR* 1983;140:325–331
43. Simon N, Franklin SS, Bleifer KH, Maxwell MH: Clinical characteristics of renovascular hypertension. *JAMA* 1972;220:1209
44. Doubilet P, Abrams H: The cost of underutilization: percutaneous transluminal angioplasty for peripheral vascular disease. *N Engl J Med* 1984;310:95

Part 9. Aortic, Iliac, and Peripheral Arterial Angioplasty

—Donald E. Schwarten, M.D., S. Murthy Tadavarthy, M.D., and Wilfrido R. Castañeda–Zúñiga, M.D., M.Sc.

Nonsurgical restoration of normal, or near normal, hemodynamics in the presence of arteriosclerotic stenotic or occlusive disease was first described by Dotter and Judkins in 1964,[1] in the first description of the procedure now known as percutaneous transluminal angioplasty (PTA). Modification of the original Dotter–Judkins coaxial Teflon catheter system was described by Staple in 1968,[2] and further modifications were described by Van Andel, who chose to use a gradually tapered catheter rather than a more cumbersome coaxial system.[3] Several theoretical benefits accrued from Van Andel's design, including a diminution in the (undesirable) longitudinal shear force on the intima, which predisposes to acute thrombosis of the angioplasty site, and elimination of the possibility of entrapment of the intima between the two coaxial catheters, causing the "snowplow effect," which also predisposes to acute postangioplasty thrombosis. One further addition to the nonballoon-type catheters was made by Zeitler, who added a sidehole for contrast injection.[4] Both the Dotter and the Van Andel types of systems were utilized extensively in Europe for PTA of midsize and relatively small arteries but were used only sparingly in the United States for a number of reasons, not the least of which was consciousness of the potential for complications in the groin because of the large puncture wounds needed in the femoral artery.

The Dotter- and Van Andel-type catheters were too small to alter the hemodynamics in the common iliac arteries. Therefore, Porstmann designed a "caged" or "corset" catheter comprising a latex balloon enclosed in Teflon strips that helped minimize the propensity of the elastic latex to deform around the lesion rather than to dilate it.[5] However, Porstmann's balloon catheter caused little change in the prevailing attitude of angiographers and surgeons toward management of arteriosclerotic occlusive disease by PTA.

In 1974, Grüntzig and Hopff introduced an angioplasty catheter with a balloon made of a relatively nonelastic material, polyvinyl chloride.[6] This balloon could be inflated to a consistent predetermined diameter over a modest range of pressures without fear of balloon overdistention and vessel rupture. The advantages of such a device are obvious: 1) the balloon exerts almost exclusively radial forces against the plaque and the arterial wall, thereby minimizing the unwanted shear forces; 2) the balloon can be placed on a smaller catheter shaft (2.5–9Fr); and 3) balloons can be made in various diameters (3.0–25.0mm at present), thus permitting dilatation of the aorta, iliac arteries, superficial and deep femoral arteries, popliteal arteries, and tibial vessels. Also, since Grüntzig's initial reports

of coronary and renal angioplasty,[7,8] other reports have confirmed the value of PTA in a wide variety of applications.[9–12]

It is now clear that polyvinyl chloride is not the ideal material for angioplasty balloons, and numerous studies are in progress to determine the ideal material as well as which balloon configuration optimizes the immediate and long-term results of PTA (see Chapter 4, Part 5 for an extensive discussion of catheter materials, properties, and actions). Today, it appears that the most widely used material is irradiated polyethylene. Polyethylene terephthalate (e.g., Mylar) materials tolerate enormous pressures (15–20 atm) with little, if any, tendency toward deformity or bursting; but whether such high pressures are necessary or beneficial in a significant percentage of patients with atherosclerotic disease remains unresolved. These high-pressure balloons may be of more value in treating nonatherosclerotic disease.

The long-term results of PTA in a variety of vessels in properly selected patients are as good as the results achieved with traditional surgical methods,[13] and the advantages of the percutaneous method are obvious. First, the procedure is safe, simple, and relatively painless. Second, in nearly all cases, the procedure can be performed with the patient in the hospital for little more than 24 hours. Third, unsuccessful angioplasty does not preclude surgical revascularization. Fourth, recurrent or worsening disease after an initially successful PTA can be managed with another angioplasty without the necessity of dealing with postoperative scarring. Finally, there is no risk of loss of sexual function as a consequence of aortoiliac angioplasty, as there is when the surgical procedures are used.

Perhaps, then, the time has come for an aggressive approach to patients with even mild lower extremity claudication who, because their symptoms are not severe or for other reasons, might not be surgical candidates. Rather than give these patients medical therapy until claudication limits their lifestyle and their disease becomes too extensive for angioplasty, so that operation is the only way to restore relatively normal hemodynamics, one should consider early accurate anatomic evaluation and, perhaps, PTA.

PATIENT SELECTION

Indications and Contraindications

Selecting patients for aortoiliac and peripheral angioplasty requires assessment of both clinical and anatomic features. Angioplasty is more dependent than is surgery on certain anatomic criteria as predictors of both primary and long-term success. Therefore, both the clinical and the anatomic indications and contraindications are discussed here.

PTA is a cooperative effort, and although the burden of performing the diagnostic and dilatation procedures falls upon the angiographer, the decision to do PTA should be made jointly by a qualified vascular surgeon, the angiographer, and, usually, an internist. It is imperative to refrain from attempting PTA where surgical cooperation is not available; although the procedure is relatively safe, complications are inevitable in any series, and the immediate availability of a capable vascular surgeon will be essential to avert catastrophes.

CLINICAL INDICATIONS

At this time, the clinical indications for PTA are essentially those guidelines observed by many moderately aggressive vascular surgeons. As a rule, patients with intermittent claudication who desire symptom relief will be considered candidates for arteriography and possible angioplasty provided that data from noninvasive studies suggest that the principal hemodynamic abnormalities are proximal to the popliteal artery.[14] However, when limb salvage is the goal, patients are considered for arteriography and angioplasty regardless of the site of disease predicted by noninvasive studies.[15]

CLINICAL CONTRAINDICATIONS

The presence of symptoms for less than six to eight weeks, or sudden worsening of lower extremity symptoms within this time, is a relative contraindication to angioplasty.[16] Because fresh thrombus is likely to be present in these cases, PTA should not be performed unless the radiologist is thoroughly familiar with thrombolytic agents and uses them before PTA to lyse any relatively fresh thrombus and so minimize the risk of downstream embolization. The patient presenting with the "trash-foot" syndrome, indicative of peripheral embolization, likewise must be considered to have at least a relative contraindication to angioplasty,[17] although some unpublished work suggests that angioplasty is an appropriate alternative to operation in some of these patients as well (BT Katzen and A Van Breda, personal communication).

ANATOMIC INDICATIONS AND PROCEDURE PLANNING

Doppler data are invaluable in planning the approach for diagnostic arteriography in anticipation of angioplasty performed either in conjunction with the arteriogram or later. Furthermore, a baseline Doppler study obtained at approximately the same time as the arteriogram, when considered in conjunction with a study obtained 24–48 hours after successful angioplasty, permits objective assessment of the immediate and long-term results of the procedure.[18]

For the authors' first 1000 lower extremity angioplasty procedures, postprocedural Doppler examinations were routinely obtained at quarterly intervals during the first year and semiannually for the next year. The efficacy of the procedure in the authors' hands is now well established, and we no longer perform such frequent noninvasive studies. Instead, patients are carefully instructed about the implications of even minor recurrent symptoms, particularly within the first year, and are asked to see their referring physician immediately for a Doppler examination should symptoms return. Certainly as a quality control measure during the development of a PTA program at an institution, it is helpful to obtain regular noninvasive examinations of the first several hundred patients for comparison with the results of reported large series.

Perhaps the single most important factor in deciding whether a patient is a candidate for PTA is the diagnostic arteriogram. No other information is as valuable as the appearance of the pathologic anatomy in predicting the likelihood of success. It stands to reason, then, that the arteriogram, whether obtained by conventional screen film techniques or by digital techniques, must be of the highest quality to permit identification of ulcerations, mural thrombus, or thread-like patent channels within high-grade stenoses if the appropriate therapeutic decision is to be made. Oblique views are needed for examination of such areas as the orifices of the common iliac arteries, the origins of the hypogastric arteries, and the bifurcation of the common femoral artery.

ANATOMIC CONTRAINDICATIONS

Certain angiographic features are said to diminish the likelihood of success or to increase the likelihood of recurrent disease at the angioplasty site. Thus, these findings may be considered relative anatomic contraindications[19,20]:

Aorta—eccentric lesions in the proximal infrarenal region, particularly those of nonatherosclerotic etiology;

Iliac arteries—stenoses longer than 2.0–3.0cm, eccentric stenoses, heavy calcification (particularly if eccentric), total occlusion of the common iliac artery, or stenosis at the origin of the common iliac artery;

Superficial and deep femoral arteries—stenoses longer than 2.0–3.0cm, occlusions longer than 10–15cm, or heavy calcification of the stenotic or occlusive lesion;

Popliteal, tibial, and peroneal arteries—long segments of disease where there is a large patent vessel at the ankle, because the latter vessel is suitable for bypass grafting, and good results are likely to be obtained, particularly in institutions where in situ grafting is utilized;

In general, at this time, the authors consider ulcerative disease in the presence of evidence of distal embolization a contraindication;

Complete occlusion of the superficial femoral artery in the presence of morbid obesity (relative contraindication);

Extensive disease in any segment of the aortoiliac or femoral vasculature, because long segments of intimal–

medial disruption predispose to recurrent disease and distal complications.

The demonstration of fresh mural thrombus is an absolute contraindication unless thrombolysis is successful. This anatomic contraindication points out the necessity for performing a diagnostic arteriogram immediately before attempting any angioplasty procedure: even an overnight interval may permit thrombus to develop in an area of high-grade stenosis in a low-flow system. If such a thrombus is overlooked, the risk of embolization is increased.

Poor runoff diminishes the likelihood of long-term benefit from PTA. Zeitler et al. found, in patients who had had a successful common iliac angioplasty, that if runoff was good to excellent, the patency rate at five years was approximately 85%, whereas in patients with poor runoff it was 50%.[21] The same limitation confronts the surgeon, however, so even if poor runoff is apparent in a patient who probably will have severe symptoms and, possibly, tissue loss, PTA may be the treatment of choice because of its simplicity and safety.

The foregoing list of anatomic contraindications must be considered in light of the patient's clinical condition; in general, they are relative contraindications. It is clear that long occluded segments of the superficial femoral artery can be recanalized using balloon catheter techniques (Fig. 4.9.1). Likewise, calcification is not always a predictor of failure, nor is eccentricity of a lesion. The radiologist must recognize that these anatomic situations are merely less than optimal for PTA; they do not preclude it. Because angioplasty failures rarely cause significant deterioration in the patient's clinical status, the authors attempt PTA in the presence of unfavorable anatomy in these circumstances:

When the patient is at high operative risk;
When preservation of a saphenous vein is desirable;
When operation would be technically compromised because of an inadequate saphenous vein;
When the patient is not expected to live much longer;
Whenever limb salvage is the primary goal; that is, when an amputation is expected, angioplasty is attempted regardless of the anatomy if for no other reason than that it may alter the level of amputation even if it is only partially successful;
As an adjunct to surgery, such as in patients who may be at high risk in a major intra-abdominal operation. Here, angioplasty of a flow-limiting aortoiliac segment lesion to provide inflow to the groin in preparation for a femoral-popliteal bypass graft, profundoplasty, or femoral-femoral bypass graft may obviate the intra-abdominal procedure.

Lesions for which the authors never perform PTA are stenoses below the knee (except for limb salvage) and occlusions of the origin of the superficial femoral artery flush with the common femoral artery bifurcation. In the

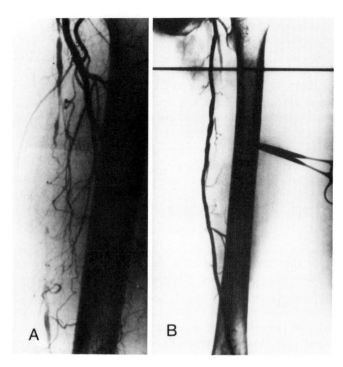

Figure 4.9.1. **A.** Complete occlusion of superficial femoral artery. **B.** Successful recanalization of long-segment occlusion of superficial femoral artery.

latter instance, there is no reasonable way to catheterize the superficial femoral artery.

LESIONS IDEAL FOR ANGIOPLASTY

The lesions that are ideal for PTA are:

Focal distal aortic stenoses of atherosclerotic origin;
1.0–2.0cm concentric, high-grade stenoses of the iliac arteries located some distance from a major bifurcation;
2.0–4.0cm stenoses or occlusions of the superficial and deep femoral arteries;
Relatively short isolated stenoses or occlusions in the popliteal and tibial arteries.

PERIPROCEDURAL PATIENT CARE

Preangioplasty Care

Well before the procedure, at a minimum, the following laboratory data should be available: blood urea nitrogen, serum creatinine, platelet count, prothrombin time, and partial thromboplastin time. If the patient has compromised renal function and a diagnostic arteriogram is obtained near the time of the planned angioplasty, the serum creatinine level should be ascertained immediately prior to PTA to ensure that the procedure is not begun on a patient with failing kidneys.

All patients receiving intravascular contrast medium should be well hydrated, so intravenous fluids should be begun the evening before angioplasty and continued at a rate of 50–100ml/hr at least until the evening after the procedure.

Patients who are to undergo PTA should be seen well in advance of the procedure and be apprised of the primary success rate for the vessel to be treated as well as of the expected long-term success rate, the complication rate at that institution, and in general of what factors influence the results. More specifically, the patient should be informed about the use of antiplatelet agents, the probable value of an exercise program (the guidelines for which are best determined by the patient's internist or cardiologist), and the necessity of abstinence from tobacco use.

It is best not to premedicate heavily if narcotic analgesics are to be used, not only because of the risk of complications but because of the value of having the patient able to communicate the degree of discomfort as the balloon is inflated within the vessel. It has been the authors' experience, as well as that of Katzen (personal communication) and others, that a patient who feels no discomfort during inflation of the balloon in the distal aorta, common or external iliac arteries, or hypogastric arteries may have an anatomically unsatisfactory result unless a larger balloon is used. Conversely, the patient who experiences excruciating pain with minimal inflation of a balloon may be at risk of excessive arterial trauma and perhaps should be treated with a smaller balloon. Therefore, the authors believe it is ideal for a patient to feel moderate discomfort and to communicate this during the procedure. Obviously, a patient under the influence of substantial doses of narcotics is not likely to be communicative.

Intraprocedural Care

BALLOON SELECTION AND USE

The many and varied effects of balloon inflation within a vessel range from initiation of an aggressive atherosclerotic process to the creation of an atonic, somewhat ectatic, vessel.[22-24] Probst and coworkers have shown that the likelihood of the vessel remaining patent after successful angioplasty is greater if the treated site is slightly greater in diameter than the adjacent normal caliber vessel.[25] This finding suggests that use of a balloon slightly larger than the actual diameter of the vessel would produce the ideal result; in practice, it is the authors' belief that the size of the balloon used should depend on the size of the nearest segment of normal caliber artery. In general, the authors use a balloon equal to the measured diameter of the nearest normal caliber segment of vessel without correction for magnification. The balloon should be slightly longer than the lesion. It is important to optimize the anatomic result because, as Tegtmeyer and colleagues have shown, recurrent stenoses are most likely after incomplete dilatation.[26] If we have performed angioplasty on a common iliac artery, for example, and find an unsatisfactory arteriographic appearance, indicating incomplete dilatation of the vessel, in a patient who experienced mild to modest discomfort during balloon inflation, the procedure is repeated with a balloon one size larger, stopping only if the patient experiences severe pain (Fig. 4.9.2).

The duration of balloon inflation may have some bearing on the outcome of the angioplasty. For example, Kaltenbach and colleagues showed that, by prolonging the inflation, "nondilatable" lesions frequently can be dilated adequately.[27] The authors routinely inflate the balloon to its maximum diameter and pressure and leave it in this state for 60–120 seconds. With this technique, a single inflation usually produces the desired result. Balloons should be inflated with a 3–12ml syringe with contrast medium diluted 1:3, because smaller syringes generate unacceptably high pressures, predisposing to balloon rupture. Intraballoon pressures should be monitored. Deflation of balloons is best performed with large-bore syringes, which can generate maximum negative pressure (see Chapter 4, Part 5).

PRESSURE MEASUREMENTS

The authors do not routinely measure pressures before angioplasty in patients with lesions that obviously are hemodynamically significant; it is only in questionable lesions that pressure measurements are of value in determining whether to perform angioplasty. Under these circumstances, pressures are measured with the patient at rest and after maximizing lower extremity flow with tolazoline (15mg intra-arterially), nitroglycerin (100µg intra-arterially), or contrast medium. The authors believe that any pressure gradient at rest is significant and that a gradient of ≥15mm Hg after flow augmentation warrants angioplasty of the offending lesion.

PHARMACOLOGIC CONSIDERATIONS

During angioplasty, all of the authors' patients are systemically heparinized. Some angiographers believe that heparin is not essential during angioplasty in high-flow vessels—e.g., the aorta and the iliac and, in many cases, the superficial femoral arteries—but the authors believe heparin is of value, not only for its properties as an anticoagulant, but because of its antithromboxane A effect and thus its antispasm properties. We therefore use this versatile drug routinely. Wolf has shown that the duration of the angioplasty procedure is adequately covered by systemic heparinization with 2500 units, which the authors use routinely except when dealing with the distal vasculature, when we occasionally use 5000 units.[28] With high-flow vessels, if postprocedure bleeding at the groin is a problem, systemic heparinization can be reversed with intravenous protamine on a milligram-for-milligram basis with allowance for the amount of heparin already metabolized. Protamine must be given slowly intravenously. The authors frequently reverse the effects of systemic heparin in patients undergoing angioplasty of large and medium-sized vessels,

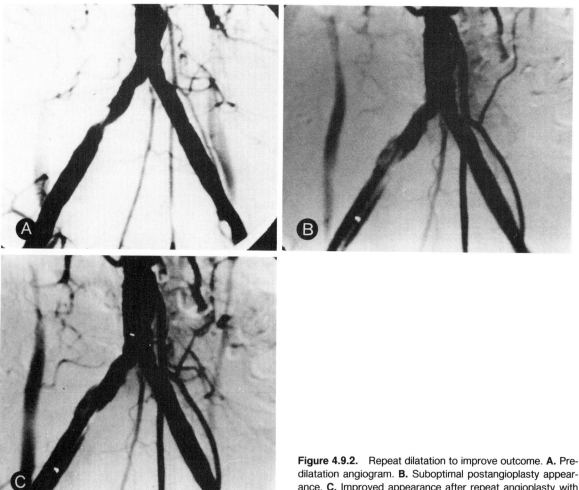

Figure 4.9.2. Repeat dilatation to improve outcome. **A.** Predilatation angiogram. **B.** Suboptimal postangioplasty appearance. **C.** Improved appearance after repeat angioplasty with larger balloon.

whereas patients undergoing angioplasty of vessels below the knee, particularly when the disease is extensive, continue to receive systemic heparin for 48–72 hours afterward. The goal is to maintain the partial thromboplastin time in the therapeutic range of 60–90 seconds. Similarly, whenever flow is compromised after angioplasty, heparin therapy is extended.

Pharmacologic manipulation plays a more important role in angioplasty than is generally appreciated, certainly a more important role than in general diagnostic arteriography. In certain circumstances, drugs other than heparin are invaluable. Useful agents include the following:

1. Lidocaine (Xylocaine);
2. Nitroglycerin (sublingual, transdermal, or as a 100μg intra-arterial bolus);
3. Sublingual or oral nifedipine (10–20mg);
4. Tolazoline (15mg bolus);
5. Papaverine;
6. Prostaglandins;
7. Intravascular verapamil (2.5mg).

Peripheral vessels are surprisingly agile structures, even those one would expect to be relatively rigid and thick-walled secondary to the arteriosclerotic process. There-

fore, it is not uncommon to see severe vasospasm obliterating the vascular lumen around the catheter in the external iliac artery, particularly in women. This phenomenon is also seen in the common femoral artery, and, to some degree, in the superficial femoral artery. Zeitler et al. have noted that significant vasospasm occurred in more than half of their patients in whom a guidewire was placed in the popliteal artery or tibial vessels.[4] To combat such catheter-induced vasospasm, the drug of first choice is nitroglycerin given as a 100μg intra-arterial bolus. This dose may be repeated several times unless systemic hypotension appears. The stimulus to vasospasm is the presence of the catheter and guidewire; once the spasm is broken with nitroglycerin or other drug and the stimulus is removed, it is unlikely that vasospasm will recur. If the operator is concerned about incomplete resolution of vasospasm, transdermal nitroglycerin may be given. Sublingual nitroglycerin also is useful, but its short duration of action makes it less effective than the transdermal form when the patient is away from the cardiovascular laboratory. In the cardiovascular laboratory, the availability and the almost immediate onset of action of intra-arterial nitroglycerin make this agent more attractive than the sublingual form.

Because of the propensity of the popliteal and tibial vessels to respond with spasm to the presence of the guidewire and catheter, the authors routinely premedicate patients scheduled for angioplasty of these vessels with 10–20mg of nifedipine unless there is a contraindication to its use. If the dose is to be given on an on-call basis, it may be given orally; if the drug is to be given when the patient arrives in the cardiovascular laboratory, it is given sublingually. Adequate blood levels are then reached in approximately 10 minutes. The duration of action of nifedipine is 4–6 hours, which is enough for even the most tedious below-the-knee procedures. Patients undergoing below-the-knee procedures also are given at least one 100μg bolus of nitroglycerin as soon as the catheter is placed in the proximal popliteal artery. Nitroglycerin is utilized liberally whenever a spasm is noted.

In the unlikely event that severe vasospasm cannot be controlled with nitroglycerin, intravascular verapamil may be given if one exercises the utmost care. Verapamil is contraindicated in the presence of congestive heart failure or bradyarrhythmias.

The authors have had little success in blocking or reversing vasospasm with papaverine or tolazoline. We have had no experience with prostaglandins as antispasm agents. Intravascular lidocaine has been utilized as an antispasm drug, but the present authors, like Wolf, believe that this drug is of little value in the vascular system, although it is of substantial value as a local anesthetic in the groin.[28] The purpose of lidocaine is to prevent pain, and it belongs where the pain is generated.

Postangioplasty Care

Postangioplasty care in patients treated for lower extremity arterial insufficiency is similar to that given after routine diagnostic arteriography. The patient who has had a groin puncture is returned to a general medical or surgical bed and maintained at bed rest with the leg extended for six hours. The groin is monitored for bleeding, vital signs are monitored, and pulses are checked at frequent, regular intervals. If it was necessary to utilize an axillary approach, the patient is likewise maintained at bed rest, with the arm kept in a sling for 24–48 hours. The axilla is monitored, and the neurologic function of the arm is checked regularly for evidence of brachial plexus dysfunction secondary to an axillary hematoma which, if not promptly cared for, could cause devastating permanent brachial plexus palsy.

ANTIPLATELET THERAPY

All patients receive salicylates for at least six months postangioplasty; the authors believe that salicylates should be maintained indefinitely. We administer 80mg of acetylsalicylic acid (ASA) once daily in combination with 50–75mg of dipyridamole. The optimum dose of ASA is uncertain, particularly when used in combination with dipyri-

damole, and the results of some current clinical studies are being awaited.

EQUIPMENT FOR ANGIOPLASTY

Dilatation Catheters

Although almost all angioplasty today is performed with balloon catheters, other angioplasty catheters are still manufactured and, in certain circumstances, are useful adjuncts. In particular, the Van Andel-type catheter should be available in the cardiovascular laboratory for special situations.

In general, three types of balloon catheters are available from various manufacturers. Balloons are constructed of polyvinyl chloride, polyethylene, or Mylar, and the shafts of the catheters are available in woven Dacron, polyethylene, and polyvinyl chloride.

Initially, the authors approached distal popliteal and tibial angioplasty with the catheters designed for coronary angioplasty. These catheters are available only in 125cm lengths, and for this reason their use is cumbersome via an antegrade puncture down the relatively short superficial femoral artery. New 60–85cm variations of these small angioplasty catheters have become available recently. Although, in the past, the Van Andel-type angioplasty system was used for these distal vessels almost exclusively, this technique has been abandoned for the small ($\leqslant$5Fr) balloon catheters.

Guidewires and Sheaths

Guidewires used for angioplasty are the same as those used for diagnostic angiography, with some additions. Which guidewire to use in a specific situation depends in part on the angiographer's preference. Versatility and the use of meticulous, gentle technique in the manipulation of these guidewires are vital in negotiating lesions, preventing subintimal guidewire passage, and achieving a successful angioplasty.

Sheaths occasionally are valuable. The authors do not routinely use them for what appear to be straightforward aortic, iliac, and femoral angioplasties. However, if the groin is scarred, if entrance through graft material is necessary, or if several catheter exchanges are expected, a sheath is used. Sheaths are routinely used for angioplasty of the vessels below the knee.

TRANSLUMINAL ANGIOPLASTY OF ABDOMINAL AORTA AND PROXIMAL ILIAC VESSELS

The feasibility of dilatation of the abdominal aorta was conceived and implemented successfully at the University of Minnesota in 1980.[29] The aortoplasty was carried out by placing two balloons across the area of stenosis in the distal abdominal aorta, using bilateral retrograde femoral artery

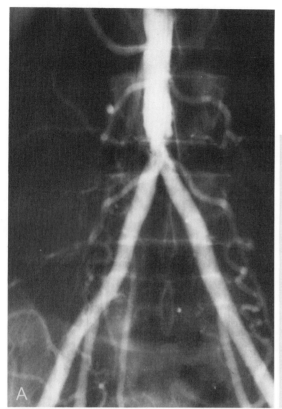

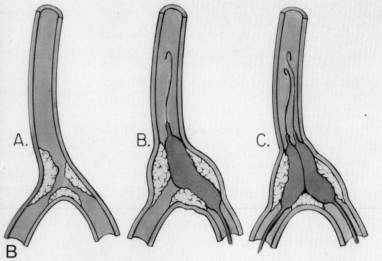

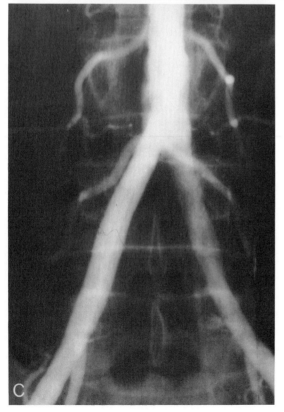

Figure 4.9.3. **A.** High-grade stenosis of distal abdominal aorta extending into the proximal segment of the common iliac arteries. **B.** Diagram illustrating possible mechanism of plaque displacement into contralateral iliac artery by single balloon inflation. **C.** Follow-up aortogram shows a widely patent lumen.

punctures (Fig. 4.9.3). This technique was used to minimize the risk of displacing atheromatous plaque into the contralateral iliac artery if only one balloon was used, which could have caused occlusion of this vessel. Later, the same technique was popularized as the "kissing balloon" technique by Tegtmeyer.[30] This technique is also used to dilate proximal stenosis of the common iliac arteries.

Dilatation of the proximal common iliac arteries has been performed in the following subsets of disease processes:

—Discrete focal abdominal aortic stenosis[30–37];
—Long diffuse aortic stenosis[31];
—Distal aortic stenosis with involvement of the proximal iliac arteries.[30,31,35,37]

Discrete, Focal Abdominal Aorta Stenosis

This disease process is predominantly seen in females at a relatively young age and is commonly associated with a history of heavy cigarette smoking, and it is less common in men.[29,33] Patients usually present with buttock and lower extremity claudication. These patients have commonly normal vessels in the lower extremities, with the only disease being the focal abnormalities in the distal abdominal aorta. Men are frequently afflicted with impotence. Sproul and Pinto suggested that women who are heavy smokers, with small hypoplastic low abdominal aorta segments, are more prone to acquire atherosclerosis in the fourth decade or later.[38] There are frequently associated abnormalities of cholesterol metabolism. Hemodynamically significant, discrete, focal aortic stenoses are best treated with aortoplasty. A nine-year follow-up of a case illustrating the clinical efficacy and patency of aortoplasty on magnetic resonance image (MRI) scanning has been published recently.[39] This patient happens to be a surgeon who refused surgery for the potential complications of aortobifemoral surgery, especially impotence.[29] Similar long-term favorable results were reported from other institutions.[30–35,37]

Yakes described focal, concentric, infrarenal aortic stenosis in four female siblings with familial immune disorders. Three of the four had varying degrees of autoimmune thyroiditis and the fourth was afflicted with rheumatoid arthritis and Sjögren's syndrome. Three of these four patients, despite good initial results, continued to demonstrate clinical obstruction and underwent a second aortoplasty.[31]

Long Diffuse Aortic Stenosis

The experience in this group of patients is very limited and, so far, only one published report has been found in the English literature.[31] Thirteen of 32 patients (41%) had a stenosis 2cm or longer. Seven of 13 patients (22%) had aortic stenoses 4cm or longer. The mean follow-up at 32

months indicated favorable results as demonstrated by mean ankle-arm index (AAI) of 1.01.

Because of the limited experience that has been reported so far in this subset of patients, it goes without saying that diffuse long stenotic lesions with calcifications and ulcerations with or without thrombi are best treated by surgery. It represents a challenge for the interventionalist to select patients with appropriate anatomy who may benefit from aortoplasty. Whenever possible, long diffuse stenosis of the distal abdominal aorta should be subjected to surgery.

Distal Aortic Stenosis with Involvement of Proximal Iliac Vessels

Transluminal angioplasty of distal aortic stenosis with involvement of the proximal segment of the common iliac arteries can be successfully managed with the kissing balloon technique. In the past decade, considerable experience has been gained and several publications attest to these facts.[29–37] As one would anticipate, the majority of these patients have associated inflow and outflow disease, mostly requiring distal reconstructive vascular surgery.

These patients are dilated with two balloons using bilateral retrograde femoral punctures. The balloons have to be long enough to include the segment of iliac artery that needs to be dilated as well as the segment of abdominal aorta requiring dilatation.

Technique of Aortoplasty

Aortoplasty is generally performed by the femoral route. The advantages are obvious when compared with the brachial or axillary approach. The diagnostic angiography is performed through the femoral artery with the stronger pulse. Even pulseless femoral arteries can be successfully cannulated using Doppler ultrasound to locate the femoral artery. The methodology is described under the section of catheterization of occluded iliac segments. Following the diagnostic angiography with a 5Fr pigtail, the morphological appearance is studied. It may require supplemental oblique angiography to evaluate the extent of iliac artery involvement. At times, typical difficulties are encountered for advancement of the guidewires through the stenotic aortic-iliac junction. This can be resolved by redirecting the guidewire with a torque-controlled catheter. A wide variety of guidewires can be used to cross the obstruction, including Bentson, movable core, long tapered straight, hydrophilic coated wires and occasionally a tight J guidewire. Extreme caution should, however, be paid during advancement of a hydrophilic coated wires. Occasionally, the wire can be subintimal; this can go unnoticed since the wire due to its slippery surface can be easily advanced subintimally, up to the level of the abdominal aorta, without feeling any significant resistance, creating,

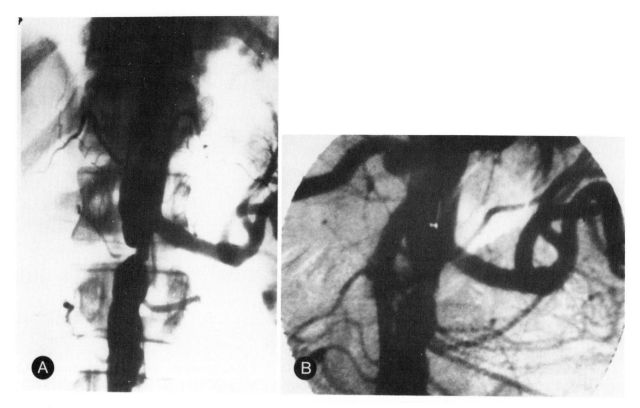

Figure 4.9.4. Stenosis of abdominal aorta before (**A**) and after (**B**) dilatation with single (15mm) aortic angioplasty catheter.

therefore, a subintimal tract. The authors prefer to use a long floppy segment Bentson wire, which is usually atraumatic, since it deflects off eccentric plaques, with minimal risk of subintimal dissection.

Prior to angiography, AAIs are obtained before and after exercise. Exercise AAIs are useful in cases with a history of exertional claudication and physical examination indicating normal or slightly weak pulses. The post-exercise AAI will definitely reveal the abnormality if the lesions are hemodynamically significant. Aspirin (325mg) is started the day before the aortoplasty is to be performed.

In the majority of institutions, the decision to dilate the aorta is made in agreement with the vascular surgeon. The morphological appearance and the pros and cons of aortoplasty versus surgery should be carefully explored prior to subjecting the patient to balloon dilatation.

Roadmapping capabilities and digital subtraction angiography greatly facilitate the procedure. The subtracted image will allow the angiographer to safely direct the guiding catheter and guidewires beyond the obstruction.

If the anatomy of the lesion dictates the use of a dual balloon technique, instead of a single balloon dilatation, the opposite femoral artery is catheterized and once the lesion is crossed, 5000 units of heparin is administered. Sizing of the balloon for effective dilatation is extremely crucial. The diameter of the dilating balloon should be equal to the diameter of the aorta above or below the level of the obstruction. Although there is an inherent magnifi-

cation of 10-20%, on cut film angiography, the measured diameter determines the size of the balloon or balloons to be used. The resultant effect is stretching of the aortic wall slightly beyond its normal size. The aorta can be effectively dilated by the introduction of one, two, or three catheters, depending on the diameter of the aorta. If the lesion is infrarenal and well above the bifurcation, a single balloon catheter of larger diameter will suffice to complete dilatation (Fig. 4.9.4). The availability of 10, 12, and 15mm balloon catheters, on 8 and 9Fr shaft diameters, greatly facilitates balloon dilation of the aorta. If the lesion involves the distal abdominal aorta and the proximal common iliac arteries, obviously the dual balloon technique has to be implemented (Fig. 4.9.5).

Kumpe described the theoretical advantage of placing three balloons across the lesion, arguing that the configuration of the inflated balloons conforms better to the shape of the aorta than two balloons placed side by side and inflated simultaneously. Obviously, this requires placement of balloon catheters from each femoral artery and from the left brachial and/or axillary artery approach.[40] The authors feel that undertaking angioplasty with more than two balloons is unnecessary, in addition to the increased risk of axillary catheterization using large balloons.

Prior to the dilation, measurements of pressure above and below the stenosis are routinely obtained. The balloons are inflated simultaneously two or three times for

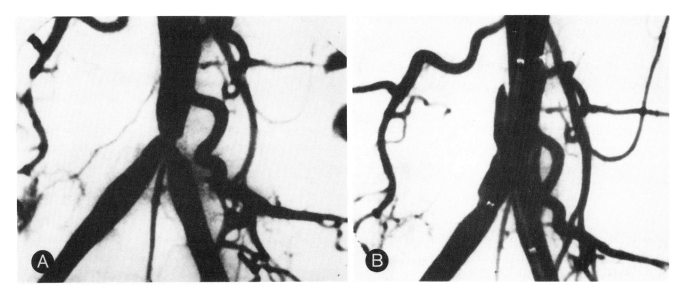

Figure 4.9.5. Appearance of distal aortic disease before (**A**) and after (**B**) dilatation with two balloon catheters.

30–45 seconds. Compression of the femoral arteries each time the balloons are deflated will help to direct any debris or emboli into the hypogastric circulation where they could be tolerated without clinical symptoms.[29]

The end point of balloon inflation is the disappearance of the waist in the balloon during inflation. Pressure measurements are routinely obtained after the aortoplasty along with follow-up arteriograms, preferably using a 5Fr catheter. The circulating heparin is reversed with protamine sulfate administered slowly. Traditionally, for each 1000 units of heparin, 10mg of protamine sulfate is required. If the procedure lasts for one hour, usually only half the initial dose of heparin is circulating; this is the amount that will need to be neutralized with protamine sulfate for effective hemostasis. Patients are placed on aspirin (325mg daily) for life and are encouraged to quit smoking and to start on a vigorous exercise program.

DISCUSSION

The revascularization of aortic iliac disease can be accomplished by surgical endarterectomy, aorto-bifemoral bypass, or by balloon aortoplasty. In surgical circles, aorto-bifemoral bypass is favored over the endarterectomy procedure. Bifemoral bypass was introduced in 1953,[39,41] and the patency rates are 80–90% at 5 years and 60–80% at 10 years, according to numerous studies.[39] The operative mortality of aorto-bifemoral procedure is 2–4%,[39] and the average hospital stay is eight days.[42] The morbidity associated with aorto-bifemoral bypass graft includes infection (2–4%), anastomotic pseudoaneurysms (1.4–8.2%), femoral neuropathy (3.4%), aortic-enteric fistulae (0.5%), and impotence. Other complications include renal failure,

local infections, peripheral embolization (trash foot), and spinal cord ischemia.[39] Impotence is one of the major complications of the bypass surgery and may occur in up to 11–30% of the patients.[43–47] It is caused by the dissection and division of parasympathetic nerve fibers at the aortic bifurcation region.

Obviously, comparisons between surgery and the limited aortic-iliac aortoplasty data are difficult due to the small number of aortoplasties that have been reported. At the time of writing, aortoplasty is indicated for discrete, focal aortic stenosis with or without involvement of the proximal iliac vessels. The experience with diffuse, long stenotic lesions is limited,[31] and therefore an endorsement of aortoplasty for this subset of patients cannot be made. Individual judgments can be made by interventionalists in cases of severely diseased, diffuse, ulcerated long stenotic lesions. A safe alternative in these patients is aorto-bifemoral bypass procedure.

Balloon aortoplasty is attractive and easy to implement. However, it requires caution. The law of Laplace indicates that for a given dilation pressure, wall tension is proportional to the vessel diameter, which means that large vessels are dilated at a lower pressure and may rupture at lower pressures.[32]

Blue Digit Syndrome

The blue digit syndrome is characterized by sudden onset of *p*ain and *p*urple discoloration of the digits in the presence of *p*alpable peripheral pulses ("3 Ps" of the blue digit syndrome").[48]

The cyanotic areas can affect the lower legs, toes, hands, or fingers and are clearly demarcated from the adjacent normally perfused skin.[49] The pathological alterations are attributed to atherotomatous and/or embolization of fibrinoplatelet aggregates.[50-52] In the past, Flory[53] and Hoye et al.[54] recognized the embolic events to the visceral organs and to the peripheral vessels stemming from the ulcerated atherosclerotic plaques. Recently, the blue digit syndrome has been discussed by Karmody et al., and they have indicated close similarities of the clinical manifestations of the blue digit syndrome and transient ischemic attacks of the brain.[55] These episodes can be termed ischemic episodes of the foot or hand. It has been stressed in surgical literature that in more than 50% of the cases, recurrences can appear and may result in amputation[52,55] Therefore, the blue digit syndrome should be treated as a limb salvage situation, as in other entities, such as rest pain or gangrene.[55]

Atherosclerotic lesions in the aorta, iliac, or femoral vessels can result in macro- or microembolization. Large mural thrombi can be a source of macroemboli and can produce acute symptoms. The thrombi that are surgically retrieved are either white or pinkish-white depending upon the degree of organization. Histologically, the white thrombus is made up of different amounts of platelets and fibrous material.[56] This clinical situation demands prompt aggressive treatment. The smaller microemboli may represent either cholesterol plaques[52] or exuberant fibrinoplatelet debris from ulcerated atheromatous plaque.[55]

These emboli breaking off from an upstream lesion can occlude the small vessels in the hand and foot. Detailed magnification angiography is required to demonstrate such lesions. However, angiography is seldom practiced in patients with blue digit syndrome with intact pulses and well perfused extremities. Cholesterol systemic embolization is presented in many different ways and has been called "the great masquerader."[49,57] Atheromatous plaque in the aorta may erode through the intima, ulcerate, and discharge cholesterol emboli into downstream distant peripheral circulation. It can cause renal failure, hypertension, gastrointestinal hemorrhage, diarrhea, transient ischemic attacks, and myocardial infarctions.[58]

Cholesterol emboli in the legs can cause microinfarcts of the skin, recognized as livedo reticularis. In patients with digital ischemia from cholesterol emboli, the peripheral pulses are intact. When the peripheral circulation is affected, it may mimic diffuse vasculitis or hypersensitivity angiitis. Cholesterol microembolizations to the lower legs can cause nocturnal aching, muscular cramps, and restless shuffling.[59] The biopsies demonstrate occlusion of arterioles with needle-shaped clefts containing cholesterol crystals.[52,54,59] Secondary to chronic inflammation, there is lymphocytic infiltration, thickening of the media and intima, and eventual fibrosis leading to end-stage fibrosis.[54,59] On the basis of clinical symptomatology alone, it is difficult to differentiate between cholesterol emboli or fibrinoplatelet aggregates causing the blue digit syndrome. Systemic cholesterol embolization is easily differentiated from unilateral blue toe syndrome on a clinical basis.

ETIOLOGICAL FACTORS

The blue digit syndrome may be seen in the following pathological states:

1. In the upper extremity, the source of emboli is aneurysms of the subclavian artery, bypass grafts, and radial and ulnar arteries. The mural thrombi secondary to compression from the cervical or anomalous first rib might generate the emboli (thoracic outlet syndrome). The atherosclerotic plaques from stenotic lesions of the subclavian arteries might also embolize to digital arteries.[60]
2. Diffuse ulcerative lesions of the abdominal aorta and iliac vessels with or without aneurysms. Stenotic and occlusive lesions of the femoral-popliteal system can also shower microemboli into the distal digital vessels accounting for the blue digit syndrome.[48,49,51,52,55,61-65]
3. Rarely, the thrombotic material in false aneurysms of the thoracic aorta can also shower emboli accounting for the blue toe syndrome manifestations.[66]
4. Nonatherosclerotic lesions such as fibromuscular dysplasia of external iliac arteries can also generate emboli.[67]

TREATMENT

The traditional treatment for blue digit syndrome has been surgical eradication of the embolic source. This includes surgical endarterectomy, arterial incision with interposition of synthetic grafts, and bypass procedures with interruption of the diseased arteries proximal to the distal anastomosis, thereby preventing further embolization through an intact arterial conduit.[48,50,52,55,61,62,65,67-69]

In patients with multilevel atherosclerotic ulcerative or occlusive disease, the treatment of peripheral ulcerated lesions on the superficial femoral or popliteal arteries prior to the eradication of central aortic disease has been recommended.[67] This is the reverse order of conventional treatment of occlusive disease where proximal lesions are bypassed first to increase the pressure head and improve the collateral flow. The reason for primary management of peripheral lesions is based on the need to treat the peripheral ulcerated lesions with viable thrombi as the source of embolization.[62]

A lateral abdominal aortogram is extremely helpful in detecting the mural thrombi or posterior aortic wall ulcers that are responsible for showering distal emboli.[56,62,64]

So far, the role of angioplasty has been limited and controversial. Kumpe et al. have recommended angioplasty to be followed by antiplatelet therapy of the offending iliac or femoral-popliteal lesions as a sole therapy of treatment in a subset of patients with certain identifiable characteristics.[49] Those patients have the following findings:

1. Few clinical episodes of microembolization;
2. No evidence for macroembolization and acute ischemia;

3. No systemic cholesterol embolization or livedo reticularis affecting the extremity;
4. Hemodynamically significant high-grade stenotic lesions (over 90%);
5. No radiographic evidence for diffuse ulcerations of the aorta;
6. Patent tibial peritoneal run-off without significant occlusive disease.[49]

The hemodynamically significant stenotic lesions cause turbulence and create shear forces that cause clumping and adherence of platelets to the vessel walls.[70]

Therefore, hemodynamic correction of the lesions without eradication or exclusion by bypass surgery may prevent recurrent emboli that may ultimately threaten the limb.[49] In a series published by Wingo et al.,[48] in at least half of the patients with blue digit syndrome, abnormal ankle-arm indices were noted. However, in this series they have also included patients with distal tibioperoneal occlusive disease. Therefore, the exact number of patients that can benefit from proximal angioplasty is difficult to determine without collection of extensive data on this subset of ischemic vascular disease. Kumpe et al. treated 10 patients with angioplasty, and 9 were clinically improved immediately with no untoward emboli.[49] One patient showed no improvement, despite angioplasty of the superficial femoral artery, because of occlusion of all the three vessels below the knee joint. Seven patients had long-term follow-up with an average of 28 months. Four patients remained stable and three exhibited hemodynamic deterioration. Out of the three patients, one underwent femoropopliteal bypass and two remained stable. One patient showed recurrent embolization two months after dilatation. The presumed source in this patient was a small infrarenal abdominal aortic aneurysm.

In a series by Brewer et al.,[63] 15 atherosclerotic lesions in a group of 12 patients were identified. These were the presumed source for the blue digit syndrome. Six of the fifteen lesions were treated with antiplatelet drugs or anticoagulation for 6–12 weeks followed by angioplasty. Three of the fifteen lesions were treated by surgery, three with long-term anticoagulation, and one with transcatheter aspiration and angioplasty. Two of the fifteen lesions that were treated with immediate anticoagulation had significant complications. Brewer et al. recommend delayed PTA, following the antiplatelet and anticoagulation therapy.[63] The rationale behind this approach is to allow the clot to organize and get firmly attached to the arterial wall. Those authors do not recommend immediate angioplasty because of the theoretical risk of distal embolization of the thrombus.

The choices for anticoagulation in high-flow stenotic lesions are aspirin and dipyridamole. This is based on the finding that the white thrombus is related to clumping of platelets. In occlusions with poor run-off, fibrin seems to

contribute to clot formation, and the most effective drugs in this situation are heparin and warfarin.[63]

The two patients that were treated with immediate fibrinolytic therapy had serious complications from systemic lytic states. The authors recommend delayed PTA following antiplatelet therapy as the safest approach.[63] Angioplasty removes the source of emboli and restores the physiologic circulation.

Common and External Iliac Artery Stenoses

The common and external iliac arteries are ideal for angioplasty. The best approach is the most direct approach, which, in most cases, is ipsilateral retrograde catheterization. As noted previously, the authors utilize Doppler data to select the approach for diagnostic arteriography. When the Doppler data indicate a common or external iliac artery stenosis, the diagnostic arteriogram is performed from the ipsilateral approach in expectation of an angioplasty procedure immediately after the diagnostic procedure provided that renal function is not severely compromised. If the diagnostic arteriogram reveals a long segment of external iliac artery that appears severely narrowed, to the degree that the lumen of the vessel is filled by the diagnostic catheter and no contrast medium is visible until the level of the common femoral artery, the diagnostic catheter is retracted over a 0.025-inch guidewire with a Y adapter, and $100\mu g$ of intra-arterial nitroglycerin is administered via the catheter at the origin of the external iliac artery. A small volume of diluted contrast medium is then injected with the catheter parked in the common iliac artery, and digital images are acquired; these usually reveal a relatively focal stenosis uncovered by the ablation of vasospasm by the nitroglycerin (Fig. 4.9.6). Once an iliac artery stenosis has been demonstrated, provided the lesion does not involve the origin of the common iliac artery or the common iliac bifurcation and clearly is hemodynamically significant, a single appropriate size balloon catheter is placed within the distal aorta after exchange over a soft guidewire for the diagnostic catheter.

With the balloon catheter in the distal aorta, 2500 units of heparin is administered intra-arterially. The soft-tip guidewire is then placed in the distal aorta below the renal arteries but well above the aortic bifurcation. The radiopaque markers designating the balloon position are placed within the stenosis, which, in the iliac system, usually is easy to locate without contrast medium because of the available bony landmarks. The balloon is inflated slowly to its maximum diameter and then to its maximum permissible pressure with diluted contrast medium and maintained in this state for one to two minutes even if there is an initial waist in the balloon that "pops." After deflation of the balloon, a documentary arteriogram should be obtained. If digital capabilities are available, a high-quality study can be obtained with a simple manual injection of contrast

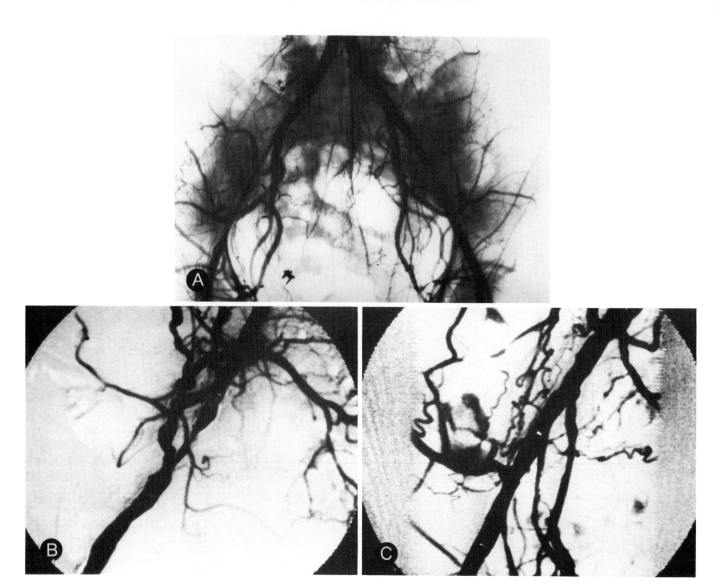

Figure 4.9.6. Spasm giving false impression of extent of disease. **A.** Apparent long-segment obstruction of external iliac artery. **B.** After relief of spasm with 100μg of nitroglycerin, focal stenosis is revealed. **C.** Postangioplasty appearance.

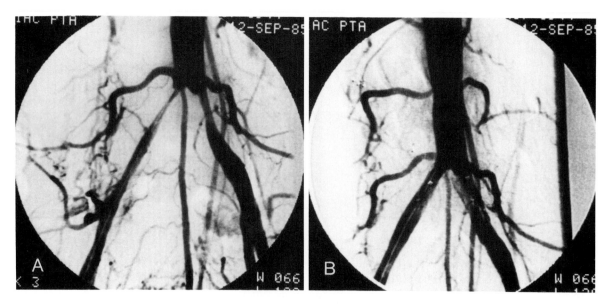

Figure 4.9.7. **A.** Long stenosis of right common iliac. **B.** Successful common iliac angioplasty; injections made by hand through angioplasty catheter.

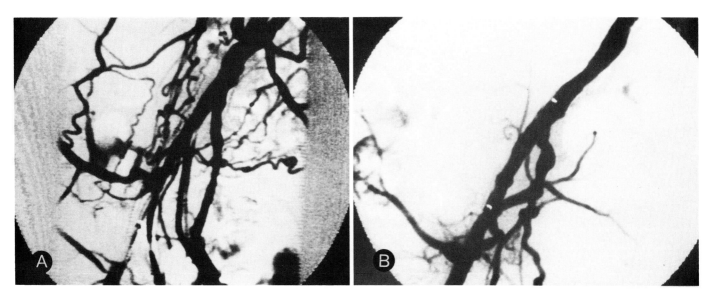

Figure 4.9.8. Digital subtraction examinations made during manual injection of contrast medium documenting appearance of external iliac lesion before (**A**) and after (**B**) angioplasty.

medium through the angioplasty catheter (Figs. 4.9.7 and 4.9.8). If digital techniques are not available, it is advisable to place a multihole catheter in the distal aorta and obtain a spot-film or cut-film arteriogram.

Never inject through an end-hole catheter in the vicinity of an angioplasty site. The risk of lifting the fractured intima-media is significant and may convert a successful angioplasty procedure into a catastrophe (Fig. 4.9.9). The documentary arteriogram should always be obtained with the catheter tip remote from the angioplasty site.

If the stenosis revealed by arteriography is of uncertain hemodynamic significance by anatomic criteria, then it is appropriate to obtain pressure measurements to confirm the significance of the lesion before angioplasty. This is accomplished by placing a 0.025-inch guidewire in the dis-

tal aorta and retracting the catheter across the stenosis into the iliac artery. Pressure measurements are particularly useful after flow augmentation to maximize any gradient that may be present. If a gradient cannot be documented, angioplasty should not be performed. There is no justification for prophylactic angioplasty of lesions without hemodynamic significance.

The authors are less likely to use pressure measurements to determine if an angioplasty procedure is complete. The goal is to create a normal, or near normal, lumen caliber, and we therefore rely on angiographic data to determine if there is need for additional dilatation. A residual stenosis of >30% in any projection in a patient who experienced only mild discomfort during balloon inflation is enough to warrant exchanging the original angioplasty catheter for

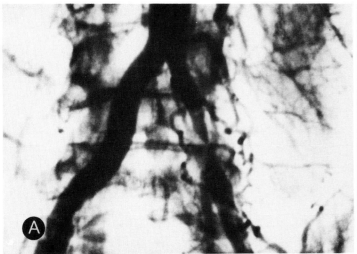

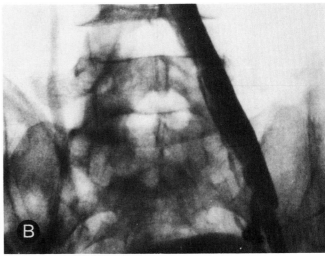

Figure 4.9.9. Complication of postangioplasty radiographic study. **A.** Preangioplasty appearance of high-grade iliac stenosis. **B.** Postangio-plasty injection of contrast medium creates extensive dissection secondary to elevation of intima-media at angioplasty site by jet of fluid.

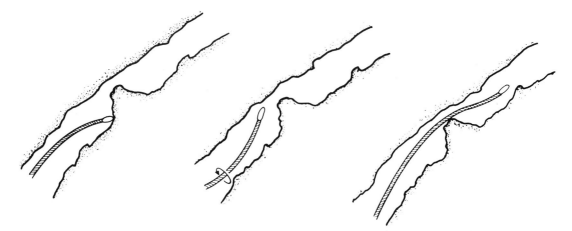

Figure 4.9.10. Use of 15mm J guidewire to negotiate simple iliac stenosis.

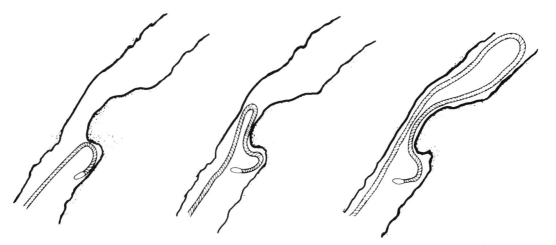

Figure 4.9.11. Bentson wire is so soft that it will deflect off eccentric, undermined lesions with little risk of intimal elevation or subintimal passage.

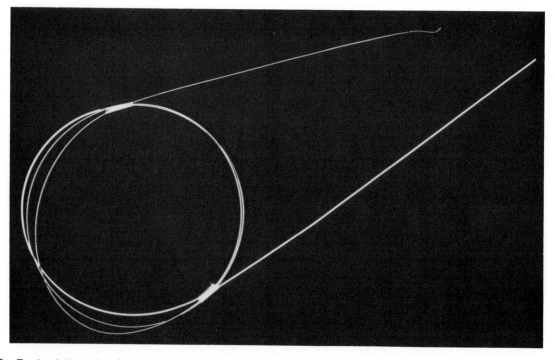

Figure 4.9.12. Torsional attenuating diameter guidewire; at base, wire is 0.035 inch; tip tapers to 0.018-inch floppy segment (Advanced Cardiovascular Systems; Mountain View, CA).

one with a balloon 1.0mm larger and repeating the procedure. In this case, it is important to inflate the balloon slowly; if the patient experiences severe discomfort, further inflation should be approached with exceptional care. Excruciating pain is highly suggestive of excessive vessel trauma, and the goal of an optimum anatomic result probably should be abandoned.

Iliac angioplasty can be a quick (<10 minutes) procedure, or it can be an extremely time-consuming, tedious procedure. Difficulties in performing iliac angioplasty are largely the result of the need to traverse complex, tortuous, ulcerated, highly diseased segments of the artery. Many solutions to this common problem have been offered. The author prefers one of the following. The initial attempt to negotiate the artery is made with a standard 0.035- or 0.038-inch 15mm J guidewire. These wires are, to some degree, "steerable" and may traverse the vessel with relative ease. If this fails, the authors generally place a simple curved catheter with a "hockey-stick" configuration in combination with a 15mm J wire and attempt to steer through the diseased segment(s) of the vessel (Fig. 4.9.10). If the vessel is severely ulcerated with multiple eccentric lesions, a Bentson wire is used in combination with the catheter because of its soft distal segment (Fig. 4.9.11). The authors have recently begun to use the Wholey steerable guidewire (Advanced Cardiovascular Systems, Mountain View, CA) to negotiate highly diseased iliac arteries and have found it extremely useful. It is available in several configurations. We would use it more often were it not for its high cost. When dealing with near occlusions and with vessels that are severely ulcerated and tortuous, the authors have used a combination of the hockey-stick catheter and a guidewire tapered from 0.035 inch at its base to 0.018 inch at its distal 4.0cm segment (Advanced Cardiovascular Systems). This tip is not of the traditional

"safety wire" configuration but has a densely opaque platinum tip. It is ultrasoft and appears to be the least traumatic guidewire available today (Fig. 4.9.12), but, again, its expense precludes its routine use. When all else fails, this guidewire may salvage the procedure. An alternative to the tapered wire is a combination of a 0.018-inch floppy platinum-tip guidewire as the core of an "injectable" guidewire (USCI, Billerica, MA). This guidewire is used in a 0.038-inch configuration, providing the needed rigidity for the passage of iliac angioplasty catheters.

Negotiation of complex pathologic anatomy in the iliac system or femoral-popliteal-tibial system is greatly facilitated by digital roadmapping.

Lesions at the orifice of the common iliac artery may be dealt with using a single balloon catheter and the ipsilateral retrograde approach (Fig. 4.9.13). However, many of these lesions resist angioplasty, and it appears that placement of a second, contralateral balloon catheter and simultaneous inflation of the two balloons in the orifices of the common iliac arteries buttresses the balloon on the diseased side, helping to create the desired intimal-medial cleft and produce a successful angioplasty (Fig. 4.9.14). The authors have not encountered occlusion of the nonstenotic common iliac artery when using the ipsilateral approach with a single catheter for a common iliac artery orifice lesion, although published experiences would indicate that this occurs.[71] If the radiologist is concerned about the risk of occluding the contralateral iliac artery, it may be reasonable to pass a small diagnostic catheter into the distal abdominal aorta from the contralateral vessel to provide access in the event that angioplasty of one iliac artery orifice results in occlusion of the opposite side. With this access, any occlusion can be reversed quickly merely by exchange for an angioplasty catheter and simultaneous balloon inflation within the iliac artery orifices.

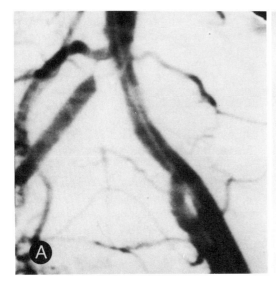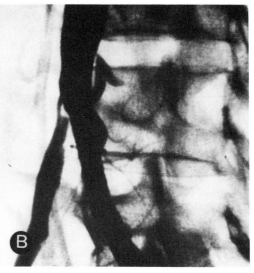

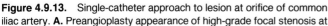

Figure 4.9.13. Single-catheter approach to lesion at orifice of common iliac artery. **A.** Preangioplasty appearance of high-grade focal stenosis at orifice of common iliac artery. **B.** Appearance after angioplasty with single catheter from ipsilateral approach.

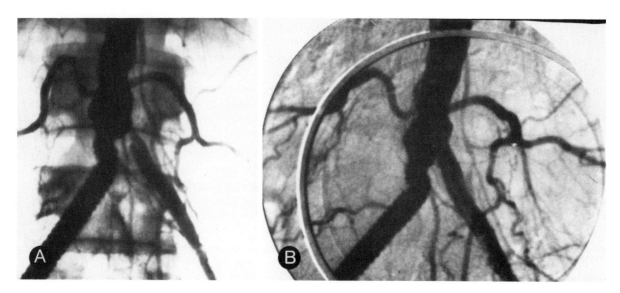

Figure 4.9.14. Two-catheter approach to lesion at orifice of iliac artery. **A.** Preangioplasty appearance of iliac orifice lesion. **B.** Appearance after angioplasty utilizing bilateral catheters.

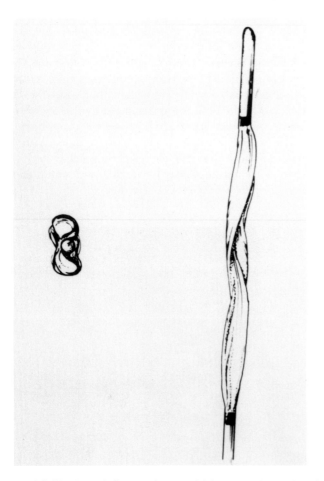

Figure 4.9.15. Large balloons, when not tightly wrapped around shaft of catheter, will have "wings," which are designed to be tightly wrapped in clockwise or counterclockwise fashion around shaft. This will minimize trauma at puncture site.

Upon completion of an iliac angioplasty, it is the authors' habit to reverse part of the effect of the systemic heparinization. This is accomplished, as previously noted, with intravenous protamine, allowing for a 30% drop in heparin activity within the first hour after its administration.

Insertion and removal of the large-caliber balloon catheters should be done with considerable care. The catheter should be inserted and extracted while suction is applied with a large-bore syringe to ensure that the balloon hugs the catheter shaft as tightly as possible. Some manufacturers wrap the "wings" of the balloon around the catheter shaft and designate that catheter as wrapped for clockwise or counterclockwise insertion. Be aware of the design of the catheter of your choice, and if it is appropriate to rotate it as it is passed through the groin tissue and vessel wall, be sure it is being rotated in the proper direction (Fig. 4.9.15).

Hypogastric Artery and Common Iliac Bifurcation

Angioplasty at any bifurcation may create a noncolinear intimal-medial cleft that spirals an intimal flap into the orifice of the untreated vessel, causing a temporary, or even a permanent, occlusion (Fig. 4.9.16). In the case of the common iliac artery bifurcation, the authors feel that it is optimal to protect the hypogastric artery even if it does not have a significant stenosis at its origin. To do this, angioplasty is accomplished by bilateral retrograde catheterization of the common femoral arteries. On the ipsilateral side, the appropriate size balloon catheter is placed within the stenosis using bony landmarks as guide. The contralateral femoral artery is catheterized with a catheter suitable for passage of a guidewire and catheter system around the

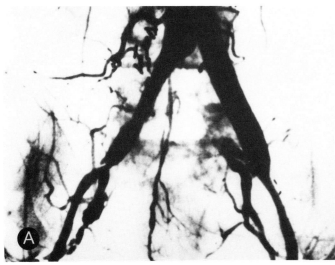

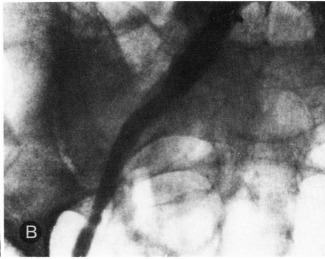

Figure 4.9.16. Insufficient extent of dilatation leading to arterial occlusion. **A.** Preangioplasty arteriogram demonstrating stenosis at bifurcation of common iliac artery in patient after aortoiliac bypass surgery. **B.** Failure to perform angioplasty on both the hypogastric and iliac arteries results in occlusion of hypogastric artery.

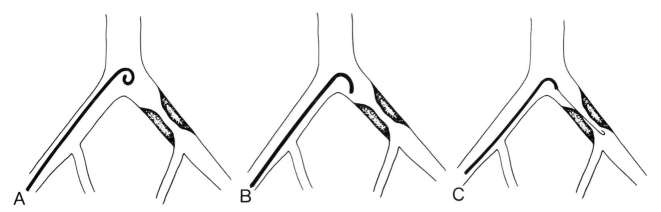

Figure 4.9.17. Use of pigtail catheter to engage contralateral iliac orifice.

aortic bifurcation. This crossover technique can be accomplished in at least three ways:

1. A pigtail catheter is used to engage the orifice of the contralateral common iliac artery. The guidewire is then passed down the contralateral iliac system.[72] Occasionally, it may be passed directly into the hypogastric artery, greatly facilitating quick placement of a balloon catheter there (Fig. 4.9.17).

2. A Simmons-type curved catheter is used to engage the contralateral common iliac artery origin after the catheter has been reformed in a more proximal branch of the abdominal aorta or in the descending thoracic aorta.[73] However, the primary segment of the Simmons catheter may not be long enough to facilitate passage into the hypogastric artery (Fig. 4.9.18). Therefore, we prefer to:

3. Form a loop with a cobra catheter[74] and use this in conjunction with a Bentson wire to negotiate the orifice of the contralateral common iliac artery and ultimately the hypogastric artery (Fig. 4.9.19).

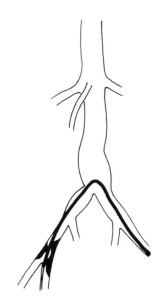

Figure 4.9.18. Use of Simmons-type catheter to engage a contralateral iliac orifice.

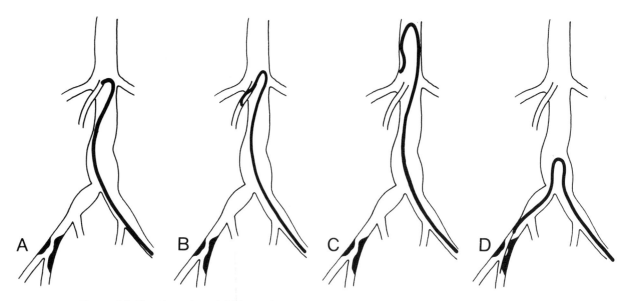

Figure 4.9.19. Formation of Waltman loop with cobra catheter to engage contralateral iliac system.

Once the hypogastric artery has been entered, if the aortic bifurcation is not extremely acute, a heavy-duty, 15mm, 0.038-inch J guidewire is placed in the hypogastric artery. Angioplasty of the diseased common iliac bifurcation is performed, and a control arteriogram is obtained using digital techniques and injecting through the angioplasty catheter while a guidewire is left in the hypogastric artery (Fig. 4.9.20). If there is no evidence of compromise of the orifice of the hypogastric artery, the procedure is considered complete, heparinization is reversed, and the catheters are removed. If there is a stenosis of the hypogastric artery, or if there is evidence of compromise of the hypogastric artery after angioplasty of the iliac bifurcation, an appropriate size balloon catheter is placed around the aor-

tic bifurcation over the heavy-duty guidewire and inflated simultaneously with the catheter in the common iliac artery bifurcation. Digitally acquired images are again reviewed, and if the angioplasty result is satisfactory, heparinization is reversed and the catheters are removed as previously described (Fig. 4.9.21).

If the aortic bifurcation is acute and the contralateral approach is being used for whatever reason—be it for hypogastric angioplasty or because the angiographer desires, for anatomic reasons, to approach a common external iliac artery this way—the authors find either the Amplatz wire (Cook, Inc., Bloomington, IN) or the Wholey wire to be very helpful. The stiffness of the shaft of these wires greatly facilitates passage of catheters around an

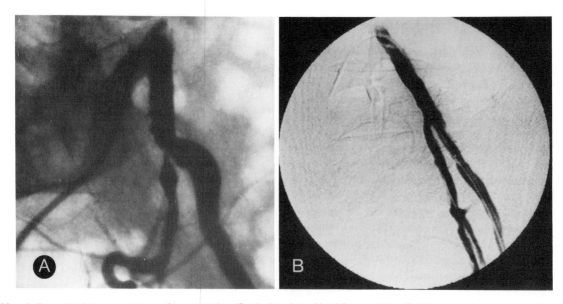

Figure 4.9.20. **A.** Preangioplasty appearance of hypogastric orifice lesion viewed in oblique position. **B.** Intra-angioplasty examination with guidewire in hypogastric artery and angioplasty catheter retracted.

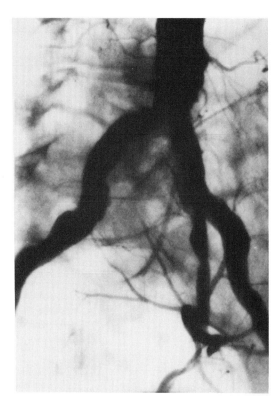

Figure 4.9.21. Postangioplasty appearance of a common iliac bifurcation-hypogastric orifice lesion.

acute aortic bifurcation. The Wholey wire offers the additional advantage of being steerable and permitting relatively easy negotiation of stenotic lesions.

When the contralateral approach is used for iliac disease in general, and the catheter tends to buckle into the abdominal aorta rather than to follow the guidewire

around the aortic bifurcation, if the guidewire can be advanced to the groin, manual compression of the common femoral artery will entrap the guidewire and reduce the likelihood of such buckling (Fig. 4.9.22).

When the contralateral approach is used for angioplasty of the common iliac bifurcation and there is a rigid stenosis at the hypogastric origin, the balloon placed ipsilaterally may be inflated gently at the orifice of the common iliac artery and pulled down slightly to force the hypogastric catheter through the stenotic origin (Fig. 4.9.23).

The interventional radiologist is uniquely equipped to revascularize the hypogastric system for patients who suffer hip and buttock claudication.[75] In addition, angioplasty of the proximal hypogastric artery or its pudendal branch has, in a few patients, helped in the management of vasculogenic impotence.[76] It is unreasonable to perform angioplasty at the common iliac bifurcation and to ignore a diseased hypogastric artery.

Occluded Common Iliac Arteries

There is significant controversy as to the role, if any, of PTA in the management of occluded iliac arteries. A recent publication of Piotrowski et al. concluded that aortobifemoral bypass graft is the treatment of choice for unilateral iliac artery occlusion, even though a hemodynamically significant occlusion is not present on the contralateral

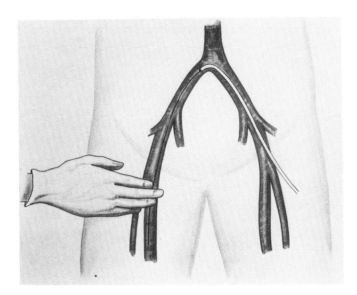

Figure 4.9.22. Entrapment of guidewire at groin by manual compression provides more rigid track for catheter to follow and decreases likelihood of buckling in aorta.

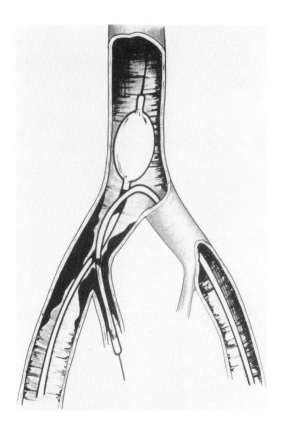

Figure 4.9.23. Gentle traction on ipsilateral catheter with balloon inflated forces contralateral catheter to pass into hypogastric artery.

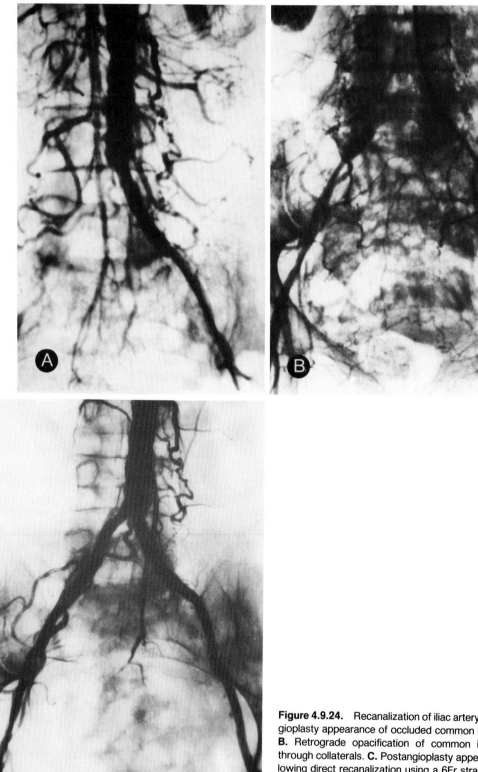

Figure 4.9.24. Recanalization of iliac artery. **A.** Preangioplasty appearance of occluded common iliac artery. **B.** Retrograde opacification of common iliac artery through collaterals. **C.** Postangioplasty appearance following direct recanalization using a 6Fr straight Teflon catheter advanced in combination with a Rosen guidewire through the occluded segment.

side. This recommendation was done on the face of a morbidity of 34% and a mortality of 3%, with patency rates of 89% at five years with an open superficial femoral artery (SFA) and of 72% with a closed SFA.[77] Percutaneous recanalization with a guidewire and catheter followed by balloon angioplasty has a primary success rate of 66% and a three-year patency rate of 85%.[78] No complications were reported. In Schwarten's experience with 100 patients, primary success was obtained in 60% with no complications. It is clear that an attempt to recanalize and dilate the occluded iliac artery is warranted before the patient is subjected to the risk of a surgical procedure.

Technique

Puncture of the "pulseless" common femoral artery in the presence of occlusive or stenotic iliac disease can be accomplished with relative ease by:

Palpation of the nonpulsatile thick-walled artery (in slender patients);
Fluoroscopic observation of the femoral head and puncture of the artery, which is almost always located over the medial third of the femoral head. Any calcification in the vessel wall may facilitate the puncture;
Doppler localization of the vessel[79]; or
Injection of contrast medium, if a catheter is present in the distal aorta from a diagnostic procedure performed via the contralateral approach, to cause collateral opacification of the common femoral artery, which can then be punctured. Roadmapping is also very useful to guide the puncture.

Schwarten reports success in approximately 60% of attempted direct recanalizations using the Rosen guidewire introduced by the ipsilateral approach in combination with a straight Teflon catheter. The catheter and guidewire are advanced as a unit through the occluded segment (Fig. 4.9.24). Failure to achieve recanalization is almost invariably secondary to subintimal passage of the guidewire, which has not, in the author's hands to date, caused significant complications.

Failure to recanalize is also due to the inability to advance the balloon catheter over a guidewire across the stenosis. A technique to circumvent this technical problem was described by Gaines, Loose, and Saibil.[80–82] Bilateral punctures enable placement of sheaths in both common femoral arteries. Using a sidewinder catheter to cross the obstruction, a guidewire is negotiated across the obstruction in the iliac artery and the wire is then advanced into the catheter placed from an ipsilateral approach. In the Saibil and Loose report, the ipsilateral wire is then pushed forward into the abdominal aorta.[80,81] Subsequently, the kissing balloon technique is used to dilate. In Gaines' technique,[82] the contralateral wire is advanced until it exits through the introducer sheath, establishing a wire loop. The kissing balloon technique is used to dilate. This technical modification is useful in those cases in which attempts

to recanalize the occluded iliac artery resulted in subintimal dissection.[82] Ginsburg proposed a modification to the wire-loop approach, by using a snare to trap a wire passed across an area of occlusion, subsequently pulling the wire across the contralateral femoral sheath.[83] This technical modification of the wire loop is recommended in those cases in which a wire can be passed across the occluded segment, but a balloon catheter cannot be advanced over the wire. With a through and through wire a balloon can be pulled across the obstruction without much effort.[83]

Ring et al. have reported contralateral embolization during attempts at direct recanalization of occluded common iliac arteries.[84] Schwarten has not seen this problem in >100 patients in whom he has performed direct recanalization. He, however, attempts the procedure only in patients with what appear to be relatively straight iliac arteries with short-segment occlusions and relatively nondiseased distal abdominal aortas (Fig. 4.9.24).

Although the authors have had modest success with direct recanalization of the occluded common iliac artery, the incidence of contralateral embolization cannot be ignored. Thus, it would seem that the best approach to angioplasty of the occluded common iliac artery is to catheterize the contralateral common femoral artery, place a 4–5Fr Simmons catheter in the abdominal aorta, wedge its tip in the orifice of the occluded vessel, and infuse a thrombolytic agent in an attempt to uncover the stenosis, which may be suitable for angioplasty (Fig. 4.9.25).[85] It goes without saying that this should not be attempted unless the angiographer is thoroughly familiar with the use of thrombolytic agents.

Using thrombolytics, Motarjeme reported an increased success rate in recanalizing occluded iliac arteries from 25 to 81%.[86] Debulking of iliac artery occlusions after recanalization with the Simpson atherocath prior to PTA has been reported by Maynar et al.. The success rate at two years was 70%.[87] Rees et al. discussed the use of balloon expandable stents in the management of complete occlusion of the iliac artery following successful recanalization.[88] Long-term follow-up showed a patency rate of 90%. One acute occlusion due to thrombosis of the stent was successfully treated with thrombolytics.[88]

Common Femoral Artery

Lesions of the common femoral artery are frequently related to previous surgery. When atherosclerosis is present, the lesions are frequently thick, heavily calcified, and eccentric and may not yield optimally to balloon angioplasty. In contrast, lesions at graft anastomoses are usually caused by intimal hyperplasia and respond readily to angioplasty.

Transluminal angioplasty of the common femoral artery usually requires a contralateral approach with passage of a catheter around the aortic bifurcation using one of the methods previously described. This approach is not unrea-

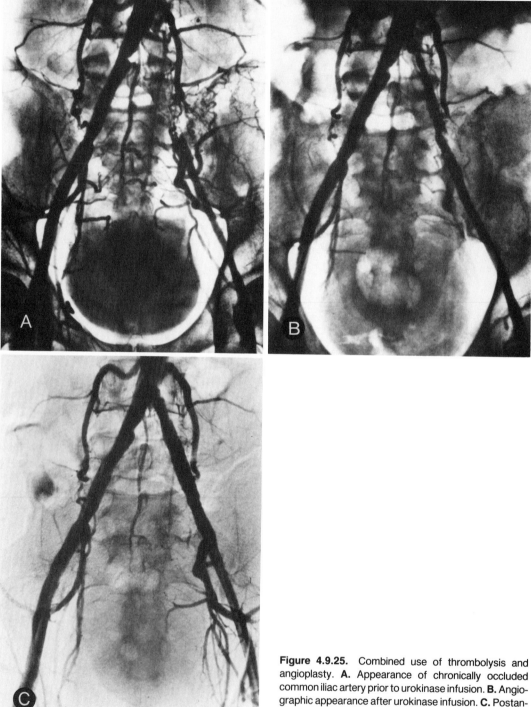

Figure 4.9.25. Combined use of thrombolysis and angioplasty. **A.** Appearance of chronically occluded common iliac artery prior to urokinase infusion. **B.** Angiographic appearance after urokinase infusion. **C.** Postangioplasty arteriogram. (Courtesy of Barry T. Katzen, M.D.)

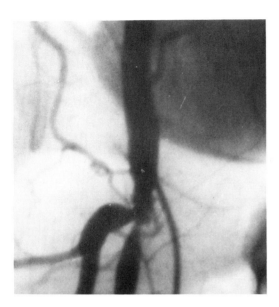

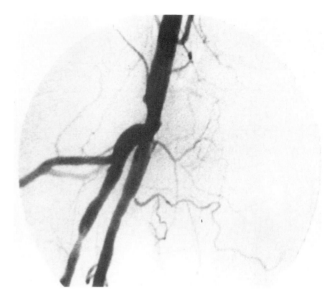

Figure 4.9.26. Dilatation at common femoral bifurcation. Preangioplasty appearance of common femoral bifurcation lesion.

Figure 4.9.27. Postangioplasty appearance; two balloon catheters were used.

sonable for stenotic disease of the proximal and mid-common femoral artery, particularly in patients who are high surgical risks. The authors are reluctant to undertake angioplasty of the bifurcation of the common femoral artery with a single catheter because of the potential for occlusion of either the superficial or the deep femoral artery if the procedure creates a nonlinear intimal-medial cleft (Figs. 4.9.26 and 4.9.27). The occluded common femoral artery is not suitable for angioplasty because it is unlikely that the forces necessary to traverse the occlusion can be generated via the contralateral approach, inasmuch as the catheter tends to buckle into the abdominal aorta when forward force is applied in the groin.

Surgical management of common femoral artery disease is a well established procedure that usually can be done at low risk.[89] Thus, it seems unwise to attempt angioplasty of this vessel in most circumstances.

Superficial and Deep Femoral Artery Stenoses

The optimal approach to stenoses of the superficial and deep femoral arteries is an ipsilateral antegrade common femoral puncture, which may be the most difficult maneuver for the interventional radiologist with little experience. The difficulties are related to:

—Patient's obesity;
—Shorter segment of common femoral artery (normally, it measures between 2 and 4cm);
—Too high and steep puncture above the inguinal ligament, resulting in uncontrollable bleeding;
—A lower puncture below the common femoral bifurcation which may result in a pseudoaneurysm formation.[90]

Several techniques have been proposed to enter the common femoral artery in an antegrade fashion with the

sole purpose of advancing the guidewire into the superficial femoral artery for PTA. These techniques will be summarized briefly.

Antegrade puncture requires that the skin of the abdominal wall be entered above the inguinal ligament, whereas the needle enters the common femoral artery below the ligament (Fig. 4.9.28). In obese patients, this can be extremely difficult; it is frequently helpful to retract the panniculus cephalad and medially. For angiographers beginning their experience, it may be beneficial to observe the groin area fluoroscopically with the needle poised for puncture to ascertain the level at which the needle tip will enter the artery in order to avoid puncturing the vessel proximal to the inguinal ligament. Puncture below the

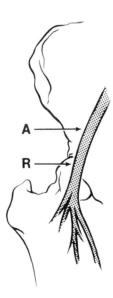

Figure 4.9.28. Bony landmarks and their relations to skin entrance sites for antegrade (*A*) and retrograde (*R*) punctures.

Figure 4.9.29. Comparative angles for needle approach for antegrade (*A*) and retrograde (*R*) punctures.

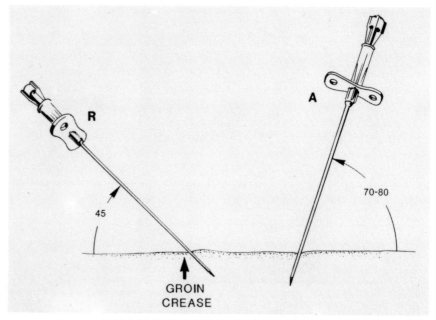

common femoral bifurcation increases the risk of a groin hematoma. Of necessity, the angle of puncture of the common femoral artery is steeper when using the antegrade than the retrograde approach (Figs. 4.9.29*A,B*). Once the common femoral artery has been entered, it is helpful to depress the hub of the needle against the abdominal wall to elevate the tip when it is the angiographer's desire to enter the superficial femoral artery. If the needle hub is not depressed, the natural tendency of the guidewire will be to enter the deep femoral artery (Fig. 4.9.30).

Because all of these maneuvers need to be done under fluoroscopy, the possibility of exposing the operator's fingers to direct radiation should be kept in mind during the procedure. Tight coning of the fluoroscopy field, partial protection with lead gloves and utilization of roadmapping techniques for guiding the wire into the superficial femoral artery are some helpful recommendations.

The common femoral artery is usually 2–4cm long and lies anterior to the head of the femur, below the inguinal ligament. The artery usually bifurcates at the level of the inferior margin of the femoral head, and below its bifurcation it is unprotected posteriorly by the bony pelvis. The artery should be entered above its bifurcation; effective hemostasis can then be achieved by compressing the vessel against the femoral head. The transition of the external iliac artery into the common femoral artery occurs below the inguinal ligament. The demarcation can be identified on angiograms by noting the origins of the inferior epigastric and deep circumflex iliac artery, immediately above the ligament. Anatomically, the inguinal ligament demarcates the caudal extension of the peritoneal cavity, and extends from the anterosuperior iliac spine to the pubic tubercle. The external inguinal crease does not represent the inguinal ligament and therefore cannot be used as a landmark for the puncture technique. The bifurcation of the common femoral artery occurs at the same level in 3.5%, below the crease in 20%, and above it in 76.5% of the cases.[91]

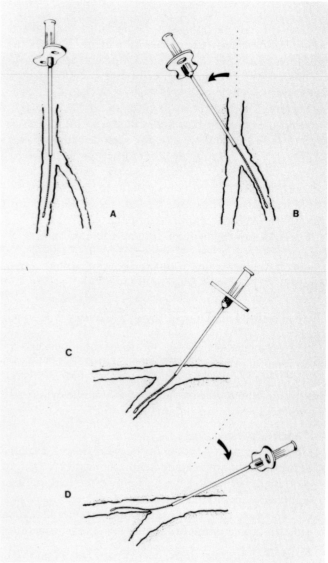

Figure 4.9.30. Manipulations of needle hub permit angiographer to direct needle tip toward superficial or deep femoral artery.

In cases of high bifurcation of the common femoral artery, only a short segment of the common femoral artery can be punctured safely. In such situations, direct puncture of the superficial femoral artery is recommended.[92] Hemostasis can be safely achieved in these cases by compressing the superficial femoral artery against the femoral head. Placement of a guidewire into the superficial femoral artery from the contralateral approach facilitates the puncture. It can be used as a target and the needle is inserted along the course of the target wire. It is recommended to separate the deep and superficial femoral arteries by placing the patient in ipsilateral anterior oblique position prior to the puncture.[92]

Antegrade catheterization of the superficial femoral artery can be accomplished by utilizing a movable-core straight or J guidewire.[93] If the wire enters the deep femoral artery, a 5.0Fr vessel dilator or a short 45° angle catheter is advanced over the wire. Under fluoroscopy, the catheter is withdrawn to the common femoral artery level aided by the injection of short bursts of contrast medium or by digital roadmapping. The core of the wire is withdrawn about 10cm, and the wire is advanced until the softer, outer spring coil falls into the superficial femoral artery. The core is readvanced to stiffen the guidewire and then the dilator or the short guiding catheter is advanced over the wire.

A directional needle with a closed pencil-point tip and a distal sidehole has been proposed by Hawkins et al., as another method of placing the guidewire into the superficial or deep femoral arteries.[94] The needle is either 18-, 19-, or 20-gauge, the vessel is entered at an angle of approximately 90°, and both walls are punctured. Slow withdrawal into the lumen is identified by the exit of blood, and then a guidewire is advanced into the superficial femoral artery. The authors claim that advancement of guidewires or catheters is not difficult at a 90° angle of entry. The 90° exit angle minimizes the risk of subintimal injury, which can occasionally be encountered with standard bevelled needles. If the wire seeks the deep femoral artery, it is simply retracted and the needle is torqued in such a fashion that the exit angle points anteromedially toward the origin of the superficial femoral artery.

In difficult cases, a retrograde puncture can be utilized to direct an accordion catheter into an antegrade position.[95] A 4.0Fr accordion catheter, with a long distal tip and designed with a sidehole 10cm from the tip, is used. A monofilament is strung in a continuous loop, and when it is retracted the sidehole is oriented 180° from the direction of the catheter tip.[95] The catheter is retracted until the sidehole is in the common femoral artery just above the puncture site. A stiff 0.018-inch mandrel guidewire can be advanced until it exits through the sidehole in the U-shaped segment of the catheter. Once the guidewire enters the superficial femoral artery, the accordion catheter is removed and the appropriate guiding or balloon catheter is advanced. The authors believe that this technique protects the operator's hands from radiation hazard. The 4.0Fr catheter is equivalent to the diameter of an 18-gauge needle; the smaller diameter easily accommodates to tight curves and reforms into a U shape with retraction of the monofilament.

A needle set with a preshaped catheter has been proposed as another method of catheterizing the superficial femoral artery in an antegrade fashion. This set consists of a 19-gauge needle with a stylet and a short 30° preshaped catheter.[96] The catheter is loaded onto the needle, the puncture is made in the usual fashion, and its location is determined with contrast injections. The needle is retracted and the catheter is rotated into an anteromedial direction to seek the superficial femoral artery. This rotation is facilitated by designing the catheter with a wing-like steering base.

Saddekni et al. proposed a modified Cope dilator for antegrade catheterization of the superficial femoral artery.[97] Following the antegrade puncture, it is not unusual for the guidewire to seek the deep femoral artery, in spite of every effort being made to advance it into the superficial femoral artery. The modified Cope introducer has both an end hole and a sidehole about 6cm from the distal end. The introducer is preshaped into a hockey stick configuration. The introducer is advanced over the wire into the deep femoral artery. The sidehole is oriented anteromedially opposite the bend in the introducer. The introducer is gradually withdrawn until the sidehole reaches the common femoral artery and faces the superficial femoral origin. The location should be confirmed by the injection of contrast material. A tight 1.5mm J guidewire or a Bentson floppy-tipped wire is then advanced through the sidehole into the superficial femoral artery. This system has been used by many interventionalists with great success.

A retrograde puncture can be converted to an antegrade catheterization of the superficial femoral artery by the utilization of a sidewinder catheter.[98] The loop of the sidewinder catheter can be reformed in the aortic arch and it is withdrawn into the common iliac artery with the tip facing the lateral wall. This avoids inadvertent entry into the hypogastric artery which originates medially. As soon as the catheter reaches the common femoral artery, the tip is rotated medially and the catheter is withdrawn slowly. The tip of the catheter advances into the origin of the superficial femoral artery. This concept has been further modified by the introduction of a loop catheter with a long tip.[99] On the same principles, a double-curved triangular catheter with a primary curve of 135° and a secondary curve of 35° was introduced.[100] This catheter easily reforms into the abdominal aorta and has little tendency to re-open the loop in the iliac artery. In cases of failure of entry into the superficial femoral artery by antegrade methods, a retrograde catheterization via the popliteal artery was proposed by Tonnensen et al.[101] Antegrade approach can become difficult or fail in obese patients, stenotic or occluded origins of the superficial femoral artery, and in patients with high origins of the superficial femoral artery. In cases of proxi-

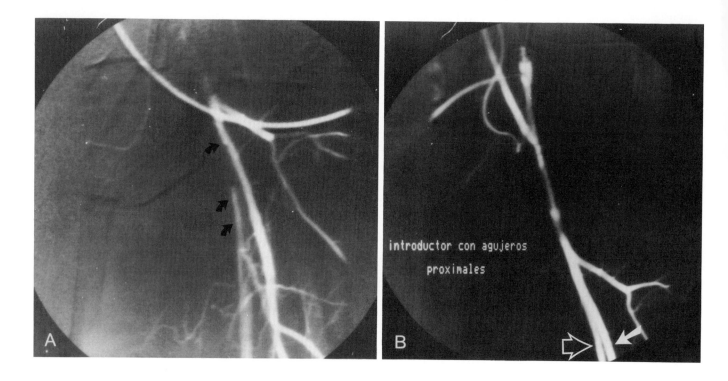

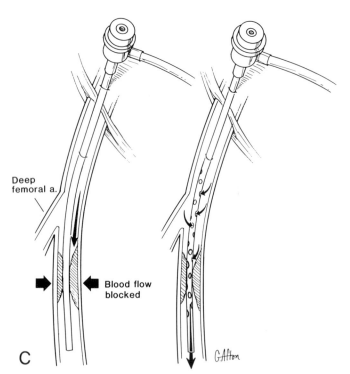

Figure 4.9.31. **A.** Sheath placement through a high-grade stenosis of the proximal superficial femoral artery causes complete block of blood flow *(arrows).* **B.** Sheath with sideholes allows flow through the sheath into the distal superficial femoral artery. **C.** Diagrammatic representation of complete occlusion caused by placement of sheath through area of high-grade stenosis of the proximal superficial femoral artery *(left).* Flow preservation using sheath with sideholes *(right).*

mal stenosis of the superficial femoral artery, the catheter or sheath placement across the area of narrowing can cause total obstruction of blood flow (Fig. 4.9.31*A*). In these cases a modified sheath with sideholes can be used to allow flow of blood through the sheath into the distal femoral artery (Fig. 4.9.31*B*).

Popliteal Artery Puncture

Retrograde catheterization of the superficial femoral artery through a popliteal approach might facilitate the advancement of guidewires or laser probes in cases of failure of an antegrade catheterization.[101-103]

The femoral arteries are catheterized from the contralateral groin approach and the patient is placed in a prone position. The puncture of the popliteal artery is technically easy if it can be seen fluoroscopically by contrast injections of the femoral artery. The roadmapping is extremely useful in these situations.

The popliteal artery lies in the popliteal fossa and is separated anteriorly from the femur and the knee joint by muscles. On its lateral aspect, superiorly is the biceps femoris muscle and below is the lateral head of the gastrocnemius. On its medial aspect, superiorly, is the semimembranosus, and, inferiorly, is the medial head of the gastrocnemius. Posteriorly, the artery is covered by the semimembranosus superiorly and the gastrocnemius inferiorly. The midsegment of the popliteal artery is separated from the skin by fat and is crossed from lateral to medial by the tibial nerve and the popliteal vein. The vein is interposed between the artery and the posteriorly placed nerve.

The artery can be entered if the puncture is made in the medial aspect of the fossa above the knee joint. The tibial nerve and the popliteal vein can be avoided since they cross the artery from lateral to medial at the inferior aspect of the popliteal fossa.

The skin over the vessel is infiltrated with Xylocaine and a small incision is made. The vessel is entered, using a 19-gauge thin-wall needle and preferably using a single-wall puncture. A 0.025-inch guidewire can be advanced through the needle and a 5Fr working sheath is placed in the vessel lumen. Hemostasis after angioplasty may be difficult because of the deeper placement of the vessel and the loose tissue around the artery.[101-103] In 2 of 50 angioplasties carried out using a popliteal approach, two painful hematomas were encountered.[11]

The hematomas are a potential problem and may be minimized by neutralizing the effects of heparin with protamine sulfate following a successful procedure.[101]

Deep Femoral Artery

Angioplasty of the deep femoral artery should be performed using an ipsilateral or contralateral approach. Uncommonly, an axillary or brachial approach is necessary. Dacie described the use of a retrograde ipsilateral femoral artery approach.[104] This approach is indicated when a PTA from an ipsilateral approach is unsuccessful, because of obesity, high division of the common femoral artery close to the inguinal ligament, or postoperative scarring of the groin. A sharp-angled aortic bifurcation and severely diseased and tortuous iliac vessels make a contralateral approach difficult or impossible.[104] If the ipsilateral retrograde femoral approach is used, the arterial puncture must be at a sufficient distance from the PTA site so as not to dilate the arterial entry site during balloon inflation.[104] Renal tip balloon catheters are preferred which have the balloon located as close as possible to the tip, thus minimizing the chance of trauma to distal branches of the deep

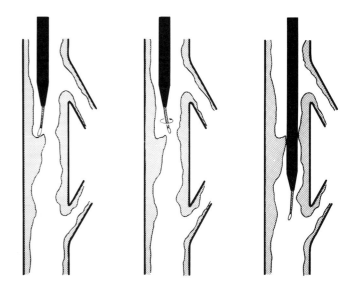

Figure 4.9.32. Use of 15mm J-curve guidewire to negotiate superficial femoral stenosis.

femoral artery beyond the treated area. One should give careful consideration to deep femoral angioplasty when that artery is the sole collateral source in a nonthreatened limb in a patient with an occluded superficial femoral artery. Angioplasty of the deep femoral artery also may be a useful adjunct to iliac angioplasty, particularly in high-risk patients with peripheral ischemia.[105,106]

Bony landmarks may be of some help in angioplasty of the superficial and deep femoral arteries, as may be calcification observed at fluoroscopy. When these landmarks are not available for locating the stenotic lesion, it is necessary to place towel clips or other opaque markers at the site of the stenosis, as determined by the injection of a small volume of contrast medium through the first dilator placed in the vessel to be treated. An opaque ruler also may be used to mark the lesion(s).

Once the stenosis has been located in either the superficial or the deep femoral artery, crossing the lesion with a guidewire is undertaken. As in the iliac system, our first choice is the 15mm, 0.035- or 0.038-inch J guidewire (Fig. 4.9.32).[20] This somewhat steerable wire frequently negotiates uncomplicated stenoses with surprising ease. Alternatives include the Bentson wire, the Wholey wire, and the Amplatz wire. The authors have found the previously described 0.035-inch wire tapered to a 0.018-inch soft platinum tip useful in negotiating extremely high-grade ulcerated lesions, where the risk of subintimal wire passage is high (Fig. 4.9.33).

After the stenosis has been negotiated, a catheter with a balloon of appropriate diameter and length is advanced over the guidewire and positioned within the lesion. The guidewire is removed, and a small volume of contrast medium is injected to ensure intraluminal position. Heparin is administered, and the guidewire is reinserted and parked in the distal superficial femoral artery or the distal

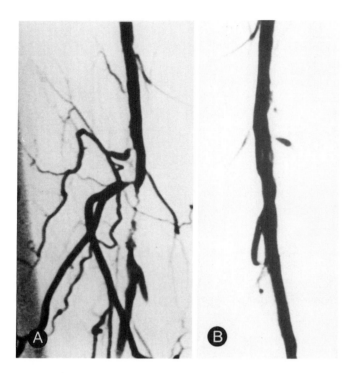

Figure 4.9.33. Dilatation of irregular segment lesion. **A.** High-grade irregular segment superficial femoral artery stenosis negotiated with torsional attenuating diameter guidewire. **B.** Postangioplasty appearance.

deep femoral artery. The balloon is inflated slowly to its maximum diameter with diluted contrast medium and then to its maximum pressure, and inflation is maintained for 60–120 seconds. If a standard end hole angioplasty catheter is used and the angiographer desires to document the appearance of the angioplasty site before removing the dilating system, a 0.025-inch guidewire may be parked in

the distal vessel during the angioplasty. Alternatively, after angioplasty, the dilating catheter may be retracted and, with the use of a Y adapter, contrast medium can be injected manually and digital images are acquired to assess the immediate appearance of the vessel (Fig. 4.9.34). If the result is satisfactory, the system can be removed, the heparin reversed, and hemostasis obtained at the groin. If the result is not satisfactory, the catheter can be advanced over the 0.025-inch wire to a point distal to the angioplasty site. The wire is then replaced with a larger diameter wire to facilitate exchange for an angioplasty catheter with a larger balloon or for a catheter permitting higher pressures for repetition of the procedure. It is essential that a guidewire be left well distal to the angioplasty site until the angiographer is certain that the procedure is complete (Fig. 4.9.35), because any attempt to recross a freshly dilated site risks intimal dissection and vessel occlusion.

When dealing with multiple stenoses in the same vessel, all of the lesions should be negotiated with the guidewire; angioplasty should begin with the most distal lesion, working toward the most proximal lesion. More than one catheter may be necessary because of the increasing diameter of the vessel.

Two angioplasty catheters are available that permit injection of contrast medium without the necessity of inserting a 0.025-inch guidewire. Barth's design[107] has two sideholes distal to the balloon and a relatively long catheter tip (Fig. 4.9.36).[72] He believes that this catheter is useful, not only for postangioplasty angiographic checks, but also for negotiating lesions while injecting contrast medium. The other catheter, devised by Ricketts, has a sidehole proximal to the balloon (Fig. 4.9.37). Simple use of a side-arm adapter over a conventional 0.035- or 0.038-inch

Figure 4.9.34. Appearance of focal superficial femoral artery stenosis before (**A**) and after (**B**) angioplasty.

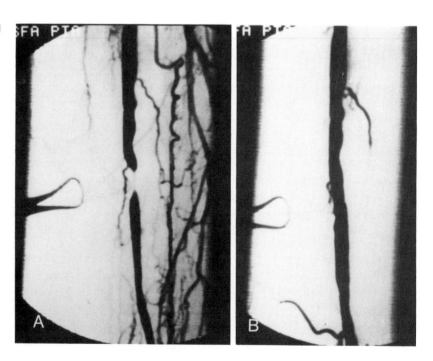

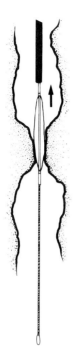

Figure 4.9.35. If balloon is not centered precisely, it may retract or advance spontaneously during inflation. For this reason, among others, it is always wise to leave guidewire well distal to angioplasty site until procedure is complete.

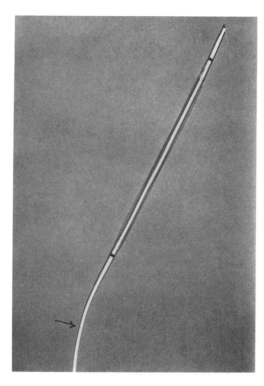

Figure 4.9.37. Angioplasty catheter with sidehole proximal to balloon *(arrow).*

guidewire also permits injection of contrast medium, which will exit through the sidehole and provide adequate images of the angioplasty site, particularly if digital techniques are used.[108] In this way, the anatomic result can be ascertained before catheter removal.

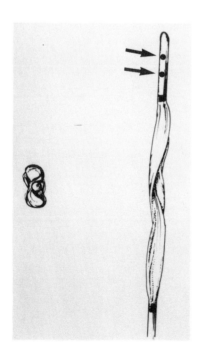

Figure 4.9.36. Angioplasty catheter with sideholes distal to balloon *(arrows).*

Occasionally, it is nearly impossible to advance the angioplasty catheter over a conventional guidewire through an extremely tight, rigid femoral artery stenosis; the catheter and guidewire buckle in the groin, and no forward progress can be made. This is a particular problem in the obese patient. In this circumstance, it may be helpful to:

Insert a sheath into the femoral artery to provide additional support for the catheter to prevent buckling in the groin;

Use a heavy-duty Amplatz- or Wholey-type guidewire for additional support;

Manually support and compress the groin tissues;

Advance a heavy-duty guidewire into the popliteal artery and then manually compress the artery, entrapping the guidewire and providing a more rigid system for the catheter to follow.

The same maneuvers may be helpful if the initial insertion of the angioplasty catheter is difficult, e.g., because of groin obesity or scar tissue. If these measures fail, it may be useful to attempt PTA with a Van Andel-type catheter, which has a more rigid shaft.

Rarely, it is necessary to approach femoral artery stenoses contralaterally around the aortic bifurcation. Any of the techniques for passing a catheter around the bifurcation can be employed. A catheter with a longer shaft may be necessary to reach a distal lesion. In general, the authors avoid this approach.

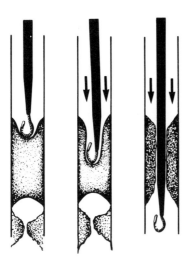

Figure 4.9.38. Method of advancing guidewire-catheter combination through superficial femoral artery occlusions.

Occluded Superficial Femoral Arteries

Successful angioplasty of occluded superficial femoral arteries requires ipsilateral antegrade femoral artery puncture, inasmuch as it generally is impossible to achieve the desired forward forces from the contralateral approach because of catheter buckling in the abdominal aorta. Antegrade catheterization is performed, and a 6Fr straight Teflon catheter is advanced into the proximal superficial femoral artery over a flexible-tip guidewire. The proximal and distal limits of the occluded segment are identified with opaque markers or other landmarks.

Several methods for recanalizing occluded segments of the superficial femoral artery have been described, including attempts to pass a Bentson- or a Newton-type straight guidewire through the occluded segment and the use of a movable core straight guidewire, alternately advancing and retracting the core to stiffen the tip of the wire as it passes through the occluded segment. The authors prefer to use a Rosen-type guidewire advanced as a unit with a catheter through the occluded segment (Fig. 4.9.38), because we have tried all the above-mentioned methods and believe that the incidence of subintimal passage is lowest with the Rosen wire-catheter combination. Once the occluded segment has been bridged, the guidewire is removed, and, after confirmation of the position of the catheter tip with a small volume of contrast medium, heparin is administered. The guidewire is inserted and parked in the distal superficial femoral artery, and the procedure is completed as when dealing with a simple stenosis (Fig. 4.9.39). As with previously described procedures, after completion of the angioplasty, the heparin is usually partly reversed unless runoff is poor or a low-flow state exists, and hemostasis is obtained at the groin.

ARTERIAL OCCLUSIVE DISEASE
BELOW THE KNEE

Up until now, angioplasty below the knee has been reserved for patients with threatened limbs.[109-116] The introduction of steerable guidewires and low-profile balloon catheters along with the administration of potent vasodilators has vastly improved the technical results and

Figure 4.9.39. Appearance of occluded superficial femoral artery before (**A**) and after (**B**) recanalization and angioplasty.

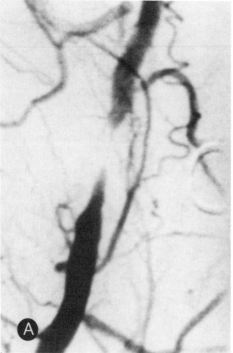
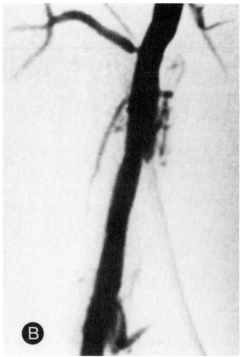

clinical outcome. Because of this, there has been a tendency lately, in selected cases, to perform angioplasty in the tibioperoneal vessels for lifestyle-limiting claudication.[109] It has also been recommended in patients with severe claudication (Stage IIB Fontainne Classification) to improve the outflow following proximal recanalization.[110] The experience is, however, limited, and a larger volume of data is necessary to support the performance of small vessel angioplasty in patients with severe claudication. Strict criteria are needed, however, since complications of infrapopliteal angioplasty have potentially severe consequences. Zeitler noted a high incidence of popliteal artery vasospasm during angioplasty of the popliteal artery and its branches and suggested the use of lidocaine intra-arterially to minimize or eliminate vasospasm.[117] Transluminal angioplasty in the infrapopliteal vessel was performed initially with Van Andel-type dilators. The use of these dilators produced effective recanalization; however, there was an unacceptable degree of shear force, denuding long segments of intima, which predisposed to acute postangioplasty thrombosis and later to a high incidence of recurrent disease.

The development of low-profile balloon catheters similar to the coronary balloons that can accommodate a 0.014–0.018-inch guidewire with a soft platinum tip has facilitated the management of small vessel disease below the knee.[109–114]

The interventionalist should carefully screen and select the patients who may benefit from the recanalization procedure. Anatomic indications for infrapopliteal angioplasty include:

1. Single or multiple focal stenoses;
2. Short (less than 4cm) occlusions.

The anatomical contraindication to infrapopliteal angioplasty is the presence of long segmental occlusions with a patent vessel distally.[118] Frequently, limb salvage recanalization involves dilatation of all the stenotic or occluded vessels.[110]

Materials and Methods

Whenever possible, diagnostic angiography should be performed from the contralateral femoral approach, preferably utilizing balloon occlusion technique for exquisite detail.[119] The contraindications to angioplasty include morbid obesity, acute ischemia, and, obviously, a nonthreatened limb. The clinical indications for angioplasty are the presence of ischemic rest pain, ischemic ulcerations or gangrene, and an ankle-brachial index of less than 0.4. Infrapopliteal angioplasty is performed with 4.3Fr catheters with balloon diameters of 2.0–3.5mm used in conjunction with a steerable 0.018-inch platinum-tipped guidewire.

Routinely, 10–20mg of sublingual nifedipine is administered prior to the procedure. After the superficial

femoral artery is cannulated, 5000 units of heparin is administered intra-arterially. Supplemental heparin is administered at 2000 units/hr, if the procedure is prolonged. For patients with infrapopliteal disease, systemic heparin therapy is maintained for 24–72 hours after the procedure. Patients are subsequently maintained on aspirin at a dose of 325mg daily.

Technique of Angioplasty

The technique of infrapopliteal angioplasty is relatively straightforward. Antegrade puncture of the common femoral artery is performed in the usual fashion and a sheath is advanced into the superficial femoral artery over a J guidewire. If there are superficial femoral or popliteal artery lesions, these should be dilated prior to the small vessel angioplasty. The presently available low-profile balloon catheters are equipped with different diameter balloons, ranging from 2 to 3.5mm. Prior to the angioplasty, a 200µg bolus of nitroglycerin is administered intra-arterially. Angiographers performing infrapopliteal angioplasty should be familiar with the use of vasodilator drugs such as:

1. Nifedipine: 10–20 mg orally or sublingually prior to the procedure;
2. Nitroglycerin: 100–200µg intra-arterial bolus as needed;
3. Transdermal nitroglycerin patches;
4. Verapamil: 2.5–5 mg.

Needless to say, patients should be carefully monitored for hypotension during the administration of vasodilators.

The low-profile catheter and the 0.018-inch guidewire are advanced together through the sheath. The location of the balloon with respect to the lesion can be determined by small injections of contrast medium through the side port of the sheath. More commonly, state-of-the-art roadmapping is used, with the real-time image superimposed on the digitally subtracted vascular image, greatly facilitating the location and crossing of the obstruction with the guidewire and balloon.[109,110]

Preshaping the distal end of the guidewire to a gentle curve facilitates the catheterization of the tibioperoneal arteries. Once the balloon is placed across the area to be dilated, the balloon is inflated to its maximum diameter and maintained at its maximum diameter/pressure for 90–120 seconds (Fig. 4.9.40). Following the dilatation, follow-up angiography is obtained, leaving the guidewire across the stenosis and retracting the balloon catheter proximal to the site of dilatation. Contrast medium is injected through the sidearm of the sheath and digital images are obtained. If a suboptimal result was obtained, redilatation can be performed by simply advancing the balloon over the guidewire or by using a larger diameter balloon. Alternatively, a balloon on the wire can be used to dilate. If several stenoses are to be dealt with, the most distal lesion is dilated first and then the more proximal lesions (Fig. 4.9.41).

Figure 4.9.40. Appearance of focal peroneal-tibial trunk stenosis before (**A**) and after (**B**) angioplasty with 3.5mm balloon.

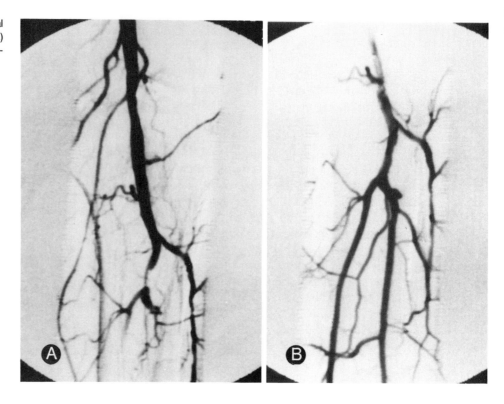

If vasospasm is a problem despite nifedipine and nitroglycerin, multiple boluses of intra-arterial nitroglycerin can be administered, bearing in mind that the patient should be monitored constantly for systemic hypotension (Fig. 4.9.42). For the rare spasm that is not relieved by nitroglycerin, intravascular verapamil may be administered if there is no contraindication to its use.

Upon completion of the procedure, the balloon catheter and guidewire are removed. Systemic heparinization is maintained for 48–72 hours.

Occlusions of the Distal Popliteal and Tibial Arteries

Angioplasty of distal vascular occlusions is considered only for limb salvage. The patient is premedicated with nifedipine, and the procedure is begun in the same fashion as for stenotic disease. Once the sheath is in the superficial femoral artery, a straight 5Fr Teflon catheter is advanced into the popliteal artery. With the catheter tip in this artery, a 100µg bolus of nitroglycerin is administered. A

Figure 4.9.41. Appearance before (**A**) and after (**B**) balloon angioplasty of multiple tibial lesions.

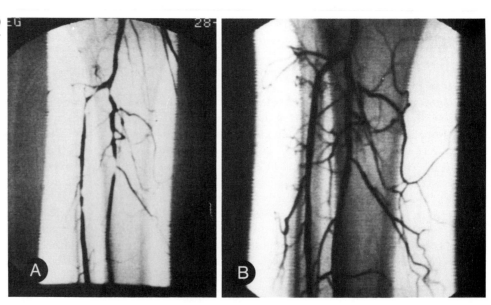

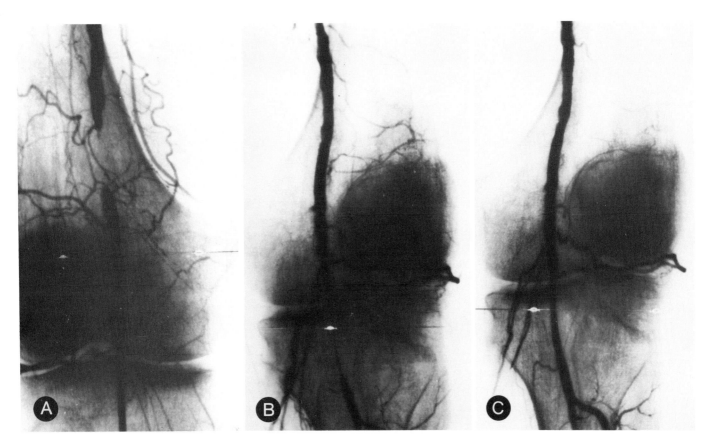

Figure 4.9.42. Spasm compromising angioplasty result. **A.** Preangioplasty appearance of short-segment occlusion of proximal popliteal artery. **B.** Severe spasm after successful angioplasty compromises angioplasty site. **C.** Marked improvement in appearance of popliteal artery after bolus of 100μg of intra-arterial nitroglycerin.

tight J small diameter guidewire is advanced together with the catheter through the occluded segment of the vessel. The guidewire is removed, and intraluminal position is confirmed with a small volume of contrast medium. Heparin is administered via the arterial catheter, and an exchange is made for the angioplasty catheter over a 0.018-inch exchange guidewire. Angioplasty is completed as in the case of stenotic disease (Fig. 4.9.43). Bifurcation lesions of the popliteal artery branches are dealt with differently. Angioplasty of a bifurcation stenosis can occlude the orifice of the adjacent vessel by raising a cleft. Therefore, guidewires are placed in each branch vessel at risk, and sequential angioplasty is carried out. On some occasions, simultaneous angioplasty of both areas of stenosis is performed.

Once again, the patient is maintained on systemic heparin for 48–72 hours.

Anastomotic and Graft Stenoses

Szilagyi et al. described the changes in reversed saphenous vein grafts used for peripheral bypass grafting.[120] Serial angiography revealed wavy narrowings of the vessel lumen that were attributed to intimal thickening, athero-sclerosis, fibrotic valves, traumatic stenoses, suture stenoses, and aneurysmal dilatation. Intimal thickening and atherosclerosis were the most common findings, with atherosclerosis appearing similar to that in native arteries. All of the lesions observed by these investigators were progressive. Angioplasty is ideal for the management of stenoses at anastomoses of aortoiliac or aortofemoral bypass grafts, at anastomoses of reverse saphenous vein bypass grafts, or stenoses within saphenous vein bypass grafts, whereas reoperation through scar tissue is technically more difficult than the original procedure and carries greater risk.

Proximal and distal anastomotic stenoses associated with aortoiliac bypass grafts are approached in the same fashion as lesions in the native iliac arteries or abdominal aorta. The distal lesions are frequently secondary to clamp injury to the native vessel and the development of intimal thickening and will yield to PTA, although dilatation may require use of a high-pressure balloon. Restenoses are common, so repeated dilatations may be necessary.

Stenoses at the distal anastomosis of an aortofemoral bypass graft can be approached from the contralateral groin around the graft bifurcation. This requires the use of a sheath for introduction of the balloon catheter. Graft

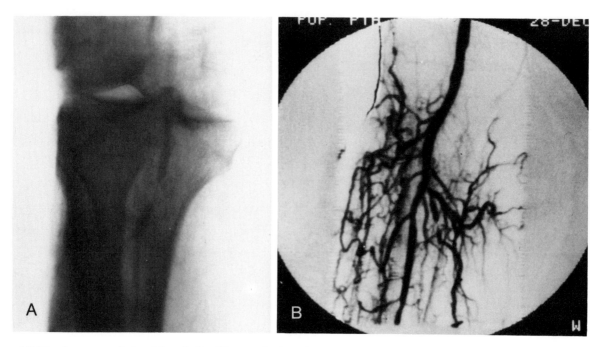

Figure 4.9.43. Appearance before (**A**) and after (**B**) recanalization of occluded distal popliteal artery and subsequent balloon angioplasty.

bifurcations are frequently acute, and it is usually technically difficult to reach the stenoses for angioplasty. Once again, the lesions may prove difficult but probably will yield, particularly when balloons of Mylar-type material are used.

Stenoses related to autogenous vein bypass grafts are suitable for angioplasty. The proper approach to a lesion at an anastomosis or within a graft depends on the location of the lesion. Proximal anastomotic lesions may be approached ipsilaterally or contralaterally, whereas lesions within the graft or at the distal anastomosis may be approached by antegrade puncture of the ipsilateral common femoral artery using a technique similar to that for stenotic disease of the native superficial femoral artery. Alternatively, the graft may be punctured directly (Fig. 4.9.44). Whenever scar tissue is traversed, a sheath is used to permit easy introduction and withdrawal of the balloon catheter.

Figure 4.9.44. Appearance of femoral-popliteal saphenous vein bypass graft stenoses before (**A**) and after (**B**) angioplasty.

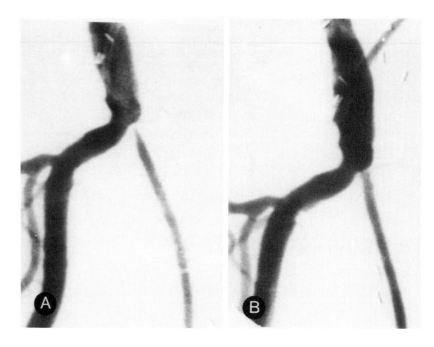

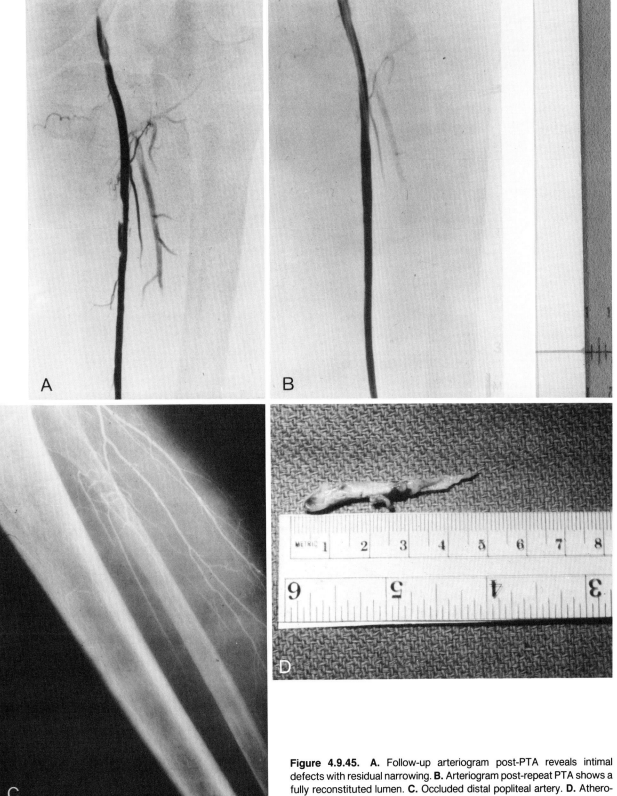

Figure 4.9.45. **A.** Follow-up arteriogram post-PTA reveals intimal defects with residual narrowing. **B.** Arteriogram post-repeat PTA shows a fully reconstituted lumen. **C.** Occluded distal popliteal artery. **D.** Atherosclerotic plaque emboli removed surgically.

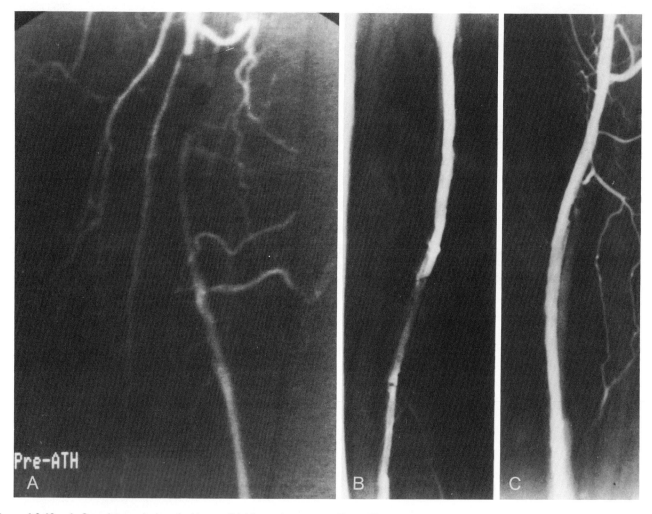

Figure 4.9.46. **A.** Complete occlusion of mid-superficial femoral artery. **B.** Post-PTA, there is a partially detached intimal flap causing obstruction. Note difference in density of contrast column. **C.** Postatherectomy, note widely patent lumen.

COMPLICATIONS OF ANGIOPLASTY

Nearly every conceivable complication has been reported, but a list of likely problems includes the following:

1. Significant groin hematomas (2–4% of angioplasty procedures)[121–124];
2. Distal embolic complications (Fig. 4.9.45) (2–5%)[121–124]; distal embolization *should not* occur except in occlusive vascular disease[121–124];
3. Elevation of intimal flaps (Fig. 4.9.46) (≤4%)[121–123];
4. False aneurysms (Fig. 4.9.47) (≤2%);
5. Arterial rupture secondary to catheter or balloon trauma (Fig. 4.9.48) (rare in the iliac artery[121–123]; approximately 3% in the superficial femoral artery);
6. Burst balloon with a circumferential tear (rare).

Hematomas at the puncture site can be minimized by consistently puncturing the common femoral artery, using the smallest suitable catheter, and using a sheath when several catheter exchanges are expected.

Distal embolization is unavoidable in attempts to recanalize occluded native vessels. The incidence can be minimized by passing through occlusions with small-bore catheters and by not undertaking direct angioplasty of possibly recent occlusions, such that fresh thrombus will be present. The appropriate management of the embolism depends on the clinical status of the leg (Fig. 4.9.45). If the limb remains viable, with intact sensation and motor function, attempts to deal with the embolism in the cardiovascular laboratory may be reasonable. Thrombolysis is unlikely to be of value, because the offending material is probably old, organized clot. However, it may be possible to aspirate the embolus into a nontapered large-bore catheter. Percutaneous Fogarty embolectomy also has been successful.[125,126] If these methods fail and the distal extremity remains viable, semiselective surgical removal may be planned. If distal embolization causes acute ischemia of the leg, spending time with percutaneous techniques is inappropriate, and the patient is best managed by urgent surgical removal of the embolism to decrease the risk of a compartment syndrome or loss of the limb.

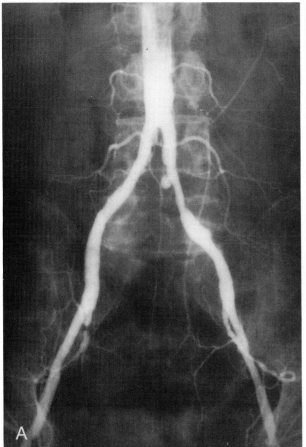

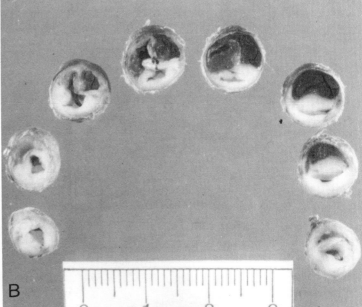

Figure 4.9.47. **A.** Long stenosis of left common iliac artery. Follow-up arteriogram one year post-PTA shows recurrence of stenosis and presence of a false aneurysm. **B.** Histopathology of artery at site of false aneurysm. Wall of aneurysm is formed by the adventitia.

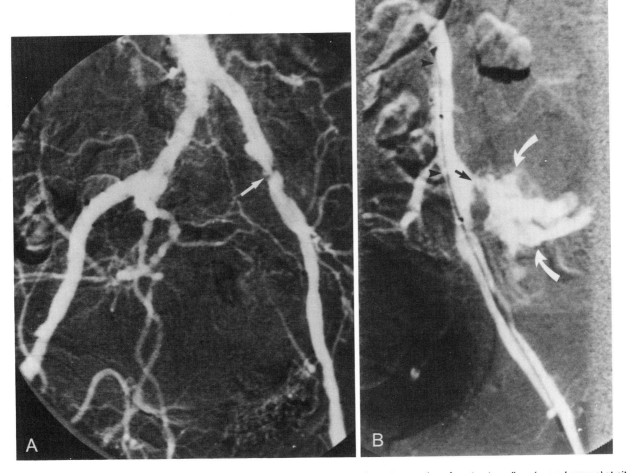

Figure 4.9.48. **A.** High-grade stenosis of iliac artery *(arrow)*. **B.** Post-PTA, note massive extravasation of contrast medium *(curved arrows)* at site of dilatation *(black arrow)*.

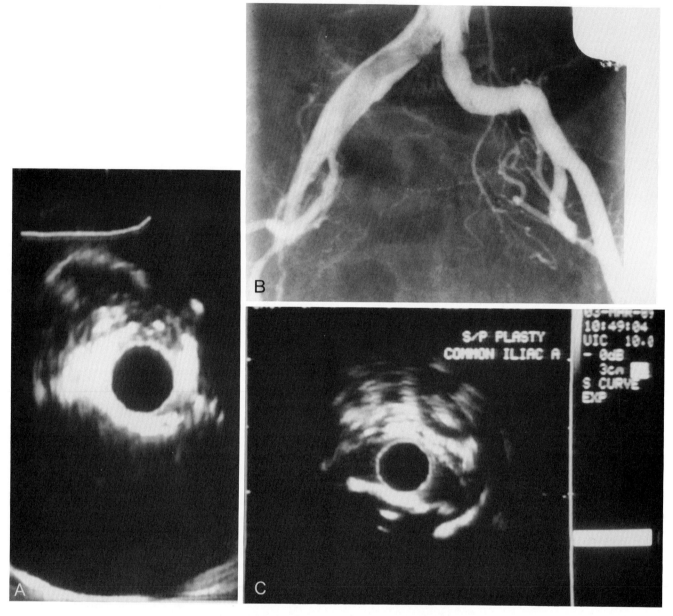

Figure 4.9.49. **A.** Intravascular ultrasound (IVUS) before PTA shows a severely narrowed lumen fully occupied by the transducer. **B.** Angiogram post-PTA shows widely patent lumen with a large intraluminal filling defect. **C.** IVUS post-PTA shows a narrowed, ellipsoid lumen. Acute thrombosis occurred 24 hours post-PTA.

Acute postangioplasty occlusion can be prevented by creating the optimum anatomic result whenever possible to maximize flow. When flow cannot be optimized, either because of a large intimal-medial disruption at the angioplasty site (Fig. 4.9.46) or because of poor runoff, systemic heparinization may avert acute thrombosis. The use of intravascular ultrasound provides valuable information about the status of the vascular lumen past the PTA, and helps to decide if adjuvant procedures are needed, such as stenting or atherectomy (Fig. 4.9.49A,B). Prevention of acute postangioplasty thrombosis is of particular value in patients with below-the-knee disease who are candidates for angioplasty for limb salvage, because these patients do not need long-term patency rates equivalent to those achieved in the more proximal vessels. That is, the goal is tissue healing, and this may occur in a relatively short time. Thereafter, even if the vessel reoccludes or restenoses, tissue breakdown will not necessarily recur.

When a balloon ruptures, the tear is usually longitudinal, and the balloon can be removed without difficulty. However, when the tear is circumferential, it is difficult to remove the balloon without excessive trauma at the site of insertion and extraction: therefore, the hub of the balloon catheter should be cut off and a sheath 1–2Fr larger than the shaft of the catheter should be inserted to permit atraumatic extraction.[127]

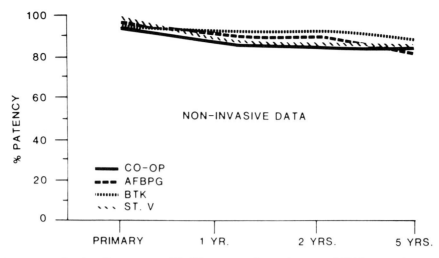

Figure 4.9.50. Results of angioplasty for short iliac stenoses. *CO-OP* = cooperative study group; *AFBPG* = aortofemoral bypass graft; *BTK* = Barry T. Katzen, M.D.; *ST. V* = St. Vincent's Hospital, Indianapolis, IN.

Occasionally, immediately after an apparently successful angioplasty, the patient's foot will appear cold, mottled, and pale, suggesting distal embolization. Before catheter removal, an angiographic check of the distal vasculature should be made. If no evidence of distal embolization is observed, a 100μg bolus of nitroglycerin should be administered through the catheter in an attempt to relieve what is probably distal vasospasm causing the "ugly foot" syndrome. Additional boluses of nitroglycerin may be necessary; occasionally, transdermal nitroglycerin is beneficial.

Restenoses may reasonably be considered a complication of angioplasty, and it appears that they are best avoided by using balloon catheters that produce the optimum anatomic result and by giving patients antiplatelet drugs postangioplasty. The patient who is motivated will refrain from cigarette smoking, will exercise appropriately, and, in general, will reduce his or her risk factors for atherosclerosis as much as possible.

RESULTS

The results of PTA are, as previously described, influenced by the preangioplasty anatomy. The five-year patency rate in initially successful procedures involving the iliac arteries with short, focal, concentric stenoses should approximate 90% given a 95% primary success rate.[128–132] When longer segments of the iliac artery are subjected to angioplasty, the primary success rate drops to approximately 89% for stenotic lesions, and as low as 33% in recanalization of occluded common iliac arteries,[131] and the 5-year patency rate drops to approximately 65% (Figs. 4.9.50 and 4.9.51).[128–132]

Short stenoses of the superficial femoral and popliteal arteries can be dilated >90% of the time and will remain patent five years later in approximately 75% of patients (Fig. 4.9.52). When longer or multiple stenoses are treated, a high primary success rate may be obtained, but

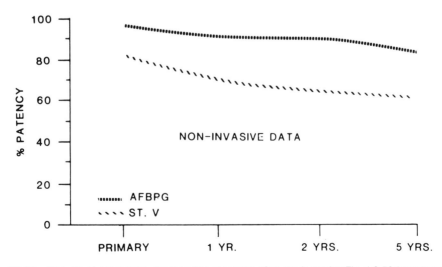

Figure 4.9.51. Results of angioplasty for long iliac stenoses. (See the legend to Fig. 4.9.50 for abbreviations.)

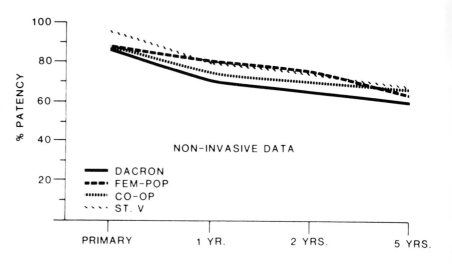

Figure 4.9.52. Results of angioplasty for short superficial femoral stenoses. *DACRON* = Dacron graft; *FEM-POP* = femoral-popliteal artery bypass graft. (See the legend to Fig. 4.9.50 for additional abbreviations.)

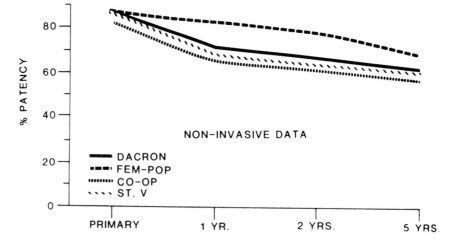

Figure 4.9.53. Results of angioplasty for long or multiple superficial femoral stenoses. (See the legends to Figs. 4.9.50 and 4.9.52 for abbreviations.)

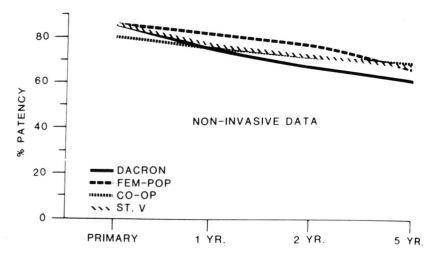

Figure 4.9.54. Results of angioplasty for short-segment occlusions in superficial femoral artery. (See the legends to Figures 4.9.50 and 4.9.52 for abbreviations.)

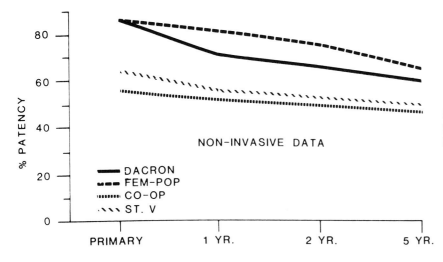

Figure 4.9.55. Results of angioplasty for long-segment occlusions in superficial femoral artery. (See the legends to Figs. 4.9.50 and 4.9.52 for abbreviations.)

the five-year patency rate varies from 45 to 75%[128-132] (Fig. 4.9.53).

Short occlusions of the superficial femoral and proximal popliteal arteries can be recanalized in 85–90% of patients and will have a 70–75% five-year patency rate (Fig. 4.9.54). When longer occlusions are dilated, the primary success rate diminishes to approximately 80% and the five-year patency rate to 60%[128-132] (Fig. 4.9.55). In the authors' experience, distal popliteal and tibial-peroneal angioplasty with the techniques described here has a primary success rate of 90% and an initial limb-healing rate of 92%.

References

1. Dotter CT, Judkins MP: Transluminal treatment of arteriosclerotic obstruction: description of a new technique and a preliminary report of its application. *Circulation* 1964; 36:654
2. Staple TW: Modified catheter for percutaneous transluminal treatment of arteriosclerotic obstructions. *Radiology* 1968; 91:1041
3. Van Andel GJ: *Percutaneous Transluminal Angioplasty: The Dotter Procedure.* Amsterdam, Excerpta Medica, 1976
4. Zeitler E, Grüntzig A, Schoop W (eds): *Percutaneous Vascular Recanalization: Technology, Application, Clinical Results.* Berlin, Springer–Verlag, 1978
5. Porstmann W: Ein neuer Korsett-Balloon-Katheter zur transluminalen Rekanalisation nach Dotter unter besonderer Berucksichtigung von obliterationen an den Beckenarterien. *Radiol Diag (Berl)* 1973;14:239
6. Grüntzig A, Hopff M: Perkutane Rekanalisation chronischer arterieller Verschlusse mit einem neuer Dilatations Katheter: Modifikation der Dotter-Technik. *Dtsch Med Wochenschr* 1974;99:2502
7. Grüntzig A, Vetter W, Meier B, Kuhlman U, Lotoff U, Sigenthaler W: Treatment of renovascular hypertension with percutaneous transluminal dilatation of renal-artery stenosis. *Lancet* 1978;1:801
8. Grüntzig A: Transluminal dilatation of coronary-artery stenosis (letter). *Lancet* 1978;1:263
9. Tegtmeyer CJ, Kellum CD, Ayers C: Percutaneous transluminal angioplasty of the renal artery: results and long term follow-up. *Radiology* 1984;153:77
10. Spence RK, Freiman DB, Gatenby R, et al: Long term results of transluminal angioplasty of the iliac and femoral arteries. *Arch Surg* 1981;116:1377
11. Grüntzig A: Percutaneous transluminal angioplasty: six years experience. *Am Heart J* 1984;107:818
12. Motarjeme A, Kiefer JW, Zuska AJ: Percutaneous transluminal angioplasty of the brachiocephalic arteries. *AJR* 1982;138:457
13. Schwarten DE: Transluminal angioplasty: overview of complications and long term results. *ARRS Categorical Course on Interventional Radiology,* April 21, 1985
14. Waltman AC, Greenfield AJ, Novelline RA, et al: Transluminal angioplasty of iliac and femoropopliteal arteries. *Arch Surg* 1982;117:1218
15. Tamura S, Sniderman KW, Beinart C, Sos TA: Percutaneous transluminal angioplasty of the popliteal artery and its branches. *Radiology* 1982;143:645
16. Greenfield AJ: Femoral, popliteal and tibial arteries: percutaneous transluminal angioplasty. *AJR* 1980;135:927
17. Katzen BT: Transluminal angioplasty of the iliac arteries, in Castañeda–Zúñiga WR (ed): *Transluminal Angioplasty.* New York, Thieme–Stratton, 1983, p 93
18. Friedman MH, Katzen BT: Noninvasive evaluation procedures, in Castañeda–Zúñiga WR (ed): *Transluminal Angioplasty.* New York, Thieme–Stratton, 1983, p 48
19. Motarjeme A, Keiger JW, Zuska AK: Percutaneous transluminal angioplasty and case selection. *Radiology* 1980; 135:573
20. Schoop W: Indications for PTA from the angiologic point of view, in Zeitler E, Grüntzig A, Schoop W (eds): *Percutaneous Vascular Recanalization.* Berlin, Springer–Verlag, 1978
21. Zeitler E, Richter EL, Roth FJ, Schoop W: *Results of Percutaneous Transluminal Angioplasty.* Berlin, Springer–Verlag, 1985
22. Block PC, Fallon JT, Elmer D: Experimental angioplasty: lessons from the laboratory. *AJR* 1980;135:907
23. Castañeda–Zúñiga WR, Formanek AG, Tadavarthy SM, et al: Mechanism of balloon angioplasty. *Radiology* 1980; 135:565
24. Castañeda–Zúñiga WR, Laerum F, Rysavy JA, Rusnak BW, Amplatz K: Paralysis of arteries by intraluminal balloon dilatation: an experimental study. *Radiology* 1982;144:74

25. Probst P, Cerny P, Owen A, Mahler F: Patency after femoral angioplasty: correlation of angiographic appearance with clinical findings. *AJR* 1983;140:1227

26. Tegtmeyer CT, Kellum CD, Ayers C: Percutaneous transluminal angioplasty of the renal artery. *Radiology* 1984;153:77

27. Kaltenbach M, Beyer J, Walter S, et al: Prolonged application of pressure in transluminal coronary angioplasty. *Catheter Cardiovasc Diagn* 1984;10:213

28. Wolf GL: Pharmacology of angioplasty. Presented at the 10th Annual Course on Diagnostic Angiography and Interventional Radiology, Society of Cardiovascular and Interventional Radiology, Orlando, FL, March 1985

29. Velasquez G, Castañeda-Zúñiga WR, Formanek A, Zollikofer C, Barreto A, Nicoloff D, Amplatz K, Sullivan A: Nonsurgical aortoplasty in Leriche syndrome. *Radiology* 1980; 134:359–360

30. Tegtmeyer CJ, Kellum CD, Kron IL, Mentzer RM: Percutaneous transluminal angioplasty in the region of the aortic bifurcation. *Radiology* 1985;157:661–665

31. Yakes WF, Kumpe DA, Brown SB, Parker SH, Lattes RG, Cook PS, Haas DK, Gibson MD, Hopper KD, Reed MD, Cox HE, Bourne EE, Griffin DJ: Percutaneous transluminal aortic angioplasty: techniques and results. *Radiology* 1989;172:965–970

32. Heeney D, Bookstein J, Daniels E, Warmath M, Horn J, Rowley W: Transluminal angioplasty of the abdominal aorta. *Radiology* 1983;148:81–83

33. Charlebois N, Saint-Georges G, Hudon G: Percutaneous transluminal angioplasty of the lower abdominal aorta. *AJR* 1986;146:369–371

34. Grollman JH, Vicario MD, Mittal AK: Percutaneous transluminal abdominal aortic angioplasty. *AJR* 1980;134:1053–1054

35. Morag B, Rubinstein Z, Kessler A, Schneiderman J, Levinkopf M, Bass A: Percutaneous transluminal angioplasty of the distal abdominal aorta and its bifurcation. *Cardiovasc Intervent Radiol* 1987;10:129–133

36. Hudon G, Bonan R, Hebert Y: Abdominal aortic angioplasty: a case report with angiographic follow-up. *J Assoc Can Radiol* 1982;33:262–264

37. Odurny A, Colapinto RF, Sniderman KW, Johnston KW: Percutaneous transluminal angioplasty of abdominal aortic stenoses. *Cardiovasc Intervent Radiol* 1989;12:1–6

38. Sproul G, Pinto J: Coarctation of the abdominal aorta. *Arch Surg* 1972;105:571–573

39. Tadavarthy AK, Sullivan WA, Nicoloff D, Castañeda-Zúñiga WR, Hunter DW, Amplatz K: Aorta balloon angioplasty: 9-year follow-up. *Radiology* 1989;170:1039–1041

40. Kumpe DA: Percutaneous dilatation of an abdominal aortic stenosis: three-balloon catheter technique. *Radiology* 1981;141:536–538

41. Crawford ES, Bomberger RA, Glaeser DH, et al: Aortoiliac occlusive disease: factors influencing survival and function following reconstructive operation over a twenty-five year period. *Surgery* 1981;90:1055–1067

42. Length of stay by operation, United States, 1985. Ann Arbor, MI, Commission on Professional and Hospital Activities, 1986, p 36

43. Dewar ML, Blundell PE, Lidstone D, et al: Effects of abdominal aneurysmectomy, aortoiliac bypass grafting and angioplasty on male sexual potency: a prospective study. *Can J Surg* 1985;28:154–159

44. Flanigan DP, Schuler JJ, Keifer T, et al: Elimination of iatrogenic impotence and improvement of sexual function after aortoiliac revascularization. *Arch Surg* 1982;117:544–550

45. Sabri S, Cotton LT: Sexual function following aortoiliac reconstruction. *Lancet* 1971;2:1218–1219

46. Miles JR, Miles DG, Johnson G: Aorto-iliac operations and sexual dysfunction. *Arch Surg* 1982;117:1177–1181

47. Berger T, Sorensen R, Konrad J: Aortic rupture: a complication of transluminal angioplasty. *AJR* 1986;146:373–374

48. Wingo JP, Nix ML, Greenfield LJ, Barnes RW: The blue toe syndrome: hemodynamics and therapeutic correlates of outcome. *J Vasc Surg* 1986;3:475–480

49. Kumpe DA, Zwerdlinger S, Griffin DJ: Blue digit syndrome: treatment with percutaneous transluminal angioplasty. *Radiology* 1988;166:37–44

50. Crane C: Atherothrombotic embolism to lower extremities in arteriosclerosis. *Arch Surg* 1967;94:96–101

51. Brenowitz JB, Edwards WS: The management of atheromatous emboli to the lower extremities. *Surg Gynecol Obstet* 1976;143:941–945

52. Kempczinski RF: Lower-extremity arterial emboli from ulcerating atherosclerotic plaques. *JAMA* 1979;241:807–810

53. Flory CM: Arterial occlusion produced by embolism from eroded atheromatous plaque. *Am J Pathol* 1945;21:549–565

54. Hoye SJ, Teitelbaum S, Gore I, Warren R: Atheromatous embolization. *N Engl J Med* 1959;261:128–131

55. Karmody AM, Powers SR, Monaco VJ, Leather RP: "Blue toe" syndrome: an indication for limb salvage surgery. *Arch Surg* 1976;111:1263–1268

56. Williams GM, Harrington D, Burdick J, White RI Jr: Mural thrombus of the aorta: an important, frequently neglected cause of larger peripheral emboli. *Ann Surg* 1981;194:737–744

57. Darsee JR: Cholesterol embolization: the great masquerader. *South Med J* 1979;72:174–180

58. Retan JW, Miller RE: Microembolic complications of atherosclerosis. *Arch Intern Med* 1966;118:534–545

59. Harvey JC: Cholesterol crystal microembolization: a cause of the restless leg syndrome. *South Med J* 1976;69:269–272

60. Banis JC, Rich N, Whelan TJ: Ischemia of the upper extremity due to noncardiac emboli. *Am J Surg* 1977;134:131–139

61. Lee BY, Brancata RF, Thoden WR, Madden JL: Blue digit syndrome: urgent indication for limb salvage surgery. *Am J Surg* 1984;147:418–422

62. Fisher DF, Clagett GP, Brigham RA, et al: Dilemmas in dealing with the blue toe syndrome: aortic versus peripheral source. *Am J Surg* 1984;148:836–839

63. Brewer ML, Kinnison ML, Perler BA, White RI Jr: Blue toe syndrome: treatment with anticoagulants and delayed percutaneous transluminal angioplasty. *Radiology* 1988;166:31

64. Kwaan JHM, Connolly JE: Peripheral atheroembolism: an enigma. *Arch Surg* 1977;122:987–990

65. Kwaan JH, Vander Molen R, Stremmer EA, Connolly JE: Peripheral embolism resulting from unsuspected atheromatous aortic plaques. *Surgery* 1975;78:583

66. Roon AJ, Sauvage LR: Blue toe syndrome: a warning sign of unsuspected vascular injury. *Surgery* 1983;93:722–724

67. Mehigan JT, Stoney RJ: Arterial microemboli and fibromuscular dysplasia of the external iliac arteries. *Surgery* 1977;81:484–486

68. Samuels PB, Katz DJ: Diagnosis and management of arterial mural thromboemboli. *Am J Surg* 1977;134:209–213

69. Schechter DC: Atheromatous embolization to lower limbs. *NY State J Med* 1979;79:1180–1186

70. Sixma JJ: Role of blood vessels, platelet and coagulation interactions in haemostasis, in Bloom AL, Thomas DP (eds): *Haemostasis and Thrombosis.* New York, Churchill Livingstone, 1981, pp 252–267

71. Velasquez G, Castañeda–Zúñiga W, Formanek A, et al: Nonsurgical angioplasty in Leriche syndrome. *Radiology* 1980;134:359

72. Bachman DM, Casarella WJ, Sos TA: Percutaneous iliofemoral angioplasty via the contralateral femoral artery. *Radiology* 1979;130:61

73. Katzen BT, Chang J, Knox WG: Percutaneous transluminal angioplasty with the Grüntzig balloon catheter: a review of 70 cases. *Arch Surg* 1979;114:1389

74. Waltman AC, Courey WR, Athanasoulis C, et al: Technique for left gastric artery catheterization. *Radiology* 1973; 109:732

75. Morse SS, Cambria R, Strauss EB, Kim B, Sniderman KW: Transluminal angioplasty of the hypogastric artery for treatment of buttock claudication. *Cardiovasc Intervent Radiol* 1986;9:136–138

76. Castaneda–Zúñiga WR, Smith A, Kaye K, Rusnak B, Herrera M, Hiller R, Amplatz K: Transluminal angioplasty for treatment of vasculogenic impotence. *AJR* 1982;139:371–373

77. Piotrowski JJ, Pearce WH, Jones DN, Whithill T, Bell R, Patt A, Rutherford RB: Aortobifemoral bypass: the operation of choice for unilateral iliac occlusion? *J Vasc Surg* 1988;8:211–218

78. Rubinstein ZJ, Morag B, Peer A, Bass A, Schneiderman J: Percutaneous transluminal recanalization of common iliac artery occlusion. *Cardiovasc Intervent Radiol* 1987;10:16–20

79. Kaufman SL: Femoral puncture using Doppler ultrasound guidance: aid to transluminal angioplasty and other applications. *AJR* 1980;134:402

80. Saibil EA, Maggisano R: Combined antegrade-retrograde catheterization of the occluded common iliac artery prior to angioplasty. *Canad Assoc Radiol* 1988;39:228–229

81. Loose HW, Ryall CJ: Common iliac artery occlusion: treatment with pull-through angioplasty. *Radiology* 1988; 168:273–274

82. Gaines PA, Cumberland DC: Wire-loop technique for angioplasty of total iliac artery occlusions. *Radiology* 1988;168:275–276

83. Ginsburg R, Thorpe P, Bowles CR, Wright AM, Wexler L: Pull-through approach to percutaneous angioplasty of totally occluded common iliac arteries. *Radiology* 1989; 172:111–113

84. Ring EJ, Freiman DB, McLean GK, et al: Percutaneous recanalization of common iliac artery occlusion: an unacceptable complication rate? *AJR* 1982;139:587

85. Auster M, Kadir S, Mitchell SE, et al: Iliac artery occlusion: management with intrathrombus streptokinase infusion and angioplasty. *Radiology* 1984;153:385

86. Motarjeme A: Thrombolytic therapy in arterial occlusion and graft thrombosis. *Semin Vasc Surg* 1989;2(3):155–178

87. Maynar M, Reyes R, Pulido DJM, et al: The Simpson atherocath in the management of complete obstructions. *RöFo* 1991;153(3):547–550

88. Rees CR, Palmaz JC, Garcia O, Roeren T, Richter GM, Gardiner G, Schwarten D, Schatz RA, Root HD, Rogers W: Angioplasty and stenting of completely occluded iliac arteries. *Radiology* 1989;172:953–959

89. Greenfield AJ: Percutaneous transluminal angioplasty of the femoral, popliteal and tibial vessels, in Athanasoulis CA, Pfister RC, Greene RE, Roberson GH (eds): *Interventional Radiology*. Philadelphia, WB Saunders, 1982

90. Rappaport S, Sniderman KW, Morse SS, Proto MH, Ross GR: Pseudoaneurysm: a complication of faulty technique in femoral artery puncture. *Radiology* 1985;154:529–530

91. Lechner G, Jantsch H, Waneck R, Kretschmer G: The relationship between the common femoral artery, the inguinal crease, and the inguinal ligament: a guide to accurate angiographic puncture. *Cardiovasc Intervent Radiol* 1988;11:165–169

92. Berman HL, Katz SG, Tihansky DP: Guided direct antegrade puncture of the superficial femoral artery. *AJR* 1986;147:632–634

93. Bishop AF, Berkman WA, Palagallo GL: Antegrade selective catheterization of the superficial femoral artery using a movable core guidewire. *Radiology* 1985;157:548

94. Hawkins JS, Coryell LW, Miles SG, Giovannet MJ, Siragusa RJ, Hawkins IF Jr: Directional needle for antegrade guidewire placement with vertical arterial puncture. *Radiology* 1988;168:271–272

95. Miles SG, Siragusa R, Hawkins IF Jr: New directional accordion catheter for converting a retrograde puncture into an antegrade catheter placement. *AJR* 1988;151:197–199

96. Kikkawa K: A new antegrade femoral artery catheter needle set. *Radiology* 1984;151:798

97. Saddekni S, Srur M, Cohn DJ, Rozenblit G, Wetter EB, Sos TA: Antegrade catheterization of the superficial femoral artery. *Radiology* 1985;157:531–532

98. Shenoy SS: Sidewinder catheter for conversion of retrograde into antegrade catheterization. *Cardiovasc Intervent Radiol* 1983;6:112–113

99. Giavroglou CE: "Retrograde" catheterization of the branches of the femoral artery: Technical note. *Cardiovasc Intervent Radiol* 1990;12:337–339

100. Patel YD: Catheter for conversions of retrograde to antegrade femoral artery catheterization. *AJR* 1990;154:179–180

101. Tonnesen KH, Sager P, Karle A, Henriksen L, Jorgensen B: Percutaneous transluminal angioplasty of the superficial femoral artery by retrograde catheterization via the popliteal artery. *Cardiovasc Intervent Radiol* 1988;11:127–131

102. Druy E: Retrograde popliteal approach to femoral percutaneous transluminal angioplasty. Presented at the Annual Meeting of the Society of Cardiovascular and Interventional Radiology. San Diego, CA, March 20, 1989

103. Katzen BT, Dake M, Zemel G: The popliteal arterial approach for complex superficial femoral intervention. Presented at RIPCV2, February 1990, Toulouse, France

104. Dacie JE, Tennant D: A new approach to percutaneous transluminal angioplasty of profunda femoris origin stenosis. *Cardiovasc Intervent Radiol* 1990;13:67–70

105. Motarjeme A, Keifer JW, Zuska AJ: Percutaneous transluminal angioplasty of the deep femoral artery. *Radiology* 1980; 135:613–617

106. Rieger H, Roth F-J, Schoop W: Results of percutaneous transluminal angioplasty of the deep femoral artery—a preliminary study, in Dotter CT, Grüntzig A, Schoop W, Zeitler E (eds): *Percutaneous Transluminal Angioplasty. Technique, Early and Late Results*. Springer–Verlag, Berlin, 1978, pp 308–311

107. Barth KH: Modified catheter for transluminal angioplasty of the femoral popliteal artery. *Radiology* 1983;149:598

108. Ricketts HJ: Presented at the Members Meeting, Society of Cardiovascular and Interventional Radiology, Napa, CA, February 1984

109. Schwarten De, Cutcliff WB: Arterial occlusive disease below the knee: treatment with percutaneous transluminal angioplasty performed with low profile catheters and steerable guidewires. *Radiology* 1988;169:71–74

110. Horvath W, Oertl M, Haidinger D: Percutaneous transluminal angioplasty of crural arteries. *Radiology* 1990; 177:565–569

111. Brown KT, Schoenbert NY, Moore ED, Saddekni S: Percutaneous transluminal angioplasty of infrapopliteal ves-

sels; preliminary results and technical considerations. *Radiology* 1988;169:75–78

112. Bakal WC, Sprayregen S, Scheinbaum, K, et al: Percutaneous transluminal angioplasty of the infrapopliteal arteries: results in 53 patients. *AJR* 1990;154:171–174

113. Casarella WJ: Percutaneous transluminal angioplasty below the knee: new techniques, excellent results. *Radiology* 1988;169:271–272

114. Becker GJ, Katzen BT, Dake M: Noncoronary angioplasty. *Radiology* 1989;170:921–940

115. Tamura S, Sniderman KW, Beinart C, Sos TA: Percutaneous transluminal angioplasty of the popliteal artery and its branches. *Radiology* 1982;143:645–648

116. Sprayregen S, Sniderman KW, Sos TA, et al: Popliteal artery branches: percutaneous transluminal angioplasty. *AJR* 1980;135:945–950

117. Zeitler E: Complications in and after percutaneous transluminal recanalization, in Zeitler E, Grüntzig A, Schoop W (eds): *Percutaneous Vascular Recanalization*. Berlin, Springer, 1978

118. Taylor LM Jr, Phinney ES, Porter JM: Present status of reversed vein bypass for lower extremity revascularization. *J Vasc Surg* 1986;3:288–295

119. Cardella JF, Smith TP, Darcy MD, Hunter DW, Castañeda–Zúñiga WR, Amplatz K: Balloon occlusion femoral angiography prior to in situ saphenous vein bypass. *CVIR* 1987;10:181–187

120. Szilagyi DE, Elliott JP, Hageman SH, et al: Biologic fate of autogenous vein grafts implanted as arterial substitutes. *Ann Surg* 1973;78:232

121. Bergqvist D, Jonsson K, Weibull H: Complications after percutaneous transluminal angioplasty of peripheral and renal arteries. *Radiology* 1987;28:3–12

122. Gardiner GA, Meyerovitz MF, Stokes KR, Clouse ME, Harrington DP, Bettmann MA: Complications of transluminal angioplasty. *Radiology* 1986;159:201–208

123. Weibull H, Bergqvist D, Jonsson K, Karlsson S, Takolander R: Complications after percutaneous transluminal angioplasty in the iliac, femoral, and popliteal arteries. *J Vasc Surg* 1987;5:681–686

124. Sniderman K, Bodner L, Saddekni S, Srur M, Sos T: Percutaneous embolectomy by transcatheter aspiration. *Radiology* 1984; 150:357

125. Hayden W: Presented at a round table discussion on distal percutaneous transluminal angioplasty. American Heart Association Annual Meeting, Washington, DC, Nov 1984

126. Train JS, Dan SJ, Mitty HA, Dikman SH, Harrington EB, Miller CM, Jacobson JH: Occlusion during iliac angioplasty: a salvageable complication. *Radiology* 1988;168:131–135

127. Tegtmeyer CJ, Bezirdjian DR: Removing the stuck, ruptured angioplasty balloon catheter. *Radiology* 1981; 139:231

128. Waltman AC, Greenfield AJ, Novelline RA, Abbott WM, Brewster DC, Darling RC, Moncure AC, Ottinger LW, Athanasoulis CA: Transluminal angioplasty of the iliac and femoropopliteal arteries. *Arch Surg* 1982;117:1218–1221

129. Zeitler E: Percutaneous dilatation and recanalization of iliac and femoral arteries. *Cardiovasc Intervent Radiol* 1980;3:207–212

130. Van Andel GJ: Transluminal iliac angioplasty: long-term results. *Radiology* 1980;135:607–611

131. Motarjeme A, Keifer JW, Zuska AJ: Percutaneous transluminal angioplasty of the iliac arteries: 66 experiences. *AJR* 1980;135:937–944

132. Graor RA, Young JR, McCandless M, Swift C, Smith JAM, Ruschaupt WF, Risius B, Zelch MG: Percutaneous transluminal angioplasty: review of iliac and femoral dilatations at the Cleveland Clinic. *Cleve Clin Q* 1984;51:149–154

Part 10. The Problems and Management of Hemodialysis Accesses

—Robert M. Zeit, M.D.

In 1987, 91,000 patients received chronic hemodialysis.[1] This represents a significant increase over prior years and reflects the inclusion of more high-risk patients in hemodialysis programs. Because of this expanded population, mortality among the dialysis population, which was once 10% annually,[2] has now increased to 20%.[3]

The quality of life and sometimes the very survival of hemodialysis patients is dependent on the performance of their arteriovenous accesses. An adequately functioning hemodialysis access should have a flow rate of at least 250–300ml/min (ideally 400–500ml/min)[4] and be able to withstand two 14-gauge needle punctures at least 150 times each year.[5] These are stringent requirements, and chronic hemodialysis patients usually experience the creation and subsequent deterioration of a series of accesses. Loss of the final access site can be fatal. It has been estimated that 18% of these individuals die because of a lack of adequate vascular access after all usable locations have been exhausted.[6]

The availability of thrombolytic enzymes, transluminal angioplasty, and vascular stenting has enabled the interventional radiologist to participate in the preservation and salvage of these accesses. Moreover, the interventional radiologist may resort to a number of extreme techniques when all conventional accesses have failed and death is otherwise inevitable. This chapter describes the historical development of hemodialysis accesses, the complications which plague them, their evaluation, and the interventional radiology techniques which can be used to restore access function.

DEVELOPMENT OF HEMODIALYSIS ACCESSES AND THEIR COMPLICATIONS

Practical hemodialysis was initiated by Kolff and colleagues in 1965.[7] However, vascular access was obtained by surgically cannulating an artery and a vein for each dialysis and ligating both vessels at the end of the session; obviously this attrition of vessels could not be long maintained. Dialysis was therefore limited to short-term use.

Scribner Shunt

Long-term patency of a glass arteriovenous shunt in heparinized patients was reported in 1949. In 1960, Quinton and coworkers developed a shunt using polytetrafluoroethylene (PTFE; expanded Teflon) for the intravascular portion of the cannulas, permitting long-term placement without a need for systemic anticoagulation.[8] Various modifications of the original rigid Teflon design were produced, eventually resulting in the Scribner shunt, in which the two intravascular PTFE components were connected by a Silastic bridge. This device made short-term hemodialysis practical. The sophistication of subsequent accesses has increased, but the difficulties encountered with the Scribner shunt still plague hemodialysis today.

Complications of the Scribner shunt, when used for chronic hemodialysis, included most commonly thrombosis and infection,[9] pseudoaneurysm formation, hemorrhage, and erosion of the overlying skin.[10] Stenosis or occlusion of inflow and outflow vessels was a major problem, as is the case today. Alignment of the Scribner cannula tips relative to the wall was critical, because an angulated cannula could traumatize the vessel wall, resulting in occlusive endarteritis and subsequent thrombosis (Fig. 4.10.1). Another consequence of improper tip placement was the creation of a "dead space," also implicated in arterial limb thrombosis.[11] Trauma caused by motion of the rigid catheter tip was thought to cause aneurysms at the site of cannulation (Fig. 4.10.2). Other factors contributing to shunt thrombosis included a circumferential arterial stenosis at the tip of the cannula, variously ascribed to the interaction of the Teflon with the surrounding endothelium, to the Bernoulli effect, or to rubbing of the cannula against the vessel wall.[12]

Ubiquitous Complications of Dialysis Accesses

Chronic hemodialysis brought with it access maintenance problems that persist to this day. The commonest is progressive stenosis of the proximal veins which, if untreated, progresses until thrombosis of the access occurs. In the Scribner shunt venous outflow stenosis (Fig.

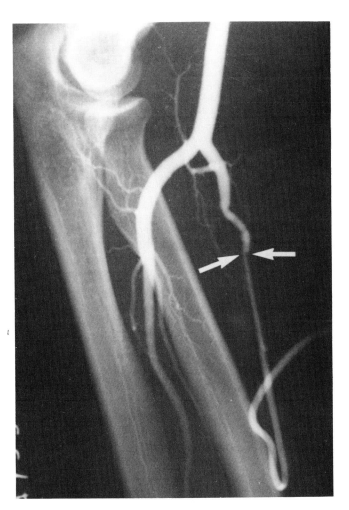

Figure 4.10.1. Scribner shunt with angulation of arterial cannula tip against vessel wall *(arrows)*. This was associated with poor shunt longevity.

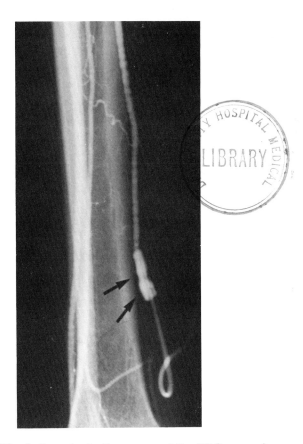

Figure 4.10.2. Scribner shunt with aneurysm at tip of Teflon cannula *(arrows)*.

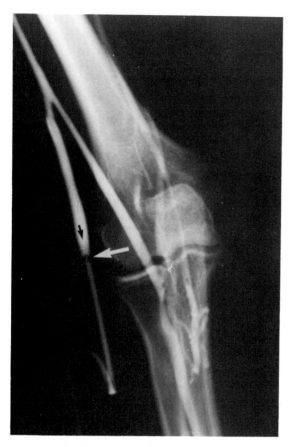

Figure 4.10.3. Scribner shunt with circumferential venous stenosis at cannula tip *(arrows)*.

4.10.3) was noted in most patients within 14 days of shunt placement.

Even today, this phenomenon remains the cause of most delayed access failures.[13] Far from being a static entity, intimal hyperplasia can occur fairly rapidly as the result of active cellular and subcellular responses to abnormally high flow.[14] Various theories of the etiology of this response have been advanced.[15]

Hypotension, usually occurring during a dialysis session, is a less common cause of thrombosis of all types of accesses. Infection occurred in 17–50% of Quinton–Scribner shunts[16] and was associated occasionally with phlebitis, embolism, septicemia, endocarditis, and pulmonary abscesses. Pseudoaneurysm formation because of the trauma of repeated needle punctures of either the native vessel or prosthetic material[9] is another complication of chronic hemodialysis first encountered with the Scribner shunt which remains a problem today.

Because of these complications the average patency of a Scribner shunt was measured in months,[10,11] with the longest reported patency being two years.[17] Because of the shunt's external location, there was a constant danger of dislodgment. Newer external devices designed for insertion into the subclavian or femoral vein, such as the Shiley and Sorenson catheters, have replaced the Scribner shunt for short-term hemodialysis.

Newer External Shunts

Twelve-French double-lumen subclavian catheters have recently become popular for short- and intermediate-term hemodialysis. They are used when it is necessary to provide emergency dialysis until a native arteriovenous fistula or surgical shunt matures sufficiently to be used, or when

Figure 4.10.4. Subclavian vein obstruction *(arrow)* after chronic catheterization.

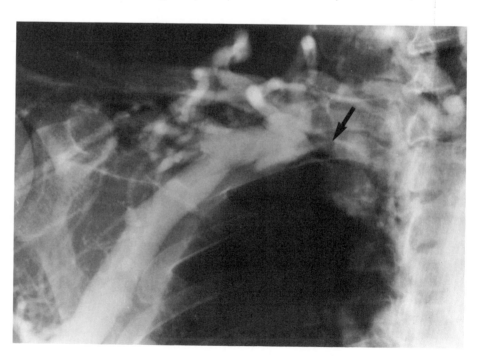

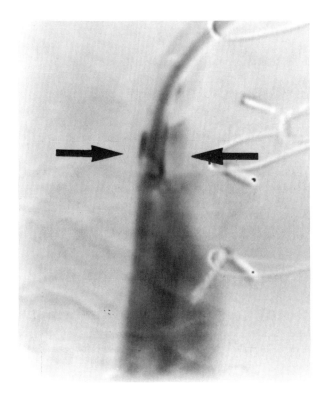

Figure 4.10.5 Thrombus at tip of double-lumen dialysis catheter *(arrows).* This was successfully lysed with 250,000 units of urokinase.

arterial or venous deficiencies preclude the use of a fistula or shunt.

Unfortunately, the use of subclavian catheters for hemodialysis may have devastating long-term complications. Subclavian stenosis is likely to occur if a catheter has been allowed to remain in the vein longer than 15 days (Fig. 4.10.4).[18] It has been theorized that this scarring is a valve responding to the trauma of catheterization.[19] Severe swelling of the ipsilateral arm appears weeks to months later. Although balloon angioplasty may sometimes[20] be successful in dilating these stenoses, as discussed below, a significant uncorrectable stenosis or thrombosis will preclude the use of that extremity for dialysis forever.[18,21]

A lesser problem resulting from prior subclavian venous catheterizations is scarring of the overlying tissues. This necessitates slight overdilatation of the tract, which, combined with the bleeding tendency of uremic patients, may result in hemorrhage. Pneumothorax is also a well documented complication of subclavian catheterization. All of these problems may be minimized by using the fine 22-gauge needle and 0.018-inch guidewire insertion sets popularized by Cope,[22] and by performing the catheterization under fluoroscopic guidance.

Complications inherent in the use of double-lumen catheters are related to the structural limitations inherent in partitioning a fairly large tube into two discrete lumens and to the stiffness of the material used. Thus, thrombosis of one or both lumens, or thrombus formation at the tip of the catheter, is commonly encountered (Fig. 4.10.5). This may be treated by thrombolytic agents, as described below.[23] Infection is a constant risk. Erythrocyte fragmentation occurs during passage through the catheter lumens. This contributes to the chronic anemia of uremic patients.

External arteriovenous accesses still have an average useful life of only three to eight months[24] and usually are used only to gain time for a more permanent access to mature.

Surgically Created Arteriovenous Fistulae

In 1966 Brescia and associates introduced a surgical arteriovenous fistula for the performance of hemodialysis, usually by anastomosing the radial artery and the cephalic vein.[25] If the patient's draining vein is able to dilate in response to the arterial inflow it can be used as the dialysis puncture site. The absence of artificial implants reduces the incidence of infection. The natural vein is more resistant to the trauma of repeated puncture than are woven prosthetics. Perhaps most important, even if the draining vein should become stenotic or thrombose, small collateral channels often hypertrophy, providing alternate routes of venous drainage and locations for needle puncture. The Brescia–Cimino fistula has been the most trouble-free and

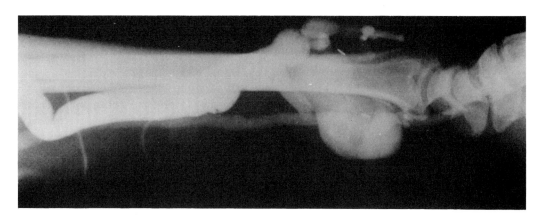

Figure 4.10.6. Venous aneurysms in Brescia–Cimino fistula.

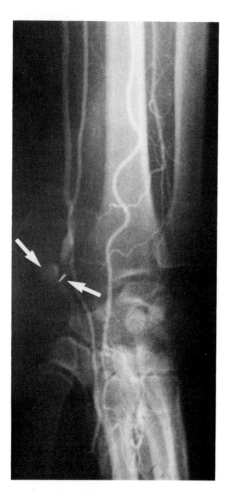

Figure 4.10.7. Pseudoaneurysm *(arrows)* of Brescia–Cimino arteriovenous fistula.

distal to the fistula or access may not get enough blood for its needs.

This siphoning off of blood is termed the "steal syndrome," and can result in digital ischemia or even gangrene.[27] The severity of the resultant ischemia, like most other vascular complications of dialysis, is more severe in diabetic patients.[28] The only treatment is to surgically reduce the inflow.

Congestive heart failure secondary to a high-output fistula has occasionally been reported.[29] It is more common in patients who have two simultaneously functioning fistulae.

Conversely, if inflow is acceptable, a stenosis or obstruction of the venous drainage may produce "venous hypertension" of the extremity caused by retention in the veins of blood under elevated pressure because of the inability of that blood to empty as fast as it flows in. Venous hypertension usually is indicated by swelling, cyanosis, and ulceration of the entire hand, but may be limited to one[4] or more[30] digits (Fig. 4.10.10). The condition also may mandate destruction of the fistula or access. This problem is all the more poignant because virtually every patient who receives a fistula or shunt for dialysis has been catheterized frequently in the subclavian vein for prior temporary dialysis (see above).

In a series of 346 fistulae reported by Giacchino and associates, arterial insufficiency of the hand, manifested by symptoms of ischemia that worsened during dialysis, appeared in three patients, and venous hypertension appeared in eight.[5] Fistulae created by side-to-side anastomosis seem more likely to result in both steal syndrome and venous hypertension than those using an end-to-end construction.

Breakdown of the outflow veins with aneurysm formation occasionally occurs in fistulae and produces atrophic changes in the overlying skin.[10]

A variant fistula, used when a Brescia–Cimino access has failed, is the "reverse fistula." Here the brachial artery is anastomosed to the basilic vein, which is then plicated cephalad. This forces blood to flow retrograde down the antecubital veins before returning through collaterals to the subclavian vein.[31]

Artificial Accesses

Only 15% of dialysis patients can utilize the Brescia–Cimino fistula. The remaining 85% must rely upon artificial shunts,[3] tubes constructed of various materials interposed between the radial or brachial artery and a large draining vein. In addition to functioning as conduits, these grafts provide sites which can be punctured during dialysis in the same manner as the dilated proximal vein of the Brescia–Cimino shunt.

The variety of materials which have been used in the creation of these shunts is far too extensive to be described in this article. Extensive review articles are available.[32] Only

longest-lived access, often having a useful life of five years or more.[1,26] However, the development of adequate venous drainage requires a period of "maturation" of the fistula, usually four weeks, before it can be used. Placement of similar fistulae in the leg is contraindicated because of the fear of leg ischemia caused by the fistula stealing blood from an inflow already compromised by arteriosclerotic disease, and the fear of venous hypertension.[10,22]

Despite the advantages of the Brescia–Cimino fistula, it is subject to the usual access complications: infection, the development of true aneurysms (Fig. 4.10.6) and pseudoaneurysms (Fig. 4.10.7),[4] thrombosis secondary to hypotensive episodes, arterial stenosis (Fig. 4.10.8), and venous intimal hyperplasia (Fig. 4.10.9).

Steal Syndrome and Venous Hypertension

Although dialysis occurs only for a few hours, a few days weekly, there is continuous flow through fistulas and accesses. This creates the possibility of complications caused by an imbalance of blood inflow and outflow. If there is too little inflow, the fistula or access will be ineffective. However, if there is excessive inflow, the extremity

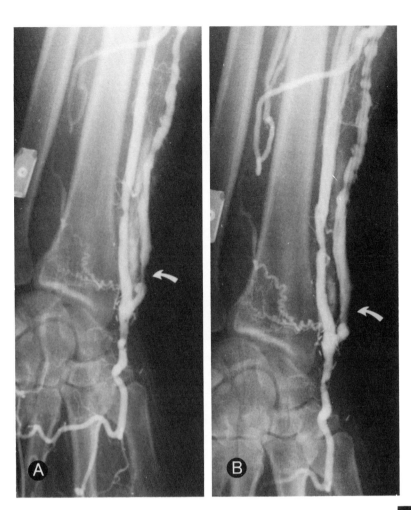

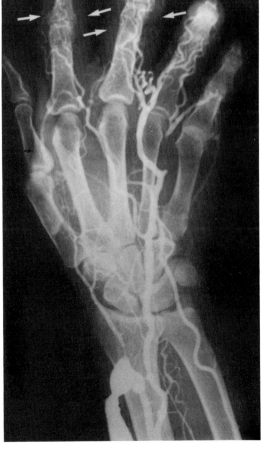

Figure 4.10.8 Brescia–Cimino shunt with intimal hyperplasia *(arrows)* 1cm from arterial anastomosis. **A.** Before dilatation. **B.** After Dotter dilatation with 7Fr sheath; good result was obtained.

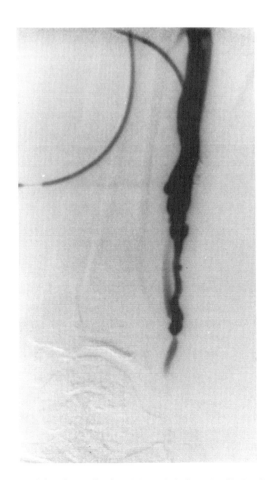

Figure 4.10.9. Stenosis of draining vein in Brescia–Cimino fistula.

Figure 4.10.10. Digital venous hypertension in patient with Brescia–Cimino fistula; note retrograde venous flow and swelling of fingers *(arrows)*.

the more widely encountered materials will be discussed here.

Both biologic materials (autogenous saphenous vein, bovine carotid artery, human umbilical vein) and artificial materials (Dacron velour, expanded polytetrafluoroethylene (E-PTFE)) have been used, sometimes in combination. All have lower patency rates and a higher incidence of complications than the Brescia–Cimino fistula. Because of this frequency of complications, their widespread use, and their amenability to treatment with thrombolytic enzymes, they are of great interest to the interventional radiologist.

Because of its success in vascular surgery, autogenous saphenous vein was regarded as a likely material for dialysis grafts. However, results were extremely poor, with only a 51% one-year graft survival rate.[24] In addition, it was difficult to free these grafts of thrombi because of the presence of valve remnants, and the grafts had a tendency to develop endothelial thickening along their entire length. The additional operative effort required for harvesting and the desire to preserve the saphenous vein for possible use later in coronary or femoral-popliteal bypass have also discouraged use of the saphenous vein.[25]

Another biologic graft material that excited considerable interest but proved unsuitable was the Sparks mandrel graft, in which living tissue was grown over Dacron mesh. In use, the Dacron fibers tended to separate, resulting in a 20% incidence of aneurysm formation. There also was a high rate of intimal hyperplasia.[35]

Bovine carotid artery modified by treatment with glutaraldehyde[36] has a better patency rate, as high as 70–80% one year after implantation.[33] However, bovine heterografts undergo degenerative changes,[37] resulting in aneurysm formation in 21% of implants[38] (Fig. 4.10.11) and loss of integrity of the entire graft wall in 9%.[33] Later bovine prostheses were covered with Dacron mesh to guard against this.

Bovine implants are also extremely susceptible to the consequences of infection, which was responsible for the loss of 38% of these grafts in one series.[39] Even a localized infection at a puncture site necessitates removal of the entire prosthesis. Moreover, thrombectomy of clotted bovine shunts is usually unsuccessful, patency being restored in less than one-third of cases.[36] Surprisingly, bovine carotid shunts are still occasionally encountered.

Human umbilical vein, once considered a promising shunt material, has proved disappointing. Rubio and DelGuercio reported an 88% patency rate four years after implantation.[40] However, subsequent studies reported a high incidence of thrombosis and infection, bacterial colonization, and aneurysm formation, with an average useful life of only 11 months.[41]

Some artificial materials have fared no better. Dacron velour gave disappointing results because of a high incidence of thrombosis and infection.[40]

The current prosthetic material of choice, by far the most widely used, is E-PTFE. Numerous studies have doc-

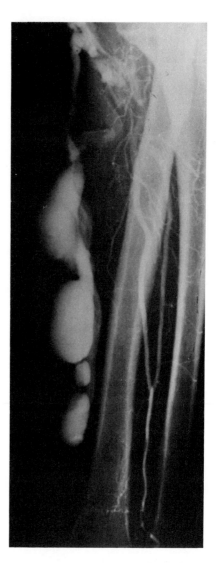

Figure 4.10.11. Bovine carotid heterograft with multiple aneurysms.

umented that this material results in longer shunt survival and diminished complications compared to saphenous vein or bovine carotid artery.[33,37,40] In part, this superiority is attributed to the unique structural and physical characteristics of E-PTFE, in which nodes of PTFE are interconnected with fibrils, resulting in 10–30μm pores that allow tissue ingrowth and eventual production of a true neointima.[42,43] These grafts also have a 17mV electronegative potential, which reduces their thrombogenicity.[42,43] The presence of a true neointima results in a higher success rate in thrombectomy of E-PTFE than in bovine grafts, 50%[44] and 32%, respectively. The E-PTFE shunts also require only half as many revisions per dialysis month as do bovine prostheses.[39] One year shunt survivals of 74% and five year survivals of 47% have been reported.[45]

Nevertheless, E-PTFE accesses are subject to the same types of complications as those shunts previously described. Early (1975–1976) E-PTFE grafts were prone to aneurysm formation.[46] Subsequent reinforcement of the E-PTFE with Dacron mesh reduced the rate of aneurysm formation far below that of bovine implants.[45] Attempts to thin the walls of PTFE shunts have shown no decrease in intimal hyperplasia but have produced an unacceptable incidence of aneurysm formation.[13] Bacterial and even fungal[47] infection of E-PTFE prostheses occurs, occasionally leading to fatal sepsis.[48] Infection constitutes about 19% of all graft complications.[49] As with all vascular accesses, the skin overlying the shunt may erode, and surgical transposition of skin or muscle[50,51] may be required to re-cover the prosthesis. Occasionally, the anastomosis between the artery and the E-PTFE shunt is too wide, causing excessive flow; the use of a tapered prosthesis reduces the likelihood of this problem.[52]

Diabetes, Lower Extremity Accesses, and Infection

Three interrelated factors deserve special mention in any review of the complications of hemodialysis accesses: diabetes, infection, and lower extremity access placement.

Hemodialysis access placement in the lower extremity is undesirable. The arterial inflow is susceptible to atherosclerotic narrowing (Fig. 4.10.12). This is exacerbated in diabetic uremic patients, who develop atherosclerosis at an

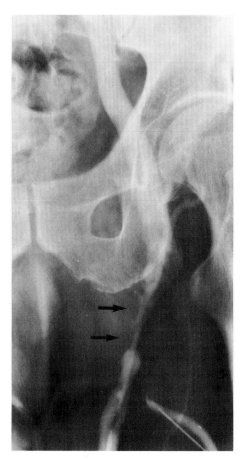

Figure 4.10.13. Venous drainage stenosis in lower extremity Gore-Tex dialysis shunt.

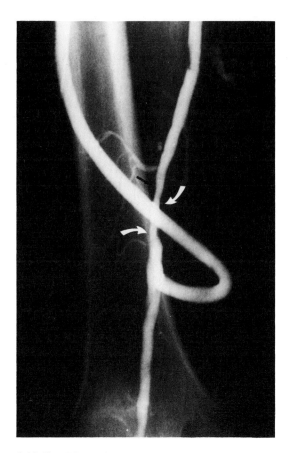

Figure 4.10.12. Atherosclerotic narrowing *(arrows)* of superficial femoral artery proximal to arterial anastomosis of lower extremity shunt. Significant narrowing of proximal artery will decrease flow through shunt.

accelerated rate[5] and experience more vascular complications than do nondiabetics.[28,44]

Lower extremity venous outflow is less developed than in the arm, and is more likely to be further compromised by thrombophlebitis. Finally, there is a greatly increased incidence of infection in lower extremity accesses of all types.[40] This is potentially life-threatening. Infection is second only to heart disease as a cause of morbidity and death in these patients,[6] and 75% of septic episodes in dialysis patients are attributable to infected vascular accesses.[53] Lower extremity accesses develop the same outflow stenoses as those in the arm (Fig. 4.10.13).

Early Warning Signs of Thrombosis

The timely treatment of stenotic lesions by angioplasty can be performed on an outpatient basis and is greatly preferable to treating a thrombosed shunt or fistula. Elevated venous resistance during dialysis should initiate a search for a correctable outflow stenosis (Fig. 4.10.14). In our institution, venous pressures over 200mm Hg at a flow rate of 300ml/min triggers such a search. Angioplasty of venous lesions can easily be performed on an outpatient basis. Saeed et al. experienced only four self-limited hema-

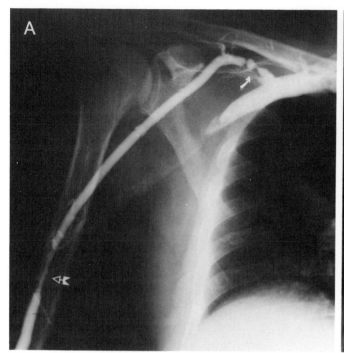

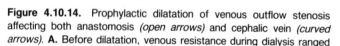

Figure 4.10.14. Prophylactic dilatation of venous outflow stenosis affecting both anastomosis *(open arrows)* and cephalic vein *(curved arrows)*. **A.** Before dilatation, venous resistance during dialysis ranged from 250–300mm Hg. **B.** After dilatation with 10mm high-pressure balloon, venous resistance dropped to 125–150mm Hg (normal range).

tomas complicating 30 venous dilatations in dialysis accesses and fistulas.[54]

If thrombosis occurs, not only is immediate treatment less likely to be successful, but long-term patency is decreased. Gmelin et al. compared the results of angioplasty in stenotic and occluded fistulas.[55] Among those fistulas treated while stenotic, the patency rate was 91% at one year and 57% after two years. If occlusion had occurred, the one-year patency rate dropped to 50% and the two-year patency rate dropped to 14%. While it is possible that the occluded fistulas had more severe disease, these figures support an aggressive program of intervention.

ANGIOGRAPHIC EVALUATION OF DIALYSIS ACCESSES

The use of angiography in the anatomic and functional evaluation of dialysis accesses coincided with their development. Initially arterial and venous opacification was used to define the anatomy for shunt and fistula placement.[56,57] Management of the complications of Scribner shunts was aided by contrast studies,[58,59] and a prospective angiographic study of Scribner shunts from the day of insertion over a period of several months documented the gradual onset of outflow stenosis.[11]

With the advent of the radiocephalic arteriovenous fistula, angiography was used in the evaluation of this access as well.[60]

The complete examination of a dialysis fistula or shunt involves the visualization of the entire blood pathway from the arterial anastomosis, through the draining veins, into the vena cava. If there is a suspected inflow problem, the entire length of the feeding artery should be visualized from its origin to the fistula or to the arterial anastomosis of the shunt. If inflow is adequate, but dialysis times are prolonged and venous resistance during dialysis is high, venous stenosis should be suspected.[3] Even if stenosis of a draining vein is found, the possibility of a second stenosis in the subclavian vein should not be overlooked.

Direct puncture of the feeding artery provides excellent visualization of the fistula or the arterial anastomosis and the draining veins[60,61] (see also Chapter 16).[4,62] Injection into the venous limb of the shunt or fistula during blockade of outflow by a tourniquet or inflated cuff produces the same result. Because it avoids the trauma of arterial puncture, the author uses the latter technique. An interesting variation of the venous approach is described by Hunter et al.[63] They cannulate Brescia–Cimino fistulae from the distal venous limb, which allows them to measure pressure gradients across the fistula or to probe the stump of an occluded fistula with a guidewire, possibly allowing percutaneous recanalization.

Both conventional[64] and real-time[65] sonography have been used to evaluate the complications of arteriovenous fistulae and prosthetic shunts. One study, comparing color Doppler sonography with digital subtraction angiography demonstrated asymptomatic arterial steals undetected by angiography.[66] However, the same study concluded that the overall sensitivity of digital subtraction angiography was greater. Thus, contrast angiography remains the primary modality in evaluating insufficient hemodialysis.

INTERVENTIONAL RADIOLOGIC SALVAGE OF DIALYSIS ACCESSES
Thrombolysis

The widespread availability of thrombolytic enzymes and percutaneous transluminal angioplasty with balloon catheters has allowed the interventional radiologist to play a significant role in the salvage of hemodialysis accesses. In 1970, Hartley and colleagues used urokinase to declot thrombosed Quinton–Scribner shunts that had not responded to the usual heparin irrigation.[67] Although the initial results were encouraging, the study was discontinued because of the cost of the enzyme. Gordon and colleagues performed transluminal angioplasty on 16 stenotic accesses, with restoration of function in ten.[68] Hunter et al. approached nine nonfunctional Brescia–Cimino fistulae from the distal venous limb, as previously described.[63] Despite the complete occlusion present in five fistulae, good results were obtained. In a series of 56 angioplasties of dialysis access fistulae, Glanz et al. treated 44 venous anastomotic stenoses, nine venous outflow stenoses, and three arterial stenoses, with initial success in 70%. Of those patients with a successful result, 80% had patent accesses after three months, 70% after six months, and 55, 50, and 33% after one, two, and three years, respectively.[69] Stenosis of the venous anastomosis and proximal outflow tract predominates over stenosis of the feeding artery by a ratio of 15:1.[3,70]

Thrombolysis of clotted dialysis accesses has been accomplished both by the continuous infusion of dilute streptokinase solution into the shunt[71,72] and by injection of streptokinase directly into the clot.[70,73] Rodkin and colleagues administered a loading dose of 40,000 units of streptokinase, followed by the hourly infusion of 5,000–7,500 units through a multihole catheter. Clinical benefit was obtained in seven of nine patients. One graft bled from previous puncture sites.[71] Graor et al. treated 50 thrombosed dialysis accesses, with a 68% success rate, by a similar infusion technique.[72]

By alternately injecting dilute streptokinase solution percutaneously into the clot and massaging the shunt, Zeit and Cope were able to declot 77% of 33 dialysis accesses.[70] Most shunts were reopened in an hour with streptokinase doses of 15,000–100,000 units, and long-term infusions of streptokinase were frequently avoided. With transluminal angioplasty after thrombolysis, 52% of the shunts treated were restored to function without surgery (Fig. 4.10.15),

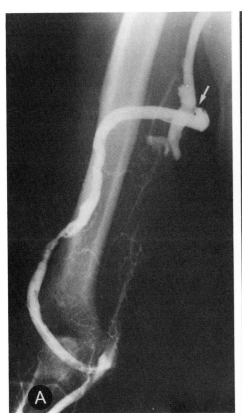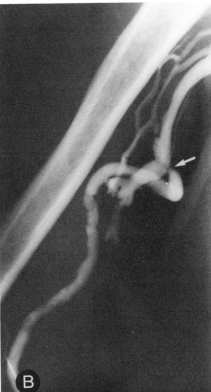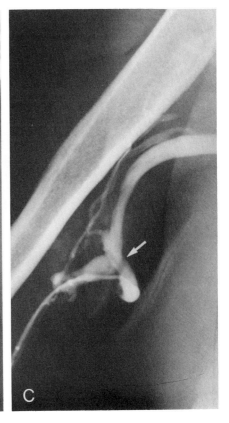

Figure 4.10.15. Thrombosed E-PTFE shunt declotted with 50,000 units of streptokinase injected over a period of 45 minutes. Balloon angioplasty was performed the following day with good result. **A.** Angiogram obtained during thrombolysis. **B.** Predilation angiogram. **C.** Postdilation angiogram. Note venous anastomosis narrowing *(arrows)* in all images.

and an additional 21% were declotted and restored to function after minor operations. Two accesses bled severely enough from sites of previous dialysis punctures to force termination of thrombolysis. A similar technique of injection of small amounts of streptokinase has been useful in declotting double-lumen subclavian dialysis catheters.[23]

Today, streptokinase has largely been supplanted by urokinase, which appears to be more effective in lysing clots, has fewer bleeding complications and has a more rapid effect.[3] Moreover, streptokinase, a nonhuman protein, produces occasional immunologic responses, usually manifested only by low fever,[72] but occasionally resulting in "serum sickness." Urokinase, a human protein, is not known to cause these reactions.

The dosage of urokinase used in thrombolysis varies greatly. High-dose protocols, exemplified by that of McNamara and Fischer[74] call for infusion of 240,000 units/hr and total doses of 2,000,000 units. Pulsed delivery systems utilize 100,000–600,000 units.[75] The author has used a protocol of 250,000 units embedded into the thrombus followed by the infusion of another 250,000 units over 90 minutes with successful thrombolysis in 67%. The quantity of enzyme used was deliberately limited to assess the efficacy of this regimen. In the absence of standardized methods of enzyme delivery and dosage, dogmatic assertions of the "correct" dose are unwarranted.

Another promising trend in thrombolysis is the development of mechanical devices for delivering forceful pulsed sprays of thrombolytic agent into clot.[75,76] One study using such a device to infuse urokinase demonstrated lysis of 46 of 47 occluded dialysis accesses.[76] More important, the mean time for complete lysis was only 63 minutes. Rapid lysis of clot may avoid the need for costly hospitalization, as will be discussed.

Thrombolysis must be complete before angioplasty can be attempted, because the introduction of a dilating catheter into a shunt containing even a small residual thrombus usually precipitates immediate total rethrombosis. Although this problem can be treated by a second course of thrombolytic enzymes, an overnight delay after initial declotting usually results in lysis of small residual clot fragments and allows uneventful angioplasty the following day. If necessary, low-dose heparin may be infused into the access to prevent rethrombosis until angioplasty can be performed.

Angioplasty

Balloon angioplasty of dialysis stenoses differs from dilatation of atherosclerotic arterial lesions. The latter usually respond to relatively low balloon pressures. Dialysis access stenoses may be due either to intimal hyperplasia, which responds to low dilatation pressures, or to scarring at a surgical anastomosis or in the subclavian vein because of prior catheterization. Dilatation of scar tissue requires ex-

tremely high balloon pressures. Dilatation of scarring is also extremely painful. Infiltration of local anesthetic into the area of dilatation brings some relief. Inflation must often be maintained for several minutes. Occasionally, scarring appears to respond, but the stenosis recurs as soon as the balloon is deflated. However, some decrease in venous resistance during subsequent dialysis usually results.

Infected accesses should not receive thrombolysis or angioplasty because of the risk of inducing sepsis and the probable necessity for eventual surgical removal.

METALLIC STENTS AFTER ANGIOPLASTY

Restenosis is a frequent occurrence after angioplasty. Glanz et al. reported a one-year patency rate of only 45% in postangioplasty dialysis shunt stenoses.[61] Various types of vascular stents have been developed to provide mechanical support to dilated vessels in the hopes of inhibiting this process. Palmaz has written a comprehensive review of these devices.[77] Most published reports deal with arterial, rather than venous, stenting.

Gunther and colleagues stented six accesses which were unimproved after thrombectomy and angioplasty.[78] Results were mixed. Three accesses (50%) rethrombosed within six weeks. After repeat thrombectomy, five of the six accesses were patent after two to six months, but intimal hyperplasia had narrowed the lumen in two. Another report described the development of stenosis in a dialysis access within 4.5 months after stenting.[79]

Another factor that may limit the utility of stents is that the stented area can no longer be punctured for dialysis purposes.[78] However, since most stenoses involve the proximal veins rather than the access itself, this may not prove to be a major problem. It is too early to judge the future utility of vascular stenting.

COMPLICATIONS OF THROMBOLYSIS AND ANGIOPLASTY

Bleeding from previous puncture sites is the most frequent complication and the greatest obstacle to success in access thrombolysis when streptokinase is used (Fig. 4.10.16). Young et al. showed that punctures in E-PTFE grafts are sealed with a collagenous plug, presumably the result of organization within a thrombus, and postulated that recently thrombosed puncture sites are themselves susceptible to fibrinolytic effects.[80] The substitution of urokinase for streptokinase has greatly diminished the incidence of bleeding complications.[76]

Other complications of thrombolysis by either infusion or direct injection include embolization of the partially lysed clot (Fig. 4.10.17)[72]; extravasation through graft interstices (usually with knitted Dacron grafts but also seen in an E-PTFE graft treated with urokinase)[81]; and septicemia if the clotted shunt is infected.

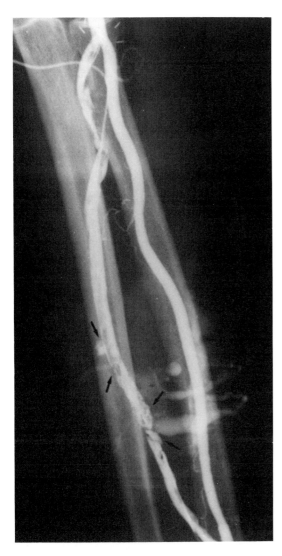

Figure 4.10.16. Extravasation from sites of multiple previous dialysis punctures *(arrows)* during streptokinase thrombolysis by direct injection.

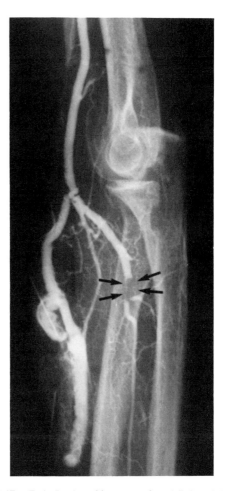

Figure 4.10.17. Embolization of fragment of partially lysed clot *(arrows)* during thrombolysis by direct injection of streptokinase. Patient remained asymptomatic.

Complications of access angioplasty include intimal shearing,[68] thrombosis,[69] and the late development of pseudoaneurysm at the catheterization site.[69] One delayed rupture of natural vein after angioplasty of a Brescia-Cimino fistula has been reported.[82]

DESPERATION INTERVENTION

Inevitably, some patients will outlive all their usable access sites. In the author's experience, occlusion or stenosis in both subclavian and iliac veins is not rare. Peritonitis or abdominal adhesions often preclude peritoneal dialysis. Catheters placed into the superior vena cava become infected or produce caval thrombosis. Renal transplantation becomes mandatory. Methods have been developed which may provide temporary access to prolong life until transplantation can be performed.

Translumbar venous catheterization has been reported in two series.[83,84] The use of a postmortem allogenic vein graft for hemodialysis in a child has also been described.[85]

ECONOMIC CONSIDERATIONS

Containing costs while maintaining quality is medicine's newest challenge. Interventional radiology has demonstrated that it has the capability to play a major role in dialysis access salvage. Thrombectomy and surgical revision are not invariably successful in salvaging an access.[43] Usually thrombectomy or surgical revision extend the useful life of the access only six months to one year.[3] Wilson cites an operative failure rate of 17%, with an additional 23% of thrombectomized and revised shunts failing within the first postoperative month.[10] Moreover, thrombectomy fails to diagnose or treat proximal venous outflow stenoses.

Nevertheless, in many institutions thrombectomy, sometimes assisted by vascular imaging, has been resurrected and has supplanted enzymatic thrombolysis.[78,86] Surgery is claimed to be more rapid and is usually less expensive than thrombolytic protocols requiring overnight hospitalization. This is especially true if institutional policy requires intensive observation of patients receiving thrombolytic therapy. Thrombolytic therapy costs of $2500 per day have been reported.[76]

If thrombolysis is to remain a viable economic alternative in dialysis patients, rapid outpatient treatment protocols must be developed. Because urokinase has a more rapid onset of action than streptokinase, and a biologic half-life of only 14 minutes,[3] costly hospitalization may be avoided by using this drug. Graor found that, considering all cost factors, treatment with urokinase was only $11 more expensive than with streptokinase.

Angioplasty of stenoses, however, is a relatively inexpensive outpatient procedure. Moreover, when concomitant angiography will disclose otherwise unsuspected stenoses or obstructions.

DISCUSSION AND CONCLUSIONS

The interventional radiologist is able to treat the stenosed access shunt cheaply, easily, and usually, successfully. Even a modest radiographic improvement may translate into several months or even years of additional use (Fig. 4.10.18). Once an access has thrombosed, however, the prognosis for return of function depends on the underlying cause. For example, accesses that have clotted because of hypotension or excessive postdialysis compression respond well to thrombolysis.[70] Shunts that thrombose because of an underlying stenosis may be declotted and used for some time, but their ultimate longevity will depend on the ability to treat the underlying stenosis by angioplasty or surgery. Accesses that fail within the first few weeks probably suffer from technical problems (Fig. 4.10.19),[88] and although they, too, may be usable after thrombolysis, eventual surgical revision is inevitable.

No systematic study of shunt survival after thrombolysis and angioplasty or angioplasty alone has yet been published. However, numerous such shunts have remained useful longer than a year,[68,72] and the patient in Figure 4.10.14 has had years of trouble-free use of his shunt. It is therefore apparent that significant benefit may be obtained by nonoperative treatment.

In this review, the historical development of dialysis accesses and their problems have been outlined. Although some of the complications described are beyond the ministrations of the interventional radiologist, many, including the common venous outflow stenosis, are treatable by transcatheter techniques. With methods now readily avail-

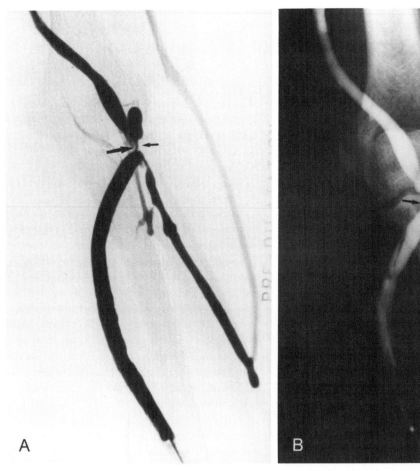

A

B

Figure 4.10.18. Dilatation of venous outflow stenosis after streptokinase thrombolysis. Only modest radiographic improvement was obtained, but shunt has functioned without further difficulty for 31 months. **A.** Before dilatation; marked outflow stenosis *(arrows)*. **B.** After dilatation; considerable residual narrowing is still present *(arrows)*.

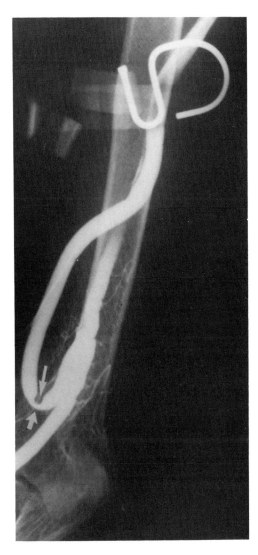

Figure 4.10.19. Kinking of E-PTFE shunt *(arrows)* produced occlusion nine days after implantation. Shunt was declotted with 25,000 units of streptokinase. Surprisingly, shunt remained open for one month and was used for dialysis during that period. Surgical revision was performed after reclotting.

able, and with the close cooperation of clinical colleagues, radiologists can effect significant improvements in access longevity.

References

1. Kennedy J, Stewart D: Interventional coronary arteriography. *Annu Rev Med* 1984;35:513–534
2. Codini M: Management of acute myocardial infarction. *Med Clin North Am* 1986;70:769–790
3. Bell WR: Update on urokinase and streptokinase: a comparison of their efficacy and safety. *Hosp Formul* 1988;23:230–241
4. Gilula LA, Staple TW, Anderson CB, Anderson LS: Venous angiography of hemodialysis fistulae. *Radiology* 1975;115:555
5. Giacchino JL, Geis WP, Buckingham JM, et al: Vascular access: long term results, new techniques. *Arch Surg* 1979;114:403
6. Wilson SE: Complications of vascular access, in Wilson SE, Owens ML (eds): *Vascular Access Surgery.* Chicago, Year Book Medical Publishers, 1980, p 185
7. Kolff WF: The first clinical experience with the artificial kidney. *Ann Intern Med* 1965;62:608
8. Quinton W, Dillard D, Scribner BH: Cannulation of blood vessels for prolonged hemodialysis. *Trans Am Soc Artif Intern Organs* 1960;6:104
9. Pendras JP, Smith MP: The Silastic-Teflon arterio-venous cannula. *Trans Am Soc Artif Intern Organs* 1966;12:222
10. Haimov M: Vascular access for hemodialysis. *Surg Gynecol Obstet* 1975;141:619
11. Moskowitz H, Gerber NA, McDonald HP Jr, et al: Angiographic study of arteriovenous shunt in hemodialysis patients. *Radiology* 1969;93:72
12. Glashan RW, Walker FA: A histological examination of veins used in artificial arteriovenous (Quinton–Scribner) shunts. *Br J Surg* 1968;55:189
13. Baste JC, Midy D, Albert M, et al: L'utilisation des prothèses Impra a paroi fine dans l'abord vasculaire en hémodialyse chronique. *J Chir (Paris)* 1989;126:232–241
14. Sottiurai VS, Yao JST, Batson RC, et al: Distal anastomotic intimal hyperplasia: histopathologic character and biogenesis. *Ann Vasc Surg* 1989;3:26–33
15. Okuhn SP, Connelly DP, Calakos BA et al: Does compliance mismatch alone cause neointimal hyperplasia? *J Vasc Surg* 1989;9:35–45
16. Foran RF, Golding AL, Treiman RL, DePalma JR: Quinton–Scribner cannulas for hemodialysis: review of four years' experience. *Calif Med* 1970;112:8
17. Mandel SR: Vascular access in a university transplant and dialysis program. *Arch Surg* 1977;112:1375–1380
18. David D, Petersen J, Feldman R, et al: Subclavian vein stenosis: a complication of subclavian dialysis. *JAMA* 1984;252:3404–3408
19. Daniell SJN, Dacie JE: Percutaneous transluminal angioplasty of brachiocephalic vein stenoses in patients with dialysis shunts. *Radiology* 1988;169:280–81
20. Daniell SJN, Dacie JE: Failure of percutaneous transluminal angioplasty in symptomatic subclavian vein thrombosis complicating subclavian vein cannulation for haemodialysis. *J Intervent Radiol* 1987;2:113–116
21. Watlington J, Contes G, Yium J, et al: Arm edema due to subclavian vein occlusion and vascular access placement in maintenance hemodialysis patients with previous subclavian vein temporary catheters (abstract). 33rd Annual Scientific Meeting of the National Kidney Foundation. New York, Grune and Stratton, 1983, p 33
22. Cope C: An improved fine needle catheter introducing set for safer central vein cannulation. *Parent Enteral Nutr* 1983;7:296
23. Caruana RJ, Raja RR, Zeit RM, et al: Thrombotic complications of indwelling central catheters used for chronic hemodialysis. *Am J Kidney Dis* 1987;9:497–501
24. Butt KMH, Riedman EA, Kountz SL: Angioaccess. *Curr Probl Surg* 1976;13:1–14
25. Brescia MJ, Cimino JE, Appel K, et al: Chronic hemodialysis using venipuncture and surgically created arteriovenous fistula. *N Engl J Med* 1966;275:1089
26. Haimov M, Burrows L, Casey JD, Schupak E: Vascular access for hemodialysis: experience with 214 patients: special problems and causes for early and late failures. *Proc Eur Dial Transplant Assoc* 1973;9:173
27. Matolo W, Kastigir B, Stevens L, et al: Neurovascular complications of brachial arteriovenous fistula. *Am J Surg* 1971;121:716
28. Buselmeier TJ, Najarian JS, Simmons R, et al: A-V fistulae

and the diabetic: ischemia and gangrene may result in amputation. *Trans Am Soc Artif Intern Organs* 1973;19:49

29. Ahern D, Maher J: Heart failure as a complication of hemodialysis arteriovenous fistula. *Ann Intern Med* 1972;77:201

30. Swayne LC, Manstein C, Somers R, Cope C: Selective digital venous hypertension: a rare complication of hemodialysis arteriovenous fistula. *Cardiovasc Intervent Radiol* 1983;10:61

31. Geis WP, Giacchino JL, Iwatsuki S, et al: The reverse fistula for vascular access. *Surg Gynecol Obstet* 1977;144:901

32. Guidoin R, Couture J, Assayed F, et al: New frontiers of vascular grafting. *Int Surg* 1988;73:241–49

33. Haimov M, Burrows I, Schanzer H, et al: Experience with arterial substitutes in the construction of vascular access for hemodialysis. *Cardiovasc Surg* 1980;21:149

34. Giardet RE, Hacket RE, Goodwin NJ, et al: Thirteen months' experience with the saphenous vein graft arteriovenous fistula for maintenance hemodialysis. *Trans Am Soc Artif Intern Organs* 1970;16:285

35. Beemer RK, Hayes JF: Hemodialysis using a mandril grown graft. *Trans Am Soc Artif Intern Organs* 1973;19:43

36. Chintz JL, Yoloyama T, Bower R: Self-sealing prosthesis for arteriovenous fistula in man. *Trans Am Soc Artif Intern Organs* 1972;18:452

37. Tellis VA, Kohlberg WI, Bhat DJ, et al: Expanded polytetrafluoroethylene fistula for chronic hemodialysis. *Ann Surg* 1970;189:101

38. Mohaideen AH, Tanchaija S, Avram MM, Mainzer RA: Arteriovenous access for hemodialysis utilizing polytetrafluoroethylene grafts. *NY State J Med* 1980;80:190

39. Anderson CB, Sicard GA, Etheredge EE: Bovine carotid artery and expanded polytetrafluoroethylene grafts for hemodialysis vascular access. *Surg Res* 1980;29:184

40. Rubio PA, DelGuercio LRM: Vascular access: methods, maintenance and management of complications. *Infect Surg* 1985;26:355

41. Gill F, Guzman R, Guidoin R, et al: An histo-morphological evaluation of ninety surgically excised human umbilical vein grafts. *J Biomed Mater Res* 1989;23:363–380

42. Sabanayagam P, Schwartz AB, Soricelli RR, et al: A comparative study of 402 bovine heterografts and 225 reinforced expanded PTFE grafts as AVF in the ESRD patient. *Trans Am Soc Artif Intern Organs* 1980;26:88

43. Shack RB Neblett W, Richie RE, Dean RH: Expanded polytetrafluoroethylene as dialysis access grafts: serial study of histology and fibrinolytic activity. *Am Surg* 1977;44:817

44. Anderson CB, Etheredge EE, Sicard GA: One hundred polytetrafluoroethylene vascular access grafts. *Dial Transplant* 1980;9:237

45. Tordoir JMH, Herman JMMPH, Kwan TS, et al: Long-term follow-up of the polytetrafluoroethylene (PTFE) prosthesis as an arteriovenous fistula for haemodialysis. *Eur J Vasc Surg* 1987;2:3–7

46. Mohr LL, Smith LL: Polytetrafluoroethylene graft aneurysms: a report of five aneurysms. *Arch Surg* 1980;115:1467

47. Pasternak BM, Samson R, Karp MP: Fungal infection of a vascular prosthesis. *Surgery* 1979;85:586

48. Rendl KH, Prenner KV: The redo-surgery of expanded polytetrafluoroethylene (PTFE) arteriovenous fistulae for hemodialysis. *Vasc Surg* 1984;18:261

49. Palder SB, Kirkman RL, Whittemore AD, et al: Vascular access for hemodialysis: patency rates and results of revision. *Ann Surg* 1985;202:235–239

50. Hodgkinson DJ, Shepard GH: Coverage of exposed Gore-Tex dialysis access graft with local sublimis myocutaneous flap. *Plast Reconstr Surg* 1982;69:1010

51. McKenna PJ, Leadbetter MG: Salvage of chronically exposed Gore-Tex vascular access grafts in the hemodialysis patient. *Plast Reconst Surg* 1988;82:1046–1049

52. Rosental JJ, Bell DD, Gaspar MR, et al: Prevention of high flow problems of arteriovenous grafts. *Am J Surg* 1980;140:231

53. Dobkin JF, Miller RH, Steigbigel NH: Septicemia in patients on chronic hemodialysis. *Ann Intern Med* 1978;88:28

54. Saeed M, Newman GE, McCann RL, et al: Stenoses in dialysis fistulas: treatment with percutaneous angioplasty. *Radiology* 1987;164:693–97

55. Gmelin E, Winterhoff R, Rinast E: Insufficient hemodialysis access fistulas: late result of treatment with percutaneous balloon angioplasty. *Radiology* 1989;171:657–660

56. Chintz J. Onesti G, Brest AH, Swartz C: Radiography of A-V shunt in hemodialysis. *JAMA* 1969;207:2286

57. Wing AJ, Jones NF, Lea–Thomas M, Thompson AE: Peripheral angiography of arms and legs as aid to planning shunt and fistula operations. *Proc Eur Dial Transplant Assoc* 1971;7:510

58. Dathan JR, Thompson JMA, Worthington BS: Angiographic studies of Quinton–Scribner arterio-venous cannulae. *Br Med J* 1969;4:20

59. Snalley RH, Klinger EL Jr, Blakeley WR: Angiographic evaluation in external arteriovenous shunt management. *AJR* 1969;107:434

60. Hurwich BJ: Brachial arteriography of the surgically created radial arteriovenous fistula in patients undergoing chronic intermittent hemodialysis by venipuncture technique. *AJR* 1968;104:394

61. Glanz S, Bashist B, Gordon DH, et al: Angiography of upper extremity access fistulae for dialysis. *Radiology* 1982;143:45

62. Anderson CB, Gilula LA, Sicard GA, Etheredge EE: Venous angiography of subcutaneous hemodialysis fistulae. *Arch Surg* 1979;114:1320

63. Hunter DW, So SKS, Castañeda–Zúñiga WR, et al: Failing or thrombosed Brescia-Cimino arterio-venous dialysis fistulae: angiographic evaluation and percutaneous transluminal angioplasty. *Radiology* 1983;149:105

64. Kottle SP, Gonzalez AC, Macon EJ, Fellner SK: Ultrasonographic evaluation of vascular access complications. *Radiology* 1978;129:751

65. Scheible W, Skram C, Leopold GR: High resolution real-time sonography of hemodialysis vascular access complications. *AJR* 1980;134:1173

66. Middleton WD, Picus DD, Marx MV, et al: Color Doppler sonography of hemodialysis vascular access: comparison with angiography. *AJR* 1989;152:633–39

67. Hartley LCJ, Ellis FG, Rendall M. et al: The use of urokinase in Scribner shunts. *Br J Urol* 1980;42:246

68. Gordon DH, Glanz S, Butt KM, et al: Treatment of stenotic lesions in dialysis access fistulae and shunts by transluminal angioplasty. *Radiology* 1982;143:53

69. Glanz S, Gordon D, Butt KMH, et al: Treatment of stenoses by transluminal angioplasty. *Radiology* 1984;152:637

70. Zeit RM, Cope C: Failed hemodialysis shunts: one year of experience with aggressive treatment. *Radiology* 1985;154:353

71. Rodkin RS, Bookstein JJ, Heeney DJ, Davis GR: Streptokinase and transluminal angioplasty in the treatment of acutely thrombosed hemodialysis access fistulae. *Radiology* 1983;149:425

72. Graor RA, Risius B, Young JR, et al: Low dose streptokinase for selective thrombolysis: systemic effects and complications. *Radiology* 1984;152:35

73. Zeit RM: Clearing of clotted dialysis shunts by streptokinase injection at multiple sites. *AJR* 1983;141:1053

74. McNamara TO, Fischer JR: Thrombolysis of peripheral arterial and graft occlusions: improved results using high-dose urokinase. *AJR* 1985;144:769–775

75. Bookstein JJ, Fellmeth B, Roberts A, et al: Pulsed-spray pharmacomechanical thrombolysis: preliminary clinical results. *AJR* 1989;152:1097–1100

76. Kandarpa K, Drinker PA, Singer SJ, et al: Forceful pulsatile local infusion of enzyme accelerates thrombolysis: in vivo evaluation of a new delivery system. *Radiology* 1988; 168:738–744

77. Palmaz JC: Balloon-expandable intravascular stent. *AJR* 1988;150:1263–1269

78. Gunther RW, Vorwerk D, Bohndorf K, et al: Venous stenoses in dialysis shunts: treatment with self-expanding metallic stents. *Radiology* 1989;170:401–405

79. Zollikofer CL, Largiader I, Bruhlmann WF, et al: Endovascular stenting of veins and grafts: preliminary clinical experience. *Radiology* 1988;167:707–712

80. Young AT, Hunter DW, Castañeda–Zúñiga WR, et al: Thrombosed synthetic hemodialysis access fistulae: failure of fibrinolytic therapy. *Radiology* 1985;154:639

81. Becker GJ, Holden RW, Rabe FE: Contrast extravasation from a Gore-Tex graft: a complication of thrombolytic therapy. *AJR* 1984;142:573

82. Bourne EE: Late venous rupture after angioplasty of an arteriovenous dialysis fistula. *AJR* 1988;150:797–798

83. Denny DF Jr, Greenwood LH, Morse SS, et al: Inferior vena cava: translumbar catheterization for central venous access. *Radiology* 1989;170:1013–1014

84. Lund GB, Lieberman RP, Haire WD: Translumbar inferior vena cava catheters for long-term venous access. *Radiology* 1990;174:31–35

85. Brynitz S, Alsbjorn B, Iversen-Hansen R: Post-mortem allogenic vein for graft as vascular access in chronic haemodialysis. *Lancet* 1988;2:900–901

86. Smith TP, Cragg AH, Castañeda F, et al: Thrombosed polytetrafluoroethylene hemodialysis fistulas: salvage with combined thrombectomy and angioplasty. *Radiology* 1989; 171:507–508

87. Graor RA, Young JR, Risius B, et al: Comparison of cost-effectiveness of streptokinase and urokinase in the treatment of deep vein thrombosis. *Ann Vasc Surg* 1987;II:524–528

88. Rohr MS, Browder W, Frentz GD, McDonald JC: Arteriovenous fistulae for long term dialysis. *Arch Surg* 1978; 113:153

Part 11. Vascular Access for Long-term Hemodialysis: Preoperative Evaluation and the Management of Failing and Thrombosed Accesses

—Samuel K. S. So, M.B., B.S, and David W. Hunter, M.D.

The first section of this part provides a synopsis of the basic principles and choice of access for long-term hemodialysis. The second section deals with the role of radiographic evaluation in assisting the surgeon in the preoperative and postoperative assessment of the patient and with the management of the complications–associated with each access device.

BASIC CONSIDERATIONS

Vascular access is appropriately described as the Achilles heel of dialysis patients, because problems associated with these accesses are a significant cause of morbidity and even death.[1–3] Nonetheless, if the initial access is carefully tailored to the needs of the individual patient, high long-term patency rates usually can be achieved with few complications.

Surgeons strive to provide reliable vascular accesses without compromising the perfusion of the extremity. The access should provide adequate flow for efficient dialysis with the greatest likelihood of long-term function and the fewest complications. The initial access should be constructed with the most distal suitable vessels in order to preserve valuable proximal lengths of vessels for future access needs. Together with the nephrologist, the surgeon must make sure that the type of access is matched to the needs of the patient and the capabilities of the particular dialysis unit. Therefore, the surgeon must be familiar with the needs of the patient and with the advantages, limitations, and possible complications of each type of access procedure and type of dialysis. Access procedures for immediate (short-term) and long-term hemodialysis are often different and require different strategies.[4,5]

Long-term hemodialysis accesses, such as the Brescia–Cimino fistula and bridge grafts, usually must mature for three weeks before being used. Therefore, an access route must be chosen for all patients with end-stage renal disease in whom a need for maintenance dialysis is expected within a few months. Such planning will minimize the need for a temporary access procedure to be added to that required for maintenance hemodialysis. If a temporary subclavian or internal jugular hemodialysis catheter is required, it must be placed in the contralateral side in order to minimize the risk of catheter-associated thrombosis or stenosis of the ipsilateral central vein.

CHOICE OF ACCESS FOR LONG-TERM HEMODIALYSIS

A low incidence of complications, high long-term patency rates, and patient acceptance are the key features of an ideal angioaccess for long-term hemodialysis (Fig. 4.11.1). The direct arteriovenous (DAV) Brescia–Cimino fistula, introduced in 1966, is constructed between the distal radial artery and the cephalic vein and is still the best access for long-term hemodialysis.[2,4–6] Its complications are minor and few. For example, in 1049 patients followed for more than one year, the chances of hospitalization for an access-related problem was 5 times greater in patients with shunts or bovine grafts than in patients with Brescia–Cimino fistulae.[2] The one-year and three-year cumulative patency rates are estimated at 85–90% and 60–85%, respectively.[7–9] If the distal vessels are unsuitable for an access, the next best choice is a DAV fistula higher in the forearm, such as between the proximal radial artery and the cephalic vein or an adjacent suitable superficial vein. The external Scribner shunt, introduced by Quinton et al. in 1960, is now seldom used for long-term hemodialysis because of its low long-term patency rate.[8,10]

In patients who have no suitable forearm vessels, the best access is usually an antecubital direct arteriovenous fistula between the brachial artery and the cephalic or median cubital vein or a bridge graft. However, a proximal DAV fistula[11] is suitable only for patients with a patent and easily accessible upper arm cephalic vein. The normally deeply seated basilic vein is generally unsuitable for dialysis unless extensive dissection is performed to elevate it to a

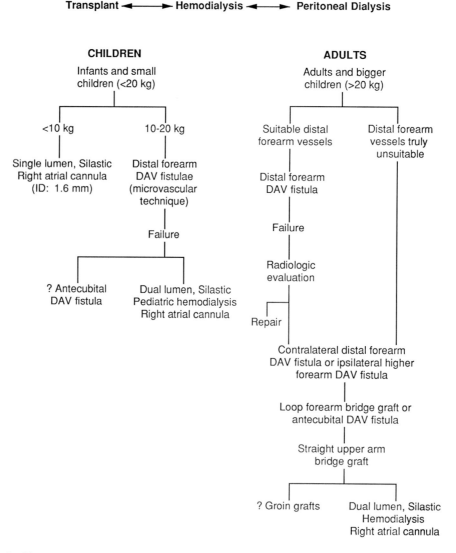

Transplant ⟷ Hemodialysis ⟷ Peritoneal Dialysis

Figure 4.11.1 A practical guide to access selection for long-term hemodialysis. (Modified from So SKS: General principles of access surgery, in Simmons RL, Finch ME, Ascher, NL, Najarian JS (eds): *Manual of Vascular Access, Organ Donation, and Transplantation*. New York, Springer-Verlag, 1984, pp 3–87.)

superficial subcutaneous position for easy puncture by dialysis needles.

For patients with no suitable vessels for a forearm or an antecubital DAV fistula, either a straight (radial artery–antecubital vein) or looped (brachial artery–antecubital vein) forearm bridge graft can be used. There is no ideal graft material, but in most dialysis centers expanded polytetrafluoroethylene (E-PTFE) has performed better than any other material, including autogenous veins, as determined by the patency and complication rates.[4,12–14] Because the distal radial artery is frequently unsuitable for graft placement, the authors prefer to use the loop forearm graft from the brachial artery to an antecubital vein. If no suitable antecubital vein is available, an excellent alternative is a straight brachial artery to basilic or axillary vein bridge graft.

Bridge grafts in the groin are associated with a high incidence of infectious complications and should be considered only for the rare patient who has no suitable vessels in the arms and in whom peritoneal dialysis is not feasible.[3] Even then, these grafts may be unnecessary if the dual-lumen Silastic long-term hemodialysis catheter can be used.[4,15]

In children weighing between 10 and 20kg, the authors advocate a similar approach with minor modifications. Microvascular techniques are mandatory in the construction of DAV fistulae in young children. Distal forearm DAV fistulae in these small children usually require four to eight weeks to mature. In small children, a relatively short length of vein is available for needle puncture, and since repeated punctures often cause venous stenoses, use of single-needle dialysis may help to prolong the problem-free lifespan of these small fistulae. Small children will often tolerate a distal ulnar artery-basilic vein fistula when no suitable radiocephalic vessels are found. The short, narrow extremities of small, thin children render them poor candidates for bridge graft placement, and groin grafts should be avoided because of the high incidence of infection and leg swelling.

For infants weighing <10kg, long-term access is a difficult problem.[16] Distal forearm fistulae have a high early failure rate and may take four months to mature,[17] so internal access is limited to antecubital DAV fistulae and bridge grafts placed in the groin. Many dialysis centers prefer peritoneal dialysis for these tiny infants. Since June 1980, the authors have taken a new approach to this problem: hemodialysis with a Hickman catheter (internal diameter, 1.6mm) or the larger bore (2.0mm) Silastic catheter placed in the right atrium.[4,18–20] This method creates a painless and reliable access for dialysis and spares the peripheral vessels for future access sites. The catheter is usually left in place until the child is sent home after renal transplantation. Children who might not receive an allograft for some time—e.g., because of a high antibody titer—can be maintained on hemodialysis with the Silastic catheter until they are big enough for a more suitable angioaccess.

CHOICE OF ACCESS SITE

When selecting a vascular access site, the following factors should be taken into consideration.[4,21] First, the non-dominant arm is chosen preferentially if the vessels are equally suitable bilaterally. Second, the most distal site is chosen so a longer segment of the proximal vessel can be used for needle puncture and the proximal vessels can be preserved for future revision if necessary. Third, use of the groin vessels should be avoided because the incidence of infection is extremely high, and septic complications in the groin can cause serious morbidity and even death. Fourth, use of the more proximal major arteries for access generally increases the risk of ischemic complications and high-output cardiac failure. Fifth, use of extremities with poor collateral circulation should be avoided. Also, the popliteal artery and the brachial artery at the bifurcation are particularly vulnerable to ischemic complications and should be avoided as vascular access sites. Sixth, when hemodialysis is required in a patient whose long-term access site is not ready for use, a temporary access, such as a subclavian venous cannula, should be placed in the opposite extremity to avoid compromising the venous outflow of the long-term access. Seventh, the thin-walled veins on the volar surface of the forearm are generally unsuitable for construction of a DAV fistula. Finally, patients with two functioning AV fistulae are at a higher risk of congestive heart failure.

Venipunctures *must* be prohibited above the wrist of the arm chosen for access. While the patient is in the hospital, the chosen extremity could be kept in Ace wraps and labeled so that other medical staff members do not accidentally use it for injections or venipunctures.

PREOPERATIVE EVALUATION

It cannot be overemphasized that the key to creating a long-lasting reliable access for hemodialysis is careful planning. This includes obtaining a thorough medical and surgical history, with particular attention to past access procedures; a thorough physical examination of the arterial and venous system bilaterally; and, if necessary, a preoperative venogram or duplex sonography. This information provides a map of the patient's available vasculature and helps the surgeon select the best site as well as the best form of access. A high incidence of primary nonfunction is frequently a hallmark of poor planning rather than of poor surgical technique.

The arterial system is assessed simply by palpation of the brachial, radial, and ulnar pulses in both upper extremities. The possibility of limb ischemia after arterial interruption is evaluated by selective occlusion of the major vessels and by performing the Allen test to check the adequacy of collateral perfusion to the hand. To perform the Allen test, both the ulnar and the radial arteries are occluded at the wrist by the thumbs of the examiner. The hand is then drained of blood by repeated digital flexion. Color should return to all the fingers within six seconds after each artery is individually released.[22] If digital circulation returns promptly after release, either artery can be ligated safely. In the authors' experience, any artery with a palpable pulse, even if the vessel is calcified, generally provides adequate blood flow and is suitable for construction of a DAV fistula. A preoperative brachial or axillary arteriogram is both hazardous and unnecessary.

The venous system is often the limiting factor in determining flow through any AV fistula. The veins must be assessed by applying a tourniquet over each extremity. Even though a distal vein is distended, a more proximal stenotic segment may be present. Therefore, it is extremely important to palpate and percuss the vein along its entire length to check for proximal stenosis that can result from previous venipuncture or cannulation. In difficult circumstances, a preoperative venogram or duplex sonography will identify the caliber of the veins and help to rule out proximal stenosis and obstruction. A preoperative venogram is particularly useful in the evaluation of children and in adult patients who have bilateral venipuncture bruises along their forearms and antecubital fossae. A venogram is also useful in assessing patients who have had indwelling subclavian vein or jugular vein catheters, who may have developed thrombosis or stenosis of the subclavian or innominate veins. An AV fistula inadvertently placed on the side with a tight stenosis or thrombosis of the central veins will quickly fail or cause severe venous hypertension.

To minimize the risk of nephrotoxicity in the uremic patient, it is important to use the minimum amount of intravenous contrast medium in performing the venogram. In the authors' experience, the veins of the arm are best evaluated as shown in Figure 4.11.2. Access to the venous system is obtained by cannulation of a superficial vein over the dorsum of the hand. A rubber tourniquet or blood pressure cuff is then placed around the upper arm to occlude venous outflow, so that the vessels can be filled with just 10–20ml of 30% diatrizoate. Anteroposterior and lateral views of the forearm and upper arm vessels are then obtained. As the tourniquet is released, rapid sequential films or cinefluorograph (cine) radiographs should be taken of the upper arm or shoulder to rule out a more proximal lesion. Proximal obstruction may either be evident radiologically or be suggested by a delay in the clearance of the contrast medium. In recent years duplex sonography of the proximal veins has become the procedure of choice in preoperative evaluation of patients who are not yet dialysis-dependent. However, if subclavian vein stenosis is suspected, venography is still the most reliable test since satisfactory examination of the proximal part of the subclavian vein located behind the clavicle remains difficult by ultrasound.

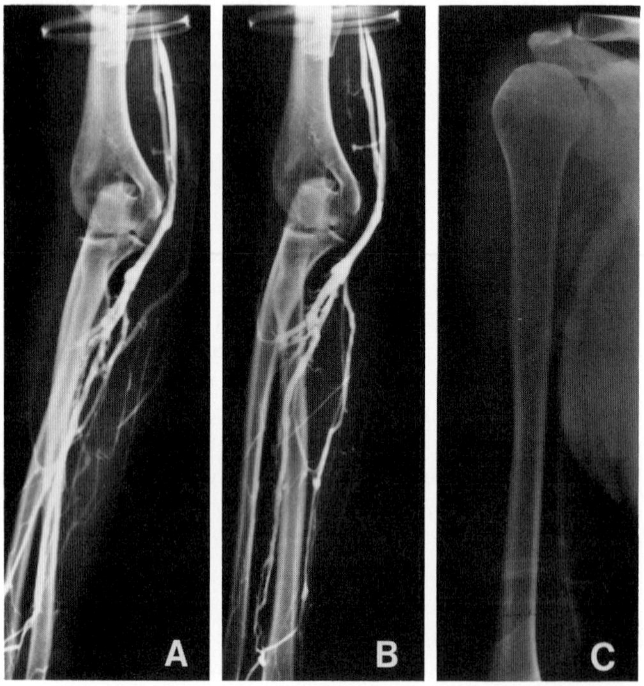

EVALUATION AND MANAGEMENT OF ACCESS PROBLEMS

Complications related to the vascular access are the most frequent cause of hospitalization of patients on long-term hemodialysis. In a one-year, five-center study of 1049 patients on dialysis for at least three months, 26% of the initial hospitalizations were necessitated by access problems. In addition, patients with xenogeneic bridge grafts or external prosthetic shunts had a 5-fold greater frequency of hospitalization than did patients with autogenous DAV fistulae.[2]

Access-related complications can be minimized if the patient is thoroughly evaluated preoperatively and if the procedures are well planned and carefully performed. However, all dialysis staff members and physicians must be aware of the possible complications so they can be recognized early and treated promptly to prevent both access loss and morbidity.

There are, essentially, five complications: infection, bleeding, aneurysm, partial or complete obstruction, and hemodynamic problems.[1,4] Infection is the second most common cause of access failure. The principle in the management of access-related infection is prevention; it is important to give prophylactic antibiotics and to use strict aseptic techniques in access surgery and whenever invasive radiologic procedures are used. Bleeding is primarily a problem of external AV shunts; fatal hemorrhage may

Figure 4.11.2. A venogram of the upper extremity can be obtained with minimum contrast medium by using a tourniquet to occlude the venous outflow. After anteroposterior (**A**) and lateral (**B**) views of the forearm and arm have been obtained, proximal venous runoff is assessed by rapid sequential films or cine radiographs of the upper arm and shoulder (**C**) as the tourniquet is released.

result from disconnection of the external cannulas. Brescia–Cimino fistulae may appear aneurysmal, with dilated, tortuous veins, but these rarely reach a size that requires excision. True aneurysms are uncommon in E-PTFE grafts, although repeated traumatic punctures may create a small hole in the graft, leading to formation of a pseudoaneurysm. Arterial insufficiency following creation of an AV access is uncommon if the adequacy of collateral perfusion has been carefully assessed preoperatively and if the diameter of the bridge graft does not exceed 6mm. Ischemic complications are best assessed by physical examination and Doppler studies[4]; contrast studies are seldom indicated.

The most common cause of access failure is thrombosis, which is often preceded by increasing problems during dialysis, such as difficult cannulation, withdrawal of clots, and high venous resistance or poor arterial flow. In addition, patients with AV communications may have a diminished bruit or thrill.

Radiographic evaluation is invaluable in the management of a failing access, because it helps confirm the presence and locate the site of the lesion. Simple roentgenograms of the chest confirm the positioning of right atrial Silastic hemodialysis catheters. Contrast study via the fistula or graft is the best way to assess the lumen of the access

device and the caliber of the venous outflow. Assuming that the study is carefully planned, reliable information can be obtained with a low risk and a small volume of contrast medium. Needle puncture of the graft or fistula for radiologic study is no more invasive than needle puncture for dialysis and almost always yields more useful information than does ultrasonography. Operative angiography is absolutely necessary during repair of the occlusive defects.

Radiocephalic and Autogenous Direct AV Fistulae

The Brescia–Cimino internal fistula is the best access for maintenance hemodialysis because of its low incidence of complications and the high long-term patency rate.[2,7–9] Ideally, the distal radial artery is directly anastomosed to the distal cephalic vein just above the wrist so a long segment of arterialized cephalic vein can be used for cannulation by dialysis needles. Because thrombosis is still the most common cause of early failure, the authors prefer to use the side-to-side anastomosis described by Brescia et al., because it produces the highest blood flow[23] (Fig. 4.11.3). However, some surgeons prefer to construct an end-to-side or end-to-end fistula with ligation of the distal cephalic vein and radial artery to minimize the risk of distal extrem-

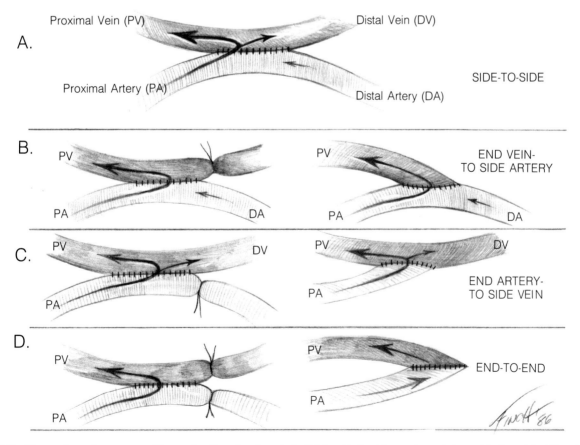

Figure 4.11.3. Types of anastomoses used in construction of radiocephalic fistula; side-to-side anastomosis is used in the original Brescia–Cimino fistula.

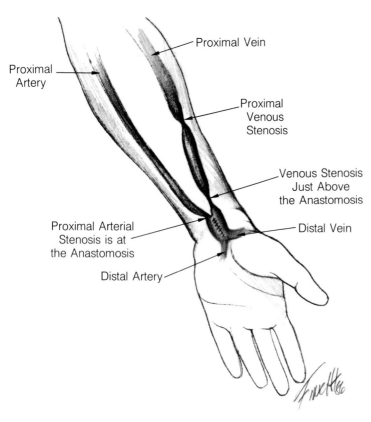

Figure 4.11.4. Common lesions found in association with failing or thrombosed Brescia–Cimino fistula.

ity venous hypertension or arterial steal (Fig. 4.11.3).[24–26] Direct AV fistulas can also be created at the level of the antecubital vein, or the cephalic vein or basilic vein; at the level of the wrist between the ulnar artery and basilic vein; and at the anatomic "snuff box" between the radial artery and cephalic vein.

Failure of a DAV fistula is often signaled by difficulties in dialysis, with low flow rates or high venous resistance; an apparent diminution of the thrill or bruit; or failure of a recently created fistula to mature despite the presence of a thrill or bruit. Some patients with a stenosis in the proximal outflow vein may suffer venous hypertension, characterized by swelling of the arm and hand distal to the fistula which may be associated with stasis ulceration and throbbing pain over the thumb.[24,25] The common causes of failing Brescia–Cimino fistulae are stenoses of either the proximal artery or the vein at or just above the anastomosis or stenoses of the proximal vein at the dialysis needle puncture sites (Fig. 4.11.4).[4,27–30] The most common problem, stenosis of the vein just above the anastomosis, can be the result of a technical error, a fibrous band, or intimal hyperplasia from turbulent flow. Stenosis of the artery at the anastomosis is often the result of technical error.

EVALUATION OF FAILING DAV FISTULAE

It is most important and informative to analyze the clinical information and perform a thorough physical exami-

nation. Insight into the problem is often obtained by talking to the dialysis staff. It is helpful to remember that high venous resistance during dialysis is suggestive of proximal venous stenosis or occlusion of the major venous outflow channel, whereas poor arterial flow is indicative of proximal arterial stenosis or stenosis of the fistula distal to the arterial needle. Venous hypertension with swelling of the hand is usually associated with proximal venous stenosis or occlusion. Loss of the thrill and bruit on compression of the distal vein below a side-to-side direct AV fistula is a sign of proximal venous obstruction. If the thrill is replaced by a prominent pulsation, venous runoff is probably compromised.

With these data alone one can often locate the lesion, and they are of utmost value to the access surgeon or the radiologist. For example, the patient in Figure 4.11.5 had a normal venous fistulogram up to the elbow; but because he had high venous pressure during dialysis, contrast flow was followed above the elbow, revealing complete occlusion of his major venous outflow tract.

A failing fistula is best evaluated by a venous fistulogram.[4,5,27–29] A clear picture of the vessels is usually obtained with a small amount of contrast medium if both arterial and venous flow are temporarily occluded in the upper arm with a tourniquet. Although Glanz and associates used the brachial artery and reported few complications,[30] the present authors prefer to cannulate the distal vein of the fistula, which allows easy access to both the proximal artery and the vein for balloon angioplasty[27,31–33] (Fig. 4.11.6). Furthermore, even if stenosis develops at the puncture site, flow through the fistula will not be compromised. In an end-to-side fistula when the distal vein has been ligated, the distal artery or the proximal vein can be cannulated.

The authors do fistulograms of failing Brescia–Cimino fistulae on an outpatient basis after obtaining permission to perform percutaneous balloon dilation if it proves appropriate. A blood pressure cuff is placed close to the axilla, and the extremity is prepared with antiseptic solution and draped from the hand to 6cm above the elbow. After venous distention has been obtained by inflating the cuff to 60mm Hg, the distal vein of the fistula is punctured with a 19-gauge butterfly infusion needle 3–5cm below the fistula (Fig. 4.11.6). The cuff is then deflated, and the needle is replaced with a 5Fr angiocatheter threaded over a 0.022-inch guidewire to avoid inadvertent displacement of the needle during subsequent manipulation. The catheter is advanced 2–3cm beyond the puncture site so that the tip lies below the level of the proximal vessels of the fistula. Small doses of contrast medium are infused to verify the catheter position and to make a preliminary assessment of the proximal venous anatomy. A cine fistulogram is made with 15–30ml of 30% contrast medium (60% diatrizoate in a 1:1 dilution) infused at the rate of 2–5ml/sec with the blood pressure cuff inflated 20mm Hg above systolic pressure to obtain arterial as well as venous filling. Rapid clear-

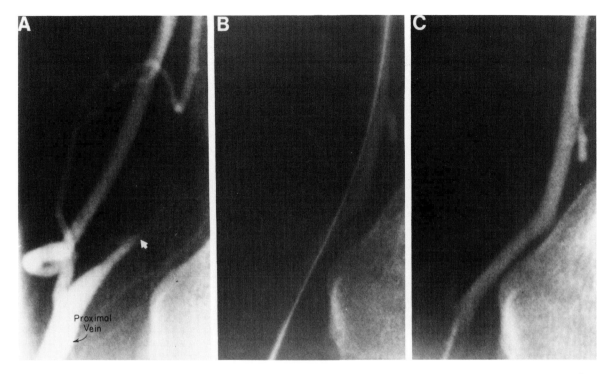

Figure 4.11.5. Patient was evaluated because high venous resistance was persistently encountered at dialysis. **A.** Cine fistulogram shows high proximal venous stenosis with occlusion above the elbow at the site where the patient normally applied a tourniquet to train the fistula *(arrow)*. **B.** Occlusion has been traversed by the guidewire. **C.** Normal caliber vessel after balloon angioplasty.

ing of the contrast when the cuff is deflated and the anatomic distribution distinguish the arteries from the veins. Oblique and lateral views are obtained by rotation of the arm slowly through 90° to evaluate lesions that may otherwise be obscured by contrast-filled vessels. One or two injections may be necessary. The vessels should be traced to the axilla to avoid overlooking a proximal stenosis (Fig. 4.11.5).

This technique is simple and no more invasive than is venipuncture of the fistula for dialysis. A cine fistulogram with video recording permits a more dynamic study with instant replay and reduces the expense.

Pressure gradients are measured across the fistula to assess the functional significance of any stenoses and to reveal any lesions not appreciated on angiography (Fig. 4.11.7). The lesions most difficult to assess by contrast study are those at the junction of the proximal vessels and the anastomosis. For this reason, the authors now routinely measure the pressure within the fistula by positioning the catheter just below the proximal vessels. This value is compared with the systemic cuff pressure; a pressure gradient of ≥20mm Hg suggests significant proximal arterial stenosis. The catheter is then positioned in the proximal artery, and pullback pressures across the fistula are measured to confirm the presence of a significant gradient and the site of narrowing. Pullback pressures are also measured across the fistula from the proximal vein and across gross stenotic lesions. Although a gradual change in pressure may occur without indicating a lesion, an abrupt change of >20mm Hg is considered significant. Pressure gradient

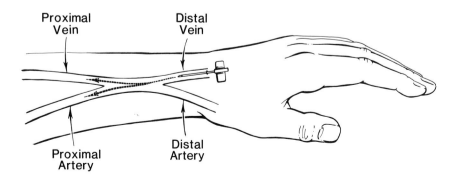

Figure 4.11.6. Cine fistulography and manipulation through distal vein of fistula provides easy access to fistula, proximal artery, and vein. Furthermore, if stenosis occurs at a distal artery or vein, it has almost no functional significance.

Figure 4.11.7. Value of pressure gradient measurement. **A.** Pressure measurements across a seemingly insignificant arterial stenosis *(arrows)* show impressive gradient of 110mm Hg. **B.** After balloon dilation of the proximal artery, there is marked morphologic improvement as well as a drop in pressure gradient to only 20mm Hg. The systolic pressure at the fistula or the proximal vein rose from 40 to 130mm Hg after dilation. *PV* = proximal vein; *PA* = proximal artery.

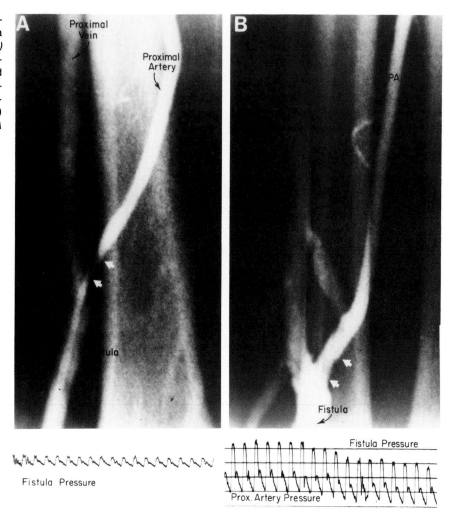

measurement is an essential part of the evaluation and may predict the outcome of the dilation.

On completion of the contrast study and pressure measurements, the vascular access surgeon should review the findings with the radiologist and plan therapy.

PERCUTANEOUS TRANSLUMINAL ANGIOPLASTY

If dilation of the stenotic lesion is chosen, 5000 units of heparin is given intravenously through the catheter placed proximal to the stenotic segment. The stenosis is then repeatedly stretched with Teflon dilators as large as 8Fr that are passed over a 0.038-inch guidewire. A Grüntzig catheter with a 4–10mm balloon is then centered across the stenosis, and several (usually 4–6) inflations to 4–6 atm are performed at 1.5-minute intervals until the narrowing around the balloon is relieved (Figs. 4.11.5, 4.11.7, and 4.11.8). The result is assessed by contrast injection and pullback pressure measurements. Successful dilation is invariably accompanied by the return of a prominent thrill or bruit.

In the authors' experience, transluminal angioplasty will salvage a failing fistula caused by proximal venous or arterial stenosis and is well tolerated by the patient, with no need for hospitalization.[27,33] Complications are few and often minor, and dialysis can be resumed immediately after the procedure,[27] although as a precaution against traumatic restenosis, the authors generally request to the dialysis staff not to insert the needles directly over the dilated segment for at least two weeks. In contrast, critical stenosis near the anastomosis of an end-to-end fistula is difficult or impossible to dilate and should be managed by surgical revision and an operative fistulogram. Also, if more than two dilations are required within 12 months, surgical revision is recommended: venous patch angioplasty, interposition graft, or reconstruction of the fistula just proximal to the stenosis.[4,34]

DIRECT DAV FISTULA THROMBOSIS

When a bruit or thrill can no longer be detected over the fistula, thrombosis has occurred. The standard treatment for a previously well functioning fistula is surgical exploration, thrombectomy with Fogarty balloon catheters, and, if necessary, revision of the fistula.[4,32,34] After clot removal, an intraoperative fistulogram is essential to locate any unsuspected stenotic lesions which predispose the fistula to thrombosis. These lesions can be treated by balloon

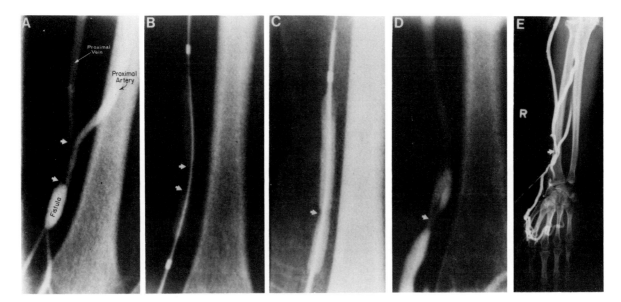

Figure 4.11.8. Balloon angioplasty of AV fistula. **A.** Cine fistulogram shows tight proximal venous stenosis *(arrows).* **B.** Deformity of balloon at site of stenosis. **C.** Correction of balloon deformity with progressive and repeated dilation. **D.** Significant morphologic improvement after dilation. **E.** Follow-up angiography with portable equipment at dialysis six weeks later shows that dilated proximal vein has remained wide open.

angioplasty or surgical repair.[27] However, if the fistula thrombosed immediately after or within a few days of surgery because an unsuitable vein or artery was chosen, re-exploration and attempts to evaluate the fistula radiologically are usually futile. It is wise to obtain a venogram to plan for a new access at a different site.

Arteriovenous Bridge Grafts

If a Brescia–Cimino fistula cannot be constructed, a looped forearm graft is a well accepted alternative. The U-shaped graft is positioned in a subcutaneous tunnel to allow easy access for cannulation by dialysis needles, and the ends of the graft are anastomosed end to side to the brachial artery and an antecubital vein (median cubital, cephalic, or basilic vein). In patients who have no suitable antecubital veins, a straight bridge graft between the brachial artery and the axillary or basilic vein is an excellent alternative (Fig. 4.11.9). All newly constructed bridge grafts should be allowed to heal for three weeks to minimize the risk of early failure due to bleeding and infection.[1,4]

There are two types of graft materials. Biologic grafts include autogenous or homologous saphenous vein, bovine carotid artery, and human umbilical cord veins.[14] These grafts are more susceptible to the formation of aneurysms, and, over time, the incorporation of the graft into the adjacent soft tissues makes revision difficult or impossible. Infected biologic grafts, with the exception of autogenous saphenous vein, generally require removal, so these grafts have a relatively poor salvage rate. The autogenous saphenous vein graft is the least susceptible to infection, but it has a high incidence of diffuse stenosis and aneurysm formation.

Among the synthetic graft materials, E-PTFE is the most popular graft material in North America.[4,12,13,35] Despite the propensity of prosthetic material to infection, suture line disruption is rare compared with bovine grafts. The graft withstands repeated needle punctures, has a low incidence of aneurysm formation, and is relatively easy to revise because it can be removed easily from its fibrous tract. Arterial-arterial bridge grafts enjoyed a brief popularity but were abandoned because of aneurysm formation and the risks of ischemic and embolic complications.

Stenosis at or just above the venous anastomosis is a common finding in failing bridge grafts no matter what material was used (Fig. 4.11.10). Stenosis probably results from the intimal damage with reactive hyperplasia caused by the turbulence associated with the progressive increase in flow over time. Critical stenosis can be managed with a trial of transluminal angioplasty, although the venous anastomotic narrowing associated with bridge grafts often resists dilation and often recurs if it does respond.[36] It is important to stress that all invasive procedures in patients with bridge grafts, as with other types of dialysis access, must be performed with appropriate antibiotic coverage and strict aseptic techniques.

Operative repair is the best treatment for a thrombosed bridge graft. Because the most common lesion is a stenosis near the venous anastomosis,[32,36,37] the authors advocate making an incision at the venous end of the graft to perform thrombectomy and an intraoperative contrast study. After the stenosis has been located, it can be repaired by patch angioplasty or bypassed by a short-segment interposition graft. Intraoperative balloon angioplasty may be useful in some cases, particularly when a high proximal venous stenosis is found. The authors do not recommend use of fibrinolytic agents such as streptokinase and uroki-

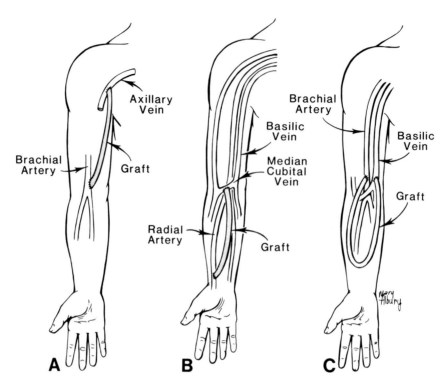

Figure 4.11.9. Common types of bridge grafts used for long-term hemodialysis.

nase because of the resulting need for many days of hospitalization for infusion and monitoring and because of the risk of infection and bleeding through old needle punctures in the graft[37] (Fig. 4.11.11).

Arteriovenous External Shunts

Although the artificial kidney was invented in 1944,[38] its clinical application was restricted for the next 16 years by the lack of a reliable vascular access. The breakthrough came in 1960, when Quinton, Dillard, and Scribner introduced the Teflon–Silastic AV shunt.[10] The Scribner shunt and other external AV shunts are seldom used for long-term hemodialysis now, however, because they are plagued by relatively low long-term patency rates as a result of infection and clotting, the average shunt lifespan in an adult being 7–10 months.[39] Nonetheless, the Scribner shunt is still effective for temporary hemodialysis and may be indicated when placement of a subclavian cannula for short-term hemodialysis is considered hazardous or difficult.[4] Use of the Scribner shunt requires ligation of the distal artery and vein, and preoperative assessment therefore must include the Allen test of the adequacy of collateral perfusion. The common sites for shunt placement are the radial artery and cephalic vein above the wrist and the saphenous vein and posterior tibial artery above the ankle.

The Scribner shunt has two components, a radiolucent Teflon vessel tip and a silicone rubber shunt cannula. An appropriate size vessel tip is tied to the shunt cannula

before being secured within the lumen of the vessel (Fig. 4.11.12). The two ends of the shunt cannulas are then brought out through separate incisions and connected externally with a straight or a T-shaped connecting piece. Patency is ensured if a bruit or a thrill is detected over the proximal vein. A clotted shunt is easily recognized, because blood separates into distinct serum and red cell layers in the external tubing.

Stenosis at the vessel-Teflon tip junction due to excessive motion or angulation of the tip is the most frequent finding in a thrombosed shunt or a shunt inadequate for dialysis. Any clots are removed by aspiration with a syringe and, if necessary, a small polyethylene catheter is passed beyond the obstruction to flush out the clots with heparinized (10 units/ml) saline as the catheter is withdrawn.[4] A shuntogram can be obtained using 10–20ml of 30% diatrizoate infused through the arterial or venous cannula after temporarily occluding the proximal flow with a tourniquet applied to the upper arm (Fig. 4.11.13). Infusion through the artery must not be forceful, or retrograde cerebral embolization can result. If the shuntogram shows a critical mechanical obstruction, surgical revision is the best treatment. If only residual thrombus is seen, however, the clot can be removed by further aspiration and flushing with a polyethylene catheter or by gentle Fogarty thrombectomy. After declotting the shunt, the authors prefer to use an intermittent or continuous heparin infusion until the next dialysis session, the heparin being infused directly into the shunt through a T-shaped connector.

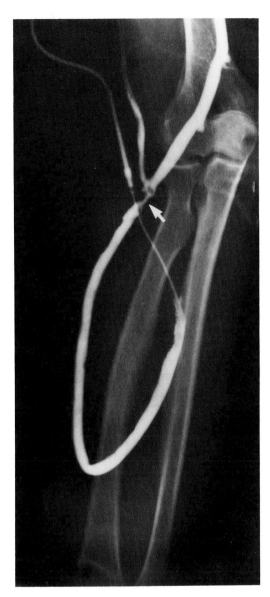

Figure 4.11.10. High venous resistance during dialysis caused by tight stenosis *(arrow)* at venous anastomosis of an E-PTFE bridge graft.

Right Atrial Cannulas

Dual-lumen cannulas positioned in the right atrium are becoming more common as access for both immediate and long-term hemodialysis. The more rigid polyethylene or polyurethane catheters are inserted percutaneously through the internal jugular or subclavian vein and have largely replaced the Scribner shunt for immediate or short-term dialysis.[40] Cannulation of the internal jugular veins is preferable since the subclavian catheters have been associated with a high incidence of subclavian stenosis or thrombosis, rendering the corresponding upper extremity unsuitable for future hemodialysis access. The less thrombogenic and more flexible silicone rubber catheters with internal diameters of 1.6mm (regular Hickman catheter)

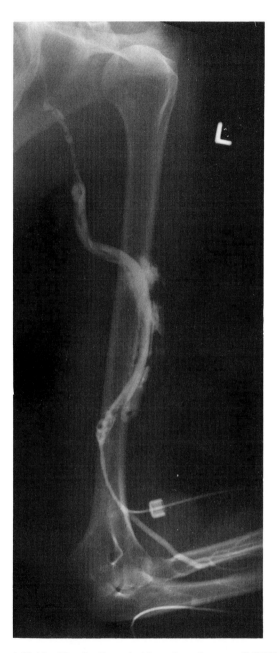

Figure 4.11.11. Bleeding through old puncture sites on an E-PTFE graft after infusion of streptokinase; note tight stenosis at venous anastomosis.

and 2.0–2.6mm, as well as the large dual-lumen catheter, can be used for long-term dialysis. The dual-lumen silicone rubber catheters are particularly useful in managing adult patients in whom almost all the available vessels in the arms have been exhausted in previous access procedures and in those who are likely to suffer ischemic complications if the proximal arteries are used.[15] The smaller single-lumen silicone rubber Hickman catheter is invaluable as a reliable and painless access for dialysis in small children.[18–20] In infants, the silicone rubber dialysis catheters are positioned through a direct cut-down into the anterior facial or internal jugular veins[4] (Fig. 4.11.14). In older children and

A.

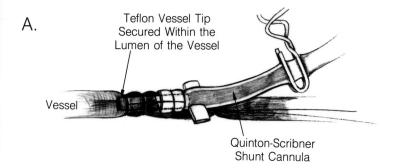

Teflon Vessel Tip Secured Within the Lumen of the Vessel

Vessel

Quinton-Scribner Shunt Cannula

B.

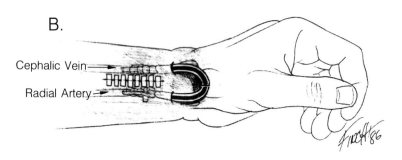

Cephalic Vein

Radial Artery

Figure 4.11.12. In the construction of a Scribner shunt, both the distal artery and vein are ligated.

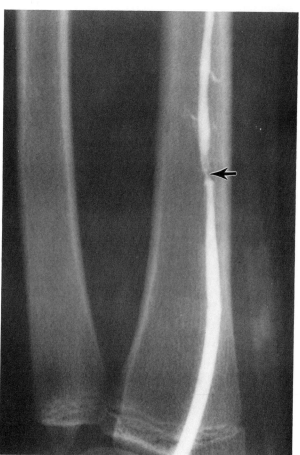

Figure 4.11.13. Shuntogram through venous cannula showing stenosis at the Teflon tip-vessel junction and partial occlusion with thrombus *(arrow)*.

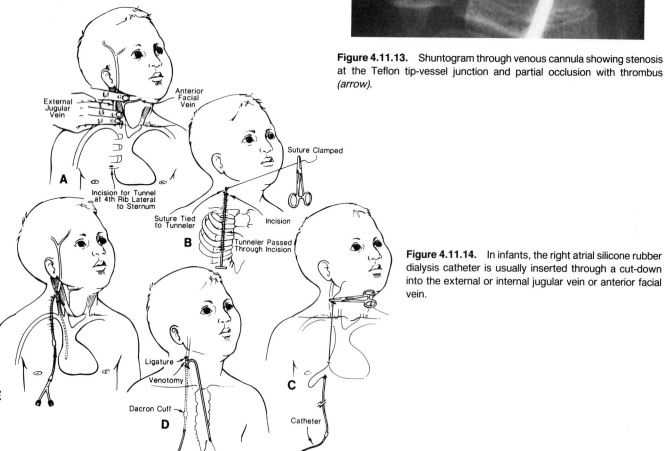

Figure 4.11.14. In infants, the right atrial silicone rubber dialysis catheter is usually inserted through a cut-down into the external or internal jugular vein or anterior facial vein.

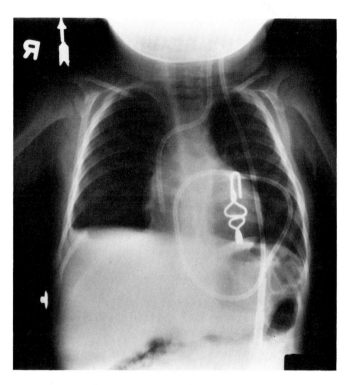

Figure 4.11.15. Chest film obtained after catheter placement to check position of radiopaque catheter in right atrium and to rule out pneumothorax and hemothorax.

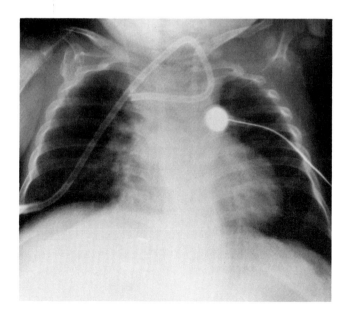

Figure 4.11.16. Acute angulation of catheter tip against superior vena cava may occur when catheter is introduced through left-sided vessels; this catheter must be repositioned immediately to prevent erosion of the vessel.

adults, the dual lumen, Silastic hemodialysis catheters can be safely inserted percutaneously into the internal jugular or subclavian vein using a Seldinger technique combined with the end of a Teflon peel-away sheath.[41]

Flow inadequate for efficient dialysis may occur when: 1) the catheter is too small for the patient; 2) the catheter tip is not positioned correctly in the right atrium; 3) the lumen of the catheter is compromised by a tight suture; or 4) the catheter is kinked along its subcutaneous course. A roentgenogram of the chest is essential after catheter placement to assess the position and course and to rule out technical complications such as pneumothorax or hemothorax (Fig. 4.11.15). Radiologic evidence of acute angulation of the catheter against the superior vena cava is sometimes seen when the catheter is introduced from the left side (Fig. 4.11.16). These catheters must be repositioned to prevent erosion of the catheter tip through the vena cava. Thrombosis of the silicone rubber catheters does not appear to be a significant problem as long as the catheter is aspirated and then filled with heparinized saline every 6–12 hours. When the catheter does become obstructed by thrombosis, and the clot cannot be dislodged by aspiration, infusion of several milliliters of urokinase solution (5000 units/ml), or a volume just great enough to fill the catheter every 8 hours, often lyses the clot within 24–48 hours.[4]

References

1. Wilson SE: Complications of vascular access procedures, in Wilson SE, Owens ML (eds): *Vascular Access Surgery.* Chicago, Year Book Medical Publishers, 1980, p 185
2. Hirschman GH, Wolfson M, Mosimann JE, Clark CB, Dante ML, Wineman RJ: Complications of dialysis. *Clin Nephrol* 1981;15:66
3. Morgan AP, Knight DC, Tilney NL, Lazarus JM: Femoral triangle sepsis in dialysis patients: frequency, management, and outcome. *Ann Surg* 1980;191:460
4. So SKS: Access for dialysis, in Simmons RL, Finch ME, Ascher NL, Najarian JS (eds): *Manual of Vascular Access, Organ Donation and Transplantation.* New York, Springer–Verlag, 1984, pp 3–87
5. So SKS, Sutherland DER: Vascular access procedures, in Najarian JS, Delaney JP (eds): *Advances in Vascular Surgery.* Chicago, Year Book Medical Publishers, 1980, p 185
6. Brescia MJ, Cimino JE, Appel K, Hurwich BJ: Chronic hemodialysis using venipuncture and a surgically created arteriovenous fistula. *N Engl J Med* 1966;275:1089
7. Kinneart P, Vereerstraeten P, Toussaint C, Van Geertruyden J: Nine years' experience with internal arteriovenous fistulas for haemodialysis: a study of some factors influencing the results. *Br J Surg* 1977;64:242
8. Ishihara AM: The current state-of-the-art for vascular access in hemodialysis. *Controv Dialysis* 1980;1:9–29
9. Reilly DT, Wood RFM, Bell PRF: Prospective study of dialysis fistulas: problem patients and their treatment. *Br J Surg* 1982;69(9):549
10. Quinton WE, Dillard D, Scribner BH: Cannulation of blood vessels for prolonged hemodialysis. *Trans Am Soc Artif Intern Organs* 1960;6:104

11. Gracz KC, Ing TS, Soung LS, Armbruster KFW, Seim SK, Merkel FK: Proximal forearm fistula for maintenance hemodialysis. *Kidney Int* 1977;11:71

12. Haimov M, Slifkin R: Experience with the PTFE graft in the construction of vascular access for hemodialysis, in Kootstra G, Jorning PJG (eds): *Access Surgery.* Lancaster, MTP Press, 1983, p 113

13. Sabanayagam P, Schwartz AB, Soricelli RR, Lyons P, Chinitz J: A comparative study of 402 bovine heterografts and 225 reinforced expanded PTFE grafts as AVF in the ESRD patient. *Trans Am Soc Artif Intern Organs* 1980;26:88

14. Akhondzadeh L, Wilson SE, Williams R, Owen ML: Infection of materials used in vascular access surgery: an evaluation of Dacron, bovine heterograft, Teflon, and human umbilical vein grafts. *Dialysis Transplant* 1980;9:697

15. McGonigle DJ, Schrock LG, Hickman RO: Experience using central venous access for long-term hemodialysis: a new concept. *Am J Surg* 1983;45:571

16. Buselmeier TJ, Santiago EA, Simmons RL, Najarian JS, Kjellstrand CM: Arteriovenous shunts for pediatric hemodialysis. *Surgery* 1971;70:638

17. Bourquelot P, Wolfeler L, Lamy L: Microsurgery for hemodialysis distal arteriovenous fistulas in children weighing less than 10kg. *Proc Eur Dialysis Transplant Assoc* 1981;18:537

18. Mahan JD Fr, Mauer SM, Nevins TE: The Hickman catheter: a new hemodialysis access device for infants and small children. *Kidney Int* 1983;24:694

19. So SKS, Mahan JD Jr, Mauer SM, Sutherland DER, Nevins TE: Hickman catheter for pediatric hemodialysis: a 3-year experience. *Trans Am Soc Artif Intern Organs* 1984;30:619

20. Nevins TE: A new Hickman catheter for hemodialysis access in children (abstract). *Trans Am Soc Artif Intern Organs,* 1984

21. Humphries AL, Nesbit RR, Caruana RJ, Hutchins RS, Heimburger RA, Wray CH: Thirty-six recommendations for vascular access operations: lessons learned from our first thousand operations. *Am Surg* 1981;47:145

22. Kamienski RW, Barnes RW: Critique of the Allen test for continuity of the palmar arch assessed by Doppler ultrasound. *Surg Gynecol Obstet* 1976;142:861

23. Forsberg G, Forsberg L, Lindstedt E, Westling H, White T: Side-to-side, side-to-end, end-to-end anastomosis for Cimino–Brescia fistula: preliminary report of a randomized study, in Kootstra G, Jorning PJP (eds): *Access Surgery.* Lancaster, MTP Press, 1983, p 21

24. Butt KMH, Friedman EA, Kountz SL: Angioaccess. *Curr Probl Surg* 1976;13:3

25. Wood RFM, Reilly DT: Hyperemia of the hand in side-to-side arteriovenous fistulas, in Kootstra G, Jorning PJG (eds): *Access Surgery.* Lancaster, MTP Press, 1983, p 147

26. Bussell JA, Abbott JA, Lim RC: A radial steal syndrome with arteriovenous fistula or hemodialysis. *Ann Intern Med* 1971;75:387

27. Hunter D, So SKS, Castañeda–Zúñiga W, Coleman C, Sutherland DER, Amplatz K: Angiographic evaluation and percutaneous transluminal angioplasty in failing or thrombosed Brescia–Cimino arteriovenous dialysis fistulas. *Radiology* 1983;149:105

28. Gilula LA, Staple TW, Anderson CB, Anderson LS: Venous angiography of hemodialysis fistulas. *Radiology* 1975; 115:555

29. Lawrence PF, Miller FJ, Minean DE: Balloon catheter dilatation in patients with failing arteriovenous fistulas. *Surgery* 1985;89:439

30. Glanz S, Bashist B, Gordon DH, Butt K, Adamsons R: Angiography of upper extremity access fistulas for dialysis. *Radiology* 1982;143:45

31. Heidler R, Zeitler E, Gessler U: Percutaneous transluminal dilatation of stenosis behind A-V fistulas in hemodialysis patients, in Zeitler E, Grüntzig A, Schoop H (eds): *Percutaneous Vascular Recanalization.* New York, Springer–Verlag, 1978, pp 142–144

32. Bone GE, Pomijzl MJ: Management of dialysis fistula thrombosis. *Am J Surg* 1979;138:901

33. So SKS, Castañeda–Zúñiga, WR, Hunter D, Sutherland DER, Amplatz K: Percutaneous transluminal angioplasty in failing arteriovenous fistula, in Kootstra G, Jorning PJP (eds): *Access Surgery.* Lancaster, MTP Press, 1983 p 225

34. Silcott GR, Vannix RS, DePalma JR: Repair versus new arteriovenous fistulae. *Trans Am Soc Artif Intern Organs* 1980;26:99

35. Palder SB, Kirkman RL, Whittemore AD, Hakim RM, Lazarus JM, Tilney NL: Vascular access for hemodialysis: patency rates and results of revisions. *Ann Surg* 1985;202:235

36. Tortolani EC, Tan AHS, Butchart S: Percutaneous transluminal angioplasty: an ineffective approach to the failing vascular access. *Arch Surg* 1984;119:221

37. Young AT, Hunter DW, Castañeda–Zúñiga WR, So SKS, Mercado S, Cardella JF, Amplatz K: Thrombosed synthetic hemodialysis fistulas: failure of fibrinolytic therapy. *Radiology* 1985;154:639

38. Kolff WJ, Berk HTJ: The artificial kidney: a dialyser with a great area. *Acta Med Scand* 1944;117:121

39. Cross AS, Steigbigel RT: Infective endocarditis and access site infections in patients on hemodialysis. *Medicine* 1976;55:453

40. Dorner DB, Stubbs DH, Shadur CA, Flynn CT: Percutaneous subclavian vein catheter hemodialysis impact on vascular access surgery. *Surgery* 1982;91:712

41. Linos DA, Mucha P Jr: A simplified technique for the placement of permanent central venous catheters. *Surg Gynecol Obstet* 1982;154:248

Part 12. Balloon Angioplasty Restenosis: Intimal Proliferation and Chronic Elastic Recoil

—Bruce F. Waller, M.D., Charles M. Orr, M.D., Cass A. Pinkerton, M.D., John D. Slack, M.D., James W. VanTassel, M.D., and Thomas Peters, M.D.

Since its introduction in 1977,[1] coronary balloon angioplasty has become widely accepted as a nonsurgical form of therapy for acutely or chronically obstructed coronary arteries. Despite the widespread use of coronary balloon angioplasty, advances in angioplasty technology, improvements in operator techniques, and over 90% primary success rates in dilation, restenosis at the angioplasty site is the major problem limiting the long-term efficacy of this procedure. The frequency of restenosis ranges from 17 to 47% depending on variations in definitions of restenosis: clinical, angiographic, physiologic, anatomic, and statistical.[2-10] Several previous studies have been conducted to determine various factors which might predispose to or be associated with restenosis: 1) angiographic-hemodynamic factors (e.g., number of angioplasty sites, pre- and post-dilation diameters, changes in transstenotic pressure gradients); 2) lesion characteristics (diffuse, long, eccentric, calcified); 3) the presence or absence of intimal flaps or dissection); 4) clinical factors (e.g., gender, presence or absence of unstable angina pectoris, diabetes mellitus, smoking); and 5) technical factors (e.g., number of balloon inflations, duration, and pressure of balloon inflations, balloon:vessel size ratio). This chapter describes previously reported[11] clinical, morphologic, and histologic changes late (730 days) after clinically successful coronary balloon angioplasty in 20 necropsy patients and classifies the restenosis lesion into two categories. This part also reviews 41 previously reported necropsy patients with coronary angioplasty restenosis lesions.[12-16]

CARDIOVASCULAR PATHOLOGY REGISTRY ACCESSION

Between September 1982 and June 1990, hearts from 20 necropsy patients with previous coronary balloon angioplasty procedures were entered into the Cardiovascular Pathology Registry. Hearts were obtained from 11 hospitals in 7 states.

Medical records including results of cardiac catheterization, coronary angiography, and balloon angioplasty were reviewed for each patient.

MORPHOLOGIC LOCALIZATION OF THE ANGIOPLASTY SITE

The artery and site of previous balloon angioplasty were identified from the balloon angioplasty procedure report.

In some cases, the coronary arterial tree was perfused with 10% formalin at 100mm Hg pressure for 24 hours prior to coronary artery sectioning. The artery of angioplasty was excised from the heart (intact vessel if previously uncut, or in pieces if previously sectioned into transverse sections) and radiographed for calcific deposits. The study vessel was then serially cut into transverse cross-sections from its origin to its most distal point. The area of previous angioplasty was serially step-sectioned in order to localize the precise area(s) of previous angioplasty injury and to avoid missing any areas of focal intimal proliferation.

Of the 20 angioplasty coronary arteries studied, 266 coronary segments were cut and stained histologically (three stains each), and 20 angioplasty sites from these arteries were serially sectioned yielding 8–12 additional sections per angioplasty artery. Percent cross-sectional area luminal narrowing by atherosclerotic plaques, intimal proliferation, or both was histologically determined by using the internal elastic membrane as the outer border of the true coronary lumen. Luminal area reductions were classified into four subgroups: 0–25%, 26–50%, 51–75%, and 76–100%.

CLASSIFICATION OF ECCENTRIC VERSUS CONCENTRIC LESIONS

The residual coronary lumen at the angioplasty site was classified as *concentric* or *eccentric*. If atherosclerotic plaque was distributed along the entire circumference of the artery, the cross-sectional coronary lumen was located centrally and was termed "concentric." If atherosclerotic plaques failed to involve the entire coronary artery circumference, leaving a variable arc of disease-free wall, the residual cross-sectional lumen was termed "eccentric." The site of previous angioplasty was classified as concentric or eccentric based upon the initial atherosclerotic plaque distribution and not upon any superimposed intimal fibrous proliferation tissue or thrombus. Old, underlying atherosclerotic plaque was clearly discernible from new and/or superimposed intimal proliferation tissue by the use of specialized histologic stains.

CLINICAL DATA

Table 4.12.1 summarizes certain clinical information in the 20 necropsy patients undergoing coronary balloon angioplasty greater than 30 days prior to death. All pro-

Table 4.12.1. Certain Clinical Parameters in 20 Necropsy Patients with Restenosis Late (>30 Days) after Clinically Successful Coronary Balloon Angioplasty

Parameter	Number
1. Ages (years) [mean]	33–63 [49]
2. Gender (men:women)	18 (90):2 (10)
3. Interval of Restenosis (months) [mean]	1.6–24.1 [8.2]
4. Arteries of Restenosis:	
Left anterior descending	14 (70)
Right	5 (25)
Left circumflex	1 (5)
5. Clinical Symptoms of Restenosis:	
Angina	12 (60)
Acute myocardial infarction	2 (10)
Sudden death	6 (30)
6. Mode of Death	
Cardiac	14 (70)
a. Acute myocardial infarctions = 2	
b. Sudden death = 6	
c. After coronary bypass = 6	
Noncardiac	6 (30)

Table 4.12.2. Certain Morphologic Observations in 20 Necropsy Patients Late (>30 Days) after Clinically Successful Coronary Balloon Angioplasty

Parameter	Number
1. Type of Lumen at Restenosis Site:	
Concentric	10 (50)
Eccentric	10 (50)
2. Type of Lesion at Restenosis Site:	
Intimal proliferation	12 (60)
Atherosclerotic plaque only	8 (40)
3. Evidence of Previous Angioplasty Injury	9 (45)[a]
4. Intimal Proliferation Plus:	
Calcium	2 (10)
Lipid	1 (5)
5. Possible Mechanism of Restenosis:	
Smooth muscle proliferation	12 (60)
Chronic elastic recoil	8 (40)

[a]All in restenosis lesions with intimal proliferation present.

cedures were clinically successful in that symptoms of myocardial ischemia were relieved and final diameter reduction at the angioplasty site was ≤30% (ranging from luminal irregularities to 30%). The interval from balloon angioplasty to morphologic examination ranged from 1.6 months to 24.1 months (average 8.2 months). Fourteen patients had restenosis under 12 months, five patients had restenosis between 12 and 24 months, and one patient was studied at 24.1 months. Clinical symptoms of restenosis occurred in 16 (80%). Four patients (20%) had no clinical evidence of restenosis. Patients with clinical evidence of restenosis had shorter intervals from angioplasty to death compared with those without clinical symptoms (7.0 versus 13.1, $p < 0.05$).

MEDICATIONS AFTER ANGIOPLASTY

Each of the 20 patients had some type of pharmacologic therapy postangioplasty: nitrates, β-blockers, calcium channel blockers, aspirin, dipyridimole, warfarin, or steroids. Five patients used aspirin alone, the remaining 15 patients had used two or more drugs. *No specific correlation existed between the interval of restenosis and the type of pharmacologic therapy employed.* Two patients were treated with warfarin and one patient received a course of prednisone (10mg/day) tapering over one month.

MODE OF DEATH

Of the 20 patients, 14 (70%) had a *cardiac* mode of death: 2 (10%) with recurrent angina and subsequent fatal acute myocardial infarction; 6 (30%) with sudden coronary death (2 with preceding angina), and 6 (30%) had recurrent angina and underwent coronary artery bypass surgery and died shortly thereafter. The remaining six (30%) patients

had *noncardiac* causes of death: three with neoplastic disease, two auto accident victims, and one with a fatal stroke. Of the six patients with noncardiac causes of death, four had no clinical evidence of myocardial ischemia and two had recurrent angina pectoris.

NECROPSY DATA (TABLE 4.12.2)

Of the 20 angioplasty coronary arteries examined, gross evidence of the angioplasty site was present in 14 (70%) arteries, all of which had "whitish" material on the luminal surface corresponding to intimal proliferation. In the remaining 6 (30%) arteries, no gross evidence of previous angioplasty was identified. These angioplasty sites appeared as typical atherosclerotic plaques. Of the 20 balloon angioplasty sites, 10 (50%) were concentric and 10 (50%) were eccentric. Correlation of the interval of restenosis with the type of lumen disclosed no significant difference in the timing of restenosis: concentric, 1.6–20 months (average 8.13); eccentric, 2.0–24 months (average 8.2). Comparing various intervals of restenosis timing also failed to disclose significant differences in concentric versus eccentric plaques: <6 months: 1.6–5.0 months (average 3.7); 2.0–5.5 months (average 3.9); 6–12 months: 6.8 months, 7.4 months; >12 months: 17.2–20 months (average 18.2); 12.1–24.1 months (average 16.9), respectively. *Thus, restenosis was similar in eccentric versus concentric lesions.* Restenosis in eccentric lesions was similar in frequency whether the interval of restenosis was less than six months or greater than one year after balloon angioplasty.

TYPE OF LESION AT THE RESTENOSIS SITE (FIGS. 4.12.1–4.12.8)

Histologic analysis of the angioplasty sites disclosed *intimal proliferation* which was responsible for the restenosis in 12 (60%) patients (Table 4.12.2, Figs. 4.12.1–4.12.5). Of

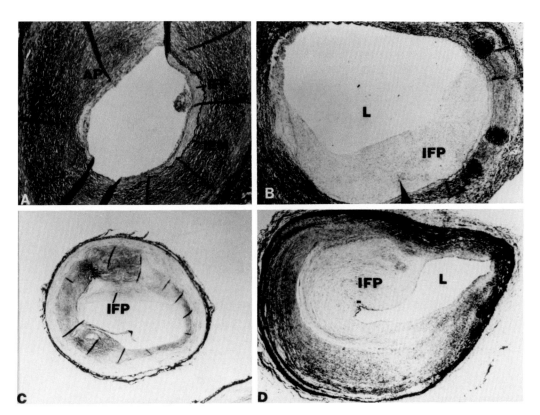

Figure 4.12.1. Intimal proliferation at restenosis sites. Sites of balloon angioplasty restenosis showing intimal fibrous proliferation (*IFP*) of various degrees. **A.** Patient showing mild, concentric IFP at 1.6 months. **B.** Patient showing eccentric IFP at 2.0 months. **C.** Patient showing IFP in the right coronary artery at 3.7 months. **D.** Patient showing IFP at 5.5 months after angioplasty. Magnification ×12 (**A,B**), ×4 (**C**), ×8 (**D**). Elastic-tri-chrome stains. *AP* = atherosclerotic plaque; *IEM* = internal elastic membrane; *L* = lumen. (From Waller BF, Pinkerton CA, Orr CM, VanTassel JW, Slack JD: Morphologic observations late (>30 days) after clinically successful coronary balloon angioplasty: an analysis of 20 necropsy patients and literature review of 41 necropsy patients with coronary angioplasty restenosis. *Circulation* 1991;83, in press.)

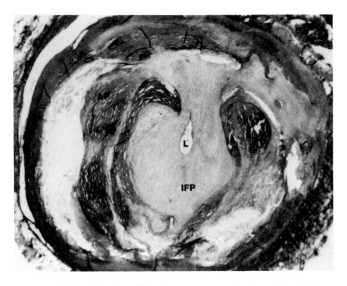

Figure 4.12.2. Intimal proliferation at restenosis sites. Intimal fibrous proliferation (*IFP*) at the site of balloon angioplasty in the proximal left anterior descending coronary artery 4.3 months after dilation. *Arrows* indicate previous dilation cracks. Magnification ×10, elastic-trichrome stain, *AP* = atherosclerotic plaque, *L* = lumen. (From Waller BF, Pinkerton CA, Orr CM, VanTassel JW, Slack JD: Morphologic observations late (>30 days) after clinically successful coronary balloon angioplasty: an analysis of 20 necropsy patients and literature review of 41 necropsy patients with coronary angioplasty restenosis. *Circulation* 1991;83, in press.)

the 12 sites with intimal proliferation, 9 (75%) had some evidence of previous intimal or intimal-medial "tears," "cracks," or "breaks." Histologic analysis of the remaining eight (40%) angioplasty sites disclosed typical *atherosclerotic plaques* (Fig. 4.12.6). Of these eight sites, six were eccentric atherosclerotic lesions with a variable arc of disease-free or nearly disease-free wall (Fig. 4.12.6). None of these eight sites had evidence of previous angioplasty injury (crack, break, tears) or healed modification of previous injury. The atherosclerotic plaque was uniformly consistent without histologic evidence of a new, immature luminal layer. The plaque was uniformly densely fibrotic with occasional calcific deposits. *Thus, no evidence of new or accelerated atherosclerotic plaque was observed in these eight angioplasty sites.* The arc of disease-free wall contained medial layers of normal thickness without evidence of scar or atrophy.

CLINICAL PATHOLOGIC CORRELATIONS

Morphologic and histologic observations at the angioplasty restenosis sites permit separation of the patients into two distinct subgroups: 1) intimal proliferation with or without evidence of healed angioplasty injury, and 2) atherosclerotic plaques without evidence of previous ligation injury (Fig. 4.12.7).

Figure 4.12.3. Intimal proliferation at restenosis sites. Photomicrographs of intimal fibrous proliferation (*IFP*) from various sites of balloon angioplasty restenosis. Several areas of previous ''cracks'' *(arrows)* are now ''coated'' by the IFP. IFP is histologically distinct from underlying atherosclerotic plaque (*AP*). *L* = lumen. (From Waller BF, Pinkerton CA, Orr CM, VanTassel JW, Slack JD: Morphologic observations late (>30 days) after clinically successful coronary balloon angioplasty: an analysis of 20 necropsy patients and literature review of 41 necropsy patients with coronary angioplasty restenosis. *Circulation* 1991;83, in press.)

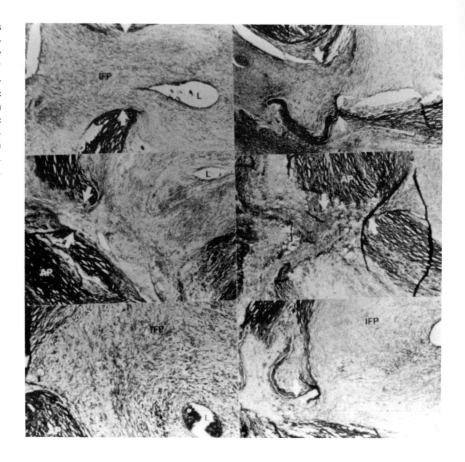

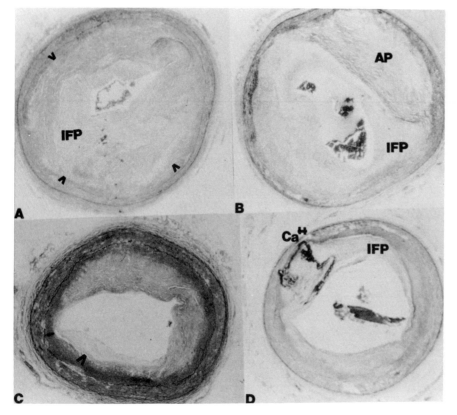

Figure 4.12.4. Intimal proliferation at restenosis sites. Sites of restenosis from previous coronary balloon angioplasty showing varying degrees of intimal fibrous proliferation (*IFP*) *(arrowheads).* **A.** IFP severely narrowing the angioplasty site at 4.4 months. **B.** Concentric IFP at the angioplasty site 4.8 months after dilation. This patient was treated with a short course of steroids following angioplasty. IFP is histologically similar to that in other patients without steroid treatment. **C.** IFP at 17.3 months in a patient *without* clinical restenosis and a noncardiac death. **D.** IFP at 20 months. Note the calcific deposits (*Ca*$^{++}$) within the IFP. Magnification ×10. Elastic-trichrome and hematoxylin and eosin stains. (From Waller BF, Pinkerton CA, Orr CM, VanTassel JW, Slack JD: Morphologic observations late (>30 days) after clinically successful coronary balloon angioplasty: an analysis of 20 necropsy patients and literature review of 41 necropsy patients with coronary angioplasty restenosis. *Circulation* 1991;83, in press.)

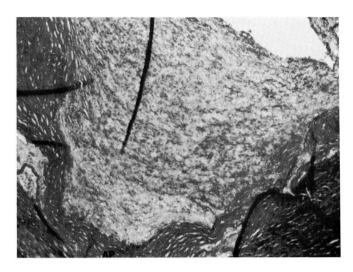

Figure 4.12.5. Photomicrograph showing characteristic features of intimal fibrous proliferation: relatively cellular but "loose" matrix, numerous smooth muscle cells, fibroblasts, reticulum, and elastic fibers. This intimal coating is distinctly different from the underlying atherosclerotic plaque (*AP*) which contains dense fibrous tissue, absence of smooth muscle cells and cholesterol clefts. Magnification ×80. Elastic-trichrome stain.

Intimal Proliferation

In the study reported by Waller et al.,[11] 60% of restenosis angioplasty lesions had intimal proliferation. The proliferation was histologically similar despite differences in the interval of restenosis (early versus late), the type of postangioplasty medical therapy (nitrates versus blockers versus aspirin), the artery of angioplasty, the presence or absence of recurrent myocardial ischemia, or the type of death (cardiac versus noncardiac). The amount of proliferation tissue appeared greater in lesions with evidence of previous intimal-medial angioplasty injury compared to lesions with intimal injury only. The most widely accepted theory for the development of fibrocellular intimal proliferation involves responses from damaged vessel endothelium and media.[2,4−7,10] Major participants in this response appear to be smooth muscle cells in the media and diseased intima and platelets. With plaque disruption, localized deposition of platelets occurs with subsequent release of thromboxane A_2, further platelet deposition and subsequent release of growth factors such as platelet-derived growth factor. Vessel endothelium also releases various growth factors such as endothelial and fibroblast growth

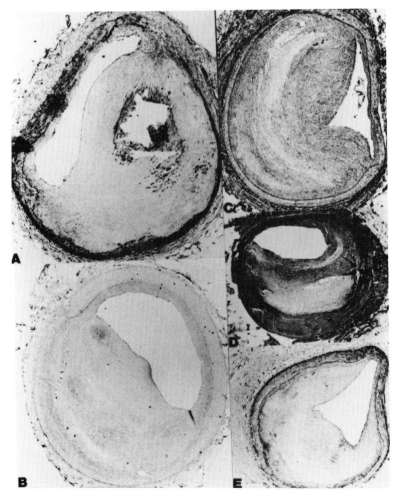

Figure 4.12.6. Atherosclerotic plaques only at sites of restenosis. Each of these sites of previous balloon angioplasty shows no intimal fibrous proliferation and no evidence of previous balloon injury ("cracks, breaks, tears") or healed version. Instead, each is an eccentric atherosclerotic plaque with a variable arc of disease-free or nearly disease-free wall. Elastic recoil of the overstretched eccentric wall is the likely mechanism of restenosis in these patients. Note the medial thickness is normal in the eccentric wall. The patients in **B, C,** and **E** had clinical symptoms of restenosis. Magnification ×10. Elastic-trichrome stains. (From Waller BF, Pinkerton CA, Orr CM, Van-Tassel JW, Slack JD: Morphologic observations late (>30 days) after clinically successful coronary balloon angioplasty: an analysis of 20 necropsy patients and literature review of 41 necropsy patients with coronary angioplasty restenosis. *Circulation* 1991;83, in press.)

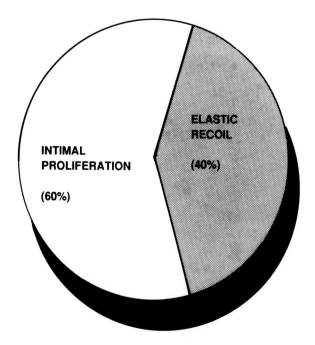

Table 4.12.3. Summary of Clinical and Necropsy Features of Previously Reported Patients (1979–1989) with Restenosis Late (>30) after Coronary Balloon Angioplasty

1. Number of Studies (Refs 12–26)	15
2. Number of Patients	41
3. Number of Coronary Sites	44
4. Ages (years) [mean]	33–72
5. Artery of Restenosis	
Left anterior descending	68%
Right	1%
Left circumflex	1%
Diagonal	3%
Left main	3%
6. Lumen Type (11/44 sites)	
Concentric	2/11
Eccentric	9/11
7. Changes at Angioplasty Site	
Intimal proliferation	69%
Atherosclerotic plaques only	31%

Figure 4.12.7. Diagram showing frequency of two mechanisms of restenosis lesions in 20 necropsy patients. (From Waller BF, Pinkerton CA, Orr CM, VanTassel JW, Slack JD: Morphologic observations late (>30 days) after clinically successful coronary balloon angioplasty: an analysis of 20 necropsy patients and literature review of 41 necropsy patients with coronary angioplasty restenosis. *Circulation* 1991;83, in press.)

factors. This process appears to result in migration, proliferation, and alteration of the vessel wall smooth muscle cells with fibrocellular tissue accumulation.

A review of previously published reports describing *late* findings after coronary balloon angioplasty[12–26] (Table 4.12.3) discloses 41 necropsy patients with 44 lesions. In 29 lesions (69%), the angioplasty site contained various amounts of intimal proliferation. The interval from angio-

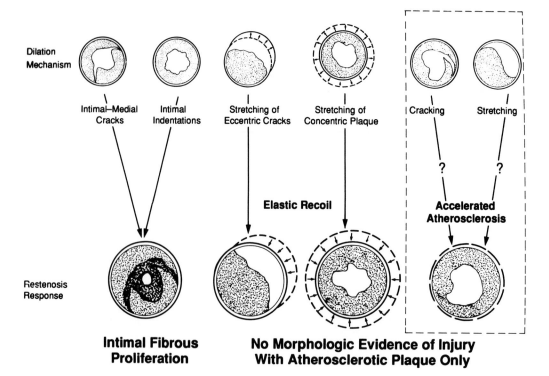

Figure 4.12.8. Diagram showing mechanisms (cracking, stretching, or both) of balloon angioplasty and the two major subgroups of restenosis lesions: those with intimal fibrous proliferation and those with no morphologic evidence of injury (elastic recoil). "Accelerated atherosclerosis" is an unlikely explanation for the latter subgroup. (From Waller BF, Pinkerton CA, Orr CM, VanTassel JW, Slack JD: Morphologic observations late (>30 days) after clinically successful coronary balloon angioplasty: an analysis of 20 necropsy patients and literature review of 41 necropsy patients with coronary angioplasty restenosis. *Circulation* 1991;83, in press.)

plasty to death ranged from two months to nine months (Table 4.12.3).

Atherosclerotic Plaques without Intimal Fibrous Proliferation

In the study by Waller et al.,[11] eight (40%) restenosis angioplasty sites had atherosclerotic plaques only—*without* superimposed intimal fibrocellular proliferation, *without* evidence of previous angioplasty injury, and *without* evidence of newly developing atherosclerotic plaque. Six of the eight patients in this subgroup had clinical evidence of myocardial ischemia. Of the eight late angioplasty lesions, six were eccentric and two were concentric. The arc of disease-free wall in the six eccentric lesions had histologically normal-appearing media without atrophy and without scar. In contrast, the media of the diseased wall segments were atrophied and focally scarred. This observation suggests that disease-free wall segments may be dynamic segments reacting to various mechanical, neurogenic, or vasoactive stimuli (i.e., capable of stretch and elastic recoil).

The absence of morphologic signs of previous dilation injury or intimal proliferation tissue in this subgroup of previously dilated patients can be explained in at least two ways: 1) *stretching* of diseased wall (concentric lesions) or disease-free wall (eccentric lesions) during the initial procedure with subsequent elastic recoil (restenosis); 2) progression of atherosclerotic disease ("accelerated atherosclerosis") (Fig. 4.12.8). We have been one of the earliest groups to suggest that gradual elastic recoil of overstretched vessel wall may represent an important subgroup of restenosis lesions following balloon angioplasty.

In review of previously reported necropsy patients with late coronary balloon angioplasty sites, about one-third of the sites were described as showing "atherosclerotic plaque only" (Table 4.12.3). The specific type of coronary lumen was not provided in most of these studies.[12-26]

Although acute elastic recoil shortly after balloon angioplasty is a generally well recognized mechanism of abrupt narrowing, chronic elastic recoil as a mechanism of late luminal narrowing is not well appreciated. Possible explanations for chronic recoil of overstretched eccentric segments involve recovery from temporary or permanent injury to medial smooth muscle cells. Temporarily dysfunctional ("stunned") smooth muscle cells over a period of weeks to months may eventually regain their function, thereby setting the stage for late recoil. On the other hand, acute injury of the smooth muscle cells during dilation may result eventually in replacement rather than repair of these cells. Replacement with normally functioning smooth muscle cells over a period of weeks to months may permit recoil on a late basis.

The absence of morphologic signs of previous balloon angioplasty in necropsy patients with restenosis also may be interpreted as indicating "acceleration" or "progression" of underlying atherosclerotic plaque.[27,28] Two histologic features in the present study indicated that this is an unlikely explanation: 1) the atherosclerotic plaque is densely fibrotic with focal calcific deposits indicating mature atherosclerotic lesions, and 2) the inner (luminal) layers of the atherosclerotic plaque are histologically similar to the outer layers of the plaque (i.e., no evidence of "new" versus "old" plaque). It is conceivable that many months or years after balloon angioplasty, intimal proliferation tissue "changes" or "converts" or "degenerates" to typical atherosclerotic plaque by incorporation of lipid. In our two oldest restenosis lesions, calcific deposits were noted in the intimal proliferation tissue. In one case, lipid accumulation had occurred. The possibility that mural thrombus becomes incorporated into the underlying plaque and later changes to atherosclerosis also is unlikely in that none of the earlier angioplasty sites (2.7 to 3.4 months) with plaques only had any residual or partial mural thrombus.

CONFIRMATION OF NECROPSY RESTENOSIS FINDINGS IN THE LIVING PATIENT WITH ANGIOPLASTY RESTENOSIS

An interventional device used in the treatment of obstructed coronary arteries is the Simpson atherectomy device. This device alters luminal obstruction by removal of obstructing material.[6] Frequently, the atherectomy device has been used to treat balloon angioplasty restenosis lesions. Tissue removed from angioplasty restenosis sites falls into three categories[29] (Fig. 4.12.9): 1) intimal proliferation, 2) atherosclerotic plaque with or without thrombus, and 3) thrombus only. The intimal proliferation tissue removed in the living patient is grossly and histologically identical to angioplasty restenosis tissue observed in necropsy patients. Atherosclerotic plaques removed from restenosis sites may correlate with the second group of restenosis lesions described here—eccentric or concentric atherosclerotic plaque without intimal proliferation. The initial angioplasty mechanism in this instance would include inadequate or superficial dilation of the lesion, eccentric or concentric vessel wall stretching, or both. Thus, atherectomy samples obtained from living patients with angioplasty restenosis are identical to restenosis tissue found in necropsy patients (Fig. 4.12.10). The frequency of intimal proliferation samples obtained from atherectomy coronary restenosis sites is slightly less than that reported in the present study.

RELATIONSHIP BETWEEN CORONARY BALLOON RESTENOSIS AND PERIPHERAL ARTERY RESTENOSIS

Mechanisms of balloon angioplasty (cracking, breaking, and stretching) in the coronary arteries also occur within

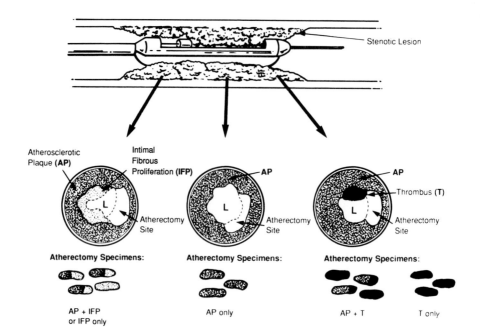

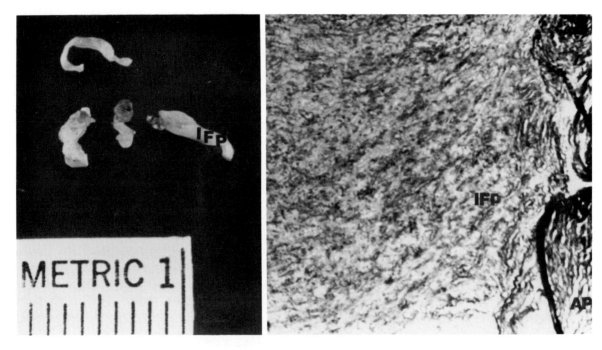

Figure 4.12.9. Explanations for angioplasty restenosis tissue removed by atherectomy. (From Waller BF, Pinkerton CA: "Cutters, scoopers, shavers, and scrapers"—the importance of atherectomy devices and clinical relevance of tissue removed. *J Am Coll Cardiol* 1991, in press.)

peripheral arteries undergoing dilation procedures. Specific information concerning the mechanism and type(s) of restenosis tissue at sites of previous peripheral balloon angioplasty have been evaluated from atherectomy sam-

ples. Johnson and associates[30,31] have histologically evaluated arterial samples excised at peripheral atherectomy from 218 peripheral arteries in 100 patients. Of the 218 lesions, 170 were de novo (primary) stenosis, 48 were from

Figure 4.12.10. Coronary atherectomy specimen from a restenosis lesion in the left anterior descending artery. *Left,* the whitish material is intimal fibrous proliferation (*IFP*) tissue. The darker material is atherosclerotic plaque (*AP*). *Right,* histologically, the IFP material is identical to that seen in necropsy patients with IFP restenosis and to that reported from peripheral atherectomy restenosis lesions. (From Waller BF, "Crackers, breakers, stretchers, drillers, scrapers, shavers, burners, welders, melters"—the future treatment of atherosclerotic coronary artery disease? A clinical-morphologic assessment. *J Am Coll Cardiol* 1989;13:969–987.)

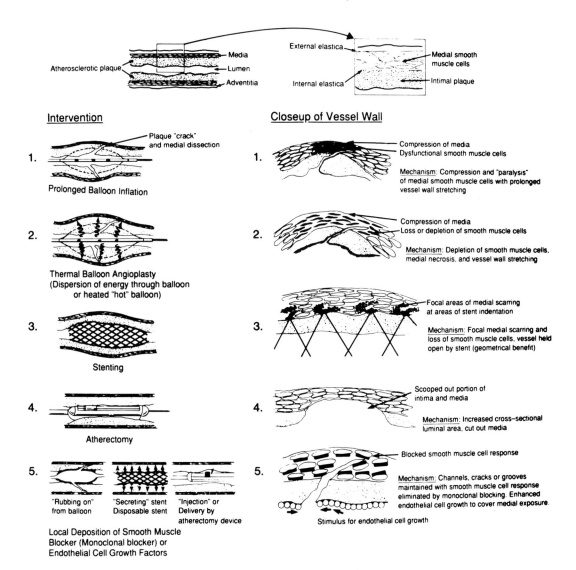

Figure 4.12.11. Diagram showing various interventional devices and techniques in delaying or preventing angioplasty restenosis. The use of the various devices and techniques depends in part upon the anatomic substrate of restenosis. (From Waller BF, Pinkerton CA, Orr CM, Van-

Tassel JW, Slack JD: Morphologic observations late (>30 days) after clinically successful coronary balloon angioplasty: an analysis of 20 necropsy patients and literature review of 41 necropsy patients with coronary angioplasty restenosis. *Circulation* 1991;83, in press.)

restenosis lesions following previous balloon angioplasty (*n* = 15), following atherectomy (*n* = 29), and after combined angioplasty and arthrectomy (*n* = 4). Histologic diagnoses fell into two major categories: *atherosclerotic plaque plus thrombus* and *intimal hyperplasia*. Of the primary stenoses excised, all had atherosclerotic plaque, fibrous thickening, and/or thrombus. *None* had intimal proliferation present. In contrast, tissue excised from restenosis lesions consisted of *atherosclerotic plaque plus thrombus without intimal hyperplasia* in 12 (25%) and *intimal hyperplasia* in 36 (75%). The former group was not histologically different from the de novo atherosclerotic plaque. In addition, intimal proliferation lesions were similar to the coronary artery restenosis lesions described above, and the restenosis lesions after angioplasty and after atherectomy were identical.

IMPLICATION OF MORPHOLOGIC FINDINGS RELEVANT TO THE THERAPY OF ANGIOPLASTY RESTENOSIS LESIONS

Treatment strategies for balloon angioplasty restenosis depend primarily upon the morphologic-histologic response at the angioplasty site. If the lesion consists of intimal proliferation tissue, various mechanical, pharmacologic and/or immunologic approaches may be undertaken (Fig. 4.12.11). If, alternatively, the restenosis lesion represents recoil of an overstretched arc of disease-free wall, other treatment strategies including thermal dilation ("pyroplasty") and "anti-recoil" pharmacologic therapy may be useful.[6-9]

References

1. Grüntzig AR, Myler RK, Hanna EH, Turina MI: *Circulation* 1977;84(suppl 11):55–56 (abstract)
2. Myler RM, Shaw RE, Stertzler SH, Clark DA, Fishman J, Murphy MG: Recurrence after coronary angioplasty. *Cath Cardiovasc Diag* 1987;13:77–86
3. Haudenschild CC: Restenosis. Basic considerations, in Topol EJ (ed): *Textbook of Interventional Cardiology.* Philadelphia, WB Saunders, 1990, pp 344–362
4. Califf RM, Ohman EM, Frid DJ, Fortun DE, Mark DB, Hlatky MA, Herndon JE, Bengtson JR: Restenosis: the clinical issues, in Topol EJ (ed): *Textbook of Interventional Cardiology.* Philadelphia, WB Saunders, 1990, pp 363–394
5. Blackshear JL, O'Callaghan WG, Califf RM: Medical approaches to prevention of restenosis after coronary angioplasty. *J Am Coll Cardiol* 1987;9:834–848
6. Waller BF: "Crackers, breakers, stretchers, drillers, scrapers, shavers, burners, welders, melters"—the future treatment of atherosclerotic coronary artery disease? A clinical-morphologic assessment. *J Am Coll Cardiol* 1989;13:969–987
7. Waller BF, Orr CM, Pinkerton CA, VanTassel JW, Pinto RP: Morphologic observations late after coronary balloon angioplasty; mechanisms of acute injury and relationship to restenosis. *Radiology SCVIR Special Series* 1991, in press
8. Waller BF, Pinkerton CA: Coronary balloon angioplasty restenosis: definitions, pathogenesis, and treatment strategies. *J Intervent Cardiol* 1991, in press
9. Waller BF: PTCA: Mechanisms of dilatation and causes of acute and late closures. *Cardiovasc Rev Report* 1989;10:35–47
10. Liu MW, Roubin GS, King SB: Restenosis after coronary angioplasty. Potential biologic determinants and role of intima hyperplasia. Point of view. *Circulation* 1989;79:1374–1387
11. Waller BF, Pinkerton CA, Orr CM, VanTassel JW, Slack JD: Morphologic observations late (>30 days) after clinically successful coronary balloon angioplasty: an analysis of 20 necropsy patients and literature review of 41 necropsy patients with coronary angioplasty restenosis. *Circulation* 1991, in press
12. Grüntzig AR, Senning A, Siegenthaler WE: Nonoperative dilatation of coronary-artery stenosis. *N Engl J Med* 1979;301:61–68
13. Essed CE, Van Den Brand M, Becker AE: Transluminal coronary angioplasty and early restenosis. Fibrocellular occlusion after wall laceration. *Br Heart J* 1983;49:393–396
14. Hollman J, Austin GE, Grüntzig AR, Douglas JS, King SB: Coronary artery spasm at the site of angioplasty in the first 12 months after successful percutaneous transluminal coronary angioplasty. *J Am Coll Cardiol* 1983;6:1039–1045
15. Giraldo A, Esposo OM, Meis JM: Intimal hyperplasia as a cause of restenosis after percutaneous transluminal coronary angioplasty. *Arch Pathol Lab Med* 1985;109:173–175
16. Schneider J, Grüntzig A: Percutaneous transluminal angioplasty: morphologic findings in 3 patients. *Pathol Res Pract* 1985;180:348–352
17. de Morais CF, Lopes EA, Checchi H, Arie S, Pileggi F: Percutaneous transluminal coronary angioplasty—histopathological analysis of 9 necropsy cases. *Virchows Arch A* 1989;410:195–202

18. Duber C, Jungbluth A, Rumpelt H–J, Erbel R, Meyer J, Theones W: Morphology of the coronary arteries after combined thrombolysis and percutaneous transluminal coronary angioplasty for acute myocardial infarction. *Am J Cardiol* 1986;58:698–703
19. Bruneval P, Guermonpres J–L, Perrier P, Carpentier A, Camilleri J–P: Coronary artery restenosis following transluminal coronary angioplasty. *Arch Pathol Lab Med* 1986; 110:1186–1187
20. Ueda M, Becker AE, Fujimoto T: Pathological changes induced by repeated percutaneous transluminal coronary angioplasty. *Br Heart J* 1987;58:635–643
21. Morimoto S–I, Sekiguchi M, Endo M, Horie T, Kitasume H, Kodama K, Yamaguchi T, Ohno M, Kurogane H, Fujino M, Shimizu Y, Mizuno K, Chino M: Mechanism of luminal enlargement in PTCA and restenosis: a histopathological study of necropsied coronary arteries collected from various centers in Japan. *Jpn Circulation J* 1987;51:1101–1115
22. Kohchi K, Takebayashi S, Block PC, Hiroki T, Nobuyoshi M: Arterial changes after percutaneous transluminal coronary angioplasty: results at autopsy. *J Am Coll Cardiol* 1987; 10:592–599
23. Walley VA, Higginson LAJ, Marguis J–F, Williams WL, Morton BC, Beanlands DS: Local morphologic effects of coronary balloon angioplasty. *Can J Cardiol* 1988;4:17–24
24. Potkin BN, Roberts WC: Effects of percutaneous transluminal coronary angioplasty on atherosclerotic plaques and relation of plaque composition and arterial size to outcome. *Am J Cardiol* 1988;62:41–50
25. Gravanis MB, Roubin GS: Histopathologic phenomena at the site of percutaneous transluminal coronary angioplasty: the problem of restenosis. *Human Pathol* 1989;20:477–485
26. Morimoto S–I, Kajita A, Sekiguchi M, Endo M, Itoh N: Autopsy findings in a case where PTCA percutaneous transluminal coronary angioplasty was successful but where the patient died seven months later of a non-associated cause. *Heart Vessel,* 1991, in press
27. Waller BF, McManus BM, Gorfinkel HJ, Kishel JC, Schmidt ECH, Kent KM, Roberts WC: Status of the major epicardial coronary arteries 80 to 150 days after percutaneous transluminal coronary angioplasty: analysis of 3 necropsy patients. *Am J Cardiol* 1983;51:81–84
28. Waller BF, Pinkerton CA, Foster LN: Morphologic evidence of accelerated left main coronary artery disease: a late complication of percutaneous transluminal angioplasty of the proximal left anterior descending coronary artery. *J Am Coll Cardiol* 1987;9:1019–1023
29. Waller BF, Pinkerton CA: "Cutters, scoopers, shavers, and scrapers"—the importance of atherectomy devices and clinical relevance of tissue removed. *J Am Coll Cardiol* 1991, in press
30. Johnson DE, Hinohara T, Selmon MR, Braden LJ, Simpson JB: Primary peripheral arterial stenosis and restenosis excised by transluminal atherectomy: a histopathologic study. *J Am Coll Cardiol* 1990;15:419–425
31. Johnson DE: Directional peripheral atherectomy: histologic aspects of a new interventional technique. *J Vasc Intervent Radiol* 1990;1:29–33

LASER-ASSISTED ANGIOPLASTY

Part 1. Laser Physics, Spectrum of Available Lasers, and Laser Safety

—Edward J. Grogan, C.C.E.

INTRODUCTION

In 1960, Dr. Theodore H. Maiman and associates at Hughes Aircraft Company in Culver City, CA, developed the first laser device utilizing ruby crystals as their lasing medium.[1] Since that date, lasers have been developed for numerous applications. This chapter seeks to present the reader with a basic understanding of laser physics as well as some insight into the functional design of current laser systems utilized for angioplasty. In addition, we shall discuss general guidelines to ensure safe applications of this new technology in the patient care environment.

LASER PHYSICS—ATOMIC THEORY

The structure of an atom is such that at any given time the atom exists in an energy state dependent upon the number of orbiting electrons and their distance from the nucleus of the atom. As the distance between nucleus and orbiting electron increases, so does the atom's defined energy state. The lowest energy level is defined as the resting or ground state of the atom. It is in this state that the radius of electron orbit is at its minimum.

Electrons orbiting about the nucleus of an atom may change energy levels by atomic absorption or emission of energy. If an orbiting electron absorbs energy, $\Delta E_{0 \to 1}$, in the form of heat, light, or an electric field, a transition will occur such that it will make a "quantum leap" into a more distant orbit. The atom, once in its resting energy state, E_0, will assume an excited state with an increased energy level, $E_1 = E_0 + \Delta E_{0+1}$ (Fig. 5.1.1). Within a short period of time (on the order of 10^{-8} second), however, the electron will spontaneously drop to a lower level, as the atom no longer remains in its excited state with energy, E_1, but seeks to return to its ground state, E_0. The atom emits, in the form

of a photon, a bundle of energy $\Delta E_{1 \to 0}$ equal in magnitude to the absorbed energy (Fig. 5.1.1). This is known as spontaneous emission of radiation by an atom and was hypothesized by Bohr in the 19th century.

Spontaneous emission may also occur between two excited levels such that a bundle of energy, $\Delta E_{2 \to 1}$ is emitted (Fig. 5.1.2).

In the early 1900s, Albert Einstein hypothesized that if atoms in their excited states ($E_1 = E_0 + \Delta E_{0 \to 1}$) prior to spontaneous decay were bombarded by photons of precisely the same energy, $\Delta E_1 = \Delta E_{0 \to 1}$, as was initially absorbed to achieve excitation, that excited electrons would move to a lower state and emit a photon of energy $\Delta E_{1 \to 0}$, equal in magnitude to ΔE_1. The stimulating photon, rather than being absorbed, would instead also be propagated to produce a net result of two photons of equal energy traveling in the same spatial and temporal phase (Fig. 5.1.3). This is known as stimulated emission of radiation and is the principle upon which the laser is based.[2-4] (Note: LASER = Light Amplification by Stimulated Emission of Radiation.)

LASER BEAM PRODUCTION

For a sustained stimulated emission to occur, and thus a sustained beam of laser light to be produced, a "population inversion" must be achieved such that a majority of atoms exist in their excited state. This condition is produced by "pumping" energy into a laser medium so as to produce spontaneous emissions of photons which then collide with other atoms in their excited state, stimulating them to emit an additional photon. These photons then collide with other transitional atoms and a chain reaction of stimulated emission occurs. To maintain this state, energy must be continually supplied to the laser medium

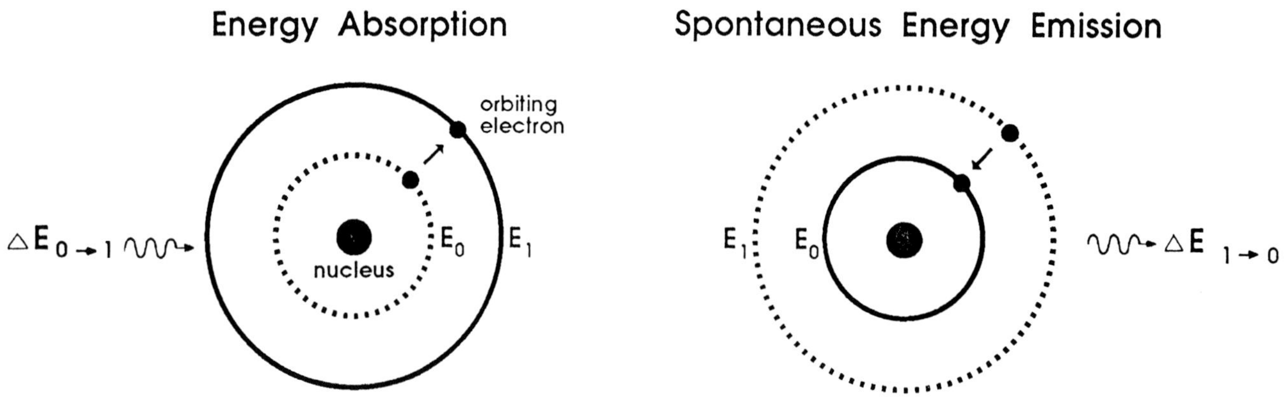

Energy Absorption

Spontaneous Energy Emission

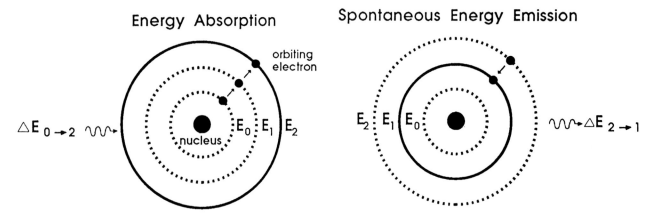

Figure 5.1.1.   Spontaneous emission of radiation.

Energy Absorption

Spontaneous Energy Emission

Figure 5.1.2.   Spontaneous emission of radiation.

being excited. Gas lasing mediums use electrical power (DC or RF electric fields), whereas liquid or solid lasing mediums require optical power produced by a xenon flash lamp or other lasers.

Since a fine beam of laser light is desired, the random directional movement of spontaneous and stimulated emissions must be changed to a uniform direction. This requires an amplification scheme (Fig. 5.1.4) incorporating a laser tube (optical or resonant cavity) designed such that photon propagation parallel to the axis of the tube is reflected back through the axis of the medium causing more atoms in their excited state to emit photons. Carefully aligned mirrors are placed at both ends of the laser tube. The lasing effect is amplified with photons resonating back and forth along the axis of the optical cavity. One of the mirrors is designed to be 100% reflective while the other is designed to partially transmit the laser beam out of the resonant tube. The energy from spontaneous photon emissions nonparallel to the axis of the tube is lost in the form of heat. Air or water cooling systems will often be incorporated into the design of the laser system to dissipate this lost energy and to prevent laser tube damage.

Optical delivery systems which are used to transmit laser energy from the output of the laser tube to the point of application are currently of two primary designs: 1) flexible delivery systems utilizing a focusing lens and fiberoptic bundles, and 2) rigid delivery systems utilizing a hollow waveguide or an articulating arm assembly consisting of a series of mirrors, hollow tubes, and "elbow" joints.[5-7]

Stimulated Energy Emission

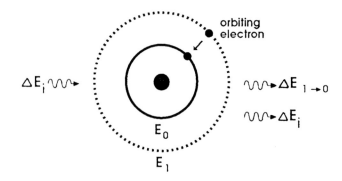

Figure 5.1.3.   Stimulated emission of radiation.

Basic Laser System Design

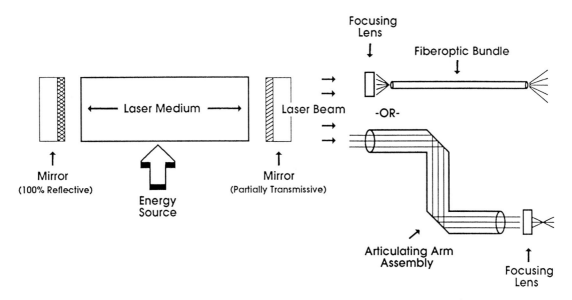

Figure 5.1.4. Basic laser system design.

Properties and Characteristics of Laser Energy

Laser radiation possesses three unique characteristics: coherence, collimation, and monochromaticity.

Coherence refers to the phenomenon that all electromagnetic radiation in the form of photons emitted from the laser tube are in phase with each other both in time and in space. Thus, the effect on the amplitude of the waves is additive, and superimposng individual photons provides for maximum power yield.[8,9]

Collimation refers to the fact that photons exiting the laser cavity do not appreciably diverge from one another as they travel outward. The path of the laser beam is such that all photons travel parallel to one another at the output of the laser tube. This accounts for the remarkable directionality of laser light. For example, NASA has fired a high-power Nd-glass laser from the earth to the moon, producing a spot size about 0.5 mile in diameter. This divergence is small in comparison to the approximate 240,000-mile distance between the earth and moon.[10]

Monochromaticity signifies that all emitted laser photons are of discrete wavelengths as all photons originate from discrete energy level transitions.[11] Whereas white light from a regular light bulb emits photons of numerous wavelengths, the unique characteristic of monochromaticity provides that a laser can be selected for a discrete wavelength to have a designated tissue effect during a medical procedure. Current medical lasers operate in the ultraviolet to infrared portion of the electromagnetic spectrum (Table 5.1.1).[12,13]

Table 5.1.1. The Electromagnetic Spectrum

Radiation	Wavelength
Cosmic	10^{-8} μm
X-ray	10^{-4} μm
Ultraviolet	10^{-2} to 0.4 μm
HeCd	0.325 μm
Excimer:	
XeCl	0.308 μm
XeF	0.351 μm
Optical	0.4–0.7 μm
Argon	0.488 μm (Blue)
	0.514 μm (Green)
532 YAG	0.532 μm (Green)
Krypton	0.531 μm (Green)
	0.568 μm (Yellow)
Tunable dye (optical spectrum)	0.4–0.7 μm
Coumarin	0.480 μm (Blue)
Helium neon	0.630 μm (Red)
Gold vapor	0.630 μm (Red)
Krypton	0.647 μm (Red)
Ruby	0.694 μm (Red)
Infrared	1.0–10^2 μm
Nd-YAG	1.064 μm
Ho-YLF	2.06 μm
Er-YAG	2.94 μm
CO_2	10.6 μm
Microwave	10^4 μm
TV and FM radio	10^6 μm
Shortwave radio	10^7 μm
AM radio	10^9 μm

Laser Energy Interaction with Tissue

Electromagnetic radiation interacts with objects in primarily one of four manners: transmission, reflection, scattering, or absorption. It is important to note that for laser energy to exert any effect on tissue, the energy must be absorbed. Reflection or transmission, though important in various applications, will not render any significant effect on incident tissue. Scattering will result in absorption over a larger area such that its effect is more diffuse than direct absorption.[14]

The way in which tissue absorbs laser energy, and thus the net effect of interaction, is determined by the characteristics of the laser beam (wavelength, energy density, fluence) as well as the characteristics of the incident tissue. We shall look at these considerations in detail.

Wavelength

Absorption characteristics vary with wavelength for different tissues. An analysis of absorption versus wavelength for water, hemoglobin, and melanin (substances most abundant in various tissues) is illustrated in Figure 5.1.5.[15] Generally, the greater the degree of absorption, the greater the tissue effect. Likewise, the degree of "scattering" is also wavelength-dependent.

Energy Density

Energy density is a most important factor in determining tissue effect of incident laser energy. Generally speaking, the greater the energy density of the laser beam, the greater the tissue effect.[16] The energy density of the laser beam is determined by two factors—exposure time and power density—and is determined as follows:

$$\text{Energy Density} = \text{Exposure Time} \times \text{Power Density}$$

As we see, tissue effect may be increased by increasing the exposure duration or by increasing the power density.

Power density, termed irradiance, refers to the amount

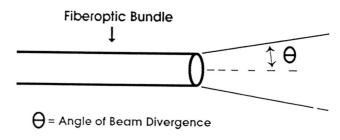

θ = Angle of Beam Divergence

Figure 5.1.6. Beam divergence from a fiberoptic bundle.

of power per unit surface area directed toward tissue during a single pulse. Power density is calculated as follows:

$$\text{Power Density} = \text{Power/Cross-sectional Area}$$

Greater tissue effect may be obtained by either increasing the power setting on the laser or by decreasing the cross-sectional area of the incident beam.

In those angioplasty applications where laser energy is incident upon tissue, it is important to understand this concept of power density and its effect on tissue. Optical delivery systems most common to laser angioplasty applications require delivery of laser energy via fiberoptics incorporated into the design of flexible catheters. Laser energy propagates through the fiberoptic bundle from the output of the laser tube via a series of numerous reflections off the sides of the fiberoptic strand and eventually exits the catheter at some point with its output beam not in collimated form, but in a divergent manner (Fig. 5.1.6). It is important to note that for a given power setting on the laser, tissue effect will decrease as the distance from catheter to tissue to be "lased" increases, since the cross-sectional area of the laser beam necessarily increases (and thus the power density decreases) due to the divergent nature of the laser beam output.[17]

Fluence

The term fluence refers to the rate at which laser energy is delivered to tissue, and also has great bearing upon tissue effect. In general, the higher the fluence, the more precise tissue effects will be realized. For example, since energy density equals power density multiplied by exposure time, 100 joules of energy/cm^2 delivered at different rates could yield different tissue effects as illustrated in Figure 5.1.7.[18]

We see that increased peak power (fluence) results in decreased effect on underlying tissue and increased effect upon incident tissue.

Laser energy may be delivered to tissue not only in a continuous mode of operation, but may also be delivered in a pulsed mode (Fig. 5.1.8).

Let us define several concepts associated with pulsed laser energy:

Activation time (t) = Duration of pulse
Cycle time (T) = Interval between onset of consecutive pulses
Frequency (f) = Number of pulses per second = $1/T$

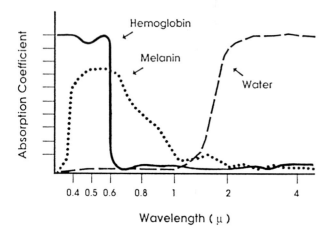

Figure 5.1.5. Absorption characteristics vs. wavelength.

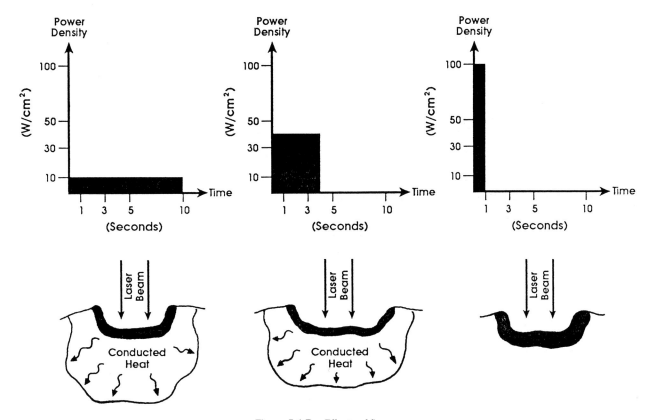

Figure 5.1.7. Effects of fluence.

Duty cycle (%) = Percent "on" time of laser = $(t/T) \times$ 100%

Peak power (P_{pk}) = Maximum power during energy application

Average power (P_{av}) = ($P_{pk} \times$ Duty cycle) = peak power $\times$ pulse width $\times$ pulse frequency

Just as with single pulse delivery, maximum precision may be realized in pulsed mode (with a given average power available) by maximizing the fluence via selection of output with highest peak power at the shortest pulse width.

To summarize, in order to determine tissue effect resultant from incident laser energy, we need to know not

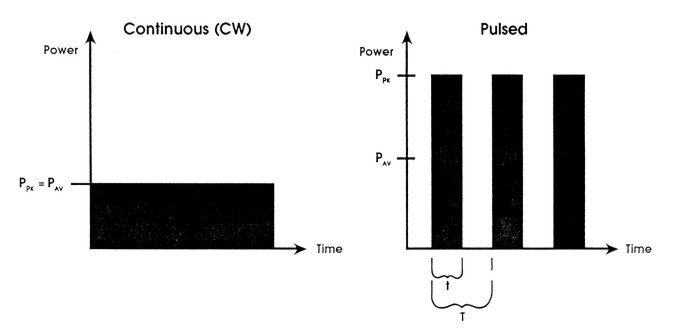

Figure 5.1.8. Continuous vs. pulsed mode of energy delivery.

the tissue type to be lased, but also the following characteristics of the laser energy to be applied:

1. Wavelength—to determine tissue absorption;
2. Energy Density—determined by exposure time, peak power, and cross-sectional area of the incident laser beam;
3. Fluence—determined by peak power density, pulse width, and pulse rate.

MODES OF ABSORPTION

Three basic mechanisms of absorption of laser energy have been observed: photothermal, photoplasma, and photochemical.

The photothermal mechanism is the most commonly observed for continuous wave and low peak-power pulsed lasers in the optical and infrared spectrum. In this mechanism, absorbed photons are converted to heat and the temperature of the tissue rises to 60 °C, where protein denaturization and cell necrosis occurs. As laser energy continues to be applied, temperature rises until it exceeds 100 °C, where vaporization begins to occur and tissue is ablated. The photothermal mechanism presents perhaps the least precise mode of absorption in that thermal conduction may result in damage to surrounding tissue.

The photoplasma mechanism is observed resultant from the use of very high peak-power pulsed lasers such that a dielectric breakdown of material occurs producing a local plasma and resultant shockwave effect resulting in precise tissue ablation.

The photochemical mechanism is observed from the use of high peak-power short pulse ultraviolet wavelengths such that molecular bonds are directly broken resulting in precise tissue ablation.[19]

SPECTRUM OF AVAILABLE LASERS

While the FDA has approved the use of a limited number of laser systems for angioplasty applications at the time of this writing, the vast majority remain investigational. It is important to keep in mind that what is written today about the spectrum of available lasers may become outdated within a short period of time as technology evolves rapidly in an effort to develop a useful tool for the percutaneous treatment of vascular disease.

ARGON LASER SYSTEMS

A very high electrical current is passed through the argon gas lasing medium to produce excited argon ions and stimulated emission of photons with wavelengths in the blue-green portion of the optical spectrum. Specifically, argon lasers are designed to produce primarily two discrete wavelengths of 0.488 and 0.514μm. These discrete wavelengths are highly absorbed by hemoglobin and melanin and exhibit an intermediate scattering effect. Argon systems are currently designed to deliver laser power up to 20 watts continuous wave (CW) in continuous or pulsed fashions via fiberoptics. Generally, because the argon laser is highly inefficient in production of optical energy, special electrical hookups are required for operation. In addition, elaborate water cooling systems are often required to prevent excessive heat build-up in (and consequent damage) to the laser tube.[20,21]

At present, two argon laser systems have been approved by the FDA for general use in the peripheral vasculature (still investigational in coronary vessels). One system (Trimedyne Optilase 900) incorporates a 12-watt argon laser source and utilizes two types of delivery systems. The "Laserprobe" and "LaserCath" catheters incorporate an optical fiber coupled to a metallic cap in which laser energy (4–12 watts) is applied to heat the metal cap in order to thermally ablate tissue.[22,23] The "Spectraprobe" catheter (investigational) combines thermal and optical delivery by incorporating an optical fiber coupled to a metallic cap with a recessed sapphire crystal which enables 18% of the total energy to be emitted through a small window at the distal end of the catheter.

The other approved argon laser system (GV Medical Lastac System II) incorporates use of a 20-watt argon laser source coupled to a control monitor and an optical fiber control handle. The delivery system incorporates an optical quartz fiber, a balloon, an irrigating lumen, and an optical assembly at the distal tip which diverges the delivered laser energy (multiple 10-watt exposures for 2–10 seconds) to a 40° cone angle (in a clear fluid medium). Whereas a bare fiber might diverge the beam 5° (to produce a 10° cone angle), in a clear fluid medium the increased divergence of the Lastac system more quickly increases the diameter of area of ablation and dissipates the intensity of the beam as distance from catheter tip increases so that beyond 3mm from the fiber tip, power density falls below the threshold for tissue ablation. The centering, dilating balloon coaxially aligns the fiber tip within the arterial lumen and the delivery of a heparinized saline irrigating solution clears blood and contrast medium from the fiber tip.[24]

One other argon laser system is currently undergoing investigation. This system provides for thermal angioplasty in a temperature-controlled manner, utilizing a 16-watt argon laser source (HGM 20-S) and a delivery system (HGM PLAC) incorporating an optical fiber coupled to a metallic tip (a platinum/iridium sphere) with a thermocouple junction to allow continuous monitoring and adjustment of tip temperature (typically set from 300–400 °C).

EXCIMER LASER SYSTEMS

The excimer laser, or rare-gas halide laser, operates in the ultraviolet region of the electromagnetic spectrum. The high-power pulsed output is achieved via a high voltage, pulsed electric discharge through a gas mixture containing one inert gas (helium, neon, or argon), another inert rare gas (xenon or krypton) and a halogen compound (hydrogen chloride or fluorine). The term excimer is derived from "excited dimer" and refers to an ionic bond that is created by the halogen ion and the inert rare gas ion in their excited states. The wavelengths produced by the various excimer lasers include $0.193\mu m$ (ArF), $0.222\mu m$ (KrCl), $0.308\mu m$ (XeCl), and $0.351\mu m$ (XeF). Peak powers of up to several hundred kilowatts per pulse are delivered in pulse durations ranging from 10 to 250 nanoseconds. These high bursts of energy account for the photochemical molecular dissociation mechanism observed in tissue interaction, as use of the excimer laser allows for precise ablation of incident tissue without thermal conduction to surrounding tissue.[25]

At present, only the "long-pulse" XeCl excimer laser produces laser energy of sufficient magnitude to efficiently ablate tissue which may also be transmitted through high-purity silica-based flexible fiberoptics and, thus, is the only excimer laser currently undergoing investigation. This "long-pulse" XeCl excimer laser system (AIS Dymer 200+) provides direct irradiation with laser energy of high fluence (peak power to hundreds of kilowatts, pulse width of 200 nanoseconds) and energy density of 35–60mJ/mm²/pulse, at a repetition rate of 20–30Hz. For total occlusions, a delivery system is available in which an external balloon is utilized to center the fiber within the vessel. Contact ablation within the blood field prevents the propagation of laser light from the region of the fiber end, thereby preventing laser ablation of any part of the vessel not in direct contact with the fiber tip.[26]

PULSED DYE LASER SYSTEMS

A pulsed dye laser system utilizes a liquid lasing medium in which optical energy (via the use of a flash lamp or another laser) excites the liquid dye medium, adjusted to produce a specific wavelength in the optical spectral region.[27]

One such laser (Medilase System 4000) currently undergoing investigation utilizes flash lamp excitation of a coumarin dye solution to produce high power (150kW), short duration (1 microsecond) pulses (energy of 150mJ/pulse) with a wavelength of 480 nm in order to remove plaque via a combination of both photothermal and photoacoustic effect. This pulsed dye laser is guided by an integrated angioscope and aimable laser fiber system. A low-power HeNe laser is used as an aiming beam, and a motorized catheter positioner is controlled by the system's computer to precisely aim the laser toward the obstruction as directed by the physician.[28]

ND-YAG LASER SYSTEMS

Nd-YAG is a shortened version of neodymium-yttrium-aluminum-garnet. The solid lasing medium for this laser consists of a yttrium aluminum garnet crystal doped with

1–3% neodymium ions. The active medium (neodymium) is excited with a xenon flash lamp to provide laser energy in the near infrared spectrum (wavelength = $1.06\mu m$). This wavelength is highly absorbed by tissue protein and exhibits a relatively high scattering effect when delivered in continuous wave (CW) or low peak-power pulsed modes of operation. Nd-YAG "solid-state" CW lasers are currently designed to deliver, via fiberoptics, laser power up to 140 watts in continuous mode or pulsed fashion. Like the argon laser, the CW Nd-YAG laser is very inefficient in its production of laser energy, and often requires a specialized electrical hook-up as well as an elaborate water cooling system for its laser tube. A low-power (2–5 milliwatts) helium neon gas laser with output wavelength in the visible spectrum ($0.63\mu m$) is typically aligned with the Nd-YAG laser at its output to serve as an aiming beam.[29]

At present, CW Nd-YAG lasers are utilized in varying investigational angioplasty techniques. One system (Trimedyne Cardiolase 4000 or Optilase 1000), approved by the FDA for general use in the peripheral vasculature (still investigational in coronary vessels), utilizes an Nd-YAG laser source (40W for Cardiolase 4000; 60W for Optilase 1000) together with the Laserprobe and LaserCath delivery systems (the Spectraprobe delivery system is still investigational) in much the same manner as with Trimedyne's Optilase 900 argon laser system, as previously discussed.

Two Nd-YAG laser systems are currently investigational. One system utilizes a 60W Nd-YAG laser source (SLT CL-60) together with a delivery system incorporating an optical fiber coupled to a focusing sapphire tip (Surgical Laser Technologies). This focusing tip protects the laser fiber from charring as frequently occurs during laser emissions in blood and provides for precise tissue ablation.[30,31]

A second investigational application involves the use of a CW Nd-YAG laser (Quantronix System 1500) with a delivery system (USCI/Bard Spears Laser Balloon) in which laser energy is transmitted radially through a balloon transparent to the laser's wavelength. Laser energy is applied during final balloon inflation of an otherwise conventional balloon angioplasty procedure to coagulate tissues thermally within the artery wall in order to achieve two primary tissue effects—to fuse disrupted tissue elements such as plaque-arterial wall separations and to reduce elastic recoil.[32]

"SMART LASER" SYSTEM

One major concern in utilizing laser technology in the coronary vessels is the risk of vessel perforation. One firm (MCM Laboratories) is addressing this concern via development of a "smart laser" system consisting of a "treatment laser" used in conjunction with a "diagnostic laser," optical delivery and feedback system, and computer to provide for safe application of laser energy in order to avoid damage to the vessel wall. The diagnostic laser (a HeCd gas laser with ultraviolet wavelength of 325nm, and low power of 2mW) is pulsed through a fiberoptic channel, causing target tissue to fluoresce. The evoked fluorescence is transmitted back through the same fiber, where a beam splitter directs it to an optical analyzer, enabling determination of tissue type. The treatment laser (currently investigating the use of various high-fluence, pulsed solid-state lasers in the near infrared spectrum) is then enabled if the optical analyzer determines incident tissue does not represent normal vessel wall. Both the diagnostic and treatment lasers are pulsed in alternate fashion to ensure safe delivery of laser energy.[33]

FUTURE DEVELOPMENTS

Two presently available laser system—the CO_2 and the super-pulsed Nd-YAG—might find application in angioplasty applications in future years given advancements in fiberoptic technology development.

CO_2 gas lasers are currently designed to deliver laser power to 100W in a continuous wave mode at a wavelength of $10.6\mu m$ in the infrared region of the electromagnetic spectrum. A low-powered helium-neon (HeNe) gas laser is aligned to the output of the CO_2 laser to serve as an aiming beam. While CO_2 lasers are currently used in other medical specialties for precise tissue ablation (the $10.6\mu m$ wavelength is highly absorbed by water and exhibits a relatively low scattering effect), the CO_2 laser's wavelength cannot be efficiently transmitted through presently available flexible fiberoptics.[34]

Nd-YAG lasers have also been designed to produce "super pulses" of laser energy via "Q-switching." These systems generally incorporate an intracavity fast shutter between the lasing medium and one of the mirrors. With the shutter closed, the energy contained in the lasing medium will be pumped to a level far above the lasing threshold with the shutter open, as the population inversion can be made much larger than before. The result, upon releasing the shutter, is a single, short (10–20-nanosecond duration) high-power pulse on the order of up to 1 megawatt of power. This high-power pulse produces a photoplasma effect when incident upon tissue and results in high precision tissue ablation. Unfortunately, the same dielectric effect which precisely ablates tissue also damages fiberoptics, and so the laser energy cannot presently be delivered to tissue via flexible catheters.[35–37]

Laser systems undergoing current development (in addition to those already mentioned) include the holmium-YLF (Ho-YLF), the erbium-YAG (Er-YAG), and other solid state lasers. The Ho-YLF laser produces a wavelength of laser energy in the near infrared spectrum at $2.06\mu m$, which can be transmitted through currently available silica-based fibers. Energy is emitted as high-power pulses with pulse durations of approximately 100 microseconds. Efficiency of plaque ablation is superior to current argon and CW Nd-YAG lasers as the absorption coefficient for plaque at this wavelength is greater and increased fluence leads to improved precision. The Er-YAG laser produces energy with a wavelength also in the near infrared spectrum at $2.9\mu m$, with high-power pulses delivered in 100-microsecond bursts. The wavelength produced provides excellent ablation efficiency but cannot be efficiently transmitted via flexible silica fibers.[38]

A relatively new breakthrough in quantum physics research has led to the development of a prototype "free electron" laser which could potentially be tuned to a broad range of discrete wavelengths enabling use of one device for ablation, welding, coagulation, etc. of numerous tissue types. Development of this versatile product into a useful clinical tool is projected into the 21st century.[39]

Research and development efforts in the near future will focus primarily upon delivery systems which will enable safe and effective utilization of medical lasers for angioplasty applications. Research will continue in the development of fibers that will more efficiently transmit laser energy in the ultraviolet and infrared spectrums to enable investigation of the use of the ArF, KrCl, and XeF excimers, CO_2 and Er-YAG lasers. Development of specialized optical lens tips will provide for the ability to focus or defocus the laser energy at the output of the catheter. Modifications to catheter design will enable better placement of the catheter tip within the vessel.

Research will also focus on improvements to the "smart laser" design concept. Multifiber catheters could be designed in which individual fibers are responsible for fluorescence plaque identification and subsequent laser ablation for a given tissue zone, providing for selective topographic vaporization of sclerotic plaque.[40] Incorporation of ultrasound technology into "smart laser" catheter tip design may provide for increased safety, as information would be provided not only about the surface of incident tissue but also about tissue depth. Such information may prove valuable when the laser beam is removing tissue close to the vessel wall and would enable production of three-dimensional images of the artery during the angioplasty procedure.[41]

LASER SAFETY

The American National Standards Institute (ANSI) has developed guidelines for the safe design and use of medical laser systems.[42,43] This section will briefly summarize these guidelines as they apply to the angioplasty suite.

Hazard Classification

The Radiation Control for Health and Safety Act (RCHSA) and the Federal Laser Product Performance Standard establish a classification scheme (Table 5.1.2) for lasers in which the laser's class determines the kind of controls, performance features, and labeling requirements. The manufacturer is responsible to properly classify the product.

Table 5.1.2. Hazard Classification

Class	Control Measures	Medical Surveillance
1	Not applicable	Not applicable
2a	Applicable	Not applicable
3a	Applicable	Not applicable
3b	Applicable	Applicable
4	Applicable	Applicable

Administrative Controls

Institutional administrative controls are required to ensure safe implementation. These include the designation of a Laser Safety Officer (LSO) responsible for the establishment and surveillance of appropriate laser safety control measures and the formation of a Laser Use Committee to govern laser activity and establish use criteria. Committee membership would consist of a physician representative from each specialty utilizing laser technology, the designated Laser Safety Officer, and other support personnel. The committee typically approves all facility users after receipt of a formal protocol and standard operating procedures.

Equipment Controls

Manufacturers are required to incorporate equipment controls in the design of their Class 3 and Class 4 laser systems. These include incorporation of a protective housing for the laser tube to limit laser radiation exposure, interlocks on equipment covers to guard against electrical and optical hazards, a keyswitch master interlock, a guarded footswitch, and application of warning labels. Beam delivery disconnect features are required such that disconnection of a delivery system (i.e., optical fibers) from a laser source shall not permit excess laser radiation to directly exit from the laser system. A beam stop attenuator is required to prevent output emission when the laser system is on standby. (Note: It is important to disable output emission via turning off the footswitch enable control and/or by closing the mechanical safety shutter during interims when laser energy is not required for treatment.) An audible or visual warning associated with delayed emission of laser radiation is also required.

LASER TREATMENT CONTROLLED AREA

A "Laser Treatment Controlled Area" is to be defined in which certain safety measures are to be implemented. This typically would include the procedure suite and possibly any remote viewing areas. The controlled area is defined by the limits of the "Nominal Hazard Zone" (NHZ) as determined by the LSO. The NHZ describes the area within which the level of direct, reflected, or scattered radiation, during normal operation, exceeds the maximum permissible exposure limit, and may be determined by

information supplied by the manufacturer, by measurement, or by using the NHZ equations referenced in the ANSI standard.

Laser treatment controlled areas for Class 3b and Class 4 laser systems require the following:

1. Appropriate warning signs posted;
2. Supervised and only occupied by authorized personnel;
3. Direct supervision by an individual knowledgable in laser safety;
4. Location such that access to the area by spectators is limited and requires approval;
5. A potentially hazardous beam must be terminated by a beam stop of an appropriate material;
6. Only diffusely reflective materials in or near the beam path, where feasible;
7. Personnel who regularly require entry must be adequately trained, provided with appropriate protective equipment, and required to follow all applicable administrative and procedural controls;
8. All windows, doorways, etc. must be either covered or restricted in such a manner as to reduce the transmitted laser radiation to levels at or below the appropriate ocular MPE limit;
9. The laser system must be stored or disabled (key removed) when not in use to prevent unauthorized use;
10. The shutter mechanism must be closed during standby periods;
11. An emergency shut-off switch provided to enable rapid shutdown of the laser system.

Personal Protective Equipment

Eye protection must be worn by all persons within the NHZ (including the patient) to prevent possible exposure to hazardous laser radiation. Corneal or retinal burns, depending upon wavelength, are possible from acute exposure; and corneal or lenticular opacities or retinal injury may be possible from chronic exposure to excessive levels.[44]

Per the standard, the optical density (OD) of lens filters must meet or exceed that specified by the laser manufacturer for all applicable wavelengths of emitted laser energy. In addition, all laser protective eye wear should be clearly labeled with the optical density and wavelength for which protection is afforded, should be comfortable, and should prevent exposure to hazardous peripheral radiation. Periodic inspection should be made of protective eye wear to ensure satisfactory conditions to include inspection of attenuation material for pitting, crazing, cracking, or discoloration, inspection of frame for mechanical integrity, and inspection for light leaks that could permit hazardous intrabeam viewing. An appropriate protocol would be to require that applicable eye wear be worn any time the

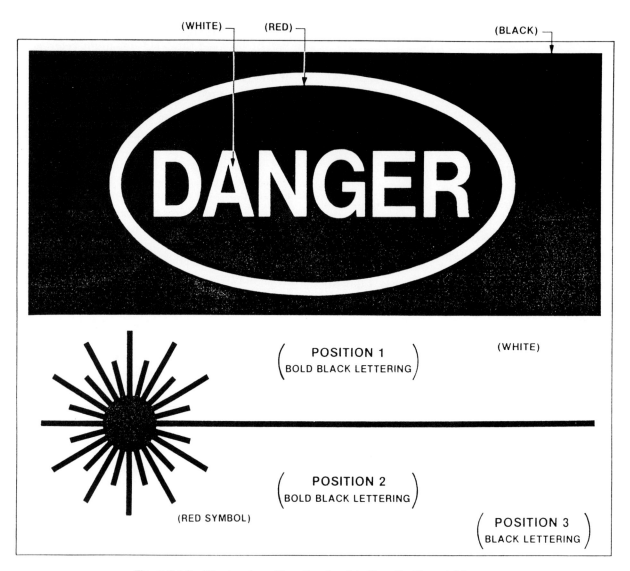

Figure 5.1.9. Warning sign—Class 2 and certain Class 3a, 3b, and 4 lasers.

mechanical beam stop is in its open position to enable laser energy output.

Where personnel may be exposed to levels of radiation that clearly exceed the maximum permissible exposure for skin, consideration should be given to the use of protective clothing. Where personnel may be subject to chronic skin exposure from scattered ultraviolet radiation, skin protection should be provided even at levels below the MPE for skin.

Warning Signs

Warning signs are placed at all entrances to the laser treatment area. The design of the sign should be in accordance with Figure 5.1.9.[45] Position 1 should indicate precautionary instructions such as, "Laser in Use—Eye Protection Required," and in addition, the following: "Laser Radiation—Avoid Direct Eye Exposure" (Class 3a

laser systems); "Laser Radiation—Avoid Eye or Skin Exposure to Direct or Scattered Radiation" (Class 4 laser systems). Position 2 should indicate type of laser or emitted wavelength, pulse duration if appropriate, and maximum output. Position 3 should indicate the class of the laser system.

Laser Safety and Training Programs

All laser support personnel (technicians, nurses, service personnel) must receive adequate training appropriate to their role to include basic laser physics, laser safety considerations, and operation of the applicable laser systems.

Establishing physician credentials requires attendance at a laser principles and safety course to include basic laser physics, laser tissue interaction, discussions of the clinical specialty field, and hands-on experience with lasers. In addition, preceptorship training is required in which the physician observes and assists an experienced operator in the specialty area involved.

Medical Surveillance

Health care personnel who work routinely in a laser system environment should have a baseline eye examination prior to working in the laser environment, to include an ocular history and inspection of visual acuity, macular function, and contrast sensitivity. Should ocular function in any of the tests prove abnormal, then a funduscopic examination would be required. Incidental health care personnel whose work makes it possible (but unlikely) that they will be exposed to laser energy should have a baseline eye examination to include an ocular history and inspection of visual acuity. Eye examination should be performed prior to working with lasers, immediately after a suspected abnormal exposure of the eye, for specific eye complaints possibly related to laser energy exposure on an individual basis, and at the termination of work in the laser environment. The results of all eye examinations should be discussed with the employee, and complete eye examination records should be retained for a minimum of 30 years.

Electrical Safety

It is recommended that the laser system be accepted, certified, listed, labeled, or otherwise determined safe by a qualified testing laboratory, such as, but not limited to, Underwriters Laboratories, Inc., or Factory Mutual Corporation.

Fire Safety

The laser shall not be used in the presence of flammable or combustible chemicals such as anesthetics, preparation solutions, drying agents, ointments, methyl methacrylate, or other plastic resins. Only nonflammable, flame-resistant surgical drapes should be used.

Toxic Gases

The majority of medical lasers in use today which utilize gas lasing mediums require gas sources which do not pose a hazard to operating personnel in terms of toxicity. (As with most pressurized gas cylinders, there always exists the hazard of displacement of room air in a nonventilated room.) Excimer lasers, however, do require a toxic gas source. The "long-pulse" XeCl excimer laser requires use of hydrogen chloride, an extremely corrosive gas with strong fumes. Inhalation of HCl can cause pulmonary edema and skin contact causes severe tissue irritation. The established OSHA threshold limit value for exposure is 5 parts/million.

Control measures include, but are not limited to, metic-

ulous handling (the most important), the use of a specialized gas cabinet enclosure for storage and gas delivery, the installation of exhaust fume hoods with direct venting to outside the facility located directly above the storage of HCl, points of HCl gas hookup to the laser, or locations where the HCl cylinders are changed, storage of HCl gas mixtures in a dedicated room with direct ventilation to the outside, and separate from the storage of gases which are flammable or oxidizing agents (fire code), and the use of a gas mask (with a halogen filter) and gloves when changing HCl cylinders.[46]

I would like to thank Ric Colegrove, a graphic artist from Delray, Florida, for contributing to the technical illustrations for Chapter 5, Part 1.

References

1. Vassiliadis A: *Lasers and Tissue Effects*, Colorado Springs, Xanar, 1982, p 13
2. Vassiliadis A: *Lasers and Tissue Effects*, Colorado Springs, Xanar, 1982, pp 4–6
3. Fuller TA: The physics of surgical lasers. *Lasers Surg Med* 1980;1:6–8
4. Huether SE: How lasers work. *AORN J* 1983;38,2:209
5. Vassiliadis A: *Lasers and Tissue Effects*. Colorado Springs, Xanar, 1982, pp 10–12
6. Fuller TA: The physics of surgical lasers. *Lasers Surg Med* 1980;1:8–9
7. Huether SE: How lasers work. *AORN J* 1983;38:2:209–211
8. Absten GT: *Fundamentals of Laser Surgery*. Grove City, OH, Paul Rogers Company, 1983, pp 7–8
9. Janssen WD: *Fundamentals of Laser Surgery*. Columbus, OH, Grant Hospital Laser Center, p. 7
10. Absten GT: *Fundamentals of Laser Surgery*. Grove City, OH, Paul Rogers Company, 1983, p 9
11. Janssen WD: *Fundamentals of Laser Surgery*. Columbus, OH, Grant Hospital Laser Center, p 7
12. Huether SE: How lasers work. *AORN J* 1983;38,2:207–208
13. Laudenslager JB: Laser fundamentals, in White RA, Grundfest WS (eds): *Lasers in Cardiovascular Disease*. Chicago, Year Book Medical Publishers, 1987, pp 7–26
14. Absten GT: *Fundamentals of Laser Surgery*. Grove City, OH, Paul Rogers Company, 1983, p 9
15. "Absorption Coefficients" slide. Sharplan Lasers, Allendale, NJ
16. Janssen WD: *Fundamentals of Laser Surgery*. Columbus, OH, Grant Hospital Laser Center, pp 11–12
17. Ready JF: Laser technology: the new energy source. *Lastext* 1988;1,2:6
18. "The Importance of High Powers" slide. Sharplan Lasers, Allendale, NJ
19. Laudenslager JB: Laser fundamentals, in White RA, Grundfest WS (eds): *Lasers in Cardiovascular Disease*. Chicago, Year Book Medical Publishers, 1987, pp 27–29
20. Fuller TA: The physics of surgical lasers. *Lasers Surg Med* 1980;1:9
21. Huether SE: How lasers work. *AORN J* 1983;38,2:212–213
22. Sanborn TA, Haudenschild CC, Garber GR, et al: Angiographic and histologic consequences of laser thermal angioplasty: comparison with balloon angioplasty. *Circulation* 1987;75,6:1281–1286
23. Sanborn TA, Greenfield AJ, Guben JK, et al: Human percu-

taneous and intraoperative laser thermal angioplasty: initial clinical results as an adjunct to balloon angioplasty. *Vasc Surg* 1987;5,1:83–90

24. Nordstrom LA, Castañeda–Zúñiga WR, Young EG, et al: Direct argon laser exposure for recanalization of peripheral arteries: early results. *Radiology* 1988;168:359–364

25. Laudenslager JB: Laser fundamentals, in White RA, Grundfest WS (eds): *Lasers in Cardiovascular Disease*. Chicago, Year Book Medical Publishers, 1987, pp 25–29

26. Laudenslager JB: Excimer lasers adapt to angioplasty. *Laser Focus/Electro-Optics* May, 1988

27. Vassiliadis A: *Lasers and Tissue Effects*, Colorado Springs, Xanar, 1982, p 17

28. Company Profile: Medilase, Inc. *Angioplasty Technology Update Newsletter*. Strategic Business Development, Inc., 1990;1(1):3–4

29. Fuller TA: The physics of surgical lasers. *Lasers Surg Med* 1980;1:10

30. Geschwind HJ, Blair JD, Mongkolsmai D, et al: Development and experimental application of contact probe catheter for laser angioplasty. *J Am Coll Cardiol* 1987;9,1:101–107

31. Fourrier JL, Brunetaud JM, Prat A, et al: Percutaneous laser angioplasty with sapphire tip. *Lancet* 1987;105

32. Spears JR: Percutaneous transluminal coronary angioplasty restenosis: potential prevention with laser balloon angioplasty. *J Am Coll Cardiol* 1987;60:61B–64B

33. Miller DL: Fluorescence-guided laser angioplasty: the probe and treat laser system. *Vascular Interventional Laser: Physics, Safety, and Clinical Applications Course*. SCVIR Annual Meeting, 1989

34. Vassiliadis A: *Lasers and Tissue Effects*, Colorado Springs, Xanar, 1982, pp 15–16

35. Wyard SJ: *Solid State Biophysics*, New York, McGraw-Hill, 1969, pp 377–384

36. Vassiliadis A: *Lasers and Tissue Effects*. Colorado Springs, Xanar, 1982, pp 21–22

37. Young M: *Optics and Lasers: An Engineering Physics Approach*, New York, Springer-Verlag, 1977, pp 151–166

38. Leon MB, Smith PD, Bonner RF: Laser Angioplasty Delivery Systems, in White RA, Grundfest WS (eds): *Lasers in Cardiovascular Disease*. Chicago, Year Book Medical Publishers, 1987, pp 51–54

39. Gallivan M: "Star Wars" laser may alter the future of surgery. *Hospitals* 1986;60,18:90

40. Leon MB, Smith PD, Bonner RF: Laser angioplasty delivery systems, in White RA, Grundfest WS (eds): *Lasers in Cardiovascular Disease*. Chicago, Year Book Medical Publishers, 1987, p 60

41. Leon MB, Smith PD, Bonner RF: Laser angioplasty delivery systems, in White RA, Grundfest WS (eds): *Lasers in Cardiovascular Disease*. Chicago, Year Book Medical Publishers, 1987, p 58

42. *American National Standard for the Safe Use of Lasers*, ANSI Z136.1-1986, Toledo, The Laser Institute of America, 1986

43. *American National Standard for the Safe Use of Lasers in Health Care Facilities* ANSI Z136.3-1988, Toledo, The Laser Institute of America, 1988

44. Smith JF (ed): *Laser Safety Guide*, Toledo, The Laser Institute of America, 1988, p 1

45. *American National Standard for the Safe Use of Lasers in Health Care Facilities*, ANSI Z136.3-1988, Toledo, The Laser Institute of America, 1988, pp 21–22

46. Lorenz AK: Gas handling safety for laser makers and users. *Lasers and Applications*, March 1987

Part 2. Lasers in Peripheral Vascular Disease

—Charitha C. Fernando, B.H.B., MB.CHB., Andrew H. Cragg, M.D., Tony P. Smith, M.D., Flavio Castañeda, M.D., Wilson Greatbatch, Ph.D., T. J. Bowker, M.A., M.R.C.P., and Wilfrido Castañeda–Zúñiga, M.D., M.Sc.

INTRODUCTION

Since the first working laser was constructed in 1960,[1] lasers have been applied to numerous disease states and their value has been well demonstrated. The use of lasers in the treatment of vascular disease, however, is a relatively recent phenomenon.

Over the past several years, there has been tremendous interest in development of new technology to treat atherosclerotic vascular disease. The impetus for this has arisen from several factors including: 1) demonstration of the long-term efficacy of balloon angioplasty as an alternative to surgery, 2) rapid proliferation and application of angioplasty procedures to the treatment of coronary artery disease, and 3) recognition by scientists and industry that a large market exists for new technology which would improve on the results of balloon angioplasty.

With the refinement of existing catheter technology, it occurred to numerous investigators that remote delivery of laser energy via catheter-based quartz fibers could potentially allow percutaneous obliteration of atherosclerotic plaque, thereby achieving vessel recanalization without surgery or balloon angioplasty. The major potential advantage to this type of approach was that by removing plaque from the blood vessel, rather than redistributing it, as occurs with angioplasty, one would achieve a better long-term result.

During the early 1980s, a number of investigators began developing delivery systems for various laser sources in order to accomplish percutaneous laser angioplasty.[2–9] Some of this work has matured into clinical studies and Food and Drug Administration (FDA) approval of laser devices. However, difficulty in harnessing laser energy for angioplasty has slowed development of the technique. In addition, major questions remain about the efficacy of any laser angioplasty system given the high cost and mixed results which have been obtained to date. To illustrate the present state of development of laser angioplasty, it may be useful to review briefly what is currently known about laser sources, catheter delivery systems, and experimental and clinical results.

LASER

A laser consists of a tubular chamber with mirrors at each end. The medium within this may be gaseous, such as carbon dioxide, argon and the excitable dimers (excimer), xenon chloride and xenon fluoride, or solid, for example neodymium-yttrium-aluminum-garnet (Nd-YAG).

The electrons in the medium are excited by an external energy source. As the electrons return to ground state, a photon, whose wavelength is determined by the medium, is released. Creation of standard waves by reflection of this light between the mirrors allows for coherence and high intensity.

At one end of the tube, not all the light is reflected. One percent of the beam, which is parallel to the tube, is released. This emitted light can be directed by an optical fiber to sites of atheroma.

CHARACTERISTICS OF LIGHT

The events at the tissue-light interface depend on the parameters of the light beam and the nature of the tissue. The energy (E) of the beam will be proportional to its frequency (F) ($E = HF$ where H = Planck's constant) and inversely proportional to its wavelength (λ) ($E = H \div \lambda$, $C = \lambda \times F$; where C = velocity of light). The beam may be emitted continuously and the resultant energy (fluence) measured in joules per square centimeter, or high peak energies may be delivered by short pulses of radiation.

PHOTO TRANSFORMATIONS

The photo physical principles governing the light and tissue transformations have been reviewed by Boulnoy.[10] The three basic transformations are photothermal, photochemical, and photoablative. The electromechanical mode of interaction occurs at very high energies and is not involved in endovascular laser therapy. Photothermal interactions are the predominant mode of interaction of continuous wave lasers and involve conversion of light energy to thermal energy. Photochemical transformations occur where the laser wavelength matches the excitation bands of tissue molecules, chromophores or photosensitizers. The energies involved are sufficiently high to disrupt chemical bonds. Photoablative interactions occur where vaporization of the tissue results in the dissociation products of transformation occupying a larger volume than the original solid, and these are therefore released from the solid. The ablated tissues are thereby vaporized.

ARGON LASERS

Argon lasers produce continuous wave green light at 488 and 514.4nm. They are similar to x-ray tubes in that they are inefficient energy converters, for example, requiring a 23kW generator to produce a 17W laser beam (Optilase 900).[11]

Argon gas is the active medium for this type of laser which produces coherent, monochromatic light in the visible range of the spectrum, particularly 488 and 514nm. Advantages of argon lasers as a source for laser angioplasty include: (*a*) the ability to lase in a blood field, (*b*) the ability to easily transmit argon light down an optical fiber and (*c*) the fact that argon lasers are readily available and economical to operate. Disadvantages which have been demonstrated in experimental and clinical work to date include: (*a*) relatively low peak energy of the argon beam which results in thermal tissue destruction and charring at the lasing site[12]; (*b*) continuous wave output which adds to the thermal effect of the laser source; and (*c*) difficulty in controlling the depth of ablation which has required shielding or capping of the argon laser output to prevent vessel perforation.

Special wiring and cooling facilities are also required, so these lasers are usually not portable.[11] Although the laser beam is readily transmitted by optical fibers, up to 2W of energy may be lost by the fiber and associated couplings.[11]

As there is insufficient time for tissue cooling and the 2.5keV photon energy is below the threshold required to directly break peptide and carbon bonds,[13] the principal interaction is photothermal. The nature of the tissue damage does not differ if a bare fiber or a heated metal tip is used.[14] A central crater results at the site of lasing, with a concentric zone of thermal injuries seen 1mm distant from this.[15] Gross charring is seen at the perimeter of the crater, with a superficial zone of coagulative necrosis and an adjacent zone of lacunae formation.[16,17] Thrombus formation has been observed at the center,[16] and an elevated thrombogenicity index has been documented.[17] Although the extent of platelet adhesion may not be great,[18] re-endothelialization has been shown to occur within 60 days.[18] Strikwerda et al.[19] demonstrated that tissue ablation occurs at a threshold intensity of $2.5W/m^2$ and fluency of 3.2 joules/mm^2. At lower intensities, ablation was inconstant and greater coagulative necrosis was seen at the surrounding tissue. Tissue ablation was most efficient at 5.1 joules/m^2. In this study, histological evidence of coagulative necrosis was not seen at this fluence.

As argon laser light is absorbed by hemoglobin, the transmission characteristics are different in saline and blood.[20] Greater beam divergence and broader arterial damage is seen in blood, although the laser beam penetration in blood is less than that in saline.[20] Argon laser light can be used to vaporize human clot. In vitro studies[21,22] showed that clot rich in red cells is vaporized by argon laser emission, but red cell pool clot is not able to be lysed.

ND-YAG LASERS

There is broad experience with Nd-YAG lasers in other areas of medicine such as ophthalmology. Therefore, because of their availability, they have been fairly extensively investigated as sources for laser angioplasty.

Neodymium-yttrium-aluminum-garnet (Nd-YAG) lasers (1064nm, 5032nm, and 288nm) may be operated in continuous or pulsed modes. Pulsed radiation seems to be preferable for atheroma ablation because thermal effects on the irradiated vessel are reduced when compared to continuous wave radiation.[23,24] This is likely due to a combination of shorter wavelength pulses (higher energy) and the fact that interpulse time allows for more efficient cooling than can occur with continuous radiation. In practice, most Nd-YAG laser angioplasty systems operate in the continuous mode. While a higher power output is achieved than with the argon source, there is considerable thermal damage which again limits the usefulness of Nd-YAG as a free beam source.

Advantages of Nd-YAG lasers, therefore, include ready availability, higher power output than other sources, and relatively easy transmission down optical fibers. Disadvantages include deep, relatively nonspecific tissue penetration and thermal effects related to continuous wave delivery.

Geschwind et al.[25] have shown in vitro that tissue vaporization occurs at 360–600 joules with power intensities of 12 watts at the fiber tip. Tissue vaporization is optimal in a dilute blood perfusate, as this light is poorly transmitted in saline. Thermal effects can be minimized in vitro by cooling with a dilute blood perfusate. However, thermal effects usually dominate, and peripheral coagulative necrosis and vaporization is seen and is similar to that which occurs with an argon laser.[26] In the pulsed mode, thermal tissue damage can be considerably reduced,[27] but high power densities are required and transmission at these energies by the available optic fibers may be difficult.[28]

CARBON DIOXIDE LASERS

Carbon dioxide lasers operate at 1064nm in the continuous mode utilizing silver chloride optical fibers. Eldar et al.[29] have demonstrated the feasibility of atheroma ablation, and that peripheral charring thermonecrosis, coagulative changes, and acoustic injury occur. CO_2 lasers produce a reduction in platelet number and function, which could reduce thrombogenicity.[30] The energy is highly absorbed by water and biological tissues, resulting in a narrow zone of thermal injury.

EXCIMERS

Excimer lasers have sparked considerable interest as a laser angioplasty source since they appear to remove many of the disadvantages which have plagued more conventional laser sources such as argon and Nd-YAG.

Excimer lasers such as xenon chloride (308nm) and xenon fluoride (351nm) operate in short pulses (10–250 nanoseconds) and wavelengths (200–400nm). They generate high peak energies which offer several advantages over continuous wave lasers. The high energies enable disruption of molecular bonds, resulting in photochemical ablation. In contrast to continuous wave laser, calcified lesions can be ablated.[31] The combination of high-energy, pulsed radiation produces clean tissue ablation without significant thermal effects.[32,33] This is in part due to the increased cooling time because of larger interpulse duration.[16] Decreasing this cooling time results in an increase of the thermal effects.[34] Thermonecrosis distant from the crater of ablation is not seen.[16,35,36] Faster healing of laser sites, with reduction of inflammation, is claimed.[16] Although excimer laser light is absorbed by blood tissue, ablation through 5mm of blood has been successful.[35] In addition, excimer light appears to have a very short zone of ablation which means that the device can be operated as a free beam laser with a lower risk of laser-induced vessel perforation than with argon or Nd-YAG sources.[37]

However, perforation has not been eliminated as a cause of technical failure,[35] but satisfactory acute success is reported.[38] Adequate delivery of energy for tissue ablation has so far required the use of larger diameter and stiffer fibers.[31]

There are disadvantages to the excimer laser, however, which have hampered its introduction into the laser angioplasty field. The lasers are large and relatively cumbersome to operate. The high peak power can make transmission down optical fibers difficult.[39] Excimer light does not transmit well through blood which requires a blood-free lasing field. Finally, excimer lasers are expensive, which adds to the cost of the revascularization procedure itself.

DYE LASERS

Dye lasers contain an active medium to which a dye has been added to control the wavelength of light emitted. Murray[40] has demonstrated that using coumarin 504 as the dye, 504nm laser light in one-microsecond pulses is able to selectively ablate fatty, fibrous, and calcified plaque with a minimum of adjacent thermal tissue damage. Although clinical experiences are limited, Geschwind et al.[41] have demonstrated the ability to recanalize occluded arteries, but perforation remained a problem.

FIBEROPTIC CONDUCTORS

Glass fibers for fiberoptic systems are made of a core with a high index of refraction coated by a cladding with a lower index of refraction. Because of this design, light is continually bent from the periphery toward the core and cannot escape unless it encounters some discontinuity such as a scratch or a slag inclusion. Fibers may be made entirely of glass or of plastic-cladded silica or plastic. Fiberoptics for therapeutic lasers use all-glass construction, because plastics would be destroyed at the power levels necessary.[42] Connectors for optical fibers are a problem, inasmuch as any discontinuity will instantly develop destructive temperatures. Ideally, the ends to be joined should be polished, mated, and fused. A number of mechanical connection schemes are commercially available, but one must exercise great care in using them, because a loose connection or a spot of dirt could destroy the connector and the fiber.

The CO_2 infrared laser has been limited to open procedures because of the absence of satisfactory nontoxic fiberoptics to guide the laser beam to closed areas. However, infrared-transmitting glasses may become the next generation of optical communications, and if this happens, medical usage will soon follow.[43]

A number of new fibers have been suggested. Poulain described a heavy-metal fluoride glass (HMFG) that transmits well in a $2.5\mu m$ window but not at $10.6\mu m$.[44] Polycrystalline fibers extruded from KRS-5 (thallium bromoiodide) transmit at $5-20\mu m$ and have losses of 1db/km at $10.6\mu m$. Chalcogenide glasses (As_2S_3) have historically been good for short runs.[45] Unfortunately, thallium and arsenic are probably too toxic for medical work.[42] White describes KRS-5 chalcogenide fibers by Galileo, based on Texas Instruments 1173 glass, which have been drawn in diameters as small as $25\mu m$.[45] Transmission is good in the $8-12\mu m$ (CO_2 laser) range.

CARDIOVASCULAR APPLICATIONS OF ANGIOPLASTY

Lasers have been used to measure coronary blood flow, to map the propagation of myocardial depolarization, and to ablate atrioventricular conduction tissue. However, most of the interest has been in their use to recanalize blood vessels, either alone or in conjunction with balloon angioplasty. Initial results appear promising, in that with the additional assistance of balloon angioplasty, several investigators achieved some improvement in patency in approximately 90% of patients.[46]

PROBLEMS AND QUESTIONS

Before laser or laser-assisted angioplasty can be considered for routine use, numerous questions need to be answered.

What Type of Energy Should Be Delivered?

The power, exposure time (pulse duration), and wavelength of the laser energy determines the immediate damage to the vessel wall, which presumably differs depending on the nature of that wall, e.g., normal or atherosclerotic tissue. Studies of these factors, the physical mechanisms of laser ablation and the optical and thermal properties of atherosclerotic and healthy vascular tissue have provided a large volume of information. However, more experimentation is needed to find new laser sources with more true tissue specificity in order to enhance the ability to ablate atheroma, while at the same time reducing perforation risk. In addition, laser sources capable of complete atheroablation are required in order to improve on the results of the currently available systems, which provide mainly a way to recanalize vascular obstruction. Without adequate removal of atheromatous material, laser recanalization systems are no more than a glorified experimental guidewire.

What Is the Best Way to Deliver Laser Energy?

Several variables are involved in answering this question. One group of variables concerns the orientation of the laser fiber in relation to the target tissue. For example, the core diameter of the optical fiber determines the diameter of the beam as it strikes the target (spot size), which, in turn, determines the power density at each set of energy parameters. There also are questions about the proximity of the optical fiber to the target: the closer the tip, the smaller the spot and thus the greater the power density. At the same time, it must be remembered that the optical fiber can easily perforate a vessel, either mechanically or by lasing. It was in an attempt to avoid this complication that balloon catheter systems have been designed to maintain the optical fiber in the center of the vessel lumen.[47] Spectroscopic feedback has been used in attempts to improve the efficiency of detection of atheroma and, therefore, decreasing the risk of perforation. Improvements in the technique are, however, needed to improve efficiency of atheroma removal. A better solution to the guidance problem is the use of intravascular ultrasound (IVUS) to guide the laser atheroablation. In its present form, however, IVUS can only provide information about the structures located at almost 90° to the transducer. Forward scanning is needed for laser atheroablation guidance. Side viewing scanning with IVUS is of help to determine the amount of rendered plaque. Finally, the effect of intra-arterial fluid cannot be ignored, especially for laser wavelengths readily absorbed by hemoglobin.

The second group of delivery variables involves the delivery system itself. Most percutaneous laser treatments have been delivered by classic angiographic techniques with fluoroscopic monitoring. An alternative system, still in the early stages of development, involves passage of a fine intravascular endoscope (angioscope) through which the optical fiber of the laser is passed. This technique necessitates removal of most of the blood from the operating field. Production of such an instrument has proved to be a significant challenge. The use of angioscopes has not proved of great value, since one can only see what is in front of one's self, but one cannot see through the obstacle; therefore one cannot prevent perforation. A third option, already mentioned, is the use of a laser-heated metal cap to ablate the lesion.[46,48]

How Can the Uptake of Laser Energy by Atheroma Be Enhanced?

It would be ideal if atheroma and normal vascular tissue differed in their optical absorption characteristics or could be made to do so. Some preliminary results are encouraging.[49,50] For example, tetracyclines localize in atherosclerotic tissue, presumably because of their interaction with calcium. Hematoporphyrin derivative also is taken up selectively by atheroma and has been an effective enhancer of the action of a tunable-dye laser driven by an argon laser in animal models. Unfortunately, animal models of atherosclerosis differ considerably from the human disease, so the clinical applicability of these findings is in doubt. In vitro, fluorescein and Sudan Black enhance the action of argon lasers on atherosclerotic arteries.

How Dangerous Is the Debris Created by Laser Angioplasty?

Two by-products of laser treatment must be considered: vaporization products and particulate debris. Available information suggests that neither will be a significant problem.[47] For example, Nordstrom et al. isolated the products of in vitro laser application to human atheroma and found that ambient air and CO_2 were the most abundant vaporization products. Tetrafluoroethylene was present in concentrations of 100ppm, and there were trace amounts of short carbon chain gases such as ethane.[47] Most of the particles were in the $10-20\mu m$ range and had little or no cytotoxicity. No toxic reactions or embolizations have been apparent in the clinical trials of laser angioplasty.

Is There Significant Long-term Damage to the Vessel Wall?

In atherosclerotic rabbits fed an atherogenic diet, lasers can damage the vascular wall. Application of 3–6J to aortic plaques invariably caused damage to the medial layer of the vessel wall, and in follow-up studies areas of aneurysmal dilatation were apparent. Histologically, these outpouchings were thinned, necrotic, and disorganized.[51,52] Again,

there is some question of the applicability of these findings to the human disease, because rabbit atheroma is considerably softer than the human type. Application of heat through a metal cap to recanalize vascular obstructions has resulted in recurrences of disease, not only at the original site of vascular obstruction, but at sites immediately proximal and distal to the site of thermal recanalization.

LASER ENERGY DELIVERY SYSTEMS

The simplest method of laser energy delivery is with a bare fiber. These are most often constructed of quartz silica, with silver chloride used for excimer lasers. Fiber diameters range from 10 to $1000\mu m$, with larger fibers being stiffer. The use of a bundle of small fibers enables delivery of more energy while preserving flexibility. There are two main problems with the use of bare fibers: The perforation rate using a bare fiber is unacceptably high, and the amount of plaque ablated was insufficient to use the technique as sole therapy.[53,54] As such, most research into development of laser delivery systems over the past several years has focused on finding a solution to the above problems, particularly the problem of vessel perforation. A brief review of the results of several different laser delivery systems follows.

BARE FIBERS

Quartz silica fibers, which form the basis of all laser angioplasty systems, are quite efficient at delivering laser energy from the source to the target. Given a 20–30% power loss at the distal tip of the fiber, it is still possible to generate high fluences at the target site or plaque. Because the cone angle or degree of beam divergence at the fiber tip is quite small, however, laser light delivered in this fashion is very concentrated, which means that a relatively small hole is created in the target tissue by the incident beam. In addition, since the power of the beam is concentrated in a small area, the depth of penetration tends to be difficult to control. These difficulties have been demonstrated in experimental studies which have generally shown an inability to completely remove an atherosclerotic stenosis without an unacceptably high perforation rate.[55,56] These findings were confirmed in preliminary clinical trials with a bare fiber delivery system which demonstrated a 50% recanalization rate and an 18% perforation rate.[57]

The use of bare fibers, however, is associated with a higher rate of perforation.[58,59] Perforation is caused both by the mechanical effect of advancing the fiber and by the laser energy. Using an argon thermal probe, Tobis et al.[60] showed that the fiber is mechanically deflected from hard calcific plaque and can then advance between the intima and media before perforating the adventitia. The initial studies, using bare fiber with excimer lasers, suggest that these may be associated with a lower incidence of perforation.[61] To reduce the incidence of perforation, several modifications have been made to the laser delivery system. Of these, "hot-tip" thermal laser angioplasty has received the most clinical attention.

FIBER TIP MODIFICATION

To reduce the risk of vessel perforation which occurred frequently with bare fibers, numerous modifications of the distal fiber tip have been proposed. The best known of these is the "hot-tip" device in which a metal cap is crimped on the end of a fiber[62] (Fig. 5.2.1). The laser light then is absorbed by the metal cap which causes rapid heating of the metal. In air, the cap can reach 300–500 °C; however, tissue temperatures are generally between 100 and 200°C.[63] When contact is made with noncalcified plaque, the probe is capable of thermally ablating tissue within a narrow zone of the tissue-probe interface.

The purpose of this device is to recanalize occluded peripheral blood vessels which cannot be traversed with conventional guidewire and catheter techniques. As such, the device represents an adjunct to conventional balloon angioplasty.

Sanborn et al. have reported good clinical results with this device. Primary angiographic and clinical success was achieved in 21 of 22 stenoses (95%) and 78 of 107 occlusions (73%).[64] Others, however, have reported less favorable results. Perler et al. reported a 15-month patency of 7% in 47 laser-treated femoropopliteal occlusions.[65] Matsumoto et al. recently reported their results using an argon or YAG hot-tip laser to treat 148 lesions in 137 patients.[66] They reported an overall immediate success rate of only 53%. Their success rate in treating stenoses and segmental occlusions was 61%. Their perforation rate was 6% and the amputation rate was 10%. These results are inferior to those obtained with conventional guidewire/balloon angioplasty techniques. Interestingly, Morgenstern et al. have recently reported a 91% technical success rate for treatment of femoropopliteal occlusions with guidewire/balloon recanalization which is as good or better than results reported with laser-assisted balloon angioplasty.[67]

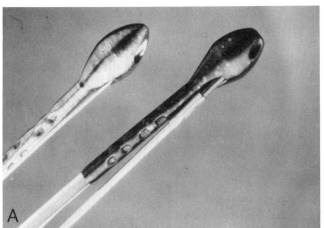

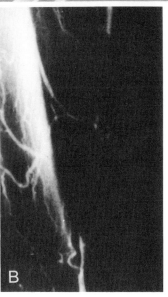
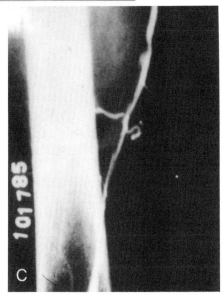
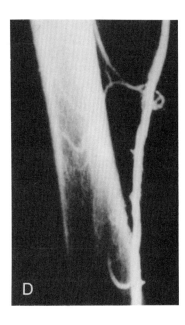

Figure 5.2.1. **A.** Hot tip laser probes. **B.** Complete occlusion of right superficial femoral artery with distal reconstitution. **C.** Post-hot tip recanalization. Note irregular lumen. **D.** Postangioplasty marked increased lumen diameter.

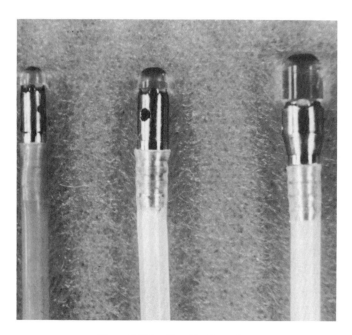

Figure 5.2.2. Sapphire tip probes.

plasty.[67] This seems to confirm the anecdotal experience of most experienced angiographers, that most occluded peripheral vessels can be recanalized successfully with a catheter and guidewire alone. As such, the value of laser recanalization in this setting is dubious.

Other investigators have studied the effect of sapphire contact probes (Fig 5.2.2). Recanalization of occluded femoropopliteal segments has been reported in 74–88% of cases (Fig 5.2.3), without a clear difference between the metal and sapphire tips.[68,69] Still other tip modifications such as quartz optical assemblies to increase beam divergence have been successfully used to recanalize occluded vessel segments in association with conventional balloon angioplasty.[70]

Other approaches to the problem include expansion of the fiber tip and the use of lenses (sapphire tip). At the distal end of the fiber,[71,72] combinations of metal cap and lens systems, such as the hybrid laser (Figs. 5.2.4 and 5.2.5), have also been used[73] (Fig. 5.2.6).

ROLE OF LASER IN THE TREATMENT OF PERIPHERAL VASCULAR DISEASE

Laser energy may be used to recanalize occlusions furnishing a channel to enable balloon dilatation (laser-

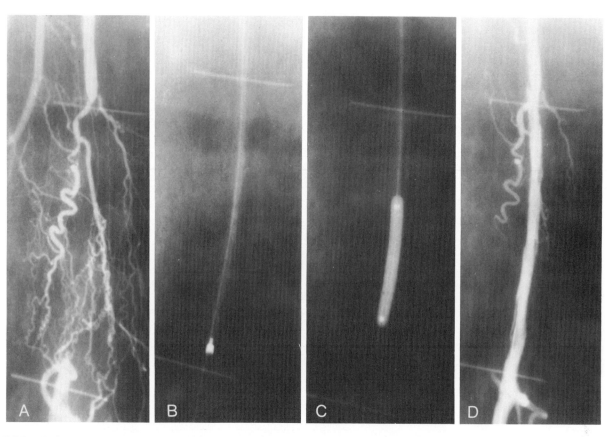

Figure 5.2.3. **A.** Complete occlusion of superficial femoral artery. **B.** Sapphire probe has been advanced through the obstruction. **C.** Balloon dilatation postrecanalization. **D.** Postprocedure arteriogram; widely patent lumen. (Reproduced from Lammer J: Sapphire probe laser assisted angioplasty, in *Percutaneous Revascularization Techniques.* New York, Thieme Medical Publishers, in press.)

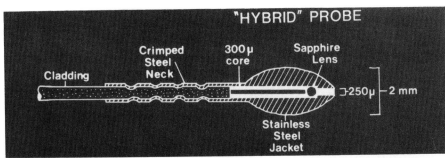

"HYBRID" PROBE

Cladding
Crimped Steel Neck
300 μ core
Sapphire Lens
Stainless Steel Jacket
250 μ
2 mm

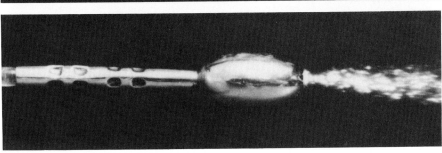

Figure 5.2.4. Hybrid laser probe with sapphire lens allowing passage of laser energy through the tip of the probe.

Figure 5.2.5. Crater produced by hybrid probe. Note difference in diameter of recanalization created by the laser beam versus the metal cap.

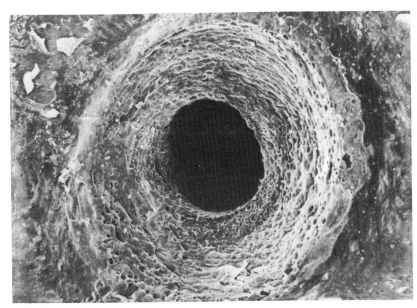

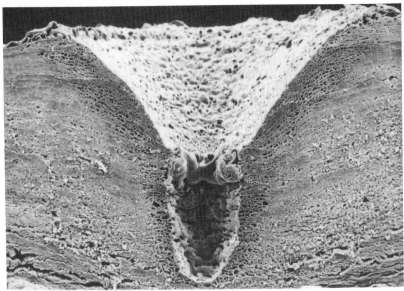

Figure 5.2.6. **A.** Complete occlusion of superficial femoral artery. **B.** Post-hybrid laser probe recanalization. Note irregular lumen. **C.** Graph of temperature/time during lasing. **D.** Post-balloon angioplasty; widely patent lumen. (Reproduced from Abela G: Hybrid laser angioplasty, in *Percutaneous Revascularization Techniques*. New York, Thieme Medical Publishers, in press.)

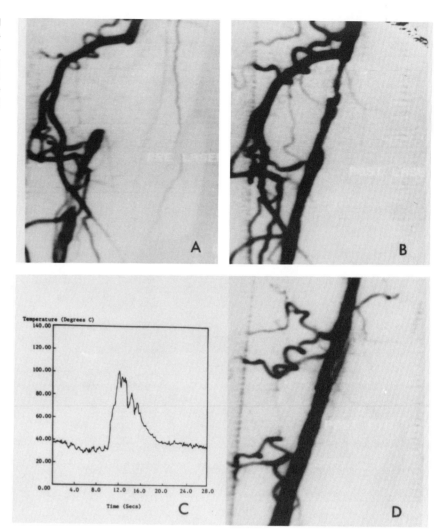

assisted balloon angioplasty), as sole therapy of stenosis and occlusions (sole laser angioplasty), as an adjunct to angioplasty by welding the fractured intima to the arterial wall, and as selective ablation by plaque modification (Fig. 5.2.7).

LASER RECANALIZATION

Laser recanalization must be compared with the standard technique for recanalization of vascular occlusions. Interventional radiologists have achieved a high rate of recanalization of occlusions using the wire and catheter techniques.[67,74] Once an occlusion has been traversed, angioplasty can be performed. The success rate for traversing occlusions has been improved in recent times, in part due to the increased experience of interventional radiologists, and in part due to the larger array of wires and catheters available.[67,75]

In comparison to laser, catheter and wire techniques offer simplicity, a reduction in the size of the arterial sheath required, and are considerably cheaper. Morgenstern et al.[67] were able to achieve recanalization in 86% of occlusions 5–10cm in length and in 95% of lesions 1–4cm in

length. Technical success rates of 74–91% have been reported by other authors.[74,76–78] In clinical practice, therefore, the laser would be used where recanalization with the wire has been unsuccessful. Although laser recanalization rates of up to 90% are quoted,[75,79,80] most of these authors have not attempted recanalization with a wire beforehand. No randomized comparison of laser and catheter techniques in recanalization is currently available. Leon et al.[81] have used fluorescence-guided laser to recanalize lesions following an unsuccessful attempt by standard techniques. Recanalization was achieved in 83% of lesions averaging 8.4cm in length.[81] Subsequent balloon dilatation was possible in 53% of cases. Six of ten lesions were recanalized by Harrington et al.[82] and eight of eleven by Cumberland et al.[79] using a hot-tip laser. Eleven of fourteen lesions, not treatable by catheter and wire, were recanalized by Lammer using a hot-tip and sapphire lens.[83] Matsumoto et al.[84,85] showed that successful recanalization decreased with lesion length, and, in particular, that total superficial femoral artery (SFA) occlusions were unlikely to be successfully treated by laser. Increased length and calcification led to an increase in the perforation rate.[82,84,85]

Perforation can be reduced by maintaining the laser in

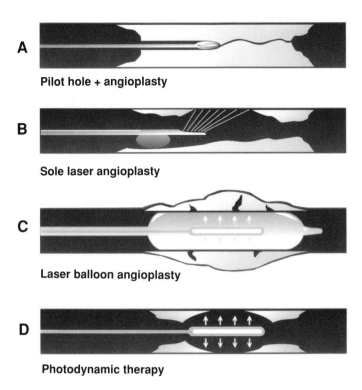

Figure 5.2.7.   Concepts in laser angioplasty. **A.** Most clinical laser angioplasty research now focuses on use of a modified optical fiber to create a small pilot hole in an obstructed vessel prior to balloon angioplasty. The efficacy of this concept is unproved. **B.** More favorable laser sources, such as excimer or tunable dye, may allow plaque ablation without the need for modification of the fiber tip or subsequent balloon angioplasty. **C.** Laser irradiation through an inflated balloon causes "welding" of fractured plaques and decreased elastic recoil. Potential, but unproved, advantages include decreased abrupt closure and lower restenosis rates compared with conventional balloon angioplasty. **D.** Chemical modification of plaque may allow more rapid and selective laser angioplasty. This technique could theoretically produce plaque regression in diffusely diseased vessels.

a coaxial position.[86] This can be accomplished by placing it within a balloon catheter (Fig 5.2.8). Using such a technique, perforation was limited by Nordstrom et al.[75] to three instances in 53 procedures. Seeger et al.[88] showed that proximal occlusions were less likely to be recanalized than mid- and distal SFA lesions. Recanalization of small vessels has also been shown by Sanborn.[89]

LASER-ASSISTED BALLOON ANGIOPLASTY

The currently available data do not suggest that balloon dilatation of occlusions or stenosis following recanalization with laser confers improved patency in comparison to recanalization with a wire. The suggested theoretical improvement in long-term patency conferred by laser recanalization in comparison to recanalization by wire due to removal rather than displacement of atheroma and reduced platelet adherence and fibrocellular proliferation have yet to be proved in clinical practice.[59] Especially in long stenosis and occlusions, not all laser recanalized lesions can subsequently be successfully dilated by balloon. Matsumoto[84] was able to perform angioplasty on 55% of lesions successfully recanalized by laser, and Leon's results are similar.[81]

Balloon dilation of stenoses and occlusions has been shown to have a five-year patency rate of 50–87% in the iliac arteries,[78,90–95] and 50–70% in the femoral popliteal artery. These results are satisfactory in clinical practice and a valuable alternative to surgery. Long-term patency rates at the tibial vessels are still awaited, but Schwarten[96] has shown satisfactory healing of 82% of lower limb ulcers at two years after angioplasty of the tibial vessels. Surgical bypass procedures in the pelvic vessels are associated with higher morbidity and mortality in comparison to angio-

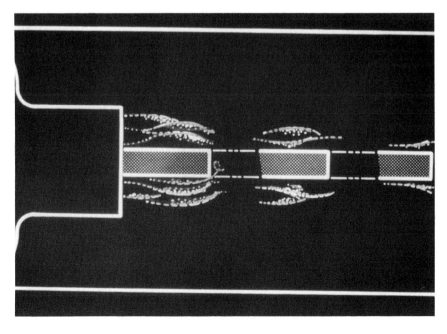

Figure 5.2.8.   LASTAC coaxial argon laser delivery system. The inflated balloon keeps the fiber in the center of the vessel.

plasty;[97] although morbidity and mortality are less in surgical bypass of the femoropopliteal vessels, the patency rates are comparable to angioplasty of short occlusions when autogenous saphenous vein is used.[74,98,99] In contrast, angioplasty of long occlusions (7–10cm) is disappointing.[85,94,100]

To date, the use of lasers to recanalize and allow balloon dilatation of long lesions with hot-tip and sapphire probes has been disappointing[59] with reocclusion rates of 60–90%[82,88,101,102] at one year. Laser thermal injury and charring, with an increase in thrombogenicity, has been suggested as a causative factor.[101]

However, using a pulsed-dye laser and spectroscopic guidance,[93,103] a 75% patency rate for lesions greater than 15cm, at 13 months, has been achieved. A 64% patency rate at three years was achieved by Pilger,[70] using an Nd-YAG laser with a sapphire contact probe.

A high incidence of complications is reported with the use of contact probes. These include perforation and dissection reported at 46% by Harrington et al.[82] and 33% by Wright et al.[102] using a hot-tip, 33% by Seeger[88] using a metal cap with sapphire tip, and 14% by Lammer[83] using both sapphire and hot-tip. Bleeding requiring transfusion has been reported in up to 9%[82] of cases and may, in part, be due to the need to make a shallow antegrade puncture at the groin, and to the requirement of at least an 8Fr sheath, with heparinization. Entry of the artery above the inguinal ligament increases the likelihood of hemorrhagic complications, as compression is difficult. Clinically significant distal embolization has been reported to occur in up to 30% of cases,[104] but other authors report a much lower incidence.[58,82,105]

If laser recanalization is unsuccessful, a significant proportion of patients may be rendered hemodynamically worse by the procedure. In 9 of 21 technical failures reported by Perler et al.[101] using a hot-tip laser, there was extension of the occluded segment. Eleven of 69 patients in Harrington's[82] series were hemodynamically worse after the procedure, and 5 of these required urgent operative intervention.

Thus, it is evident that the value of laser is in the treatment of short occlusions, which cannot be recanalized by catheter and wire techniques, and thereby allowing balloon angioplasty. The clinical benefit of recanalization by laser to enable angioplasty of the longer lesions has yet to be demonstrated. Where autogenous vein is available for bypass, this is preferred.[82,106] However, where the patient's condition or the absence of autogenous vein precludes successful surgical therapy, it would appear reasonable to attempt percutaneous therapy with the assistance of laser.

SOLE LASER THERAPY

As sole laser therapy results in a small lumen size (of 2–3.5mm), and poor long-term patency,[84] with the possible exception of the tibial vessels, subsequent balloon angioplasty is invariably required.

Although the data on sole laser therapy of the tibial vessels is limited (Fig. 5.2.9), Sanborn[89] has shown technical feasibility, with success in 14 of 16 patients. Harrington,[82] however, demonstrated patency of only 25% at one year.

LASER WELDING/BALLOON ANGIOPLASTY

An innovative system has been designed by Spears,[107] who placed a cylindrical defusing tip of a $300\mu m$ fiber inside an angioplasty balloon, which delivers laser light radially at the sites of contact with the arterial wall (Fig. 5.2.10). Tissue temperatures of 90–120°C are reached, which results in welding of the dehiscence between the intima and media following balloon angioplasty with a reduction in elastic recoil. Damage to smooth muscles may also contribute to reduction in recoil following thermal balloon dilatation.[107]

The application of laser energy to the blood vessel wall in a radial fashion through an inflated angioplasty balloon has been postulated to have several important, potentially beneficial, effects.[108,109] 1) Thermal "welding" of the dehisced plaque elements could reduce the incidence of acute closure after conventional balloon angioplasty. 2) Elastic recoil of the dilated vessel may be reduced due to medial coagulation. 3) Atherogenesis may be reduced by thermal destruction of smooth muscle cells.

These concepts have been tested experimentally with favorable results[110] and they are now being investigated in clinical trials. We have investigated the same principle using hot water in the angioplasty balloon with similar results.[111]

Other laser guidance systems include the use of angioscopy[112] (Fig. 5.2.11) and in the coronary circulation, the use of ultrasound. Perforation has, however, not been eliminated by these techniques.

PLAQUE MODIFICATION/PHOTODYNAMIC THERAPY

The concept of modifying the spectral properties of atherosclerotic plaque to allow selective ablation by laser light is an intriguing one which has been investigated by several groups. Murphy–Chutorian et al. showed that physiologic levels of tetracycline would be preferentially taken up in plaque.[34] Since tetracycline selectively absorbs light in the red range (peak, 355nm), a laser which operates at or near this wavelength will be more strongly absorbed by tetracycline-treated plaque. This finding has been confirmed by Crass et al. using an excimer laser operating at 35nm.[113] Other plaque modifiers such as hematoporphyrin derivative (HPD) and exogenous carotenoids have shown promise for selective plaque destruction; however, clinical application of these drugs has not been successful.[114,115]

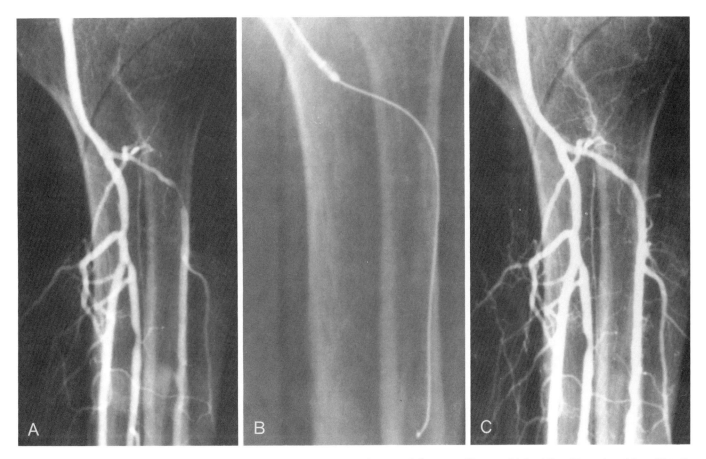

Figure 5.2.9. **A.** High-grade stenosis of anterior tibial artery. **B.** A guidewire has been passed across the stenosis. The laser catheter is being advanced over the wire. **C.** Post-laser-assisted angioplasty. Note increased diameter with a small intimal flap. (Reproduced from Mitty H: Tibial-sole angioplasty, in *Percutaneous Revascularization Techniques*. New York, Thieme Medical Publishers, in press.)

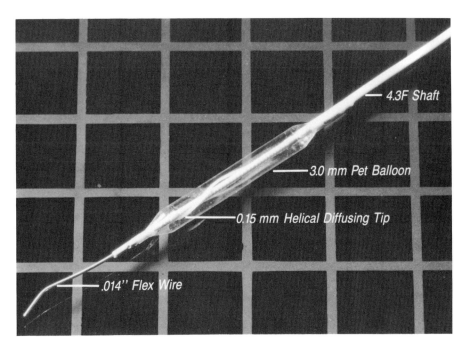

Figure 5.2.10.   Spears laser balloon.

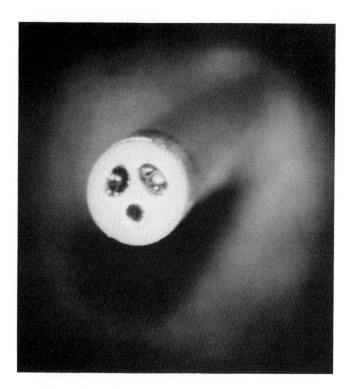

Figure 5.2.11. Medilase angioscope-laser delivery system.

In photodynamic therapy, differences in light absorption by normal arterial wall and atheroma is used to advantage. This differential absorption of light is maximal at 450–500nm for lipid atheroma,[116,117] and 600–690nm for calcified plaque, but occurs over a wide spectral range, between 440 and 1070nm. Ingestion of exogenous chromophores, such as β-carotene and tetracycline, which are incorporated into atheroma, enhances the differential effect and has been used experimentally to increase the safety of lasers.[116]

The difference in absorption of light by atheroma in normal arteries is also used in fluorescence-guided laser angioplasty. Here, the energy delivery of the active laser is computer controlled by the wavelength of the light reflected from the arterial wall. In a typical fluorescence-guided system,[117] light of 325nm is delivered through the optic fiber, and lasing only occurs if the reflected light, which also travels down the same fiber, is characteristic of atheroma.

FUTURE DIRECTIONS

A discussion of the state of the art of laser angioplasty in the 1990's would not be complete without reference to the technical limitations of present laser systems and the political ramifications of laser angioplasty.

During the past 10 years or so, there have been great changes in the American medical system which have altered the way that physicians treat patients with vascular disease. For most physicians and administrators, medicine is now a market-driven, competitive industry which responds quickly to the demands of the consumer (the patient). The cardiovascular market is one of the most profitable and competitive markets in medicine today. The boom in cardiovascular intervention really began when cardiologists began performing coronary angioplasty. The explosive growth of this technique spurred the development of numerous industries to support this procedure.

As with any competitive and lucrative market, new technology formed the cornerstone of any company which wished to enter the market or stay competitive. Patients have benefited from this competition by innovation and refinement of vascular technology. Because of media attention, it is often the patients themselves who demand new, sometimes unproven, technology in their treatment.

As the American medical system becomes more competitive, physicians now find themselves in direct competition with their colleagues for patients. This competition, which is, in part, driven by a surplus of physicians and changes in reimbursement patterns, has become fierce among cardiovascular specialists and has resulted in "foraging" of one specialty into the domain of another in order to garner new patients.

Unfortunately, the laser angioplasty industry has developed in this atmosphere and has to a large extent come to embody the negative aspects of this competitive environment. This has occurred for several reasons.

First, the technological potential of medical lasers is indisputable. This has been quite effectively communicated to the public and there now exists an "aura" about lasers that patients find irresistible. This fact, in combination with the demand for technical innovation in the cardiovascular market, has created a powerful incentive for development of laser angioplasty.

Second, early development of laser angioplasty systems did not meet the expectations of the investigators who developed them. The hope that laser light could "clean out" a blood vessel quickly and efficiently has not been realized. This has created a great deal of skepticism on the part of many individuals in the cardiovascular field.

Third, early laser devices which received FDA approval based on demonstration of safety have demonstrated little efficacy in the hands of most practitioners. Despite this, however, the devices have found their niche as a marketing tool to garner patients. This has created tremendous cynicism about lasers and, in concert with the general climate of competition in the cardiovascular field, it has fueled the estrangement of the previously collegial specialties of cardiology, interventional radiology, and vascular surgery.

Despite the problems which exist between cardiovascular specialists in the 1990s, it seems clear that the role of interventional vascular therapy will continue to expand. Cardiovascular laser therapy is in its infancy and it is not yet clear what role it will play. Ethical investigation of the merits of any new technology should continue to be the gold standard by which we practice.

CONCLUSIONS

Despite the extensive clinical use of laser to treat peripheral vascular disease, many fundamental questions concerning the clinical role of laser remain unanswered. Prospective randomized studies are needed to assess if laser- assisted angioplasty confers improved patency in comparison to balloon angioplasty.[59,118-121] Similarly, it remains to be shown that laser recanalization of long occlusions, which cannot be treated by catheter and wire techniques, is a viable alternative to surgery.

It is possible that new methods of laser energy delivery, different wavelengths, larger probes, and improved guidance systems will, in the future, enable ablation of atheroma with a reduced complication rate.

Laser may enable percutaneous therapy for patients with peripheral vascular disease who are unlikely to benefit from standard techniques, but further clinical research is required before general usage can be scientifically advocated.

References

1. Maiman TH: Stimulated optical radiation in ruby. *Nature* 1960;187:493-494
2. Abela GS: Laser recanalization: a basic and clinical perspective. *Thorac Cardiovasc Surg* 1988;36:137-141
3. Choy DSJ: History and state-of-the-art of lasers in cardiovascular disease. *Laser Med Surg News Advances* 1988;34-38
4. Grundfest WS, Litvack F, Hickey A, et al: The current status of angioscopy and laser angioplasty. *J Vasc Surg* 1987; 5:667-672
5. Isner JM, Clarke RH: Laser angioplasty: unraveling the Gordian knot. *J Am Coll Cardiol* 1986;7:705-708
6. Lee G, Chan MC, Reis RL, Argenal AJ, Low RI, Mason DT: Potential applications of lasers in the management of cardiovascular diseases. *J Intervent Cardiol* 1988;1:59-74
7. Litvack F, Grundfest WS, Papaioannou T, Mohr FW, Jakubowski AT, Forrester JS: Role of laser and ablation devices in the treatment of vascular diseases. *Am J Cardiol* 1988;61:81G-86G
8. Sanborn T: Laser angioplasty: what has been learned from experimental studies and clinical trials? *Circulation* 1988;78:769-774
9. Spears JR: Percutaneous laser treatment of atherosclerosis: an overview of emerging techniques. *Cardiovasc Intervent Radiol* 1986;9:303-312
10. Boulnoy JL: Photophysical processes in recent medical laser developments: a review. *Lasers Med Sci* 1986;1:147-166
11. Smithson PH, Jenes WD, Murphy E: Installation requirements for an argon laser angioplasty system. *Br J Radiol* 1989;62:71-73
12. Grundfest WS, Litvack IF, Goldenberg T, et al: Pulsed ultraviolet lasers and the potential for safe laser angioplasty. *Am J Surg* 1985;150:220-226
13. Ross FW, Bowker TJ: The physical properties of tissue ablation with excimer lasers. *Med Instrum* 1987;21:226-230
14. White RA, White GH, Vlasak J, et al: Histopathology of human laser thermal angioplasty recanalization. *Lasers Surg Med* 1988;8:469-476
15. Garret L, Ikeda R, Theis JS, et al: Acute and chronic complications of laser angioplasty: vascular wall damage and formation of aneurysms in the atherosclerotic rabbit. *Am J Cardiol* 1984;53:290-293
16. Higginson LA, Farrel EM, Walley BM, et al: Arterial response to excimer and argon laser irradiation in atherosclerotic swine. *Lasers Med Sci* 1989;4:85-92
17. Ragimov SE, Belyaev AE, Vertepaia IA, et al: Comparison of different lasers in terms of thrombogenicity of the laser-treated vascular wall. *Lasers Surg Med* 1988;8:77-82
18. Abela GS, Crea F, Seeger JM: The healing process in normal canine arteries and in atherosclerotic monkey arteries after transluminal laser irradiation. *Am J Cardiol* 1985;56:983-988
19. Strikwerda S, Bott-Silverman C, Ratlitt NB, et al: Effects of varying argon ion laser intensity and exposure time on the ablation of atherosclerotic plaque. *Lasers Surg Med* 1988;8:66-71
20. Fenech A, Abela GS, Crea F, et al: Comparative study of laser beam characteristics in blood and saline. *Am J Cardiol* 1985;55:1389-1392
21. Garret L, Chan MC, Seckinger DL: Argon laser radiation of human clots differential photoabsorption in red cell rich and red cell poor clots. *Thromb Process Res* 1985;38:561-565
22. Garret L, Ikeda RM, Stobbe D, et al: Effects of laser irradiation on human thrombosis. Demonstration of the linear dissolution-dose relation between clot vent and energy intensity. *Am J Cardiol* 1983;52:876-877
23. Deckelbaum LI, Isner JM, Donaldson RF, et al: Reduction of laser-induced pathologic tissue injury using pulsed energy delivery. *Am J Cardiol* 1985;56:662-667
24. Gibson PH, Holten D, Smith SC, et al: Absence of thermal tissue injury using a pulsed mode Nd-YAG laser (abstr). *Circulation* 1985;72(suppl 3):1605
25. Geschwind HJ, Tiesseire B, Boussignac G, et al: Laser angioplasty of arterial stenosis. *Cardiovasc Intervent Radiol* 1986;9:313-317
26. Grundfest WS, Litvak IF, Goldenberg T, et al: Pulsed ultraviolet lasers and the potential for safe laser angioplasty. *Am J Surg* 1985;150:220-226
27. Deckelbaum LI: Laser angioplasty. *Intervent Cardiol Clinics* 1988;6:345-356
28. Litvack F, Grundfest WS, Papainoannou T, et al: Role of laser and thermal ablation devices in the treatment of vascular disease. *Am J Cardiol* 1988;61:81G-86G
29. Eldar M, Battler A, Neufeld HN: Transluminal carbon dioxide laser catheter angioplasty for dissolution of atherosclerotic plaques. *J Am Coll Cardiol* 1984;3:135-137
30. Eldar M, Gal D, Djaldetti M, et al: Carbon dioxide laser effect on platelet function and surface ultrastructure in-vitro. *Lasers Surg Med* 1988;8:259-263
31. Wollenek G, Laufer G, Grabenwoger F: Percutaneous transluminal eximer laser angioplasty in total peripheral artery occlusion in man. *Lasers Surg Med* 1988;8:464-468
32. Grundfest WS, Litvack F, Forrester JS, et al: Laser ablation of human atherosclerotic plaque without adjacent tissue injury. *J Am Coll Cardiol* 1985;5:929-933
33. Grundfest WS, Litvack F, Doyle L, et al: Comparison of in-vitro and in-vivo thermal effects of argon and excimer lasers for laser angioplasty (abstr). *Circulation.* 1987;74(suppl 2):813
34. Murphy-Churtorian D, Kosek J, Mok W, et al: Selective absorption of ultraviolet laser energy by human atherosclerotic plaque treated with tetracycline. *Am J Cardiol* 1985;55:1293-1297
35. Isner JM, Doval ALD, Steg PJ, et al: Percutaneous in-vivo

excimer laser angioplasty results in two experimental animal models. *Lasers Surg Med* 1988;8:223–232

36. Isner JM: Excimer laser angioplasty: pygmalion makes it to the ball. *Lasers Surg Med* 1988;8:447–449

37. Cross FW, Bowker TJ: The physical properties of tissue ablation with excimer lasers. *Med Instrum* 1987;21:226–230

38. Grundfest W, Litvack F, Hestrin L, et al: Percutaneous peripheral excimer laser angioplasty. *Circulation* 1989; 80:97 (abstracts of the 62nd scientific session)

39. Forrester JS, Litvack F, Grundfest W, et al: The excimer laser: current knowledge and future prospects. *J Intervent Cardiol* 1988;1:75–80

40. Murray A, Crocker PR, Wood RM: The pulsed dye laser and atherosclerotic vascular disease. *Br J Surg* 1988;75(4):349–351

41. Geschwind HJ, Dubois–Rand EJ, Shafton E, et al: Percutaneous pulsed laser-assisted balloon angioplasty guided by spectroscopy. *Am Heart J* 1989;1147–1151

42. Haavind R: Lighting the way with lasers. *High Technology* 1985;5:39

43. Tick PA, Thompson DA: IR fibres: at the frontier. *Photon Spectra* 1985;19:65

44. Poulain M: The paths ahead for fluoride fibres. *Photon Spectra* 1985;19:68

45. White P: Chalcogenide fibres make their debut. *Photon Spectra* 1985;19:70

46. Litvack F, Grundfest W, Beeder C, Forrester JS: Laser angioplasty: status and prospects. *Semin Intervent Radiol* 1986;3:75

47. Nordstrom LA, Castañeda–Zúñiga WR, Grewe DD, Schoster JV: Laser enhanced transluminal angioplasty: the role of coaxial fiber placement. *Semin Intervent Radiol* 1986;3:47

48. Sanborn TA, Faxon DP, Haudenschild CC, Ryan TJ: Experimental angioplasty: circumferential distribution of laser thermal energy with a laser probe. *J Am Coll Cardiol* 1985;5:934

49. Dougherty TJ, Kaufman JE, Goldfarb A, Weiskaupt KR, Boyle D, Mittleman A: Photoradiation therapy for treatment of malignant tumors. *Cancer Res* 1978;38:2628

50. Kelley JF, Snell ME: Hematoporphyrin derivative: a possible aid in the diagnosis and therapy of carcinoma of the bladder. *J Urol* 1976;115:150

51. Gerrity RG, Loop FD, Golding LAR, Erhart LA, Argenyl ZB: Arterial response to laser operation for removal of atherosclerotic plaques. *J Thorac Cardiovasc Surg* 1983;85:409

52. Abela G, Franzini D, Crea F, Pepine CJ, Conti CR: No evidence of accelerated atherosclerosis following laser radiation (abstract). *Circulation* 1984;70(suppl II):323

53. Anderson HV, Zaatari GS, Roubin GS, et al: Steerable fiberoptic catheter delivery of laser energy in atherosclerotic rabbits. *Am Heart J* 1986;111:1065–1072

54. Anderson HV, Zaatari GS, Roubin GS, Leimgruber PP, Gruntzig AR: Coaxial laser energy delivery using a steerable catheter in canine coronary arteries. *Am Heart J* 1987;113:37–47

55. Crea F, Abela GS, Fenech A, et al: Transluminal laser irradiation of coronary arteries in live dogs: an angiographic and morphologic study of acute effects. *Am J Cardiol* 1986;57:171–174

56. Isner JM, Donaldson RF, Funai JT, et al: Factors contributing to perforations resulting from laser coronary angioplasty: observations in an intact human postmortem preparation of intraoperative laser coronary angioplasty. *Circulation* 1985;72(suppl 2):191–199

57. Ginsburg R, Wexler L, Mitchell RS, Profitt D: Percutaneous transluminal laser angioplasty for treatment of peripheral vascular disease: clinical experience with 16 patients. *Radiology* 1985;156:619–624

58. Cumberland DC, Taylor DI, Procter AE: Percutaneous laser angioplasty initial clinical experience. *Ann Radiol* 1986;29(2):215–218

59. Cragg AH, Gardiner GA, Smith TP: Vascular applications of laser. *Radiology* 1989;172:925–935

60. Tobis J, Smolin M, Mallory J, et al: Laser assisted thermal angioplasty in human peripheral artery occlusions. Mechanism of recanalization. *JACC* 1989;13:1547–1554

61. Litvak F, Margolis J, Grundfest W: Percutaneous excimer laser coronary angioplasty in lesions not well suited for P.T.C.A. *Circulation* 1989(80);suppl II:1010 (abstract)

62. Lee G, Ikeda RM, Chan MC, et al: Dissolution of human atherosclerotic disease by fiberoptic laser-heated metal cautery cap. *Am Heart J* 1984;107:777–778

63. Welch AJ, Bradley AB, Torres JH, et al: Laser probe ablation of normal and atherosclerotic human aorta in-vitro: a first thermographic and histologic analysis. *Circulation* 1987;76:1353–1363

64. Sanborn TA, Cumberland DC, Greenfield AJ, Welch CL, Guben JK: Percutaneous laser thermal angioplasty: initial results and one-year follow-up in 129 femoropopliteal lesions. *Radiology* 1988;168:121–125

65. Perler BA, Osterman FA, White RI Jr, Williams GM: Percutaneous laser probe femoropopliteal angioplasty: a preliminary experience. *J Vasc Surg* 1989;10:351–357

66. Matsumoto T, Okamura T, Rajyaguru V: Laser arterial disobstructive procedures in 148 lower extremities. *J Vasc Surg* 1989;10:169–177

67. Morgenstern BR, Getrajdman GI, Laffey KJ, Bixon R, Martin EC: Total occlusions of the femoropopliteal artery: high technical success rate of conventional balloon angioplasty. *Radiology* 1989;172:937–940

68. Lammer J, Pilger E, Karnel F, Horvath W, et al: Austrian multicenter trial for laser angioplasty: 2-year results (abstr). *Radiology* 1988;169(P):139

69. Lammer J, Karnel F: Percutaneous transluminal laser angioplasty with contract probes. *Radiology* 1988;168:733–737

70. Nordstrom LA, Castañeda–Zúñiga WR, Young EG, Von Seggern KB: Direct argon laser exposure for recanalization of peripheral arteries: early results. *Radiology* 1988;168:359–364

71. Pilger E, Lammer J, Stark J: Laser angioplasty in peripheral arterial occlusion: three-year follow-up. Abstracts of the 62nd Scientific Session of the American Heart Association. *Circulation* 1989;80:1641

72. Decker–Dunn D, Christensen A, Vincent G: Multi-fiber gradient index lens laser angioplasty probe. *Lasers Surg Med* 1990;10:85–93

73. Anna–Maria B, Cumberland DC, Myler RK: Peripheral arterial occlusions initial results from percutaneous angioplasty with a hybrid probe. *Radiology* 1990;174:447–449

74. Martin EC, Fankuchen EI, Karlson KB, et al: Angioplasty for femoral artery occlusion: comparison with surgery. *AJR* 1981;137:915–919

75. Nordstrom LA, Young EG: Direct laser recanalization of occluded superficial femoral and iliac arteries: primary success rate and low complication rate. *Semin Intervent Radiol* 1988;5:276–278

76. Levy JM, Hessel SJ, Horsley WN, et al: Value of laser assisted angioplasty in the community hospital. *Radiology* 1989;170:1017–1018

77. Zeitler E: Percutaneous dilatation and recanalization of iliac and femoral arteries. *Cardiovasc Intervent Radiol* 1980;3:207–212

78. Waltman AC, Greenfield AJ, Novelline RA, et al: Transluminal angioplasty of the iliac and femoral popliteal arteries. *Arch Surg* 1982;117:1218–1221

79. Cumberland DC, Sandborn TA, Tayler DI, et al: Percutaneous laser thermal angioplasty: initial clinical results with the laser probe in total peripheral artery occlusion. *Lancet* 1 1986;1457–1459

80. McCowan TC, Ferris EJ, Barnes RW, et al: Laser thermal angioplasty for the treatment of obstruction of the distal superficial femoral or popliteal arteries. *AJR* 1988;150:1169–1173

81. Leon MB, Almagor Y, Bartorelli AL, et al: Fluorescence-guided laser assisted balloon angioplasty in patients with femoro-popliteal occlusions. *Circulation* 1990;81:143–155

82. Harrington ME, Schwartz ME, Sandborn TA, et al: Expanded indications for laser-assisted balloon angioplasty in peripheral arterial disease. *J Vasc Surg* 1990;11:146–155

83. Lammer J, Karnel F: Percutaneous transluminal laser angioplasty with contact probes. *Radiology* 1988;168:733–737

84. Matsumoto T, Okamura T, Rajyaguru V: Laser arterial disobstructive procedures in 148 lower extremities. *Vasc Surg* 1989;l0:169–177

85. Matsumoto T, Rajyaguru V, Okammura T: Laser recanalization, laser assisted balloon angioplasty, and laser angioplasty. *Surg Gynecol Obstet* 1989;169:195–198

86. Castañeda–Zúñiga WR: Coaxiality of optical fiber during transluminal laser-assisted angioplasty. *Semin Intervent Radiol* 1988;273–276

87. Nordstrom LA, Castañeda–Zúñiga WR, Lindeke CC: Laser angioplasty controlled delivery of argon laser energy. *Radiology* 1988;167:463–465

88. Seeger JM, Abela GS, Silverman SH, et al: Initial results of laser recanalization in lower extremity arterial reconstructions. *Vasc Surg* 1989;9:-7–10

89. Sanborn TA, Mitty HA, Train JS: Infrapopliteal and below knee popliteal lesions: treatment with sole laser thermal angioplasty. *Radiology* 1989;172:89–93

90. Schwarten DE: Aortic, iliac and peripheral arterial angioplasty, in Castañeda–Zúñiga WR, Tadavarthy SM (eds): *Interventional Radiology.* 1st ed. Baltimore, Williams & Wilkins, 1988, p 268

91. Spence RK, Friedman DB, Gotenby R, et al: Long-term results of transluminal angioplasty of the iliac and femoral arteries. *Arch Surg* 1981;116:1377–1386

92. Becker GJ, Katzen B, Dake M: Noncoronary angioplasty. *Radiology* 1989;170:921–940

93. Ewes RC, White RI, Murray RR, et al: Long-term results of superficial femoral artery angioplasty. *AJR* 1986;146:1025–1029

94. Kreple VM, Van Andle GJ, Van Erp WFM, et al: Percutaneous transluminal angioplasty of the femoral popliteal artery: initial and long-term results. *Radiology* 1985;156:325–328

95. Tamura S, Sniderman KW, Beinart C, Sos TA: Percutaneous transluminal angioplasty of the popliteal artery and its branches. *Radiology* 1982;143:645–648

96. Schwarten DE, Cutcliff WB: Arterial occlusive disease below-the-knee treatment with percutaneous transluminalangioplasty performed with low-profile catheters and steerable guidewires. *Radiology* 1988;169:71–74

97. Tadavarthy AK, Sullivan WA, Nicoloff D, et al: Aorta balloon angioplasty: 9-year follow-up. *Radiology* 1989;170:1039-1041

98. Darling RC, Linton RR: Durability of femoral popliteal reconstructions. *Am J Surg* 1972;123:472–479

99. DeWeese JA, Rob CG: Autogenous venous grafts 10 years later. *Surgery* 1977;82:775–784

100. Murray RR, Hewes RC, White RI, et al: Long segment femoro-popliteal stenosis: is angioplasty a boom or a bust? *Radiology* 1987;162:473–476

101. Perler BA, Osterman FA, White RA, et al: Percutaneous laser probe femoropopliteal angioplasty: a preliminary experience. *J Vasc Surg* 1989;10:351–357

102. Wright GJ, Belkin M, Greenfield AJ: Laser angioplasty for limb salvage observations on early results. *Vasc Surg* 1989;10:29–38

103. Geschwind HJ, Dubois–Rande JL, Boussignac G: Early and long-term results after guided pulsed laser balloon angioplasty of totally occluded arteries. Abstracts of the 62nd Scientific Session of the American Heart Association. *Circulation* 1989;80(suppl II):581

104. Katzen BT: Complications of "hot tip" laser-assisted angioplasty. *Circulation* 1988;78(suppl II):417

105. Sanborn TA, Greenfield AJ, Gaben JK, et al: Human percutaneous and intraoperative laser thermal angioplasty—initial clinical results as an adjunct to balloon angioplasty. *J Vasc Surg* 1987;5:183–190

106. White R, White GH: Laser thermal probe recanalization of occluded arteries. *J Vasc Surg* 1989;9:594–604

107. Spears JR: Percutaneous laser treatment of atherosclerosis: an overview of emerging techniques. *Cardiovasc Intervent Radiol* 1986;9:303–312

108. Ward H: Laser recanalization of atheromatous vessels using fiber optics. *Lasers Surg Med* 1984;4:353–363

109. Spears JR: Percutaneous transluminal coronary angioplasty restenosis: potential prevention with laser balloon angioplasty. *Am J Cardiol* 1987;60:61B–64B

110. Jenkins RD, Sinclair N, Anand R, et al: Laser balloon angioplasty: effect of tissue temperature on weld strength of human postmortem intima-media separations. *Lasers Surg Med* 1988;8:30–39

111. Gleason T, Cragg AH, DeJong SC, Smith TP: Results of thermal balloon angioplasty in a canine model (abstr). 75th Scientific Assembly and Annual Meeting of the Radiological Society of North America, 1989

112. Rees MR, Aschley S, Gehani AA, et al: Percutaneous angioscopy of sapphire tip laser angioplasty. Abstracts of the 62nd Scientific Session of the AHA. *Circulation* 1989;80:1638

113. Smith TP, Cragg AH, Landas SK: Plaque modification with tetracycline: enhanced tissue ablation during excimer lasing (abstr). 75th Scientific Assembly and Annual Meeting of the Radiological Society of North America, Nov 1989

114. Spears JR, Serur J, Shropshire D, Paulin S: Fluoresence of experimental atheromatous plaques with hematoporphyrin derivative. *J Clin Invest* 1983;71:395–399

115. Prince MR, Deutsch TF, Shapiro AH, et al: Selective ablation of atheromas using a flashlamp-excited dye laser at 465 nm. *Proc Natl Acad Sci USA* 1986;83:7064–7068

116. Prince MR, Deutsch TF, Mathews-Roth MM, et al: Preferential light absorption in atheromas. *Clin Invest* 1986;78:295–302

117. Leon MB, Lu DY, Prevosti LG, et al: Human arterial surface fluorescence atherosclerotic plaque identification and effects of laser atheroma ablation. *J Am Coll Cardiol* 1988;12:94–l02

118. Sanborn TA, Greenfield AJ: Response to peripheral angioplasty need for organized clinical trials. *Radiology* 1989;172:943

119. Mclean GK, Burke DR, Marinelli DL: Comment on the clinical appropriateness of an emerging technology. *Radiology* 1989;172:941–942

120. Strandnes DE, Barnes RW, Katzen B, Ring EJ: Indiscriminate use of laser angioplasty. *Radiology* 1989;172:945–946

121. SCVIR position statement on thermal laser angioplasty. *Radiology* 1989;172:944

6

PERCUTANEOUS ATHERECTOMY

—Wilfrido R. Castañeda–Zúñiga, M.D., M.Sc., Manuel Maynar, M.D., Joseph W. Yedlicka, Jr., M.D.,
David W. Hunter, M.D., S. Murthy Tadavarthy, M.D., Marcos A. Herrera, M.D., Patricia E. Thorpe, M.D.,
and Kurt Amplatz, M.D.

Balloon angioplasty, the standard percutaneous approach to palliation or definitive treatment of vascular stenosis, has evolved since 1964.[1] Angioplasty of focal lesions in the iliac and femoropopliteal regions has good long-term results on the order of 80–90% in the iliac arteries and 60–70% in the superficial femoral arteries.[2-4] On the other hand, long-term patency following recanalization and angioplasty of complete occlusions of the iliac and femoral arteries is 90 and 50–60%, respectively.[2-4]

The degree of disease, location of the lesion, association of tandem disease, and quality of distal vascular bed are all factors which influence immediate results and long-term outcome in both percutaneous and surgical peripheral vascular procedures.[2-4]

Designs for atherectomy devices have been conceived out of frustration with the limitations of conventional angioplasty, especially with the poor long-term results obtained in the management of total arterial occlusions.

The ideal atherectomy device has not been designed. Possibly, no one instrument can circumvent all the disadvantages of balloon angioplasty and provide the desired clinical and angiographic results. With angioplasty, we attempt to restore adequate blood supply by increasing the intraluminal diameter with barotrauma. This is done by fracture of the atheromatous intima rather than by removal of the atherosclerotic plaque, as in atherectomy. Atherectomy catheters attempt to remove plaque with minimal injury to the vessel, no significant distal embolization and a low incidence of restenosis. Ideally, the devices should be used percutaneously. However, in order to sufficiently increase the lumen without adjunctive balloon dilatation, larger diameter devices are necessary. In addition, devices incorporating a motor drive connected to a rotating shaft do not work well when an acute angle of entry into the artery is present. In large patients, therefore, a percutaneous approach is often not optimal for a good operational angle. A surgical cut-down can be helpful for access with large-bore atherectomy catheters requiring large sheaths or in obese patients. However, the politics of joint procedures requiring cooperation with the vascular

surgeon can be understandably complex in and of themselves. However, working together we gain the strength inherent in collective and cooperative efforts to treat patients with peripheral vascular disease with devices offering better long-term patency.

Thus, it is becoming increasingly clear to those of us who treat peripheral vascular disease that a concert of technical tools and adjunctive therapies is available. The successful use of any device may depend more on patient selection and choice of an appropriate approach than the mere availability of the technology. As limb salvage and/or clinical improvement are the primary goals of peripheral vascular therapy, it is important to keep in mind that successful use of a given device or combination of devices is measured by long-term outcome and not by immediate results. As we are learning, long-term outcome depends on the pattern of the patient's disease, the pathology, the judgment and technical competence of the physicians, and then the technology of the atherectomy device per se.

It should be emphasized that atherectomy devices are complementary, not competitive. The best approach to a given lesion or series of lesions is a thoughtful combined approach using the best technology suited for diagnosis and treatment. Selection of a suitable sequence of devices and therapies, including thrombolysis pre- and postatherectomy, requires knowledge of the strengths and weaknesses of each device as well as an understanding of the patient's pathology. For example, rotational devices have been shown to be superior in removing calcified plaque, whereas the laser is known to be very effective in penetrating organized thrombus, which is not calcified. Thus, in lieu of the perfect all-purpose instrument, the ideal approach is one which can best utilize the devices available in the angiography suite in the most suitable sequence determined by the pathology and patient's overall clinical status. Continued application of any device should be based on careful clinical follow-up designed to evaluate how well the device or combination of devices contributes to the satisfactory outcome. The initial technical success should be correlated to the eventual clinical success or lack thereof. Such a category of data is still forthcoming on all of the devices currently available.

MECHANICAL RECANALIZATION DEVICES

These are devices whose purpose is to recanalize segmental vascular obstructions. Their main indication is to help the recanalization in those cases where conventional angiographic recanalization techniques have failed. It has been demonstrated that if balloon angioplasty is attempted in patients with severe ischemia, about 90% of those lesions under 10cm long, and only 10% of those longer than 10cm, can be crossed with a guidewire.[5] More commonly, reported failure rates for peripheral vascular procedures fall between 10 and 20%, with most of the failures to recanalize occurring in complete occlusions.[2,4,6] For coronary angioplasty, the failure rate varies from 8% for stenosis to 33% for occlusions.[7]

Several devices have been designed to try to overcome the difficulties of recanalizing vascular occlusions. Mechanical recanalizing devices are devices that are power-driven and that by rotation at low or high speed or by pulsating create a channel through an area of vascular occlusion. The following devices are included:

Low-speed recanalizing devices:
—Vallbracht slow rotational recanalizing wire;
—Zeitler pulsating wire;
—Wholey reperfusion atherolytic wire.
High-speed recanalizing atheroablating devices:
—Kensey dynamic angioplasty catheter.
—Pfeifer milling catheter.
—Auth rotational atherectomy catheter.
—Ultrasonic atherolysis.

All of these devices typically create a channel as large as the rotating part by laterally displacing or ablating atheromatous-thrombotic occlusions, and, characteristically, no tissue is extracted.

PERCUTANEOUS ATHERECTOMY DEVICES

Included in this group of devices are several ingenious instruments designed to excise atheromatous lesions, either stenoses or complete vascular occlusions. Among them are:

—Bard rotary atherectomy system (BRAS);
—Simpson directional atherectomy catheter;
—Transluminal extraction catheter (TEC).

Typically, these devices create a channel of a diameter equal to that of the catheter tip by excising and removing atheromatous-thrombotic material. The Simpson directional atherectomy catheter is the only atherectomy device that allows one to restore the vessel lumen to its full dimensions.

EMERGING TECHNOLOGIES

Two emerging technologies are included: the Kaliman atherectomy catheter and the pullback atherectomy catheter.

ATHERECTOMY DEVICES AND ADJUNCTIVE TECHNIQUES

It is clear that atherectomy devices and adjunctive techniques including angioplasty and thrombolytic therapy are complementary and not competitive. In order to provide the best possible solution to peripheral vascular disease that requires intervention, one should have at hand a number of different technologies. As we know, from the natural history of superficial femoral artery disease alone, the presence of a lesion does not mandate treatment. When a patient becomes sufficiently symptomatic to warrant intervention, either percutaneously or surgically, the best combination of available technology should be employed. In order to ascertain the optimal approach, given the patient's clinical status and goals of the procedure, a team approach is recommended for analysis of the situation. Following accurate noninvasive studies and diagnostic angiography, a careful evaluation should address whether or not the lesion or lesions require treatment. If they do, then the procedure of choice should be that which affords the best clinical outcome in the context of the patient's overall medical status. For example, a young patient presenting with limiting claudication might undergo a percutaneous procedure in order to spare the saphenous vein in view of his life expectancy and the possibility that the vein might be required for cardiac bypass surgery or subsequent peripheral graft. In addition, younger patients treated with percutaneous procedures who stop smoking may eventually show that the long-term outcome of percutaneous procedures equals or exceeds the patency rates for venous grafts. On the other hand, a patient who shows a pattern of diffuse disease with poor runoff, may benefit from a combination of proximal atherectomy and/or angioplasty and in situ vein grafting rather than total lower extremity atherectomy-angioplasty. The combination of possibilities and optimization of patient outcome, not immediately but long-term, resides in the marriage of abilities contributed by the interventional radiologist, vascular surgeon, and attending physician. Adjunctive medical therapy cannot be ignored after treating structural occlusions with either surgery or vascular percutaneous interventional procedures.

Therefore, it is not sufficient to be able to own the devices as well as the referral rights to the patients in whom such procedures can be performed. Sophisticated and thoughtful analysis of the device applications must be performed. In addition, it is mandatory that all physicians performing angioplasty or atherectomy maintain accurate records regarding complications and long-term patency. Our ability to continue to perform these procedures and improve these procedures with the evolution of technique, technology, and clinical judgment depends on an accurate recording of the efficacy of these devices in the current clinical setting. The medical community cannot and should not tolerate anything less than responsible use of these devices and maintenance of high standards of safety in their application. Although the new atherectomy devices have been developed in a climate of competitive high technology, marketed with Wall Street glitz, we as physicians are guardians of the patient's trust and confidence. These devices are not competitive, they are complementary, and they should only be used when clinical circumstances provide a setting in which they can be used with optimal success. Faster manipulation of the device to minimize the time of arterial occlusion, and, most often, adjunctive thrombolytic therapy, is indicated to either prevent or treat associated thrombosis.

References

1. Dotter CT, Judkins MP: Transluminal treatment of atherosclerotic obstruction. *Circulation* 1964;30:654–657
2. Murray RR, Hughes RCH, White RI Jr, et al: Long segment femoropopliteal stenoses: is angioplasty a balloon or bust? *Radiology* 1987;162:473–476
3. Hewes RC, White RJ Jr, Murray RR, et al: Long-term results of superficial femoral artery angioplasty. *AJR* 1986; 146:1025–1029
4. Krepel VM, van Andel GJ, van Erp MFM, Breslau PJ: Percutaneous transluminal angioplasty of the femoropopliteal artery: initial and long-term results. *Radiology* 1985;156:325–328
5. Mosley JG, Gulati SM, Raphael M, Marston A: The role of percutaneous transluminal angioplasty for atherosclerotic disease of the lower extremities. *Ann R Coll Surg Engl* 1985;67:83–86
6. Wholey MH, Smith JA, Godlewski P, Nagurka M: Recanalization of total arterial occlusions with the Kensey dynamic angioplasty catheter. *Radiology* 1989;172:95–98
7. Detre K, Holubkov R, Kelsey S, Cowley H, Kent K, Williams D, et al: Percutaneous transluminal coronary angioplasty in 1985–1986 and 1977–1981: the National Heart, Lung and Blood Institute Registry. *N Engl J Med* 1988;318:265–270

Part 1. Low-speed Rotational Angioplasty

—Cristian Vallbracht, M.D., Dieter Liermann, M.D., Ingeborg Prignitz, M.D., Christa Paasch, M.D., Helmut Landgraf, M.D., Wolfgang Beinborn, M.D., Jürgen Kollath, M.D., Franz Josef Roth, M.D., Werner Schoop, M.D., and Martin Kaltenbach, M.D.

Histopathologic studies have shown that vascular occlusions are caused in most cases by ulcerated atherosclerotic plaques, with a superimposed thrombotic occlusion. The thrombus causing the final occlusion, because of its age, is less organized than the older segments of the obstruction. This area is the softest part of the obstruction and allows the passage of instruments, if it can be found, which may be difficult, due to the typical eccentricity of the residual vascular lumen.[1,2]

A clear risk of dissecting into the subintimal plane exists when trying to recanalize segments of vascular occlusion with angiographic guidewires, unless this path of least resistance is found.[1,2] Attempts to recanalize with conventional angiographic technique segments of vascular occlusion have a reported failure rate varying from 10 to 33% for peripheral and coronary procedures.[3–6] These failed attempts can be due to a simple failure to cross the area of obstruction, but more commonly the failure is related to the creation of a subintimal tract and/or wall perforation. Even when the operator successfully re-enters the true vascular lumen, after a subintimal passage, the results of transluminal angioplasty in these cases in the short- and long-term are unsatisfactory.

Based on these observations, Vallbracht designed a blunt-tip, low-speed rotational recanalizing wire. The advantages of such a device are purported to be minimal adhesive friction, thus facilitating advancement of the

wire, not only through straight but also along vascular bends and the transmission of any resistance from distal to proximal.[1] These properties are the cause of the low tendency to produce subintimal dissection and the low incidence of vascular perforations associated with recanalization procedures with this device.[1] The device differs from high-speed rotation techniques[2,7] not only on the speed of rotation, but in the fact that the high-speed techniques are geared to producing atheroablation, as opposed to the Vallbracht device whose aim is to displace tissue laterally as well as causing a tissue volume reduction by squeezing fluid out.[8]

DESCRIPTION OF THE DEVICE

The Vallbracht device is an electrically driven, 6.6Fr catheter, made of four 0.2mm steel-coiled wires, with an inner lumen to allow the injection of contrast or drugs and a blunt olive-shaped tip (Fig. 6.1.1). The powered unit is battery operated (9 volt battery), with speeds ranging from 0 to 550 rpm with a potentiometric speed control which guarantees a smooth adjustment (Fig. 6.1.2).

TECHNIQUE

Either a retrograde puncture for iliac lesions or an antegrade puncture for femoropopliteal lesions is used to gain

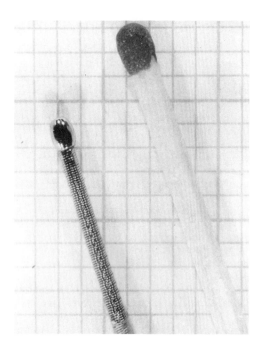

Figure 6.1.1. Rotating catheter consisting of 4 × 0.2mm V₂A-steel coiled wires covered with a highly flexible Teflon shrinking tube and an olive-shaped, blunt tip (see difference in size compared with a match).

access and place a check-flow introducer sheath. The recanalizing catheter is passed through the sheath under fluoroscopic control, until the level of obstruction is reached. Digital roadmapping is then used to guide the recanalization procedure. The power unit is turned on and the obstructed area is crossed using slow rotational speed in the order of 100–200 rpm (Figs. 6.1.3 and 6.1.4). During advancement of the catheter, slight axial thrusts are used to search for the path of least resistance, the so-called "soft point." Once the occlusion is passed, intraluminal passage is confirmed by the injection of contrast medium. An exchange wire is then passed through the central lumen

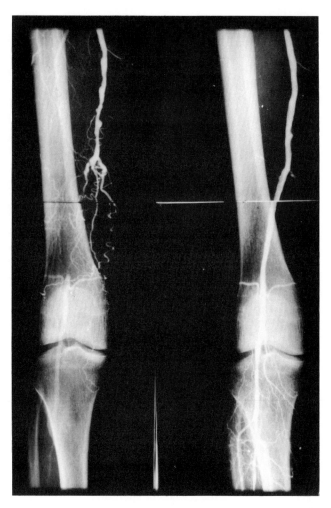

Figure 6.1.3. Chronic occlusion of the superficial femoral artery (length 11cm). *Left,* before the procedure; *right,* after reopening with low-speed rotational angioplasty and balloon dilatation.

to complete the luminal reconstitution by using an angioplasty balloon.

RESULTS

Similar success rates have been reported by Liermann in 250 patients with an 80% success rate in femoropopliteal vessels and a 60% success rate in iliac vessels.[9]

The primary success rate for recanalizing femoropopliteal occlusions dropped, however, to 65% when the occlusion was unsuccessfully manipulated with catheter and guidewire techniques, more than four weeks prior and to 25% when the previous manipulation occurred within four weeks of the Vallbracht procedure.[1,9]

COMPLICATIONS

No instances of perforations have been reported.[1,9] Dissection has occurred in 7% of the cases, and there was one instance of distal embolization without clinical consequences.[1,9]

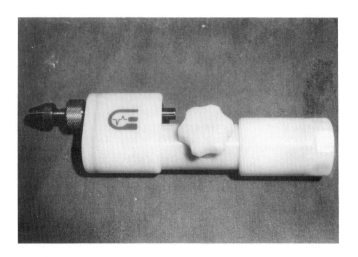

Figure 6.1.2. Battery-driven electric motor. The 9V battery is placed in a sterilized compartment with a screw fixture.

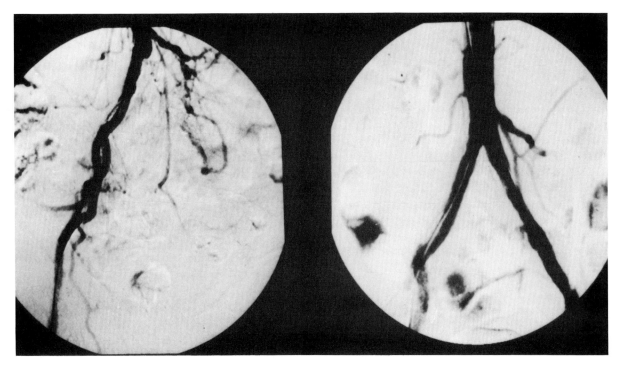

Figure 6.1.4. Chronic occlusion of the left common iliac artery. *Left,* before the procedure; *right,* after reopening with low-speed rotational angioplasty and balloon dilatation (guidewires in both sides).

CONCLUSIONS

Recanalization of occluded vessels using the low-speed rotational catheter with an overall success rate of 88% for femoropopliteal occlusions and 58% for iliac occlusions seems to be a safe and effective procedure, particularly as a primary recanalization tool, since the success rate drops significantly when prior manipulations are performed using conventional angiographic techniques.[1,9] This device is not currently under evaluation in the United States, and its use has been limited in Europe to a few centers.

References

1. Vallbracht C, Liermann D, Prignitz I, Paasch C, Landgraf H, Beinborn W, Kollath J, Roth F–J, Schoop W, Kaltenbach M: Recanalization of chronic occlusions: Low-speed rotational angioplasty, in Zeitler E, Seyferth W (eds): *Pros and Cons in PTA and Auxiliary Methods.* Berlin, Springer–Verlag, 1989, pp 101–110
2. Kensey K, Nash J, Abrahams C, Zarins CK: Recanalization of obstructive arteries with a flexible, rotating tip catheter. *Radiology* 1987;165:387–389
3. Murray RR, Hughes RCH, White RI Jr, et al: Long segment femoropopliteal stenoses: is angioplasty a balloon or bust? *Radiology* 1987;162:473–476
4. Krepel VM, van Andel GJ, van Erp MFM, Breslau PJ: Percutaneous transluminal angioplasty of the femoropopliteal artery: initial and long-term results. *Radiology* 1985;156:325–328
5. Mosley JG, Gulati SM, Raphael M, Marston A: The role of percutaneous transluminal angioplasty for atherosclerotic disease of the lower extremities. *Ann R Coll Surg Engl* 1985;67:83–86
6. Wholey MH, Smith JA, Godlewski P, Nagurka M: Recanalization of total arterial occlusions with the Kensey dynamic angioplasty catheter. *Radiology* 1989;172:95–98
7. Ritchie JL, Hansen DD, Vracko H, Auth D: In vivo rotational thrombectomy. Evaluation by angioscopy. *Circulation* 1986;74(suppl II):1822 (abstr)
8. Kaltenbach M, Beyer J, Klepzig H, Schmidtz L, Huber K: Effect of 5 kg/cm² pressure on atherosclerotic wall segments, in Kaltenbach M, Grüntzig A, Rentrop K, Bussman WD (eds): *Transluminal Coronary Angioplasty and Intracoronary Thrombolysis.* Heidelberg, Springer–Verlag, 1984, pp 189–193
9. Liermann DD, Vallbracht C, Goethe JW: Slow rotational angioplasty in peripheral and iliac vessels. Presented at the Second Annual International Symposium on Peripheral Vascular Intervention. Miami, Jan 1990

Part 2. Zeitler Pulsating Wire

—Wilfrido R. Castañeda–Zúñiga, M.D., M.Sc.

A device for the safe crossing of severely narrowed arteries or for the recanalization of vascular occlusions, in order to subsequently perform additional revascularization procedures, such as angioplasty, directional atherectomy, etc., was described by Zeitler.[1]

The device consists of a reusable, hand-held box containing a small DC motor powered by a 1.5-volt battery (Fig. 6.2.1). A side clamp (*A*) is used to hold and vibrate a guidewire (0.014 to 0.038 inch) with a side-to-side motion. The number of strokes per minute can be varied by a potentiometer (*B*) from 100 to 3000 rpm. The length of the stroke

is about 3mm. Commercially available Teflon-coated guidewires with a straight, soft tip are used either passed directly through a check-flow introducer sheath or through a straight-tipped catheter. There are two main uses for this technique.

—Guiding:

For guiding in severely narrowed, tortuous, but not totally occluded vessels, the guidewire should extend well beyond the catheter tip (5–6cm).

—Recanalization:

For recanalization of vascular occlusions, the tip of the guidewire should extend beyond the catheter tip by only 2–3cm. Zeitler states that the length of the free part of the guidewire influences the radius of pulsation and the power of the mechanical strokes on the obstructed part of the vessel.[2]

An 89.5% primary success rate in recanalization of vascular occlusions in long chronic femoropopliteal occlusion was reported.[2] It is recommended to attempt recanalization with the pulsating guidewire as a primary recanalization procedure to enhance the chances of success.

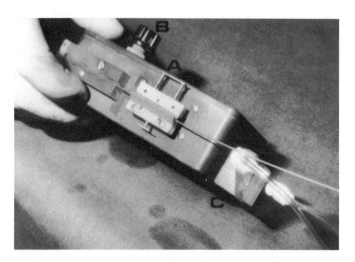

Figure 6.2.1. Zeitler pulsating wire. Hand-held power package. *A,* side clamp. *B,* potentiometer. *C,* main power switch. (Reproduced with permission from Zeitler E: The pulsating wire, in Zeitler E, Seyferth W (eds): *Pros and Cons in PTA.* Berlin, Springer–Verlag, 1989.)

References

1. Zeitler E, Richter EI, Neubauer T: Comparative studies of dynamic and laser percutaneous transluminal angioplasty. Presented at the RSNA 1987 annual meeting, Chicago, IL, Nov 1987
2. Zeitler E: The pulsating guidewire in pros and cons in PTA and auxiliary methods, in Zeitler E, Seyferth W (eds): *Pros and Cons in PTA and Auxiliary Procedures.* Berlin, Springer–Verlag, 1989, pp 129–135

Part 3. Atherolytic Reperfusion Wire Device

—Mark H. Wholey, M.D., Robert G. Levitt, M.D., and Deborah Fein–Millar, M.D.

TECHNICAL DESCRIPTION

The atherolytic wire (Medrad, Inc., Pittsburgh, PA) was designed for recanalization of total occlusions. The device consists of a 0.035-inch coil spring wire with an ellipsoid-shaped distal tip. The distal tip may be notched or unnotched (Fig. 6.3.1*A,B*). The proximal segment of the wire device is connected to a hand-held, battery-operated, motor-driven unit which rotates the wire at 600 rpm (Fig. 6.3.2). The wire passes through a conventional 5Fr catheter or any angioplasty catheter with an 0.035-inch end

hole. The wire device is used to create a "pilot-hole" through a short or long segment occlusion.[1]

INDICATIONS

Most occlusions are composed of organized thrombus superimposed on an atheromatous occlusion.[2] Commonly, the lumen can be recanalized using the conventional catheter-wire technique.[3] When excessive resistance or failure of this technique occurs, the atherolytic wire allows additional force through the segment of obstruction. The

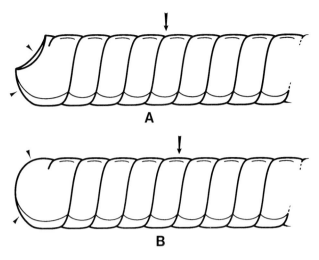

Figure 6.3.1. Atherolytic wire device consists of a 0.035-inch coil spring wire *(arrow)* with an ellipse-shaped distal tip *(arrowheads).* This tip may be notched (**A**) or un-notched (**B**).

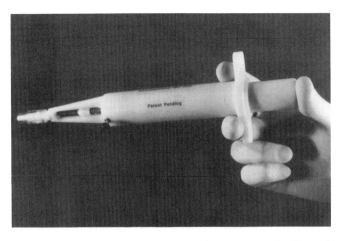

Figure 6.3.2. Self-contained battery pack for atherolytic wire. Power is activated by a button at the bottom of the plunger controlled by the operator's thumb. The wire is advanced by compressing the plunger on the syringe-like device.

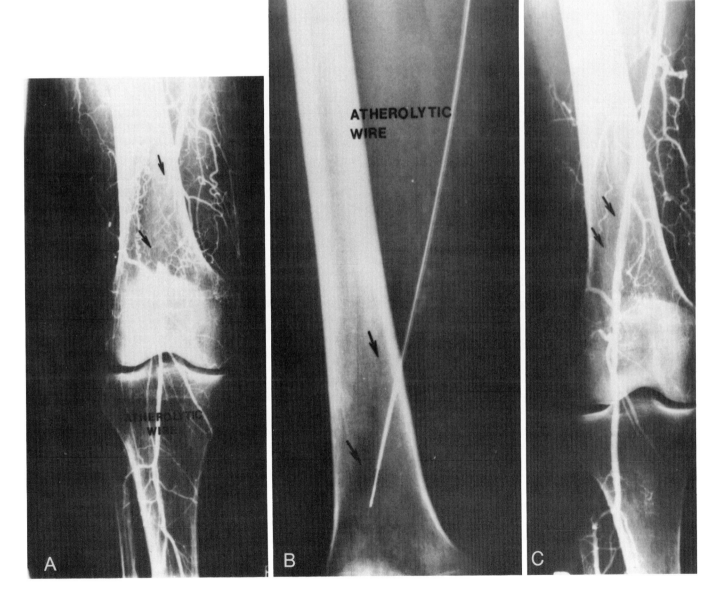

Figure 6.3.3. Occluded distal superficial femoral artery (SFA)/proximal popliteal artery (PA). **A.** Angiogram shows long segment occlusion of distal SFA/proximal PA *(arrows)* with reconstitution of distal PA by collater- als. **B.** The atherolytic wire has crossed the occluded segment. **C.** Angiogram following balloon angioplasty over atherolytic wire shows normal lumen dimension of previously occluded segment *(arrows).*

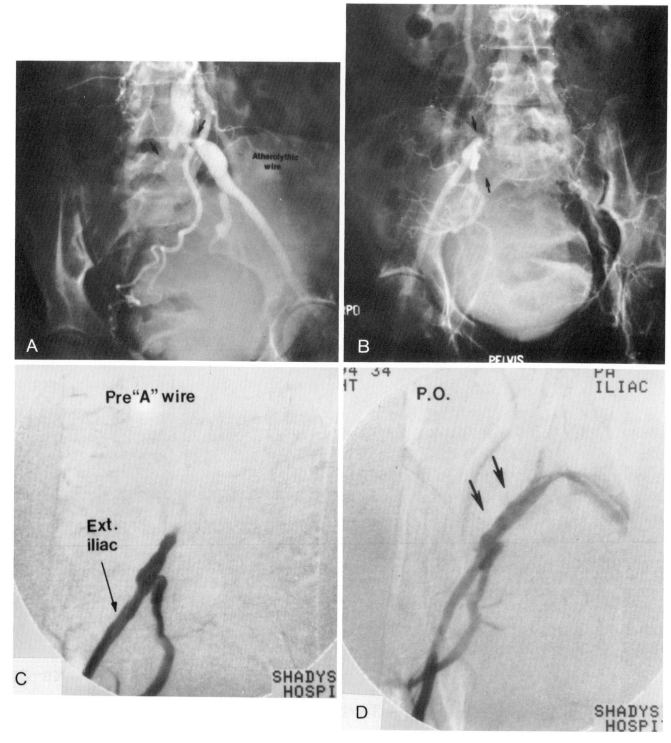

Figure 6.3.4. Occluded right common iliac artery (CIA). **A.** Aortogram shows occlusion of heavily calcified right CIA at its origin *(arrow)* and high-grade stenosis of left CIA at its origin *(arrows).* **B.** Later film from aortogram shows reconstitution of right CIA near its bifurcation *(arrows).* **C.** Digital subtraction angiogram (DSA) of reconstituted distal right CIA. An atherolytic wire was subsequently passed through the occluded right CIA segment from a retrograde left common femoral artery approach. **D.** DSA following balloon angioplasty over atherolytic wire shows normal dimension to previously occluded right CIA *(arrows).*

device is best applied in relatively straight vessels, i.e., iliac, superficial femoral, or popliteal arteries. The atherolytic wire may serve as a guide for the introduction of other recanalization devices, including atherectomy devices and conventional angioplasty balloon catheters.

TECHNICAL RESULTS

The clinical experience with the atherolytic wire is limited. Recanalization in 12 patients is reported. Eight had total occlusions of the superficial femoral artery, varying in length from 8 to 15cm. Two patients had longer than 3cm external iliac artery occlusions; and two patients had proximal 2cm common iliac artery occlusions. Eight of the twelve patients were successfully recanalized and subsequently had conventional angioplasty (Figs. 6.3.3 and 6.3.4). Four patients had calcified vascular occlusive disease which could not be crossed with the atherolytic wire.

COMPLICATIONS

Vessel dissection occurred in all four patients with calcified occlusive vascular disease which could not be recanalized. In three patients the dissections were limited, but in one patient with a common iliac artery occlusion an extensive dissection developed. Other potential complications, including vessel perforation, embolization of atherosclerotic material, and hematoma formation at the puncture site did not occur.

CLINICAL RESULTS

One-year clinical follow-up was obtained in the eight patients with successfully recanalized occlusions. Doppler studies and angiography in eight patients demonstrated continued patency in six patients and reocclusion in two patients.

CURRENT STATUS OF THE ATHEROLYTIC REPERFUSION WIRE DEVICE

The atherolytic wire device remains an investigational device. A modification of the wire is under development which would allow passage of a 0.014-inch torque-controlled coronary wire through the 0.035-inch wire. This would allow more precise positioning within the lumen of an occluded vessel and reduce the incidence of vessel dissection.

References

1. Wholey MH, Jarmulowski CR: New reperfusion devices: the Kensey catheter, the atherolytic reperfusion wire device, and the transluminal extraction catheter. *Radiology* 1989; 172:947–952
2. Wholey MH, Smith JAM: Newer atherectomy and reperfusion devices for the peripheral circulation, in Taveras JM, Ferrucci JT (eds): *Radiology: Diagnosis-Imaging-Intervention.* Philadelphia, J. B. Lippincott, 1990, pp 1–12
3. Wholey MH: A newly designed directionally controlled guidewire. *Cathet Cardiovasc Diagn* 1986;12:66–70

Part 4. Kensey Dynamic Angioplasty Catheter

—Kenneth Kensey, M.D., and Wilfrido R. Castañeda–Zúñiga, M.D., M.Sc.

In 1987, Kensey and Nash described a high-speed rotating tip catheter for recanalization of vascular occlusions.[1] The device recanalizes by ablating atheromatous plaque; typically no material is removed, and a channel as large as the rotating tip is created.

DEVICE DESCRIPTION

The Trac-Wright catheter (formerly known as the Kensey catheter) is a flexible, high-speed rotating tip catheter used for recanalization of stenotic and occluded vessels (Fig. 6.4.1).Its primary indication for use is in treating lesions unable to be passed with an angiographic guidewire. The rotating tip is essentially a blunt rotating stainless steel cam. The flexible polyurethane catheter body, available in 5 and 8Fr sizes, encloses a motor-driven cable which drives the cam at speeds of 30,000–100,000 rpm. The catheter also contains a lumen which carries pressurized fluid to the base of the cam. A combination of non-ionic contrast medium and saline solution is injected into the vessel at a flow rate of about 60ml/min. The injected contrast medium serves to identify the area of occlusion and to guide the recanalization procedure. As the rotating cam ablates atheromatous tissue, the resulting vortex created by the high-speed rotation draws in the ablated atheromatous particulate for micropulverization while the ejected fluid acts to center and cool the high-speed rotational cam.[1]

OPERATING PRINCIPLES

Safety and efficacy of the Trac-Wright catheter is based on two major assumptions:

1. Diseased tissue can be selectively pulverized based on inherent differences in its viscoelasticity, organization, and fibrous makeup; and

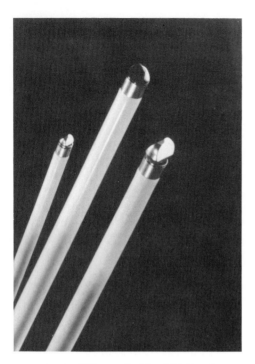

Figure 6.4.1.   Different size Trac-Wright catheters.

2. Microembolization of diseased tissue is clinically innocuous to the distal organ as shown clinically with this and other devices that microembolize tissue.[2]

ROTATING CAM

The major component of the catheter is the blunt spinning cam (Fig. 6.4.2). Since there are no sharp edges, no

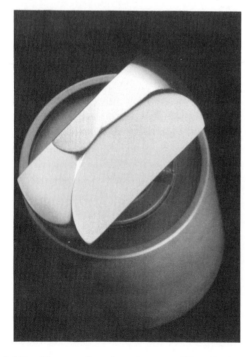

Figure 6.4.2.   Close-up view of rotating cam of Trac-Wright catheter.

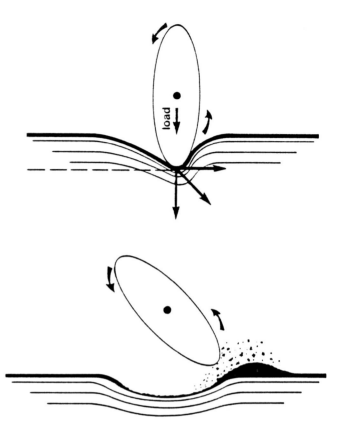

Figure 6.4.3.   Top. The degree of deformation of the arterial wall is proportional to the cam size and applied energy. **Bottom.** The difference in elastic limits enables arterial deposits to be pulverized while keeping the arterial wall intact.

cutting is involved. The shape of the cam is critical and gives the tip its ability to selectively pulverize nonviscoelastic material, based upon differences in tissue viscoelasticity between the normal arterial wall and the atherosclerotic tissue.[2] This allows the catheter to selectively pulverize atheroma while leaving the arterial wall intact.

Normal arterial walls have a high degree of elasticity which allows the tissue to yield under stress. The degree to which the tissue deforms is proportional to the cam size, the applied rotational energy, and the tissue elasticity. There is an elastic limit, however, which is defined as the amount of stress a material can withstand and still return to its original shape. Normal arterial tissue has a higher elastic limit than material such as calcium, fatty tissue, thrombus, and fibrous tissue.[2] Therefore, the stress applied by the rotating cam will surpass the elastic limits of atheromatous material (Fig. 6.4.3) earlier than the limits of the adjacent healthy elastic tissue which remains undamaged.[2]

PRESSURIZED FLUID

The high-speed rotating catheter also directs fluid jets laterally against the arterial wall. These lateral jets are important in guiding the catheter through a total occlusion, in dilating the artery, and in opening the collaterals.

The rotating tip creates a powerful vortex which in turn creates a significant negative pressure at the tip of the catheter. The vortex recirculates debris and repeatedly reduces the size of particles produced.[2]

The fluid also acts to cool and lubricate the system, allows visualization during the procedure, and allows addition of medications to the site of treatment. Traditionally, a mixture of a thrombolytic agent such as urokinase, contrast medium, and heparin is used as the perfusate. Antispasmodics could also be added to the mixture. The fluid is injected under pressure by an angiographic injector system at rates varying from 30 to 60ml/min.

PATH OF LEAST RESISTANCE

The principle of "the path of least resistance" plays an important role in guiding the working tip. Implied in this principle is the fact that total arterial occlusions have a focal area of least resistance that corresponds to that area of the artery which was last patent. Depending on the age of the obstruction, this area of least resistance would be made up of fresh and/or organized thrombus. Obviously, as the obstruction gets older, the area of least resistance becomes more fibrous or even calcified. The rotating catheter tip finds the area of least resistance through several mechanisms. Fresh thrombus is very nonviscoelastic, and since thrombus commonly fills the area of least resistance, the catheter tip will remove this area first since it is the most easily pulverized (Figs. 6.4.4 and 6.4.5). The fluid jets tend to guide the catheter to the area of least resistance (Fig. 6.4.6). The amount of pressure created by these lateral jets of fluid has been measured and is exponentially related to the revolutions/min of the tip[2] (Fig. 6.4.7). Of unknown significance is the fact that a spinning tipped catheter reduces the amount of forward friction created by the forward movement of the catheter[2] (Figs. 6.4.8 and 6.4.9). Another important component is that the catheter tip tends to vibrate when it comes in contact with a less easily pulverized surface. Bouncing of the tip or vibration deflects the tip from the hard areas into areas of least resistance[2] (Fig. 6.4.10).

In addition, rotation of the tip creates an area of high negative pressure. This negative pressure also tends to pull the catheter into the area of least resistance once a small nipple of material has been removed. The catheter tip will always be directed to this nipple, since the negative pres-

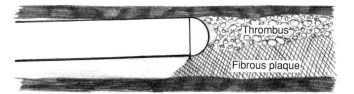

Figure 6.4.5. The area of least resistance is easily found by the Trac-Wright catheter and is removed first.

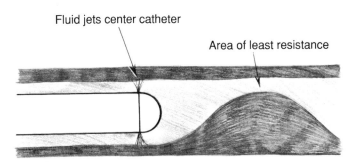

Figure 6.4.6. Fluid jets help to keep the catheter centered within the lumen of the vessel.

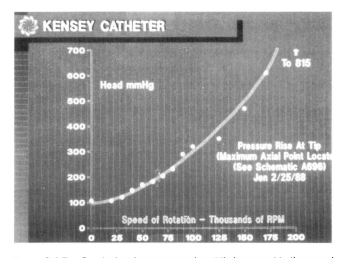

Figure 6.4.7. Graph showing pressure rise at tip in respect to the speed of rotation.

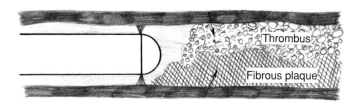

Figure 6.4.4. Recanalization of the total occlusion by differences in tissue properties.

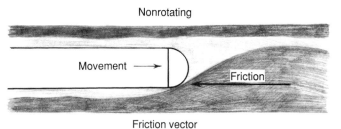

Figure 6.4.8. Diagram illustrating the degree of force required to advance through a vascular section is proportional to the forward motion of the catheter and the severity of the stenosis.

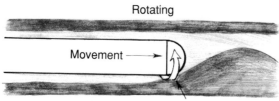

Figure 6.4.9. The force required to pass a catheter down the lumen is reduced by the rotating action of the cam with a friction vector at a right angle to the motion.

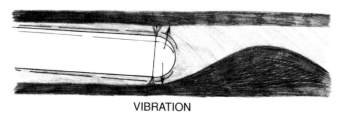

Figure 6.4.10. Bouncing of the tip helps direct the tip away from hard areas into areas of least resistance.

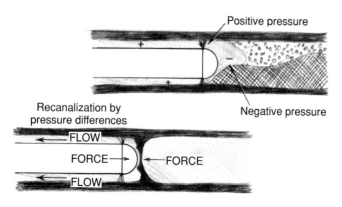

Figure 6.4.11. The vortex created by the high speed rotation of the cam creates a negative pressure that helps to center the catheter.

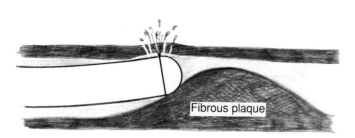

Figure 6.4.12. Extravasation of contrast medium into the wall of the artery is seen prior to perforation of the arterial wall.

sure at the tip is magnified by the shape of the occlusion[2] (Fig. 6.4.11).

These multiple forces combine synergistically to help the catheter find the area of least resistance through a total occlusion.[2]

GUIDELINES FOR USING THE DEVICE

The device is highly technique sensitive. In the hands of a skilled operator, greater than 90% technical success can be achieved in recanalizing long complete occlusions.[2] The following points should be considered when attempting a recanalization.

Extravasation of Dye

When using this catheter, extravasation of contrast medium through the arterial wall is an important safety parameter that must be watched for. If the catheter is pushed too hard or too fast through a lesion, or if the catheter deflects from an obstruction or stenosis, the catheter tip will be jammed into the arterial wall. With continued force on the tip, perforation of the arterial wall might occur. The operator who is alert and observant will note extravasation of dye occurring through the arterial wall into the soft tissues surrounding the artery before actual perforation occurs. Extravasation warns of impending perforation before actual vessel perforation occurs, allowing the operator to proceed with caution or withdraw totally and reevaluate the situation (Fig. 6.4.12).

Use of Guidewires

It is also recommended that an occlusion not be manipulated with a guidewire prior to the use of this catheter, since if the guidewire creates a false passage, an area of least resistance has been created in the arterial wall and, therefore, the Kensey catheter will always follow the false tract made by the guidewire (Fig. 6.4.13).

Recommended Speeds and Fluid Pressures

The catheter initial rotation speeds should be maintained at about 20,000 rpm with an infusion flow rate of 20–30ml/min until the lesion has been contacted by the tip. At this point, the revolutions/min are increased to 90,000, and the flow is increased to the maximum tolerated by the catheter (60ml/min). The viscosity of the fluid should be as low as possible to allow the highest flow possible. Passage of the catheter should be extremely slow with a to-and-fro motion. The operator should watch for a deflection of the tip caused by a viscoelastic lesion; i.e., the wave sign. If this occurs, the catheter should be pulled back to the non-wave state allowing the spinning tip to pulverize the deflecting lesion. The operator should be alert and

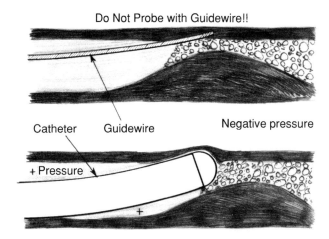

Do Not Probe with Guidewire!!

Catheter   Guidewire   Negative pressure

+ Pressure

+

Figure 6.4.13. Probing with a wire produces a subintimal tract; therefore, when the Kensey catheter is advanced, it will tend to follow the tract created by the wire.

aware of any extravasation and, prior to total recanalization, the infusion rate should be reduced to 10–20ml/min until the distal end of the lesion has been recanalized. Reducing the flow helps to reduce the risk of breaking off the distal end of the occlusion, which may cause a potentially large embolus. Once a total occlusion has been recanalized, the infusion rate and the revolutions/min are increased to their maximum to allow perfusion of the distal limb. Withdrawal of the catheter should be at the highest revolutions/min and flow rates possible.[2]

In an artery that is totally occluded with calcified material, it is important that the diameter of the catheter be as close as possible to the diameter of the artery (Fig. 6.4.14). The close fit between the catheter and the arterial wall will guide the tip through the calcified lesion. Calcium requires a great deal of rotational energy to pulverize and, therefore, much more time is needed to pulverize calcific tissue than thrombosed vessels.[2]

DISCUSSION

Several theories as to how the dynamic angioplasty catheter works have been reported,[2,3] including:

1. The device is self-centering because the fluid jets laterally delivered at the level of the rotating cam serve to keep the catheter tip centered in the vessel lumen.[1,2]
2. Hydrodilatation: The injection of fluid at rates of 30–60ml/min in a closed vascular system dilates the vascular lumen at the level of the catheter tip and thus, prevents direct contact between the rotating tip and the vascular wall, decreasing, therefore, the risk of dissection or vascular perforation.[1,2]
3. The rotating cam will not damage viscoelastic material such as the normal arterial wall, but it will readily remove dense, particularly calcific, arteriosclerotic plaque.[1,2]
4. The particles produced by the pulverization of atheromatous plaque are recirculated by the vortex produced

by the high-speed rotation of the cam, to be refragmented, with the end result being particles smaller than erythrocytes, which can therefore pass through the capillary bed.[1,2]

Experimental work by Coleman et al. revealed very little evidence of micropulverization with the majority of the particles being larger than the red cells ranging in size from a few micrometers up to 2cm.[4] The composition of the sediment collected was blood, calcific particles, hyalinized and fibrotic fragments and crystalloid material derived from the fragmented arteriosclerotic plaque.[4] The composition of this sediment varied depending on the structure of the plaque. In soft plaque, the sediment showed a background of predominant fibrous dust and cellular debris smaller than 1mm. Also present were large strips of fibrous and fibrolipoid material measuring from 10 to 2000 μm. In complex calcified plaque, the sediment showed calcified globules varying in size from 10 to 120 μm with strips of hyalinized and fibrous material varying in lengths from 50 to 800 μm.

Sections of the arterial wall showed residual atherosclerotic material in the intima in all cases. When severe circumferential calcifications were present in the intima and media, the arterial wall showed circumferential separation along the intimal-medial border. If the calcification involved only a portion of the arterial wall, the separation was only partial, adjacent to the calcified area.[4]

Using an in vitro model, Schmitz–Rode and Günther[5] put to test the different hypotheses covering the catheter's mode of action and concluded the following:

1. Self-centering of the catheter tip does not occur, because the force that the jets and the vortex exert on the vessel wall is not strong enough to achieve a coaxial placement of the tip in the lumen, even when the catheter is operated at its maximum rotation speed and injection rate. Nor is there dilatation of the vessel lumen around the catheter tip during catheter activation.
2. The existence of a vortex was confirmed, corroborating Kensey's assumption of recirculation and repeated exposure of the particles to the rotating cam.[1,2] Repeated fragmentation does indeed occur. In smaller tubular compartments, the space between the catheter and the wall was too small to allow proper development of the vortex. This was particularly true when reaching the level of the obstruction. It was concluded that with use of an alternating to-and-fro motion on the tip, a vortex can develop during catheter withdrawal.[5]
3. Pulverization of atheromatous calcified plaque showed a close relationship with the rotational speed and the forward force applied. In general, the lower the forward force applied and the higher the speed, the smaller the particles produced with particle size found between 10 and 20 μm, with the largest particles observed being more commonly around 90 μm. The duration of exposure to fragmentation by the tip did

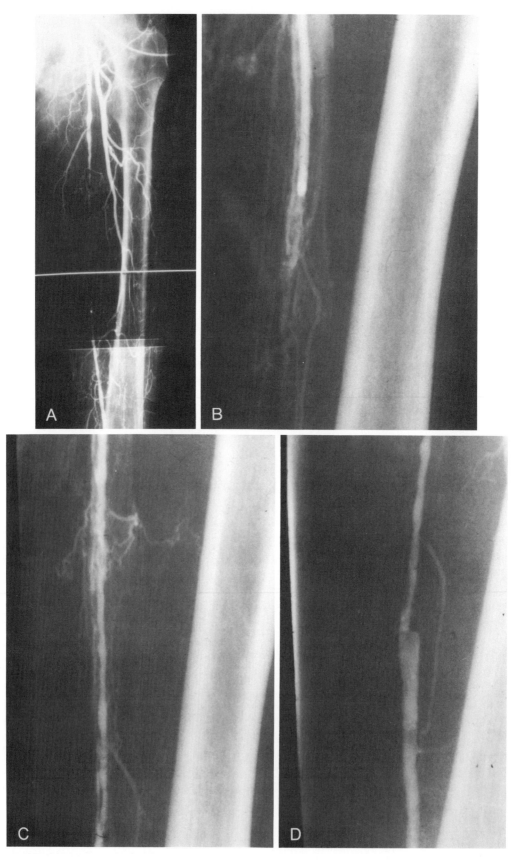

Figure 6.4.14. **A.** Complete occlusion of the superficial femoral artery with distal reconstitution of the adductor canal. **B.** During rotation of the cam, infusion of diluted contrast medium with urokinase and heparin produces intravasation of contrast medium into the wall of the vessel. **C.** Immediately after successful recanalization of occluded segment, note the irregularity of the arterial wall and persistent intravasation of contrast medium. **D.** Follow-up arteriogram 24 hours postrecanalization. Observe the irregular lumen created by the catheter and the difference in size between the recanalized lumen and the lumen of the femoral artery beyond this area of recanalization.

did not influence the particle size for atheromatous material, whereas for thrombi, particle size was reduced significantly by increased duration of exposure. There was no difference in particle size between soft, hard, or calcified plaque. The presence of tissue strips was also confirmed occasionally.[5]

Schmitz–Rode and Günther concluded that the catheter was not suitable for heavily calcified occlusions, and, because of the size of the particles, the risk of embolization needs to be considered, particularly in patients with poor distal run-off.[5]

These findings were also corroborated by Gehani who stressed again the importance of higher rotation speeds to decrease particle size.[6]

RESULTS

Wholey et al., in their initial report, described a 91% technical success but a dismal 25% clinical success rate, with four early reocclusions requiring amputation. Another patient had an amputation as a consequence of distal embolization.[3]

In a review of a combined group of patients from the United States and Europe, Miller grouped the patients in three categories:

A. Nonocclusive 1–5cm stenosis;
B. Longer than 5cm stenosis or occlusion;
C. Limb salvage patients.

Under six months' follow-up, the clinical success was 71% (A), 55% (B), and 44% (C). Technical success was 100% for stenosis and 74% for occlusions.[7]

Rees reported a technical success on 19 patients of 74% with a clinical success at one month of 67%. In 8 of 14 patients followed up with angiography at one year, the patency rate is 75% with unchanged ankle-brachial index.[8] Angioscopy demonstrated that the procedure causes multiple intimal flaps and an irregular neo-lumen with multiple loose atheromatous particles present at the end of the procedure.[8]

In Desbrosses et al.'s experience with 51 vascular occlusions, a technical success of 88% was achieved. The technical failures (12%) included two failures to cross the lesion and four vascular perforations of no clinical consequence. All failures occurred in highly calcified lesions. Early reocclusion occurred in 12% within 48 hours; there were three distal embolizations, two of them asymptomatic into the posterior tibial and one in the popliteal artery requiring a balloon embolectomy. The follow-up at 6 months showed a patency rate of 64% and at 12 months of 63%.[9]

The largest series of patients by one institution so far is that of Overlie et al. with 157 lesions treated on 113 patients. A technical success occurred in 75% of the lesions. Follow-up ranged from 0 to 28 months with a mean of 3.5 months. Overall complication included perforations in 12%, thrombosis in 2%, and distal emboli in 0.1%. They concluded that dynamic angioplasty could successfully recanalize total obstructions with acceptably low complication rates.[10]

In summary, 337 lesions have been treated, most of them occlusions with a technical success varying from 74 to 91%, a clinical success varying from 25 to 75% with the longest follow-up reported being 12 months. Complications include vascular perforations with an incidence from 4 to 12% and five distal embolizations.[1,3,7–10] Only one of these was catastrophic requiring an amputation above the knee.[3]

A final judgment is still out on this procedure that requires expert angiographic skills and a careful evaluation of the patient vascular bed before embarking on it. Considering the type of patients initially subjected to this treatment, the technical and clinical success reported are reasonable. With better selection of patients and improvements on technology soon to be introduced, including an over-the-wire catheter system and bigger rotating cams to provide a larger vascular lumen avoiding therefore the need to perform an adjunct angioplasty, better success rates and long-term results might be expected.

References

1. Kensey K, Nash J, Abrahams C, Zarins CK: Recanalization of obstructive arteries with a flexible, rotating tip catheter. *Radiology* 1987;165:387–389
2. Kensey K: Percutaneous atherectomy: Kensey catheter, technical description, in Castañeda–Zúñiga WR, Maynar M, Joffre F, Zollikofer C (eds): *Percutaneous Revascularization Techniques.* New York, Thieme, 1991
3. Wholey MH, Smith JA, Godlewski P, Nagurka M: Recanalization of total arterial occlusions with the Kensey dynamic angioplasty catheter. *Radiology* 1989;172:95–98
4. Coleman CC, Posalaky IP, Robinson JD, Payne WD, Vlodaver ZA, Amplatz A: Atheroablation with the Kensey catheter: a pathologic study. *Radiology* 1989;170:391–394
5. Schmitz–Rode T, Günther RW: Functional properties of the Kensey arterial recanalization catheter. *Invest Radiol* 1990;25:631–637
6. Gehani AA, Ashley S, Brooks SG, Stoodley K, Ball SG, Rees MR: Particles resulting from the interaction of Kensey catheter with atheromatous plaque. Presented at RIPCV 2nd International Congress, Toulouse, France, Feb 1990
7. Miller FJ: Initial European and United States experience with the Kensey catheter. Presented at the Second Annual International Symposium on Peripheral Vascular Intervention. Miami, Florida, Jan 1990
8. Rees MR, Gehani AA, Ashley S, Thorley P, Shierd K, Brooks SG, Kesten RC: Dynamic angioplasty of total occlusions using Kensey catheter. Interim analysis of results. Presented at RIPCV 2nd International Congress. Toulouse, France, Feb 1990
9. Desbrosses D, Petit H, Barrconveno D, Wenger JJ, Kieny R: Balloon assisted rotational angioplasty with catheter or Kensey in femoropopliteal occlusions. Presented at RIPCV 2nd International Congress, Toulouse, France, Feb 1990.
10. Overlie PA, Snyder SO, Wheeler JR, Matthews OA, Krajcer Z, Siragusa V, Wilbur N, Avila MH: The Kensey catheter: a mechanical recanalization device; its use in 113 patients with 157 lesions in the peripheral circulation. Presented at the American Heart Association 63rd Scientific Sessions. Dallas, TX, Nov 1990

Part 5. Pfeifer Milling Catheter

—Wilfrido R. Castañeda–Zúñiga, M.D., M.Sc.

A modification of the Kensey catheter rotating cam was used to improve performance.

According to the authors, ideally, milling performance should be smaller in the center and orthogonal to the rotational axis at the circumference. During catheter rotation, the highest circumferential speed of a hemispheric tip surface appears at the outer radius, while the velocity at the center is equal to zero. In their design, the rotating cam is a parabolic circular disk inserted vertically into a hemispheric catheter tip and rising slightly above its surface rather than at the outer radius[1] (Figure 6.5.1).

As with the Trac-Wright catheter, the main disadvantage of this device is the limited diameter of the recanalized channel. Milling catheters of different diameters for intraoperative use are available.[1] Experience with this technique is limited. The device has only been used in Europe and is not in use in the United States.

Reference

1. Pfeifer KJ, Baumgart R, Steckmeier B, Huber RM: New mechanical devices: technical modification of the Kensey rotator in Zeitler E, Seyferth W (eds): *Pros and Cons in PTA and Axillary Methods.* Berlin, Springer-Verlag, 1989, pp 221–223

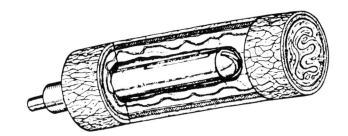

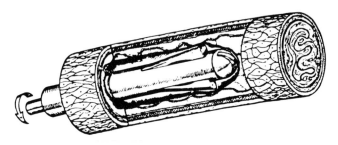

Figure 6.5.1. Milling catheter tip with variable head diameter. (Reproduced from Pfeifer KJ, Baumgart R, Steckmeier B, et al: New mechanical devices: technical modification of the Kensey rotator, in Zeitler E, Seyferth W (eds): *Pros and Cons in PTA and Axillary Methods.* Berlin, Springer-Verlag, 1989, pp 221–223.)

Part 6. Auth Rotational Atherectomy

—Patricia E. Thorpe, M.D.

INTRODUCTION

In 1987 Hansen described a high-speed, over-the-wire rotary atherectomy catheter that offered the potential for restoring patency of occluded vessels by "boring out" the atheromatous lesion and leaving a smooth, polished intraluminal surface with no intimal flaps.[1]

Multicenter clinical trials for peripheral use of the Auth Rotablator began in 1987 and continued through early 1990. To date, approximately 250 peripheral cases have been performed. Collective data submitted for FDA evaluation resulted in commercial availability of the device in November 1990.

TECHNICAL DESCRIPTION

The device consists of an elliptical rotating abrasive tip varying in diameter from 1.5 to 6.0mm. The front half of the brass burr is covered with more than 1000 microscopic diamond chips (Fig. 6.6.1). The tip is rotated by a flexible helical drive shaft at 180,000 rpm. Driven by an air turbine that is housed in a plastic casing, the drive shaft is housed in a 4Fr Teflon sheath. The only rotating part that is exposed to the vessel wall is the anterior aspect of the abrasive tip (Fig. 6.6.2A). The revolutions/min are controlled by the air pressure within the system. The compressed air pressure is controlled by a dial on the control panel. The turbine also pumps sterile saline into the plastic sheath to lubricate and cool the rotating drive shaft and burr. A 0.009-inch guidewire with a platinum tip helps to maintain the intraluminal position of the burr during rotations (Fig. 6.6.2B). The guidewire is lodged in the central hollow channel of the rotary ablation catheter. The guidewire is fixed in a stationary position during rotation of the drive shaft but can remain in position following withdrawal of the device.

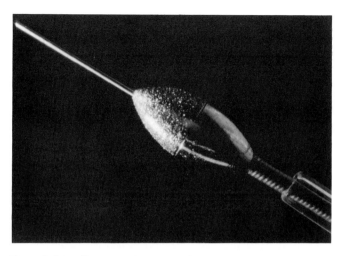

Figure 6.6.1. Close-up enlargement of the Rotablator burr as it tracks over its 0.009-inch guidewire. Hundreds of microscopic chips are embedded in the burr. When the burr rotates, each chip scoops out a microscopic amount of plaque.

MECHANISM OF ACTION

Ablation of atheromatous plaque is achieved by cleaving small divots of atheromatous/thrombotic material from the exposed surface by the elliptical burr spinning at 180,000 rpm, providing a surface speed of approximately 25msec.[2] At this speed, the diamond chips embedded on the surface of the burr can create millions of microscopic divots per second. An inherent advantage of this technique is that, because the particles are typically only around $2\mu m$ in diameter, the lumen created is extremely smooth, appearing at angioscopy as a polished surface without intimal flaps.[2]

The average length of time for passage of the device through a lesion relates to the degree of calcification, the length of lesion, and operator experience. In this series, focal, shorter lesions in the SFA averaged less than three minutes per application; longer lesions averaged five to eight minutes.

PRINCIPLE OF DIFFERENTIAL CUTTING

The strength of the Rotablator design is its cutting mechanism based on the principle of differential cutting. The diamond grinding elements take advantage of the non-elastic nature of atherosclerotic plaque.[2] The Rotablator diamond-covered surface removes fibrous, calcified and fatty atheromatous tissue which is nonelastic, sparing the elastic muscular tissue of the arterial wall (Fig. 6.6.3). The design of the Rotablator specifically addresses the pathology of the organized, calcified lesions. The mechanism of differential cutting preferentially ablates the harder non-elastic atherosclerotic material without affecting the normal intima and media and may, thereby, contribute to a decreased incidence of restenosis.[2]

The Rotablator does not stretch the arterial wall or displace plaque. It removes the plaque in millions of tiny particles which are deposited in the reticuloendothelial system. The abrasive tip creates a channel with a smooth surface as long as the cutting burr can track without undue force (Fig. 6.6.4A). Barotrauma associated with balloon inflation is thereby eliminated (Fig. 6.6.4B). This should result in fewer intimal dissections and prevent subintimal tracking. With respect to small vessels, such as those below the knee, the removal of plaque with this method decreases wall trauma and the elastic recoil associated with balloon angioplasty and, therefore, minimizes the incidence of abrupt closure and thrombosis postrecanalization.

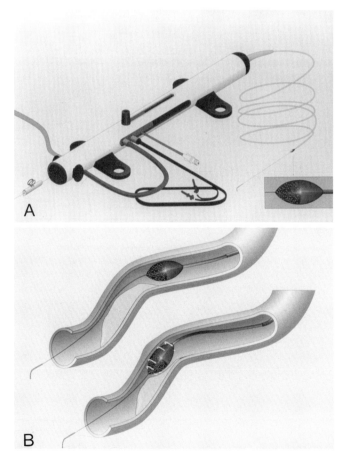

Figure 6.6.2. **A.** The Rotablator system showing the burr advancer unit, guidewire, sheath, and burr. Not shown is a small console used to control and monitor the burr revolutions/min and an air source. **B.** 0.009-inch guidewire lodged in the central hollow channel helps maintain intraluminal position of the burr during rotations.

PARTICLE SIZE

In vitro and in vivo studies have shown that the average particle size is $2\mu m$ and 90% of the particles produced are under $8\mu m$; 5% are from eight to $40\mu m$ and 5% are 40–$250\mu m$.[3,4] The size of the particles is determined by the diameter, speed, and forward pressure applied to the

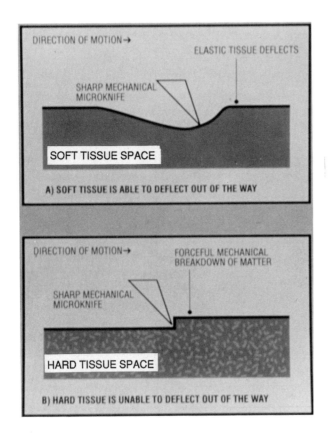

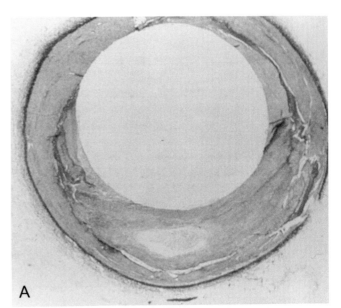

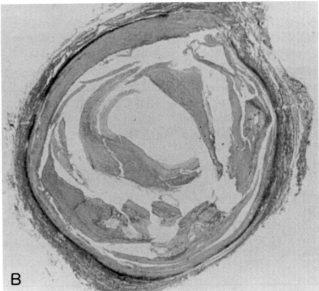

Figure 6.6.3. The Rotablator operates on the principle of differential cutting, like a cast saw. It rapidly removes inelastic plaque whether it is calcified, fibrous, or fatty. The normal vessel wall, being elastic, moves away from the rotating burr. This schematic shows how the Rotablator treats eccentric plaque in the bend of an artery. Animal and clinical studies have shown that the plaque is ablated to particles much smaller than a red blood cell. These pass out of the body via the reticulo-endothelial system.

advancing burr. The degree of fragmentation can, therefore, be changed by adjusting the size of the burr, the speed of travel across the surface, and the pressure of application.[5]

Ahn et al. demonstrated occasional disruption of internal elastic fibers, but the outer elastic fibers of the media and adventitia were intact. Scanning electron microscopy confirmed the presence of a smooth, polished surface. The junction of the treated with the nontreated segments was smooth and tapered.[6]

In vivo studies on humans demonstrated partial removal of fibrous or calcified plaque with the abraded surface being smooth and free of thrombus. The endothelium on the adjacent normal vessel wall disappeared. There was no damage to the media or adventitia and no perforations. Dehiscence of the intima and media and surface irregularities were seen when the device was used at speeds below 75,000 rpm.[7]

MATERIALS AND METHODS

During the early clinical trials, the patients referred for treatment were those with severe or "end-stage" periph-

Figure 6.6.4. A. Photomicrograph of vessel cross-section following treatment with the Rotablator. Note the smooth, polished surface. **B.** Photomicrograph of vessel cross-section following balloon angioplasty showing a rough intraluminal surface with multiple flaps.

eral vascular disease (Tables 6.6.1–6.6.3). A total of 37 patients were included in the trials. The device was used for symptomatic stenosis or occlusions in a total of 44 procedures, including 49 infrainguinal sites and two iliac lesions.

Table 6.6.1. Patient Demographics

Number of patients	37
Number of cases	44
Number of lesions	51
Males	25
Females	12
Mean age	67
Patients with at least one prior vascular procedure	21

Table 6.6.2. Patient Profile in Successful Procedures (24 Cases/24 Patients)[a]

Patient Number	Sex	Age	Previous Vascular Sx	Diabetic	Smoker	HPTN	Rest Pain	Ulcer	Gangrene
1	F	50	+	+	−	+	−	+	−
2	F	82	+	−	−	+	+	−	−
3[b]	F	80	+	−	−	+	−	+	−
5	M	71	+	−	−	+	−	−	−
6[b]	M	79	+	−	−	+	+	−	−
9[b]	F	73	−	−	+	+	−	−	−
11	M	62	−	−	−	+	−	−	−
15	F	67	−	+	−	−	+	+	−
16[b]	M	54	+	+	−	−	+	+	−
19	M	53	−	−	−	+	+	+	−
21	M	71	+	−	+	−	−	−	−
22	M	68	+	−	+	+	−	−	−
23	M	69	−	−	−	+	+	−	−
24	M	73	−	+	−	−	−	−	+
25	M	52	−	−	+	+	−	−	−
28	M	48	+	−	−	−	+	+	+
29	M	72	−	+	+	−	−	−	−
30	M	66	−	−	+	−	−	−	−
32	F	56	−	−	−	+	−	+	−
33	F	79	+	+	−	−	−	+	+
34	M	48	−	−	−	−	−	+	+
35	F	46	+	+	−	+	+	−	−
37	F	64	−	−	−	−	−	−	−
			11/24 (46%)	8/24 (33%)	6/24 (25%)	14/24 (58%)	9/24 (37.5%)	9/24 (37.5%)	4/24 (17%)

[a]Mean age all patients = 67.95 M = 16; male mean age = 67.38. F = 8; female mean age = 69.28.
[b]Repeat procedure.

Among the 44 procedures, 37 were performed on a single lower extremity, three patients had bilateral disease, and four procedures were performed on a patient who returned for a second atherectomy. In this instance, two patients had recurrent symptoms related to a new lesion and two patients became symptomatic from restenosis at the original atherectomy site. Indication for the procedure was significant claudication in 22 (59%), severe claudication (less than 100 feet) in 4 (11%) and rest pain/limb threat in 11 (30%) patients. Preprocedural evaluation for applications of the device indicated 24 patients to be favorable and 13 unfavorable or poor candidates for conven-

Table 6.6.3. Patient Profile in Procedure Failures (16 Cases/16 Patients)[a]

Patient Number	Sex	Age	Previous Vascular Sx	Diabetic	Smoker	HPTN	Rest Pain	Ulcer	Gangrene
5	M	71	+	−	−	+	−	−	−
4	M	56	+	+	+	+	−	+	−
8	F	64	−	−	−	−	−	−	−
10	F	67	+	−	−	+	−	+	−
12	M	43	−	−	+	+	−	+	−
13	M	61	−	+	+	+	−	−	+
14	M	85	+	−	−	−	+	−	−
17	M	64	+	−	−	+	−	−	−
18	F	63	+	−	+	+	−	−	−
20	M	53	+	+	+	−	−	−	−
21	M	71	+	−	+	−	−	−	−
26	M	74	−	−	−	+	+	−	−
27	F	70	−	−	−	+	−	−	−
31	M	64	+	−	−	+	−	−	−
35	M	65	+	+	−	−	+	+	−
36	M	69	−	+	−	+	−	+	+
			10/16 (63%)	5/16 (31%)	6/16 (37.5%)	11/16 (69%)	3/16 (19%)	5/16 (31%)	2/16 (12.5%)

[a]Mean age all patients = 65. M = 12; male mean age = 64.56. F = 4; female mean age = 66.

tional surgical bypass. Baseline evaluation should be complete with noninvasive studies and adequate diagnostic angiography. Follow-up data needed in order to evaluate the efficacy of the device and the procedure include 24-hour noninvasive examination, including pressure recordings and waveform analysis. As most people will not consent to follow-up angiography, particularly if they are clinically improved, it is imperative to obtain follow-up noninvasive studies at 1-, 3-, 5-, and 12-month intervals during the initial postatherectomy period. This enables the physician to monitor the patient's recovery and diagnose new lesions or restenosis.

The greatest proportion of the lesions treated were in the distal superficial femoral artery (SFA) (21 lesions, 41%) (guidewire access not possible in two SFA cases). The next largest group of arterial lesions occurred below the knee in trifurcation vessels (14 lesions, 27%). The remaining 14 lesions occurred in the popliteal artery (12 lesions, 23%) and one each in the profunda femoris and iliac arteries. A retrograde approach was used in seven patients for contralateral procedure in five patients with profunda femoris and proximal superficial femoral disease. By far, the majority of procedures were performed with an antegrade approach in the ipsilateral superficial femoral artery (86%). A slightly larger number of lesions represented occlusions[3] versus stenosis.[8]

Adjunctive angioplasty was equally distributed among patients who had a successful or unsuccessful procedure. Adjunctive balloon dilatation was performed in 21 (48%) patients overall. In 19 cases, PTA was performed following initial atherectomy, and in three cases the balloon was used before atherectomy. The percentage of adjunctive PTA procedures reflects the fact that the small ablative burr size used (1.5–3.0mm) created a pilot lumen with insufficient reduction of plaque bulk to yield a good angiographic or hemodynamic result. As such, adjunctive balloon dilatation was necessary to increase the arterial lumen. In two procedures, balloon dilatation was equal to "balloon rescue" in that a suboptimal result with the device was converted to a good clinical result with adjunctive balloon angioplasty.

TECHNIQUE

Following diagnostic angiography, one selects the most advantageous approach to the lesion or lesions based on the following considerations: An antegrade puncture is favored over a retrograde contralateral approach. A retrograde approach is suitable for an iliac lesion. Antegrade superficial femoral punctures are more difficult when the patient is obese. If the angle of entry into the vessel is too acute, it is difficult to advance the atherectomy device as well as balloon catheters. Therefore, in obese patients, a combined procedure with a vascular surgeon should be considered. Surgical exposure of the vessel is also recommended when using 14Fr sheaths required for introduction of the 4.5–6mm Rotablator burr.

Systemic administration of 10,000 units of heparin during procedures requiring large sheaths minimizes acute thrombosis. After placement of the appropriate size sheath, with a check flow valve to prevent leak of blood around guidewires and catheters, an 8Fr guiding catheter is introduced over a 0.035-inch Terumo or Bentson guidewire. A Tuohy–Borst adaptor is placed on the end of the guiding catheter. This enables intermittent contrast injection for fluoroscopic visualization. A 5Fr straight end-hole catheter is then advanced over the guidewire to the proximal aspect of the lesion (Fig. 6.6.5A). At this point, the guidewire is manipulated in order to pass through the residual lumen. Frequently, this lumen is not visible angiographically until the guidewire has passed through the lesion. The guidewire should not be forced but turned gently in multiple directions in order to seek the residual lumen. If the lumen cannot be found, 50,000 IU of urokinase can be administered directly into the proximal aspect of the lesion. It is helpful to place the tip of the 5Fr catheter within the superior aspect of the lesion to prevent flow of urokinase into collateral vessels which are generally located near this point. One may repeat the bolus of urokinase several times, if necessary, to partially remove the chronic thrombus. If necessary, a 20-minute infusion of urokinase (250,000 IU in 50ml of D5W) can be administered. Generally, this combination of guidewire manipulation and thrombolytic therapy is sufficient to allow passage of the guidewire across the occlusion. In the case of high-grade stenosis, careful manipulation with a torque-controlled guidewire and the 5Fr catheter positioned at the proximal aspect of the lesion is commonly sufficient to traverse the area of narrowing.

Once the guidewire has crossed the lesion, the 5Fr end-hole catheter is advanced distally. Ideally, one positions the distal aspect of the guidewire approximately 5–10cm below the inferior aspect of the lesion. The 8Fr guiding catheter remains above the lesion as the coaxial 5Fr catheter predilates the stenosis or occlusion.

With the guiding catheter positioned proximal to the occlusion and the 5Fr catheter traversing the lesion, the access guidewire is exchanged for the 0.009-inch exchange length guidewire which accompanies the Rotablator device. This guidewire is positioned across the lesion and the 5Fr end-hole catheter is removed. The Rotablator device is then loaded onto the guidewire and advanced through the sheath and guiding catheter to the proximal aspect of the lesion (Fig. 6.6.5B). When the burr size of the Rotablator exits the 8Fr guiding catheter, the Rotablator guidewire is sufficient to stabilize the Rotablator device during atheroablation.

Operation of the Rotablator is conducted with the foot pedal for control of the revolutions/min and saline irrigation. Visual guidance is with fluoroscopy. The audio feedback from the device passing through the lesion is helpful. Calcified lesions result in a high-pitch tone as the Rotablator ablates the lesion. Softer organized thrombus gives a lower pitched tone. The device is moved slowly but evenly

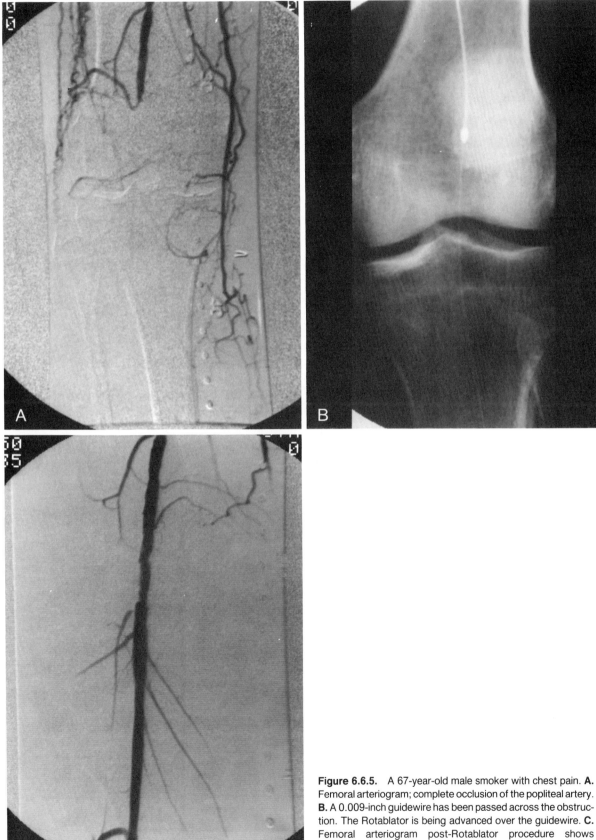

Figure 6.6.5. A 67-year-old male smoker with chest pain. **A.** Femoral arteriogram; complete occlusion of the popliteal artery. **B.** A 0.009-inch guidewire has been passed across the obstruction. The Rotablator is being advanced over the guidewire. **C.** Femoral arteriogram post-Rotablator procedure shows increased diameter at site of atheroablation with a residual stenosis of 20–30%.

through the lesion. When calcified material is encountered, the Rotablator should be used in a pulsed fashion. The Rotablator is advanced while the driveshaft is rotating. The motor is stopped and the catheter is retracted several millimeters and advanced again in a similar fashion. Heavily calcified lesions require longer periods for successful atheroablation. Constant normal saline drip irrigation accompanies application.

Selection of burr size is similar to selection of balloon size. The width of the vessel is measured above and below the lesion. Magnification should be taken into account for vessels below the knee. Larger vessels such as the distal superficial femoral artery and mid-superficial femoral can be sized without calculating the magnification factor of 20%. Additionally, after the initial successful passage of the first burr, the diameter of the abrasive tip can be increased

until the stenosis or occlusion is reduced to less than 30% narrowing of the normal arterial lumen (Fig. 6.6.6). During Rotablator exchanges, the system guidewire remains in place.

Once the Rotablator has crossed the stenosis or occlusion, the device can be removed, leaving the guidewire in place. It is not necessary to repeat the atherectomy, as the maximum diameter is achieved during the initial passage. Through the guiding catheter, contrast can be injected to evaluate the results of atheroablation with digital imaging (Fig. 6.6.5C). If a guiding catheter is not in place, contrast can be injected through the sheath side port or a 5Fr endhole catheter can be reintroduced into the superficial femoral artery. However, a Tuohy–Borst adaptor is required in order to keep the guidewire in place across the lesion.

Adjunctive balloon angioplasty can be performed at this

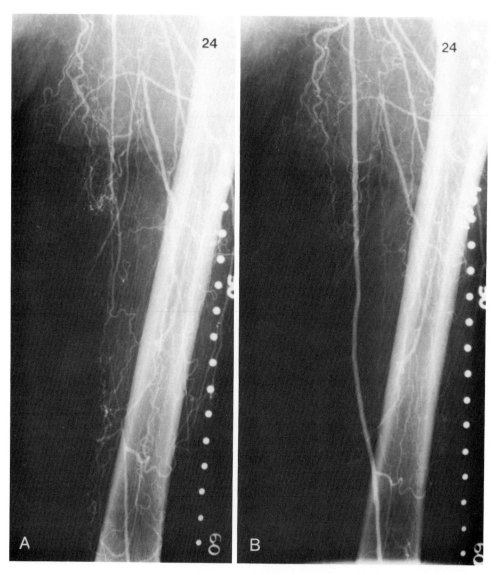

Figure 6.6.6. An 80-year-old female with previous fracture and non-healing ulcer of left foot. **A.** Femoral arteriogram reveals diffuse, severe atherosclerotic changes with areas of subtotal occlusion in the proximal SFA. **B.** Femoral arteriogram following Rotablator procedure. Note the significant increase in diameter of the entire superficial femoral artery.

point by advancing a balloon catheter over the Rotablator guidewire. It is also possible to position the 5Fr end-hole catheter across the lesion and exchange the 0.009-inch Rotablator guidewire for an exchange-length guidewire of larger caliber to perform the balloon angioplasty. If an optimal burr size has been used and the intravascular lumen is adequate, with less than 20% residual stenosis, additional balloon angioplasty is not indicated.

If distal spasm occurs, intra-arterial nitroglycerin may be administered to reverse the spasm. If thrombus develops at the atherectomy site, direct infusion of 50,000–250,000 units of urokinase is sufficient to restore flow, if not totally lyse the thrombus. At this point, a digital angiographic examination is important to exclude any evidence of intimal flap or subintimal dissection which could cause reocclusion if it is not treated with additional atherectomy or balloon angioplasty. An intimal flap can be removed with the Simpson atherectomy device or repositioned favorably with balloon dilatation.

Following digital assessment of the angiographic result, the guidewires and catheters are removed through the sheath. If the procedure has been performed percutaneously, the sheath is then removed and manual pressure is applied at the groin for hemostasis. Distal pulses are immediately recorded by palpation or Doppler to have a baseline evaluation following atherectomy.

If the procedure has been performed with surgical exposure of the proximal superficial femoral artery, the sheath is removed after placement of a purse-string suture. This prevents any need to cross-clamp the vessel and occlude flow during the vessel closure.

Heparinization should be maintained with partial thrombin time (PTT) between 50 and 90 seconds. Heparinization is recommended if the atherectomy has been performed in a small (<3mm) vessel. Before and after the procedure, the patient is given one coated aspirin per day. Other antiplatelet medications are not routinely used.

RESULTS

When evaluating a new device, one has to separate the device performance from the overall procedure. We have chosen to analyze the results in the following categories (Table 6.6.4):

1. Procedure success, device success;
2. Procedure success, device failure;
3. Procedure failure, device success;
4. Procedure failure, device failure.

The definition of procedure success is immediate angiographic and hemodynamic success, as indicated by greater than 0.15 increase in ankle-brachial index (ABI) or newly palpable foot pulses as well as less than 20% residual angiographic stenosis. These circumstances should persist greater than 24 hours for overall procedure success. Thrombosis occurring within 24 hours was deemed pro-

cedure failure even if the exact cause of failure was not determined. Device success is defined as ability to pass the Rotablator through the stenosis or occlusion without resulting in perforation, spasm or thrombosis which caused compromise of the clinical outcome. Device failure is defined as inability to pass the Rotablator through the lesion or the occurrence of subintimal dissection, perforation or associated spasm with device application. Procedure failure was recorded in all cases in which clinical decline occurred in the immediate procedure or within 24 hours following atherectomy (Table 6.6.5). Loss of pulse and ischemic changes characterize the majority of the failures. However, procedure failure was also related to significant subintimal flaps created at the time of sheath insertion in the operating room in three patients requiring conversion of an atherectomy into a surgical procedure for a bypass or surgical repair at the site of injury (Table 6.6.6).

In the Stanford clinical trials, two patients could not undergo Rotablator atherectomy because of initial failure of the guidewire to cross the lesion. Therefore, of the 42 procedures in which the Rotablator was introduced into the vessel for atherectomy, a total of 35 procedures (83.3%) were initially successful in terms of the device performance (Tables 6.6.7 and 6.6.8). However, in seven of these procedures, although the Rotablator action was successful, the procedure failed due to technical complications. In only 12% of the procedures did the device fail to cross the lesion. Analysis shows that subintimal position of the guidewire was responsible for inability to successfully perform the atherectomy. In two procedures, the device incompletely traversed the lesion, but balloon angioplasty was performed and a good clinical outcome was achieved. The majority of the cases in which device success was achieved were superficial femoral lesions. In patients in whom initial device failure occurred, 75% of the lesions were below the knee (Table 6.6.9). Thirty-seven percent of these patients had tandem lesions (Fig. 6.6.7). Nineteen percent of the lesions were greater than 7cm and 81% of these lesions were less than 7cm. Thus, as with balloon angioplasty, lesions below the knee represent a high-risk group for revascularization and successful outcome. Initial technical success related to occlusion versus stenosis shows that 79% of occlusions and 88% of stenoses were successfully traversed by the Rotablator. Analysis of the cases in which the Rotablator failed to traverse the lesion shows that a subintimal position of the guidewire, as mentioned above, was the primary reason for device failure. Among patients who had successful atherectomy with the Rotablator but subsequently experienced clinical failure, the main complication was related to subintimal dissection, subsequent thrombosis or sheath flap (Table 6.6.10). In the future, the incidence of subintimal dissection may be reduced with adjunctive preprocedure thrombolytic therapy (which can convert occlusions to high-grade stenoses) and the use of tapered steerable platinum-tipped guidewires. Technical complications resulting in procedure fail-

Table 6.6.4. Immediate Device Success (24 Patients/30 Sites/28 Procedures)[a]

Patient Number	Site	Length (cm)	% Stenosis	Pre-ABI	Post-ABI	0–12 Months FU ABI	1 Year Patency Clinical Status
1	R SFA	3	100	–	0.73	0.73	Improved/deceased
2	R SFA	3	100	0.47	0.75	0.83	Improved/mild claudication
3	L Pop	3	100	0.37	0.86	0.50	Restenosis/redo
5	L Pop/PT	5	100	0.65	0.86	–	Improved/deceased
6	R SFA	2	95	0.56	0.72	0.42	Restenosis/redo/deceased
	R SFA	4	100	0.41	–	0.32	
7	L Pop	3	95	0.56	–	–	Worse/deceased (PF disease)
8	L Tib/Per	3	99	–	–	–	Improved/deceased
9	L SFA	30	99	0.34	0.41	0.24	Restenosis/redo
11	L SFA	30	100	0.53	–	1.0	Improved
15	L SFA	15	100	0.38	0.55	0.39	Improved/mild claudication
16	R PF	2	90	0.31	0.90	0.58	Worse/new lesion/PF OK
19	R SFA	20	70	–	–	–	Improved
21	R SFA	7	100	0.71	0.71	0.96	Improved/no claudication
22	R SFA	20	90	0.37	0.68	0.55	Improved/no claudication
23	R SFA	10	100	–	0.91	0.96	Improved
24	L Pop	2	95	0.45	0.65	–	Improved initially/BKA 6 mo
25	R Pop	4	100	0.65	–	0.56	Improved
28	R SFA	13	100	0.56	0.72	0.36	Restenosis
29	L Pop/AT	10	100	0.45	0.65	–	Improved
30	R Pop	4	100	0.26	0.39	0.25	Stable
32	R SFA	5	100	–	0.52	0.71	Improved
33	L AT	2	100	–	–	–	Improved initially/BKA 6 mo
34	L SFA	1	99	–	0.83	0.96	Improved
37	L SFA	5	100	–	–	–	Improved/no claudication
3[b] RS[c]	L Pop	5	100	–	–	–	Improved
6[b] RS[c]	R Per	2	100	0.42	0.60	–	Improved
9[b] RS[b]	L SFA	20	99	–	–	–	Improved
16[b] New	R Pop	2	95	0.58	0.70	0.75	Improved

[a]FU = follow-up; PF = profunda femoris; BKA = below knee amputation.
[b]Redo.
[c]Restenosis.

Table 6.6.5. Procedure Failure (19 Sites/16 Patients/16 Procedures/3 Multiple Lesions)

Patient Number	Site	Length (cm)	% Stenosis	Pre-ABI	Post-ABI	FU ABI	Outcome
5[a]	R PT	3	99	0.57	–	–	Subintimal; balloon rescue
4[b]	R AT	2	100	0.56	0.81	–	Below knee amputation
8[c]	R SFA	3	100	–	–	–	No change
10[b]	R Per	3	90	0.65	0.89	–	Sheath flap
	R SFA	10	90	–	–	–	
12[b]	R SFA	4	100	0.81	0.49	–	Graft
13	L Per/AT	4	100	–	–	–	Graft
	L Per	2	100	–	0.48	–	
14[a]	L Per	1	90	0.43	–	–	Below knee amputation
17[a]	R Iliac	10	100	–	–	–	Aorto-femoral graft
18[b]	R SFA	30	90	–	–	–	Sheath flap
20[a]	R Pop/R Tib	3	100	0.21	0.58	0.93	Subintimal; balloon rescue
21[c]	L SFA	15	100	–	–	–	Graft
26[b]	L SFA	8	100	0.48	0.48	–	Thrombosis <7d, clinically no change
27[b]	L SFA	2	100	0.62	–	–	Sheath flap
31[b]	R SFA	20	90	–	–	–	Graft
35[a]	R Per	2	90	–	–	–	Graft
36	R AT	20	90	–	–	–	Graft

[a]6 Rotablator not successful secondary to subintimal guidewire.
[b]7 Rotablator successful but procedure failure.
[c]2 Guidewire not successful.

Table 6.6.6. Rotablator Successful/Procedure Failed

Patient Number	Vessel	Length (cm)	% Stenosis	Problem	Outcome	Comments
4	R AT	20	100	Thrombosis <7d	Vein graft-BKA	Poor runoff/no Coumadin
10	R Tib Per	3	90	Sheath flap	Venous patch	Technical problem
	R SFA	10	90			
12	L SFA	4	100	Thrombosis	Graft	Residual stenosis >20%
18	R SFA	30	90	Sheath flap	Endarterectomy	Technical problem
26	L SFA	8	100	Thrombosis <7d	Clinically no change	Refused new procedure
27	LSFA	2	100	Sheath flap	Graft	Technical problem
31	R SFA	20	90	Thrombosis	Graft	Residual stenosis 40% Distal emboli?

Table 6.6.7. Early Trial Results/Stanford 1987–1989[a]

	Device Success	Device Failure	
Procedure Success	28/42 (67%)	2/42 (5%)	30/42 (72%)
Procedure Failure	7/42 (16%)	5/42 (12%)	12/42 (28%)
Total	35/42 (83%)	7/42 (17%)	

[a]Note that the percent success is slightly lower when using total procedures, not sites, as the denominator.

Table 6.6.8. Device Success: Distribution per Atherectomy Site

Vessel	Success	Failure
SFA[ad]	22	2
POP[b]	9	1
Tibial	5	
PF/Iliac[c]	1	10
Total	37/51 (73%)	14/51 (27%)

[a]Superficial femoral artery.
[b]Popliteal.
[c]Profunda femoris.
[d]Initial guidewire access not successful.

Table 6.6.9. Distribution of Technical PTRA Success[a]

Vessel	Occlusion	Stenosis	Total	
SFA	11[b]/12	11/12	22/24	(92%)
POP	6/7	3/3	9/10	(90%)
TRI	1/5	4/10	5/15	(33%)
PF	0/0	1/1	1/1	(100%)
Iliac	0/1	0/0	0/1	(0%)
Total	18/25 (72%)	19/26 (73%)	37/51 (73%)	

[a]Defined as passage of device across occlusion or stenosis.
[b]Failure of initial guidewire acess

Table 6.6.10. Technical Complications

Distal emboli	1
Known subintimal dissection[a]	4
Sheath-related flaps[b]	3
Perforation	1
Hematoma[b]	2
Thrombosis	4
Spasm	1
Pseudoaneurysm[b]	1
Total	17

[a]Subintimal guidewire.
[b]Not directly related to device.

ure can be addressed by experience and adhering to technical recommendations when placing large sheaths in the superficial femoral artery.

The site of the lesion and the presence or absence of tandem disease, as well as the quality of run-off below the knee are major factors in determining success of atherectomy or angioplasty. In the Stanford series, 23 (42%) of all lesions were in the superficial femoral artery. In the group of immediate technical failures, including procedural complications as well as device failure, 50% of the lesions were located below the knee. However, in the initial success group only 17% of the lesions involved tibial and peroneal vessels, whereas 80% of the lesions were in the superficial femoral and popliteal arteries. If one eliminates the procedures in which technical difficulties caused procedure failure, and only considers the instances in which the Rotablator was unsuccessful or resulted in immediate clinical failure, one notes that 5 of 7 or 71% of these lesions were below the knee. The other two lesions in the Rotablator failure category included one popliteal and one iliac lesion.

In evaluating patients who subsequently had a below-the-knee amputation, within 12 months of atherectomy, one notes that the disease pattern ranged from 1cm focal occlusion to long occlusions and diffuse disease. However, in 4 of 5 (80%), the patient was diabetic or had single vessel run-off. Although the profunda femoris artery was patent and augmented in each of these cases, the atherectomy site

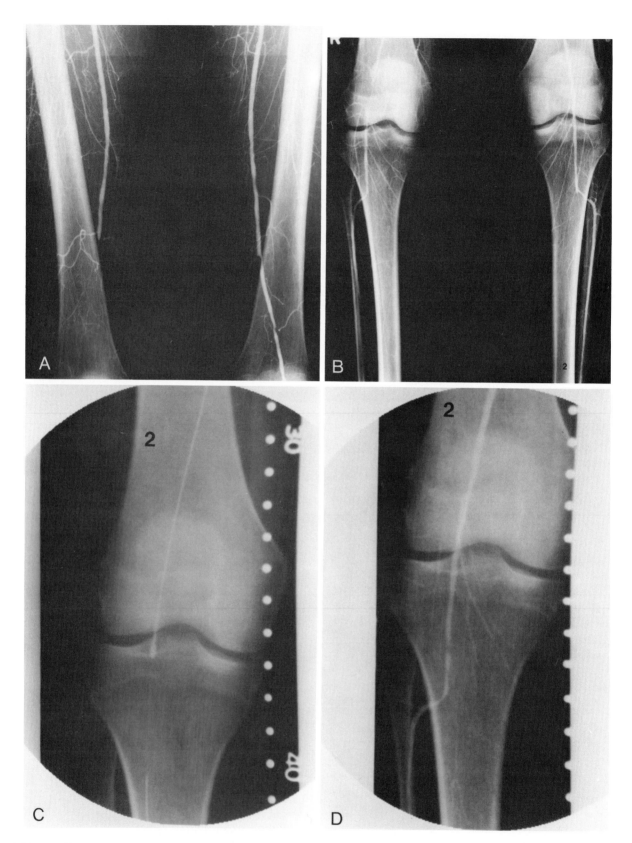

Figure 6.6.7. An 82-year-old female with rest pain. **A.** Femoral arteriogram reveals complete occlusion of the distal superficial femoral artery at the adductor canal level. **B.** Reconstitution of the popliteal artery which shows diffuse narrowing. Note a complete occlusion of the tibioperoneal trunk and a high-grade stenosis of the anterior tibial. **C.** A 0.009-inch guidewire has been placed across the obstruction and the Rotablator is advanced over the stationary guidewire. **D.** Femoral arteriogram shows recanalization of distal superficial femoral artery and residual stenosis of the distal popliteal artery.

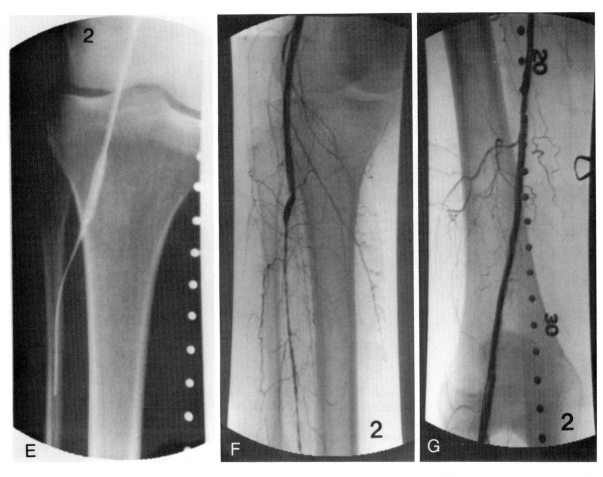

Figure 6.6.7. (*Continued*). **E.** Balloon angioplasty of popliteal and anterior tibial artery lesions. **F.** Follow-up arteriogram reveals adequate increase in diameter at site of angioplasty. **G.** Follow-up arteriogram post- angioplasty of distal superficial femoral artery shows complete luminal reconstitution.

was a tibial or peroneal vessel in four out of six lesions and the SFA and popliteal in a single instance only. Two of these patients had previously undergone a contralateral below-the-knee amputation, and four of these patients presented with nonhealing ulcers. In patients who subsequently underwent below-knee amputations, three of them required amputation immediately after the failed atherectomy procedure. Only two of the patients experienced a successful atherectomy and were able to have an interval of clinical improvement before requiring amputation at a later date. Of these two patients, one had a 2cm, 95% occlusion of the left popliteal artery and the other had a 2cm occlusion of the left tibial artery. However, the presence of advanced disease precluded long-term healing and elimination of ulceration secondary to ischemic changes.

Among the 24 patients who initially had a successful Rotablator procedure, two patients presented within 12 months with restenosis at the original site (Fig. 6.6.8). Two other patients presented with recurrent symptoms and angiographic evidence of new lesions responsible for return of symptoms. In both cases, the previous Rotablator atherectomy site was patent. Overall, follow-up of the successful procedures shows 16 patients clinically improved with continued patency at 12 months. At 24 months, 10

(42%) of the original 24 successful procedures were clinically stable or improved (Table 6.6.11).

Ahn reported results in 68 cadaver arteries with atheromatous lesions involving the superficial femoral, popliteal, and tibial arteries. Obstructive lesions were removed in 36 of 37 stenotic lesions (97%) and 18 of 31 complete occlusions (58%), for an overall efficacy of 79%.[4] Zacca reported success on all six patients attempted, with a residual stenosis of less than 30% of the normal lumen. One hundred percent patency at 3.5 months' mean follow-up was found by Doppler study and clinical evaluation in five patients with eight atherectomized lesions.[6]

Dorros reported success in 85 of 96 lesions (89%), 69 of 77 stenoses, and 16 of 19 occlusions. The arterial obstruction was significantly reduced in stenoses from 85 to 0% and in occlusions from 100 to 15%. Complications included gross hemoglobinuria without sequelae in 40 patients (65%), groin hematoma in 10 (16%), arterial spasm in 12 (20%), arterial perforation in 5 (8%), and need for arterial bypass in 2 patients (3%).[9]

Fourrier reported results in 53 long superficial femoral artery lesions treated with the Rotablator. Thirty-eight were 5–10cm in length, eleven were 10–20cm, and four were longer than 20cm. Overall success was 90.6% (48/

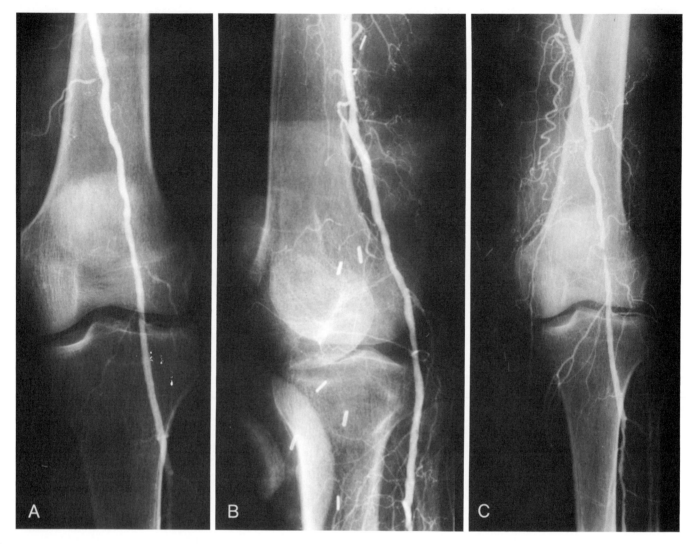

Figure 6.6.8. A 73-year-old male with history of hypertension, smoking, ABI of 0.34 preprocedure. **A,B.** Follow-up arteriogram in AP and oblique views post-Rotablator procedure shows a good result with minimal resid- ual narrowing. **C.** Repeat arteriogram six months post-Rotablator proce- dure because of recurrent claudication reveals high-grade stenosis beyond site of previous Rotablator atheroablation.

Table 6.6.11. Stanford Data: 0–24 Months' Clinical Follow-up after Successful PTRA

Clinical Status	0–6 Months	6–12 Months	12–24 Months
Improved	18 (75%)	15 (62%)	9 (37%)
Worse			
No Angiogram	1	0	0
Angiogram			
Restenosis	2[a]	1	0
New Lesion	0	1[a]	0
Thrombosis	1[a]	0	0
BKA	0	2	0
Deceased[b]	2 (8%)	2 (8%)	5 (21%)
LTFU[c]	0	1	3

[a]Repeat procedure.
[b]9/24 (37%) deceased.
[c]4/24 (17%) lost to follow-up.

53). Adjunctive angioplasty was required in 32.1% of the cases (17/53). The average initial stenosis of 91.5% was reduced to 33.8% with the Rotablator alone, and after angioplasty to 16.8%. There was only one complication requiring intervention (1.9%); a severe spasm that was resolved with balloon inflation. In short-term follow-up (two to five months), 75% were clinically improved.[10] In Buckbinder's series, 118 consecutive patients with 140 lesions were treated; 58% eccentric lesions, 34% tortuous vessels, 29% calcified, and 25% at bifurcation points. Acute success defined as less than 50% residual stenosis was achieved in 95%. The mean stenosis was reduced from 86.5 to 40.4% post-treatment. Adjunctive angioplasty was performed in 41% of patients, reducing the stenosis to 22.6%.[11] Cheirif et al. studied the effects of particles liberated during rotational atherectomy in the coronary arteries in comparison to the ischemic changes induced by coronary angioplasty and found that rotational atherectomy is as effective as coronary angioplasty (PTCA) and is associated with less evidence of ischemia than PTCA.[12] Rodriguez reported on the use of larger burr sizes (2.25 or 2.5mm) in 27 patients without adjunctive balloon angioplasty and described a substantial decrease in the percent of residual stenosis to values around $34.2 \pm 11.0\%$. Transient spasm was common and one patient had an intimal dissection.[13]

COMPLICATIONS

Complications can be separated into technical complications unrelated to the procedure and complications directly related to manipulation and operation of the device. Because the Rotablator is a coaxial system, if the guidewire successfully traverses the lesion, the incidence of device-related complications during atherectomy is very small. In the Stanford series, no distal embolization was recorded although in the collective experience from the multicenter trials, distal embolization has been recorded in two cases. The most frequent complication related to Rotablator atherectomy in the combined national series has been distal spasm. This has occurred in five cases in which papaverine was able to reverse the symptoms in two cases and in three patients, balloon angioplasty was required. In the Stanford series, irreversible spasm in the anterior tibial artery in one patient resulted in thrombosis which was not successfully reversed with thrombolysis. Subintimal tracking associated with use of the device is invariably subsequent to initial malposition of the guidewire (Table 6.6.12). Thus, the incidence of complication directly attributable to the Rotablator was approximately 5%. In the Stanford series, technical complications unrelated to the device contributed to procedure failure in seven cases. Sheath-related flaps accounted for three of these; two large hematomas occurred at the groin; one of these required transfusion and extended hospital stay. Thrombosis occurred in five patients within 24 hours after an apparently successful angiographic and hemodynamic result at the time of atherectomy. Most likely, thrombogenicity related to the atherectomy and the possibility of a subintimal dissection cannot be excluded in these cases. One pseudoaneurysm developed in a patient who underwent atherectomy via a percutaneous approach. There-

fore, technical complications were recorded in 14 of 44 (32% of the procedures) (Table 6.6.10). In addition, hemoglobinuria was recorded in five cases. Although not noted in early applications, hemoglobinuria was most often noted in cases requiring longer time for atherectomy, even though the burr size ranged from 1.75 to 4mm. Occurrence may be related to degree of back-flow from distal collaterals, thus exposing blood to the trauma of high-speed rotation. The hemoglobinuria clears spontaneously and is, in itself, generally not clinically significant. In only one case did the related decrease in hematocrit require transfusion. In the five patients in whom hemoglobinuria was reported, the average duration of rotational atherectomy was five minutes. However, some patients with long sessions did not have hemoglobinuria whereas in one focal lesion requiring only a three-minute procedure time there was mild hemoglobinuria. Analysis of the complications and modifications of the procedure has resulted in fewer difficulties in later clinical applications. Review of our experience has yielded at least three lesions which are listed below.

The Rotablator can successfully treat all lesions that can be traversed with a guidewire. This includes eccentric, calcified, ostial, diffuse, tortuous, small caliber, bifurcation, and adductor lesions. The one prerequisite for use of the Rotablator is access across the lesion with a guidewire.

The use of thrombolysis and new guidewires has improved the success of crossing vascular occlusions; the Rotablator can, therefore, be applicable in the treatment of the majority of peripheral lesions. Its coaxial design and other features of the device contribute to a predictable atherectomy result and fewer complications.

Long-term results regarding the restenosis rate associated with rotational devices are forthcoming. Initial evaluation of cases treated with the Rotablator, which eliminates the disadvantages of barotrauma as well as laser thermal injury, appear favorable. Early results reflect the fact that initial clinical trials were performed on patients with very severe disease. Many of these patients have had previous vascular procedures and have failed surgery as well as balloon angioplasty.

In summary, our results suggest that the length of the lesion is not a factor in determining success or failure of atherectomy. Since many high-grade focal stenoses have superimposed thrombus, which can propagate through the

Table 6.6.12. Rotablator Unsuccessful

Patient Number	Vessel	Length (cm)	% Stenosis	Problem	Result	Outcome
5	R Per	5	95	Could not advance	Balloon	Improved
20	R Pop	10	100	Subintimal[a]	Balloon	Improved
13	L AT	4	100	Perforation	Thrombosis	Graft
14	L Per	6	90	Subintimal[a]	Thrombosis	BKA
17	R Iliac	10	100	Subintimal[a]	Thrombosis	AFB
35	R Per	2	90	Subintimal[a]	Thrombosis	Graft
36	R AT	20	90	Spasm	Thrombosis	Graft

[a]Guidewire position.

entire length of the superficial femoral artery, the length of the occlusion is not an accurate factor in predicting outcome. Patient selection is, however, very important. A far greater number of technical and clinical failures are encountered in below-the-knee lesions. In addition, the pattern of the disease is pertinent; diffuse disease responds less well to atherectomy as in endarterectomy and angioplasty. In addition, the presence of tandem disease negatively affects long-term results, as similarly documented in follow-up studies of PTA and bypass procedures. Whether or not adjunctive balloon angioplasty will contribute to long-term patency or diminish long-term favorable outcome is still a question which has not been answered. Specifically, the incidence of restenosis associated with atherectomy, with or without balloon assistance, is a complex issue not yet resolved. Additional randomized clinical trials involving patients with comparable disease are necessary to establish an answer to this question.

References

1. Hansen DD, Auth DC, Vracko R, Ritchie JL: Rotational atherectomy in atherosclerotic rabbit iliac arteries. *Prog Cardiol* 1987;115(l)(Pt l):160–165
2. Ritchie JL, Hansen DD, Intlekofer MJ, Hall M, Auth DC: Rotational approaches to atherectomy and thrombectomy. *Z Kardiol* 1987;76(6):59–65
3. Zacca NM, Raizner AE, Noon GP, Short HD, Weilbaecher DG, Gotto AM, Roberts R: Short term follow up of patients treated with a recently developed rotational atherectomy device and in vivo assessment of the particles generated (abstr). *Circulation* 1987;76(suppl IV):IV–48
4. Zacca N, Raizner AE, Short D, Noon G, Weilbaecher D, Roehm J, Gotto A, Roberts R: First in-vivo human experience with a recently developed rotational atherectomy device (abstr) *Circulation* 1987;76(suppl IV):IV–46
5. Auth D: Micro-ablation catheters for removing cardiovascular obstructions. Presented at the New Frontiers in Cardiovascular Therapy Conference. Newport Beach, CA, Nov 1987
6. Ahn SS, Auth D, Marcus DR, Moore WS: Removal of focal atheromatous lesions by angioscopically guided high-speed rotary atherectomy preliminary experimental observations. *J Vasc Surg* 1988;7(2):292–300
7. Fourrier JL, Stankowiak C, Lablanche JM, Prat A, Brunetaud JM, Bertrand ME: Histopathology after rotational angioplasty of peripheral arteries in human beings (abstr). *J Am Coll Cardiol* 1988;II(2):109A
8. Miller FJ: Initial European and United States experience with the Kensey catheter. Presented at the Second Annual International Symposium on Peripheral Vascular Intervention. Miami, FL, Jan 1990
9. Dorros G, Iyer SS, Zaitoun R, Lewin R, Cooley R, Olson K: Acute angiographic and clinical outcome of high speed percutaneous rotational atherectomy (Rotablator). American Heart Association 63rd Scientific Sessions. Dallas Convention Center, Dallas, TX, Nov 1990
10. Fourrier JL, Dorros G, Ginsburg R, Zacca NM, Walker CM: Percutaneous peripheral rotational ablation in long lesions: multi-center experience. *Circulation* 1990;82(suppl III):309
11. Buckbinder M, O'Neill W, Warth D, Zacca N, Dietz U, Bertrand JL, Fourrier JL, Leon MB: Percutaneous coronary rotational ablation using the Rotablator: Results of a multi-center study. Abstracts of the American Heart Association 63rd Scientific Sessions. 1990;III–493
12. Cheirif BJ, Heibig J, Harris S, Staudacher R, Brown D, Quinones MA, Zacca N: Rotational ablation is associated with less myocardial ischemia than PTCA. Abstracts of the American Heart Association 63rd Scientific Sessions. Dallas Convention Center, 1990;III–493
13. Rodriguez AR, Zacca N, Heibig J, Warth D, Harris S, Staudacher R, Smith GS, Minor ST, Abukhalil JM, Raizner AE, Kleiman NS: Coronary rotary ablation using single large burr and without balloon assistance. *Circulation* 1990;82(4):suppl III:III–310

Part 7. Sonic Atherolysis

—Wilfrido R. Castañeda–Zúñiga, M.D., M.Sc., Joseph W. Yedlicka, Jr., M.D., David W. Hunter, M.D., Flavio Castañeda, M.D., Marcos A. Herrera, M.D., Manuel Maynar, M.D., and Kurt Amplatz, M.D.

Ultrasound wave energy has been used successfully in the management of genitourinary and gallbladder lithiasis with a wide safety margin. Ultrasound energy has also been used effectively in general surgery, cardiovascular surgery, and neurosurgery.[1-5]

The use of ultrasound energy for dissolution of atherosclerotic plaque was suggested by Anschuetz in 1965,[6] and its applicability for mechanical thrombectomy was described in 1976 by Trubestein.[7] Siegel's studies showed that power, strength, and length of exposure to ultrasonic energy at the levels required to ablate atherosclerotic plaque resulted in insignificant damage to normal vascular endothelium.[8-10]

As with other atherectomy devices currently in use or being evaluated, the size of the lumen created by the ultrasonic probe is directly related to the diameter of the probe tip and also to the duration of exposure to the ultrasonic energy.

Four mechanisms of action have been described:

—Direct mechanical effect;
—Cavitation;
—Thermal effects;
—Generation of microcurrents at the cellular level.[7,8,11]

Siegel believes that the main mechanism is the mechanical effect caused by the longitudinal and transverse oscillations induced by the probe with an amplitude of 15 μm and a frequency of 20kHz. These waves are strong enough to disrupt rigid noncompliant atherosclerotic plaque, but are not strong enough to cause damage to the more compliant, "normal" blood vessel wall.[12] The ultrasonic shock waves generate upon impact over the tissues, thermal energy leading to the formation of a plasma (a gaseous collection of ions and electrons) within the plaque and causing a subsequent implosion with resulting fragmentation of the plaque. When this plasma implodes, it generates up to 304kPa (3 atm) of pressure.

Local thermal injury to tissues has not been a problem in other applications of ultrasonic energy.[13] The potential problem in the intravascular applications resulting from the conversion of ultrasonic energy to thermal energy in the delivery system can be minimized by using pulsed wave energy delivery and cool perfusates.[8] The probe initially used by Siegel had the disadvantages of a lack of steering capability and of rigidity.[12] Rosenschein described a flexible, solid ultrasound transmission wire attached at its proximal end to a piezoelectric element vibrating at 20kHz. The device uses an external power generator. As with the device used by Siegel, the distal end of the ultrasound wire vibrates longitudinally with an amplitude of 150 ± 25 μm. The ultrasonic generator was operated in the pulsed mode with a 50% duty cycle to assure resonance capture. Duration of pulse was 0.5 second with an interval of 0.5 second.[14]

The size of the fragments produced varied from 0.2–8 μm (41 ± 5%); 8–30 μm in 48 ± 8% and, in the remainder, 30–100 μm. All debris produced by the ultrasonic energy was under 100 μm. In comparison, the debris produced in the control group, where the occlusion was mechanically recanalized using the same ultrasonic probe, but without the use of ultrasonic energy, the size of the debris produced was subcapillary size in 5%, over 100 μm in 47%. Histologic examination of the treated arteries revealed a clean, smooth channel. No damage to the media or adventitia was found. The percentage of luminal recanalization was found to be greater for the ultrasonically than for the mechanically recanalized arteries by a factor of 3 to 1. The incidence of arterial wall injury was greater in the mechanically than in the ultrasonically recanalized group, although this was not statistically significant.[14]

Siegel in 1989 successfully utilized the technique in seven of eight patients; four with stenosis and four with complete vascular occlusions. Residual stenosis after ultrasonic treatment was 54% in the patient with occlusions and 37% in patients with stenosis. In all patients, transluminal angioplasty was performed to achieve complete luminal reconstitution, with the residual stenosis after transluminal angioplasty being overall 20%. No instance of dissection, perforation, spasm, or distal embolization was found.[12]

In Rosenschein's experience, the ultrasonic atherectomy was successful in seven complete occlusions.[14] The angiogram of the treated arteries showed a mean recanalization of 82.5%. The recanalized lumen area and the flow were greater for ultrasonically treated than for mechanically recanalized arteries. The debris was significantly smaller for ultrasonically recanalized arteries in the order of 18.9 versus 86.7 μm. Histologically, there was no difference in the degree of arterial wall injury. Cavitation is said to be the main mechanism of ultrasonic atherectomy.[14]

Monteverde reported the first percutaneous application of ultrasonic atherectomy in 1990. He achieved success in 8 out of 10 complete occlusions with a residual stenosis of 48 ± 6%. All lesions had adjunct transluminal angioplasty with a mean residual stenosis of 11 ± 5%. No complications were reported. No restenosis at 13 ± 2 weeks was found.[15]

The relative lack of vascular wall injury with the use of ultrasonic energy is believed to be due to the differences in elasticity between the atherosclerotic plaque and the adjacent normal media.[16–18] Collagen is abundant in normal media particularly in the internal elastic lamina. Collagen in arteriosclerotic plaque is abnormal in composition and structure. This abnormal collagen structure makes plaque less elastic than arterial wall, which has normal collagen fibers.[19,20] Therefore, when ultrasonic waves at a given level of ultrasound energy impact tissues, they will exert a more disruptive effect upon the less elastic arteriosclerotic plaque than on the normal arterial wall.[19,20]

This theory of elasticity-dependent selectivity is supported by the resistance to damage by ultrasonic energy of tissues rich in collagen fibers,[21,22] and by the susceptibility of tissues poor in collagen matrix to ultrasonic energy damage.[23–26] It should be remembered, however, that if ultrasonic intensity is raised beyond a threshold level, tissue deformity and displacement can become so extreme that it can result in damage and/or disruption of both arteriosclerotic plaque and normal arterial wall.[27]

Further studies by Watkins et al. have shown that the mechanism of ultrasonic atherectomy is cavitation-induced ablation of arteriosclerotic plaque. Tissue ablation was observed only above cavitation threshold (40 watts), concurrent with production of ultrasonic pressure waves.[28] Tissue ablation rates correlated negatively with elasticity, but not with collagen content.[28]

Angioscopy showed the lumen created by ultrasonic atherectomy to be smooth in comparison to the disruption caused by transluminal angioplasty[29] or by some other devices.[30]

Conclusion

Although technological limitations such as rigidity and lack of steering capability at the present time limit the scope of applications of ultrasonic atherectomy in the management of arteriosclerotic vascular occlusions, the available data suggest that ultrasonic atherectomy may be a safe and effective method for recanalization of total vascular occlusions. Based on the elastic tissue selectivity of ultrasonic energy, a wide safety margin exists for arteriosclerotic plaque ablation, before damage to normal arterial wall can occur. It is said that with the coaxial placement of the ultrasonic probe, exact focusing and timing of application are not crucial for a successful ultrasonic atherectomy.[14]

References

1. Segura JW, LeRoy AJ: Percutaneous ultrasonic lithotripsy. *Urology* 1984;23:7–10
2. Marberger M, Stackl W, Hruby W, Krosis A: Late sequelae of ultrasonic lithotripsy of renal calculi. *J Urol* 1985;133:170–174
3. Chan KK, Watmough DJ, Hope DT, Moir K: A new motor-driven surgical probe and its in vitro comparison with the Cavitron ultrasonic surgical aspirator. *Ultrasound Med Biol* 1986;12:279–283
4. Hodgson WJB, DelGuercio LRM: Preliminary experience in liver surgery using the ultrasonic scalpel. *Surgery* 1984;95:230–234
5. Brown AH, Davies PG: Ultrasonic decalcification of calcified cardiac valves and annuli. *Br Med J* 1972;3:274–277
6. Anschuetz R, Bernard HR: Ultrasonic irradiation and atherosclerosis. *Surgery* 1965;57:549–553
7. Trubestein G, Engel C, Etzel F, et al: Thrombolysis by ultrasound. *Clin Sci Mol Med* 1976;51:697s–698s
8. Siegel RJ, Fishbein MC, Forrester J, et al: Ultrasonic plaque ablation. A new method for recanalization of partially or totally occluded arteries. *Circulation* 1988;78:1443–1448
9. Siegel RJ, DonMichael TA, DeCastro E, et al: In vivo recanalization of total atherosclerotic arterial occlusions. *Circulation* 1988; 78(suppl II):IV–1077
10. Siegel RJ, DeCastro E, Forrester JS, DonMichael TA: In vivo ultrasonic recanalization of arterial occlusion (abstr). *Circulation* 1988;78(suppl II):IV–1077
11. Bhabredier T, Lemaire V, Louis V, Merchier PA, Montalescot G, Moussallem N: Elaboration d'un système a ultrasons pour deobstruction des artères coronaires. *Arch Mal Coeur* 1989;82:377–380
12. Siegel RJ, Myler RK, Cumberland DC, DonMichael TA: Percutaneous ultrasonic angioplasty: initial clinical experience. *Lancet* 1989;772–774
13. Howards S, Merrill E, Harris S, et al: Ultrasonic lithotripsy: Laboratory evaluation. *Invest Urol* 1984;11:273–277
14. Rosenschein U, Bernstein JJ, DiSegni E, Kaplinsky E, Bernheim J, Rozenszajn LA: Experimental ultrasonic angioplasty: Disruption of atherosclerotic plaques and thrombi in vitro and arterial recanalization in vivo. *J Am Coll Cardiol* 1990;15:711–717
15. Monteverde C, Velez M, Victoria R, Nava G, Alliger H, Borges J: Percutaneous transluminal ultrasonic angioplasty in totally occluded peripheral arteries: immediate and intermediate clinical results. *Circulation* 1990;82(Suppl III):III–2694
16. Woolf N: *Pathology of Atherosclerosis.* London, Butterworth, 1982, pp 113–138
17. Blankenhorn DH, Kramsch DM: Reversal of atherosis and sclerosis: the two components of atherosclerosis. *Circulation* 1989;79:1–7
18. Rokosova B, Rapp JH, Porter JM, Bentley JP: Composition and metabolism of symptomatic distal aortic plaque. *J Vasc Surg* 1986;3:617–622
19. Keeney SM, Richardson PD: Stress analysis of atherosclerotic arteries. Proceedings of the Ninth Annual Conference, Engineering in Medicine and Biology. *Trans IEEE* 1987;EBM3:1484–1485
20. Hykes D, Hendrik WR, Starchman DE: *Ultrasound Physics and Instrumentation.* New York, Churchill Livingstone, 1985, pp 23–31
21. Hodgson WJB: Instruments and techniques: ultrasonic surgery. *Ann R Coll Surgeons Engl* 1980;62:459–461
22. Weitz J, Hodgson WJB, Localzo LJ, McElhinney RT: A bloodless technique for tongue surgery. *Head Neck Surg* 1981;3:244–246
23. Hodgson WJB, DelGuercio LRM: Preliminary experience in liver surgery using the ultrasonic scalpel. *Surgery* 1984;95:230–234
24. Brown AH, Davies PG: Ultrasonic decalcification of calcified cardiac valves and annuli. *Br Med J* 1972;143:1088–1089
25. Anschuetz R, Bernard HR: Ultrasonic irradiation and atherosclerosis. *Surgery* 1965;57:549–553
26. Trubestein G, Enget C, Etzel F, Sobbe A, Cremer H, Stumff U: Thrombolysis by ultrasound. *Clin Sci Mol Med* 1976; 51:697S–698S
27. Ernst A, Schenk EA, Gracewski SM, Wdlck TJ, Murant FG, Serrino P, Melzer RS: Can high-intensity ultrasound selectively destroy human atherosclerotic plaques and minimize residual debris size (abstr). *Circulation* 1989;80(suppl II):II–306
28. Watkins JF, Rose EA, Detwiler P, Fong JC, Sanchez JA, Coppey LJ, Cannon PJ, Rosenchein U: Mechanisms of ultrasonic angioplasty. *Circulation* 1990;82(4)(suppl III):III–219
29. Siegel RJ, Michael TAD, Belli A, Pflueger R, Myler RK, Procter A, Cumberland DC: Percutaneous ultrasound angioplasty: clinical comparison of 2 systems. *Circulation* 1990;82(4)(suppl III):III–219
30. Kensey K, Nash J, Abrahams C, Zarins CK: Recanalization of obstructive arteries with a flexible, rotating tip catheter. *Radiology* 1987;165:387–389

Part 8. Bard Rotary Atherectomy System (BRAS)

—Amir Motarjeme, M.D.

The Bard rotary atherectomy system (BRAS) is being evaluated for the management of arteriosclerotic vascular disease.[1]

The system consists of an 8Fr catheter with a 9Fr stainless-steel cutter fitted at the tip (Fig. 6.8.1). The material excised by the cutter is collected by the guidewire, which has an auger design to collect excised atheroma (Fig. 6.8.2). The wire is 0.038-inch in diameter with a soft, flex-

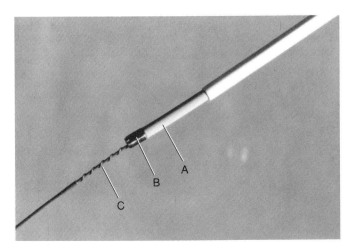

Figure 6.8.1. **A.** Atherectomy catheter. **B.** Metal cutter. **C.** System's auger guidewire.

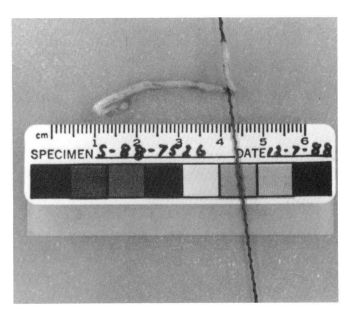

Figure 6.8.2. A 6cm-long cylindrical atheroma affixed to the wire removed from a totally occluded SFA.

ible tip. The power source is a hand-held battery driven motor with a push-button activator (Fig. 6.8.3). The power source allows two levels of speed and torque, a lower speed of 600 and a higher one of 1200 rpm. It also offers normal and high-torque selections.

A metal introducer is used to facilitate insertion of the device into the channel located on the motor drive and a Tuohy–Borst adapter is tightened around the guidewire, to prevent blood leakage, as well as to immobilize the wire during rotation of the catheter shaft.

MATERIALS AND METHODS

An antegrade puncture is required for placement of an arterial sheath into the common femoral artery. The obstruction is carefully probed and crossed with the

BRAS's wire. If the obstruction appears difficult to cross, the lesion is first negotiated with conventional guidewire-catheter technique. The angiographic wire is then exchanged for the auger wire. Once the auger wire is in place, the cutting catheter is advanced over the auger wire up to the level of the obstruction, manually or with the help of the motor drive. Before the motor drive is started, fixation of the auger wire needs to be verified by tightening of the Tuohy–Borst adapter.

The BRAS system works by excising atheroma from the arterial wall with the cutter tip and wrapping it around the auger wire. The auger guidewire across the lesion remains

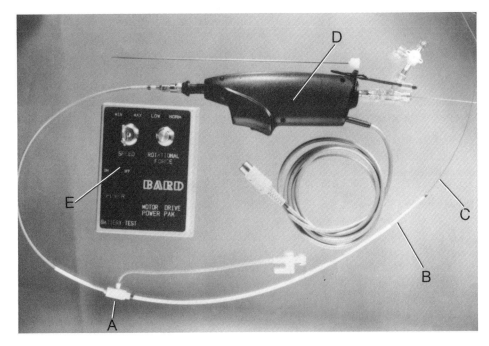

Figure 6.8.3. Bard rotary atherectomy system (BRAS). **A.** Arterial sheath. **B.** Atherectomy catheter. **C.** System's guidewire. **D.** Motor drive. **E.** Power pack.

stationary while the cutting catheter, activated by the motor drive, revolves around the wire at a speed of 600 or 1200 rpm. During these revolutions, the excised atheromas are wrapped around the wire. After the lesion is crossed, the cutting catheter remains in place while the auger wire is removed, along with the excised atheromatous material[1] (Fig. 6.8.4).

The device has been used in 40 patients: 27 males and 13 females, with ages varying from 39 to 78 years. The degree of obstruction ranged from 75 to 100%. Forty-one arteries were treated for stenosis and twelve for complete occlusions. The length of the lesions varied from 0.5 to 45cm. Thirty-eight patients had claudication while two were treated for gangrene. Thirty-four patients were smokers and twenty had diabetes. BRAS atherectomy was performed percutaneously in 39 patients while it was done intraoperatively in 1 patient. Pulse-volume recording (PVR) was performed on all patients, both before and after the procedures. All patients were anticoagulated with 5,000 units of heparin. Thirty-eight patients had an additional transluminal angioplasty while two patients were treated with BRAS atherectomy alone.[1]

Arteriograms were performed prior to and after atherectomy and also after the subsequent angioplasty. Follow-up evaluation included clinical examinations and PVR monthly initially and every three months thereafter. Six and eighteen months' follow-up arteriograms were performed on eighteen patients.

Patients in whom a long segment occlusion (longer than 10cm) was recanalized were treated with Coumadin for six months. The remainder of the patients were treated with Persantine (75 mg three times a day) and aspirin (325mg daily).

RESULTS

The results were evaluated in three groups:

1. Technical success when atheroma was excised;
2. Clinical success when the arterial lumen was improved; and
3. Failure when neither technical nor clinical success was seen.

Thirty-three patients (82.5%) had both technical and clinical success while six patients (15%) had only clinical success, presumably due to Dotterization while no atheroma was removed. Atherectomy failed in one patient (2.5%), following an unsuccessful angioplasty. Overall success rate was 97.5%.[1]

An improvement in the ankle-brachial index by at least 50% was seen in 39 patients. There were two reocclusions and five restenoses during the first year. The cumulative follow-up is 14 months, ranging from 1 to 24 months. The overall one-year patency rate for total occlusions and stenosis is only 74.5%. The angiographic examination of patients with clinical evidence of reocclusions showed,

however, progression of disease, mostly in other areas rather at the treated segments. No restenosis or reocclusions were seen after one year, and the two-year patency rate remains at 74.5%.[1]

Pathologic examination of the excised atheroma revealed absence of adventitia; intimal fragments in 60%; medial fragments in 12.5%; organized thrombus in 15%; fibromatous tissue in 12.5%; fibroadipose tissue in 2% and evidence of inflammation in 7%; 12.5% of removed atheroma was classified as calcified atheroma.[1]

COMPLICATIONS

Thromboses of the superficial femoral artery at the site of insertion of the sheath occurred in one patient and was treated successfully with intra-arterial infusion of urokinase. No distal emboli, arterial perforation, or thromboses at the site of the atherectomy were seen. There was one large local hematoma on the groin and scrotum in a patient who had a high antegrade common femoral artery puncture.[1]

DISCUSSION

Angioplasty in the treatment of peripheral vascular disease has a restenosis rate of 25–60%.[2] Angiographic evidence of intimal dissection is seen in most vessels following angioplasty. Extensive dissections are complicated with arterial occlusion.[3] It has been reported that the use of atherectomy catheters, alone or in combination with angioplasty catheters, by excising atheroma leaves a smoother lumen, and that by debulking the atheromatous lesions without damaging the media and adventitia, the long-term patency rate is increased.[4,5]

Restenosis following BRAS atherectomy was seen when sufficient atheroma was not removed and the residual stenosis, prior to angioplasty, was greater than 50%. These findings have also been experienced with the Simpson atherocath.[5] These findings support the hypothesis that the patency rate might be directly related to the bulk of atheroma removed during atherectomy.[4,5] In the BRAS series previously reported,[6] the following findings supporting this theory include:

1. Patients who were treated with BRAS atherectomy alone or in combination with angioplasty showed no evidence of progression of disease at the atherectomized segment, in comparison with those lesions treated with angioplasty alone, which showed recurrence of disease at the dilated segment (Fig. 6.8.5).
2. In addition, when all the atheromatous material was removed, the follow-up arteriograms showed an ectatic artery at the site of atherectomy (Fig. 6.8.6). The histologic appearance of restenosis of the atherectomized arteries varies from that of angioplasty, suggesting

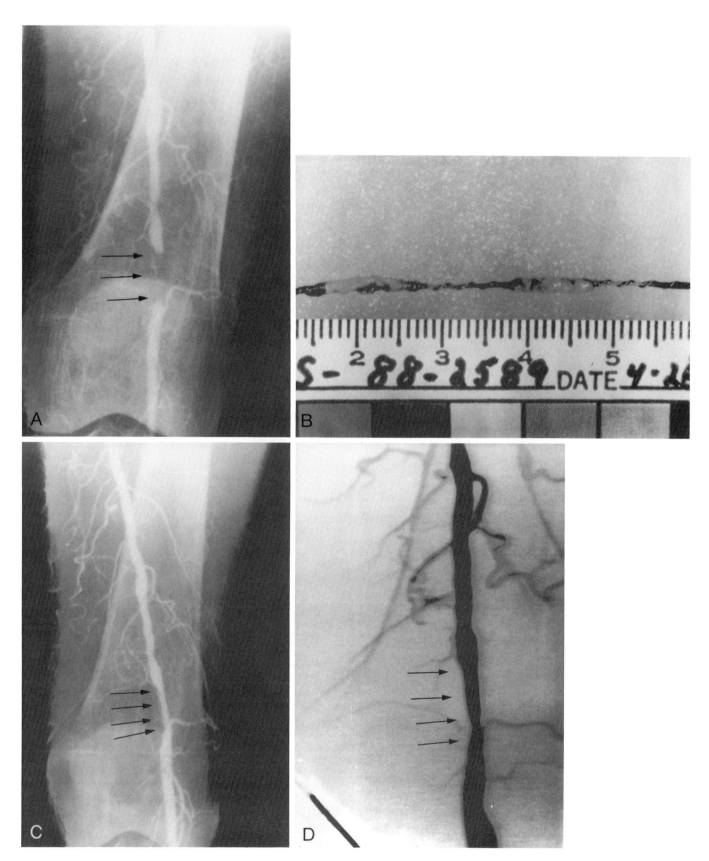

Figure 6.8.4.   **A.** A femoral arteriogram of a 72-year-old woman complaining of intermittent claudication shows a focal stenosis and a 2cm occlusion *(arrows)* of the popliteal artery. **B.** Excised atheromas. **C.** Post-atherectomy arteriogram showing residual stenosis, not greater than 50% *(arrows).* **D.** Eighteen-month follow-up arteriogram revealed no progression of disease *(arrows).*

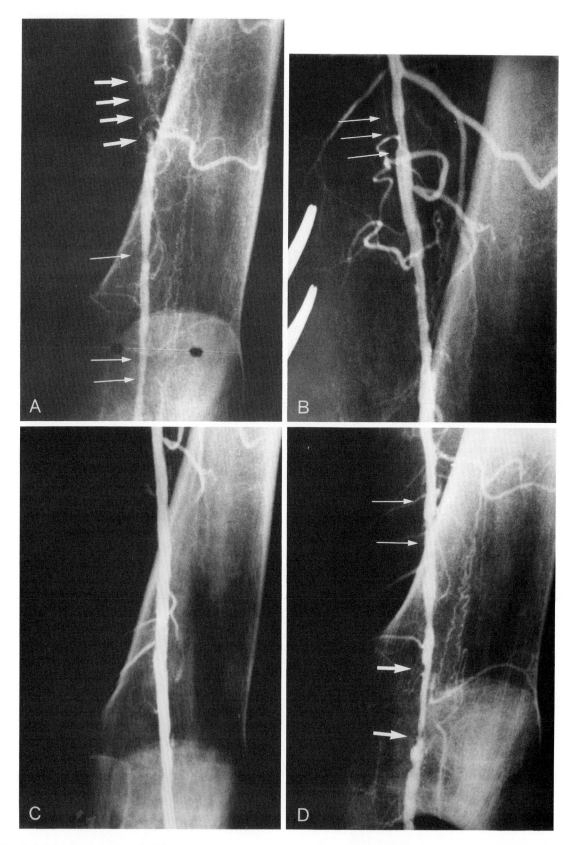

Figure 6.8.5. **A.** A femoral arteriogram of a 52-year-old man showing a 3cm total occlusion of the distal superficial femoral artery *(large arrows)* and two focal stenoses of the popliteal artery *(small arrows)*. **B.** Postatherectomy arteriogram shows recanalization of the totally occluded segment with only minimal residual stenosis *(arrows)*. **C.** Postatherectomy and PTA arteriograms showing no residual stenosis of the occluded segment and focal stenosis (treated with PTA). **D.** A six-month follow-up arteriogram showed no evidence of progression of disease where atherectomy was performed *(between small arrows)* while restenoses are seen where only PTA was performed *(between large arrows)*.

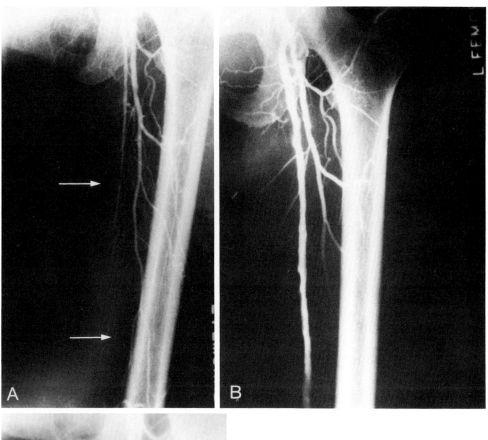

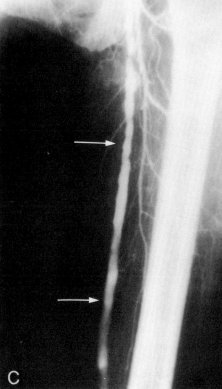

Figure 6.8.6. **A.** A femoral arteriogram showing stenosis of the proximal SFA and long segment total occlusion of the distal SFA *(between arrows)* (excised atheroma shown in Fig. 6.8.4B). **B.** Postatherectomy and PTA arteriogram. Atherectomy was only done on occluded segment. **C.** A six-month arteriogram shows patency and further dilatation of atherectomized segment *(between arrows)* while restenosis is seen in the proximal SFA where no atherectomy was done prior to PTA.

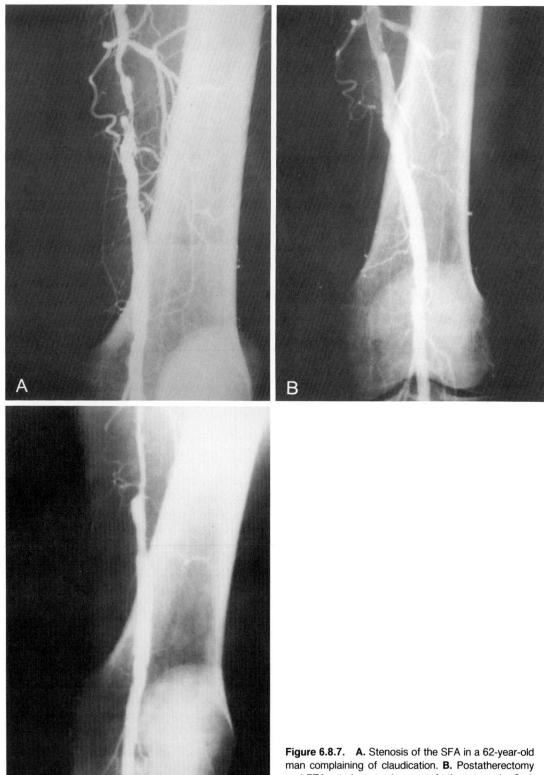

Figure 6.8.7. **A.** Stenosis of the SFA in a 62-year-old man complaining of claudication. **B.** Postatherectomy and PTA arteriogram shows no further stenosis. **C.** A six-month follow-up arteriogram showing smooth and elongated restenosis suggestive of intimal hyperplasia.

intimal hyperplasia rather than progression of atherosclerosis[4,5,7] (Fig. 6.8.7). These findings strongly suggest that the atherectomized lumen might remain patent longer than those treated with angioplasty alone.[1]

3. The BRAS atherectomy catheter system appears to be safe, fast, and simple to operate. Because of the over-the-wire capability, there is no risk of arterial perforation, as is seen with other atherectomy systems. In this series, there have not been any thromboses at the atherectomy site, or any distal emboli, either clinically or angiographically.

References

1. Motarjeme A: Bard rotary atherectomy system. Two years clinical experience. *Circulation* 1990;82(suppl III):III–610
2. Widlus D, Osterman F Jr: Evaluation and percutaneous management of atherosclerotic peripheral vascular disease. *JAMA* 1989;261:3148–3153
3. Gardiner GA Jr, Meyerovitz MF, Harrington DP, et al: Dissection complicating angioplasty. *AJR* 1985;145:627–631
4. Maynar M, Cabrera V, Reyes R, Roman M, Pulido JN, Castañeda F, Tobio R, Letourneau JG, Castañeda–Zúñiga WR: Percutaneous atherectomy with the Simpson atherectomy device in the management of arterial stenosis. *Semin Intervent Radiol* 1988;5:247–252
5. Schwarten DE, Cutcliff WB, Krok KL: The late results of femoral directional atherectomy. Presented at RIPCV-2. Toulouse, France, Feb 1990
6. Ernst A, Schenk EA, Gracewski SM, Wedlick TJ, Murant FG, Serrino P, Melzer RS: Can high-intensity ultrasound selectively destroy human atherosclerotic plaques and minimize residual debris size (abstr). *Circulation* 1989;80(suppl II):II–306
7. Vom Polnitz A, Backa D, Remberger K, et al: Restenosis after atherectomy shows increased intimal hyperplasia as compared to primary lesions. *J Vasc Med Biol* 1989; 1:283–287

Part 9. Directional Atherectomy with the Simpson Atherocath

—Manuel Maynar, M.D., Ricardo Reyes, M.D., Juan M. Pulido-Duque, M.D., Vicente Cabrera, M.D., Mariano de Blas, M.D., Carmen Garcia, M.D., José Garcia–Medina, M.D., Aracelli Cruz, M.D., and Wilfrido R. Castañeda–Zúñiga, M.D., M.Sc.

Introduction

In 1964, Dotter first described a technique for percutaneous treatment of atherosclerotic arterial stenosis using a coaxial catheter system.[1] Initially, this technique was poorly accepted in the United States; it was nonetheless extensively and successfully used by European investigators.[2,3] It was not until 1974 when Grüntzig described a nonexpandable balloon catheter that percutaneous transluminal angioplasty techniques gained widespread acceptance in the United States.[4] Since then, treatment of peripheral atherosclerotic disease has become even more aggressive and innovative with the hope that the percutaneous reconstitution of arterial flow will ultimately reduce the need for surgical revascularization or extremity amputation.

Percutaneous transluminal angioplasty results in the management of peripheral vascular disease show a five-year patency rate of 90% in the iliac arteries and 50–60% in the femoropopliteal system.[5–7] Despite improvements in balloon and guidewire technologies in recent years, the long-term patency rate following angioplasty of the femoral and popliteal arteries has not increased. Several novel approaches have been described in the past few years trying to improve these results by debulking the lesions, including mechanical devices,[8,9] laser ablation systems,[10,11] laser welding,[12] hot-tip devices,[13,14] and intravascular stents[15,16]; most of these devices are undergoing clinical trials in the United States and Europe. The rationale for the development of these devices is that removal or fracture and fixation of the atherosclerotic intima to the underlying media will leave behind a smooth lumen; theoretically, this should be associated with a lower incidence of postprocedural recurrence and complications compared with transluminal angioplasty.

The Simpson Atherocath has been used successfully by several authors to manage arterial stenoses.[17–20] The greatest potential advantage of directional atherectomy over balloon angioplasty is that it provides two mechanisms for treatment of atherosclerotic obstruction. These are the removal of the plaque by the Atherocath and a secondary dilatation of the vessel lumen by both a Dotter coaxial mechanism and the effect caused by the positioning balloon inflation.[17,21] Sharaf expressed that up to 75% of luminal improvement following directional atherectomy can be attributed to the Dotter effect.[21] This dilatation phenomenon was presumably seen in some of our cases in which a good angiographic result was obtained despite removing only a small amount of atheromatous material. The atherocath probably functions in part as a Dotter angioplasty device in these patients.

The ability to remove the plaque is probably the greatest advantage of directional atherectomy relative to angioplasty. Development of intimal flaps protruding into the arterial lumen is a common finding following balloon angioplasty.[22] This has the potential for stimulating thrombosis and intimal hyperplasia and thereby promoting a recurrence of arterial stenosis. Histologically, media has been retrieved by atherectomy in 43–64% and adventitia in 16.8–23% of lesions.[23-25] Angiographic perforation or pseudoaneurysm was present in 10.3% of the lesions with adventitial retrieval.[23] Dick reported that in 58 of 82 patients retrieval of media occurred, while adventitia was retrieved in only 26. Ectasia of the atherectomized segment was found in 10.9% of cases where media and/or adventitia was extracted.[25] It has been said that the simultaneous use of intravascular ultrasound (IVUS) can prevent vascular wall damage.[26] In its present form, it is however difficult to direct atherectomy cuts with IVUS. The recent literature relating to the use of the Simpson Atherocath describes six-month patency rates comparable to those of angioplasty.[19,20] The six-month patency rate in our series is 95%.[17] It has been reported that the results of directional atherectomy are optimized by matching the diameter of the normal artery at the stenotic site to the diameter of the Atherocath used; this will ensure that the extraction of atheromatous material will be optimized.[17] This is an important consideration since there are reports that those lesions left with a residual stenosis of more than 30% have a 28% recurrence rate at six months, in comparison with those left with a residual stenosis of less than 30% that have an 11% recurrence rate.[20]

PATIENT SELECTION

The classic indications for surgical intervention in patients with peripheral vascular disease also apply in the case of directional atherectomy, that is, lifestyle-limiting intermittent claudication, as well as more advanced stages of peripheral ischemia such as rest pain, nonhealing ulcers, and gangrene. Contraindications to directional atherectomy include acute ischemia, "trash foot syndrome," morbid obesity, and densely calcified lesions, although this is debatable. Concerning the type of lesion present, directional atherectomy can be performed in stenosis, preferably short, recurrent lesions, and retained valve cusps on in situ bypass grafts. Calcified lesions are difficult to treat as are complete obstructions, which can be treated after first recanalizing them with angiographic catheter techniques.

DEVICE

The Simpson Atherocath (DVI; Redwood City, CA) consists of a shaft with a cylindrical metal housing attached to the end of the braided double-lumen shaft (Fig. 6.9.1). The housing has a 20mm window, opposite which is a positioning balloon, designed to force the window against the atherosclerotic plaque (Fig. 6.9.2). The inflation pressure

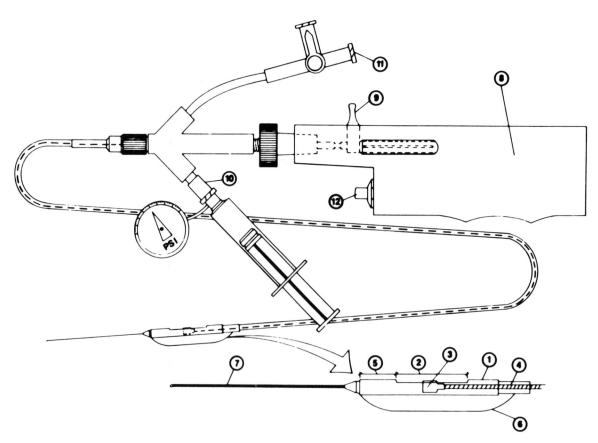

Figure 6.9.1. Diagrammatic representation of the Simpson Atherocath. *1,* metallic capsule containing cutter and storage area; *2,* window; *3,* rotating cutter; *4,* rotating shaft; *5,* storage compartment; *6,* positioning balloon; *7,* floppy wire; *8,* power pack; *9,* manual cutter advance unit; *10,* side port for balloon inflations; *11,* side port for contrast medium injection; *12,* power unit switch.

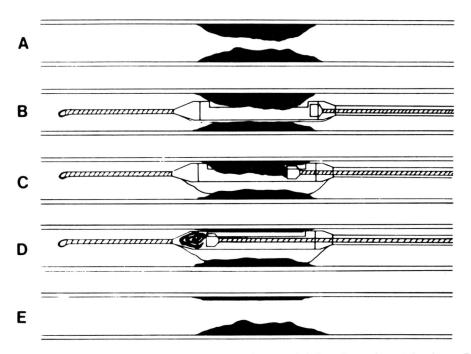

Figure 6.9.2. Diagrammatic representation of the Simpson Atherocath mechanism of cutting. *A,* atherosclerotic narrowing in a vessel. *B,* the window of the Atherocath has been placed against the plaque. *C,* the positioning balloon has been inflated, forcing the plaque into the window and the cutter is being advanced to cut the plaque. *D,* the excised atheroma has been stored in the storage compartment and the cutter is kept at the end of the capsule, holding the excised atheroma. *E,* the Atherocath has been removed, leaving a smooth, clean cut.

used is low (35 psi). Attached to the metal housing there is an extended flexible housing which serves as a collection chamber into which large amounts of atheromatous material can be deposited (Fig. 6.9.3). The disadvantage of this two-part housing is the narrowing of the lumen present at the level of the juncture of the rigid with the flexible housing. This narrowed area makes the passage of the resected atheromatous material from the rigid to the flexible housing difficult. Attached to the flexible housing there is a detachable nose cone with a fixed 0.018-inch or 0.035-inch guidewire. The flexible housing and nose cone are detachable and are available as separate parts from the manufacturer. Schwarten recommends the purchase of an additional flexible housing and nose cone if an extensive area of atheromatous material is to be removed, in order to speed up the procedure, by exchanging the flexible collection chamber filled with atheromatous material for the second one. In this form, the procedure can continue almost without interruption. In the meantime, the first collection chamber is emptied and made readily available for service.[18] The spare nose cones are useful to replace nose cones with kinked wires.

A third generation of device will soon be available with over-the-wire capability.

TECHNIQUE

Because of the catheter design, the Atherocath must be introduced through a check-flow sheath, using an ipsilateral approach, retrograde in the case of the iliac and renal artery and antegrade for the femoral, popliteal, and tibioperoneal arteries. Ideally, the puncture has to be performed as horizontal as possible to avoid kinking of the sheath, since this makes passage of the Atherocath difficult. Kinking of the sheath is a common problem in obese patients, in whom it is practically impossible to perform a horizontal puncture.

Proper sizing of the Atherocath to the arterial diameter is extremely important. The best match is one in which the Atherocath working diameter is equal to the diameter of the "normal" adjacent arterial segment to the area of obstruction. The working diameter of the Atherocath represents the diameter of the metal housing plus the diameter of the inflated positioning balloon (Fig. 6.9.4). For the currently available Atherocath sizes, the working diameters are: 7Fr, 4.8mm; 8Fr, 5.7mm; 9Fr, 6.0mm; 10Fr, 6.8mm; 11Fr, 7.7mm.

Therefore, for a given arterial diameter of 6mm, a 9Fr Atherocath should be used in order to obtain the best match possible. Undersizing of the Atherocath in respect to the arterial diameter results in incomplete atheromatous material removal and consequently a significant residual stenosis[17] (Fig. 6.9.5). As has been shown by Schwarten and Simpson, residual stenoses larger than 30% following directional atherectomy are associated with a 28% recurrence rate at six months, in comparison with residual stenoses of less than 30% which have an 11% recurrence rate.[20]

After establishing access, the patient is systemically heparinized with 8,000–10,000 IU of heparin. Vasodilators

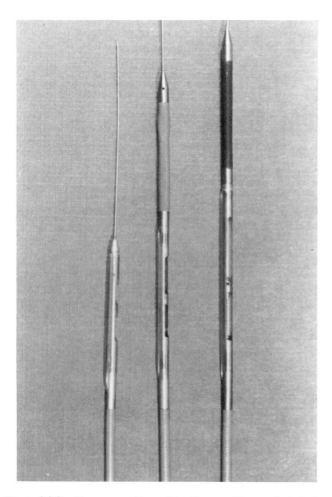

Figure 6.9.3. Three generations of the Simpson Atherocath. *Left,* first generation. *Middle,* second generation showing an extended storage compartment, but keeping the same window size. *Right,* the window length has been increased, as has the storage compartment.

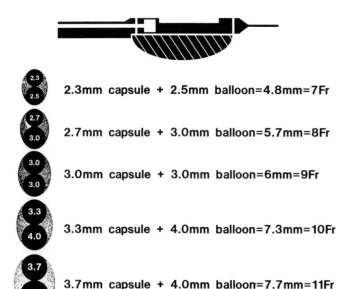

2.3mm capsule + 2.5mm balloon=4.8mm=7Fr

2.7mm capsule + 3.0mm balloon=5.7mm=8Fr

3.0mm capsule + 3.0mm balloon=6mm=9Fr

3.3mm capsule + 4.0mm balloon=7.3mm=10Fr

3.7mm capsule + 4.0mm balloon=7.7mm=11Fr

Figure 6.9.4. Diagrammatic representation of working diameter of different catheters.

can be used particularly during atherectomy of the popliteal or tibioperoneal vessels.

A digital subtraction angiogram is obtained at least in two planes to localize the lesion and study its morphologic characteristics. We are now routinely doing intravascular ultrasound before, during and after the directional atherectomy to assess in a more accurate way the type of lesion present and to monitor the removal of tissue (Fig. 6.9.6).

After passing the Atherocath through the check-flow valve, taking care to protect the leading wire with the Atherocath catheter introducer, the Atherocath is advanced under fluoroscopic control using roadmapping, until the metal housing is at the level of the lesion. While advancing or withdrawing the catheter, the cutter blade should be positioned at the distal end of the rigid metal housing. Usually with careful manipulation of the steerable leading wire and gentle catheter advancement, all lesions can be crossed. Once the lesion is crossed, the window is positioned against the atheromatous plaque and the positioning balloon is inflated to 10–20 psi forcing the plaque into the window and the cutter blade is retracted. The balloon is then inflated to 35 psi, the motor drive is activated and the cutter blade is manually advanced to cut the atheromatous plaque protruding into the window. While holding down the cutter blade, the motor is stopped, the balloon is deflated and the catheter is rotated 10–20° either clockwise or counterclockwise and the procedure is repeated until a complete 360° circuit has been completed. It is important to stress that while the balloon is deflated, the cutter blade should be held against the distal end of the metal housing to prevent escape of resected atheromatous material resulting in distal embolization. The same principle is true during withdrawal of the Atherocath from the vessel.

A completion digital arteriogram in multiple projections or an intravascular ultrasound examination or both are necessary to assess the degree of lumen reconstitution. The end point of the procedure should be to leave less than 20% residual stenosis.[17]

Intermittent small volume injections of contrast medium during the procedure help to locate areas of residual plaque. Information in this respect is also gained by observing the positioning balloon during inflation. If an indentation is present, this is a good indicator that residual atheroma is present in that location and needs to be removed.[20]

DIRECTIONAL ATHERECTOMY OF ARTERIAL STENOSES

The Simpson Atherocath has been used successfully to manage arterial stenoses.[17,19,27] The greatest potential advantage of directional atherectomy over balloon angioplasty it that it provides two mechanisms for the treatment of the atherosclerotic obstruction. These are the removal of the plaque by the Atherocath and a secondary dilatation

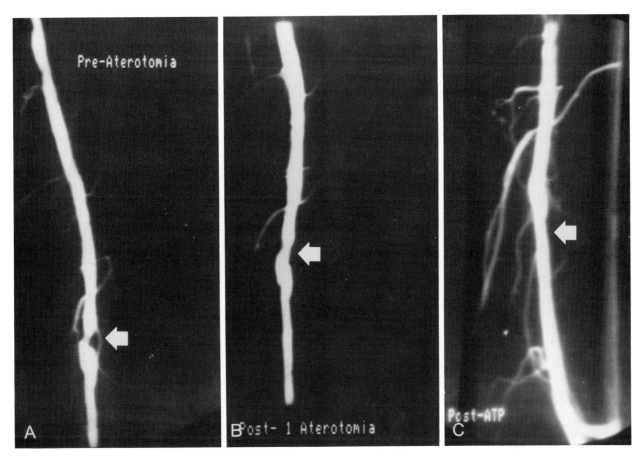

Figure 6.9.5. **A.** Femoral arteriogram showing a 60% stenosis of the mid-superficial femoral artery *(arrow).* **B.** Following atherectomy with a 7Fr Atherocath, note residual 30–35% narrowing at the site of atherectomy *(arrow).* **C.** Following balloon dilatation, note minimal residual narrowing at site of procedure *(arrow).*

of the vessel lumen by both a Dotter coaxial mechanism and the angioplasty effect caused by inflation of the positioning balloon.[17,22] This dilatation effect was seen in some of our patients in whom a good angiographic result was obtained despite removing only a small amount of atheromatous material.[17] This Dotter effect has been confirmed also by intravascular ultrasound observations after the simple passage of the Atherocath without cutting any atheromatous material.[21]

DIRECTIONAL ATHERECTOMY OF THE ILIAC VESSELS

It has already been mentioned that the results of atherectomy are optimized by matching the diameter of the normal adjacent artery at the stenotic site to the diameter of the Atherocath utilized; this will ensure that the extraction of atheromatous material is adequate.[17,27] This is an important consideration since a residual stenosis of more than 30% has a 28% recurrence rate at six months, in comparison with a residual stenosis of less than 30% that has an 11% recurrence rate.[20]

It should be noted that the compound diameter of the 7, 8, 9, 10, and 11Fr atherectomy capsule plus the inflated balloon corresponds to 4.8, 5.7, 6.0, 6.8, and 7.7mm diam-

eter, respectively. The common iliac arteries are generally larger in diameter than the largest Atherocath available (7.7mm diameter). Therefore, a good match is very difficult to obtain in the common iliac arteries (Fig. 6.9.6).[27]

The external iliac artery, because of its smaller caliber, lends itself to better results (Fig. 6.9.7). Maynar reported results of directional atherectomy in 31 patients, with 36 lesions treated. At 18 months post-procedure, a patency rate of 87% was reported.[27] Until the long-term efficacy of these devices is proved in removal of the atherosclerotic material in these larger vessels, angioplasty is the procedure of choice in the iliac arteries. It should, however, be noted that a smoother lumen is a common finding following atherectomy of the iliac artery even when it is combined with balloon angioplasty (Fig. 6.9.8). This could lead to a better long-term follow-up result.[27]

DIRECTIONAL ATHERECTOMY OF SUPERFICIAL FEMORAL POPLITEAL ARTERY STENOSIS

The initial overall patency rate for balloon angioplasty is 81.3%. However, the restenosis rate is 46% for stenosis, and 26% for occlusion of less than 7cm at two years. Lesions more than 7cm in length have a patency rate of

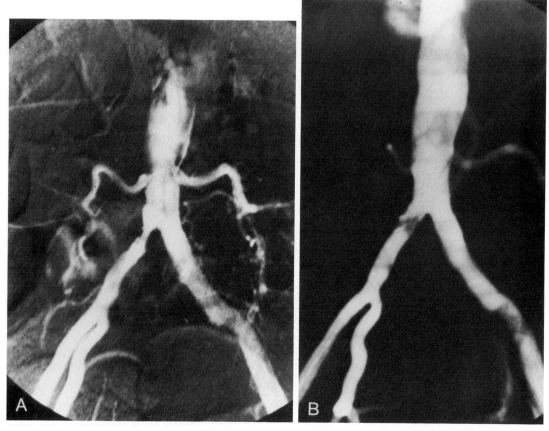

Figure 6.9.6. A. Pelvic arteriogram showing a 70% narrowing of the right common iliac with diffuse 30% narrowing of the distal common iliac. **B.** Following atherectomy and angioplasty of the right common iliac, note increase in diameter but a significant residual intraluminal defect due to incomplete removal with the Atherocath.

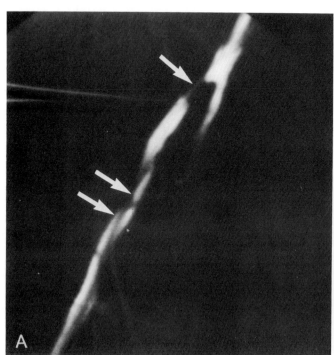

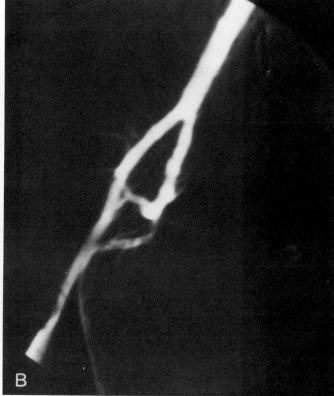

Figure 6.9.7. A. Iliac arteriogram shows a subtotal occlusion at the take-off of the right external artery, which has been recanalized with a catheter *(arrow)*. More distally, there is a 50–60% narrowing of the right external iliac artery *(paired arrows)*. **B.** Following atherectomy of the multiple lesions in the right external artery, note the marked increase in diameter with minimal residual narrowing.

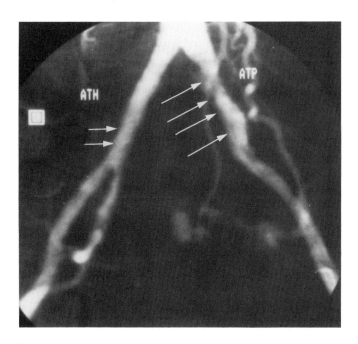

Figure 6.9.8. Pelvic arteriogram postatherectomy of the right common iliac and angioplasty of the left common iliac. Note the smooth contours of the right common iliac in contrast to the irregular appearance of the left common iliac *(arrows)*.

23% at 6 months, which drops to zero at 30 months.[5-7] It is hoped that debulking of the atheromatous lesions may improve long-term patency (Fig. 6.9.9). An initial patency rate of 95 and 92.5% with atherectomy was reported by Schwarten and Maynar at six months' follow-up.[17,18] Graor reported a 12-month patency rate for simple lesions <5cm stenotic or occlusive lesion) and of 93 and 80% for complete lesions (>5cm stenosis or occlusion).[28] Rousseau reported a three-year patency rate of 87%.[29] Reports in the cardiology literature have significantly poorer results including Iyer's report of 52 and 65% recurrence rate at 5.4 months for stenosis and occlusions, respectively, with an overall recurrence rate of 55%.[30] Von Polnitz reported a recurrence rate of 24% for residual stenosis larger than 50%. Restenosis rates are higher in concentric than in eccentric lesions and more common yet in cases of total occlusions. In addition, the mean six-month percent stenosis for all lesions was 39%.[31]

A common denominator in the Iyer and Von Polnitz series is their definition of angiographic success as a residual stenosis of less than 50%.[30,31] This contrasts markedly with the definition of success for Graor and Maynar (<20% residual stenosis) and Schwarten (<30%).[17,18,28] It is clear that the philosophical approach to residual stenosis

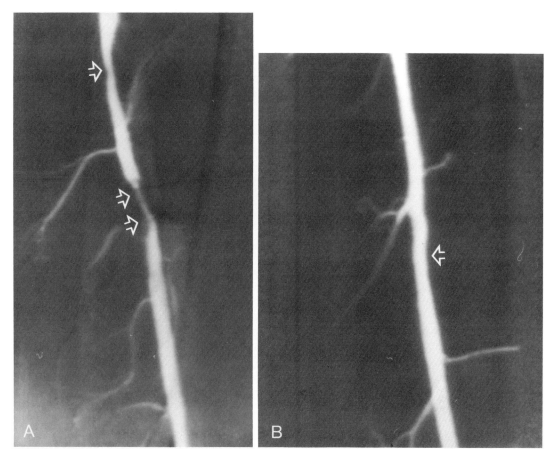

Figure 6.9.9. **A.** Femoral arteriogram showing a 50% narrowing of the mid-superficial femoral artery *(single open arrow)* and a long 70% narrowing at the junction of the mid-SFA with the distal SFA *(two open arrows)*.

B. Following atherectomy, note the excellent result with minimal 20% residual narrowing *(arrow)*.

is quite different between cardiologists and interventional radiologists. While it might be acceptable to leave a residual 40–50% stenosis in the coronary arteries (although this is arguable if one remembers the high recurrence rate of restenosis following percutaneous transluminal coronary angioplasty (PTCA)), a 40–50% residual stenosis in the peripheral circulation will commonly cause an early recurrence. The early data of Simpson and Schwarten clearly reflected this problem, with a recurrence rate of 28% at six months when a residual stenosis of more than 30% was left behind compared with a recurrence of 11% at six months, when less than 30% residual stenosis was present.[8,20] It seems, however, that certain factors such as concentric lesions, calcification, and length do affect the rate of recurrence.[30,31]

DIRECTIONAL ATHERECTOMY IN BLUE DIGIT SYNDROME

The blue digit syndrome is thought to be due to microemboli composed of fibrinoplatelet aggregates. Neither antiplatelet nor anticoagulant therapy will prevent recurrent embolization, and may actually cause further microembolization. Affected patients have focal high-grade stenoses, patent tibial run-offs, absence of atheromas in the aorta, and no history of macroembolization. The

initial treatment of choice includes percutaneous transluminal angioplasty followed by administration of platelet inhibitors.[32] Surgery is indicated in patients with recurrent microembolization after percutaneous dilatation, extensive severe ulcerating atheromatosis, or systemic cholesterol embolization.[33] Recently, Simpson and Schwarten described the use of the Atherocath in the management of a patient with a grossly ulcerated lesion of the superficial femoral artery and the blue digit syndrome[20] (Fig. 6.9.10). We have recently utilized this technique in a similar patient and feel that the technique may have promise in treating this clinical problem.

DIRECTIONAL ATHERECTOMY OF RESTENOSIS POSTANGIOPLASTY

Postangioplasty restenosis has been reported with an incidence varying from 15 to 45% at one year following coronary angioplasty.[34,35] Mechanisms advocated include: l) acute reocclusions—spasm and dissection with reclosure, thrombosis, and elastic recoil; 2) early reocclusion—fibrocellular proliferative response and elastic recoil; 3) late reocclusion—progressive atheromatous disease.[34] Recently, directional atherectomy has been used by Simpson and Schwarten in the management of restenosis following angioplasty[20,27] (Fig. 6.9.11). It is hoped that histo-

Figure 6.9.10. **A.** High-grade stenosis of superficial femoral artery with ulcerated plaque *(arrow).* **B.** Postatherectomy; note smooth lumen. **C.** Resected specimen.

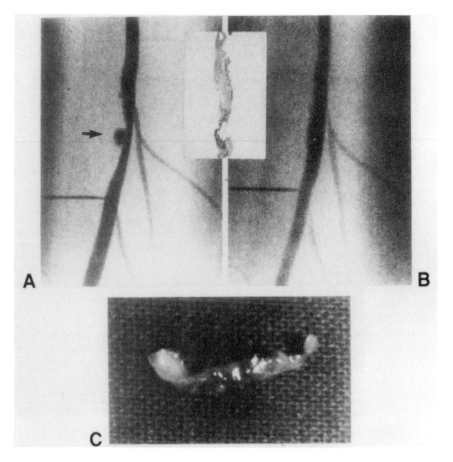

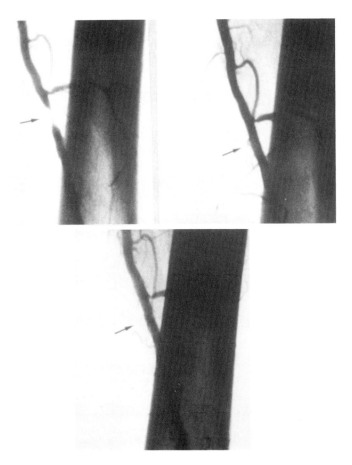

Figure 6.9.11. Top left. High-grade stenosis of superficial femoral artery *(arrow).* **Top right.** Follow-up arteriogram shows recurrence of stenosis of site of previous angioplasty. **Bottom.** Postatherectomy; note improved lumen.

logical studies from these cases will help elucidate some of the pathogenic mechanisms that mediate restenosis.

DIRECTIONAL ATHERECTOMY OF POSTANGIOPLASTY INTIMAL FLAP

In 1979, the physiopathologic basis of balloon angioplasty was established and supported by extensive microscopic and physiologic data.[22,36,37] These studies showed that partial or complete separation of the atheromatous plaque and associated rupture of the media were responsible for the increase in luminal diameter.[22] These changes were manifested angiographically by the appearance of radiolucent linear filling defects within the vessel lumen after angioplasty. These intimal flaps are commonly of little clinical significance as they are nonobstructive.[22,37] In some cases, the flaps are obstructive because of their orientation within the arterial lumen (Fig. 6.9.12). Occasionally, an intimal flap becomes detached completely from the arterial wall and embolizes distally.[38]

Nonobstructive intimal flaps are commonly shown by angiography after percutaneous balloon angioplasty. These flaps result from the fracture and partial detach-

ment of the atherosclerotic intima from the media.[39] The partially detached intima usually remains attached to the arterial wall at both its proximal and distal margins. If the proximal end detaches, the flap can become completely or intermittently obstructive by acting as a valve[39] (Fig. 6.9.12B). This, fortunately, is an unusual occurrence, as it can lead to acute postprocedural thrombosis. More commonly, these large nonobstructive intimal flaps can be the cause of delayed restenosis or occlusion.

In the past, if an obstructive intimal flap was detected during a balloon angioplasty procedure, redilatation with the balloon catheter was attempted with the hope that the intimal flap would be pressed against the arterial wall. When this maneuver was not successful, surgical revascularization was frequently required. Maynar et al. reported their experience with intimal flaps in which the obstruction to flow caused by the intimal flap was nearly complete and would have required surgical bypass (Fig. 6.9.13). The use of the Atherocath permitted removal of the obstructing intimal flap and restoration of blood flow to normal levels as indicated by the ankle-arm indices[39] (Fig. 6.9.14). Use of the directional atherectomy technique in these patients presented the potential risk of embolizing the atheromatous flap. However, these patients were already in need of a surgical bypass procedure and if peripheral embolization of large fragments occurred, the fragments could have been removed at the time of surgery. A different situation is present in those patients in whom the flaps are only partially obstructive but of sufficient severity to compromise long-term arterial patency[39] (Fig. 6.9.15). The use of the Atherocath to remove these flaps might improve long-term patency.[39]

DIRECTIONAL ATHERECTOMY OF COMPLETE OBSTRUCTIONS

Use of the Simpson Atherocath has been recommended for the treatment of atherosclerotic stenotic lesions.[17–19,27] The lack of "over-the-wire" capability has restricted its applications in the setting of complete arterial obstruction.

Based on the assumption that an atherectomy should provide better long-term clinical results than angioplasty since it removes the obstructing material, Maynar attempted to use the atherectomy device in patients with complete vascular occlusions.[40]

The Simpson Atherocath has been used successfully to recanalize complete occlusions of the iliac and femoropopliteal arteries. Directional atherectomy and angioplasty techniques were used in combination in 75% of the cases and directional atherectomy alone in 25% of the cases. Following directional atherectomy, all patients showed clinical improvement. Distal pulses returned in 64%; rest pain and/or claudication disappeared in the other 36%. Ischemic ulcers healed in the affected patients. Overall, the ankle-arm index (AAI) improved by an average of 0.43,

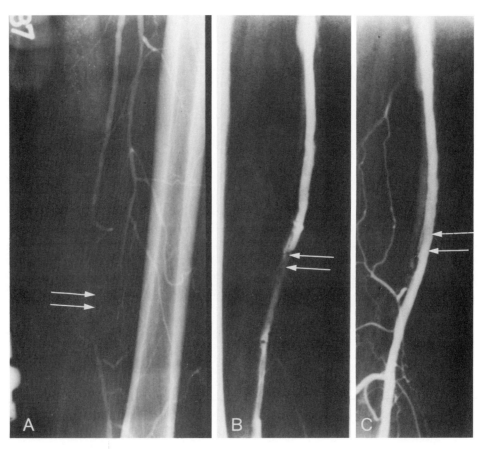

Figure 6.9.12. **A.** Left superficial femoral arteriograms show severe diffuse narrowing of the proximal, middle, and distal superficial femoral artery with a segment of complete occlusion in the distal SFA *(arrows).* **B.** Following angioplasty, there is an increase in diameter of the proximal superficial femoral artery, but a subtotal occlusion by a partially detached atherosclerotic plaque *(arrows).* Note the difference in density in the contrast medium column. **C.** Following atherectomy with removal of the occluding partially detached atheromatous plaque, note the marked increase in diameter with excellent flow of contrast medium.

with the improvement being greater (0.55) in patients in whom the luminal improvement was accomplished to a maximum of 90–100% of native luminal diameter. Seventy percent of patients have remained with stable AAI values and without change in their clinical status at 18 months' follow-up.[40]

Ankle-arm indices were obtained in all patients before, immediately after, and every six months after the atherectomy. Digital subtraction angiography was used for the preliminary angiographic assessment of the occlusions. Road mapping and conventional fluoroscopy were used to guide the recanalization of the occluded segments, as well as the subsequent directional atherectomy. Systemic anticoagulation was used during the procedure with 5000 units of heparin IV, administered after the placement of the vascular sheath. Intra-arterial nitroglycerin (bolus injections of $100\mu g$) was used liberally to prevent spasm. All patients were placed on aspirin/Persantin after the procedure.[40]

Recanalization of the occluded segment was accomplished using an antegrade approach for the superficial femoral artery and a retrograde approach for the iliac artery (Figs. 6.9.16 and 6.9.17A,B). This was done with a guidewire passed through a 6Fr straight catheter that had

both an endhole and a sidehole; this instrumentation permitted the injection of contrast during the advancement of the guidewire. After recanalization and/or angioplasty, an 0.012-inch guidewire was passed through the recanalization or angioplasty catheter and kept in place alongside the Atherocath during the entire atherectomy procedure to preserve access to the distal segment of the artery in the event of a complication[41] (Fig. 6.9.17C). In some cases, the directional atherectomy was performed immediately following the recanalization with the guidewire-6Fr catheter combination. In the remaining cases, the 6Fr catheter was replaced by a 3 or 4mm angioplasty balloon catheter for dilatation. Undersizing of the dilating balloon on the angioplasty catheter was deliberately done to facilitate removal of the intima by the Simpson Atherocath, without needing to resort to a larger diameter Atherocath[40] (Fig. 6.9.17D).

Following recanalization of the arterial lumen, an Atherocath was introduced to remove as much atheromatous/thrombotic material as was possible. The Simpson Atherocath size was selected in direct correlation to the arterial diameter immediately proximal or distal to the site of obstruction, keeping in mind that the manufacturer's specifications state that the 7, 8, 9, 10, and 11Fr atherectomy

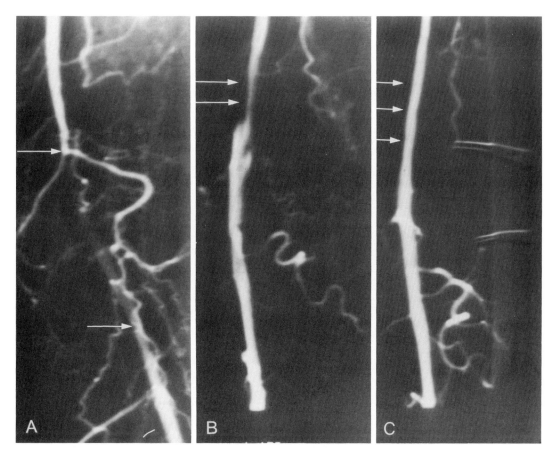

Figure 6.9.13. **A.** Left superficial femoral arteriogram shows a complete occlusion of the mid-superficial femoral artery with distal reconstitution via collaterals *(arrows)*. **B.** Following angioplasty there is a high-grade residual obstruction caused by a partially detached atherosclerotic plaque *(arrows)*. **C.** Following atherectomy the occluding, partially attached atheromatous plaque has been removed and there is improvement in flow, although there is a residual 30–40% diffuse narrowing of the proximal SFA *(arrows)*.

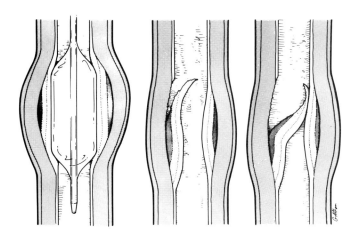

Figure 6.9.14. Diagram illustrating the mechanism of occlusion caused by a partially detached plaque. **Left.** Balloon angioplasty is performed on a high-grade stenosis in a vessel. **Middle.** After removal of the angioplasty balloon, the proximal detached segment of the plaque is hanging loose in the arterial lumen. **Right.** The force of the blood stream has pushed the partially detached plaque against the opposite arterial wall causing an obstruction of the vascular lumen.

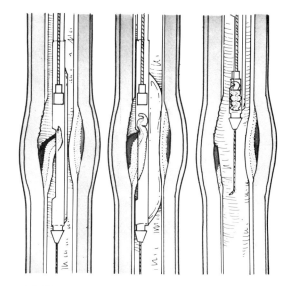

Figure 6.9.15. Diagram illustrating removal of partially detached plaque by Atherocath. **Left.** The Atherocath window has been placed against the partially detached plaque. **Middle.** The positioning balloon has been inflated, forcing the plaque into the window. **Right.** The plaque has been excised and is being removed by the Atherocath, leaving a smooth, wide-open lumen.

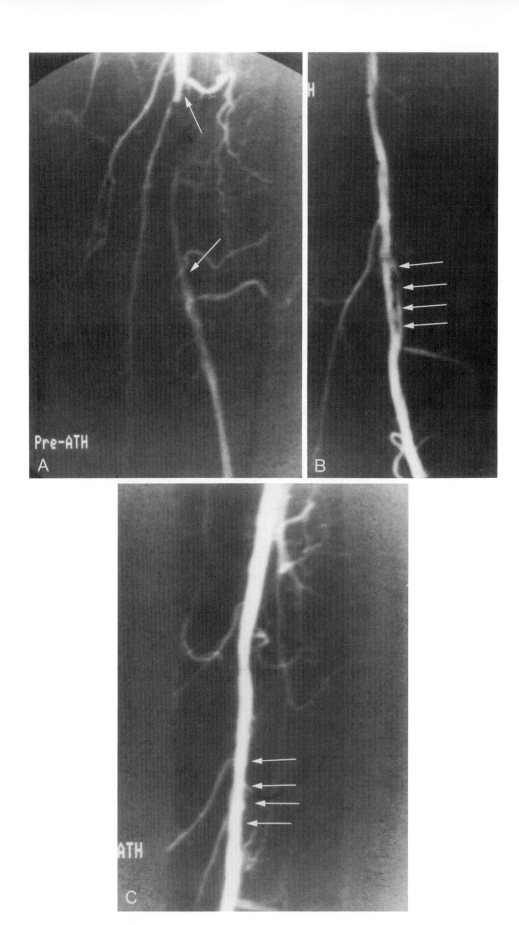

Figure 6.9.16. **A.** Left femoral arteriogram shows 100% occlusion of the mid-superficial femoral artery with distal reconstitution *(arrows)*. **B.** Superficial femoral arteriogram postrecanalization and angioplasty of the complete obstruction in the mid-superficial femoral artery shows a large intimal flap *(arrows)* with significant narrowing of the lumen. **C.** Femoral arteriogram postatherectomy of intimal flap shows a widely patent lumen with a residual 30% narrowing *(arrow)*.

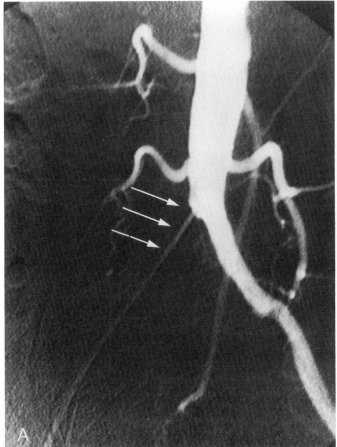

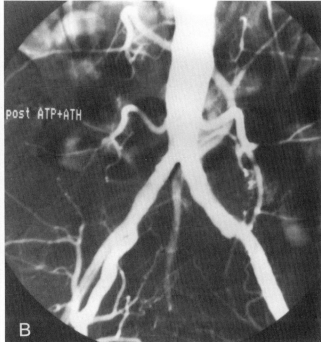

Figure 6.9.17. **A.** Pelvic arteriogram shows 100% occlusion of the right common iliac. A catheter has been passed across the area of obstruction into the abdominal aorta *(arrows)*. **B.** Repeat pelvic arteriogram postatherectomy of the obstructing lesion in the right common iliac followed by angioplasty to complement the reconstitution of the lumen shows an increase in diameter with a residual diffuse 30% narrowing of the right common iliac.

complex of capsule plus balloon inflated catheters corresponds to 4.8, 5.7, 6.0, 6.8, and 7.7mm, respectively. Use of an undersize Atherocath results in a less than optimal result. Follow-up angiography in several projections was done to evaluate the results of the procedure.[40] If needed, further passes with the same Atherocath or a larger device are used to complete the removal, trying to leave less than a 20% residual narrowing. After an initial complication in our first patient, all remaining patients were fully anticoagulated with heparin for 48 hours following the procedure.

The criteria that we used to assess radiologic success were:

1. 91 to 100% luminal reconstitution.
2. 81 to 90% luminal reconstitution.
3. 71 to 80% luminal reconstitution.
4. 61 to 70% luminal reconstitution.
5. Less than 60% luminal reconstitution.

The atheromatous material extracted was sent for histologic examination.

Following directional atherectomy all patients showed clinical improvement. In 63% of patients, including those in whom the procedure was performed without preliminary use of balloon angioplasty, there was an increase in the arterial lumen of more than 90%. Eighty-one to ninety percent luminal reconstitution was found in another 27% of patients and 60% reconstitution was accomplished in 10%. Changes in the ankle-arm index were greater in patients in whom the maximal improvement in luminal diameter was achieved (91–100%); the ankle-arm index increased an average of 0.47 points in 63%. In the patients with an increase of luminal diameter to 81–90% the ankle-arm index increased by an average of 0.40 points. When the lumen increased only by 70%, the ankle-arm index increased by only 0.30 points. Seventy percent of patients have remained clinically stable for 18 months following the procedure with no significant decrease in the Doppler indices.

The amount of material extracted was greater in the lesions where the Atherocath was of equal or larger diameter than the native artery; in these cases an average number of 19 fragments were removed. When the artery was slightly larger in diameter than the Atherocath, the average

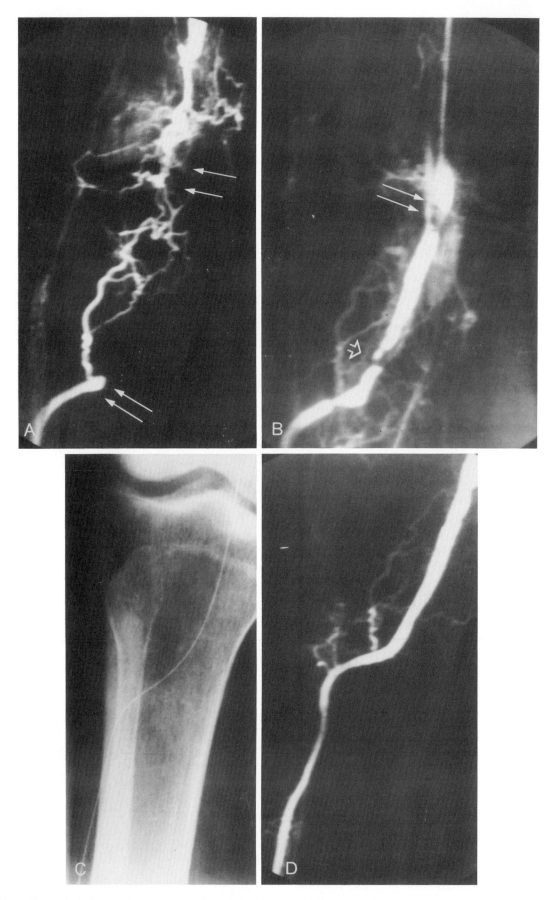

Figure 6.9.18. **A.** Femoral arteriogram showing a complete occlusion of the distal superficial femoral artery with distal reconstitution of the anterior tibial artery *(arrows)*. **B.** Following recanalization with a wire and PTA, a femoral arteriogram shows significant intraluminal filling defects *(arrows)* and a high-grade stenosis in the distal popliteal artery *(open arrow)*. **C.** A 0.012-inch guidewire has been passed into the distal anterior tibial artery. **D.** Following atherectomy of intimal defects, note significant increase in arterial diameter with excellent run-off.

number of fragments removed was 12. When the artery was definitely larger than the Atherocath diameter, the average number of fragments removed was only five. The angiographic improvement in luminal diameter tended to be better in those procedures where more material was removed.

The risk of either angioplasty or directional atherectomy procedures was not significantly increased by the use of the two techniques in combination, as was demonstrated by the absence of complications such as distal embolization or intimal dissections. The use of an 0.012-inch guidewire across the stenosis was designed as a safety precaution, maintaining vascular access in case of a significant complication, such as perforation, plaque detachment, or subintimal dissection.[40] Passage of the atherectomy catheter across a recently recanalized and dilated area was simple and relatively atraumatic, because the 0.018-inch floppy wire at the front of the catheter steers the capsule through

the lumen. Similar results have been seen in coronary angioplasty with the use of the 0.018-inch platinum tip guidewires. In the cases in whom the directional atherectomy was performed without preliminary angioplasty, the distance to be recanalized was short and the channel created after the recanalization with the guidewire and angiographic catheter was adequate to allow the direct passage of the Atherocath. Distal access was guaranteed by the placement of a 0.012-inch guidewire across the segment to be recanalized. Anticoagulation was instituted after the initial complication in this series of recanalization of complete occlusions. This contrasts with the protocol followed in the remaining atherectomy patients that we have treated for stenotic, but not completely obstructing, lesions in whom heparinization has not been necessary.[17,18]

The Atherocath size has to be directly related to the arterial diameter, as it is desirable to remove as much of the atheromatous/thrombotic material as possible. As has

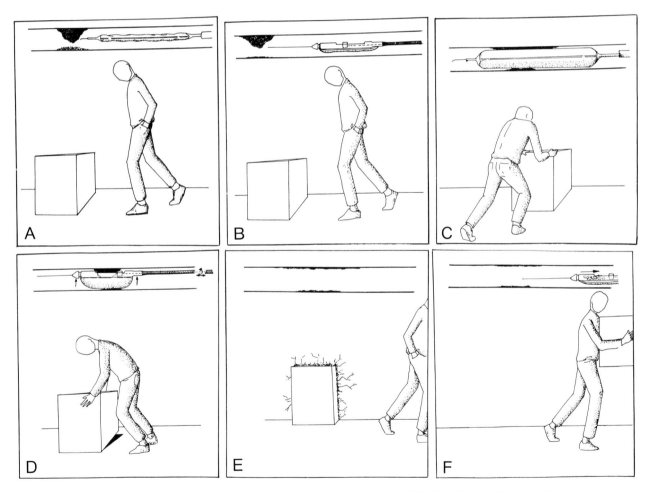

Figure 6.9.19. Diagram illustrating the difference between angioplasty and atherectomy. **A.** The angioplasty balloon approaches an obstructing atherosclerotic plaque in a vessel in the same manner as a man walking in a hallway approaches an object. **B.** The Atherocath approaches an obstructing plaque in a vessel in the same manner as a man approaches an obstacle in a hallway. **C.** The angioplasty balloon disrupts and pushes the plaque against the wall in the same manner as a man pushes an object against the wall. **D.** The Atherocath excises the plaque for subsequent removal; in the same manner, a man lifts up an object. **E.** After removal of the balloon, the atherosclerotic plaque has been impacted into the wall of the artery in the same manner that the man has impacted the object into the wall of the hallway. **F.** The Atherocath removes the excised plaque, leaving a clean vascular wall in the same manner as the man who picks up an object and walks away with it, leaving a clean wall and hallway.

been shown in a series of patients done by Simpson, the recurrence rate can be as high as 28% when a residual stenosis over 30% is left behind.[15] In our series, multiple passes of the atherectomy catheter were frequently necessary and this factor is one of the well known disadvantages of the Simpson Atherocath. This problem will, however, be partially solved by the use of the Atherocath with the extended storage space.

The long-term results obtained by transluminal angioplasty in the management of complete obstructions of the femoropopliteal system have been poor; one-year patency rates of 81% and four year patency rates of 67% have been reported for complete obstructions less than 7cm in length. For occlusions longer than 7cm, patency rates of 91% and 68% at six months and four years have been reported.[5-7] In an attempt to improve on these patency rates by debulking the lesions, the combination of two recanalization techniques, one to re-establish the arterial lumen (percutaneous angioplasty) and the other to debulk (directional atherectomy) was attempted, to remove the fractured and displaced atheromatous material and associated organized thrombus.[40] It was hoped that the removal of the intraluminal material would reduce turbulence, platelet aggregation and intimal hyperplasia and result in an improved long-term patency rate. At 18 months' follow-up, 70% of patients who have been followed up remained asymptomatic with stable ankle-arm indices.[40] Von Polnitz reported a patency rate of only 53% at six months.[31] Iyer found a 35% patency rate of 5.4 months.[42] Again, it should be mentioned here that for these two investigators, the definition of success was a residual stenosis of less than 50%.[31,42] Limitations of directional atherectomy include calcified lesions with a success rate of only 70%,[43,44] and length of lesions, with tubular lesions having a lower success rate than focal lesions.[40,43,45,46] The patency rate reported by them does not seem to be appreciably better than that of transluminal angioplasty alone. Larger and randomized series are, however, needed in order to establish the real role of directional atherectomy in this group of patients. The role of directional atherectomy in the management of complete arterial obstructions is still not well defined. We hope that the patency rates we have obtained using a combination of balloon angioplasty and atherectomy techniques can be sustained and surpass the 68% five-year patency rates currently reported for balloon angioplasty of complete occlusions in the superficial femoral and popliteal arteries.

CONCLUSIONS

Revascularization of vascular occlusions with the Atherocath removes atheromatous plaque leaving a smooth surface (Fig. 6.9.18) and also dilates the vessel lumen by the angioplasty and coaxial Dotter effects. Adequate matching of catheter to the arterial diameter optimizes positioning of the cutting capsule and also the angioplasty effect.

Other applications of the Atherocath include removal of obstructive intimal flaps, ulcerated lesions, and treatment of completely obstructing lesions. Angioscopy and intravascular ultrasound may provide valuable information for revascularization procedures not readily apparent by angiography, and may play a major role in the future of vascular interventional techniques.

References

1. Dotter CT, Judkins MP: Transluminal treatment of atherosclerotic obstruction. *Circulation* 1964;30:654–657
2. van Andel GJ: Transluminal dilatation with separate Teflon catheters, in Zeitler E, Grüntzig A, Schoop W (eds): *Percutaneous Vascular Recanalization*. Berlin, Springer–Verlag, 1978, pp 13–16
3. Wierny L, Dass R, Portsman W: Long-term results in 100 consecutive patients treated by transluminal angioplasty. *Radiology* 1974;112:543–548
4. Grüntzig A, Hopff H: Perkutane rekanalization chronischer arterieller Verschlusse mit ein neuem Dilationskatheter: Modification der Dottertechnik. *Dtsch Med Wschr* 1974; 99:2502–2505
5. Murray RR, Hughes RCH, White RI Jr, et al: Long segment femoropopliteal stenoses: is angioplasty a balloon or bust? *Radiology* 1987;162:473–476
6. Hewes RC, White RJ Jr, Murray RR, et al: Long-term results of superficial femoral artery angioplasty. *AJR* 1986;146:1025–1029
7. Krepel VM, van Andel GJ, van Erp MFM, Breslau PJ: Percutaneous transluminal angioplasty of the femoropopliteal artery: initial and long-term results. *Radiology* 1985; 156:325–328
8. Simpson JB, Zimmerman JJ, Selmon MR, Shoor PM, Cipriano PR, Martin F, McAuley BJ, Fogarty TJ, Hayden WG: Transluminal atherectomy: initial clinical results in 27 patients. *Circulation* 1986;74(suppl 2):II–203
9. Kensey K, Nash J, Abrahams C, Lake K, Zarins CK: Recanalization of obstructed arteries using a flexible rotating tip catheter (abstr). *Circulation* 1986; 74(suppl 1–II):457
10. Nordstrom LA, Dorros G: Laser enhanced angioplasty: an alternative to thermal contact plaque ablation (abstr). *Circulation* 1987;76(suppl IV):47
11. Geschwind H, Boussingnac G, Teisseire B: Percutaneous transluminal laser angioplasty in man. *Lancet* 1984;1:844
12. Jenkins RD, Sinclair ID, Arnand RK, James LM, Spears JR: Laser balloon angioplasty: effect of exposure on shear strength of welded layers of postmortem human aorta (abstr). *Circulation* 1987;76(suppl IV):46
13. Sanborn TA, Cumberland DC, Greenfield AJ, Tayler DI, Welsh CL, Guben JK, Ryan TJ: Six-month follow-up of laser probe assisted balloon angioplasty (abstr). *Circulation* 1986; 74(suppl. II):457
14. Fourrier JL: Angioplastie laser par saphir de contact: propriétés optiques et thermiques du catheter, et résultats cliniques préliminaires. Presented at RIPCV-2 Congress International, Toulouse, France, Feb 1990
15. Schatz R, Palmaz J, Garcia F, Tio F, Reuter S: Balloon expandable intracoronary stents in dogs (abstr). *Circulation* 1986;74(suppl II):458
16. Puel J, Rousseau H, Joffre F, Hatem S, Fauvel JM, Bounhourne JP: Intravascular stents to prevent restenosis after transluminal coronary angioplasty (abstr). *Circulation* 1987; 76(suppl IV):27
17. Maynar M, Cabrera V, Reyes R, Roman M, Pulido–Duque

JM, Castañeda F, Tobio R, Letourneau JG, Castañeda–Zúñiga WR: Percutaneous atherectomy with the Simpson atherectomy device in the management of arterial stenosis. *Semin Intervent Radiol* 1988;5(4):247–252

18. Schwarten DE, Cutcliff WB, Krok KL: The late results of femoral directional atherectomy. Presented at RIPCV-2, Toulouse, France, Feb 1990

19. Schwarten DE, Katzen BT, Simpson JB, Cutcliff WB: Simpson catheter for percutaneous transluminal removal of atheroma. *AJR* 1988;150:799–801

20. Schwarten D: Percutaneous atherectomy using the Simpson's atherectomy catheter. Presented at the Pros and Contras in PTA and Auxiliary Methods Symposium. Nurenberg, 1988

21. Sharaf BL, Williams DO: Dotter effect contributes to angiographic improvement following directional coronary atherectomy. *Circulation* 1990;82(suppl III):III–310

22. Castañeda–Zúñiga WR, Formanek G, Tadavarthy M, Amplatz K: The mechanism of balloon angioplasty. *Radiology* 1980;135:565–571

23. Selmon MR, Robertson GC, Simpson JB, Rowe MH, Johnson DE, Leggett JH, Hinohara T: Retrieval of media and adventitia by directional coronary atherectomy and angiographic correlation. *Circulation* 1990;82(4):III–624

24. Safian RD, Gelbfish JS, Erny RE, Schnitt S, Baim DS: Histologic findings of coronary atherectomy. *Circulation* 1990;82(suppl III):III–310

25. Dick RJ, Kunkel JF, Debowey DL: Does ectasia following directed coronary atherectomy predict the histological depth of excision? *Circulation* 1990;82(suppl III):III–623.

26. Smucker ML, Howard PF, Scherb DE, Kil D, Sarnat WS: Does intracoronary ultrasound prevent deep cuts during coronary atherectomy? *Circulation* 1990;82(suppl III):III–440

27. Maynar M, Reyes R, Cabrera V, Pulido–Duque JM, Yetano J, Castañeda F, Letourneau J, Castañeda–Zúñiga WR: Percutaneous atherectomies of iliac arteries. *Semin Intervent Radiol* 1988;5:253–255

28. Graor RA, Whitlow PL: Transluminal atherectomy for occlusive peripheral vascular disease. *J Am Coll Cardiol* 1990;15:1551–1558

29. Rousseau H, Levade M, Maquin P, Escude B, Joffre F, Raichac JJ: Peripheral atherectomy with the Simpson catheter: long-term results. Presented at RIPCV-2 International Congress. Toulouse, France, 1990

30. Iyer SS, Dorros G, Zaitoun R, Lewin RF: Angiographic follow-up after percutaneous directional atherectomy (Simpson Atherocath) for peripheral vascular disease. *Circulation* 1990;82(suppl III):III–623

31. vonPolnitz A, Norlich A, Berger H, Hofling B: Percutaneous peripheral atherectomy: angiographic and clinical follow-up in 60 patients. *J Am Coll Cardiol* 1990:15:682–688

32. Kumpe O, Zwendlinger S, Griffin D: Blue digit syndrome: treatment with percutaneous transluminal angioplasty. *Radiology* 1988;166:37–44

33. Lee BY, Bracato RF, Thosen WR, Madden JL: Blue digit syndrome: urgent indication for limb salvage surgery. *Am J Surg* 1984;147:418–422

34. Schwartz L, Bourassa MG, Lesperance J, Aldridge HE, Kazim F, Salvatori VA, et al: Aspirin and dipyridamole in the prevention of restenosis after percutaneous transluminal coronary angioplasty. *N Engl J Med* 1988;318:1714–1719

35. Holmes DR Jr., Vliestra RE, Smith HC, Vetrovec GW, Kent KM, Cowley MJ, et al: Restenosis after percutaneous transluminal coronary angioplasty (PTCA): a report from the PTCA registry of the NHLBI. *Am J Cardiol* 1984;53:77C–81C

36. Zollikofer CL, Salomonowitz E, Sibley R, et al: Transluminal angioplasty evaluated by electron microscopy. *Radiology* 1984;153:369

37. Castañeda–Zúñiga WR, Tadavarthy SM, Laerum F, Amplatz K: "Pseudo" intramural injection following percutaneous transluminal angioplasty. *Cardiovasc Intervent Radiol* 1984;7:104

38. Katzen BT, Chang J: Percutaneous transluminal angioplasty with the Grüntzig balloon catheter. *Radiology* 1979;130:623

39. Maynar M, Reyes R, Cabrera V, et al: Percutaneous atherectomy as an alternative treatment for postangioplasty obstructing intimal flap. *Radiology* 1989;170(3):1029–1032

40. Maynar M, Reyes R, Pulido JM, et al: The Simpson atherectomy catheter in the management of complete obstruction. *RöFo* 1991;153(3):547–550

41. Maynar M, Reyes R, Cabrera V, Perez GIJ, Letourneau JG, Castañeda–Zúñiga WR: Use of safety wire in atherectomy procedures for recanalization of complete arterial obstruction. *Semin Intervent Radiol* 1988;5:256–259

42. Iyer S, Zaitoun R, Dorros G: Lesion recurrence following directional atherectomy in peripheral vascular disease. *Circulation* 1990;82(suppl III):III–623

43. U.S. Directional Coronary Atherectomy Investigator Group. Directional coronary atherectomy: multicenter experience. *Circulation* 1990;82(suppl III):III–71

44. Popma JJ, De Cesare NB, Zlyad C, Cass G, Pinkerton CA, Garratt KN: Predictors of improvement in quantitative coronary dimensions following coronary atherectomy. *Circulation* 1990;82(suppl III):III–311

45. Robertson GC, Selmon MR, Hinohara T, Rowe MH, Legget JH, Braden LJ, Simpson JB: The effect of lesion length on outcome of directional coronary atherectomy. *Circulation* 1990;82(suppl III):III–623

46. Robertson GC, Selmon MR, Hinohara T, Rowe MH, Legget JH, Braden LJ, Simpson JB: The effect of lesion length on outcome of directional coronary atherectomy. *Circulation* 1990;82(suppl III):III–623

Part 10. Transluminal Endarterectomy Catheter (TEC)

—Mark H. Wholey, M.D., Robert G. Levitt, M.D., and Deborah Fein–Millar, M.D.

INTRODUCTION

Over 200,000 patients are currently being treated for inoperable peripheral vascular disease or failed prior surgery. Percutaneous transluminal angioplasty (PTA) is an important alternative to surgery in these patients. Major factors limiting its use include acute occlusion due to uncontrolled injury and a restenosis rate of 15–25% at one to two years increasing to 30–45% at four to five years.[1,2] Atherectomy was developed with the hypothesis that

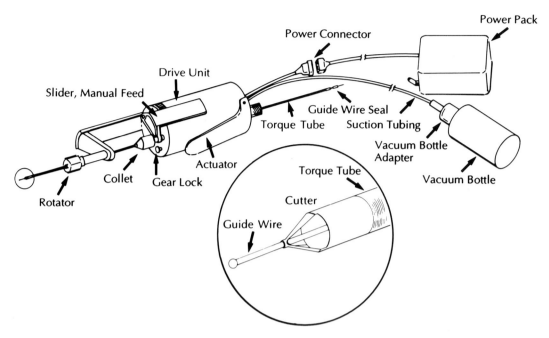

Figure 6.10.1. Diagram of components of TEC peripheral atherectomy device.

removal of plaque instead of remodeling of plaque (PTA) would result in a lower acute occlusion and restenosis rate than PTA.[3,4]

TECHNICAL DESCRIPTION

The transluminal endarterectomy catheter (TEC) (Interventional Technologies, Inc., San Diego, CA) was designed by R. S. Stack and his co-workers at Duke University.[5] This unit is the first atherectomy device for recanalization and reperfusion through total obstructions which continuously removes the debris by the vacuum effect, thereby reducing the incidence of distal embolization.[6]

The TEC system includes a cutter mounted on the distal end of a torque tube that is mounted over an 0.014-inch steerable wire (Fig. 6.10.1). The cutter consists of three blades which form the sides of a triangle (Fig. 6.10.2). The torque tube is connected to a hand-held drive assembly and power source which rotates the torque tube/cutter at 750 rpm to circumferentially resect atheromatous material from occluded or stenotic peripheral vessels (Fig. 6.10.3). The excised atheromatous material is evacuated through the hollow torque tube by an attached 125ml vacuum bottle under 1 atmosphere of negative pressure. Larger amounts of atheromatous plaque may be removed using this device. The TEC system comes in 5.0, 5.5, 6.0, 6.5, 7.0, 7.5, 8.0, 9.0, 10.0, 12.0, and 14.0Fr sizes (Fig. 6.10.4). In contrast to the Simpson atherectomy catheter, the cutter is exposed on the end of the torque tube, not protected within a catheter housing unit. Also, unlike the Simpson atherectomy catheter, the TEC does not require removal of the device (to remove excised debris) until the recanalization process is completed.

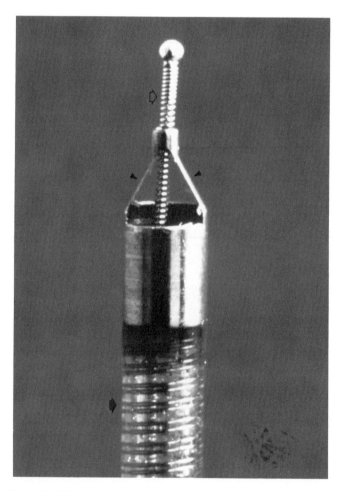

Figure 6.10.2. The TEC cutter consists of three triangular blades *(arrowheads)* mounted on the digital end of the torque tube *(closed arrow).* The IVT 0.014-inch guidewire *(open arrow)* passes through the cutter and torque tube.

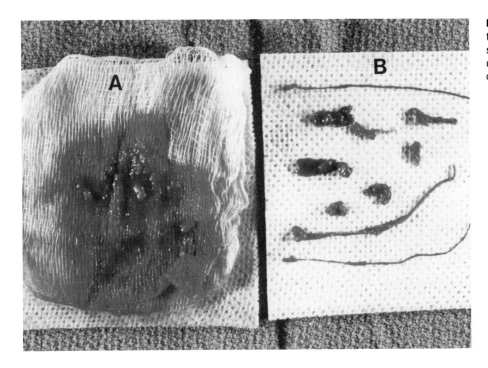

Figure 6.10.3. Atherosclerotic debris retrieved from TEC atherectomy of occluded superficial femoral artery. **A.** Debris from vacuum bottle filtered through gauze. **B.** Retrieved debris consists of several long cores.

INDICATIONS

The TEC is designed for use in stenoses or occlusions of peripheral vessels or grafts. It may also be used for percutaneous thrombectomy.[7] There is no restriction on the number, length, or severity of lesions as long as the 0.014-inch leading guidewire can be advanced across the lesion. The use of the TEC is contraindicated, whenever the guidewire cannot be positioned across the obstruction. The out-side diameter of the selected TEC device should never exceed the intraluminal diameter of the native vessel or graft immediately proximal or distal to the lesion(s). TEC atherectomy should be performed with a small French-size device initially, followed by a larger TEC device if necessary. The TEC device may be used in conjunction with other recanalization techniques including thrombolysis and PTA. Only the Interventional Technologies Inc. (IVT) 0.014-inch guidewire should be used with the TEC device.

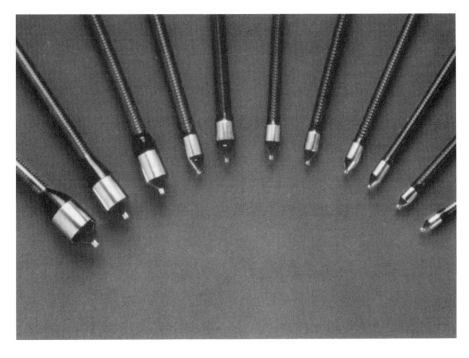

Figure 6.10.4. Different diameter TEC devices (IVT, Inc. cutter catheters) (5.0, 5.5, 6.0, 6.5, 7.0, 7.5, 8.0, 9.0, 10.0, 12.4) (5.0 = 1.7mm; 14.0 = 4.7mm).

TECHNIQUE

After the angiographic documentation of the lesion(s), an appropriately sized sheath is introduced, either retrograde or antegrade depending upon the vessel involved. One should avoid sharp angulation or kinking of the sheath to facilitate passage of the device. Five thousand units of heparin is administered intra-arterially. The IVT 0.014-inch guidewire is advanced to a position such that the flexible tip is distal to the lesion to be removed. The cutting head is then advanced over the wire to the proximal end of the lesion. The motorized drive unit provides rotational and linear feed motion to the cutting assembly while a vacuum source removes excised plaque. One hundred to two hundred micrograms of nitroglycerin is administered if the lesion is below the knee. The flow into the vacuum bottle should be monitored continuously and the vacuum bottle changed when full. The postatherectomy site is evaluated by removing the TEC device while holding the guidewire in position and injecting contrast medium through the sheath. If a larger lumen is necessary, the device is replaced with one of larger diameter and repeat atherectomy is performed. Alternatively, adjunctive PTA should be considered.

TECHNICAL RESULTS

A 16-center trial of the TEC device involving 132 patients is reported. A total of 204 lesions in this population were treated by TEC atherectomy. Slightly less than two-thirds of the lesions were short segment (<2cm) stenoses (129), while approximately one-quarter of the lesions were long segment (>2) stenoses (27) or total occlusions (48). The mean percentage stenosis was 80%. Five percent of lesions (10) were at the iliac artery level; 73.5% of the lesions (150) involved the superficial femoral artery, while 21.5% of the lesions (44) were located at or below the knee.

A TEC atherectomy was classified a technical success if a residual stenosis of less than 50% was achieved; this was accomplished in 88% of the TEC procedures (Table 6.10.1). When the residual stenosis was 30% or greater, PTA was performed. A supplemental PTA was required in 50% of the total occlusions, 40% of long segment stenoses, and 25% of the short segment stenoses.

Table 6.10.1. TEC Technical Success[a]

	No. Lesions	TEC Only	TEC + PTA	Success
Occlusion	48	24	24	41 (85%)
Stenosis ≤ 2cm	129	94	35	114 (89%)
Stenosis ≥ 2cm	27	16	11	24 (89%)
Total	204	134	70	179 (88%)

[a]Residual stenosis < 50%.

Table 6.10.2. TEC Complications in 132 Cases

Hematoma	10
Thrombosis	6
Dissection	8
Intimal flap	7
Embolization	0
Perforation	0

COMPLICATIONS

In the multicenter study, 23% of the patients had complications related to the TEC procedure (Table 6.10.2). Hematoma at the puncture site was the most frequent complication (8%). Thrombosis at the atherectomy site, dissection, and intimal flaps each occurred in approximately 5% of procedures. Regional intra-arterial urokinase restored patency in thrombotic occlusions at the atherectomy site. Intimal flaps were "tacked up" by adjunctive PTA. No distal embolization occurred in the multicenter clinical trial, but this complication has been reported in a smaller study.[8]

CLINICAL RESULTS

A six-month clinical follow-up was obtained in 50% of the 132 patients entered in the multicenter study (Table 6.10.3). This follow-up comprised 65% of the patients with lesions treated by TEC and supplemental PTA. Clinical improvement was defined by no symptoms or only mild symptoms (7–10 block claudication) in the six-month follow-up period. Restenoses or reocclusion was defined clinically by the development of moderate (three block) claudication to severe (minimal exertion) claudication or symptoms of ischemia during the six-month follow-up period. Patients with total occlusions or short segmental stenoses had good clinical results (Fig. 6.10.5); 86% of the patients with total occlusions and 77% of the patients with short segment stenoses had no symptoms or mild symptoms six months post-TEC atherectomy. Patients with long segment stenoses did poorer (Fig. 6.10.6); 50% of the patients had moderate or severe symptoms at six months (Table 6.10.4).

Patients with lesions requiring supplemental PTA following TEC atherectomy (Table 6.10.5) did not do nearly as well as the TEC-only group. In this group only the

Table 6.10.3. TEC Six-month Clinical Follow-up

	No. Patients	TEC Only	TEC + PTA
Occlusion	14	7 (50%)	7 (50%)
Stenosis ≤ 2cm	41	35 (85%)	6 (15%)
Stenosis ≥ 2cm	6	4 (67%)	2 (33%)
Total	61	46 (75%)	15 (25%)

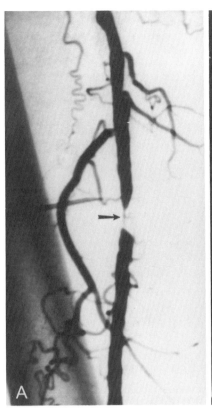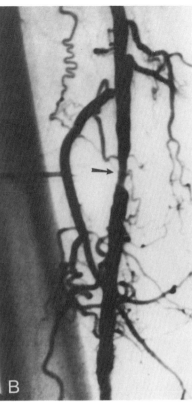

Figure 6.10.5. Short segment stenosis of superficial femoral artery (SFA). **A.** Digital subtraction angiogram reveals high-grade stenosis of SFA *(arrow)*. **B.** DSA shows improved diameter of stenotic segment *(arrow)* after passage of 7Fr TEC.

patients with total occlusions undergoing TEC and supplemental PTA (Figs. 6.10.7 and 6.10.8) had good clinical results; 71% of these patients had no symptoms or mild symptoms at six months. Patients with stenotic lesions had poor results; 50% of the patients with short segment stenoses had moderate or severe symptoms at six months and 100% of the patients with long segment stenoses had moderate or severe symptoms at six months. The poorer results of the TEC + PTA group compared to the TEC-only group are not unexpected. As noted in the Introduction, restenosis of peripheral vessels after balloon angioplasty continues to be a major problem. We have recently started using the Simpson atherectomy device to remove residual eccentric plaque following TEC atherectomy of critical stenoses, in an effort to reduce the restenosis rate (Fig. 6.10.9).

Stack's results in 51 coronary arteries revealed that the TEC was used alone in 39 patients and associated with PTA in 12 patients. Overall procedure success was 90% (less than 50% residual stenosis) (46/51). There were no com-

plications associated with the use of the TEC device.[9] Sketch reported on 63 peripheral vascular lesions in 34 patients. The primary success rate was 97%. The restenosis rate at six months was 20% (7/35). The lesion restenosis rate was 13% (4/30) for subtotal occlusions and 60% (3/5) for total occlusions. Patients with good distal runoff (2 or 3 vessels) had a 21% restenosis rate versus 100% (1/1) restenosis in patients with one vessel runoff. He concluded that TEC restenosis rates appear to be related to the extent of vessel occlusion and degree of distal disease in the vascular bed.[10] In his experience with coronary arteries, Sketch used the TEC alone in 35/44 lesions and associated PTA in nine. The primary success rate was 88%. Restenosis at six months occurred in 33% (6/18) of the patients treated with TEC alone and in 100% (2/2) of those treated with TEC plus PTA. In the lesions with restenosis post TEC atherectomy alone, those with a postprocedural residual stenosis of less than 30% had a restenosis rate of 14% (1/7), while those with a residual stenosis of more than 30%

Table 6.10.4. TEC-only Six-month Clinical Follow-up

	Mild/No Symptoms	Moderate/Severe Symptoms
Occlusion	6 (86%)	1 (14%)
Stenosis ≤ 2cm	27 (77%)	8 (23%)
Stenosis ≥ 2cm	2 (50%)	2 (50%)
Total	35	11

Table 6.10.5. TEC + PTA Six-month Clinical Follow-up

	Mild/No Symptoms	Moderate/Severe Symptoms
Occlusion	5 (71%)	2 (29%)
Stenosis ≤ 2cm	3 (50%)	3 (50%)
Stenosis ≥ 2cm	0	2 (100%)
Total	8	7

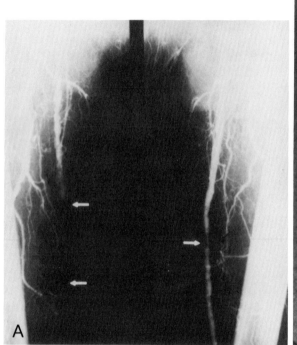

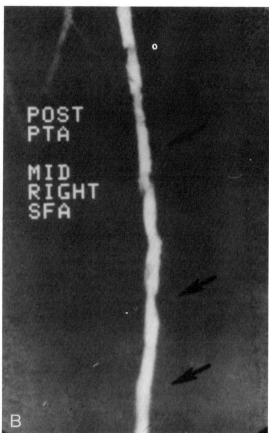

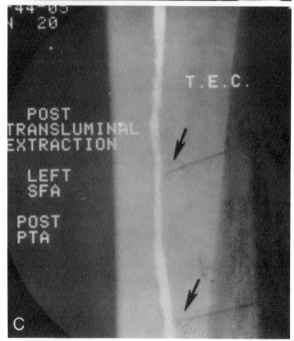

Figure 6.10.6. Long occlusion and short stenosis of superficial femoral arteries (SFA). **A.** Angiogram demonstrates long segment occlusion of calcified right superficial femoral artery *(arrows)* and short eccentric stenosis of left superficial femoral artery *(single arrow).* **B.** Digital subtraction angiogram (DSA) of long segment occlusion of right SFA *(arrows)* following 7Fr TEC atherectomy and supplemental 5mm PTA. **C.** DSA of short segment stenosis of left SFA *(arrows)* after 7Fr TEC atherectomy and supplemental 5mm PTA.

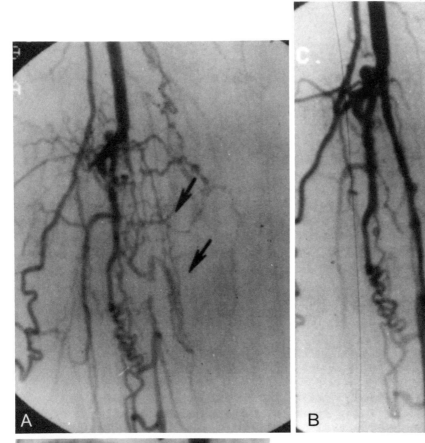

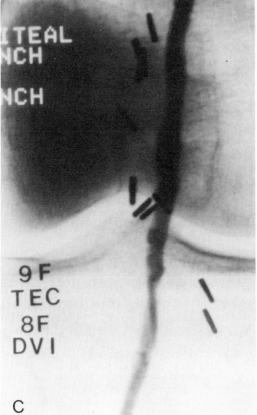

Figure 6.10.7. Occlusion of right common peroneal trunk (CPT). **A.** Digital subtraction angiogram of right CPT occlusion *(arrows).* **B.** DSA of recanalized CPT *(arrows)* after passage of 5Fr TEC. A supplemental PTA of the residual stenosis in the mid-CPT was performed.

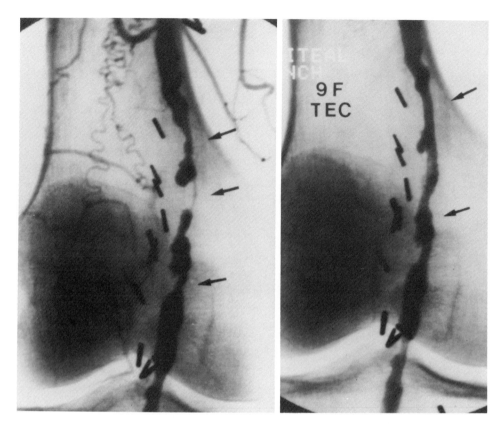

Figure 6.10.8. Multiple stenoses of vein interposition graft placed after popliteal artery aneurysm resection 7 years earlier. **A.** Digital subtraction angiogram (DSA) shows multiple high-grade stenoses and one critical stenosis of proximal vein interposition graft *(arrows)* and moderate stenoses of distal graft. **B.** Following a 9Fr TEC atherectomy, the high grade and critical stenoses are relieved *(arrows)* but moderate stenoses are still present distally. After an 8Fr Simpson atherectomy, the distal moderate stenoses were no longer present.

had a recurrence rate of 50% (6/12). Lesions treated for a previous PTCA restenosis had a 44% (4/9) restenosis rate while the restenosis rate was only 30% (3/10) for native lesions.[11]

STATUS OF TEC ATHERECTOMY

The results of the multicenter study show that TEC atherectomy is a safe and efficacious therapy for occluded peripheral vessels and short segment stenoses if no residual stenosis greater than 30% remains postatherectomy. In the TEC-only patients' follow-up studies, the patency rate for total occlusions was 85% and the clinical improvement (no symptoms/mild symptoms) for short segment stenoses was 77%; the clinical restenosis rate (moderate/severe symptoms) was 50% at six months. IVT redesigned the cutter in 1990 so that the blades are of microtome-like sharpness. Early reports show a decrease in the restenosis rate at six months.[12,13] When TEC atherectomy of a total occlusion left a residual stenosis greater than 30% requiring supplemental PTA, the combined procedure was effective; 71% of the total occlusions were patent at six months. TEC atherectomy of stenoses which required supplemental PTA was not effective; clinical restenosis developed in 50–100% by six months.

The major problem with the original TEC atherectomy device was its small working diameter. The largest 9Fr

device had a working diameter of only 3mm. In contrast, the Simpson 9Fr atherectomy catheter has a working diameter of 6mm. The small working diameter of the TEC device explains the frequent requirement for supplemental PTA. For example, a 9Fr (3mm) TEC atherectomy successfully performed on a critical stenosis or a normal-sized superficial femoral artery (6–8mm) leaves a residual stenosis of 50–60%, requiring supplemental PTA. Conversely, the smaller TEC device can fully recanalize occluded or highly stenotic vessels below the knee. These cases have been the most rewarding because threatened limb loss has been reversed (Fig. 6.10.9). The newly designed TEC devices have a diameter varying from 5.0 to 14.0Fr.

We currently recommend TEC atherectomy for total occlusions above and below the knee with supplemental PTA or Simpson atherectomy if a residual stenosis greater than 30% exists after TEC atherectomy.

References

1. Holfing B, Backa D, Lauterjung L, Polnitz AV, von Arnim TH, Jauch KW, Simpson JB: Percutaneous removal of atheromatous plaques in peripheral arteries. *Lancet* 1988; 1:384–385

2. Johnston KW, Rae M, Hogg–Johnston SA, Colapinto RF, Walker PM, Baird RJ, Sniderman KW, Kaliman P: 5-year

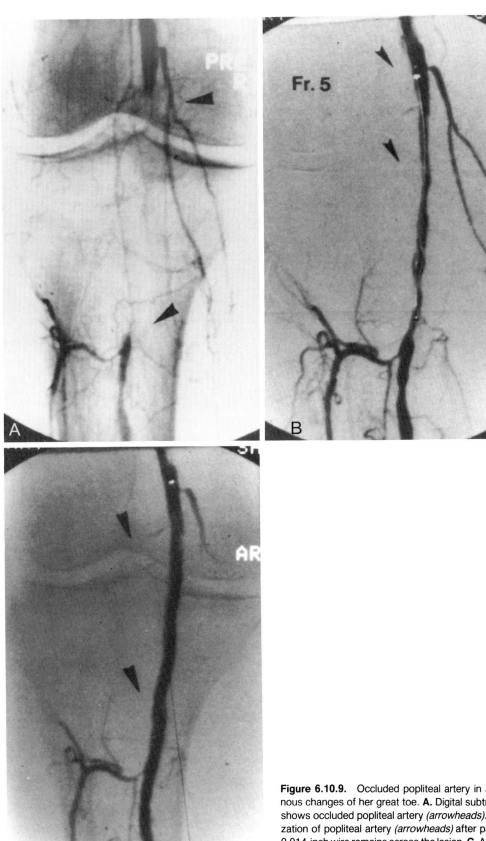

Figure 6.10.9. Occluded popliteal artery in a woman with pregangrenous changes of her great toe. **A.** Digital subtraction angiography (DSA) shows occluded popliteal artery *(arrowheads)*. **B.** DSA showing recanalization of popliteal artery *(arrowheads)* after passage of a 5Fr TEC. The 0.014-inch wire remains across the lesion. **C.** After supplemental PTA, the previously occluded popliteal artery *(arrowheads)* has normal lumen diameter.

results of a prospective study of percutaneous transluminal angioplasty. *Ann Surg* 1987;206(4):403–413

3. Hinohara T, Semon MR, Robertson GC, Braden L, Simpson JS: Directional atherectomy: new approaches for treatment of obstructive coronary and peripheral vascular disease. *Circulation* 1990;81(suppl 3)IV:79–91
4. Bates ER, O'Neill WW, Topol EJ: Percutaneous atherectomy catheters. *Cardiol Clin* 1988;6(3):373–382
5. Perez JA, Hinohara T, Quigley PJ, Lee MM, Hoffman PU, Mikat EM, Phillips HR, Stack RS: In-vitro and in-vivo experimental results using a new wire concentric atherectomy device (abstr). *Circulation* 1988;78(suppl 2):II–21
6. Wholey MH, Jarmolowski CR: New reperfusion devices: the Kensey catheter, the atherolytic reperfusion wire device and the transluminal extraction catheter. *Radiology* 1989; 172:947–952
7. Yedlicka JW Jr, Carlson JE, Hunter DW, Castañeda–Zúñiga WR, Amplatz K: Thrombectomy with the TEC endarterectomy system: an experimental study and clinical evaluation. *J Vasc Intervent Radiol*, in press
8. Graor RA, Whitlow PL: Transluminal atherectomy for occlu-

sive peripheral vascular disease. *J Am Coll Cardiol* 1990; 15(7):1551–1558

9. Stack RS, Quigley PJ, Sketch MH Jr, Stack RK, Walker C, Hoffman PU, Phillips HR: Treatment of coronary artery disease with the transluminal extraction-endarterectomy catheter: initial results of a multicenter study. *Circulation* 1989;80(suppl 2):II-583
10. Sketch MH, Newman GE, McCann RL, Himmelstein SI, Hoffman PU, Stack RS: Transluminal extraction-endarterectomy in peripheral vascular disease: late clinical and angiographic follow-up. *Circulation* 1989;80(suppl 2):II-305
11. Sketch MH, Quigley PJ, Bauman RP, Phillips HR, Stack RS: Restenosis following coronary transluminal extraction-endarterectomy. *Circulation* 1989;80(suppl 2):II-583
12. Selmon MR, Robertson GC, Simpson JB: Restenosis in peripheral transluminal atherectomy (abstr). *Circulation* 1988;78(suppl 2):II-269
13. Godlewski P: Restenosis rates in peripheral TEC-alone cases: a comparative analysis of the effect of change in the cutter manufacture procedure. Interventional Technologies, Incorporated. October 16, 1990

Part 11. Emerging Technologies: Kaliman Atherectomy Catheter

—Wilfrido R. Castañeda–Zúñiga, M.D., M.Sc.

A device for the percutaneous removal of atherosclerotic tissue was described by Kaliman et al.[1] The device consists of an 8Fr flexible polyurethane catheter with a rotating metal triangular cutting head consisting of two blades, with an opening between the blades to allow the passage of resected tissue across the catheter lumen. The cutting head is positioned on the distal end of the catheter shaft. The cutter is connected to the motor by a wire. A second wire passes through the head and serves a dual purpose: guiding wire and driving axle to help move the cutter forward, through the stenosis or occlusion. The battery-operated

motor rotates the cutter at a speed of 1000–8000 rpm. Suction is applied through a side port to remove the resected atheromatous material. Five fresh human arterial specimens with occlusions 3–5cm in length were successfully recanalized by the device. No perforations are reported.[1]

Reference

1. Kaliman JF, Wichart A, Rejlek K: Kaliman catheter for percutaneous transluminal removal of atherosclerotic tissue. *Circulation* 1990;82(suppl III):III-219

Part 12. Emerging Technologies: Pullback Atherectomy Catheter

—Wilfrido R. Castañeda–Zúñiga, M.D., M.Sc.

Denny and Fischell[1,2] reported on the use of an over-the-wire pullback atherectomy catheter on cadaver arteries. The device consists of a conical cutter and collecting chamber with an outer "closing catheter" 3.5mm in diameter, and an inner "cut-collect" catheter (2.0mm in diameter) rotated at 2000 rpm by a hand-held motor drive unit. The mean stenosis was improved from 95 ± 3 to $21 \pm 5\%$ after pullback atherectomy.[1] Results on the early use of the device on humans were reported by Denny et al.[2]

References

1. Fischell TA, Fischell RE, White RI, Chapoloni R, Wexler L: Ex-vivo and early clinical results using a new pullback atherectomy catheter (PAC). *Circulation* 1990;82(suppl III):III-415
2. Denny DF, Fischell TA, White RI, Fischell RE, Yoselevitz M, Wexler L: New "over the wire" pullback atherectomy catheter (abstr). *Radiology* 1990;177(suppl):145

New Stent Developments

—Wilfrido R. Castañeda–Zúñiga, M.D., M.Sc., and S. Murthy Tadavarthy, M.D.

Several new stent designs are currently being tested in clinical trials, mostly with coronary applications in mind. Obviously, applications in peripheral vascular disease are being overlooked because of the more profitable coronary artery market. Among these stent designs are:

—Medtronic–Wiktor stent (Part 8);
—Gianturco–Roubin stent (Part 9);
—Cordis balloon expandable stent (Part 10).

Part 1. Intravascular Stents: Experimental Observations and Anatomopathologic Correlates

—Julio C. Palmaz, M.D.

Intraluminal Stenting As the Mechanical Solution to Balloon-Angioplasty Failure

Elastic recoil and subintimal or medial dissection often limit the success of transluminal balloon angioplasty. They cause a decrease of the diameter achieved by the inflated balloon and leave irregularities on the surface of the dilated vessel causing hemodynamic disturbance and decreased flow. Balloon overdilatation of the stenotic segment has been advocated as a means to antagonize elastic recoil by maximizing the stretching of the musculoelastic media. This is very often effective but definitely increases the risk of hemorrhage by transmural rupture. An intraluminal stent placed simultaneously or immediately after balloon angioplasty prevents elastic recoil by holding the vessel open to a predetermined diameter, corrects the effects of dissection by displacing the dissected layers against the arterial wall, and provides a cylindrical lumen by forcing asymmetrical plaques eccentrically.[1] This can be accomplished by a variety of stents, some of which are already undergoing clinical evaluation.[2-6] In general, stents are metallic coils or tubular mesh that are introduced into the body via a delivery catheter in a small or constrained diameter. After reaching a desired location,

the stent expands to a larger diameter by a variety of mechanisms previously described.[2] All intravascular stents currently in use are metallic. This is dictated by the need to have relatively high radial strength with the lowest possible bulk. In addition, metals in general are radiopaque, a feature needed for precise manipulation and positioning under fluoroscopy.

The Main Goal: Endothelialization of the Stented Surface

An important feature of an intravascular stent is to have an open design, which means to have the lowest possible ratio of metal to open surface without compromising its mechanical properties. An open stent wall configuration is desirable because of the need to keep thrombogenicity of the metal surface at a minimum and to preserve as much endothelium as possible. This promotes multicentric endothelialization by allowing confluent growth of surviving endothelium between metal members.[7] Complete coverage of the treated surface by endothelium is the ultimate goal of vascular prosthetic implants because endothelium protects against low-flow thrombosis, a serious limitation of all synthetic vascular bypass materials currently in use.

The endothelium covering stents is stable, as suggested

by the mature appearance of the cells, several months following implantation in dog, rabbit, and pig arteries. This is evidenced by the spindle shape of the endothelial cells with their long axis oriented in the direction of the flow, by their flat nuclei, and by the rare blood cell elements attached to the surface when examined by scanning electron microscopy.[8] In addition, positive immunospecific stains for arterial endothelium support this assumption.[9]

Fascinating albeit unclear is the fact that rapid stent endothelialization is also observed when these devices are placed in tracks of liver parenchyma serving as portocaval shunts.[10] The origin of the endothelial cells covering shunt tracks is unclear. It may originate from hepatic capillary sinusoids, from adjacent hepatic or portal veins, or from blood-borne precursors. Despite the uncertainty about its origin, this endothelium was found to have histological and histochemical features similar to those of arterial stents.

STENT THROMBOGENICITY PRIOR TO ENDOTHELIALIZATION: THE ACHILLES HEEL

Since all metal surfaces are thrombogenic, the risk exists for a recently implanted stent to accumulate an excessive amount of thrombus to the point of occlusion. In prosthetic bypass tubular conduits, shear of the limiting flow layer with the prosthetic surface determines the amount of thrombus deposited.[11] This is a self-limiting phenomenon since a low flow situation increases thrombus deposition, narrowing the lumen and increasing flow velocity and shear. However, with critically low flow, thrombus deposition continues until complete occlusion occurs. Stents in small vessels are also at increased risk of thrombosis because of the lower shear rates and unfavorable diameter/volume relationship. The same thickness of thrombus causing significant reduction of lumen area in a small diameter vessel may not be as obstructive in a comparatively larger vessel.

The amount of laminar thrombus initially deposited on a stented surface determines the thickness of the intimal tissue that will be present later. This was demonstrated in dogs with stents placed in femoral arteries with artificially induced distal stenosis as compared to stents placed in the opposite unobstructed femoral arteries.[12] Groups of animals with stents placed in this fashion were sacrificed at regular intervals for histological examination of the stents. As expected, the amount of thrombus on the surface of the stents subjected to low flow was significantly larger than in arteries with normal flow. This thrombus was noted to be progressively replaced by fibromuscular tissue, which in turn was significantly thicker in low flow stents as compared to controls. It is obvious that when a stent is exposed to low flow or it is placed in a small vessel, increased anticoagulation and antiplatelet medication is needed to ensure patency. The effect of a few anticoagulation-anti-

platelet regimens on thrombus deposition on freshly implanted stents was studied in animals by using labeled platelets.[13,14]

Particularly effective was a combination of heparin, acetyl salicyclic acid, dipyridamole, and low molecular weight dextran. This regimen, adopted for coronary stent implantation in clinical trials, is followed by Coumarin administration for a few months by most investigators in this field.[15,16] In contrast, stent implantation in large vessels with high flow such as the iliac arteries does not require any more anticoagulation than balloon angioplasty.[17] A similar experience was observed after caval and pulmonary artery stent placements.[18,19]

Ongoing research is under way to optimize the level and duration of anticoagulation to control thrombus deposition before endothelialization occurs. This is possible by the use of markers of focal platelet activity such as the ^{99m}Tc-S12 antibody, which selectively attaches to the inner membrane of α granules of activated platelets (Centocor, Malvern, PA).[20] In addition, heparin-coated stents are currently being compared to noncoated stents regarding thrombus formation and long-term patency.

STENTING INHIBITS RECURRENT ATHEROMATOUS PLAQUE FORMATION: TRUE OR FALSE?

Stents placed in the abdominal aortas of rabbits subjected to balloon denudation and high cholesterol diet were incorporated in similar fashion to stents placed in normal rabbit aortas. The tissue covering the stent and the underlying plaque, 24 weeks following stenting, did not contain foamy macrophages and was essentially fibrous in nature, despite the maintenance of high serum cholesterol levels.[8] A possible explanation for this occurrence is the preservation of endothelium at the site of stent placement, followed by multicentric spread of endothelial cells. After this experimental observation, we had the opportunity to examine the autopsy specimen of a patient with an iliac stent placed 26 months prior to his demise from a myocardial infarction. The tissue covering the stent was fibromuscular in nature and showed no evidence of cholesterol, calcium, or necrosis. Rousseau et al. had a similar experience using a self-expandable stent.[21]

It is conceivable that stents provide a framework for fibrous tissue growth while maintaining favorable rheological conditions. This tissue would cover faltering and ulcerated atheromatous tissue avoiding thrombus formation and possible embolization. However, if biochemical or hemodynamic conditions that created the atherosclerotic plaque prior to stenting remain present, they should eventually lead to recurrence of such plaque. Failure of stenting by recurrence of the lesion within the stented lumen is therefore to be expected a few years following implantation of the device if atherogenic conditions such as cigarette smoking, high serum lipids, and hypertension persist.

FLEXIBLE VERSUS RIGID STENTS: A SUBJECT OF DEBATE

Several investigators working with intravascular stents have stressed the need for stent flexibility for ease of deployment and to accompany vessel movement when placed in segments subjected to bending such as the femoral, axillary, or popliteal arteries.[6,22] Flexibility is certainly needed to negotiate curves in delivery catheters and tortuous vessels leading to the target area. This led to a change in our stent design consisting of one or more smaller stent segments joined by a short bridge for certain applications such as coronary and renal artery stenting. However, we still believe that stents should be rigid after placement to provide a stable, nonshifting surface for endothelial growth. The assumption that dimensional change in a prosthetic surface causes increased endothelial slough, platelet and mononuclear cell attachment, and ensuing muscle cell proliferation is supported by previous work. Barra et al.[23] significantly decreased intimal hyperplasia in vein grafts by placing a perivenous mesh to render the grafts noncompliant. These authors demonstrated that the endothelium of meshed grafts was more mature and free of attached blood cells as compared to nonmeshed grafts. Thubrikar et al.[24] also emphasized the beneficial effect of relieving intramural stress by experimentally placing periarterial acrylic casts around branching points and bifurcations of large vessels of rabbits, where intramural stress was assumed to be maximal. After exposing the animal to a high-cholesterol diet, the arterial segments with surrounding rigid casts were compared to segments covered with flexible silicone casts and to uncovered arterial segments. Areas relieved of stress by the rigid casts developed less intimal thickening and fat accumulation as compared to arteries with flexible casts or to arteries not covered at all.

The importance of matching radial compliance between an artery and an interposed prosthetic conduit has been repeatedly stressed in the literature.[25] Compliance mismatch has been identified as one of the potential causes of anastomotic intimal hyperplasia in small caliber synthetic grafts. Therefore, synthetic grafts are designed in such way that their radial compliance matches that of the human arteries. Radial compliance mismatch could be present between rigid stents and adjacent artery, causing intimal hyperplasia at the transition point. However, in practice, this was not observed. Angiographic and gross examination of healed stents in arteries of animals and patients did not reveal a tendency of the intima to be thicker at the transition points between artery and stent. Whenever stent stenosis developed, the tissue causing it was generally distributed throughout the length of the stented lumen. It is possible that compliance mismatch is not relevant when rigid stents are placed in diseased vessels which are usually rendered rigid by wall thickening and calcification.

THE RESORBABLE STENT: A UTOPIAN DREAM?

In theory, resorbable suture material should be mechanically sound before wound healing occurs. After healing, it should be phagocytized without inducing chronic cellular reaction. It is conceivable that a stent of resorbable material could be constructed to keep intravascular atheromatous lesions open until the tissue replacing such stent would reorganize the vessel into a cylindrical conduit. This new tissue could then be considered a biological stent. Unfortunately, all polymeric plastic materials including the few available resorbable materials are far from having the strength characteristics needed to perform as mechanical stents with reasonable bulk. This is particularly true in small vessels where a small decrease in diameter could produce a large flow restriction. An additional concern regarding the concept of resorbable stents is the possibility of developing weakness at the level of the treated area resulting in vessel rupture or aneurysm. After months to years following stent placement, the musculoelastic elements of the stented arterial wall atrophy for lack of use.[8] After stent placement, the stress of the pulsatile blood pressure normally borne by the arterial wall is transferred to the stent, eventually causing atrophy of such wall. It is therefore conceivable that if the stent support is removed after atrophy has occurred then aneurysm or rupture could develop. This would be of particular concern in large arteries, subjected to large wall stress. Evidence to support this thought exists in previous experimental efforts at creating resorbable grafts. Aortobifemoral grafts of knitted polyglycolic acid filament were placed in pigs. Following reabsorption of the prosthetic material, aneurysms consistently developed.[26]

The idea of resorbable stents is therefore not supported by currently available materials or experimental evidence.

THE FUTURE OF STENTING

In conjunction with emerging new diagnostic and therapeutic tools, intravascular stenting offers exiting new possibilities. Stents could expand the role of other revascularization techniques such as thrombolytic therapy, atherectomy, or lasers, and its placement could be made more accurate by intravascular ultrasound and angioscopy. However, stent safety and efficacy are not completely proved. Randomized studies and five-year patency rates are not available yet. Until they are, areas in which stents represent an alternative to proved, conventional therapy, such as iliac balloon angioplasty, should be approached with caution. In contrast, the use of stents in areas for which no viable alternative is available is received with enthusiasm. This is true in percutaneous portocaval shunting in patients with bleeding esophageal varices and poor metabolic status,[27] caval,[18] portal, and hepatic vein obstruction,[28] and pulmonary branch stenosis.[29]

References

1. Palmaz JC: Balloon-expandable intravascular stent. *AJR* 1988;150:1263–1269
2. Wright KC, Wallace S, Charnsangavej C, Carrasco CH, Gianturco C: Percutaneous endovascular stents: an experimental evaluation. *Radiology* 1985;156:69–72
3. Sigwart V, Puel J, Mirkovitch V, Joffre F, Kappenberger L: Intravascular stents to prevent occlusion and restenosis after transluminal angioplasty. *N Engl J Med* 1987;316:701–706
4. Robinson KA, Roubin GS, Siegel RJ, et al: Intra-arterial stenting in the atherosclerotic rabbit. *Circulation* 1988; 78:646–653
5. Rabkin J, Matevosov AL, Gotman LN: Radiological endovascular prosthesis, in *Radiological Endovascular Surgery*. Moscow, Moscow Medicine Publisher, 1987
6. Strecker EP, Berg G, Weber H, Bohl M, Dietrich B: Experimentelle Untersuchungen mit einer neuen perkutan einfuhr baren und aufdehnbaren Gefabendoprosthese. *Fortschr Röntgenstr* 1987;147:669–72
7. Palmaz JC, Tio FO, Schatz RA, Alvarado R, Rees C, Garcia O: Early endothelialization of balloon-expandable stents: experimental observations. *J Intervent Radiol* 1988;3:119–124
8. Palmaz JC, Windeler SA, Garcia F, Tio FO, Sibbitt RR, Reuter SR: Atherosclerotic rabbit aortas: expandable intraluminal grafting. *Radiology* 1986;160:723–726
9. Palmaz JC, Kopp DT, Hayashi H, et al: Normal and stenotic renal arteries: experimental balloon-expandable intraluminal stenting. *Radiology* 1987;164:705–708
10. Palmaz JC, Sibbitt RR, Reuter SR, Garcia F, Tio FO: Expandable intrahepatic portocaval shunt stents: early experience in the dog. *AJR* 1985;145:821–825
11. Sauvage LR: Externally supported, noncrimped external velour, weft-knitted Dacron prostheses for axillofemoral, femoropopliteal, and femorotibial bypass, in Wright CB, Hosson RW, Hiratzka LF, Lynch TB (eds): *Vascular Grafting: Clinical Applications and Techniques*. Boston, Wright, 1983, pp 168–186
12. Noeldge G, Siegesstetter V, Richter GM, Bohn R, Franke M, Eckert A, Palmaz JC: Palmaz stent: Process of neointima formation in conditions of highly impaired flow. RSNA meeting, Chicago, IL, 1989
13. Palmaz JC, Garcia O, Kopp DT, et al: Balloon-expandable intraarterial stents: effect of anticoagulation on thrombus formation (abstr). *Circulation* 1987;76(suppl IV):45
14. Palmaz JC, Garcia O, Kopp DT, et al: Balloon-expandable intraarterial stents: Effect of antithrombotic medication on thrombus formation, in Zeitler E (ed): *Pros and Cons in PTA and Axillary Methods.* Berlin, Springer-Verlag, 1989
15. Schatz RA, Leon BL, Baim DS, et al: Balloon-expandable intracoronary stents: initial results of a multicenter study. AHA meeting. New Orleans, LA, 1989
16. Serruys PW, Beatt KJ, Bertrand M, et al: Restenosis rate after coronary stent implantation: angiographic assessment of the initial series. AHA meeting. New Orleans, LA, 1989.
17. Palmaz JC, Garcia O, Schatz RA, et al: Balloon-expandable intraluminal stenting of the iliac arteries: the first 171 procedures. *Radiology* 1990;174:969–975
18. Charnsangavej C, Carrasco CH, Wallace S, et al: Stenosis of the vena cava: Preliminary assessment of treatment with expandable metallic stents. *Radiology* 1986;161:295–298
19. Mullins CE, O'Laughlin M, Vick W, et al: Implantation of balloon-expandable intravascular grafts by catheterization in pulmonary arteries and systemic veins. *Circulation* 1988; 77:188–199
20. Miller DD, Boulet A, Garcia O, et al: Monoclonal S-12 antibody imaging of in-vivo platelet activation after interventional procedures in atherosclerotic rabbit arteries. American Heart Association Meeting. New Orleans, LA, 1989
21. Rousseau H, Joffre F, Raillat, Duboucher C, Glock Y, Escourrou G: Iliac artery endoprothesis: radiologic and histologic findings after 2 years. *AJR* 1989;153:1075–1076
22. Zollikofer CL, Largiader I, Bruhlmann WF, Uhlschmid GK, Marty AH: Endovascular stenting of veins and grafts: preliminary clinical experience. *Radiology* 1988;167:707–712
23. Barra JA, Volant A, Leroy JP, et al: Constrictive perivenous mesh prosthesis for preservation of vein integrity. *J Thorac Cardiovasc Surg* 1986;92:330–336
24. Thubrikar MJ, Baker JW, Nolan SP: Inhibition of atherosclerosis associated with reduction of arterial intramural stress in rabbits. *Arteriosclerosis* 1988;8:410–420
25. Abbott WM, Megerman J, Hasson JE, L'Italien G, Warnock DF: Effect of compliance mismatch on vascular graft patency. *J Vasc Surg* 1987;5:376–382
26. Bowald S, Busch C, Erikson I: Absorbable material in vascular prostheses: a new device. *Acta Chir Scand* 1980;146:391–395
27. Richter GM, Palmaz JC, Noeldge G, Siegerstetter V, Franke M, Wenz W: Der transjugulare intrahepatische portosystemische Stent-Shunt (TIPSS). *Radiologe* 1989;29:406–411
28. Palmaz JC: Development of a non-compliant balloon-expandable stent. Miami Vascular Institute meeting. Miami, FL, 1989
29. Mullins C: Personal communication. University of Texas, Houston

Part 2. Palmaz Balloon Expandable Stent

—Wilfrido R. Castañeda–Zúñiga, M.D., M.Sc., and S. Murthy Tadavarthy, M.D.

To overcome the problem of recurrence of stenosis following transluminal angioplasty Palmaz developed a balloon expandable, intravascular stent. The device was intended to allow dilatation and simultaneous placement of an intraluminal stent to support the wall, preventing elastic arterial recoil.[1] The initial design of the stent was a continuous, woven, stainless-steel $150\mu m$ diameter wire. The cross points of the wire mesh were soldered to give the stent high resistance to radial collapse.[1] Because of the 80% open design of the stent, rapid endothelialization occurred by three weeks, together with preservation of patency of side branches.[2] In contrast to animal results, the inner surface of synthetic grafts in humans does not get covered by endothelium, but by a fibrin layer.[1] The main disadvantage of the stent is its lack of longitudinal flexibility which limits its application to straight vascular segments. The stent design was changed by replacing the woven mesh with a lath design obtained by electromechanical etching of thin walled stainless steel tubing (Fig. 7.2.1). The etching produces a stent with parallel rows of staggered rectangular slots, allowing for a smaller diameter (3.1Fr), thinner walled stent (0.015mm), with a length of 30mm and an expansion range of 8–12mm.[2] When the balloon is inflated, the rectangular slots open up to form diamond-shaped spaces. Initially the stents needed to be mounted and crimped out over an 8mm/3cm-long balloon with a crimping tool. A newer low profile version of the stent is available premounted on an 8mm angioplasty balloon. Because of the tendency of the stent to slip back on the balloon, the stent-balloon assembly needs to be protected during introduction through the hemostatic valve by a stainless steel introducer. Furthermore, a 30cm-long introducer sheath needs to be used to advance the stent-balloon assembly through the artery to the level of the obstruction. Once the stent is located at the desired level, the sheath is withdrawn and the stent is expanded to the full 8mm diameter (Fig. 7.2.2). The balloon is deflated and carefully

rotated within the stent, to refold the balloon, which is then gently withdrawn over the guidewire. An angiogram and pressure measurements are obtained to assess the results. If needed, a 10mm balloon can be introduced over the guidewire to further dilate the stent in larger diameter iliac arteries.

When long segments need to be stented, multiple stents can be placed, making sure their ends are overlapped (Fig. 7.2.3). Although a guidewire or catheter can be manipulated across a freshly placed stent, it is better to keep the guidewire across the stent until it is decided that additional stents or balloon dilation are not needed. For each additional stent placement the 30mm introducer sheath needs to be repositioned by advancing it over the guidewire across the previously placed stent. When multiple stents are needed they should be placed from cephalad to caudad, with sequential stents overlapping by at least one third of the stent length.

CLINICAL RESULTS

Initial clinical trials with the Palmaz balloon expandable stent were undertaken as part of a multicenter study including institutions from the United States and Europe and were restricted to the iliac arteries. Some of the best reported results of transluminal angioplasty have been in the management of short, concentric stenoses of the iliac arteries (50–87%).[3] The results, however, are not so good when dealing with long stenoses, complete occlusions, and in patients with diabetes mellitus or poor runoff vessels, with a reported patency rate at five years of only 55%.[4-7] Initial data included 154 patients: 28 women and 126 men with an average age of 62 years. Risk factors included: diabetes mellitus in 20%; smoking in 96%; hypertension in 52%; and obesity in 17.22%. Seventy patients were classified in stage II, 36 in stage III, and 48 in stage IV. Thirty-four patients had iliac artery stenosis and twenty had complete iliac artery occlusion. Average stenosis was 79 ± 15%, the average length of the iliac artery occlusion was 6.1cm ± 2.8. The average Doppler ankle-arm index (AAI) was 0.63 ± 0.2 in stage II patients; 0.54 ± 0.17 in stage III patients, and 0.49 ± 0.25 in stage IV patients. The initial protocol included the placement of stents only to treat iliac artery stenosis or occlusion that failed to respond to conventional balloon angioplasty. Therefore, following PTA, angiographic and hemodynamic studies were obtained to assess the results of PTA. Inadequate results were defined as the presence of intimal dissection or elastic recoil producing a residual gradient of 5mm Hg or more after the injection of vasodilators (Fig. 7.2.4). Other indications for stent placement included: restenosis after previous PTA (Fig. 7.2.5) and total iliac artery occlusion (Fig. 7.2.6). Contraindications included: extravasation after PTA; tortuous iliac arteries; and dense, extensive calcifications of the iliac arteries. Relative contraindications included: iliac artery aneurysm, severe hypertension,

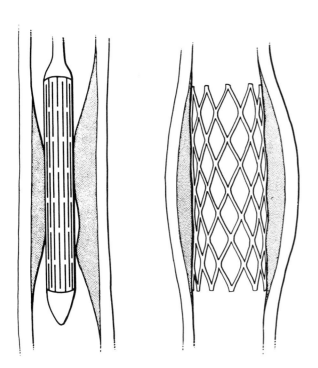

Figure 7.2.1. **Left.** Diagram of Palmaz stent mounted on angioplasty balloon, placed at the level of the stenosis. **Right.** Fully expanded stent holding lumen widely open. Balloon has been removed.

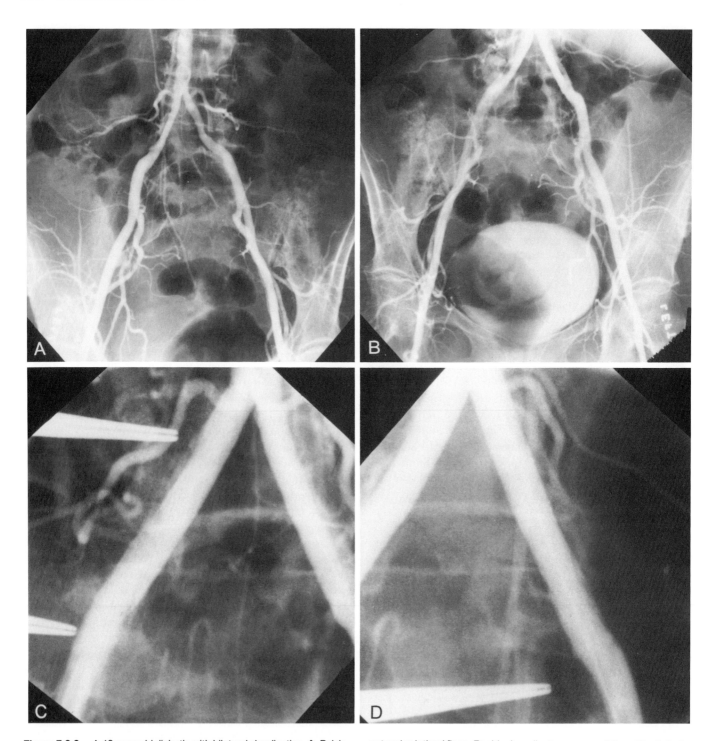

Figure 7.2.2. A 48-year-old diabetic with bilateral claudication. **A.** Pelvic arteriogram long segment stenosis of both common iliacs; 20–30mm Hg gradients were present bilaterally. **B.** Post-PTA pelvic arteriogram shows extensive intimal flaps. Residual gradients were over 20mm Hg. **C, D.** Pelvic arteriogram after placement of two Palmaz stents in both common iliac arteries shows widely patent lumens. No residual gradients.

impaired pain sensation, stenosis of the common femoral artery and poor distal runoff. One-hundred eighty-one stents were placed in the common iliac arteries and eighty in the external iliac arteries. Seventeen patients had bilateral stent placement and twenty-one patients had stents placed in the ipsilateral external and common iliac arteries. The mean pressure gradient after vasodilation measured

before stent placement was 36.4 ± 22mm Hg. The gradient fell to 1.6 ± 2.7mm Hg post-stent placement. At the latest follow-up at an average of 6 months, with a range of 1–24 months, 113 patients were asymptomatic, 25 had moderate claudication, 5 had severe claudication, 2 had rest pain, and 1 had undergone a below-the-knee amputation. When correlating these data with the clinical stage of

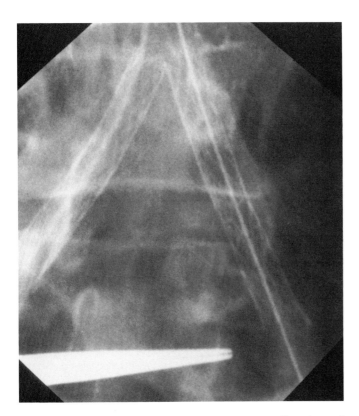

Figure 7.2.3. Overlapping stents reconstructing aortic bifurcation and both proximal common iliacs.

the disease apparent at the time of presentation, 71 patients had improved by one stage, 32 patients by two stages, and 31 patients by three stages. Eleven patients showed no initial improvement and six patients showed initial improvement with prompt recurrence of symptoms. On the early follow-up, an increase in the AAI to 0.91 ± 0.22 was found on the stage II patients; to 0.83 ± 0.22 in stage III patients and to 0.75 ± 0.21 in the stage IV patients. At the latest follow-up the reported indices were 0.90 ± 0.20, 0.85 ± 0.23, and 0.84 ± 0.28, respectively.[8,9] All stents have remained patent to the latest follow-up examination without evidence of migration or aneurysm formation. Complications related to the stent itself occurred in three patients (2%). Two of the patients had thrombosis of the stent that was successfully managed by thrombolytic infusion. The third patient had a small perforation secondary to balloon rupture during expansion. The patient had an uneventful recovery. Procedure-related complications occurred in 9.7% of patients, including groin hematoma in 3.9%, distal embolization in 2.6%, extravasation in 1.3%, pseudoaneurysm at the puncture site in 0.64%, and subintimal dissection in 0.64%.[9] Upon close examination of the results, Palmaz described a greater benefit of iliac artery stenting in patients with limbs at risk at the time of presentation, who underwent a combined iliac artery stenting and a femoropopliteal bypass procedure.[9] The absence of initial response or the early recurrence of symptoms was directly correlated to either

the presence of untreated distal disease or to the development of new lesions.[9] Patients were placed on an aspirin/dipyridamole regime for two days before the procedure and continued for three months thereafter.[8,9] Similar results were reported by Bonn et al. in 19 patients.[10] They stated that the angiographic results of stenting were uniform, independently of whether the lesion was focal or diffuse, eccentric or concentric, calcified or noncalcified, or localized to the common or external iliac arteries. In addition, the results of stenting were not affected by whether stent placement was used to treat simple vs. complex complications of PTA (such as long intimal dissection).[10] They emphasized, however, that a precise localization of the lesion by anatomic landmarks and angiography is essential, not only for planning the procedure but to prevent misplacement of stents.[10] They remarked on one of the main disadvantages of the stent, that is the large diameter of the introducer system, which excludes patients with small diameter common femoral or external iliac arteries (< 5mm), because this predisposes to thrombosis at the puncture site level.[10] Improvements in the introducer system might decrease the occurrence of this problem. Successful recanalization and stenting of completely occluded iliac arteries in 12 patients was reported by Rees et al.[11] Indications were limb salvage in seven patients and claudication in five. The AAI after stenting rose from a mean of 0.54 ± 15 to 0.94 ± 24. Transstenotic pressure gradients dropped from a mean of 42.1 ± 16.7mm Hg to 0.58 ± 1.4mm Hg. In follow-up ranging from 1 to 14 months with a mean of 7.4 months the mean AAI did not change significantly. Clinically all patients improved by one or more levels after stenting. Clinical status has remained unchanged in all, but one patient developed claudication of the contralateral leg at six months. Distal embolization occurred in two patients. Surgical embolectomy was used to manage these complications. Surgical exposure at the common femoral artery prior to PTA and stenting of completely occluded iliac arteries is suggested as a way to prevent these complications.[11]

Acute vascular occlusion following percutaneous transluminal angioplasty (PTA) has been reported in 3.8% of the cases, in a series of 224 angioplasties. Of these, 1.3% (three patients) were complications of iliac PTA and only one of these three patients (0.4%), had significant luminal compromise.[12] In the series reported by Becker the incidence of severe PTA induced dissection was 4.8%.[13] A correlation of severe intimal dissection with extensive calcification was reported by Waller[14] based on postmortem studies of PTA, and confirmed in the Becker study on angiographic findings alone.[13] In the past, vascular occlusion after PTA was managed either by trying to tack the intima against the wall by a repeat balloon inflation, leaving the balloon inflated for several minutes, by a surgical bypass procedure, or by surgical endarterectomy. Currently, other therapeutic alternatives include stenting,[13] percutaneous atherectomy,[14] and intimal flap welding[15–17]; of these options only

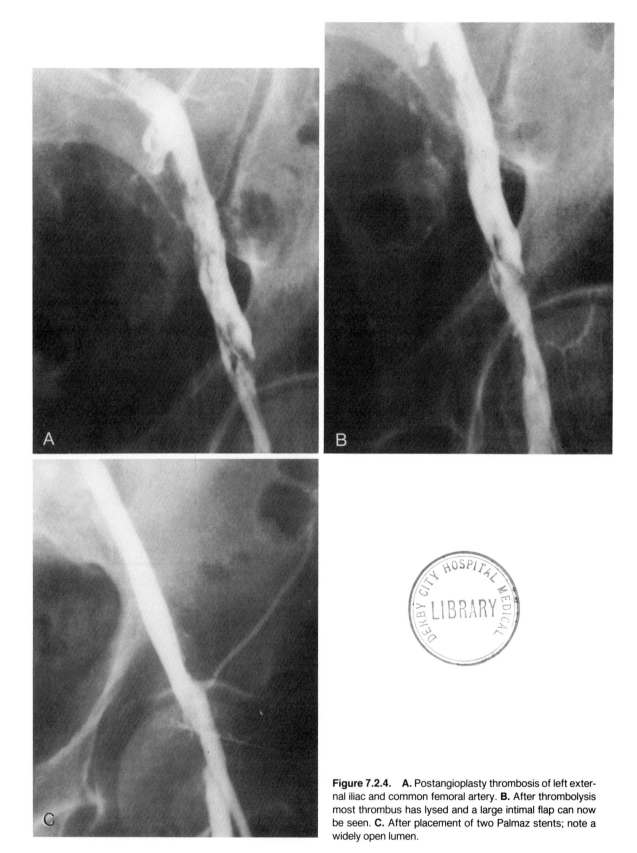

Figure 7.2.4. **A.** Postangioplasty thrombosis of left external iliac and common femoral artery. **B.** After thrombolysis most thrombus has lysed and a large intimal flap can now be seen. **C.** After placement of two Palmaz stents; note a widely open lumen.

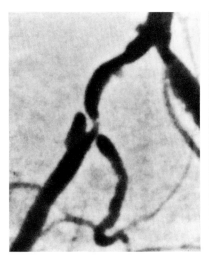 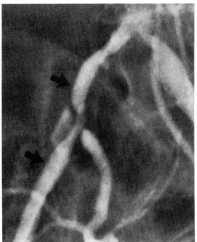 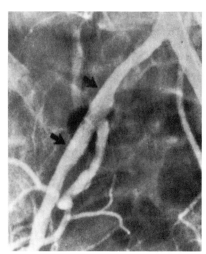

Figure 7.2.5. Left. Pelvic arteriogram depicts an eccentric, high-grade common-to-external iliac stenosis with an associated dissection created during previously performed, more distal external iliac artery PTA. **Middle.** After conventional PTA *(between the arrows)*, there is little improvement in lumen diameter and no change in the dissection. **Right.** After PTA and stent placement *(between the arrows)*, there is marked improvement in

lumen size and wall contours, with elimination of the dissection and maintenance of patency at the internal iliac artery origin. (Reproduced with permission from Bonn J, Gardiner GA, Shapiro MJ, Sullivan KL, Levin DC: Palmaz vascular stent: initial clinical experience. *Radiology* 1990; 174:741–745)

atherectomy is currently approved by the FDA. The other devices are under investigational protocols. Because of the diameter of the iliac arteries, atherectomy has only a limited role in the management of these complications.[14]

Stenting is without a doubt the best therapeutic option (Fig. 7.2.4). The management of angioplasty-induced dissection in the iliac arteries by intraluminal stenting was reported by Becker et al. in 12 iliac arteries.[12] Stents were placed at the time of angioplasty procedure in six vessels and as a separate procedure in the other six. An average of three stents per vessel was used. On angiographic follow-

up at a mean of 12.9 months on seven patients, only one stent showed evidence of intraluminal narrowing and in another patient clinical deterioration occurred despite a patent stent lumen.[13] Similar successful results with stenting of post-PTCA-induced intimal flaps was reported by Haude.[18]

Polymer coating of the Palmaz–Schatz stent has been reported to decrease the occurrence of vascular spasm following stent implantation. The coating also decreases local platelet deposition. These two effects of polymer coating can therefore decrease the risk of stent thrombosis.[19] The

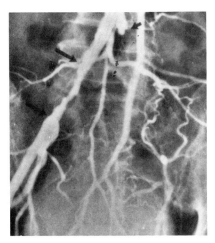 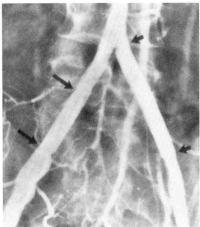 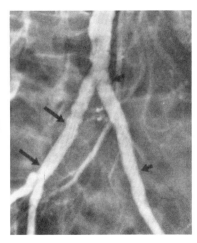

Figure 7.2.6. Left. Initial arteriogram reveals a chronic left common iliac artery occlusion *(short arrow)* and a long-segment right common iliac artery stenosis *(between the long arrows)*. **Middle.** Subsequent arteriogram shows the result after recanalization and placement of two stents in tandem in the left common iliac artery *(between the short arrows)* and a single stent in the right common iliac artery *(between the long arrows)*. **Right.** Arteriogram one year after the initial procedure demonstrates the

durability of the original result (PTA and stent placement *between the short arrows* and *between the long arrows*), with only minimal formation of neointima in the distal aspect of the left common iliac artery. (Reproduced with permission from Bonn J, Gardiner GA, Shapiro MJ, Sullivan KL, Levin DC: Palmaz vascular stent: initial clinical experience. *Radiology* 1990;174:741–745.)

purported decrease of the restenosis rate with the use of the Palmaz-Schatz stent in the coronary arteries is reportedly related to the improved initial results, rather than to a decrease in myointimal regrowth.[20] Delayed restenosis beyond six months is uncommon after intracoronary stenting. Stent implantation does not appear to delay, however, the temporal course of the restenosis process.[21] In a study of 50 of 186 patients with restenosis following stent implantation, Levine reported that due to the firm incorporation of the stent into the arterial wall four to six months after placement, the artery tends to exhibit a plastic rather than an elastic behavior. This finding might contribute to a safe and effective redilation, since the neointima might be able to stretch rather than fracture. Twenty-two patients were redilated, with reduction of luminal stenosis from 81 ± 12% to 9 ± 13%. Only one patient had a dissection following PTCA.[22] Recently the Palmaz stent has been used to manage patients with hypertension due to ostial renal artery stenosis. Rees reported 24 patients of a mean age of 64 ± 9 years, with a mean duration of hypertension of 9.7 ± 10.7 years. Initial technical success (residual stenosis < 30%) was obtained in 23 patients. Mean stenosis before PTA was 75 and 44% before stenting. In 17 patients with follow-up, up to 1 month with a mean of 6.8 months, cure or improvement of hypertension occurred in 14 patients (82%); 4 of 7 patients showed a decrease in creatinine of 15% or more. Restenosis was angiographically demonstrated in 3 of 13 patients at a mean of 7.3 months.[23] Application of the stent in other areas, including the creation of portocaval shunts,[24] and in congenital heart disease has been recently described.[25,26]

Stenting with the Palmaz stent has been proved safe and effective in the iliac arteries; disadvantages such as its lack of flexibility and the large size of the introducer system limit its application at this time. These problems may be overcome by design improvements in the future.

References

1. Palmaz JC, Sibbitt RR, Reuter SR, Tio FO, Rice WJ: Expandable intraluminal graft: a preliminary study. *Radiology* 1985;156:73–77
2. Palmaz JC, Sibbitt RR, Tio FO, Reuter SR, Peters JE, Garcia F: Expandable intraluminal vascular graft: a feasibility study. *Surgery* 1986;99(2):199–205
3. Palmaz JC, Ritcher GM, Noeldge G, et al: Intraluminal stents in atherosclerotic iliac artery stenosis: a preliminary report of a multicenter study. *Radiology* 1988;168:727–731
4. Doubilet P, Abrams HL: The cost of underutilization: percutaneous transluminal angioplasty for peripheral vascular disease. *N Engl J Med* 1984;310:95–102
5. Johnston KW, Rae M, Hogg–Johnston SA, et al: Five-year results of a prospective study of percutaneous transluminal angioplasty. *Ann Surg* 1987; 206:403–413
6. Zeitler E, Richter EI, Roth FJ, Schopp W: Results of percutaneous transluminal angioplasty. *Radiology* 1983;146:57–60
7. Kalman PG, Johnston KW: Outcome of a failed percutaneous transluminal dilation. *Surg Gynecol Obstet* 1985;161:43–46
8. Palmaz JC, Garcia O: Cardiovascular radiology: newer percutaneous interventional techniques. *Circulation* 1990;82(suppl III):III–102
9. Palmaz JC, Garcia OJ, Schatz RA, Rees CR, Roeren T, Richter GM, Noeldge G, Gardiner GA Jr, Becker GJ, Walker C, Stagg J, Katzen BT, Dake MD, Paolini RM, McLean GK, Lammer J, Schwarten DE, Tio FO, Root HD, Rogers WR: Placement of balloon-expandable intraluminal stents in iliac arteries: first 171 procedures. *Radiology* 1990;174:969–975
10. Bonn J, Gardiner GA, Shapiro MJ, Sullivan KL, Levin DC: Palmaz vascular stent: initial clinical experience. Radiology 1990;174:741–745
11. Rees CR, Palmaz JC, Garcia O, Roeren T, Richter GM, Gardiner G Jr, Schwarten D, Schatz RA, Root HD, Rogers W: Angioplasty and stenting of completely occluded iliac arteries. *Radiology* 1989;172:953–959.
12. Gardiner GA Jr, Meyerovitz MF, Stokers KR, Clouse ME, Harrington DP, Bettmann MA: Complications of transluminal angioplasty. *Radiology* 1986;159:201–208
13. Becker GJ, Palmaz JC, Rees CR, Ehrman KO, Lalka SG, Dalsing MC, Cikrit DF, McLean GK, Burke DR, Richter GM, Noeldge G, Garcia O, Waller BF, Castañeda–Zúñiga WR: Angioplasty-induced dissections in human iliac arteries: management with Palmaz balloon-expandable intraluminal stents. *Radiology* 1990;176:31–38
14. Maynar M, Reyes R, Cabrera V, et al: Percutaneous atherectomy as an alternative treatment for postangioplasty obstructive intimal flaps. *Radiology* 1989;170:1029–1031
15. Lee BI, Becker GJ, Waller BF, et al: Thermal compression and molding of atherosclerotic vascular tissue using radiofrequency energy: implications for radiofrequency balloon angioplasty. *J Am Coll Cardiol* 1989;13:1167–1175
16. Spear JR: Percutaneous transluminal coronary angioplasty restenosis: potential prevention with laser balloon angioplasty. *Am J Cardiol* 1987;60:61B–64B
17. Spears JR, Reyes VP, James LM, Sinofsky EL: Laser balloon angioplasty: initial clinical experience (abstr). *Circulation* 1988;78(suppl II):II–296
18. Haude M, Erbel R, Straub U, Dietz U: Intracoronary stent implantation in patients with symptomatic dissections after balloon angioplasty—short- and long-term results. Circulation 1990;82(suppl III):III-658
19. Bailey SR, Guy DM, Garcia OJ, Paige S, Palmaz JC, Miller D: Polymer coating of Palmaz-Schatz stent attenuates vascular spasm after stent placement. *Circulation* 1990;82(suppl III):III-541
20. Ellis S, Fischman D, Hirshfeld J, Savage M, Goldberg S, Erbel R, Cleman M, Teirstein P, Schatz R: Mechanism of stent benefit to limit restenosis following coronary angioplasty: regrowth vs. larger initial lumen? *Circulation* 1990; 82(suppl III):III-540
21. Savage M, Fischman D, Ellis S, Leon M, Cleman M, Teirstein P, Walker C, Hirshfeld J, Schatz R, Goldberg S: Does late progression of restenosis occur beyond six months following coronary artery stenting? *Circulation* 1990;82(suppl III):III-540
22. Levine MJ, Clemen MW, Schatz RA, Buchbinder M, Erbel R, Baim DS: Management of restenosis following Palmaz-Schatz intracoronary stenting: multicenter results. *Circulation* 1990;82(suppl III):III-560
23. Rees CR, Palmaz JC, Becker GJ, Ehrman KO, Richter G, Noldge G, Katzen BT, Dake M: Palmaz stenting of atheromatous lesions involving the ostium of the renal artery. *Circulation* 1990;82(suppl III):III-404
24. Palmaz JC, Sibbitt RR, Reuter SR, Garcia F, Tio FO: Expandable intrahepatic portacaval shunt stents: early experience in the dog. *AJR* 1985;145:821–825

25. Mullins CE, O'Laughlin MP, Vick GW III, Mayer DC, Myers TJ, Kearney DL, Schatz RA: Implantation of balloon-expandable intravascular grafts by catheterization in pulmonary arteries and systemic veins. *Circulation* 1988; 77(1):188–199

26. O'Laughlin MP, Perry SB, Lock JE, Mullins CE: Implantation of balloon-expandable intravascular stents in patients with congenital heart disease. *Circulation* 1990;82(suppl III):III-658

Part 3. Self-expandable Intravascular Stent: Long-term Results in the Iliac and Superficial Femoral Arteries

—Francis Joffre, M.D., Hervé Rousseau, M.D., and Rami Chemali, M.D.

Because of the limitations of percutaneous transluminal angioplasty (PTA), mainly failure secondary to intimal dissection, elastic recoil of the stenosis, and restenosis estimated to be around 30% at the femoropopliteal level[1] and 10% at the iliac level,[2] new therapeutic procedures have been developed. These new methods tried to improve on the results of PTA and to widen its indications. Among the new methods are atherectomy,[3] mechanical recanalization,[4] laser angioplasty,[5] and percutaneous stenting.[6-14] Dotter, in 1969, described the concept of percutaneous intravascular stenting in an attempt to maintain arterial patency after PTA.[6] Since then different types of stents have been developed and used clinically.[7-14] In this section we will discuss the self-expandable stent.

TECHNICAL DESCRIPTION

The self-expandable stent is composed of 20 filaments (surgical grade stainless-steel alloy), each $75\mu m$ in diameter, woven into a tubular braid configuration (Fig. 7.3.1). The 77% macroporosity of the device permits rapid endothelialization and good patency of collateral vessels bridged by the stent. The filament crossing points are not welded but are free to pivot over each other. The stent can

therefore be longitudinally stretched to a smaller diameter and will spontaneously recover its original diameter when released into the vascular lumen, because of the spring characteristics of the individual filaments. This also makes the stent resistant to collapse when subjected to extrinsic compression, since the cylindrical braid will spring back. This is not the case with the balloon expandable stents, which will stay collapsed if extrinsically compressed. When mounted in its stretched, small diameter format on the delivery catheter, the stent is constrained by a rolling membrane that the operator can retract progressively. As the stent is deployed from the catheter, it expands radially, molding itself to the vessel wall, its longitudinal flexibility allowing perfect adaptation to vessel curvature. As long as the stent is partially within the noninflated membrane, it can be pulled back if placement is incorrect, and, if necessary, it can be removed through the introducer sheath. Forward advancement of the stent is not possible once the stent is partially deployed.

The release of the stretched stent leads to a spontaneous return to the initial shape the diameter and length of which are predetermined. The stent is loaded at the distal end of the delivery catheter. The caliber of the delivery catheter varies according to the stent diameter (5–9Fr). The introducer catheter can be used over guidewires 0.014–0.035 inch in diameter. Different diameters (5–14mm) and lengths of stents are available. The delivery catheter is highly flexible, permitting advancement through tortuous vessels. The catheter tip is very flexible in spite of the presence of the mounted stent.

TECHNIQUE

The implantation technique is analogous to that of PTA since the device can be delivered percutaneously through a sheath over conventional guidewires and under local anesthesia.

For iliac implants, catheterization is achieved mainly via the ipsilateral femoral retrograde approach, but the contralateral access is possible. For femoral lesions the ipsilateral femoral antegrade approach is used except for proximal lesions which need a contralateral access.

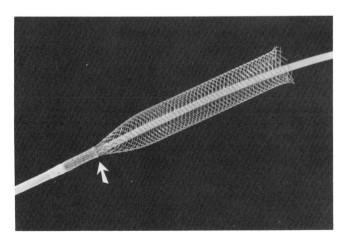

Figure 7.3.1. Photograph of a "Wallstent" endoprosthesis; withdrawal of the sheath allows progressive release of the stent *(arrow)*.

With self-expandable stents PTA is always performed before stenting; attempts to achieve placement without dilatation were mostly unsuccessful. Implantation is performed under fluoroscopic guidance.

The diameter of stents used varied between 5 and 10mm. The diameter is chosen to be slightly (15%) greater than the diameter of the native artery, to generate additional radial pressure against the vessel wall and prevent migration. The stent length is selected to allow coverage of the entire diseased segment. If necessary for long lesions, several stents can be slightly overlapped in order to cover the affected segment. Immediate angiographic and pressure measurement controls are necessary to assess the result of the procedure and as a baseline study for future follow-up studies.

Follow-up of the patients includes clinical examination and Doppler determination of the systolic ankle-arm index, at 1, 6, and 12 months.

Angiographic control is performed, if possible, at 1, 6, and 12 months. Acetylsalicylic acid (300mg/day) and dipyridamole (75mg three times per day) are given 24 hours before implantation and for 6 months afterward. During implantation, 5000 IU of heparin is given intra-arterially, as well as dextran. Intravenous heparin is continued 24 h after placement followed by oral anticoagulation for two months, particularly in cases of poor distal runoff following femoral implants.

RESULTS

Immediate Results

The Toulouse group experience consists of 24 patients with 27 iliac lesions and 40 patients with 43 femoropopli-

teal lesions, with a follow-up greater than six months.[15,16] The indications for iliac implants were mainly angioplasty failures and/or complex lesions: post-PTA restenosis (11 cases), occlusion (8 cases), iliac dissection (2 cases), and failed PTA (6 cases). The mean diameter of the stents used was 8mm (range 6–10mm) and in most cases a single prosthesis was sufficient. The length of the arterial segments covered by the stents ranged from 4 to 14cm (mean of 7cm). Mean stenosis was 80%. At the femoropopliteal level, the indications were similar: failed PTA (17 cases); occlusions with a mean length of 6cm (23 cases); miscellaneous (adventitial cyst, 1 case; bypass stenoses, 2 cases). Ten patients with femoropopliteal lesions had implantation without initial PTA. Stent diameter varied from 5 to 8mm. The length of the stents varied from 23 to 65mm. Fontaine Stage II disease was present in 78% of cases, Stage III in 11%, and Stage IV in 11%. Seventy percent of the lesions were located in the superficial femoral artery, 16% in the popliteal artery, and 14% in the femoropopliteal area. In 75% of the cases the lesions were 3–7cm long; in 25% of cases, they were longer than 7cm with a maximum length of 30cm. Mean stenosis was 80%. All but one case of an adventitial cyst were atherosclerotic lesions.

Implantation was successful in all cases: misplacement was rare and mainly related to the low radiopacity of the stent especially in lesions located close to the origin of the iliac artery. In these cases it was necessary to place another stent in the appropriate site. No migration or traumatic dissection occurred. Angiographic studies showed a smooth vascular lumen, the stent eliminating the residual stenoses and subintimal dissection secondary to PTA (Fig. 7.3.2). Hemodynamically, patients after stenting showed a greater improvement in comparison to patients following PTA alone (Figs. 7.3.3 and 7.3.4). The main collateral ves-

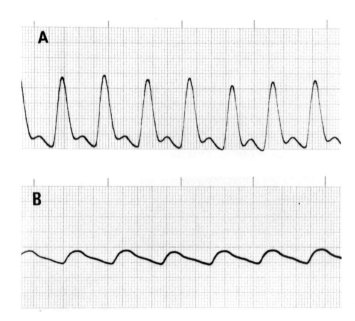

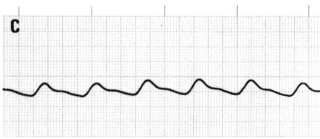

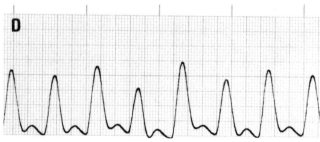

Figure 7.3.2. Hemodynamic studies reveal improvement of pressures distal to the stenosis after stenting. **A.** Aortic pressure. **B.** Femoral pressure before PTA. **C.** Femoral pressure after PTA. **D.** Femoral pressure after stenting.

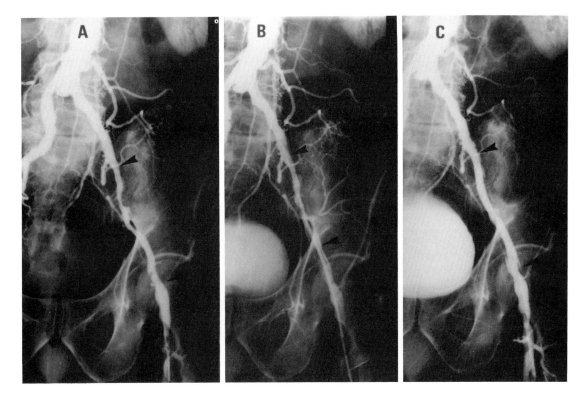

Figure 7.3.3. **A.** Angiogram shows a severe, extensive, and ulcerated lesion of the left external iliac artery *(arrowheads).* **B.** After PTA, note important residual stenosis *(arrowheads).* **C.** After placement of two stents *(arrowheads);* note excellent patency.

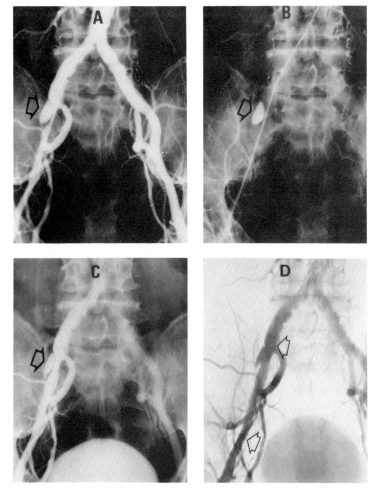

Figure 7.3.4. **A,B.** Angiograms with tight stenosis of external iliac artery, with large ulceration *(arrows).* **C.** After dilatation, note residual stenosis *(arrow).* **D.** Control at one month; the ulceration has partially disappeared and the patency is excellent *(arrow).*

sels crossed by the stent remained patent in 90% of the cases.

Among the 10 femoropopliteal lesions stented without a initial PTA, a 20–30% residual stenosis after stenting was present in five patients. In all cases, results of clinical and Doppler evaluation showed improvement.

Early in our experience, some cases of acute thrombosis occurred. Iliac thrombosis (three cases) occurred in two cases with poor distal runoff and in one case of previous iliac artery dissection. There were 10 femoropopliteal thromboses, of which 3 occurred immediately after implantation and responded to urokinase. Six thromboses occurred within a month after implantation, usually within 6–15 days. One patient received a bypass and five were treated medically. Five of these ten thromboses occurred in patients who had not undergone PTA before stenting. Only two thromboses were in lesions greater than 5cm in length. Among these 10 cases, only 1 case occurred in a patient treated with Coumadin. The first few weeks after implantation represent a critical period in which thrombotic occlusions can occur. Based on this experience we are currently using oral anticoagulants for two months until endothelialization has occurred.[15]

Late Results

The follow-up of these patients ranges from 6 to 46 months (Fig. 7.3.5). In the absence of early complications, late angiographic studies showed the presence of a thin, clear band on the inner surface of the stent corresponding to intimal proliferation. This hyperplasia remained stable with time and did not appear to progress after the third month. No case of iliac restenosis occurred in this group of patients but a multicenter study involving 100 patients, our own patients included, showed three symptomatic restenoses, between 30 and 50% within the stent (two cases) and at the extremities of the stent in one patient where the stent did not cover the entire lesion. This last case emphasizes the need to cover the entire segment treated by angioplasty with the stent.[15]

Among the 40 patients with stents on the femoropopliteal segments, 5 patients developed a symptomatic stenosis greater than 50%. The restenosis appeared at the extremities or inside the stent, within three to six months. Atherectomy was performed as a treatment of the stenosis in two of these cases using a Simpson Atherocath. The material recovered showed evidence of intimal proliferation (Fig. 7.3.6). Three other patients showed a stable (with a mean follow-up of 23 months) asymptomatic restenosis ranging from 30 to 50%. The anticoagulant therapy had no influence on the occurrence of restenosis. However, seven of eight cases occurred after the stenting of long lesions (longer than 5cm).[16]

In four cases, stenotic lesions developed away from the stented area and were presumed to be associated with progression of atheromatous disease in patients who had made no attempt to reduce their risk factors.

Including the early thrombosis at the beginning of this

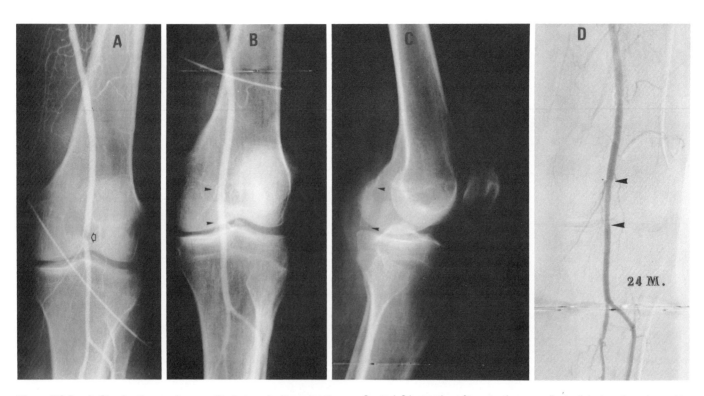

Figure 7.3.5. **A.** Simple atheromatous popliteal stenosis *(arrow)* at the level of the knee. **B.** Control after stenting without PTA: excellent patency without residual stenosis. **C.** Lateral view showing the stent *(arrows).* **D.** Control 24 months after stenting: excellent clinical and angiographic result.

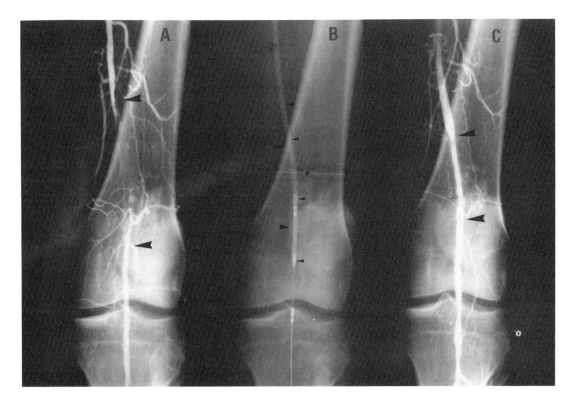

Figure 7.3.6. **A.** Angiography, six months after stenting, shows occlusion of the stented area *(between arrows)* caused by intimal hyperplasia and thrombosis. **B.** Recanalization and treatment with the Simpson catheter. **C.** Control after treatment.

experience, which declined strikingly with increasing experience, the overall long term patency is about 90% for iliac arteries lesions and 70% for femoropopliteal lesions.

DISCUSSION

PTA represents a considerable improvement in the management of peripheral vascular disease. Recurrence at variable rates remains, however, a significant problem. The presence of important longitudinal dissection secondary to PTA and/or persistent post-PTA stenosis seems to be the main factor in recurrence.

On the basis of the histologic appearance of arterial lesions treated by PTA and the results of experimental animal studies, it appears that two essential phenomena play an important role in restenosis: 1) the formation of a thrombus that progressively organizes to create a fibrous plaque; 2) intimal hyperplasia created by fibrocellular proliferation.[17,18] Both are related to the intimal lesions caused by PTA. In addition, retrospective clinical studies have shown that two other factors play important roles in restenosis with a persistent pressure gradient.[19] Van Andel showed that the long-term patency rate was 75% when the intraluminal surface was smooth and 66% when it was irregular, 80% with short lesions, and 55% with long lesions.[1,2]

The concept of using an intraluminal stent to splint the wall following PTA was described by Dotter in 1969 using an open coil spring stent.[6] He showed that open coil construction permits prompt fibroblastic development with rapid formation of a new, firmly anchored, autogenous lining surface.[6] Multiple innovative designs have been suggested, including metallic memory stent,[8] balloon expandable stent,[13] and self-expandable stent.[14] All these different kinds of stents have the same goals: 1) to avoid immediate recoil of the stenosis; 2) to reduce the pressure gradient; 3) to achieve a smooth luminal surface; and 4) consequently to decrease the frequency of restenosis. Most reports on the early clinical experience have shown immediate good results with pressure gradient reduction and excellent patency.[15,16,20,21]

Among the multiple stents available, the self-expandable stent seems to have some advantages in comparison with other types. The thinness of its filaments gives it flexibility, which allows it to be introduced through tortuous narrowed arteries over a guidewire; thus the femoral contralateral access is possible. Because of its flexibility and spring action it can be implanted at flexion areas (popliteal artery) without distortion, lumen deformation, or collapse. The small caliber of the metallic filaments allows fast endothelialization which is influenced by the thickness of the metallic elements. The lack of stent rigidity allows a progressive smooth transition, without abrupt changes of caliber between the healthy artery and the stent. Fitting the stent to the lesion is easy due to the multiple combinations of lengths (from 2 to 7cm) and diameters (from 4 to 14mm); long segments can be stented by overlapping multiple stents. Rousseau et al. used, in the femoropopliteal segment, one stent in 64% of the cases, two to three stents in 32%, and more than three in 5% of the cases.

As with most other stents the "Wallstent" has low radiopacity which causes problems for exact positioning of the stent in obese patients, and particularly for lesions near an ostium or a bifurcation.

The "two step" placement, 1) PTA and 2) stenting, does not seem to be a disadvantage in comparison to balloon expandable stents. On the contrary, it avoids overuse of stenting; it is considered that stent implantation is not necessary when a good hemodynamic and angiographic result post-PTA is obtained. If a stent is necessary, the placement of the "Wallstent" is very easy and fast.

The occurrence of early thrombosis or late restenosis is not necessarily related to the type of stent used. However, it is difficult to compare the results of the different stents, particularly in the femoropopliteal segment, since only the Wallstent has been used in a significant number of patients in this arterial segment.[17,21]

The experimental thrombogenicity of the "Wallstent" is comparable to that reported by other authors.[12] Despite the use of heparin, platelet anti-aggregating agents, and dextran, the rate of early thrombosis is high compared with that of PTA alone. The main responsible factors seem to be: 1) poor distal runoff; 2) residual narrowing or dissection at the ends of the stent, when the length of the stent is insufficient; 3) residual stenosis when stenting is used without PTA; 4) insufficient anticoagulation. With good stent placement, good patient selection, and good anticoagulation, the thrombosis rate has decreased significantly over the past two years. Nevertheless, it is important to carefully monitor the patient for the first month after stent placement. Early thrombosis can be detected and successfully treated by thrombolysis.

Restenosis is a more difficult problem, but its incidence is low and it occurs mainly in the femoropopliteal segment. The possibility of successfully treating these restenoses with the Simpson Atherocath and balloon dilation with a satisfactory follow-up beyond six months has been reported.[21,22]

Günther reported results in 45 patients. Forty patients were classified as Stage IIB, four as Stage IIA, and one as Stage III. Thirty-one patients had lesions of the iliac arteries and fourteen had lesions of the superficial femoral artery (SFA). Twenty-six patients had arterial occlusions (iliac artery in six and the SFA in ten). Nineteen patients had arterial stenosis, 15 in the iliac artery and 4 in the SFA. The length of the stenosis ranged from 1 to 4cm in 15 patients, 4 to 8cm in 3, and was 27cm in 1 patient. The length of the total occlusions ranged from 1 to 20cm. The indication for stenting was failure of PTA in 26 patients with occlusions and 11 with stenosis. Seven had recurrence post-PTA and one had recurrence with an aneurysm at the site of PTA. Six-millimeter stents were used in the SFA and 7–12mm stents in the iliac arteries. All patients improved after stenting with the mean ankle-arm index (AAI)

increasing from 0.6 to 0.92. Complications included early stent occlusion and transient thromboembolism in two. At the latest follow-up 40 of 45 patients had patent stents with AAI of 0.89 (range 0.4–1.1). Intimal hyperplasia was seen in three SFA and one iliac artery. Two of the SFA intimal hyperplasia were treated with PTA and one by atherectomy.[21] Günther, as well as Rousseau, also advised against the use of stents in the femoropopliteal segments[16,21] except in cases of failed PTA that might lead to deterioration of the patient's clinical status. Vorwerk reported the mechanical recanalization of occluded iliac arteries in 48 of 68 patients, followed by underdilation and stenting. Recanalization failed in 20 patients. Thirty-seven lesions were in the common iliac, 23 in the external iliac, and 8 in the combined common iliac-external iliac arteries. An ipsilateral approach was used in all but three patients. Early reocclusion occurred in two patients; the patency rate at six months was 93.3%. Only one embolic episode occurred.[23] Vorwerk assumed that the use of the stent helps to stabilize the mural thrombus.[23]

Because of the possibility of recurrence and although early clinical experience with self expandable stents or stents in general is very promising,[15,16,20,21] the use of stenting has to be limited to selected cases.

The unknown long-term results and the cost of the procedure are other arguments for the careful selection of patients. Systematic implantation after every PTA is not indicated. On the other hand, implantation only in recurrence after PTA is the opposite extreme. We suggest an intermediate attitude which consists of stenting following an unsatisfactory result after PTA with residual stenoses greater than 30% and/or important intimal dissection with great risk of early thrombosis. These complications are sometimes seen following PTA of simple stenoses, but are more often seen following PTA of complex lesions. These latter lesions have been considered until now as poor indications for PTA. Among them are total obstructions, long ulcerated stenoses, and calcified lesions. It is clear now that stenting dramatically improves the immediate and late results of these lesions in the iliac arteries. This is not totally true for femoropopliteal lesions for which, at the present time, we use only stenting for immediate failure of PTA.

External vascular compression, like cystic adventitial degeneration of the popliteal artery, popliteal artery entrapment, and thoracic outlet syndrome, which are poor indications for PTA, may have a nonsurgical solution, with stenting, but additional data are still required for these lesions.

After more than three years of clinical use and even though supplementary studies are necessary, it seems that arterial stenting is a very promising method. The main advantage of stenting is the possibility of treating complex iliac lesions with reasonable success. Other promising applications of self-expandable stents include the management of stenotic lesions of veins and bypass grafts.[24–26] Rousseau reported successful management of 26 stenoses in 20 patients with hemodialysis shunts. Nineteen percent recurrence was seen at six months and 35% at one year due to intimal hyperplasia.[25] Zollikofer treated one native iliac vein and two vein grafts successfully.[24]

Conclusion

The experimental results obtained with the "Wallstent" are to a great extent similar to those obtained with other types of prostheses.[12-14] These results can be summarized as follows:

1. The implantation is very easy;
2. The fitting of the stent to the arterial wall is excellent;
3. No migration of the stent has been noted;
4. The microscopic studies have not shown host reaction or inflammatory reaction.

The essential phenomenon is the fast development of a neointima which covers the filaments within four weeks.[5] Ninety percent of the collaterals which stand through the stent remain patent.

The benefits offered by stents have applications in the management of PTA complications and in expanding the indications of PTA to complex lesions, which until now were considered untreatable with balloons, and to other lesions such as extrinsic compression of both arterial and venous channels. Stent technology has room for improvement, particularly in the area of control of intimal hyperplasia. Some day Dotter's dream of percutaneous grafting may become a reality.

References

1. Krepel VM, Van Andel GL, Van Erp WFM, Brelau PJ: Percutaneous dilation of femoral artery: initial and long term results. *Radiology* 1985;156:325–328
2. Van Andel GJ, Van Erp WFM, Krepel VM, Bresleau PJ: Percutaneous transluminal dilatation of the iliac artery: long term results. *Radiology* 1985;156:321–323
3. Simpson JB, Zimmerman JJ, Selmon MR, et al: Transluminal atherectomy: initial clinical results in 27 patients. *Circulation* 1986;74(suppl 2):457
4. Kensey KR, Nash JF, Abrahams C, Zarins C: Recanalization of obstructed arteries with a flexible rotating tip catheter. *Radiology* 1987;165:387–389
5. Abela GS, Norman SJ, Cohen DM, et al: Laser recanalization of occluded atherosclerotic arteries in vivo and in vitro. *Circulation* 1985;71:403–411
6. Dotter C: Transluminal expandable nitinol coil stent grafting: long term patency in the canine popliteal artery. *Invest Radiol* 1969;4:329–332
7. Dotter C, Buschmann RW, McKinney MK, Rösch J: Transluminal expandable nitinol coil stent grafting: preliminary report. *Radiology* 1983;147:259–260
8. Cragg A, Lund G, Rysavy J, Castañeda F, Castañeda–Zúñiga WR, Amplatz K: Non surgical placement of arterial endo-

prosthesis: a new technique using nitinol wire. *Radiology* 1983;147:261–263
9. Maas D, Demiere D, Deaton D, Largiader F. Transluminal implantation of self-adjusting expandable prosthesis: principles, techniques and results. *Prog Artif Organs* 1983;2:979–987
10. Wright KC, Wallace S, Charnsangavej C, Carrasco CH, Gianturco C: Percutaneous endovascular stents: an experimental evaluation. *Radiology* 1985;156:69–72
11. Rousseau H, Puel J, Joffre F, Sigwart V, Duboucher C, Imbert C, Knight C, Kropf L, Wallsten H: Self expanding endovascular prosthesis: an experimental study. *Radiology* 1987;164:709–714
12. Palmaz JC, Sibbitt RR, Reuter SR, Tio FO, Rice WJ: Expandable intraluminal graft: a preliminary study. *Radiology* 1985;156:73–77
13. Rousseau H, Joffre F, Raillat CH, et al: Self-expanding endovascular stent in experimental atherosclerosis: work in progress. *Radiology* 1989;170:773–778
14. Sigwart V, Puel J, Mirkovitch V, Joffre F, Kappenberger L: Intra-vascular stents to prevent occlusion and restenosis after transluminal angioplasty. *N Engl J Med* 1987;316:701–706
15. Raillat Ch, Rousseau H, Joffre F, Roux D: Treatment of iliac artery lesions by using the Wallstent endoprosthesis: midterm results. *AJR* 1990;154:613–616
16. Rousseau H, Raillat CH, Joffre F, Knight C, Ginestet MC: Treatment of femoro-popliteal stenoses by means of self expandable endoprostheses: midterm results. *Radiology* 1989;172:961–964
17. Essed CE, Van Den Brand M, Becker AE: Transluminal coronary angioplasty and early restenosis: fibrocellular occlusion after wall laceration. *Br Heart J* 1983;49:393–396
18. Faxon DP, Sanborn TA, Weber VJ: Restenosis following transluminal angioplasty in experimental atherosclerosis. *Arteriosclerosis* 1984;4:189–195
19. Colapinto RF: Long term results of iliac and femoro-popliteal angioplasty, in Dotter CT, Grüntzig A, School W, Zeitler E (eds): *Percutaneous Transluminal Angioplasty*. Berlin, Springer-Verlag, 1983, pp 202–206
20. Palmaz JC, Richter GM, Noeldge G, et al: Intraluminal stent in atherosclerotic iliac artery stenosis: preliminary report of a multicenter study. *Radiology* 1988;168:727–731
21. Günther RW, Vorwerk D, Bohndorf K, et al: Iliac and femoral artery stenoses and occlusion: treatment with intravascular stents. *Radiology* 1989;172:725–730
22. Vorwerk D, Günther RW: Removal of intimal hyperplasia in vascular endoprostheses managed by combined use of atherectomy and balloon dilatation. *AJR* 1990;154:617–619
23. Vorwerk D, Günther RW. Mechanical revascularization of occluded iliac arteries with use of self expandable endoprosthesis. *Radiology* 1990;175:411–415
24. Zollikofer CL, Largiader I, Bruhlman WF, Uhlschmid GK, Marty AH: Endovascular stenting of veins and grafts: preliminary experience. *Radiology* 1988;167:707–712
25. Rousseau H, Morfaux V, Joffre F, Ton–That H, Goodable C, Bartoli P, Yong Y: Treatment of hemodialysis arteriovenous fistula stenosis by percutaneous implantation of new intravascular stent. *J Intervent Radiol* 1989;4:161–167
26. Günther RW, Vorwerk D, Klose KC, Bohndorf K, Kistler D, Mann H, Sieberth HG: Self expanding stents for the treatment of a long venous stenosis in a dialysis shunt: case report. *Cardiovasc Intervent Radiol* 1988;12:29–31

Part 4. Strecker Intravascular Flexible Tantalum Stent

—Ernst–Peter Strecker, M.D., Dieter Liermann, M.D., Hellmut R. D. Wolf, M.D., Beate Schneider, M.D., Nikolaus L. Freudenberg, M.D., Klemens H. Barth, M.D., and Michael Westphal, M.D.

The patency rate of transluminal angioplasty is influenced by a number of factors, including acute thrombosis, intimal and medial dissection, arterial recoil due to the inherent elasticity of the arterial walls, and intimal hyperplasia. All of these factors can contribute to the acute or chronic development of recurrent vascular occlusion. In an attempt to improve on the failures of transluminal angioplasty, a balloon expandable flexible tantalum intraluminal vascular stent was developed and implanted in patients with atherosclerotic, stenotic, or occluded iliac or femoropopliteal arteries.

DESCRIPTION OF THE STENT

The tantalum balloon expandable stent consists of a knitted, tubular, flexible, metal wire mesh tube. Because of its loose structure of connected wire loops, the stent shows longitudinal and radial flexibility. It has been said that since knitting forms a looser fabric than weaving, this stent design has a greater flexibility than the Wallstent[1] (Fig. 7.4.1). The dimensions are determined by the number and size of loops (1.5–2.5mm) and the inside diameter depends on the diameter of the core. All the parameters regarding the dimensions of the stent can be changed at will. The stent is mounted on an angioplasty balloon. Like the Palmaz stent, Strecker's stent has no spring action of its own. It needs to be passively expanded over a balloon up to six times its collapsed introducing dimensions to a predetermined diameter, and has no tendency to increase its diameter after placement, in contrast to the self-expandable stents.[2–10] To prevent displacement of the stent over the balloon caused by friction with the introducer sheath or with the inner arterial wall, the stent is attached by silicone sleeves to the balloon at both ends of the stent. After balloon expansion the silicone sleeves will roll back from the expanding balloon unto the catheter shaft and will thus release the prosthesis (Fig. 7.4.2*A,B*).

The loops are made of tantalum (99% pure). To decrease thrombogenicity, the wire is chemically electropolished. By this process the oxide film on the metal surface is fully removed and microscopic irregularities are eliminated. These measures ensure that the metal oxidation that will occur in the bloodstream will lead to a "uniform" oxide film surface.[3] The thin layer of inert tantalum pentoxide which creates an electrically negative surface charge will prevent the adhesion of platelets which are negatively charged as well.[11]

The advantage of tantalum over stainless-steel and other alloys includes better radiopacity which allows good visualization under fluoroscopy and the fact that tantalum can be regarded as an optimal, biologically inert material. Long-term studies of orthopedic implants and surgical clips did not show any corrosion.[12,13] In addition, implanted

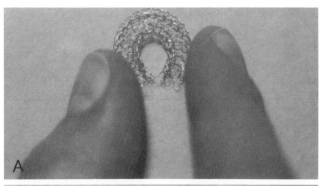

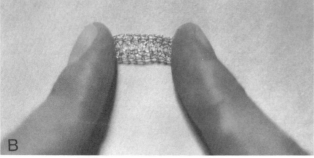

Figure 7.4.1. Expanded knitted tantalum stent. **A.** The balloon expanded vascular stent consists of loosely connected metallic loops and is therefore flexible and pliable. **B.** The vascular stent is elastic; within certain limits, it is compressible in longitudinal and radial fashion.

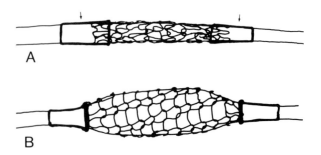

Figure 7.4.2. Diagram of the balloon stent assembly. **A.** Nonexpanded state. The knitted stent is compressed longitudinally with primarily loosely connected loops to prevent longitudinal shortening after expansion. It is held on the balloon by radial tension. In addition the stent is fixated by silicone sleeves at the catheter shaft proximal and distal to the balloon overlapping the ends of the stent preventing any stent dislocation during introduction. **B.** Half-expanded balloon. The wire loops have been widened by deformation and are almost firmly intersecting. The silicone sleeves are shortened and rolled backward leaving the stent free for implantation.

tantalum stents are not disturbed by magnetic fields, nor do they disturb magnetic resonance imaging. Magnetic resonance angiography techniques can be used to evaluate vascular patency in the presence of tantalum stents, whereas, in contrast, stainless-steel implants will create signal loss appearing as black holes within the image.[14]

Because of its design, the final length of the stent will depend on the degree of balloon expansion. An enlargement of stent diameter from 2 to 7mm causes a shortening of 50%. To prevent such degree of stent shortening, the stent is mounted on the balloon with significant compression longitudinally from both ends, with loops of the wire mesh almost completely overlapping each other.

A comparison of the shortening of a tantalum stent, longitudinally stretched, with the shortening of a stent longitudinally compressed, reveals that the latter type will also shorten to a certain extent with balloon expansion, although the degree of shortening is reduced by half. The percentage of decrease of stent diameter after completion of balloon dilatation caused by the arterial elastic recoil is demonstrated in Figure 7.4.3. The percentage of decrease in the stent diameter caused by the elastic recoil can be reduced by redilatation with increasingly larger balloon diameters or it can be compensated by choosing a nominal stent size that exceeds the diameter of the actual lumen by at least 0.5–1mm. This percentage is the known recoil of the artery with the implanted tantalum stent following balloon expansion.[1] The actual effect of elastic recoil is actually negligible. At maximum balloon expansion to 9mm, the amount of radial recoil of the stent itself is extremely low (1%).[1]

One of the main points of concern about flexible implantable stents is the unknown reaction of the moving vessel wall to a flexible stent as opposed to a rigid stent.[15] Experimental animal data have not shown any evidence of

luminal compromise at the stent site up to 12 months for either flexible[16] or rigid stents.[15]

The reaction of the normal canine arterial wall to the stent was evidenced by a progressive buildup of cells inside the implant during the first eight weeks corresponding to thrombosis and smooth muscle cell proliferation. The media outside the stent showed a progressive atrophy. As a result of the stent implantation, there was an increase in wall rigidity; the initial thickening caused by the proliferation of smooth muscle cells causes a hemodynamically nonsignificant narrowing of the lumen. This process is the same for large and small arteries.[1,6,7,17] In Barth's experience the buildup of neointima was higher over the distal end of the stent.[1] Similar findings were reported by Sutton.[8]

A disadvantage common to all balloon expandable stents appears to be the collapsability of the stents, when extrinsically compressed. However, deformation of the stents implanted into femoral or popliteal arteries has never occurred, either in experimental animals or in human patients.

STENT IMPLANTATION TECHNIQUE

The procedure is performed using a percutaneous approach to place an 8Fr sheath. Systemic heparinization is achieved with 5,000–10,000 units of heparin. The stenosis or occlusion is first balloon-dilated. During passage of the stent through the hemostatic valve of the introducer sheath, the stent-balloon assembly is protected by a 5cm piece of thin-walled Teflon tubing. The tubing is pulled back to allow hemostasis after the stent has been advanced into the sheath. Accurate positioning of the stent before expansion is verified with respect to reference points: external metallic markers or road mapping. Balloon inflation expands the stent and the lesion simultaneously. Any residual narrowing either cranially or caudally is corrected by balloon dilation or by placing a second stent. If additional stents are implanted, they should overlap the first by several millimeters. Inflation pressure values of at least 5 atm are required to ensure proper stent expansion and release.

After stent expansion the balloon is deflated and carefully withdrawn to prevent stent dislocation.

All patients are placed on intravenous heparin titrated to keep the partial thromboplastin time 2–3 times normal for two days in iliac arteries and for three days in femoro-popliteal arteries. Aspirin (325mg/day) is given immediately after the procedure and continued indefinitely thereafter.

MATERIALS

Forty-six men and ten women (median age of 61 years, range: 38–81) were treated with the balloon expandable tantalum stent. Thirty-nine patients received one stent, 14

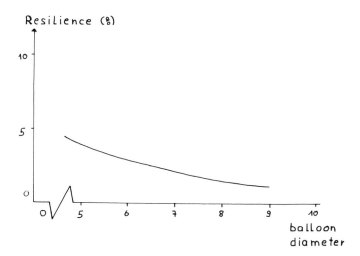

Figure 7.4.3. Resilience (elastic springback) of a knitted tantalum stent after radial balloon dilatation versus increasing balloon diameter. The elastic springback decreases with radial expansion and amounts to 1% at a diameter of 9mm.

received two stents, 1 received three stents, and 3 received four stents. Twenty femoropopliteal and 35 iliac lesions were treated with a total of 75 stents. The lesions had a median length of 5cm (range 0.5–50cm).

Atherosclerotic cardiovascular disease risk factors included diabetes mellitus (11%), high blood pressure (30%), and a history of prolonged cigarette smoking (91%).

If necessary, PTA of additional ipsilateral lesions was performed. Five patients had rotational angioplasty and thrombolysis performed prior to stent placement, one patient had percutaneous aspiration thromboembolectomy and fibrinolysis, and one patient had an occluded iliopopliteal bypass graft which was stented.

The four indications for stent placement were: restenosis after previous PTA (23 patients); poor initial PTA result with residual stenosis (33 patients); initial occlusion (18 patients); and intimal flaps (17 patients). Several patients had multiple indications.

RESULTS

Primary Results

ANGIOGRAPHIC SUCCESS

The mean stenosis pre-procedure as evaluated by angiography was 84%, which was improved to 49% after balloon angioplasty and further reduced (range 20–0%) immediately after stent placement (Fig. 7.4.4*A–C*). The pre-procedure to post-PTA improvement and the post-PTA to post-stent improvement were both statistically significant ($p < 0.0001$ according to the Wilcoxon signed-rank test). There was no thrombosis due to stent implantation during the first three months after placement.

HEMODYNAMIC SUCCESS

Hemodynamic results were measured by the determination of the Doppler ankle-arm indices (AAI), pre- and postprocedure in 26 lesions. The median AAI improved from 54% pre-procedure to 89% after stent placement. The pre- to post-Doppler AAI improvement was significant ($p < 0.0001$ according to the Wilcoxon signed rank test). Fifty-five of the lesions were successfully treated by hemodynamic criteria (Fig. 7.4.5*A,B*).

One lesion improved by less than 0.15 Doppler AAI and was considered as a hemodynamic failure. However, this case was successful by angiographic criteria. Also, this patient had a clinical follow-up and had improved by one level, according to the classification of Fontaine.

CLINICAL SUCCESS

The clinical improvement was correlated to the Fontaine classification.

   I. No symptoms;
 IIA. Claudication at >250 meters;
 IIB. Claudication at <250 meters;
 III. Rest pain;
 IV. Tissue loss.

In all patients initially successfully treated, clinical function improved by a mean of 1.9 levels (range 1–3 stages according to the Fontaine classification).

Long-term Follow-up

The six-month (range five to nine months) control angiography mostly performed by intravenous digital subtraction angiography revealed satisfactory results in patients treated with iliac artery stents. There was no restenosis or reocclusion within, proximal or distal to the stent. The internal surface of the stent was covered by a thin smooth endothelial layer (Fig. 7.4.4*D*).

Four patients with infrainguinal stents showed restenosis, occurring four to seven months after implantation. Typically, narrowing within the middle portion of the stents was found with both ends of the tubular stents remaining widely open.

The stent narrowings were treated by repeat balloon angioplasty, directional atherectomy, or laser angioplasty. Tissue specimens obtained by atherectomy revealed intimal hyperplasia combined with thrombosis.

Doppler-sonographic AAI determinations were performed up to 36 months after iliac artery stent treatment. The follow-up curves reveal in all patients good results without any decline of the indices (Fig. 7.4.5). In contrast, four patients with distal superficial femoral artery stents showed recurrent disease (Fig. 7.4.5).

LONG-TERM CLINICAL SUCCESS

Iliac artery stents with a maximum observation time of 36 months showed that the primary improvement obtained immediately after stent placement remained unchanged in all patients during the observation period.

The results were not as good in infrainguinal stents. The four patients with restenosis had a clinical deterioration of their initially improved symptoms with a clinical Stage IIB according to Fontaine.

DISCUSSION

The incidence of acute occlusions following PTCA is reported around 4–6%.[18–20] Many of these occlusions are due to intimal flaps. It is possible to reopen acute occlusions due to intimal flaps through the use of directional atherectomy[21] or with the use of stents.[22] In the Strecker series, five patients had large intimal flaps compromising blood flow following PTA. In all cases a successful resolution was achieved by stent placement. Stents can also improve the geometry of bypass graft anastomoses in cases where the graft is kinked.

Residual stenoses of 30% or greater are known to result in higher restenosis rates.[19] Stent placement greatly

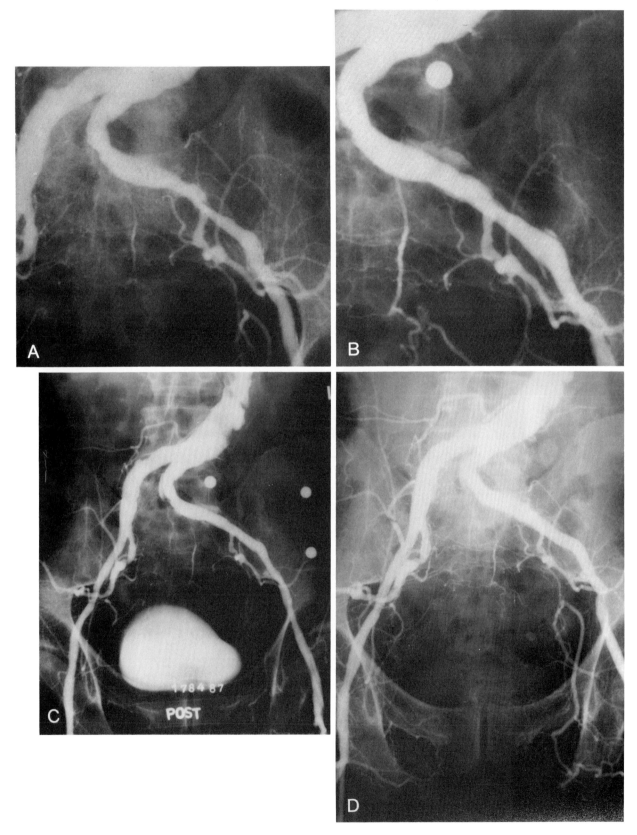

Figure 7.4.4.   A. Severe atherosclerotic stenosis with lifestyle-limiting claudication of the left external iliac artery. **B.** There is a considerable amount of residual stenosis after PTA due to elastic arterial wall recoil although overdilatation was performed. **C.** The result is optimized by the implantation of a flexible tantalum stent. **D.** 45 weeks after stent implantation the internal surface of the treated arterial segment is covered with a thin tissue layer corresponding to a neointima.

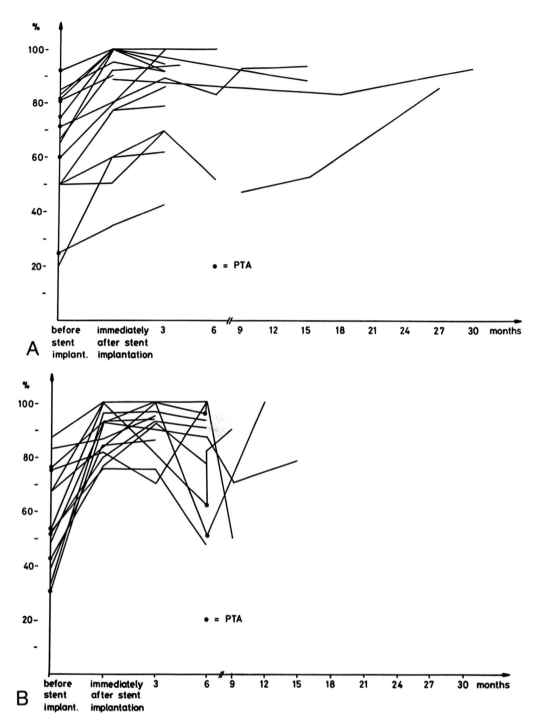

Figure 7.4.5. Long-term follow-up of Doppler ankle-arm indices. **A.** The follow-up curves of patients with iliac artery stents reveal no decline of the indices (maximum observation time being 30 months). **B.** The follow-up of patients with stented femoral arteries showed in four patients a decline of their indices which corresponded to their restenoses within the stent demanding a repeat angioplasty.

reduces residual stenosis post-PTA to less than 2%. Therefore it is possible that stents can improve the long-term patency rate in comparison to PTA, where there is always a residual lumen reduction after balloon dilatation. There is a risk of restenosis secondary to intimal hyperplasia and local thrombosis until the formation of a functionally mature neointima on the inner stent surface occurs; there-fore all patients should be treated with aspirin postprocedure.[23,24]

Liermann reported a two-year patency rate of 100% for iliac artery stenting and 100% patency rate for the proximal femoral artery at one year. Because of a 25% restenosis at six months in distal superficial femoral artery stenting, lesions in this area are only stented if there is a large intimal flap following PTA or when PTA fails to dilate leaving a residual stenosis of at least 40%.[25]

Placement of flexible balloon expandable tantalum stents optimizes the geometrical end result following balloon dilatation.[23,25,26] In addition, because the expandable stent opposes elastic recoil there is no need for overdilatation. The smooth and regular lumen obtained with the stent decreases or prevents the development of luminal irregularities after angioplasty. These irregularities disturb normal blood flow patterns creating turbulences and pressure gradients.

The knitted prosthesis offers a high degree of mechanical flexibility. Therefore, this stent can be introduced through curved arteries and over the aortic bifurcation. The stent can maintain its configuration after expansion, since the loosely connected loops, made of tantalum wire filaments, are elastic within certain limits. Percutaneously implanted expandable stents will improve PTA results and may extend the indications for PTA. More experience is necessary to determine the indications for this new therapy of occlusive atherosclerotic vascular disease in the iliac and femoral arteries.

References

1. Barth KH, Virmani R, Strecker EP, Savin MA, Lindisch D, Matsumoto AH, Teitelbaum GP: Flexible tantalum stents implanted in aortas and iliac arteries: effects in normal canines. *Radiology* 1990;175:91–96
2. Dotter CT, Buschmann RW, McKinney MK, Rösch J: Transluminal expandable nitinol coil stent grafting: preliminary report. *Radiology* 1983;147:259–260
3. Cragg A, Lund G, Rysavy J, Castañeda F, Castañeda–Zúñiga WR, Amplatz K: Non-surgical placement of arterial endoprostheses: a new technique using nitinol wire. *Radiology* 1983;147:261–263
4. Maass D, Zollikofer CL, Largiader F, Senning A: Radiological follow-up of transluminally inserted vascular endoprostheses: an experimental study using expanding spirals. *Radiology* 1984;152:659–663
5. Palmaz JC, Windeler SA, Garcia F, Tio FO, Sibbitt RR, Reuter SR: Atherosclerotic rabbit aortas: expandable intraluminal grafting. *Radiology* 1986;160:723–726
6. Duprat G Jr, Wright KC, Charnsangavej C, Wallace S, Gianturco C: Self-expanding metal stents for small vessels: an experimental evaluation. *Radiology* 1987;162:469–472
7. Rousseau H, Puel J, Joffre F, et al: Self-expanding endovascular prosthesis: an experimental study. *Radiology* 1987;164:709–714
8. Sutton CS, Oku T, Harasaki H, et al: Titanium-nickel intravascular endoprothesis: a 2-year study in dogs. *AJR* 1988;151:597–601
9. Palmaz JC, Richter GM, Noeldge G, et al: Intraluminal stents in atherosclerotic iliac artery stenosis: preliminary report of a multicenter study. *Radiology* 1988;168:727–731
10. Palmaz JC, Tio FO, Schatz RA, Alvarado R, Rees C, Garcia O: Early endothelialization of balloon-expandable stents: experimental observations. *J Intervent Radiol* 1988;3:119–124
11. Sawyer PN, Stanczewski B, Srinivasan S, Stempak JG, Kammlott GW: Electronmicroscopy and physical chemistry of healing in prosthetic heart valves, skirts and struts. *J Thorac Cardiovasc Surg* 1974;67:25
12. Kylberg F: The use of tantalum clips in general surgery. *Acta Chir Scand* 1975;141:242–244
13. von Holst H, Collins P, Steiner L: Titanium, silver, and tantalum clips in brain tissue. *Acta Neurochirurgica* 1981;56:239–242
14. Matsumoto AH, Teitelbaum GP, Barth KH, Carvlin MJ, Savin MA, Strecker EP: Tantalum vascular stents: in vivo evaluation with MR imaging. *Radiology* 1989;170:753–755
15. Schatz RA, Palmaz JC, Tio FO, Garcia F, Garcia O, Reuter SR: Balloon-expandable intracoronary stents in the adult dog. *Circulation* 1987;76:450–457
16. Roubin GS, Robinson KA, King SP, et al: Early and late results of intracoronary arterial stenting after coronary angioplasty in dogs. *Circulation* 1987;76:891–897
17. Palmaz JC: Balloon-expandable intravascular stent. *AJR* 1988;150:1263–1269
18. Crowley MJ, Dorros G, Ralsey SF, vanRoden M, Detro KM: Acute coronary events associated with percutaneous transluminal angioplasty. *Am J Cardiol* 1989;53:12C
19. Holmes DR, Holubkov R, Vlietstra RE, et al: Comparison of complications during percutaneous transluminal angioplasty from 1977 to 1981 and from 1985 to 1986: the National Heart, Lung, and Blood Institute Percutaneous Transluminal Coronary Angioplasty Registry. *JACC* 1988;12:1149–55
20. Meyorovitz MF, Friedmann PL, Ganz P, et al. Acute occlusion developing during or immediately after percutaneous transluminal coronary angioplasty: nonsurgical treatment. *Radiology* 1988;169:491–494
21. Maynar M, Reyes R, Cabrera V, et al: Percutaneous atherectomy as an alternative treatment for post-angioplasty obstructing intimal flap. *Radiology* 1989;170(3):1029–1032
22. Becker GJ, Palmaz JC, Rees CR, et al: Angioplasty induced dissection in human iliac arteries: management with Palmaz balloon expandable intraluminal stents. *Radiology* 1990;176:31–38
23. Strecker EP, Romaniuk P, Schneider B, Westphal M, Zeitler E, Wolf HRD, Freudenberg N: Perkutan implantierbare, durch Ballon aufdehnbare Gefässprothese: erste kleinishe Ergebnisse. *Dtsch Med Wòchenschr* 1988;113:538–543
24. Austin GE, Ratliff NB, Hollman J, Tabei S, Phillips DF: Intimal proliferation of smooth muscle cells as an explanation for recurrent artery stenosis after percutaneous transluminal angioplasty. *J Am Coll Cardiol* 1985;6:369–375
25. Liermann DD, Strecker EP, Kollath J: Implantation of he Strecker stent in peripheral and curved vessels: indication and first result. Presented at RIPCV-2; Toulouse, France, Feb, 1990
26. Triller J, Mahler F, Thälmann R: Die vasculäre Endoprothese bei femoro-poplitealer Verschlusskrankheit. *Fortschr Röntgenstr* 1989;150:328–334

Part 5. The Rabkin Nitinol Coil Stent: A Five-Year Experience

—Joseff E. Rabkin and Vladimir G. Germashev

Percutaneous transluminal angioplasty (PTA) has been advocated as an effective method for restoration of vascular flow to organs and tissues by treating vascular obstructions. According to different authors, the rate of restenoses after PTA can reach up to at 41.1% at two years and, for smaller vessels, up to 68.6%.[1–14]

The implantation of a steel device in the form of spiral was described by Dotter in 1969.[15] In 1983, Cragg and Dotter described simultaneously[16,17] the use of nitinol stents in the vascular lumen. However, technical problems with the devices, in particular the need to heat the alloy to 60°C in order to restore its form, hampered its introduction into the clinical field.[16,17]

An endovascular stent made of nitinol (37°C) was developed at the National Research Center of Surgery of the USSR[12,18,19] (Fig. 7.5.1A). A nitinol spiral stent made of nickel and titanium alloy possesses a thermal-shape memory and meets all medical and technical requirements including biological compatibility, corrosion resistance, lack of thrombogenicity, nonpyrogenicity, and self-fixation to the vascular wall. The stent can be easily introduced through a 7–9Fr angiographic catheter when it is cooled and straightened (Fig. 7.5.1B). Similar to a porous shunt, it permits ion exchange and allows for endothelialization.[20–27] Histologic studies demonstrated a fine, nonadhesive, nonthrombogenic intima coating the stent without any signs of intimal hyperplasia.

In a five-year period, 295 stents were placed in 268 patients in different anatomic zones[12,13,26] (Table 7.5.1). All implantations were performed percutaneously using a femoral approach. In case of the brachycephalic arteries, the transaxillary approach was used in three out of five cases.

Endovascular stent implantation was performed through an angiographic catheter following balloon dilatation. The choice of stent size is based on the angiographic

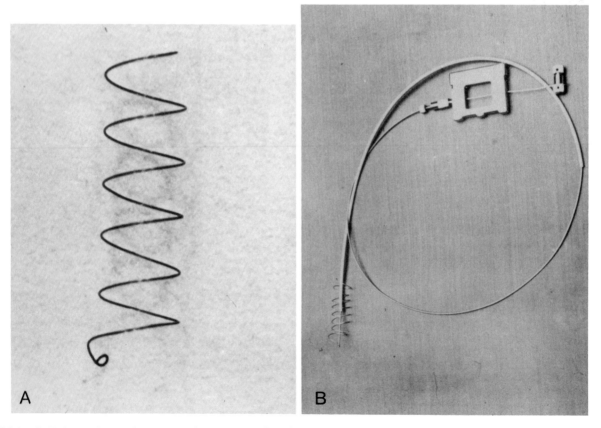

Figure 7.5.1.   **A.** Endovascular metal stent with a form memory effect. **B.** Anterior border of the stent is attached to the conductor; distal cone has a fixing device.

Table 7.5.1. Localization and Type of Stent Implantation

	No. of Patients	Bifurcation Stent	Single Stent After Recanalization and PTA	After Laser Recanalization	After Kensey Recanalization	Multiple Stents	No. of Stents
Common iliac	69	4	55	8		2	75
External iliac	53		45	5		3	56
Common femoral	3		3				
Superficial femoral	90		60	20	10	8	106
Popliteal	24		19	5		1	26
Subclavian	13		9	4			13
Brachiocephalic branch	2	2		4			2
Renal	14		11	3			14
Total	268	4	204	45	10	14	295

data, taking into account the diameter of the normal adjacent artery (Fig. 7.5.2). The stent diameter must be larger than the normal arterial diameter by 0.15–0.20mm. The length of the stent is dictated by the length of the lesion and varies from 0.5 to 3.5cm. In two cases, the implanted stents were 100mm in length. The procedure, including dilatation, stent placement, and postimplantation angiographic control took 45 minutes on average.

The most common lesions treated were atherosclerotic in 232 cases (86.7%), nonspecific arteritis in 28 cases (10%), and fibromuscular dysplasia in 8 cases (3.3%). The period from onset of symptomatology to stent placement ranged from 6 months to 12 years, and the ages of the patients varied from 21 to 72 years; 76.6% of the patients had severe associated diseases including heart disease in 125 patients, diabetes in 65 patients, and cerebrovascular problems in 14 patients. Combinations of the above-mentioned diagnoses were registered in 20.0% of the cases.

Aspirin is given two days before the procedure, in dosages varying from 125 to 250mg/day, and continued thereafter. During the procedure, dextran and 5,000–10,000 units of heparin were given intra-arterially.

The pre- and postimplantation evaluation included duplex ultrasound, radioisotope scintigraphy (RISG), and angiography, as well as the clinical evaluation of the patients. Follow-up was done immediately and at 12 months or earlier, if the clinical situation so indicated, by angiography and noninvasive methods.

The results were classified as follows: 1) good; 2) satisfactory; 3) without effect; 4) deterioration. A good result

Table 7.5.2. Results of Nitinol Stent Placement

	Immediate Results 1–7 Days				Late Results 1–3 Years				3–5 Years			
	No. of Stents	Good	Satisfactory	Deterioration	No. of Stents	Good	Satisfactory	Deterioration	No. of Stents	Good	Satisfactory	Deterioration
Common iliac	75 25.4%	75 100%	—	—	50	48 96.0%	2 4.0%	—	30	29 96.6%	—	1 3.4%
External iliac	56 100%	56 100%	—	—	38	35 92.1%	3 7.9%	—	20	19 95.0%	1 5%	—
Common femoral	3 1.01%	3 100%	—	—	2	2 100%	—	—	1	1 100%	—	—
Superficial femoral	106 35.9%	78 73.6%	—	28 26.4%	80	52 65.0%	8 10%	20 25%	45	25 55.5%	10 22.2%	10 22.2%
Popliteal	26 8.59%	17 65.3%	—	9 24.7%	18	9 50%	—	9 50%	10	5 50%	—	5 50%
Subclavian	13 4.32%	13 100%	—	—	9	9 100%	—	—	6	6 100%	—	—
Brachiocephalic branch	2 0.67%	2 100%	—	—	2	2 100%	—	—	1	1 100%	—	—
Renal	14 4.62%	14 100%	—	—	10	9 90.0%	1 10.0%	—	7	6 85.7%	1 14.3%	—
Total	295 100%	258 88.8%	—	37	209	186 88.9%	14 6.6%	29 4.5%	120	92 76.6%	12 10%	16 13.4%

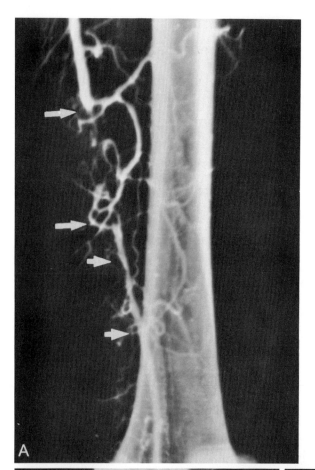

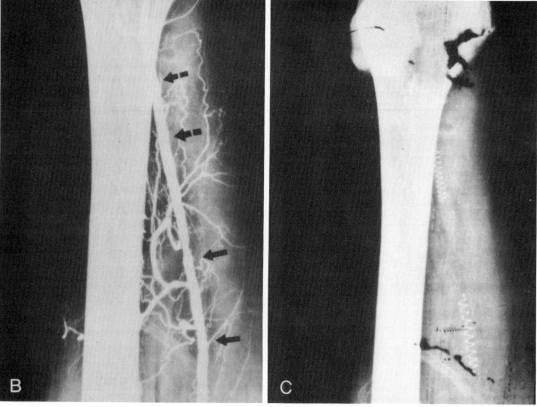

Figure 7.5.2. **A.** The arteriogram of the left femoral artery. Occlusion at the middle third *(long arrows)* and stenosis at the distal third of the superficial femoral artery *(short arrows)*. **B.** Double endovascular stent. **C.** Follow-up angiogram. Note a wide-open lumen.

was manifested by the presence of distal pulses, restoration of ankle-arm indices to normal or near normal values, normal perfusion in the radioisotope studies, lack of difference in temperatures between the extremities, angiographic evidence of normal caliber, and patency of the vessel at the site of former stenosis or occlusion. In addition, the patient should not manifest any evidence of intermittent claudication and/or skin trophic changes.

Satisfactory results were manifested by increased physical tolerance, intermittent claudication at 750–1000m, absence of trophic lesions in the lower extremities, lack of marked difference in skin temperature, and stable ankle-

arm indices with no significant difference from the opposite extremity.

In follow-up varying from six months to five years in 209 patients, analysis of the data (Table 7.5.2) showed that the success of the procedure depended on the location of the lesion. The best results were obtained for iliac (Fig. 7.5.3), brachycephalic and renal arteries (Fig. 7.5.4). In the distal arteries, superficial femoral, or popliteal arteries, the procedure was less effective, depending on the status of the distal vascular bed. The majority recurred early, within the first six months following stent placement.

Stent thrombosis was more commonly seen in patients

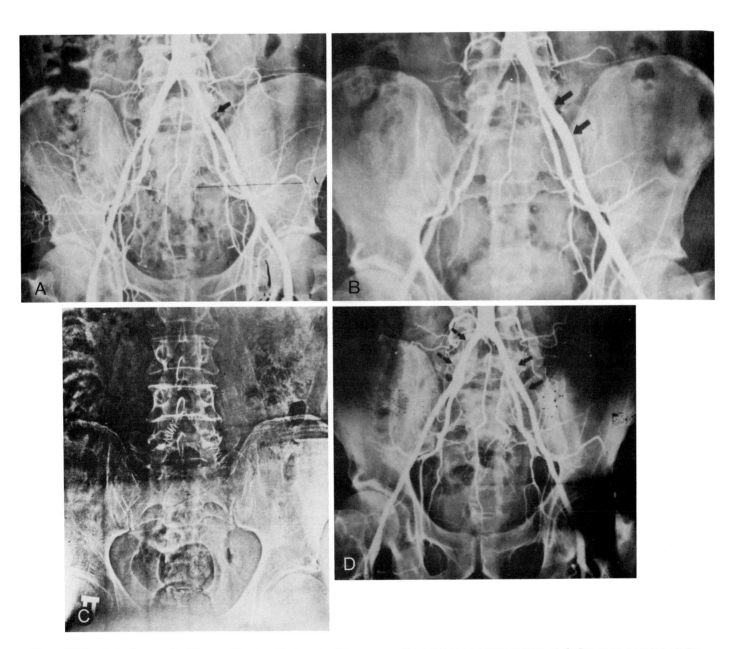

Figure 7.5.3.   **A.** Angiogram of a 56 year-old male with stenosis of the left external iliac artery *(arrow).* **B.** Angiogram of the same patient two years later. Patent lumen at the site of the stent. Stenosis of the right common iliac artery is now present *(arrows).* **C.** Stents are seen in both iliac arteries. **D.** Follow-up angiogram shows stents in both iliac arteries; three years on the left, two years on the right. Both vessels are widely patent.

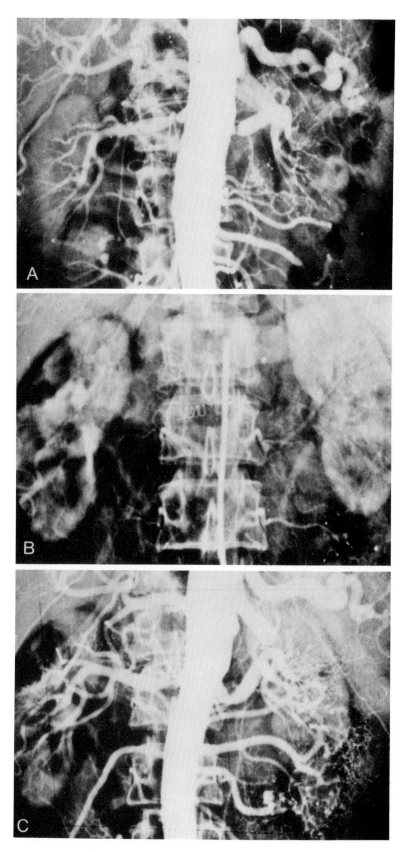

Figure 7.5.4. **A.** The angiogram of a 39-year-old male with renovascular hypertension. Bilateral stenosis of the renal arteries is seen. **B.** Bilateral angioplasty and right renal artery stenting were performed. The stent is seen in the right renal artery. **C.** Angiogram after bilateral angioplasty and stent placement on the right.

with diabetes mellitus with severe peripheral vascular disease. Acute thrombosis also occurred as the result of incorrect manipulations during stent implantation into the external femoral artery in five cases and in two popliteal arteries. Clinical deterioration after initial clinical success was registered in 30 cases, 9 of which required emergency surgery; 17 patients were operated on 6–18 months following implantation. There were no complications resulting in amputation of the extremity or patient's death related to the stent implantation.

CONCLUSIONS

1. Stent implantation is a safe, atraumatic, painless method of revascularization.
2. The nitinol stent is biocompatible.
3. A high clinical success rate of 82.7% for arteries in all locations is possible.
4. Unsatisfactory results are obtained in the superficial femoral and popliteal arteries.
5. In case of acute thrombosis of the artery, urgent or elective surgery is required. The results of surgery are not affected by stent placement.
6. No fatal outcome or amputation following stent implantation were seen.
7. Indications for stent implantation are:
   a. Restenosis or reocclusion after angioplasty for atherosclerotic disease;
   b. Stenotic occlusions in case of fibromuscular dysplasia, arteritis, extrinsic vascular compression restenosis;
   c. Stenoses of the anastomoses of vascular grafts to restore their patency.

References

1. Dotter CT: Transluminal angioplasty: a long view. *Radiology* 1980;135(3):561–564
2. Galichia JP, Bajaj AR, Vine DL, et al: Subclavian artery stenoses treated by transluminal angioplasty: six cases. *Cardiovasc Intervent Radiol* 1983;6(2):78–81
3. Grüntzig A, Hopff H: Percutane rekanalisation chronischer arterieller Verschlusse mit einem neuen Dilatationskatheter: Modifikation der Dotter-Technik. *Dtsch Med Wschr* 1974;99:2502–2505
4. Greenfield AJ: Femoral, popliteal and tibial arteries: percutaneous transluminal angioplasty. *AJR* 1980;135:927–934
5. Motarjeme A, Koifer J, Zurka A: Percutaneous transluminal angioplasty of the brachycephalic arteries. *AJR* 1982;138:457–462
6. Samson RH, Sprayregen S, Veith FG, et al: Management of angioplasty complications, unsuccessful procedures and early and late failures. *Ann Surg* 1984;199(2):234–240
7. Spence RK, Freiman DB, Catenby R, et al: Long-term results of transluminal angioplasty of the iliac and femoral arteries. *Arch Surg* 1981;116:1377–1386
8. Velasques G, Castañeda–Zúñiga WR, Formanek A, et al: Nonsurgical angioplasty in Leriche syndrome. *Radiology* 1980;134:359–360
9. Wierny L, Plass R, Porstmann W: Long-term results in 100 consecutive patients treated by transluminal angioplasty. *Radiology* 1974;112:543–548
10. Zeitler W, Schoop W, Zahnow W: The treatment of occlusive arterial disease by transluminal catheter angioplasty. *Radiology* 1971;99:19–26
11. Rabkin JK: Roentgenoendovascular surgery. *Roentgenoendovascular Surgery: Abstracts of VII All-Union Symposium for Angiography.* Moscow, 1987, pp 5–11
12. Tarakanov YP, Zvirin GE, Kuleshov VI, et al: Immediate and long-term results of endovascular balloon dilatation. *Proceedings of the All-Union Conference on Urgent Problems in CardioVascular Surgery.* Vilnius, Lithuania, 1986, pp 78–80
13. Cumberland DC. Percutaneous transluminal angioplasty: a review. *Clin Radiol* 1983;34:25–30
14. Dotter CT, Krippaehne WW, Judkins MP: Transluminal angioplasty in atherosclerotic obstruction of femoral popliteal system. *Am Surg* 1964;35:453–459
15. Dotter CT: Transluminally placed coil springs and artery. *Invest Radiol* 1969;4:329–332
16. Dotter CT, Buschmann RW, McKinney NK, Rösch J: Transluminal expandable nitinol coil stent grafting: preliminary report. *Radiology* 1983;147:259–260
17. Cragg A, Lund G, Rysavy J, Castañeda F, Castañeda–Zúñiga WR, Amplatz K: Nonsurgical placement of arterial endoprostheses: a new technique using nitinol wire. *Radiology* 1983;147:261–263
18. Rabkin JK: Revascularisatin par implantation d'une prothese radioendovasculare. Radiologie interventionelle en pathologie cardiovasquaire (abstr). Toulouse, 1988
19. Rabkin JK, Zajmovsky VA, Khmelevskaja YI, et al: Experimentally based first clinical experience in endovascular prosthetics. *Radiology Herald* 1984;4:59–64
20. Vitjugov IA, Kotenko VFV, Ghunter VV, Günther VV, et al: Tissue response to implantation of the devices from nickel titanium for osteosynthesis, in *Superelasticity, Shape-Memory Effect and Its Application in New Technologies.* All-Union Scientific Conference. Tomsk, 1985, p 143
21. Zajmovsky VA, Kolupajeva TL: Uncommon properties of ordinary metals. Moscow, Science: Nauka, 1984, p 192
22. Kurdjumov VA, Khandros LG: Thermoresistant balance of the phases in martensite conversion. *Rep USSR Acad Sci* 1949;66(2):211–215
23. Kotenko VV, Zakluchajeva VN, Günther VE, et al: Nickel content in the organs and muscles of dogs in experimental implantations of nickel-titanium alloy TN-lo, in *Superelasticity, Shape-Memory Effect.* Tomsk, 1985, p 147
24. Dzhoraev IG: Applications of RED for treatment of arterial stenoses and occlusions of extracranial brain vessels and arteries of the upper extremities. *Proceedings of the All-Union Conference of Young Scientists and Specialists:* "Urgent problems of prophylaxis and treatment of cardio-vascular diseases." Moscow, 1987, p 57
25. Litvinov AP: Effect of RED in stenosed renal arteries in patients with arterial hypertensin, in *Urgent Problems of Cardio-Vascular Surgery.* Proceedings of the All-Union Conference of Cardio-Vascular Surgeons. Vilnius, Lithuania, 1986, pp 57–58
26. Procubovsky VI, Koshkin VM, Farber AJ: Immediate and long-term results of RED in obliterating lesions of the arteries of the extremities, in *Roentgenoendovascular Surgery.* Abstract of the VII All-Union Symposium. Moscow, 1985, pp 49–51
27. Rabkin JK, Matevosov AL, Shechter YI: RED of subclavian artery. *Thorac Surg* 1988;2:76–78

Part 6. Gianturco Stents in the Venous System

—Charitha C. Fernando, B.H.B., MB.ChB., Josef Rösch, M.D., David W. Hunter, M.D., Joseph W. Yedlicka, Jr., M.D., Wilfrido R. Castañeda–Zúñiga, M.D., M.Sc., and Kurt Amplatz, M.D.

INTRODUCTION

Venous stenoses are often resistant to dilatation by angioplasty due to extensive fibrosis or extrinsic compression. Expandable stainless-steel wire stents designed by Gianturco have been successfully placed as endoprostheses in the biliary tree,[1] tracheobronchial tree,[2] and the venous system.[3–12] The stents are cylindrical wire structures which range in diameter from 0.05 to 3.5cm. Made of stainless-steel wire, bent in a zig-zag fashion, they are introduced in compressed form through a small diameter (8–14Fr) sheath. On release, they expand to dilate the narrowed vascular lumen.

STENT CONSTRUCTION

The stents are made in various diameters and lengths (Cook, Inc., Bloomington, IN); 0.025–0.03cm diameter wire is used to manufacture stents 1 to 1.5cm long, and wire 0.036–0.041cm in diameter is used for stents from 1.5 to 2.5cm in diameter. Stents 3cm in diameter are made of 0.046cm wire, and those 4cm in diameter are made of 0.05cm wire.[10]

The expansile force exerted by the stent increases with a larger number of legs in the stent, a greater angle of the leg bends, and with an increased diameter of the wire used.

The force decreases with the increased length of the stent.[10]

Several modifications of the original design have been made.[10] The bends of the wire legs may be soldered to form eyes which are then connected by surgical suture (Fig. 7.6.1). The suture assists in maintaining even expansion of the stent when released. A wire skirt can be added to one or both ends of the stent (Fig. 7.6.2). This reduces the tendency of the stent to migrate forward when released. If a single skirt is used, this should be placed at the distal portion of the stent which is released first.[10]

Small hooks and spikes orientated in the direction of stent introduction also assists in stabilizing the stent.[6]

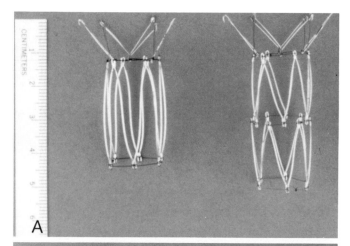

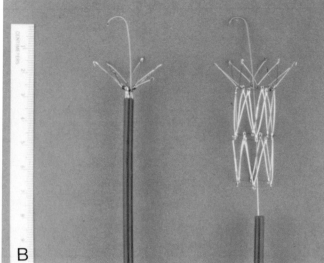

Figure 7.6.2. **A.** Gianturco–Rösch stent. A wire skirt was added to the ends of the stent. **B.** Gianturco–Rösch stent as it exits from the introducer sheath.

Figure 7.6.1. Gianturco–Rösch stent. The bends of the wire legs have been soldered to form eyes which are then connected by surgical suture.

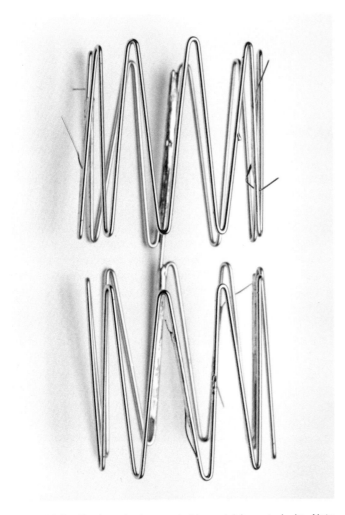

Figure 7.6.3. Tandem stent connected by a stainless-steel wire. Note spikes added to prevent slippage of the stent.

As the expansile force of a single stent is reduced with increasing length, when long lesions are treated, two or more stents can be combined. The two components of the "Tandem" stent may be connected by a monofilament suture or by a stainless steel wire (Fig. 7.6.3).[11] This configuration reduces stent slippage, enables a greater expansile force to be exerted, and also allows for flexibility.

TECHNIQUE

The venous access site should be chosen to minimize potential thrombus formation at the puncture site due to a more proximal residual stenosis that might persist after stenting or hemorrhagic potential when the access site is in very close proximity to the stenosed vascular segment. Therefore, for iliac or common femoral venous stenosis, the right internal jugular vein approach is preferred. This approach is also suitable for stenting the superior or inferior vena cava. Postprocedural thrombosis of the internal jugular vein is usually of no clinical consequence. The stiff Teflon sheath used for stent delivery is difficult to use across the bifurcation of the inferior vena cava. Preprocedural duplex Doppler ultrasound is useful to verify patency of the access site.

The stenosis is usually first dilated with an angioplasty balloon catheter. A 9–14Fr sheath, depending on the diameter of the stent to be placed, is advanced to the lesion. A stent 40–50% larger than the diameter of the adjacent normal vein is chosen. The stent is compressed and placed within the sheath with a wire passing through its lumen. The stent is pushed forward by a blunt thick wall pushing catheter to the distal end of the sheath, which is placed at the level of the venous stenosis.

The pusher is then held in place while the introducing sheath is slowly withdrawn, releasing the stent and allowing its expansion. A little modification of the stent position is possible when the stent is only partially extruded from the sheath; however, once completely released, it is not possible to alter the stent position.

Ideally, the mid-portion of the stent should be placed at the level of the mid-portion of the stenosis. Upper and lower skirts should be lodged in the normal vessel, above and below the stenosis. If several stents are to be placed, the most distal stent should be placed first with a 20–30% overlap between stents. The Gianturco stent will continue to expand to its maximum diameter over time[9]; however, they may also be balloon dilated once in position, although care must be taken not to dislodge the stent.[11]

Movement of the stent away from the center of the stenosis is a problem reported by many authors.[6,8,10,11] This occurs when the stent is squeezed into an area of greater luminal diameter by a stenosis (akin to squeezing a melon seed). Slippage requires the placement of further stents and prolongs the procedure time. Slippage can be reduced by careful selection of stent length and diameter, and the use of Tandem stents, skirts, and barbs.[10]

We routinely use heparin during the procedure and chronically anticoagulate the patients with oral Coumadin, if at all possible. Antibiotics have not proved necessary.[11]

HISTOLOGY

Animal and human studies have shown that in 4–12 weeks the stent is incorporated into the venous wall. A neointima covers the stent. The hooks of the skirt become lodged in the wall with areas of fibrosis and thickening at these sites. Side branches are not occluded.[3,8,10]

GIANTURCO STENTS IN THE SUPERIOR VENA CAVA

Superior vena cava syndrome secondary to lung carcinoma extending to the mediastinum is most often treated by radiation therapy. There is, however, a recurrence rate of 10–19%.[13] Superior vena caval compression in these patients with cancer can be caused by tumor recurrence, postradiation fibrosis, and superimposed thrombosis. Two patients with carcinoma of the lung and superior vena caval syndrome with recurrence after radiation therapy were successfully treated by Rösch et al.[7] In one patient, a 1.8cm diameter, 2cm long double-bodied stent with a single skirt which had three hooks was placed in the superior vena cava. At six-month follow-up, this patient was asymptomatic, and venography at two months showed satisfactory stent expansion and venous flow (Fig. 7.6.4). Because of the strength of the stent, initial incomplete expansion (Fig. 7.6.5A,B) might be followed by full expansion over time (Fig. 7.6.5C).

Charnsangavej et al.[6] placed four barbless stents, each 3cm in diameter and 3cm long, in the right innominate vein and superior vena cava of a patient with superior vena caval syndrome due to carcinoma of the trachea. Although the patient's symptoms were relieved, she died three weeks later from sepsis due to myelosuppression secondary to chemotherapy.

Putnam et al.[9] treated one patient with a superior vena caval thrombosis and stenosis with urokinase followed by the placement of two modified Gianturco stents. The 1.5cm diameter, 1.5cm stents with a single skirt were used. The initial stent slipped, and a third, 4cm-long, 1.5cm-diameter stent, also with the skirt, was placed across the stenosis. This stent was satisfactory in position and the patient remained asymptomatic at two months. Urokinase was also used to treat thrombosis of the superior vena cava in a patient with lung carcinoma treated by the same group. They placed a single, double-bodied stent with a skirt at one extremity within the superior vena cava in good position and the patient's symptoms abated at 24 hours, and he remained free of symptoms at one month.

Although balloon dilatation of the superior vena cava prior to stent placement has been performed without complication, we advise caution, as an acute exacerbation of the superior vena caval syndrome can occur. In one instance, this led to seizure activity which necessitated the termination of the procedure.[11] Another patient in whom we had placed four Gianturco venous stents at the superior vena cava developed seizure activity unrelated to balloon dilatation and subsequently developed electromechanical dissociation and could not be resuscitated. The procedure had been protracted due to stent slippage.

INFERIOR VENA CAVAL GIANTURCO STENTS

Charnsangavej et al.[6] used Gianturco stents to treat an inferior vena caval stenosis due to a retroperitoneal leiomyosarcoma; three, 3cm-long stents were placed across the

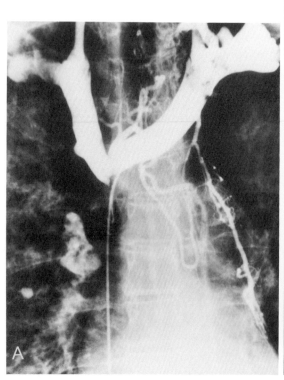
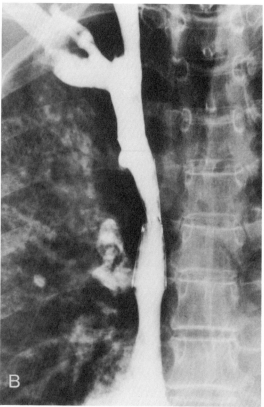

Figure 7.6.4. Patient with lung carcinoma and superior vena caval syndrome. **A.** Complete occlusion of superior vena cava. A catheter has been passed across the obstruction. Thrombus is seen in the subclavian vein.

B. Post-stenting cavogram shows a widely patent SVC, although there is incomplete expansion.

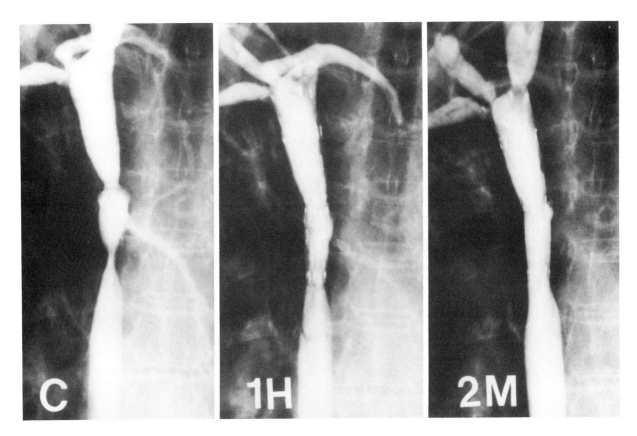

Figure 7.6.5. Postradiation fibrosis in patient with history of lung carcinoma presenting with SVC syndrome. **Left.** Two areas of high-grade stenosis of the SVC. **Middle.** Post-stenting cavogram shows a widely patent SVC. **Right.** Two-month follow-up shows further expansion of the stent.

stenosis. One stent migrated to the right ventricle. A bird's nest filter was therefore placed in the inferior vena cava to prevent migration of the other stents, and additional stents of larger diameter (3cm) were placed across the stenosis. The patient's leg edema resolved; she had no symptoms or signs attributable to the stent in the right ventricle. She died five months later with progression of the retroperitoneal tumor. At autopsy, the inferior vena cava, although encased in tumor, was patent with no clot formation within the stents.[6]

These authors reported their experience in stenting the inferior vena cava of seven dogs, who had an inferior vena caval stenosis created by percutaneous alcohol injection.[6] Four dogs were successfully stented, and at four months, when sacrificed, there was no clot formation at the stent, the luminal diameter was maintained, and side branches were patent.

Slippage occurred in two of seven dogs. In one, the proximal portion of the stent remained in the nonstenotic portion of the inferior vena cava, and the distal portion of the stent was incompletely expanded within the region of stenosis. Another dog had an occluded inferior cava prior to attempted stent placement. This stent could not restore the vena caval lumen and perforated the inferior vena cava with a resulting retroperitoneal abscess.

Eight of eight skirted stents placed in the inferior vena

cava of swine by Uchida et al.[10] were shown to be patent at venography at 4–12 weeks. Rösch has successfully stented the inferior vena cava in a patient with chronic occlusion following radiation (Fig. 7.6.6).

We have successfully placed a 3mm-diameter Gianturco stent at a stenotic proximal inferior vena caval anastomosis in a patient with a liver transplant. Prior urokinase was used to lyse extensive thrombosis of the inferior vena cava. Balloon dilatation had improved the stenosis, but as a 70% stenosis remained following dilatation, the stent was placed. Even though a good expansion was seen on the anteposterior projection (Fig. 7.6.7A) compression of the stent by the large, edematous lumen was seen in the lateral projection (Fig. 7.6.7B). Furui described the use of the stent in nine patients with caval obstruction, in six due to tumor compression and in three with Budd–Chiari syndrome.[12]

PELVIC VENOUS STENOSIS TREATED WITH GIANTURCO STENTS

We have treated 11 pelvic venous stenoses in 10 patients with 25 venous stents (Fig. 7.6.8). Five patients had pelvic malignancies, and three patients were treated for benign disease.

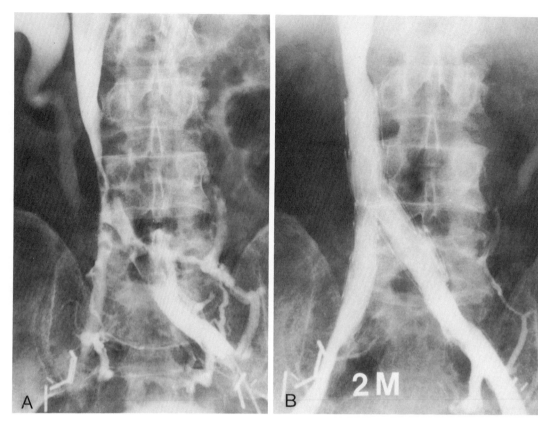

Figure 7.6.6. Patient with an occluded inferior vena cava due to post-radiation fibrosis. **A.** Inferior vena cavogram shows high-grade stenosis of the low inferior vena cava with thrombus. **B.** Post-dilatation and stenting cavography shows a widely patent inferior vena cava and common iliac veins.

The stents were manufactured in our laboratory after the design by Gianturco.[3] Twelve stents were single-bodied, 2cm in diameter and 2.5cm long. Six stents were triple Tandems with three bodies connected by a rod. Four double Tandem stents were used.

Slippage was principally a problem of single-bodied stents with 8 of 12 of these slipping. Only two of seven Tandem stents slipped. All patients had an improvement of symptoms shortly following stent placement.

Four patients developed thrombus at the stent. In two patients, this occurred one month following withdrawal of Coumadin therapy due to elevated liver function tests. In one patient, the ipsilateral common femoral vein was used to insert pelvic venous stents. Complete dilatation was not possible. This patient developed leg edema and thrombus at the stent 10 days following the procedure. The final failure occurred in a patient with multiple vein grafts for venous insufficiency. Although a 7.5cm-long stenosis was stented following balloon dilatation, a residual stenosis was noted. This patient developed nonocclusive thrombus at the stent site.

The remaining four patients have continued relief from symptoms, with follow-up ranging from 6 weeks to 14 months.[11]

A GIANTURCO STENT IN THE PORTAL VEIN

One single bodied Gianturco venous stent and one double Tandem stent were placed in a portal venous stenosis (Fig. 7.6.9). The stenosis was at the site of portal venous anastomosis in a patient with a liver transplant. Four single-bodied Gianturco stents had previously been used to treat a stenosis at the common bile duct.

Portal venography at six weeks demonstrated stent patency with a good luminal diameter.

GIANTURCO STENTS IN PERCUTANEOUS PORTOCAVAL ANASTOMOSIS

Portocaval anastomosis may be established percutaneously by passing a catheter from the inferior vena cava or hepatic venous radicles through the hepatic parenchyma to a portal venous radicle.

Rösch et al.[8] have used Gianturco stents to maintain patency in these channels. If well positioned, patency is maintained for four to six weeks; however, intimal proliferation and ingrowth of hepatic parenchyma decreases the luminal diameter and eventually results in occlusion.

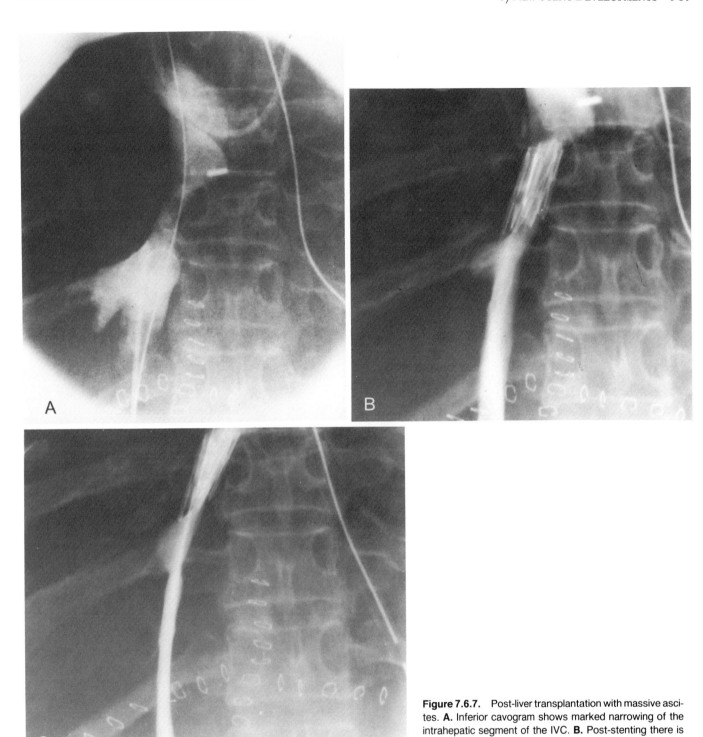

Figure 7.6.7. Post-liver transplantation with massive ascites. **A.** Inferior cavogram shows marked narrowing of the intrahepatic segment of the IVC. **B.** Post-stenting there is increased diameter of the IVC. **C.** Oblique radiograph shows anteroposterior compression of the IVC.

SUMMARY

Gianturco–Rösch stents offer great promise for treatment of resistant venous stenosis and stenosis due to extrinsic compression. Slippage has been a problem with the unmodified stent, but should be reduced with careful selection of appropriate stent characteristics and use of the recent modifications.[10] Clinical experience to date has shown symptomatic improvement in treating stenosis of the superior and inferior vena cava and pelvic veins in a small number of patients. The results of further clinical studies are awaited before widespread use can be advocated.

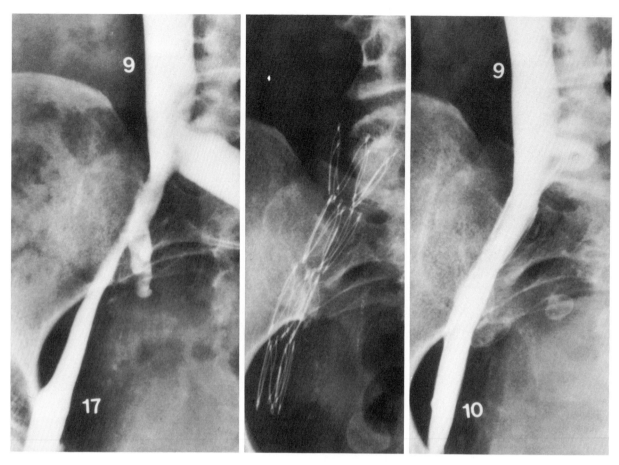

Figure 7.6.8. Postradiation fibrosis with right lower extremity edema. **Left.** Iliac venogram. Long, severe narrowing of the right iliac vein. **Middle.** Post-stenting film shows a widely expanded stent. **Right.** Iliac venogram shows almost complete restoration of the venous lumen.

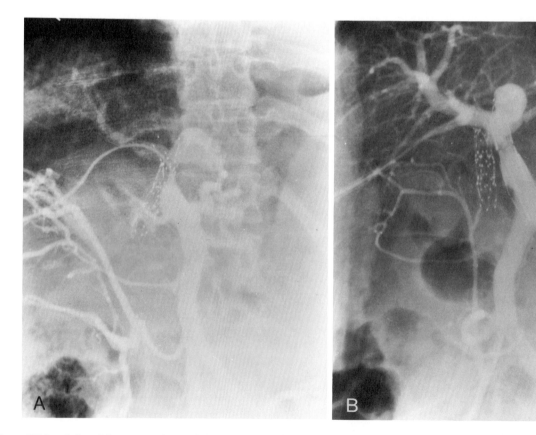

Figure 7.6.9. **A.** A portal venogram demonstrates an anastomotic portal vein stenosis. Four Gianturco stents are seen within the common bile duct. **B.** Following stent placement in the portal vein, there is good antegrade flow and an adequate luminal diameter is maintained.

References

1. Coons HG: Self-expanding stainless-steel biliary stents. *Radiology* 1989;170:979–983
2. Wallace MJ, Charnsangavej C, Ogawa K, Carrasco H, Wright KC, McKenna R, McMurtrey M, Gianturco C: Tracheobronchial tree: expandable metallic stents used in experimental and clinical applications. Work in progress. *Radiology* 1986;158:309–312
3. Wright KC, Wallace S, Charnsangavej C, Carrasco CH, Gianturco C: Percutaneous endovascular stents: an experimental evaluation. *Radiology* 1985;156:69–72
4. Charnsangavej C, Wallace S, Wright KC, Carrasco CH, Gianturco C: Endovascular stent for use in aortic dissection: an in vitro experiment. *Radiology* 1985;157:323–324
5. Rollins N, Wright KC, Charnsangavej C, Wallace S, Gianturco C: Self-expanding metallic stents: preliminary evaluation in an atherosclerotic model. *Radiology* 1987;163:739–742
6. Charnsangavej C, Carrasco CH, Wallace S, Wright KC, Ogawa K, Richli W, Gianturco C: Stenosis of the vena cava: preliminary assessment of treatment with expandable metallic stents. *Radiology* 1986;161:295–298
7. Rösch J, Bedell JE, Putnam J, Antonovic R, Uchida B: Gianturco expandable wire stents in the treatment of superior vena cava syndrome recurring after maximum-tolerance radiation. *Cancer* 1987;60:1243–1246
8. Rösch J, Uchida BT, Putnam JS, Buschman RW, Law RD, Hershey AL: Experimental intrahepatic portacaval anastomosis: use of expandable Gianturco stents. *Radiology* 1987;162:481–485
9. Putnam JS, Uchida BT, Antonovic R, Rösch J: Superior vena cava syndrome associated with massive thrombosis: treatment with expandable wire stents. *Radiology* 1988;167:727–728
10. Uchida BT, Putnam JS, Rösch J: Modification of Gianturco expandable wire stents. Technical Note. *AJR* 1988;150:1185–1187
11. Moradian GP, Hunter DW, Castañeda F, Castañeda–Zúñiga WR, Amplatz K: Clinical experience with the placement of Gianturco vascular stents in the venous system. Presented to the Radiological Society of North America. November, 1989
12. Furui S, Sawada S, Irie T, Makita K, Yamauchi T, Kusano S, Ibukuro K, Nakamura H, Takenaka E: Hepatic inferior vena cava obstruction: treatment of two types with Gianturco expandable metallic stents. *Radiology* 1990;176:665–670
13. Perez CA, Presant CA, Van Amburg AL: Management of superior vena cava syndrome. *Semin Oncol* 1978;5:123–134

Part 7. The Maass Double-helix Stent

—Christoph L. Zollikofer, M.D., Dierk Maass, M.D., and Francesco Antonucci, M.D.

In 1980, Maass developed a transluminal vascular endoprosthesis. The initial design consisted of spiral surgical steel alloy coils made from wire (0.3–0.5mm diameter).[1,2] Because of problems with migration and/or thrombosis,[2] a double-helix spiral stent made from metal bands of a heat-treated alloy (0.10–0.15mm thick and 1.5mm wide, with diameters from 12 to 35mm) was developed[2,3] (Fig. 7.7.1). Under tension, these spirals had a smaller tilting momentum and therefore allowed higher expansion ratios (relationship between relaxed and minimal diameter). A special introducer allowed the insertion, expansion, tightening, and release of the spirals under fluoroscopy via an arteriotomy or venotomy (Fig. 7.7.2). With the 7mm introducer, stents of 12–35mm diameter could be placed. For smaller vessels, stents of 12–15mm diameter mounted on a 4mm introducer were available. The pressure exerted by the expanding spirals on the vascular wall could be planned in advance or calculated in retrospect.[3] Light microscopy and scanning electron microscopy of the aorta and vena cava of dogs and calves showed that intimal proliferation started within the first postoperative days. After 2–3 weeks, the metal was almost completely covered by neointima. This process was completed after approximately six weeks and no further changes were visible (Fig. 7.7.3). A combination of intimal proliferation and microthrombi was found more frequently in the veins. These thrombi became organized and smooth. Further experiments showed that expansion pressures of 1000mm Hg in the aorta and 300mm Hg in the vena cava were tolerated without any damage to the vessel wall. Side branches of the aorta or the vena cava remained patent even when they were crossed by several spiral coils (Fig. 7.7.4).

CLINICAL APPLICATIONS

Because this prosthesis had been designed for larger vessels such as the aorta or the vena cava, the new technique was first used intraoperatively via a surgical cutdown. Double-helix Maass spirals have been used clinically since 1982. In two patients with dissecting aneurysms of the thoracic aorta, such stents were implanted into the descending aorta intraoperatively (Fig. 7.7.5). With further improvements of instrumentation, this technique may offer the unique feature of treating dissecting aneurysms nonsurgically as these two preliminary intraoperative experiences have shown.

More than 20 patients received the Maass spiral to relieve extrinsic compression of the inferior vena cava, at the time of surgical treatment for Budd–Chiari syndrome (Fig. 7.7.6) with the so-called Senning operation.[4,5] In spite of the operative recanalization of the hepatic veins, the massively hypertrophied caudate lobe of the liver frequently compresses the vena cava postoperatively causing inferior vena caval obstruction. Using the Maass spiral, this problem can be solved.[5,6]

Maass stents have been implanted in patients with

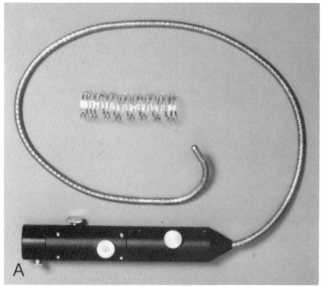

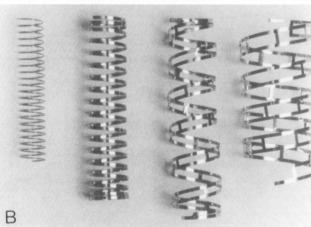

Figure 7.7.1. **A.** Introducing instrument with released double-helix spiral. The instrument is highly flexible with a bidirectional steering tip. Controls located at the handle release the spiral at its target site by retorsion. **B.** Different types of implanted spiral springs. (Reproduced with permission from Maass D, Zollikofer CL, Largiader F, et al: Radiological followup of transluminally inserted vascular endoprostheses: an experimental study using expanding spirals. *Radiology* 1984;152:659–663.)

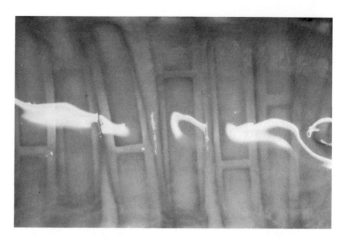

Figure 7.7.3. Specimen of dog aorta 6 weeks following stent implantation. The entire endoprosthesis is covered by a smooth, regular neointima.

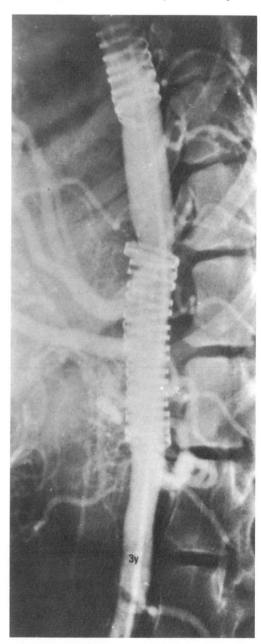

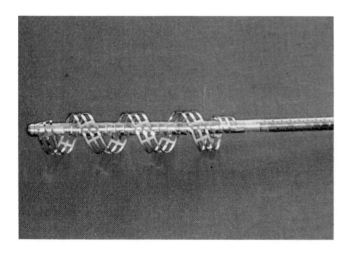

Figure 7.7.2. Tip of instrument with partially released endoprosthesis.

Figure 7.7.4. Two double-helix spirals in a canine aorta 3 years after implantation. There are no signs of obstruction of the celiac trunk and superior mesenteric artery in spite of the stent in the abdominal aorta.

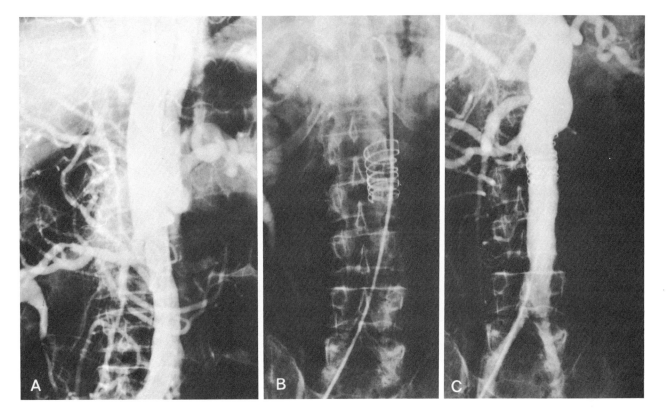

Figure 7.7.5. A 63-year-old patient with dissecting aneurysm Type B. **A.** Dissection extends to the abdominal aorta with occlusion of the left renal artery. **B.** The patient was operated on and a Dacron graft of the lower thoracic and upper abdominal aorta was used. To prevent further dissec- tion a double-helix endoprosthesis was implanted with additional external banding. **C.** Control angiogram 18 months later shows open lumen of the aorta with mild intimal hyperplasia.

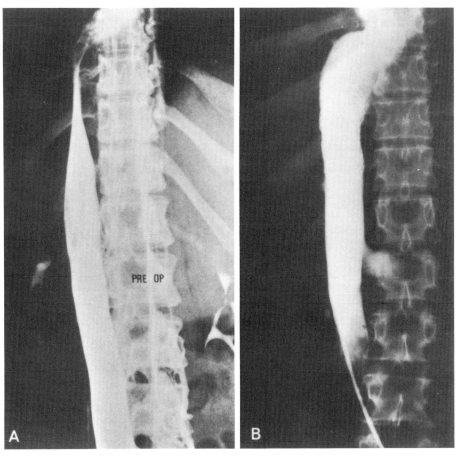

Figure 7.7.6. Patient with Budd–Chiari syndrome. **A.** Preoperative cavogram demonstrates compression of intrahepatic portion of vena cava. **B.** Cavogram of inferior vena cava 7 days after implantation of double-helix spiral shows widely patent lumen.

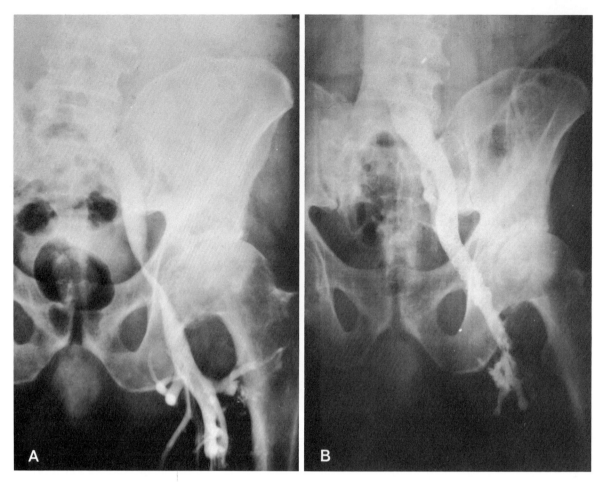

Figure 7.7.7. Patient with post-thrombotic stenosis of the external iliac vein. **A.** Venogram shows tight stenosis. **B.** Post-stenting there is a widely patent lumen.

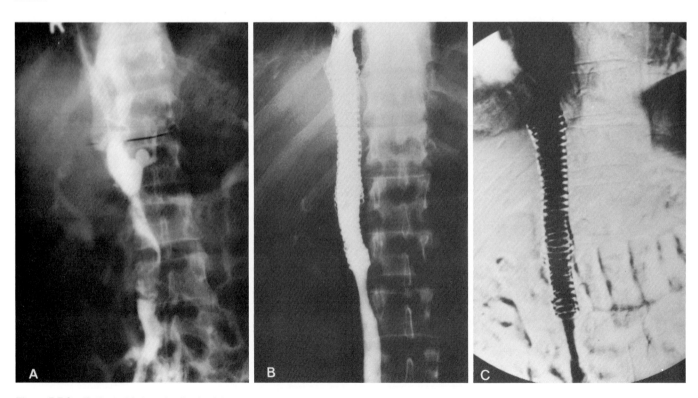

Figure 7.7.8. Patient with thrombosis of pelvic vein and the inferior vena cava. **A.** Phlebography shows clots in the infrarenal vena cava, stenosis of the suprarenal cava, and drainage via collaterals. **B.** There is free flow after surgical thrombectomy and two Maass spirals. **C.** Follow-up after three months shows continued patency.

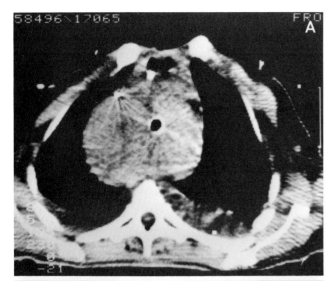

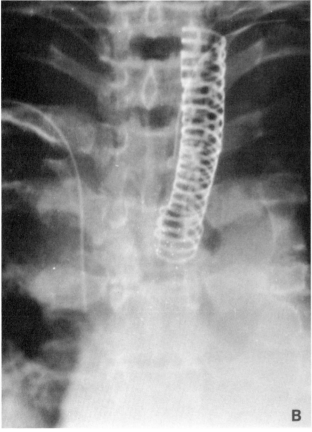

Figure 7.7.9. A 40-year-old patient with massive compression of the trachea secondary to carcinoma of the thyroid. **A.** Computed tomogram shows mediastinal tumor mass causing circular compression of the trachea. **B.** Maass spiral in the trachea with normal trachea lumen.

obstruction of the pelvic veins (Fig. 7.7.7), with excellent results in follow-up of up to 34 months.[7,8] Mechanical obstacles that cause inferior vena caval or iliofemoral thrombosis present problems that cannot be solved by thrombectomy and balloon angioplasty or other conventional means (Fig. 7.7.8). Percutaneous transluminal

angioplasty alone often fails because of the elastic recoil of the stenotic lesion. Even after surgery, success is only 50–80%[9–11] and thrombolytic treatment may not solve the problem either.[12,13] Treatment of an underlying lesion such as a venous spur, fibrotic scarring, congenital stenosis, or external tumor compression is essential but may involve major surgery or may be contraindicated in patients with malignant disease. Therefore, endoluminal stents such as the Maass stent are a promising alternative to manage these patients while avoiding major surgery. However, further improvements are necessary, particularly miniaturization of the introducing instrument for easy and safe percutaneous use. Other applications of the stent outside of the vascular system include the tracheobronchial tree (Fig. 7.7.9) and gastrointestinal tract strictures.

References

1. Maass D, Kropf L, Egloff L, Demierre D, Turina M, Senning A: Transluminal implantation of intravascular "double helix" spiral prostheses: technical and biological considerations. *ESAO Proc* 1982;9:252–256
2. Maass D, Demierre D, Deaton D, Largiader F, Senning A: Transluminal implantation of self-adjusting expandable prostheses: principles, techniques and results. *Progr Artif* 1983;15:979–987
3. Maass D, Zollikofer CL, Largiader F, Senning A: Radiological follow-up of transluminally inserted vascular endoprostheses: an experimental study using expanding spirals. *Radiology* 1984;152:659–663
4. Senning A: The cardiovascular surgeon and the liver. *J Thorac Cardiovasc Surg* 1987;93:1–10
5. Zollikofer CL: Interventionelle Behandlungsmoglichkeiten beim Budd-Chiari-Syndrom, in Friedmann G, Steinbrich W, Gross-Fengels W (eds): *Angiplastie, Embolisation, Punktion, Drainagen.* Konstanz, Schnetztor Verlag, 1989, pp 129–137
6. Ransky G, Ernest C, Jenni R, Zollikofer C et al: Treatment of Budd–Chiari syndrome by dorsocranial liver resection and direct hepatoatrial anastomosis. *J Hepatol* 1986;2:101–112
7. Jokob H, Maass D, Schmiedt W, Schild H, Oelert H: Treatment of major venous obstruction with expandable endoluminal spiral prosthesis. *J Cardiovasc Surg* 1989;30:112–117
8. Jakob H, Oelert H, Schmiedt W, Teusch P, Iversen S, Hake U, Schild H, Maass D: Initial clinical experience with an endoluminal spiral prosthesis. *Tex Heart Instit J* 1989;16:87–94
9. Hutschenreiter S, Vollmar J, Loeprecht H, Abendschein A, Rodl W: Rekonstruktive Eingriffe am Venensystem: Spätergebnisse unter kritischer Bewertung funktioneller und gefassmorphologischer Kriterien. *Chirurg* 1979;50:555–563
10. Stiegler H, Sunder-Plassman J, Becker HM: Indications and technics in pelvic and leg vein thromboses. *Chirurg* 1985;56:73–80
11. Lindhagen J, Hagland M, Harland U, Holm J, Shersten T: Iliofemoral venous thrombectomy. *J Cardiovasc Surg* 1978;19:319–327
12. Theiss W, Schlund J, Kriesmann A, Lutilsky L, Sauer E, Wirtzfeld A: Die behandlung tiefer Venenthrombosen mit Urokinase. *Klin Wochenschr* 1980;58:521–526
13. Van de Loo JCW, Kriesmann A, Trubestein G et al: Controlled multicenter pilot study of urokinase-heparin and streptokinase in deep vein thrombosis. *Thromb Haemostas* 1983;50:660–667

Part 8. Medtronic–Wiktor Stent

—Wilfrido R. Castañeda–Zúñiga, M.D., M.Sc., and S. Murthy Tadavarthy, M.D.

A sinusoidal-shaped, stainless-steel 0.279mm wire wound into an open helix (Fig. 7.8.1) makes this stent highly flexible and adaptable to vascular segments of differing diameters and lengths. Once the desired length of the stent is determined by measuring directly on the arteriogram, the required length is cut from a long stent piece and is manually crimped onto a low profile Olbert balloon (Meadox–Surgimed, Inc., Oakland, NJ). If the length of stent required is longer than the balloon, the extra portion is left lying loosely over the balloon-catheter shaft (Fig. 7.8.1). For placement, the balloon-stent assembly is advanced through a 14Fr introducer sheath into the artery to the desired location. The balloon is inflated to expand the stent, which is then fixed to the wall (Fig. 7.8.2). To help obtain fixation, the stent is expanded to a diameter slightly larger than the vessel diameter. The balloon is then deflated, and further dilatation of the trailing stent is subsequently undertaken, until the entire length of the stent has been expanded. Because of its sinusoidal configuration, the stent can be expanded to a slightly larger diameter than that of the vessel.[1] Aspirin and dipyridamole are given to block platelet function. On follow-up examination, no incidence of stent migration, perforation, thrombosis, or branch occlusion was found. Endothelialization of the stent occurred, except at side-branch orifices. Application of this stent to treat experimental dissection of the aorta in animals proved to be effective.[1] It is hypothesized by the authors that application of this stent to the management of aortic dissection is possible, and that with essentially the entire aorta stented, redissection at a new site distal to the original point of entry and aneurysmal expansion would be

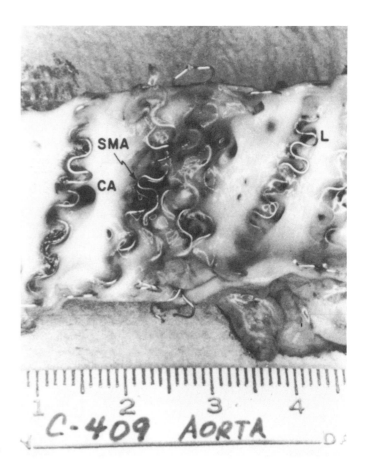

Figure 7.8.2. Aortic specimen six weeks post-stenting. Note endothelialization with preservation of side branches. *CA* = celiac axis; *SMA* = superior mesenteric artery; *L* = lumbar artery.

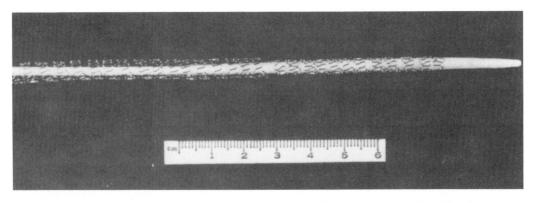

Figure 7.8.1. Stent crimped tightly over balloon *(right)*. Trailing portion lies relatively loose on shaft of balloon catheter *(left)*. (Reproduced with permission from Trent MS, Parsonet V, Schoenfeld R, et al: A balloon expandable intravascular stent for obliterating experimental aortic dissection. *J Vasc Surg* 1990;11:707–717.)

prevented.[1] Other potential applications include traumatic tears of the thoracic aorta, intimal dissection post-PTA or PTCA, prevention of embolization from ulcerated atheromatous plaques, and venous stenosis.[1] Because of the low radiopacity of the original Wiktor stent, the stainless-steel was replaced by tantalum, without an apparent effect on thrombogenicity.[2–4] The ability of the stent to be implanted in small, tortuous, continuously moving vessels has been demonstrated in animals. Stents were implanted in 17 canine coronary arteries; all stents remained patent up to six months.[2] Application to human coronary arteries has been recently reported.[3,4] In Bertrand's experience, delivery of the stent was possible in 24 of 25 attempts (96%). In the first stage of the study, four stents thrombosed, and the patients were treated with thrombolytics and/or redilatation, resulting in a limited myocardial infarction.[3] In the next seven patients, the antiplatelet and anticoagulation regimens (aspirin, dextran, heparin) were increased and no thrombotic events occurred. Follow-up by noninvasive means up to three months revealed no evidence of recurrent symptoms.[3] In a study to evaluate the morphologic changes resulting from placement of the stent in the coronary arteries, Serruys reported that implantation of the stent results in a 6-fold increase in the minimal cross-sectional area, associated with a significant reduction in length, inflow, and outflow angle of the stenosis. The stent was found to be very effective in normalizing the flow resistance of severely stenotic lesions, while respecting the natural curvature of the stenosis.[4]

References

1. Trent MS, Parsonnet V, Shoenfeld R, Brener BJ, Eisenbud DE, Novick AS, Campbell AY, Ferrara–Ryan M, Villanueva A: A balloon-expandable intravascular stent for obliterating experimental aortic dissection. *J Vasc Surg* 1990;11:707–717
2. White CJ, Ramee SR, Mesa JE, Collins TJ, Murgo JP, Wiktor D, Chokshi S: Angiographic patency of a balloon expandable tantalum coil stent in coronary and renal arteries of dogs. *Circulation* 1990;82(suppl III):III–655
3. Bertrand M, Kober G, Scheerder Y, Uebis R, Wiegand V: Initial multi-center human clinical experience with the Medtronic–Wiktor coronary stent. *Circulation* 1990;82(suppl III):III–2146
4. Serruys PW, Kober BG, De Scheerder IK, Uebis R, Wiegand V: Morphological change of coronary stenosis stented with the Medtronic–Wiktor stent: initial results from the core lab. *Circulation* 1990;82(suppl III):III–658

Part 9. Gianturco–Roubin Balloon Expandable Stent

—Wilfrido R. Castañeda-Zúñiga, M.D., M.Sc., and S. Murthy Tadavarthy, M.D.

A flexible, radiopaque balloon expandable stent for small vessels was described by Duprat et al. in 1987.[1] The stent was initially made of 0.006-inch stainless-steel wire, wrapped individually, with bends adopting a segmental U and inverted U configuration every 360° (Fig. 7.9.1). The stents are wrapped tightly over a collapsed angioplasty balloon (25mm long and 2.5mm inflated diameter). The angioplasty balloon-stent assembly is 2mm in diameter when fully expanded. The stent's dimensions are 15mm in length and 2.5mm in diameter. The stents are easily expanded to their original maximum diameter and do not show any change in diameter in follow-up angiography (Fig. 7.9.2). A 20–25% luminal narrowing was observed in all stents at eight weeks' follow-up. No vessel occlusion or migration occurred. Side branches bridged by the stent remained patent.

Endothelialization of the stent was found. The longitudinal flexibility of the stent makes this design ideal for implantation onto small, continuously moving vessels with multiple curves, such as the coronary arteries.[1] The stent has since been used in human coronary arteries.[2] The stent was successfully implanted in 42 patients. Indications for stenting were acute closure in 9 patients (21%) and threatened acute closure in 33 (79%). At a mean follow-up of 4.6 months (range 1–7 months) by angiography, restenosis occurred in 14 of 32 patients (44%) (restenosis was defined as a stenosis of more than 50%) and in 8 of 24 (33%) of Coumadin-treated patients having a single stent in their native arteries. Nine of the patients had a successful repeat percutaneous transluminal coronary angioplasty (PTCA), four had a coronary artery bypass graft and four were treated medically. Roubin concluded that coronary artery stenting for actual or threatened acute closure after PTCA is associated with an incidence of restenosis not dissimilar from that found in other PTCA subsets.[2]

References

1. Duprat G Jr, Wright KC, Charnsangavej C, Wallace S, Gianturco C: Flexible balloon-expanded stent for small vessels. *Radiology* 1987;162:276–278
2. Roubin GS, Hearn JA, Carlin SF, Lembo NJ, Douglas JS Jr, King SB III: Angiographic and clinical follow-up in patients receiving a balloon expandable, stainless-steel stent (Cook, Inc) for prevention or treatment of acute closure after PTCA. *Circulation* 1990;82(suppl III):III–191

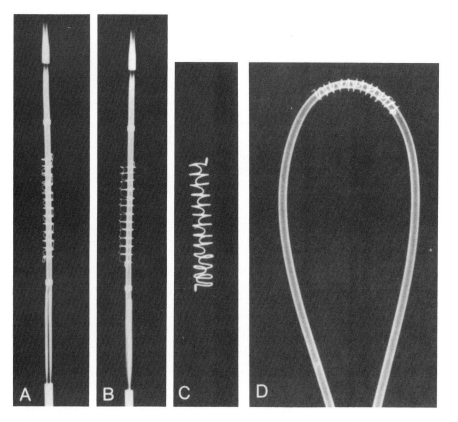

Figure 7.9.1. **A.** Gianturco–Roubin stent mounted on a balloon in the collapsed state. **B.** Stent fully expanded after balloon inflation. **C.** Expanded stent. **D.** Flexibility of the stent is shown inside the polyethylene catheter. (Reproduced with permission from Duprat G Jr, Wright KC, Charnsangavej C, et al: Flexible balloon expanded stent for small vessels. Radiology 1987;162:276–278.)

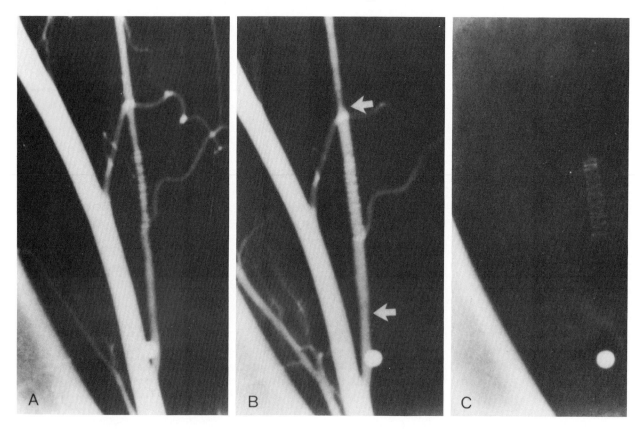

Figure 7.9.2. **A.** Plain film showing a fully expanded stent. **B.** Widely patent lumen at site of stent implant in the superficial femoral artery. *Arrows* point to the dilated arterial segment at the site of balloon inflation. **C.** Six weeks' follow-up arteriogram shows a 25% luminal narrowing within the stent. (Reproduced with permission from Duprat G Jr, Wright KC, Charnsangavej C, et al: Flexible balloon expanded stent for small vessels. *Radiology* 1987;162:276–278.)

Part 10. Cordis Balloon Expandable Stent

—Wilfrido R. Castañeda–Zúñiga, M.D., M.Sc., and S. Murthy Tadavarthy, M.D.

A highly flexible, radiopaque tantalum balloon expandable stent has been tried in laboratory animals. Deployment was successful in 73 of 79 attempts (92%). Follow-up of up to one year revealed all stents to be patent. No significant stenosis within or at the end of the stents was reported and preservation of side branches crossed by the stent was found.[1]

Reference

1. Gammon RS, Chapman GD, Bauman RP, Muhlestein JB, Overman AB, Desper JS, MacGregor DC, deCoriolis PE, Stack RS: The Cordis balloon-expandable stent: implantation features and long-term follow-up in an animal model. *Circulation* 1990;82(suppl III):III–541

FIBRINOLYTIC THERAPY

—Gary J. Becker, M.D., and Robert W. Holden, M.D.

The discovery of streptokinase (SK) by Tillett and Garner[1] and the elucidation of its interaction with the human fibrinolytic system by Sherry[2] have led to a wide variety of clinical applications. Fibrinolytic therapy has produced dramatic successes, dismal failures, and serious, even life-threatening, hemorrhage. A lack of predictive laboratory tests has made the hemorrhagic complications difficult to avoid. In this chapter, the authors provide the reader with insight into fibrinolysis: past, present, and future.

PATHOPHYSIOLOGY OF THROMBOSIS AND FIBRINOLYSIS

To understand fibrinolysis and thrombolysis, one must first grasp the core concepts in thrombosis. (The terms "fibrinolysis" and "thrombolysis" are almost interchangeable. When one uses thrombolytic therapy, one lyses the fibrin component of thrombi, not the cellular components. However, these terms are not completely interchangeable because of the difference between thrombus and blood clot. Blood clot may be formed in vitro, whereas thrombi are in vivo products of the coagulation cascade. Therefore, although one can produce fibrinolysis of an in vitro clot or an in vivo thrombus, one cannot produce thrombolysis of an in vitro clot.) Welch defined a thrombus as a solid plug formed in the living heart or blood vessels from constituents of blood.[3] Thrombosis is the process of thrombus generation. Venous and arterial thrombi have distinctive structures. Arterial (white) thrombi, which form in a higher flow circulation, are characterized by closely packed, aggregated platelets and a small amount of fibrin, whereas venous (red) thrombi consist primarily of a fibrin-red blood cell coagulum. Mixed thrombi—a white head with a red tail—are frequently found in stenotic arteries. The pathologic events leading to thrombosis are different in the arterial and venous circulations.

Arterial Thrombosis

Atheromatous roughening of the arterial endothelium can produce thrombosis, particularly where accompanying stenosis and altered blood flow are involved. Under such circumstances, platelets adhere, aggregate, and initiate thrombosis. Moncada and Vane,[4] Bunting et al.,[5] and others have shown the importance of prostaglandin endoperoxide metabolism to both the homeostatic condition of normal blood flow and under conditions of disease.

Prostaglandin endoperoxide metabolism occurs in both platelets and endothelial cells. In the latter, the endoperoxides (substrate) are converted by prostacyclin synthetase to prostacyclin (PGI_2), which is the most potent known inhibitor of platelet aggregation. It is also a disaggregator of extant platelet clumps and a potent vasodilator. Platelets utilize the same endoperoxides to synthesize thromboxane A_2 (TXA_2), which induces platelet aggregation[6-9] and constricts arterial smooth muscle.[10] This constriction may result from the opening of cellular calcium entry channels when TXA_2 binds to its receptor sites.[11] Obviously, vascular patency cannot be maintained when the TXA_2 mechanisms predominate. How can an injured vessel produce a hemostatic plug in its outer wall if PGI_2 synthesis predominates in this location? Interestingly, PGI_2 probably does not predominate under such circumstances. Not only does the vascular injury promote platelet aggregation and TXA_2-mediated events, but the ratios of proaggregatory and antiaggregatory elements are different in the various layers of the vessel wall.[12] That is, proaggregatory elements increase in concentration from the endothelium to the adventitia, whereas prostacyclin synthetase progressively decreases from the intima to the adventitia.

Although this balance is important in normal vessels, conditions are altered in the presence of atheroma. Atherosclerotic plaques contain lipid peroxides,[13] which are potent selective inhibitors of prostacyclin synthesis.[12,14] This factor alone could tip the balance in favor of TXA_2 and result in thrombosis. It has been shown in a few patients that plaques may be incapable of producing sufficient quantities of prostacyclin.[15] Differences between early and advanced plaque have not been demonstrated. Therefore, it would seem that even in early lesions, the normal protective mechanism of prostacyclin production is absent.

Venous Thrombosis

In the venous system, Virchow's triad of factors predisposing to thrombosis—changes in the vein wall, venous stasis (abnormally increased contact time of venous blood with the endothelium), and a hypercoagulable state[16]—has endured. Morphologic changes in the vessel wall are less important in venous thrombosis than they are in arterial thrombosis. We know this is true because most deep venous thromboses begin in the absence of a primary acute intimal lesion or inflammatory process.[17,18] Therefore, the term "deep venous thrombosis" (DVT) is preferable to "thrombophlebitis." Thrombus formation usually starts in the apex and vein wall of a valve pocket, but the thrombus is not attached to the valve cusp.[18,19] Growing out of the pocket and into the main channel, the thrombus produces turbulence, which increases fibrin formation and the entrapment of red blood cells. With increasing obstruction, stasis becomes nearly complete, and rapid and extensive proximal and retrograde thrombosis ensues. Edema, venous distention, pain, and tenderness result. The soleal veins of the calf are the most frequent sites of early venous thrombosis,[20,21] and stasis is the most important predisposing factor.[22]

What about the role of hypercoagulable states? In 1947, Astrup and Permin described the existence of a chemical agent in tissue which is capable of activating plasminogen.[23] Subsequently, it has been shown that human veins have a highly fibrinolytic endothelium, whereas arteries are low in fibrinolytic activity. Astrup later postulated that an imbalance between the fibrinolytic mechanism and the coagulation pathways may be causative in venous thrombosis.[24] It is now known that blood vessels are the main source of tissue plasminogen activator (tPA), and tissue culture studies have shown that plasminogen activator is synthesized and stored in endothelial cells.[25] It also appears that plasminogen activator is continuously released from normal endothelial cells into the bloodstream[26] and that, immunologically, vascular plasminogen activator is the same as tPA.[27,28] The absence of tPA in valve pockets[29] and its presence in the remainder of the venous endothelium may explain why thrombi originate in valve sinuses yet remain unattached to the vein wall as they propagate. There is evidence for fibrinolytic "shutdown" postoperatively,[30] in that a decrease in circulating tPA has been reported in patients with postoperative DVT. It is possible that this is related to a lack of activity, because exercise increases fibrinolytic activity by causing a release of tPA.[26] Other studies have revealed decreased plasminogen activator in the blood and venous walls of patients with recurrent DVT.

INTERRELATED HOMEOSTATIC MECHANISMS

Coagulation and Fibrin

Notwithstanding the obvious importance of the balances described above, they are not the sole mechanisms maintaining normal blood flow and the vascular response to injury or disease. The coagulation mechanism (clotting cascade), which involves the sequential activation of at least 13 different factors, is extremely important. Figure 8.1 is a simple representation of both the intrinsic and the extrinsic coagulation pathways. The extrinsic pathway is activated when tissue substances from outside the bloodstream, known as thromboplastin, are exposed to the bloodstream after vascular injury. The intrinsic pathway is activated when factor XII is converted to active form (XII$_a$). The latter process, which can be demonstrated in blood isolated from tissues (for example, in a test tube), also occurs in vivo. Excellent discussions of the complex interrelations between the coagulation pathways and the kallikrein and complement systems may be found in most standard textbooks of internal medicine.

Whatever the initial stimulus (intrinsic or extrinsic), the final common pathway of the two cascades is the conversion of soluble fibrinogen to fibrin by the action of the enzyme thrombin. Insoluble fibrin forms the matrix for hemostatic plugs in instances of vascular injury and the matrix which solidifies thrombi in the process of thrombosis. Fibrin also provides the framework for the reparative connective tissue. Upon this framework, healing proceeds, with fibroblastic proliferation and ingrowth of capillaries.

If the activated coagulation mechanisms were allowed to operate unchecked, the entire human circulation might coagulate after a single vascular injury. This is avoided, at least in part, through the action of various plasma coagulation factor inhibitors. These include α_2-macroglobulin, α_2-antiplasmin, antithrombin III, α_1-antitrypsin, and C1 inactivator.[31] The coagulation mechanism may also be inhibited by various other means[32]: 1) dicoumarols, which are vitamin K antagonists which interfere with the hepatic synthesis of the vitamin K-dependent clotting factors (II, VII, IX, and X); 2) heparin, which blocks the action of thrombin on fibrinogen; 3) antiplatelet agents such as acetylsalicylic acid and dipyridamole, which decrease platelet function; 4) fibrinolytic agents such as urokinase and streptokinase (mechanism to be discussed); and 5) certain snake venoms, which cause fibrinogen depletion.

Fibrin and Fibrinolysis

Another system providing a balance against the formation of fibrin, the fibrinolytic system, is the major topic of this chapter. The principal function of this system is to maintain the fluidity of blood by dissolving the fibrin in arterial and venous thrombi. In normal persons, there is a constant dynamic balance between fibrin formation and dissolution. Fibrin dissolution, a proteolytic process, results in the formation of soluble fibrin degradation products or FDPs (fragments X, Y, D, and E). The process is mediated by plasmin, a relatively nonspecific plasma protease formed from the zymogen (inactive precursor) plas-

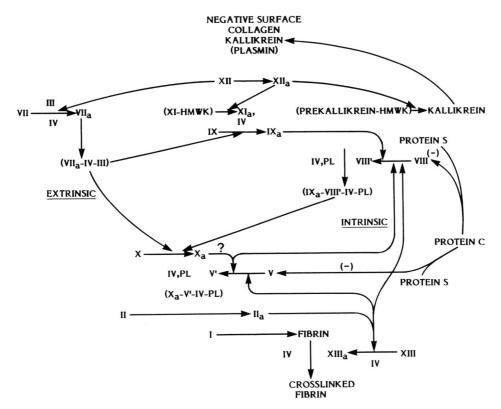

Figure 8.1. Extrinsic and intrinsic coagulation cascades. Inactive clotting factors are denoted by *Roman numerals;* activated clotting factors are indicated by *Roman numeral plus subscript "a."* Active complexes are enclosed in *parentheses.* A *prime sign* (') after clotting factor V or VIII signifies special form with enhanced activity. The identities of the clotting factors are listed below. All factors promote coagulation with the exceptions of proteins C and S. Protein C inhibits factors V and VIII, and protein S serves as a cofactor in this inhibition. These inhibitory functions are indicated by a *minus sign* (−). *I:* Fibrinogen; *II:* Prothrombin; *III:* Tissue factor; *IV:* Calcium (Ca^{pp}); *V:* Proaccelerin (labile factor); *VI:* Not assigned; *VII:* Proconvertin (stable factor); *VIII:* Antihemophilic factor; *IX:* Christmas factor; *X:* Stuart factor; *XI:* Plasma thromboplastin antecedent; *XII:* Hageman factor; *XIII:* Fibrin-stabilizing factor; Prekallikrein; *HMWK:* High molecular weight kininogen; von Willebrand factor; Protein C; Protein S; *PL:* phospholipid.

minogen (Fig. 8.2). Normally, plasminogen is found in the circulation in concentrations of 12–25mg/dl, whereas plasmin is not detectable.[31] The latter may, however, be detected in certain disease states.

Several substances promote the initial conversion of

plasminogen to plasmin. These include: urokinase (UK), which is produced by the human kidney and circulates as a trace protein; plasma activators; tissue activator (tPA); and bacterial enzymes, such as SK. Plasma activator is present in the circulation in increased concentrations in response to exercise, physical trauma, shock, ischemia, and chemicals such as nicotinic acid and epinephrine. Part of the balance provided against these activators derives from a number of inhibitors present in endothelial cells[33,34] and in plasma.[35−37] Furthermore, the plasma protein α_2-antiplasmin is a potent inhibitor of plasmin, and there are other, less rapidly acting, ones such as α_2-macroglobulin and α_1-antitrypsin.[31]

Importantly, there are significant influences of the activated fibrinolytic system on the coagulation cascade. The nonspecific protease plasmin cleaves not only fibrin, but also factors V and VIII and fibrinogen. Thus, plasmin exerts a direct anticoagulant effect. In addition, FDPs have their own inhibitory effect on the clotting cascade, which amplifies the anticoagulant effect.

Plasminogen, which has a high affinity for fibrin, probably becomes intimately bound within thrombi during the

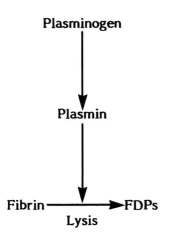

Figure 8.2. Final common pathway in fibrinolysis.

polymerization of fibrin. Because plasma activator and tPA also have high fibrin affinity, the binding processes bring plasminogen substrate close to activator molecules, which tends to localize the process of plasmin generation to sites where fibrinolysis is needed. The activators UK and SK are not nearly so specific, and as a result, administration of these agents frequently results in activation of large amounts of circulating (unbound) plasminogen, with production of high levels of circulating plasmin. The rare patients with congenital abnormalities of the fibrinolytic system have enhanced our understanding of these processes.[38-45] A few patients with recurrent DVT have proved to have functionally defective plasminogen,[38,39] and others have a familial defect in the synthesis or release of plasminogen activator from vascular endothelial cells.[40,41] Congenital deficiency of α_2-antiplasmin leads to excessive fibrinolysis,[42-44] and a hemorrhagic disorder caused by excessive plasminogen has been described.[45]

It is apparent that the fibrinolytic mechanism is protective. However, in many instances of intravascular coagulation (DVT, arterial thrombosis), this endogenous mechanism is inadequate to restore patency of the involved blood vessel. Efforts to hasten or amplify the fibrinolytic process have led to the administration of exogenous fibrinolytic agents.

STREPTOKINASE AND UROKINASE

Streptokinase

Streptokinase is a single-chain, antigenic protein product of β-hemolytic streptococci. Teleologically, streptococci are able to survive and proliferate in the face of the human healing process in part because of their capacity to synthesize this substance. Streptokinase, when coupled with human plasminogen, results in the formation of plasmin, which dissolves fibrin in the reparative framework, preventing the infection from being walled off.

Alkjaersig et al. elucidated the mechanism of clot lysis by plasmin in 1959,[46] and in the same year, Johnson and McCarty reported the lysis of human clots by intravenous infusion of SK.[47] The latter report marked the beginning of first-generation fibrinolytic therapy, a generation of high-dose intravenous systemic administration for lysing thrombi and thromboemboli remote from the site of infusion.[48]

The mechanism of action of SK is shown diagrammatically in Figure 8.3. Basically, SK forms a one-to-one stoichiometric complex with plasminogen. This enzymatically active complex controls the conversion of additional plasminogen molecules to plasmin. Plasmin is then available to lyse the fibrin component of thrombi. In addition, SK may form active complexes with plasmin molecules. With increasing dose or duration of therapy, the active SK-plasminogen complexes are gradually replaced by SK-plasmin active complexes, which are also capable of activating plasminogen. Importantly, SK does not have the high affinity for fibrin characteristic of plasma activator and tPA; therefore, it activates not only the plasminogen molecules within thrombus, but also those circulating in the plasma. This activity creates high levels of circulating plasmin, with all of the aforementioned effects on the coagulation cascade.

Urokinase

In 1946, Macfarlane and Pilling first isolated UK from human urine.[49] The work of Sherry et al. helped bring the substance into clinical use.[50] It is a protein product of the normal human kidney which is found in trace quantities in the circulation and is available commercially for exogenous administration as a fibrinolytic agent. Commercial laboratories derive the substance from cultures of human fetal kidney cells.

The mechanism of action of UK is diagrammed in Figure 8.4. Unlike SK, UK does not form active complexes with plasminogen in order to produce its fibrinolytic effect. Rather, it acts directly on plasminogen to produce plasmin. Importantly, like SK, it does not have the high affinity for fibrin that is characteristic of plasma activator and tPA. Therefore, it also activates circulating plasminogen mole-

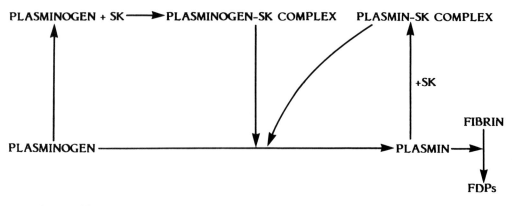

Figure 8.3. Mechanism of action of SK. As plasmin becomes more plentiful and plasminogen is depleted, the SK-plasminogen active complexes are replaced by SK-plasmin active complexes.

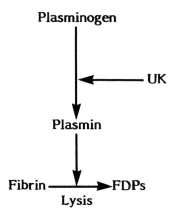

Figure 8.4. Mechanism of action of UK. UK is a nonantigenic, enzymatic protein that does not require formation of active complexes in order to activate plasminogen.

cules to produce plasmin. The action of circulating plasmin, in turn, results in the anticoagulant effects described above. When the circulating plasmin level is high, its effects on the coagulation cascade are evident, and the fibrinogen level is decreased (normal approximately 350–400mg/dl), a "systemic fibrinolytic state" is said to exist.

Streptokinase and Urokinase: A Comparison

The most obvious, and one of the most significant, difference between SK and UK is that the former is a foreign and therefore antigenic protein, whereas the latter is human derived. The antigenicity of SK has had important clinical manifestations (to be described below), whereas UK has had no such ill effects. The prevalence of SK antibody in the general population led Verstraete et al. to investigate and eventually to describe a standard dosage regimen that includes a 250,000-unit bolus administered over 0.5 hour (an amount sufficient to neutralize existing SK antibody in approximately 90% of the population) prior to initiating the continuous intravenous systemic infusion.[51] In addition, because of its antigenicity, SK retreatment within six months is not advisable because of the potential for an anamnestic immune response. UK, on the other hand, may be readministered at any time. SK is slightly pyrogenic, whereas UK is nonpyrogenic. SK has a half-life of 10–12 minutes (not the same as the fibrinolytic half-life that results from its administration), and UK has a half-life of 11–16 minutes. There is evidence that SK produces a slightly higher fibrinogenolytic:fibrinolytic ratio than does UK.[52] Both produce markedly higher ratios than does tPA, as one would expect from the more specific mechanism of action of the latter. The ratios are important in that the higher one resulting from SK would seem to indicate that SK is more likely than UK to produce a systemic fibrinolytic state and therefore is conceivably more likely to cause hemorrhage when administered in therapeutically similar amounts. Clinical experience with local infusion methods since 1981 has indeed shown more hem-

orrhagic complications with SK than with UK.[53–55] The likelihood of hemorrhagic complication is also related to infusion duration. In an effort to hasten lysis with increasing enzyme concentrations while minimizing hemorrhagic complications, high dose-rate, short infusion duration UK protocols have become a favorite method. SK is stable when stored at room temperature, but UK must be stored at 4°C until use. Finally, and importantly, UK costs approximately six times as much as SK on a per unit basis. Worse still, most UK regimens require far more units than do comparable SK regimens (four times as many units in most low-dose local regimens and three to four times as many in the systemic or intravenous regimens). These factors combine to make UK therapy as much as 24 times as expensive as therapeutically similar SK therapy. Manufacturers have recently increased the availability of UK by increasing their production capacity.

CLINICAL EXPERIENCE

First-generation Therapy

In two previous works, the cumulative clinical experience with SK and UK was described as having evolved in generations.[48,53] The first generation of therapy was characterized by high-dose intravenous infusion of fibrinolytic agents aimed at lysing thrombi or thromboemboli that usually were remote from the site of infusion. SK was used for a variety of vascular occlusive problems in this early period,[56–58] but the true momentum in first-generation therapy developed only when the National Institutes of Health (NIH) formed its Committee on Thrombolytic Agents. This committee identified UK, derived from human urine and recently purified sufficiently,[59] as the most suitable thrombolytic agent for clinical trials.

Large-scale investigation into the clinical use of UK and SK came when the National Heart, Lung, and Blood Institute (NHLBI) began the first national cooperative trial comparing UK with heparin in the treatment of pulmonary thromboembolic disease (Urokinase Pulmonary Embolism Trial; UPET).[60] This multicenter study used pulmonary angiography, perfusion lung scanning, and hemodynamic measurements in the right side of the heart and the pulmonary circulation to assess the rate and degree of dissolution of emboli. UK-treated patients received an intravenous loading dose of 4400 units/kg and a maintenance infusion of 4400 units/kg/hr for 12 hours. Heparin-treated patients received a loading dose of 165 IU/kg and a maintenance infusion of 22 IU/kg/hr. There were 160 patients. At the end of the 12 hours, all patients received heparin in therapeutic doses for at least five days, and then oral anticoagulants. In the follow-up period, patients had interval histories, physical examinations, and lung scans at 3, 6, and 12 months. Trial results revealed: 1) greater resolution of emboli with UK; 2) greater return of blood pressures toward normal with UK; 3) greater return of perfusion (by lung scanning) with UK; and 4) greatest improvement in patients with large pulmonary emboli.

Subsequently, the Urokinase–Streptokinase Pulmonary Embolism Trial (USPET) was undertaken.[61] In this multicenter study, UK, administered with two infusion durations (12 and 24 hours), was compared with SK. The results revealed no significant differences between UK-treated and SK-treated patients with respect to the measures used in the UPET trial.

Although UPET and USPET did not examine the long-term differences between fibrinolytic-treated and heparin-treated patients with pulmonary embolic disease, other studies did. In 40 patients without heart or lung disease who had pulmonary emboli, Sharma et al. proved that heparin-treated patients have abnormally low pulmonary capillary blood volumes both in the immediate convalescent period and at one-year follow-up,[62] whereas patients in the fibrinolytic group have normal pulmonary capillary blood volumes at both of these times. The significance of these measurements is not yet fully appreciated. It may well be that recurrent pulmonary emboli in patients with compromised pulmonary capillary volumes cause higher morbidity and mortality rates than similar recurrences in patients with normal pulmonary capillary blood volumes. It may also be that patients with abnormally low pulmonary capillary blood volumes have limited capacity for capillary recruitment and therefore have an inherent inability to respond to stresses such as exercise and illness (e.g., myocardial infarction with pulmonary edema). These hypotheses have not been adequately tested.

If thrombolytic agents are responsible for all of the beneficial effects described above, why did their use ever fall into disfavor? The answer is simply that physicians typically weigh the risk:benefit ratios of all forms of therapy, and many believe that the risks of hemorrhage attending systemic fibrinolytic therapy outweigh the potential benefits. This feeling stems principally from the UPET results, so it is essential to examine these findings in more detail; they provided the impetus for second-generation fibrinolytic therapy.

In the UPET study, a "moderate" hemorrhage was said to be loss of 500–1500ml with an associated decrease in hematocrit of 5–10 points. A "severe" hemorrhage was a loss of >1500ml with a hematocrit decrease of >10 points or a transfusion requirement of more than 2 units of blood. The frequency of moderate or severe hemorrhage was 27% for the heparin-treated group and 45% for the UK-treated group. Since the numbers of moderate hemorrhages were similar, the difference was accounted for almost entirely by a higher incidence of severe hemorrhage in the UK-treated patients. However, the UPET protocol was invasive by design (pulmonary angiography, arterial blood gas studies, etc.), and hemorrhage from the resulting puncture sites was definitely responsible for the difference in the overall incidences of hemorrhagic complications in the two groups. Stated simply, the incidence of spontane-

ous hemorrhage was the same (19%) in both groups. It seems that in the absence of invasive procedures, there is no difference in hemorrhagic complications between heparin-treated and UK-treated patients. However, when one examines the spontaneous hemorrhages that occurred in UPET, it is clear that the proportion of severe ones is higher in the UK-treated group than in the heparin-treated group (88 and 53%, respectively). One may conclude that *systemic doses* of fibrinolytic agents are more dangerous than systemic doses of heparin.[63] Bleeding complications occurred with equal frequency in all three study groups of USPET (UK for 12 hours, UK for 24 hours, SK for 24 hours).

Second-generation Therapy

In an effort to avoid hemorrhagic complications while effectively dissolving thrombi and thromboemboli, Dotter et al. began to use a transcatheter method of directing SK into peripheral vascular occlusions at a dose rate of approximately 1/20th the systemic dose rate (5,000 units/hr without a loading dose instead of 100,000 units/hr following a 250,000-unit loading dose).[64] As little as 1% of the usual systemic dose was given to some of their 17 patients, 15 of whom had lower extremity arterial occlusions and two of whom had upper extremity occlusions. Treatment lasted from less than one day to two weeks. The best results were achieved in patients with recent occlusions.

Even in this earliest series, the authors recognized several important features of the local infusion method. First, they realized that lysis is not curative. In most instances, it merely restores patency and uncovers an underlying structural problem that requires treatment. Indeed, Dotter et al. treated several of their patients with transluminal dilatation after identifying an underlying stenosis. Second, those authors cautioned readers about the potential for remote hemorrhages, particularly intracerebral ones, even with the local method. Third, they suggested that indwelling arterial lines may encourage thrombus formation along the catheter shaft, a problem that has since proved significant.[65]

Although the report of Dotter et al. initiated second-generation therapy—a generation of percutaneous transcatheter low-dose fibrinolytic therapy given by the interventional angiographer and the intensive care unit (ICU) nurses—enthusiasm was lacking until Katzen and van Breda reported its use in the peripheral vasculature[66] and Rentrop et al. reported a relatively high-dose, short-duration form of therapy for coronary artery occlusion.[67]

In the past few years, a number of authors have described the efficacy and complications of the local infusion method. The following sections review these reports, noting the indications, methods, and results according to anatomic region or specific type of vessel treated. Contraindications, complications, and laboratory monitoring are dealt with in separate sections that follow.

Abdominal Aorta and Lower Extremities

It would be counterproductive to list all of the different methods utilized and presumptuous to detail a "preferred" method for local transcatheter fibrinolytic therapy for thrombotic and thromboembolic occlusive disease of the legs. Instead, the basic methods used in the earliest series will be explained, and important variations on those themes will be covered by brief descriptions.

The series of Katzen and van Breda included 12 patients, 8 of whom were treated for common iliac or more distal lower extremity arterial occlusions through a 5Fr catheter with 5000 units/hr of SK in 50 ml of normal saline.[66] Five of these eight patients subsequently underwent percutaneous transluminal angioplasty (PTA), and most of the eight had a good long-term result. The authors used simultaneous heparin in two of their patients, but bleeding complications supervened, and the heparin infusions were terminated. Most importantly, Katzen and van Breda emphasized the need for proper patient selection. For example, they stated that fibrinolytic therapy should be reserved for patients tolerating their ischemia, whereas those who are not tolerating their ischemia are better candidates for operation. The present authors have found this concept invaluable when discussing therapeutic options with the vascular surgeons. Obviously, in other anatomic areas, such as the coronary circulation (and potentially in the cerebral vasculature), this concept does not apply as intuitively as it does in the extremities.

Totty et al. described 26 infusions in 22 patients. Nineteen patients (22 infusions) were treated for lower extremity arterial occlusions, 13 of which followed PTA.[68] The authors used SK (19 infusions) in doses ranging from 2,500 units/hr (one patient) to 10,000 units/hr, with 5,000 units/hr being used most frequently; UK was used in doses ranging from 40,000–80,000 units/hr in the remaining patients. Of the 13 PTA-associated infusions, 8 produced complete or nearly complete lysis, whereas 5 resulted in partial lysis, with only one of the latter patients requiring no further treatment. Of the 10 lower extremity infusions for spontaneous thrombi or thromboemboli, 9 resulted in partial lysis, but none produced complete lysis. The authors concluded that low-dose fibrinolytic therapy has a definite role in PTA-associated vascular occlusions but a less well-defined, perhaps adjunctive, role (together with operation) in spontaneous occlusions.

Becker et al. reported 57 local infusions in 50 patients in their original series.[69] They used 5,000 units/hr of SK in most patients and 20,000 units/hr of UK in two. In order to avoid catheter-related thrombosis (to be discussed), they simultaneously administered enough heparin by intravenous infusion to maintain the partial thromboplastin time (PTT) at 1.5 times normal. Catheters as small as 3Fr were occasionally introduced coaxially through larger angiographic catheters for the infusion, and catheters as large as 6.5Fr were frequently used alone. The coaxial system was generally used when the popliteal or trifurcation branches were occluded; in these instances, the larger angiographic catheter was withdrawn to the most proximal position possible. Patients were managed in the surgical ICU and monitored by physical examination, bedside Doppler examinations, and serial angiograms made via the infusion catheter in the angiography suite. When partial lysis was observed, a catheter exchange was made over a guidewire (following rescrubbing and administration of local anesthetic), and the new catheter was advanced to the level of occlusion. Only 16 of these infusions were performed for occlusion of native arteries in the legs. In each case, the catheter was positioned within or as near to the thrombus as possible. Partial lysis occurred in 50% of the infusions, complete lysis in 25%, and no lysis in 25%. The relatively small success in these vessels led the authors to postulate that native arterial occlusions have many collateral or alternate egress pathways for the fibrinolytic solution. This hypothesis also seemed to explain the small success in hemodialysis fistulae and veins in contrast to the great success in dialysis shunts and in lower extremity grafts, which have no branches. These results alerted the authors to the importance of placing the infusion catheter within the occlusion. It now seems that such intrathrombus positioning is important not only in avoiding loss of fibrinolytic agent through collateral channels but also in increasing the surface area of thrombus exposed to the fibrinolytic solution and thus hastening thrombolysis.

Hess et al. reported their use of a modified technique for low-dose intra-arterial infusion in 136 patients with lower extremity arterial occlusions.[70] Their technique involved positioning a double-lumen polyvinyl balloon catheter in the occluded vessel with the tip embedded 1cm into the thrombus or thromboembolus (eight of their patients were thought to have embolic occlusions). One to three milliliters of SK (1,000 units/ml in normal saline) were then injected. After 5–15 minutes, the catheter was advanced under fluoroscopy, and the procedure was repeated. This continued until the catheter reached the patent lumen distal to the occlusion. Residual stenoses were detected by angiography through the infusion catheter and treated with PTA. The total dose of SK required per patient ranged from 4,000–180,000 units. Patients were given acetylsalicylic acid, 500mg two or three times daily, after the initial treatment. Ninety-four recanalizations were achieved in 136 attempts (69%), but only 70 (51%) lasted two weeks according to follow-up angiography. The cumulative patency rate at 16 months was still close to 50%, however. Importantly, the method of Hess et al. requires less SK than those techniques previously reported, which may help lower the frequency of hemorrhagic complications secondary to the systemic fibrinolytic state. In addition, the procedure times were considerably shorter than those reported by others (1–5 hours). Another important observation was that patients with chronic occlusions (six months or longer) still had a 50%

recanalization frequency with the new method, whereas acute occlusions responded with an 80% frequency. The success indicated for chronic occlusions is higher than expected on the basis of the previous literature but agrees with Rabe et al.'s observation that SK can lyse chronic fibrin deposits.[71]

In the series of 159 infusions reported by Graor et al., patients were divided into groups with atherosclerotic occlusions, postprocedural occlusions, and peripheral arterial emboli.[72] The number of infusions performed for lower extremity native arterial occlusions is unclear. Atherosclerotic occlusions were opened in 56% of cases and postprocedural occlusions in 79%, and arterial emboli were lysed in 70%. Infusions were made through 5Fr endhole catheters embedded in the occlusions; heparinization was not used. Empiric cefamandole antibiotic prophylaxis was used (1g intravenously every 6 hours throughout treatment and for 24 hours afterward). Clinical estimates of the durations of the occlusions were from one hour to one year. Infusion durations ranged from 12 to 120 hours.

Dardik et al. reported their experience with SK in 38 patients, 9 of whom were managed with local infusions for lower extremity native arterial occlusions.[73] Although all infusions were begun at 5,000 units/hr, the dose rates were sequentially increased to 15,000 units/hr and continued for 48–72 hours in slow responders. Recanalization was achieved in all of these patients, and a distal bypass operation was subsequently required in only one.

In his article on the complications of intra-arterial use of SK, Lang reported 35 patients treated for lower extremity vascular occlusions, 23 of whom had occlusions in native arteries rather than grafts.[74] The SK dose of 5000 units/hr was infused through a 5Fr catheter embedded in the occlusions, with heparin (200–1000 units/hr) being given to maintain the PTT at 1.5–2.0 times normal. The catheters were advanced as lysis proceeded until patency was completely restored. Sixteen of the 23 infusions resulted in complete lysis.

In the series of Mori et al., 50 infusions of SK were made for a variety of thrombotic and thromboembolic conditions.[75] Of these, 24 involved treatment for native arterial occlusions in the legs. The most common regimen was a local infusion of SK at 5000 units/hr plus simultaneous heparin infusion at 250–500 units/hr. Infusions were terminated when: 1) significant lysis had occurred; 2) no lysis was observed after 24–48 hours; 3) the symptoms worsened; or 4) hemorrhagic complications supervened. Infusion durations were 1–20 hours. Although clinical benefit from SK infusion alone was observed in only approximately half the cases, combinations of SK plus operation or SK plus PTA produced clinical benefit in another 30%. Therefore, some benefit was obtained by approximately 80% of the patients, with slightly better results being noted for embolic occlusions than for thrombotic ones.

On the basis of evidence that high-dose local UK infusion for a short time is efficacious for coronary thrombolysis,[76] McNamara and Fischer used a similar high-dose regimen in 93 peripheral arterial and graft occlusions in 85 patients.[77] The method involves infusing 4000 units/min of UK until antegrade blood flow is re-established, and then 2000 units/min until lysis is complete. Although the authors did not separate their results according to graft versus native artery infusions, they did report clinical improvement in 75 (81%) of the patients. After an initial experience with catheter-related thrombosis (two of seven patients early in the series not treated with concomitant heparin), McNamara and Fischer began to use simultaneous heparin infusion in dose rates sufficient to maintain the PTT at approximately 3 times normal, after which the frequency of catheter-related thrombosis decreased to 3%. Those authors also found a low frequency of hemorrhagic complications and, of course, no allergic complications. The lower frequency of hemorrhage probably reflects the importance of the lower fibrinogenolytic:fibrinolytic ratio that UK has relative to SK. The authors concluded that the high-dose local UK regimen is superior to all local SK regimens previously used. This infusion regimen has now become the most popular one used by interventional angiographers in the United States.

Finally, Bean et al. recently reported successful treatment of a patient with a four-week history of Leriche syndrome by means of local SK infusion and PTA.[78] They used the blind femoral angiogram technique[79,80] to catheterize the aorta retrograde. After an arteriogram revealed thrombotic occlusion of the distal abdominal aorta, they infused SK at 5000 units/hr for 26 hours until lysis was complete and stenosis of the aorta due to atherosclerotic plaque was identified. A PTA was performed using two balloon catheters ("kissing balloon" technique).

Representative cases of local thrombolytic therapy for occlusion of native arteries in the legs are illustrated in Figures 8.5 and 8.6.

A method was proposed by Sullivan et al.[81] to accelerate the rate of thrombolysis. The technique consists of the intrathrombus deposition of either low- or high-dose urokinase utilizing a coaxial method. A diagnostic 5 or 6Fr catheter is advanced to the proximal end of the occlusion. In a coaxial fashion, either a 3.0Fr Teflon or an open-ended guidewire steered by an internal 0.018 platinum coronary-type wire, is advanced through the thrombus.

Urokinase mixed with 10–20ml of saline is injected into the thrombus as the catheter or open-ended guidewire is being withdrawn.

Sullivan et al. have laced the thrombus with two different boluses of urokinase. A low dosage of 52,000 IU was used in 28 patients and a high dose of a 230,000 IU in 21 patients. The results showed that in the high-dose group, thrombolysis was achieved in 10.4 hours vs. 36.6 hours in the low-dose group.

A 3-fold increase in the speed of thrombolysis was therefore demonstrated in the high-dose group. In spite of using a large dose to lace the thrombus, the total dose required

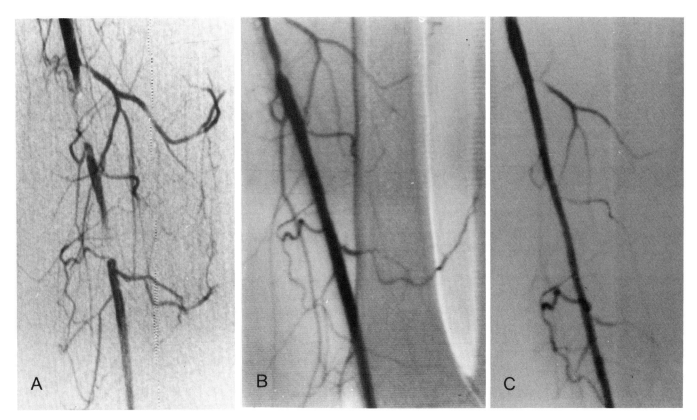

Figure 8.5. Patient with acute lower extremity ischemia. **A.** Initial digital subtraction angiogram shows two segments of superficial femoral artery (SFA) occlusion. **B.** After 24 hours of local UK at 20,000 units/hr plus intra- venous heparin, repeat angiogram shows patency of SFA and ather- omatous plaque in region of previous occlusion. **C.** SFA after PTA of ste- notic segment.

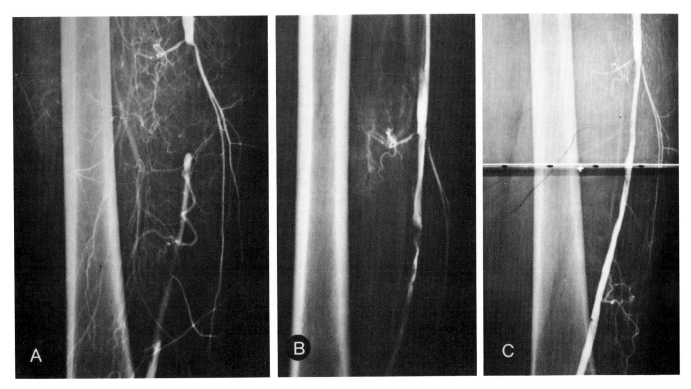

Figure 8.6. A 49-year-old diabetic man with acute right lower extremity ischemia complicating long-standing claudication. **A.** Initial right lower extremity arteriogram shows superficial femoral artery occlusion. **B.** After 1 day of transcatheter SK at 5000 units/hr plus intravenous heparin, most of thrombus has been lysed, and an underlying stenosis is identified. **C.** Angiogram after PTA.

to achieve lysis is reduced by 54% in the high- vs. the low-dose group.

The incidence of major complications was 22.9% in the low-dose group and 8.7% in the high-dose group. Distal embolization as a result of catheter advancement through the thrombus is not higher than in other series and only 3.4% of cases required surgical embolectomy. The rapid lysis is attributed to the faster conversion of plasmin into plasminogen within the thrombus. The plasmin in the thrombus has a longer life than in the circulation, because in the presence of fibrin it is protected from its inhibitor α_2-antiplasmin.

Strife reported on eight neonates treated with fibrinolytic therapy.[82] Six of them had aortic thrombosis associated with an umbilical catheter. Two received streptokinase in doses ranging from 1,000 to 5,000 units/kg as a loading dose with a maintenance dose varying from 400 to 1,200 units/kg. Five of the six received urokinase in doses varying from 4,400 to 10,000 units/kg as a loading dose and 4,000–20,000 units/kg as a maintenance dose. Two other patients had peripheral arterial thrombosis; one had a complete lysis and one had a partial lysis only. The duration of the fibrinolytic therapy ranged from 4 hours to 9 days (mean 3.5 days). Four of the patients received concomitant heparin therapy. Four of the six patients with aortic thrombosis had complete lysis, and partial lysis occurred in two.

The treatment of aortic thrombosis secondary to umbilical artery catheters is controversial. In 26% of neonates, thrombosis is detected on sonography but only 29% are symptomatic. The management of symptomatic infants includes medical, surgical, and fibrinolytic therapies.

Because of the small number of infants treated with fibrinolysis, there are no established dosage criteria or data on proved efficacy and risk of major complications. The recommended dose of streptokinase is 300–1000 units/kg/hr; and urokinase in 4000–5000 units/kg/hr. Concomitant heparinization is recommended with an initial bolus of 50 units/kg and a maintenance of dose of 20 to 25 units/kg/hr.

The one complication of intracranial hemorrhage in a premature infant is a major complication. This event may not be related to the thrombolytic administration since it has been reported in up to 56–71% of premature babies at the time of autopsy.

THROMBOLYSIS IN CHRONIC OCCLUSION

Thrombolysis of long segment chronic occlusions prior to angioplasty has been attempted recently. It is based on the assumption that occlusions of more than a few centimeters are secondary to thrombosis superimposed over a high-grade stenosis or short segment occlusion.[83] Prolonged infusions commonly result in clot maceration, facilitating therefore the recanalization of long segment occlusions. Using this approach, Motarjeme has achieved higher patency rates than using mechanical recanalization fol-

lowed by PTA.[83] Wilms used a protocol in occlusions longer than 3cm which required the infusion of low doses of streptokinase at a rate of 5000 units/hr along with 400 units of heparin into the clot. The infusions lasted between 4 and 62 hours with a mean of 18 hours. The catheter was advanced farther down the thrombus as the lysis continued to progress under fluoroscopic guidance. The primary success in 64 patients was 77% for the native arteries and 80% for short segments of less than 10cm as compared with 40% for long segment occlusions. The cumulative patency rates at the end of the first and second years were 87 and 82%, respectively.[84]

Distal embolization was noted in 3% of patients. The low embolic rate was attributed to the presence of chronic organized thrombus as opposed to poorly organized thrombi in acute occlusions.[84]

Lammer published their experience in treating chronic occlusions of iliac and femoral popliteal vessels in 136 patients. The mean length of occlusions were 12.5cm with a maximum of 65cm. They injected 2500 units of streptokinase into the thrombus in a pulsed fashion in 90 patients. In 32 patients, 4000 units of urokinase was used every five minutes. The underlying stenotic lesions were treated with balloon angioplasty. The recanalization process is stopped when there is antegrade flow in spite of residual thrombi. Following recanalization, heparin is continued at a dose of 1000 units/hr for three days. The initial success rate was 78% with early recurrent thrombosis in 10% of the patients. The two years cumulative patency rate after recanalization was 81%.[85]

Lupattelli reported their experience with selective intra-arterial infusions of urokinase in chronic arterial occlusions. They treated 21 patients with occlusions 2–12 months old and a length ranging from 7–18cm. A 5Fr catheter tip was embedded into the proximal segment of the occlusion and a bolus of 50,000 units of urokinase is deposited into the thrombus. Urokinase is then infused at a rate of 50,000 units/hr, along with heparin, 800 units/hr.[86]

Thrombolysis was achieved in 85% of patients, and in 15 patients the underlying stenosis was treated by balloon angioplasty. Complications included embolization into the tibial vessels in two patients. Two patients reoccluded within four weeks. The authors have concluded that improved long-term results can be obtained by lysing the chronic thrombus and correcting the underlying stenosis.[86] Hans Hess from Munich reported on his six years of experience in treating 564 peripheral arterial occlusions in 554 patients.[87] Favorable conditions for a successful lysis include nonorganized fibrin and lysable material that allows a catheter to be placed within the thrombus. No systemic hemorrhage effects were noted.

Of 472 thrombotic occlusions older than six months, 254 (+ = 38%) were successfully treated, with a cumulative patency of 58.8% after five years.

Of 92 embolic occlusions present for two months or

more, 59 (64%) were recanalized with a cumulative patency of 89.5% after five years.

The authors have recommended thrombolytic therapy if it meets the following criteria:

a. Thrombi of varying ages up to 6–8 months resulting from complications of balloon angioplasty can be treated.
b. Surgical embolectomy is the treatment of choice for embolic occlusion of larger vessels in arms, abdominal aorta, iliac and common femoral arteries.
c. Popliteal graft occlusions up to 11 weeks old can be efficiently lysed with thrombolytic therapy.

GRAFTS

Twenty-one infusions reported in Becker et al.'s initial series were for graft occlusions.[69] They were most successful in this group, with complete lysis occurring in 15 patients and partial lysis in an additional 4. In some patients, stenoses were identified at graft anastomotic sites and a few of these were treated with PTA. Figures 8.7 and 8.8 are illustrations of two patients with graft occlusions treated with local fibrinolysis. As stated above, the high degree of success noted in this group was attributed to the lack of collateral pathways or alternate egress channels available to divert the fibrinolytic solution.

The present authors' experience is not unique. In the series of Wolfson et al., 27 infusions of SK were given for a variety of thrombotic and thromboembolic conditions.[88] Graft occlusions lysed faster than native arterial ones (35 hours and 62 hours, respectively) and more frequently (7 of 9 cases versus 11 of 18). Most patients were treated with local infusions of 5000 units/hr. Those authors also believed that concomitant heparin administration was important in preventing catheter-related thrombosis.

None of the patients in the original series of Dotter et al.[64] was treated for graft occlusion, nor were the patients reported by Katzen and van Breda,[66] with the exception of one with an occluded dialysis graft. The latter case is discussed under "Hemodialysis Accesses." In their series, Hess et al. did not state that any patients were treated for graft occlusions.[70]

Four of the infusions reported by Totty et al. were for graft occlusion, and although all patients had some clinical improvement, only three had angiographically demonstrable improvement.[68] In the series of Dardik et al., 26 of the 38 patients had graft thromboses. Sixteen were treated with intra-arterial SK and the remainder with intravenous SK; lysis occurred in five of the former and three of the latter.[73] In Lang's series, thrombolytic therapy was most efficacious in cases of thrombosed synthetic grafts (11 of 12).[74] Of the 50 local infusions in the series of Mori et al., 10 were performed for thrombosed arterial bypass grafts to the lower extremities. Although SK infusion alone was beneficial in only 30%, SK plus operation or SK plus PTA proved beneficial in another 20%.[75] Of the 93 infusions in the series of McNamara and Fischer, 22 were performed for occlusions of grafts to the legs, but it is impossible to ascertain from the data the percentage resulting in complete lysis.[77]

In the series of Graor et al., 35 patients were treated for graft thrombosis. Of these, 11 were Dacron aortic bifurcation grafts, 12 were polytetrafluoroethylene (PTFE) grafts, and 12 were saphenous vein grafts in the legs. Although these patients were grouped with three post-PTA occlusions, for a total of 38 postprocedural occlusions, the results in this category were remarkable, with 79% of patients achieving thrombolysis—complete dissolution of thrombus and clinical improvement.[72]

The most recent experience indicates that the first line of treatment for occluded grafts is thrombolysis. Advantages of thrombolytic therapy include:

1. It uncovers the underlying stenotic lesion at the anastomotic sites or in the native vessels that have contributed to the occlusion.
2. The anatomical detail obtained by arteriography is helpful for the surgical repair or during a percutaneous angioplasty.
3. It is less traumatic compared with mechanical extraction by Fogarty catheters.
4. Thrombi in small vessels distal to the graft anastomosis are better managed by thrombolytics, compared with a surgical thrombectomy.
5. Thrombolytic therapy converts an emergency on an elective procedure.[89–93]

In the series of Gardiner et al., 72 peripheral bypass grafts in 62 patients were treated by the intra-arterial infusion of thrombolytic therapy.[92] Urokinase was the thrombolytic agent in 43 cases with a 84% success rate, and streptokinase was tried in 29 cases with a 48% success rate. The superiority of urokinase was clearly established. The overall graft patency at the end of one year was 60% by applying life table analysis.[92]

Vein grafts showed a higher patency rate (77%) with an average patency of 16 months compared with a 45% patency for prosthetic grafts at 14 months.[92] The most significant factor related to long-term patency is the presence or absence of a lesion that can be corrected either by surgery or angioplasty.

The one-year patency of grafts with anatomic lesions is 86% vs. 37% in grafts without detectable lesions.[92] In the same series, there was a 25% incidence of complications that required intervention. Complications included proximal and distal embolization, hematomas at the puncture site, transient pulmonary edema, stroke myocardial infarction, septicemia and bleeding in 10% of the cases.[92]

In the series of Durham et al., 71 urokinase infusions were performed in 53 patients.[91] Although clot lysis was achieved in 75% of grafts, antegrade flow was established in only 66%, owing to the presence of severe outflow occlusive disease. The median patency rate of grafts was five

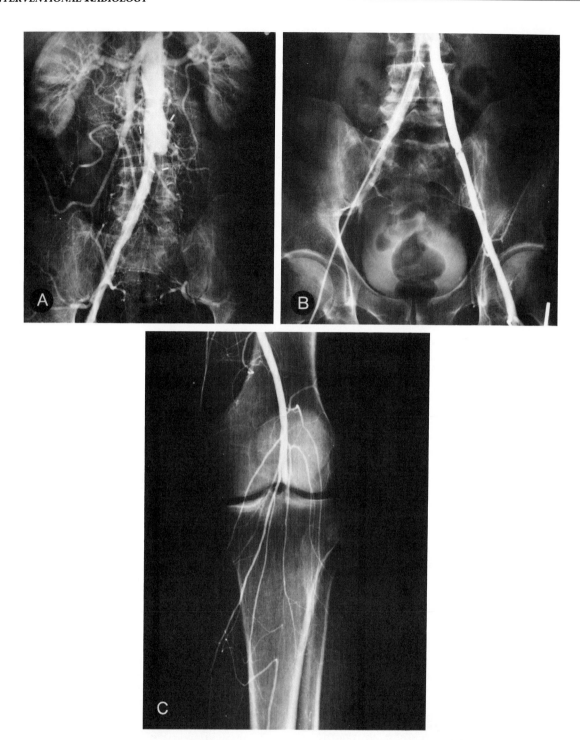

Figure 8.7. This 56-year-old man with a 5-year-old knitted Dacron aortobi-iliac graft presented with new left lower extremity ischemia. **A.** Initial angiogram discloses complete occlusion of left limb of graft. A catheter was placed over the bifurcation into the occlusion, and SK infusion of 5000 units/hr was started. The patient also received heparin. **B.** Angiogram through infusion catheter after 19 hours of SK shows patency of left limb of graft and stenosis at distal anastomotic site. **C.** This angiogram, also made after 19 hours of SK, shows complete midpopliteal occlusion (embolic). **D.** Angioplasty was performed, and this angiogram was made. **E.** After PTA, 3Fr coaxial catheter was placed into popliteal occlusion, and SK infusion was restarted. **F.** Angiogram after another 24 hours shows patency of popliteal and trifurcation arteries.

months, following thrombolytics and adjunctive therapy with 75% limb salvage at one year.[91] The long-term patency rate of infrainguinal grafts is comparable to thromboembolectomy and patch grafting but they are definitely inferior to surgical reconstruction (median patency rate is 20 months for above-the-knee bypasses). The long-term patency results are inferior to the reported suprainguinal graft reconstruction. The success rate of 75% clot lysis is comparable to that in other series.[92,93] There is 23% major complication rate. The complications included bleeding

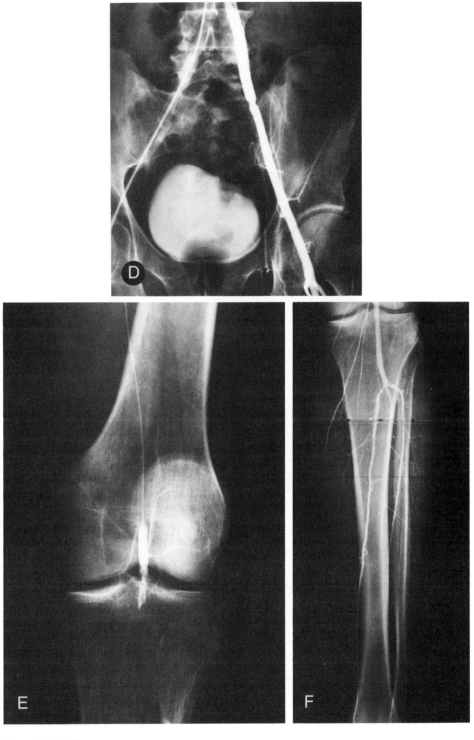

Figure 8.7 (D–F).

requiring surgical evacuation and transfusion. There were incidents of pericatheter thrombosis and distal emboli that required surgical embolectomy and continuation of uro-kinase infusion. There were strokes and periprocedural cardiac death.[91]

Risius et al. published their experience utilizing recombinant human tissue-type plasminogen activator (rt-PA) as a thrombolytic agent in 25 patients.[94] Among 25 patients,

13 had arterial occlusions (11 thrombotic and 2 embolic) and the other 12 had thrombosed bypass grafts.[89] The rt-PA was infused at the rate of 0.1mg/kg/hr through an indwelling catheter either in the occluded graft or in the native artery.

Thrombolysis was achieved in 23 of 25 patients (92%) in a time frame of 1 to 6.5 hours, with an average period of 3.6 hours. Twelve of 23 patients (52%) required additional

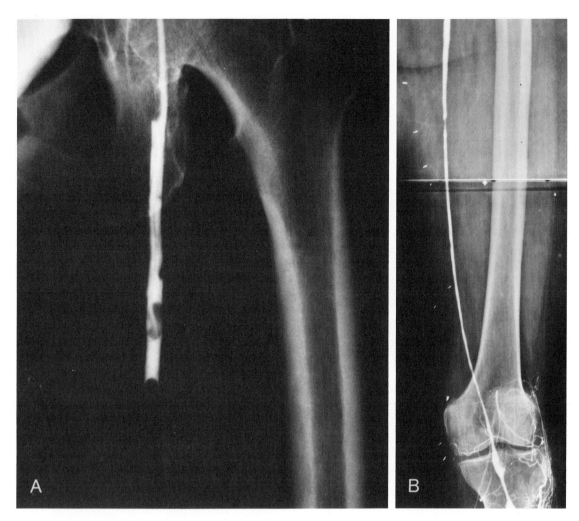

Figure 8.8. A 72-year-old woman with occluded saphenous femoropopliteal graft. **A.** Initial angiogram showing occlusion. **B.** Angiogram after local SK and intravenous heparin shows graft patency and severe midgraft stenosis that was probably responsible for thrombotic occlusion.

procedures, such as percutaneous transluminal angioplasty, revision of graft anastomosis, and endarterectomy to maintain patency of recanalized arterial segments. Concomitant anticoagulation was not administered.[94]

In three patients (12%), small hematomas at the puncture site were noted. One patient died of intracranial hemorrhage, 48 hours following the termination of rt-PA infusion. The patient was on a full dose of heparin and, the authors believed, bleeding could not be attributed to rt-PA.

The authors concluded that rt-PA is a potent fibrin-specific thrombolytic agent that achieves rapid thrombolysis without major complications in a short period of time.

UPPER EXTREMITIES

In the original series reported by Dotter et al., two patients were treated for vascular occlusions in the hands and arms.[64] The first was a patient with a two-week history of occlusion in the left digital arteries of uncertain etiology, who was treated with SK 5000 units/hr administered via a transfemoral catheter positioned in the brachial artery.

There was no change in the clinical findings or the angiographic appearance after 19 hours of infusion. The second was a patient with an ulnar artery occlusion treated with 2500 units/hr SK administered via a transaxillary catheter positioned in the brachial artery. There was no change after 23 hours of infusion, and no surgical or other confirmation of the presence of thrombus or thromboembolus was ever obtained.

Only one patient in the original series of Katzen and van Breda was treated for vascular occlusion of an arm vessel. The patient had mitral valve disease and an embolic occlusion of the left distal brachial artery. The offending thromboembolus was lysed with 7 hours of transcatheter local SK at 5000 units/hr.[66]

None of the patients in Becker et al.'s original series of 57 infusions was treated for upper extremity arterial occlusion,[69] but Totty et al. had two upper extremity cases in their series.[68] The first was an 80-year-old woman with an axillary artery thrombus and symptoms of one day's duration who was treated with transcatheter SK at 5,000 units/hr for 90 hours. Although this treatment lysed the thrombus, small brachial thrombi or thromboemboli required surgical removal. The second patient was a 45-year-old woman who presented with right axillary, brachial, radial, and ulnar occlusions and symptoms of one week's duration. Despite treatment with SK 10,000 units/hr for 45 hours that lysed the axillary thrombus, the patient ultimately required amputation below the elbow.

None of the patients in the large series of Hess et al.[70] was treated for upper extremity arterial occlusions, and it is impossible to ascertain from the data of Dardik et al.[73] whether any of their patients was treated for this problem. It appears from Lang's report that none of his patients was treated for upper extremity arterial occlusions.

Mori et al. treated one patient for axillary artery thrombosis, two for brachial artery emboli, and three for emboli to the hand, but it is impossible to ascertain their success in these cases because of the manner in which the data are grouped.[75] It can be stated that considering arterial thrombi as a group (upper and lower extremity data together) in this series, only 24% of the patients had no clinical benefit; considering arterial emboli as a group, only 10% had no clinical benefit. Likewise, although McNamara and Fischer had several patients who were treated for upper extremity arterial occlusions, because of the method of grouping the data, the exact number and treatment results are not evident.[77] Eighteen of the 27 patients of Wolfson et al. were treated for native arterial rather than graft occlusions, but in this study, too, the number of upper extremity cases is not specified.[88] The number of patients with upper extremity arterial occlusions likewise cannot be ascertained in the series of Graor et al.[72]

Tisnado et al. reported the use of local SK infusion in the treatment of hand ischemia.[95] This series has now been expanded to include nine cases of acute and one case of chronic hand ischemia treated with local SK infusion.[96] The authors make the following important points. First, most cases of hand ischemia are caused by atherosclerotic occlusion, emboli, or trauma, whereas only a small number are due to Raynaud's disease, connective tissue disorders, or thoracic outlet syndrome.[97–102] Second, although two-thirds of cases are due to occlusions proximal to the wrist, which are potentially amenable to operation, the remaining one-third are due to occlusion of the small arteries of the hand and fingers, a type in which surgical reconstruction is often difficult or impossible.[102–104] Spasm is rarely an important factor, and cervicodorsal sympathectomy is of little value. Third, occlusive disease limited to the midpalm and fingers is not amenable to vascular surgery, and the results of conservative therapy with vasodilators, anticoagulants, and dextran have been disappointing; many of these patients eventually require amputation.[102] In one previous report, nine patients with arterial occlusions in the arm were treated with local SK using a technique much like that of Hess et al., described earlier in this chapter. The SK (1000 units) was infused by hand injection every 1–3 minutes, and the catheter was advanced stepwise through the occlusion until the patent distal segment of the artery was reached.[105]

The method of Tisnado et al. involves complete upper extremity angiography, including arch aortography, as an initial step. A 5Fr transfemoral selective catheter is used for the SK infusion, and the catheter is advanced to the distal brachial artery for infusion of all forearm arteries or to the level of the distal brachial artery occlusion if one is present. This avoids placement of the catheter directly in the forearm vessels, which are small and prone to spasm. In addition, it permits simultaneous infusion of all three forearm arteries. Pharmacoangiography using 25–50mg of tolazoline, 50mg of papaverine, 0.1mg of nitroglycerin, or 50–100mg of lidocaine is used to identify fixed vascular occlusions. Vasodilators are not needed when initial forearm angiography demonstrates intraluminal filling defects. Tisnado et al. typically use a loading dose of SK of 50,000 units administered through the catheter over 30 min, but other investigators have not used loading doses in local low-dose therapy. In fact, some believe strongly that the concept of loading doses is diametrically opposed to the principal aim of fibrinolytic therapy—successful lysis without induction of a systemic fibrinolytic state. The SK infusion is then continued at 5,000 units/hr in the ICU. Heparin is administered concomitantly in doses sufficient to maintain the PTT at 1.5 times normal. Follow-up arteriograms are obtained every 6–12 hours through the infusion catheter. In the present authors' experience, angiograms with portable equipment in the ICU are often inadequate for assessing fibrinolytic therapy and are less likely to detect complications such as catheter-related thrombosis than is a conventional study in the angiography suite.

During the infusion, patients may experience transient pain and changes in pulse, color, and temperature in the extremity. All of these findings are probably due to distal emboli, which tend to lyse with continued infusion, and are identical to findings in the present authors' original series. Importantly, Tisnado et al. relate that clinical improvement in the hand may precede angiographic evidence of lysis by a day or more. After fibrinolytic therapy and catheter removal, patients are maintained on heparin for 1–3 days and then on oral anticoagulants for 3–6 months. To date, Tisnado et al. have treated nine patients with acute and one patient with chronic hand ischemia successfully. None of the patients required further vascular procedures to restore flow to the hand. In the few instances of tissue loss in the hand or digital amputations, it was believed that SK decreased the extent of amputation necessary. The authors concluded that local low-dose SK infusion should be considered the treatment of choice for patients with hand ischemia who are not candidates for vascular reconstruction because of the anatomic distribution of disease.

Recently, Rapaport et al. reported the successful use of an aggressive approach combining vasodilators, intra-arterial SK, and simultaneous heparin to salvage a vein graft and an acutely ischemic reattached index finger.[106]

Widlus has recently reported his six years experience with upper extremity ischemia in eight patients. One patient was treated with streptokinase and the other with urokinase. The causes of obstruction included: atherosclerosis, thoracic outlet compression, subclavian artery aneurysm thrombosis, brachial artery cut down, cardiac emboli secondary to atrial fibrillation, and aortocarotid subclavian kink.[107]

In most instances, a high dose of 250,000 units/hr for 2 hours, followed by 40,000 to 125,000 units/hr was directly administered into the thrombus.

Patients that were treated soon after the onset of the ischemic symptoms had complete thrombolysis compared to the patients that were treated late after the onset of symptoms.

Percutaneous transluminal angioplasty corrected the underlying stenosis in three patients. Thrombolytic therapy was successful in all patients and none of them required amputations.

A case of subclavian artery thrombosis resulting in digital ischemia secondary to thoracic outlet syndrome has been successfully treated with intra-arterial urokinase.[108]

About 4 to 12% of cases of thoracic outlet syndrome patients present with subclavian vein or artery thrombosis. In Hunter's experience, 24–48 hours of therapy has produced significant clearing of subclavian and brachial thrombi. The underlying stenosis of the subclavian vein has then been corrected by transluminal angioplasty, but surgical treatment was recommended for correction of thoracic outlet syndrome.[109]

HEMODIALYSIS ACCESSES

In Becker et al.'s series, 14 patients underwent local fibrinolytic therapy for occluded dialysis accesses.[69] The six patients with fistulae were treated with the local transcatheter method described earlier in this chapter, whereas the eight patients with shunts received SK infusions of 5000 units/hr directly into the shunt and therefore did not require a catheter or simultaneous heparinization. Although complete lysis occurred in only six patients overall, there was a great discrepancy between the results for shunts (six patients had complete lysis) and those for fistulae (five patients had no change). The authors interpret this outcome as further support for the hypothesis that

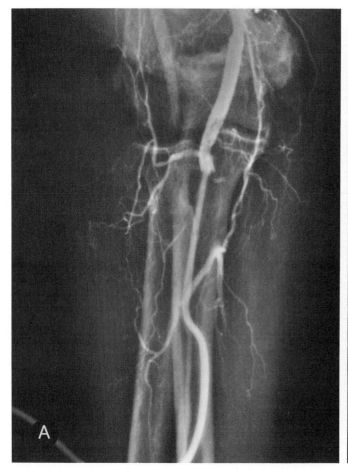
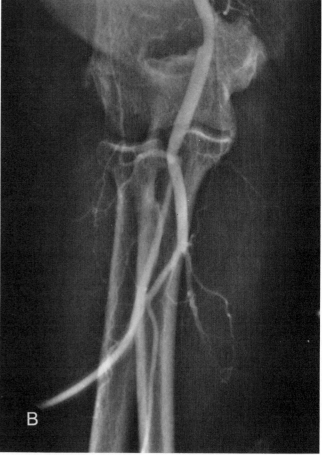

Figure 8.9. A 50-year-old woman with diminished flow through arterial limb of dialysis shunt. **A.** Preliminary study shows no common interosse-ous artery. **B.** Study after local SK through shunt without concomitant heparin shows normal common interosseous artery.

local therapy is less effective when there are numerous alternative egress channels. Figure 8.9 illustrates a representative case from this series.

In the series of Katzen and van Breda, one patient was treated for an occluded dialysis access.[66] After successful fibrinolysis, an underlying stenosis was identified. The series of Totty et al. included a single case of a thrombosed forearm dialysis access shunt. Nearly complete lysis was achieved with 19 hours of SK local therapy, and no further treatment was necessary.[68] Mori et al. treated nine patients for dialysis access thrombosis.[75] Therapeutic benefit was derived from SK alone or in combination with PTA or operation in seven cases. Ten of the patients of McNamara and Fischer were treated for occluded forearm dialysis accesses,[77] but from the presentation of the data, the degree of success cannot be ascertained.

In the series of Graor et al., 50 patients were treated for thrombosed hemodialysis fistulae.[72] Lysis was successful in 68% overall and in 84% of occlusions no more than four days old. The issue of the response to fibrinolytic therapy as a function of the duration of vascular obstruction is considered below.

Zeit reported an unusual approach to fibrinolysis for clotted dialysis accesses.[110] In two patients with thrombosed PTFE hemodialysis fistulae, following failure of more conventional infusion methods, SK was infused locally through needles placed in the occluded portion of the shunts. In one patient, a stenosis of the venous anastomosis identified after successful thrombolysis was managed with PTA.

Rodkin et al. reported their experience with local SK infusion for thrombosed PTFE dialysis accesses in nine occlusions in eight patients.[111] After diagnostic angiography, the vessels were treated through a catheter positioned in the proximal portion of the occlusion. In most cases, 40,000 units of SK were infused over 20 minutes and patients were then maintained on 5,000–7,500 units/hr in the ICU. Lysis was achieved in all but one case, and definite clinical benefit was obtained in seven of the eight patients. Three patients also underwent PTA.

Davis reported 90% success of thrombolysis followed by angioplasty of the underlying stenosis. This in turn resulted in a functional graft for hemodialysis without intervening surgery for longer than 6 months in 62% of cases.

This was achieved by depositing highly concentrated urokinase and macerating the thrombus with a crossed double catheter technique. The loop-shaped catheters are advanced into the arterial and venous ends of the dialysis graft simultaneously to macerate the thrombus, and a dose of 100,000–150,000 units of urokinase is deposited through each catheter.

The infusion is then continued at a rate of 2000 units/ min through each catheter along with the systemic administration of heparin. Lysis is achieved within a few hours and the underlying venous stenosis is overdilated with an 8mm balloon. The mean lysis time was 86 minutes, which compares very well to the 3.6 hours quoted in other series.[112]

The longest duration of manual compression for hemostasis was 8 minutes. When angiography reveals other lesions such as proximal arterial or distal venous stenosis, kinks or aneurysmal dilatations, appropriate endoluminal or surgical revision can be carried out.

Young et al. reported dismal results in treating seven episodes of acute thrombosis of PTFE dialysis fistulae in five patients.[113] After diagnostic angiography, patients underwent local transcatheter infusions of SK at dose rates ranging from 2,500–10,000 units/hr. Patients were monitored in an ICU and examined by angiography at eight-hour intervals. Infusions were terminated following either successful thrombolysis or the appearance of pain and swelling. The only two patients whose infusions resulted in lysis also underwent PTA, and only one PTA was successful. Therefore, all patients ultimately required additional surgical intervention except for one who began peritoneal dialysis when failed PTA of the venous anastomosis resulted in immediate rethrombosis.

PULSED SPRAY PHARMACOMECHANICAL THROMBOLYSIS

An enhanced method of thrombolysis has been proposed by Bookstein et al. It consists of the forceful spraying of a thrombolytic agent such as urokinase into the thrombus in short pulses along with systemic heparinization.[114]

The combination of mechanical disruption of the clot by the advancement of the infusion catheter and the spraying of the fibrinolytic agents into the thrombus reduced clot lysis time and decreased the risk of hemorrhage.

The method consists of placing a 5.0Fr end-hole catheter over a guidewire that was previously placed across the occlusion. The end hole of the catheter is occluded with a 0.032-inch beaded wire. The side holes are placed in a spiral fashion at 1cm intervals and its length is determined by the length of the thrombus. The side holes are punctured with a No. 27 or No. 30 needle. The urokinase is injected through the side arm sheath of a Tuohy–Borst adaptor at a concentration of 25,000 units/ml. About 150,000 units of urokinase are sprayed over a period of 10–15mm in 0.2ml increments with a tuberculin syringe.[114] A prototype air-driven piston syringe to replace the manual injections is being developed to achieve improved pulsatile injections with almost a nearly square wave pressure pulse.[114] The catheter is rotated by 90° and is periodically advanced to mechanically macerate the clot and to improve the homogeneous distribution of the thrombolytic agent.

This technique was employed in 41 patients with 47 thrombotic occlusions. Complete lysis was achieved in 46 of 47 occlusions with a mean completion time of 63 minutes, being 36 times faster than other reported thrombolytic protocols.[114] The complications included small distal emboli in one case and three cases of hematomas. The distal emboli were successfully lysed with further thrombolytic therapy.

Along the same lines, Kandarpa proposed a method using the forceful pulsatile local infusion of thrombolytics to accelerate thrombolysis.[115] By disrupting the clot the surface area for enzymatic action is increased, while at the same time it increases the clot-bound plasminogen for activation.[115] The accelerated thrombolysis benefits the patients by reducing the expense and morbidity associated with prolonged infusions.

The system is based on the principles of injecting short, rapid, high velocity injections of thrombolytic agents through a 3.0Fr catheter with a prototype injector.[115] Animal experiments were carried out on thrombosed inferior vena cava (IVC) of rabbits. The thrombolytic effect achieved with this method is statistically superior than with the constant infusion methods. The average percentage of lysis by weight was 54% in the pulsatile infusion group and 26% in the constant infusion group.[115]

The effect of initial penetration with the guidewire is very important with accelerated thrombolytic method, since statistically no difference was found in animals with or without guidewire penetration of thrombus.

Ten patients were subjected to thrombolysis by the accelerated method. The success rate was 90%. The duration of complete thrombolysis was 18 hours ± 14. Following thrombolysis, seven of eight patients underwent percutaneous transluminal angioplasty. The total infusion time was shorter than that of conventional constant infusion methods.[115]

New Techniques

Thrombolysis with a multiple side hole infusion catheter (EDM catheter, PSG-ACS, Mountain View, CA).

A 4.7Fr multiple side-hole catheter, with the side holes distributed over a length of 6–18cm and an end hole has been recently designed and used for thrombolysis. Its major advantage is the elimination of the need to reposition the infusion catheter, common with the single end-hole infusion catheters, thereby reducing the angiographic room time.[116]

The catheter is placed through a 5Fr sheath in an antegrade fashion for infusion of the superficial femoral artery. The end hole accommodates a 0.018-inch guidewire. The four side holes communicate with a single infusion port. For infusions in the iliac and common femoral system, the catheter is placed over a wire from the contralateral approach.

The length of the occlusion is measured from the arteriogram and the side holes are positioned in such a way that they straddle the occlusion and adequate perfusion of the thrombus can be anticipated. The duration of the infusion and the success rates of thrombolysis are not dramatically different from the standard infusion systems.[117] The catheter minimized, however, the complications of catheter exchanges, since it eliminated catheter reposition.

Mesenteric Arteries

Flickinger et al. reported a patient with a superior mesenteric artery embolic occlusion due to atrial fibrillation who was treated with local low-dose transcatheter SK infusion.[118] The patient was thought to be a poor operative candidate because of poor cardiopulmonary status, including three previous myocardial infarctions. At the time of diagnostic angiography, ischemic bowel symptoms had been present for only three hours. Although the infusion was started at 5,000 units/hr, a repeat arteriogram after three hours of therapy showed minimal improvement, and the catheter was advanced and the infusion rate increased to 10,000 units/hr. After much clinical improvement and evidence of significant thrombolysis on the 60-hour angiogram, the dose rate was decreased to 5,000 units/hr. After a total of 80 hours of infusion and resolution of the symptoms, angiography showed nearly normal vessels, and the infusion was terminated. The authors emphasized that patients with findings of bowel infarction require rapid diagnosis and surgical intervention but that certain patients with ischemic bowel may respond nicely to local SK infusion.

Pillari et al. reported a patient with congestive heart failure and transvenous pacing who had embolic occlusions of both the celiac artery and the superior mesenteric arteries.[119] Bilateral transfemoral catheters were placed selectively, one in the celiac artery and the other in the superior mesenteric artery. Each catheter provided an infusion dose rate of 5000 units/hr of SK, and the patient's ischemic bowel recovered without surgical intervention.

With so few cases reported, the role of fibrinolytic therapy in the management of ischemic bowel has not yet been adequately defined.

Local SK has been successful in treating hepatic artery thrombosis resulting from intra-arterial chemotherapy.[120]

Renal Arteries

One patient in the series of Katzen and van Breda underwent local transcatheter SK infusion for renal artery occlusion. Successful lysis in this case allowed subsequent PTA.[66] Three patients in the series of Dardik et al. were treated with local transcatheter SK for acute renal artery thrombosis. All achieved successful thrombolysis, and all required PTA for correction of an underlying stenosis.[73] One of the patients in the series of Mori et al. was treated for embolic occlusion of a renal artery, but the results are not evident from the grouping of the data.[75] Lang's series includes four patients with occluded synthetic aortorenal grafts and one patient with an occluded renal artery in a cadaveric allograft kidney who were treated with local transcatheter SK. Although the author does not specify the percentage of responders in this group, he does state that his greatest degree of success was in patients with thrombosed synthetic grafts (lysis in 11 of 12 cases).[74]

As with mesenteric thrombolysis, the experience with local transcatheter renal artery thrombolysis is not sufficient to define its role.

VEINS

There is much information attesting to the value of systemic SK therapy for acute DVT of the legs.[58,121–131] These studies indicate that SK improves the potential for early restoration of normal blood flow in addition to preventing thrombus extension and embolization and make systemic SK therapy appear more attractive than anticoagulation with heparin. However, little has been done to evaluate local (second-generation) therapy with SK and UK in venous occlusive disease, and most of the available information is anecdotal. The following sections review much of the accumulated clinical experience.

Lower Extremities

The present authors' experience with second-generation therapy in lower extremity DVT is entirely anecdotal. They have treated two patients, both of whom had extensive iliofemoral and calf DVT. The first was treated with a dorsal pedal vein infusion of SK at 5000 units/hr and semi-upright positioning. The patient suffered mild superficial phlebitis on the dorsum of the foot but had no improvement on his venogram the following day, so the infusion was terminated. The second patient was treated as follows. A transfemoral arterial catheter was passed over the aortic bifurcation and into the contralateral common femoral artery (ipsilateral to the venous thrombi). An infusion of 5000 units/hr of SK was started, and the patient was observed in the ICU. Tourniquets were applied at the ankle and knee in an effort to promote deep venous drainage and routing of the fibrinolytic solution. There was no clinically or radiographically demonstrable benefit.

Inferior Vena Cava (IVC)

Greenwood et al. reported a patient with Budd–Chiari syndrome following viral perimyocarditis.[132] Peritoneoscopy with liver biopsy revealed dilatation of central lobular sinusoids and fibrosis surrounding the central lobular veins, but no evidence of cirrhosis. Computed tomography (CT) and inferior venacavography disclosed intraluminal filling defects in the IVC between the level of the renal veins and the right atrium. Urokinase was given through the IVC catheter as a local infusion in large doses, the patient being given 308,000 units (4,400 units/kg) as a loading dose and then 4,400 units/hr as a continuous infusion (systemic doses). After 55 hours of infusion, there was marked improvement in flow in the IVC. The patient's pain, ascites, and edema rapidly resolved.

Prior to this report, SK had been used to treat hepatic vein thrombosis in a patient on oral contraceptives.[133] Pulmonary emboli occurred. Because of this potential for life-threatening pulmonary emboli during thrombolytic ther-

apy,[134] the danger of such emboli must always be considered. However, Greenwood et al. cite evidence that the risk of this complication does not appear higher for thrombolytic therapy than for treatment with heparin alone, at least in peripheral DVT.[132]

Superior Vena Cava (SVC)

In 1981, SK treatment of a patient with idiopathic SVC thrombosis was reported.[135] The largest experience with local low-dose thrombolytic therapy using SK in cases of SVC occlusion has been reported by Graor et al., who successfully treated six patients with this problem.[72] All of the occlusions were <72 hours old. Catheters were introduced through an arm vein and positioned within the most distally occluded segment.

The danger of pulmonary embolization during thrombolytic therapy for SVC obstruction should parallel that of IVC obstruction.

Axillary and Subclavian Veins

This is one area in the venous system in which local transcatheter low-dose fibrinolytic therapy is rapidly becoming the treatment of choice. Idiopathic axillary and subclavian vein thrombosis is known by a variety of names, including "gouty phlebitis," "spontaneous subclavian vein thrombosis," "effort thrombosis of the subclavian vein," and "primary axillary-subclavian vein thrombosis." Since Paget originally described the disease,[136] none of the available therapeutic options, including bed rest, bed rest with anticoagulation, thrombectomy, thrombectomy with rib resection, and stellate ganglion blockade, have proved entirely satisfactory.[137,138] Chronic disability may result from pain with use of the arm (venous claudication), recurrent swelling, or nonfatal pulmonary emboli (5–10%).

Becker et al.'s original small series of patients treated with transcatheter local thrombolytic therapy for this disorder[139] has expanded to 11 patients,[140] and review of the clinical entity and this experience is in order. Primary axillary-subclavian vein thrombosis is an entity distinct from subclavian vein thrombosis secondary to central venous catheterization, malignancy, and other causes. Two-thirds of the patients are male and 40 years of age or less. Two-thirds give a history of unusual or vigorous exercise prior to the onset of symptoms. In Becker et al.'s series, all patients had better than average upper extremity strength, and most were able to relate a particularly strenuous or unusual exercise that led to thrombosis. Weight lifting was common. Cyanosis of the extremity (which may be present only upon exertion), swelling, and prominent venous collaterals about the shoulder and anterior chest are important physical findings, which were present, to various degrees, in these patients. There are two venographic patterns. One is a long-segment obstruction of the axillary and subclavian veins, and the other is a short-segment obstruction of the axillary-subclavian venous segment at the level of the first rib-clavicle junction anteriorly.

Catheterization of an antecubital vein in a patient with significant upper extremity edema can be time-consuming and frustrating. The difficulty can be overcome by injecting the contrast medium into a hand vein, then puncturing the antecubital vein under fluoroscopic guidance. Once the vein has been cannulated, a guidewire is positioned in the subclavian vein at the level of occlusion and followed with a 5Fr catheter for venography and infusion. Patients with recent streptococcal infection or a high SK antibody titer are poor candidates for SK therapy. One of the authors' patients initially treated with SK suffered propagation of the thrombus but then responded promptly when the infusion solution was changed to UK. These problems, and the fact that 3 of their 11 patients had drug-related fevers while on SK, make them feel that UK is the drug of choice for this condition.

Once the catheter has been embedded within the thrombus, UK at 20,000 units/hr is started via infusion pump. A second infusion pump is required for concomitant intravenous heparin administration at a dose rate sufficient to maintain the PTT at 1.5 times normal. Progress is monitored with serial transcatheter venograms in the radiology department. In all of the present authors' cases, complete or nearly complete lysis was achieved using these methods. Figure 8.10 illustrates one of the cases.

Importantly, in each case, after successful thrombolysis, they were able to demonstrate irregularity, stenosis, or both phlebographically in the subclavian vein at the first rib-clavicle junction anteriorly. The authors have hypothesized that this abnormality is the important structural causative factor in this disorder and therefore have chosen to call it by another name: the "thoracic inlet syndrome." The anatomic (Fig. 8.11) and functional etiologic factors in the development of this syndrome are not completely understood. Subclavian and axillary vein compression by the costocoracoid ligament, subclavius muscle, and clavicle against the first rib may all be important. Stasis, recurrent trauma, and venospasm have been implicated. Regardless

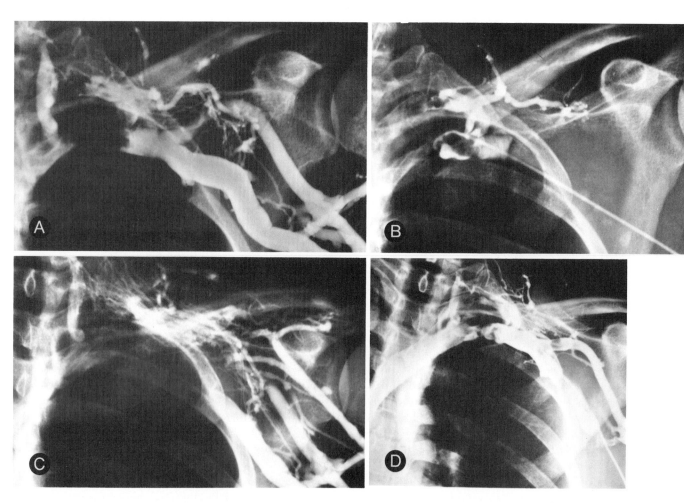

Figure 8.10.   This 35-year-old amateur weight lifter presented with left upper extremity swelling and pain after attempting to lift his car from underneath. **A.** Venogram shows short-segment subclavian vein occlusion in the region of first rib-clavicle junction anteriorly. **B.** Catheter tip positioned in occlusion for local SK. **C.** Venogram after SK shows worsened occlusion. Patient's SK resistance (blood drawn before infusion started) was later found to be markedly elevated, so infusion was changed to UK. **D.** After local UK, thrombus has been almost entirely cleared, and residual stenosis is identified in the typical location (first rib-clavicle junction anteriorly). Patient subsequently underwent venous bypass.

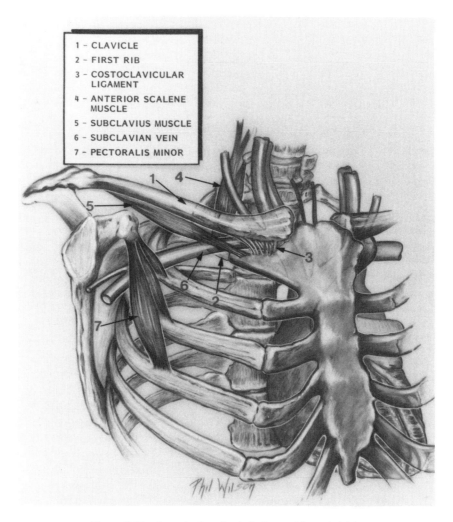

1 - CLAVICLE
2 - FIRST RIB
3 - COSTOCLAVICULAR
    LIGAMENT
4 - ANTERIOR SCALENE
    MUSCLE
5 - SUBCLAVIUS MUSCLE
6 - SUBCLAVIAN VEIN
7 - PECTORALIS MINOR

Figure 8.11.   Important anatomic features of thoracic inlet.

of the precise mechanisms involved, the venographic abnormality is consistently present.

Two patients in this series with only small stenoses improved symptomatically after fibrinolytic therapy and were maintained for a time on oral anticoagulants as outpatients. One had PTA of the subclavian vein, which resulted in venographic evidence of partial resolution of the stenosis. Five underwent venous bypass procedures, the efficacy of which has not yet been determined. Three had significant residual stenosis but have had no further treatment except oral anticoagulants. Perivascular fibrosis and mural abnormalities in the subclavian vein were found consistently in the patients who went to surgery. None of the patients in this series had hemorrhagic complications or clinical evidence of pulmonary emboli.

Patients with venous infusion catheters frequently suffer local inflammatory reactions to the catheter, fibrinolytic agent, or contrast medium. Reactions may be manifest as pain and local tenderness with or without rubor. Some authors have suggested simultaneous administration of corticosteroids to alleviate or prevent this problem, but the present authors have no experience with this.

Central Venous Lines

Double-lumen Hickman central venous catheters have been used for long-term access for transfusions and chemotherapy in patients with malignancy (JJ Reilly Jr, DL Steed, PS Ritter, unpublished data). Although a twice-daily flush with heparin solution usually preserves patency, occlusions do occur, and fibrin sheaths around the catheter tip and shaft may prevent effective venous access.[140,142]

Zajko et al. reported a series of 16 episodes of Hickman catheter occlusions in 14 patients.[143] In three instances, a mechanical problem was responsible; in the remaining 13, venography performed by direct injection of contrast medium into the catheter disclosed a fibrin sheath occluding its distal end. In each of these 13 instances, SK infusion was started using 3000 units/lumen/hr. This was continued for 12 hours, at which time venography was repeated. In 12 cases, venography revealed catheter patency. In the remaining case, infusion was continued for another 12 hours without therapeutic benefit. In this case, the catheter had been occluded for longer than two weeks.

Although others have used fibrinolytic therapy to

restore patency to central venous catheters, the results are difficult to assess because venography was not used.[144,145]

PULMONARY ARTERIES

Human Studies

The large experience with systemic (first-generation) fibrinolytic therapy for pulmonary thromboembolic disease (PTE) that resulted from UPET and USPET was described previously. Recently, several authors have described their experiences with transcatheter local fibrinolytic therapy for PTE.

Barbarena reported 11 patients who were treated with local transcatheter UK for acute PTE.[146] All patients had had symptoms for <12 hours. All had symptoms of acute PTE, but only one presented with shock. Six PTE were postoperative events (3–26 days). All patients underwent pulmonary angiography with an 8Fr, 100cm NIH cardiovascular catheter positioned in the main trunk of the pulmonary artery regardless of the location or suspected location of the embolus. Follow-up angiograms to assess therapeutic benefit were obtained at 48 hours in nine patients, at 24 hours in one, and at 72 hours in one. Infusions of UK were made through the angiography catheter, which was not moved after the diagnostic study. A loading dose of 2700 units/kg was administered over 5–10 minutes, and then a continuous infusion of 2700 units/kg/hr was maintained for 12 hours. Longer infusions were not attempted because data from UPET do not suggest that longer systemic UK infusions provide additional benefit. After fibrinolytic therapy, all patients were given intravenous heparin. All 11 patients improved clinically, and 9 improved electrocardiographically. One patient who showed evidence of only partial improvement on ECG later underwent embolectomy. Angiographically demonstrable improvement, assessed by the objective scoring method of Miller et al.,[147] was seen in all cases, with a somewhat greater improvement noted in perfusion than in the grade of obstruction. Complications, which were frequent in this series, are discussed below.

Vujic et al. treated three patients who had severe pulmonary emboli using full heparinization in combination with transcatheter low-dose SK.[148] In each case, the diagnosis was confirmed by angiography and the decision to use SK instead of operation was made because of severe or terminal underlying disease. Two patients had only acute emboli and one had had recurrent emboli over a three-week period. Pulmonary angiography and SK infusion were accomplished using a 6.7Fr Grollman pulmonary angiography catheter placed via a transfemoral approach. In one case, the catheter was positioned as near to the embolus as possible, in another within the embolus, and in the remaining patient, who had large bilateral emboli, at the bifurcation of the main pulmonary artery. The dose rate of SK was 10,000 units/hr, and simultaneous heparin was administered intravenously at 1,000 units/hr. Pulmo-

nary artery pressure and arterial PaO_2 were monitored, and shrinkage of the embolus was evaluated by follow-up pulmonary arteriography. All three patients responded favorably to this regimen. In the first case, the pulmonary artery pressure decreased from 40/19mm Hg before treatment to 22/12mm Hg after 16 hours of treatment, while the PaO_2 increased from 56 to 76 torr within 6 hours. In the second case, the pulmonary artery pressure decreased from 56/24 to 35/22mm Hg by 6 hours and 32/16mm Hg by 30 hours, while the PaO_2 went from 40 torr on 100% FiO_2 to 69 torr on 40% FiO_2. In the patient with recurrent emboli the PaO_2 increased from 38 to 85 torr after 16 hours of infusion. Although the pulmonary artery pressure did not change significantly in this patient, it had been only minimally elevated before treatment (28/10mm Hg).

The authors of this report make several interesting points about the method and their findings, as well as about the findings of others. They state that direct delivery of SK to the embolus enhances SK-plasminogen interaction by minimizing exposure of the drug to antibodies and endogenous inhibitors. At the same time, bleeding due to systemic fibrinolytic states can be avoided, because the drug can be given at much lower dose rates. The authors also think that patients with severe obstruction due to PTE have faster and more extensive lytic responses to local therapy, because severe obstruction provides more time for SK-plasminogen interaction. (As we shall see, more rapid lysis is not necessarily better lysis.) Finally, Vujic et al. think that mechanical fragmentation of the embolus by the catheter tip may enhance the lytic response by creating a larger surface for SK-plasminogen interaction.[148]

Of the 159 patients in the series of Graor et al., 10 were treated for severe pulmonary emboli involving a main or two or more lobar pulmonary arteries.[72] This experience has now expanded to include 13 patients.[149] In 10, emboli were <72 hours old; in 3, they were 1 week old. Mean pulmonary artery pressures were elevated (>30mm Hg), and all patients were hemodynamically unstable and in need of 100% FiO_2 to maintain normal arterial oxygenation. The first 10 had pulmonary angiography and local SK infusion through a 6Fr Grollman pulmonary angiography catheter or a 7Fr cardiovascular catheter at 5,000–10,000 units/hr plus concomitant systemic heparinization until the next daily pulmonary angiogram. At angiography, if no lysis had occurred, SK was discontinued. If lysis was incomplete and there were no signs of bleeding, the heparin was discontinued and the SK dose rate was increased to 100,000 units/hr. Infusions were continued until there was complete lysis or lack of further progress. In the last three patients, SK was started at 100,000 units/hr without systemic heparinization. If follow-up angiography showed either complete or no lysis, the infusion was terminated, whereas if angiography disclosed partial lysis, the infusion was continued at the same dose rate until lysis was complete. All patients received conventional anticoagulant therapy after the SK regimen was completed. As in the other patients, these patients received intravenous cephalosporins every 6 hours during and for 24 hours after therapy. Patients were monitored with Swan–Ganz catheters in the ICU.

Lytic therapy was successful in 11 of these 13 patients. Blood pressures, pulse, and respiratory rates returned to normal, and patients became increasingly comfortable. These clinical signs of improvement occurred between 6 and 18 hours after the start of local SK. By 24 hours, pulmonary artery pressures and arterial PaO_2 were normal or near baseline. One of the failures was in a patient eight days postresection of an abdominal aortic aneurysm; this patient's low-dose infusion was terminated when a retroperitoneal hemorrhage occurred. In the high-dose group, two of the three patients had complete lysis, one after 24 hours of therapy and the other after 48 hours. The remaining patient was a treatment failure who eventually required embolectomy. Seven of the 11 successfully treated patients had follow-up ventilation-perfusion lung scans showing complete resolution of the perfusion abnormalities.

Figure 8.12 illustrates the use of local fibrinolytic therapy in a patient with PTE.

Animal Studies

Over the past two years, Holden et al. have developed an animal model for comparing systemic and local fibrinolytic therapy for PTE.[150] Although the details of this work are not relevant here, a few of the salient features must be described, if only to temper enthusiasm for local fibrinolytic therapy in the pulmonary circulation. The authors' model involves adult New Zealand White rabbits, transcatheter embolization of autologous clot prepared in vitro, and a multiparametric assessment of the effects of fibrinolytic infusions. Animals were treated with high-dose SK infused in a peripheral vein, in the pulmonary artery with the catheter tip above the clot, or in the pulmonary artery with the catheter tip embedded in the clot.

All pulmonary arterial infusions (intraclot and above the clot) resulted in more rapid and thorough lysis (more lysis of intraluminal clot within the time of the experiment) than did peripheral intravenous infusions. Although rapid lysis would appear to be desirable, this is not necessarily the case. These results indicate that rapid lysis with intraclot infusion produces extensive obstruction of small pulmonary vessels, with obliteration of capillary perfusion (Fig. 8.13), in contrast to the relatively preserved pulmonary capillary perfusion that may be seen with intravenous infusion. The return of pulmonary capillary perfusion in obstructed portions of the lung in some of the animals during continued infusion suggests that blockade of small pulmonary vessels is an intermediate phenomenon resulting from fragmentation of clot during infusion and that perfusion is restored as clot fragments are lysed. It is impor-

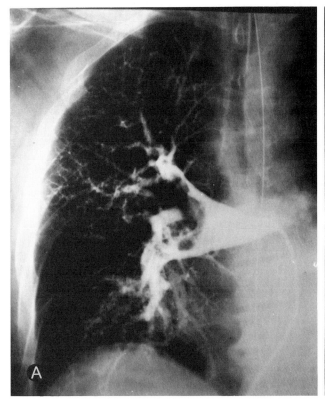
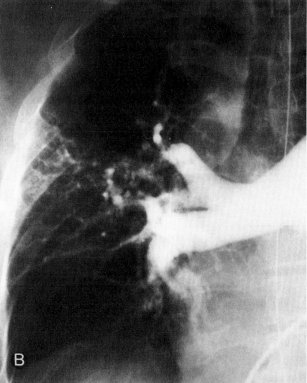

Figure 8.12. Patient with severe pulmonary embolus. **A.** Initial pulmonary angiogram reveals large embolus at bifurcation of right pulmonary artery. Note that upper lobe perfusion is intact. **B.** Angiogram after 24 hours of local SK at 60,000 units/hr shows that extensive lysis has occurred. However, note lack of perfusion in right upper lobe. This change is probably due to fragmentation and peripheral embolization.

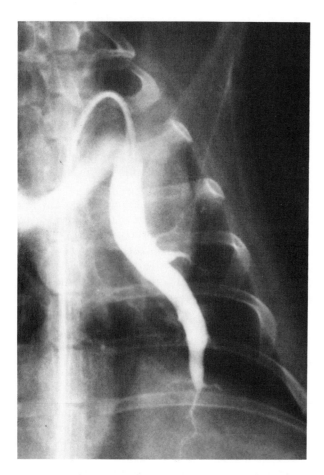

Figure 8.13. Rabbit pulmonary angiogram after 4.5 hours of transcatheter infusion of a total of 125,000 units of SK. Extensive rapid fibrinolysis has resulted in dissolution of all previously visible clot in left main pulmonary artery. Note absence of pulmonary capillary perfusion; this is caused by fragmentation of the clot as a result of rapid lysis.

tant to remember, however, that many patients probably cannot tolerate this extent of capillary blockade even for a short time. The critical point is that although fibrinolytic therapy for PTE can be lifesaving, there are instances in which it can be life threatening.

It appears from this model that one of the most important differences between central (pulmonary artery) infusions and peripheral (intravenous) infusions is the higher enzyme concentration bathing the clot with the former. Rapid fibrinolysis produced by infusion of higher enzyme concentrations increases the frequency of clot fragmentation, whereas the slower fibrinolysis produced by lower enzyme concentrations creates more soluble FDPs and relatively little pulmonary capillary blockade. There are many patients with lung disease, a diminished pulmonary capillary bed, or elevated right-sided intracardiac pressures who probably cannot tolerate clot fragmentation with pulmonary capillary blockade even as an intermediate phase. In these patients, the authors suggest monitoring right atrial and pulmonary artery pressures during therapy.

These findings and the limited clinical experience with second-generation fibrinolytic therapy in PTE serve to underscore the fact that the role of this method in the pulmonary arterial circulation is just beginning to be defined.

CORONARY ARTERIES

Since the original report of Rentrop et al. on the use of local fibrinolytic therapy for coronary occlusion,[67] many additional series have appeared in the literature.

Coronary artery thrombosis is present in approximately 90% of patients with acute myocardial infarction (AMI).[151] Prior to the elucidation of this fact, there was no pathophysiologic basis for taking aggressive measures to alleviate coronary obstruction in cases of AMI. Rather, most treatments focused on administering coronary vasodilators, decreasing myocardial oxygen demand, and improving myocardial oxygenation. Although the first use of selective SK administration for coronary occlusion was reported in 1960,[152] the method did not gain wide acceptance because of several problems. First, the reported success of those first authors was not documented by angiography. Second, the hemorrhagic risks were thought to be unacceptably high. Third, even though it was known that coronary angiography could easily be used to document coronary occlusion and resolution, most investigators were reluctant to subject their patients to coronary angiography in the acute phase of AMI.

In 1976, Chazov et al. reported the first angiographically documented selective fibrinolysis-mediated coronary recanalization.[153] Widespread enthusiasm developed after the report of Rentrop et al.[67] Because most interventional radiologists do not do selective coronary thrombolysis, and because the literature is too extensive to review thoroughly in this chapter, only a few comments will be made on this topic.

Patients selected for intracoronary thrombolysis must present within the first few hours of the onset of symptoms of AMI for there to be any likelihood of myocardial salvage by coronary recanalization. The procedure requires a 24-hour on-call emergency angiography team, and a backup cardiovascular surgical team is advisable, if not essential. Once the diagnosis is established by electrocardiogram (ECG) and clinical impression, the patient is moved to the catheterization laboratory as quickly as possible. During that time, oxygen, nitroglycerin, and other standard supportive measures are given.

According to the methods outlined by Paulin and Als,[154] patients are given 5,000 units of prophylactic heparin intravenously, and selective coronary catheterization, with or without preliminary ventriculography, is performed for diagnostic angiography in both coronary arteries in at least two projections via a transfemoral approach. Repeat angiography after 0.2mg of intracoronary nitroglycerin has been given documents the fixed nature of the occlusion. Following a hand-injected bolus of 20,000 units of SK in 20ml, Paulin and Als use a continuous intracoronary infusion of 4,000 units/min (4ml/min) administered via infusion pump. Signs of improvement include abatement of symptoms, lowering of ST segments on continuous ECG monitoring, mild hypotension, and new onset of arrhythmias. These indicators of success generally occur within 0.5 hour of the start of the infusion.

Other specific actions can be taken during the 0.5-hour delay, including placement of a mobile γ camera for ventricular function studies, repeat full 12-lead ECG, etc. Angiographic monitoring is achieved by selective injections of contrast medium at 15-minute intervals. If patency is re-established but flow velocity is less than normal, the infusion is slowed to 2,000 units/min (2ml/min). Generally, this can be continued for as long as an hour without exceeding a total dose of 250,000 units. After the fibrinolytic infusion is completed, a complete coronary arteriogram is performed. Repeat ECG and assessment of left ventricular function by radionuclide scanning can be done at this time as well. Heparinization is continued, and the patient is sent to the ICU with the sheath still in place at the puncture site; this provides hemostasis in the immediate post-treatment period and provides immediate easy access if repeat coronary arteriography becomes necessary.

In the experience of Paulin and Als, as well as that of others, successful reperfusion (not identical to myocardial salvage) occurs in approximately 70–75% of cases.[154] Often, the flow is slow initially, possibly indicating distal emboli in the coronary circulation that lyse with continued infusion. It has been known for some time that this occurs during fibrinolytic therapy for other types of thromboembolic disease, and there now is evidence that it also occurs with significant frequency in the coronary circulation.[155] In the report of Paulin and Als, reperfusion was said to be complete when the velocity and pattern of contrast flow in the involved vessel paralleled that in uninvolved coronary arteries. When flow appeared ineffective or incomplete, the authors were able to demonstrate persistent defects on thallium-201 myocardial scans.

Successful reperfusion often leads to the discovery of underlying stenosis, just as it does in the peripheral vasculature, and some of these lesions are amenable to percutaneous transluminal coronary angioplasty (PTCA). Definitive measures, such as coronary bypass grafting and PTCA, must be applied to individual patients on the basis of the clinical circumstances, expected outcomes, and analysis of treatment alternatives. Angioplasty may be considered in the immediate postfibrinolysis period if clinical and ECG evidence of persistent ischemia is present.

Predischarge follow-up angiography, practiced by many, often discloses further resolution of an area of "stenosis." This finding probably indicates continued lysis of thrombus that is adherent to the vessel wall immediately after treatment.

What is the correlation between reperfusion and myocardial salvage? Coronary occlusion leads to decreased myocardial contractility within minutes,[156] yet short-ived occlusions do not necessarily damage myocardial cells.[157,158] In dogs, hypokinesia can persist for 30 minutes

after restoration of coronary flow in instances of transient occlusion ("stunned myocardium"),[159] and the longer the duration of occlusion, the smaller the degree of recovery after re-establishment of normal flow. In the same canine models, occlusions for ≥6 hours are followed by little if any myocardial recovery. Paulin and Als suggest, however, that these results cannot readily be extrapolated to coronary occlusion in man, because of the usual presence there of atheromatous disease and variably developed collaterals. That is, it is theoretically possible that patients with atherosclerotic coronary disease would be able to tolerate longer durations of coronary occlusion than the dogs because of the presence of these collaterals.

There is evidence that left ventricular function studies are not as sensitive for determinating the degree of myocardial salvage as is thallium-201 myocardial scanning.[160]

Currently, local thrombolytic therapy for AMI must be viewed as being in the stage of clinical investigation. Nevertheless, strong support for its use may be found in the results of the Western Washington Randomized Trial in which 250 patients who were treated with selective intracoronary SK had a significant reduction in group 30-day mortality.[161] High-dose intravenous SK infusion for AMI has its proponents[162] and must be considered seriously as an alternative to second-generation therapy, especially in view of the fact that only a minority of hospitals have the cardiac catheterization laboratories needed to institute the selective method. Nonetheless, although the results of intravenous infusion are encouraging, they have not been as favorable as those achieved with the selective method.

Recently, results of clinical trials using tPA for AMI have been reported.[163,164] Although the percentage of patients responding has been extremely high, hemorrhagic complications have occurred.

CENTRAL NERVOUS SYSTEM

Investigators are working on methods of infusing UK directly into acutely occluded middle cerebral arteries in humans with the aid of flow-directed balloon catheters. Although these endeavors to recanalize acutely occluded carotid arteries appear exciting, one must remember that acute cerebral reperfusion may carry a high morbidity and mortality rate as a result of cerebral hemorrhage.[165]

To test the potential of local fibrinolytic therapy in acute carotid occlusion resulting from operation or angiography, Eskridge et al. recently studied transcatheter local fibrinolysis in a canine model of acute carotid occlusion.[166] They found the risk of hemorrhage from reperfusion to be unacceptably high, and it is with these data in mind that they discourage the use of local fibrinolytic therapy for acute carotid occlusion. Perhaps further studies will not corroborate this impression, but, for now, extreme caution is recommended.

In a recent study with New Zealand White rabbits, Narayan et al. tested the safety and efficacy of UK in lysing intracranial hematomas.[167] Using stereotactically guided equipment, the authors injected clotted human blood into the frontal lobes and lateral ventricles of these animals. A direct injection of 50,000 units of UK was then given to the test animals and saline was administered to the controls. Hematomas were lysed in 90% of the experimental animals, whereas only 14% of the control hematomas were lysed. The possible future application of this method in neurosurgery or in CT-guided interventional neuroradiology is unclear.

LABORATORY MONITORING

In first-generation fibrinolytic therapy with SK or UK, a systemic fibrinolytic state, characterized by conversion of circulating plasminogen to plasmin, is required for success. This is not to say that activation of plasminogen that is bound within the thrombus or embolus is inadequate; rather, the method of administration and the doses required entail generalized plasminogen activation. Remember that circulating plasmin is a nonspecific protease, which cleaves and inactivates not only fibrin, but also fibrinogen, factors V and VIII, and other proteins. This has an obvious anticoagulant effect. Remember, too, that FDPs resulting from cleavage of fibrin and fibrinogen have their own inhibitory effect on the coagulation cascade. This, in turn, results in further anticoagulation. In second-generation therapy, on the other hand, one attempts to activate the plasminogen that is bound within the thrombus or embolus, and a systemic fibrinolytic state is therefore considered a side effect. The available laboratory tests for monitoring the fibrinolytic state have been reviewed in detail by Ramchandani and Soulen.[168] A summary is provided here.

Free circulating plasmin may be measured directly by radioimmunoassay (RIA), by the fibrin plate method, or by euglobulin lysis time. The RIA is complex and not widely available. The fibrin plate method takes 16–20 hours, making it impractical for guiding clinical decisions. Therefore, euglobulin lysis time is the most widely utilized direct method. In this test, acidification of the patient's blood precipitates fibrinogen and the fibrinolytically active plasma components (euglobulin precipitate). Thrombin is added to the precipitate, and the clot lysis time is measured. A normal value is 3–4 hours; during fibrinolytic therapy, the time is usually much less than 1 hour. Although it is sensitive, the euglobulin lysis test is an exacting method and is not widely available on a 24-hour basis. Therefore, indirect tests are often indicated.

The blood fibrinogen level is the most useful and widely used indirect test. Since fibrinogen is a major substrate of plasmin that can be measured, it provides a useful index of fibrinolytic activity. Whereas normal levels are approximately 300–400mg/dl, most experts believe that 100mg/dl is required for adequate hemostasis. In this test, thrombin is added to a sample of the patient's blood, and thrombin clotting time is measured; the value obtained is inversely proportional to the fibrinogen concentration. A normal thrombin time must be within 5 seconds of control, and typical control values are 18–22 seconds. This test can be utilized in most cases of systemic fibrinolytic therapy, but if the patient is receiving local therapy with heparin, the test is invalid, because heparin increases the thrombin (clotting) time.

A second useful indirect test is the measurement of FDPs. These products accumulate in the blood during systemic fibrinolytic therapy and are specific for lysis of fibrinogen or fibrin by plasmin. A normal value is $<10\mu g/ml$. One must appreciate an interrelation between the laboratory measures; increased FDPs prolong thrombin time through their anticoagulant effect.

The PTT is insensitive in detecting a systemic fibrinolytic state but is a good screen for the intrinsic coagulation pathway. The authors have recently used only the PTT, measured every four hours, to monitor patients on local low-dose fibrinolytic therapy given concomitant heparin to prevent pericatheter thrombosis. The authors attempt to keep the PTT at approximately 1.5 times normal, whereas others attempt to keep it even higher (2.0–3.0 times normal). If the PTT is longer than desired, the heparin infusion rate is decreased or the heparin is replaced with saline until the next measurement but the SK or UK infusion rate is not altered. It should be remembered that during administration of this combination form of therapy, there generally is a decrease in the dose rate of heparin required to maintain the PTT at the desired value because of the anticoagulant effects of plasmin and FDPs.

Why are the fibrinolytic values not measured in such cases? There are two reasons. First, there are insufficient data showing that abnormal values correspond to a tendency for patients to hemorrhage. Second, as detailed above, in the presence of heparin, the common measures are rendered invalid. The reptilase clotting time can be used to monitor the systemic fibrinolytic state in the presence of heparin anticoagulation, but it is expensive and not readily available, particularly on a 24-hour basis.

To reiterate, no single laboratory test is a reliable predictor of the degree of lysis or of the likelihood of a hemorrhagic complication.[169–171] Therefore, the laboratory tests used to assess the systemic fibrinolytic state can only warn of severe hypofibrinogenemia and fibrinolysis.

It is probably useful to obtain certain laboratory data before beginning fibrinolytic therapy. A complete blood count, including platelets, plus PT and PTT constitutes a readily available standard screen. In addition, if SK is to be used, an anti-SK antibody titer (SK resistance test) can be obtained. In systemic fibrinolytic therapy, it is desirable to neutralize existing antibody before starting the maintenance infusion. This was the logic that led to the development of the loading dose concept. A 250,000-unit bolus of SK administered over 30 minutes is sufficient to neutralize existing antibody in approximately 90% of patients.[51] The intravenous systemic maintenance infusion can then begin.

Such a large bolus seems counterproductive in cases of local therapy, and in fact, the importance of anti-SK antibody in such cases is poorly understood. However, the authors have seen patients fail on local SK infusion yet respond beautifully to UK infusion and therefore suspect that anti-SK antibodies can influence the outcome of this therapy. Obviously, patient selection is important: one need not measure SK resistance in a patient recently (within the preceding six months) treated with SK to know that UK is the preferred drug.

COMPLICATIONS

The hemorrhagic complications of systemic infusion of fibrinolytic agents have been amply covered already; this section deals with the complications of local infusion.

The reader need only review the variety of second-generation treatment regimens to appreciate the complexity in understanding the complications and the frequencies of their occurrence. Palaskas et al. have reviewed this topic,[63] and the information in the following sections derives from their work, as well as from a review of several series.

Hemorrhage

It is safe to say that local transcatheter fibrinolytic therapy has not done away with hemorrhagic complications, even though it was hoped that it might. However, it probably has reduced their frequency. In the original series of Dotter et al., 17 patients received SK at the rate of 5000 units/hr, and 4 had significant bleeding complications.[64] Although this frequency seems to compare favorably with that in UPET (45%), Dotter et al. did not report data on hemoglobin or hematocrit, so there may have been undetected bleeding. This deficiency is noted in almost all reports of second-generation therapy. Importantly, hemorrhage during fibrinolytic therapy is usually due to dissolution of hemostatic plugs at sites of recent vascular trauma, although gastrointestinal, intracranial, and retroperitoneal bleeding and other serious hemorrhagic complications can occur.

Feissinger et al. identified six intracranial hemorrhages or emboli and 18 other bleeding complications in a series of 194 patients treated with systemic UK.[172] They also reported a series of 25 patients treated with local UK[173] in whom there were no serious hemorrhagic complications, although three patients bled slightly from the catheter insertion site. In the series of 12 local infusions reported by Katzen and van Breda, two patients who bled at the puncture site did so only after the addition of heparin, and the bleeding ceased when heparin was stopped.[66] In the series of 26 local infusions reported by Totty et al., SK was used in dose rates of 2,500–10,000 units/hr and UK in dose rates of 40,000–80,000 units/hr. All five patients with serious complications had bleeding at the catheter insertion site, although only two required transfusion with

packed red cells or whole blood. In this series, cryoprecipitate was administered to patients whose fibrinogen levels dropped to <100mg/dl.[68]

In Becker et al.'s original series of 57 local infusions plus concomitant intravenous heparin, significant hemorrhagic complications occurred in 12.2% of the patients, and only one of these patients required an operation because of the bleeding. One of the other major hemorrhages was intracerebral, but it developed in a patient whose markedly prolonged PTT had gone unrecognized for an inordinately long time. Three of the serious hemorrhages were gastrointestinal. Another 14% of patients suffered minor hemorrhagic complications not necessitating intervention.[69]

In the series of Hess et al., whose method requires a total SK dose much lower than in most other methods, only 3 of 136 patients receiving local infusion had hematomas at the catheter insertion site. No serious hemorrhagic complications occurred.[70] In the series of 159 local infusions reported by Graor et al. serious hemorrhagic complications, defined as those necessitating blood transfusion or operation or resulting in clinical deterioration, occurred in 17 patients (10.7%). Only 3.8% of these hemorrhages were at sites remote from the catheter insertion. Another 27 patients (17%) had slight bleeding at the catheter entry site.[72]

In the series of 50 local infusions of SK reported by Mori et al. minor bleeding, usually from the arterial puncture site, occurred in 30% of patients, and serious hemorrhage necessitating transfusion or operation occurred in 8%.[75] Only three hematomas (one retroperitoneal) occurred in the 38 infusions (28 local) reported by Dardik et al.[73] In a series of complications reported by Lang, 7 of 35 patients had bleeding at the catheter entry site.[74] In the series of 27 infusions reported by Wolfson et al., only one patient had a serious hemorrhagic complication. Slight bleeding not mandating discontinuation of SK occurred in another two patients.[88] In the series of 93 high-dose local UK infusions reported by McNamara and Fischer, significant bleeding necessitating transfusion occurred in 4%.[77]

It is clear that there can be hemorrhagic complications of local transcatheter fibrinolytic therapy. When they occur, they are most frequently at the catheter insertion site. Other, more serious, local and remote hemorrhages occur during local therapy with a much lower frequency. Particular attention should be paid to the methods of Hess et al. because it appears that their use of a smaller total dose of fibrinolytic agent results in a very small frequency of bleeding complications.[70]

Local fibrinolytic therapy must sometimes be given when hemorrhage ensues or when laboratory results dictate use of local therapy without concomitant heparin. When overt hemorrhage occurs during local transcatheter SK or UK infusion, the drug should be stopped and catheter patency maintained with saline infusion. Cryoprecipitate or fresh-frozen plasma (3–6 units) should be administered. For continued unresponsive bleeding, ε-aminocaproic acid (Amicar) can be given; it inhibits plasminogen activator and may stimulate antiplasmin. The initial dose is 5g followed by hourly doses of 1.0–1.25g to maintain the plasma level at 0.13 mg/ml. Obviously, packed red blood cells or whole blood should be administered in many of these cases.

Allergic Reactions

No serious allergic reactions to local low-dose SK and UK have been reported, but anaphylactic reactions have occurred with systemic SK. Local SK infusions may result in nausea, vomiting, and mild hypotension. A case of serum sickness syndrome caused by local low-dose SK infusion has been reported.[153] Allergic reactions are not expected with UK.

Fever

Fever may occur in 10–40% of patients receiving local SK. Fever occurred with approximately this frequency in the present authors' series of patients treated for axillary and subclavian vein occlusion. However, in their experience and that of others,[63] fever is truly a minor complication associated with no other ill effects and is easily managed with antipyretics. With local transcatheter therapy, sepsis must be excluded as an etiology for any fever, and blood probably should be cultured.

Distal Emboli

Distal embolizations during transcatheter local infusion for thromboembolic disease have been reported in most of the large series reviewed in this chapter. Emboli also occur with systemic intravenous infusion therapy. They are probably secondary to uneven dissolution, which weakens the thrombus in certain areas, resulting in fragmentation. In peripheral embolization, the patient may suffer abrupt onset of pain or paresthesia. Cyanosis or pallor and coolness may be noted in the extremity, and pulses may be diminished or absent. Such emboli have been demonstrated angiographically in some of these patients. Fortunately, these emboli usually dissolve with continued fibrinolytic infusion, although in some cases, they must be surgically removed.

Emboli remote from the thrombus being treated have been reported with systemic infusion therapy, so the potential for such phenomena cannot be ignored. For instance, patients with embolic occlusion of a leg secondary to mural thrombi or other cardiac etiology may release additional emboli to other portions of the systemic circulation during fibrinolytic therapy. Sicard et al. recently reported four patients who had pulmonary emboli during or shortly after local infusion therapy.[175] One explanation offered by those authors is that the emboli may have originated in DVT partially lysed during the infusion. The

other possible explanation is that the pulmonary emboli may be due to a relatively hypercoagulable state.[176]

Catheter-related Thrombosis

Although catheters indwelling for such maneuvers as vasopressin infusion do not often cause thromboembolic complications, those placed for fibrinolytic therapy often do. This may be simply because the diminished flow proximal to the occlusion enhances the potential for thrombus formation around the catheter shaft. Eskridge et al. reported a 26% frequency of this phenomenon in 57 local infusions.[65] Although other authors report a lower incidence, many of the evaluations were performed by hand injection of contrast medium and a single film obtained in the ICU. The present authors' arteriograms are all performed in the angiography suite with multiple films, and they believe that pericatheter thrombosis is much more likely to be detected with this method.

Concomitant heparin administration for prevention of this complication has already been discussed. Pilla et al. described a modification of the local transcatheter infusion technique that also may help prevent pericatheter thrombosis.[177] Those authors use a 5Fr Teflon sheath and a coaxial 2.5Fr catheter for their infusions. The smaller catheter may prove less thrombogenic for two reasons. First, it provides less surface area for thrombus formation than does a standard 5.0–7.0Fr angiographic catheter. Second, the smaller diameter may cause less diminution of flow in the vessel proximal to the occlusion. Small heparin-bonded catheters for infusion are available.

Extravasation through Graft Interstices

This phenomenon may be seen on serial angiograms (Fig. 8.14) during local fibrinolytic therapy with either SK or UK.[71] The authors' first report of this problem included four patients with occluded knitted Dacron grafts, all of whom were treated with SK and none of whom became symptomatic during infusion. Since one of these grafts was 6 years old, it was apparent to us that SK can lyse long-term fibrin deposits in the "pseudointima" of grafts. There is much other supportive evidence that SK is efficacious in chronic occlusions.[178,179] Additional reports have confirmed that both UK and SK can permeate graft interstices; that PTFE grafts, like Dacron ones, are susceptible; and that the angiographic findings of permeation may also be associated with symptomatic perigraft hematoma formation.[180,181] In one of Becker et al.'s patients with a PTFE graft, a hematoma formed in the popliteal fossa during low-dose transcatheter UK therapy.[180] Figure 8.14 illustrates contrast extravasation through graft interstices. The authors suggest that patients with angiographic evidence of extravasation, particularly those with aortofemoral or aortoiliac grafts, undergo CT examination to search for an "occult" hematoma. In some patients, it is likely that hema-

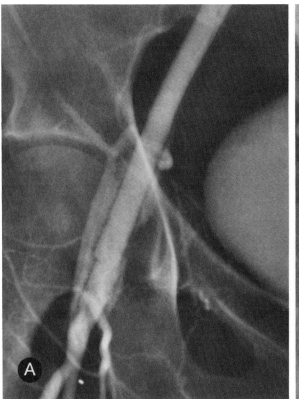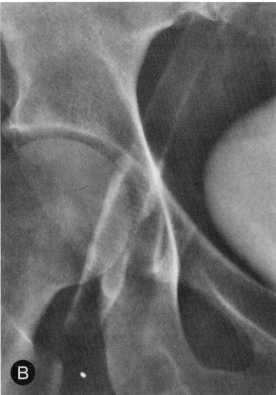

Figure 8.14. A 50-year-old woman with a 16-month-old Dacron aorto-bifemoral graft. **A.** After 28 hours of right graft limb SK infusion for graft thrombosis, extravasation of contrast medium through the graft is seen.

B. Later phase of same angiogram sequence; negative cast of graft is result of extravasated contrast medium.

toma will be found, and fibrinolytic therapy may have to be stopped.

Myoglobinuria and Renal Failure

Lang's article on the complications of intra-arterial use of SK reminds us that reperfusion of ischemic-necrotic muscle achieved by operation or other means of revascularization, including fibrinolytic therapy, can lead to the "crush syndrome."[74] This syndrome is characterized by shock, myoglobinuria that may cause renal failure, hyperkalemia, and cardiac conduction abnormalities, including bundle branch block, complete heart block, and asystole. In 17 patients who presented with neither ischemic necrosis nor compartment syndrome in the involved extremity, Lang observed no instances of myoglobinuria. However, significant myoglobinuria did occur in 10 of 18 patients who presented with compartment syndrome. Fasciotomy appears efficacious but may not prevent myoglobinuria once perfusion has been re-established. Three patients in this series whose myoglobinuria intensified after thrombolytic therapy developed acute tubular necrosis. Lang concluded that attempts at limb salvage by means of revascularization when tissue is already compromised are unjustified and carry an unacceptable risk of renal complications as well as a threat to the patient's life.

CONTRAINDICATIONS

Most of the contraindications to fibrinolytic therapy relate to the risk of hemorrhage. Some relate to the allergenic potential of SK. See Table 8.1 for a complete list of contraindications.

Table 8.1. Contraindications to Fibrinolytic Therapy

Hemorrhagic
    Recent major operation
    Recent gastrointestinal bleeding
    Severe hypertension
    Hemostatic defects
    Diabetic hemorrhagic retinopathy
    Cerebrovascular disease
Embolic
    Subacute bacterial endocarditis
    Left-sided cardiac thrombus
Allergic (SK)
    Known allergy to SK
    Recent SK infusion
    Recent streptococcal infection
    Rheumatic fever
    Post-streptococcal glomerulonephritis

THIRD-GENERATION THERAPY: PRESENT AND FUTURE

There are several formidable challenges in fibrinolytic therapy today. First, it needs to be less invasive. Second-generation therapy has brought both improvements in the results and a lower frequency of hemorrhagic complications, but the methods still lead to a significant frequency of hemorrhage and to new complications, such as pericatheter thrombosis, not seen with first-generation therapy. Second, one or more "magic bullets" are needed which, upon intravenous or oral administration, will lyse thrombi without creating high levels of circulating plasmin (third-generation therapy). With such agents, thromboembolic disorders could be treated effectively yet the systemic fibrinolytic state and its accompanying hemorrhagic complications could be avoided. In addition, the setting for patient management would once again be the medical ward instead of the angiography suite and the ICU. Third, the magic bullets need to be widely available and affordable so they can be used on an emergency basis. For instance, such agents might be administered intravenously by ambulance crews or other emergency specialists to abort myocardial infarctions or cerebrovascular accidents. Finally, radiologists need to keep up with all the changes in medicine that are relevant to their practice and use their growing knowledge to increase their participation in overall patient management. The latter challenge is fundamental to interventional radiologic practice.

The preceding challenges have been addressed to some extent and continue to be addressed in biochemical and microbiologic research laboratories around the world. Tissue plasminogen activator is a magic bullet capable of lysing remote thrombi upon intravenous administration without inducing a systemic fibrinolytic state. Its fibrinogenolytic:fibrinolytic ratio is markedly lower than that of UK in vitro.[182] This highly specific activity is related to its great affinity for fibrin-bound plasminogen and its relatively low affinity for circulating free plasminogen (Fig. 8.15). tPA has been isolated from normal human tissues,[183] as well as from the culture fluid of a cell line derived from human melanoma.[184] The derivation of tPA from melanoma is a tedious, time-consuming, and expensive process, with an extremely low yield. Therefore, researchers have sought other sources. Recently, the protein was purified and sequenced so that its messenger RNA (mRNA), together with reverse transcriptase, could be used to generate the DNA sequence that codes for the enzyme. Armed with the sequence, investigators produced a plasmid, which, when inserted into *Escherichia coli*, directed synthesis of a polypeptide with the same fibrinolytic activity as authentic human tPA.[185] This recombinant DNA product has coronary fibrinolytic activity similar to that of tPA in a canine model of coronary occlusion.[163] The biosynthetic

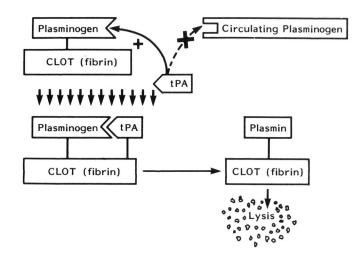

Figure 8.15. Mechanism of action of tPA. This agent's specific affinity for fibrin-bound plasminogen is probably due to a conformational difference between fibrin-bound and circulating free plasminogen. This special affinity allows the formation of a trimolecular complex between tPA, plasminogen, and fibrin. The activity of this complex results in fibrinolysis. The observable consequences of lack of activation of circulating plasminogen include very little circulating plasmin and no systemic fibrinolytic state.

process or one like it has provided larger quantities of tPA for clinical use.

Weimar et al. used melanoma-derived tPA to lyse iliofemoral and renal vein thrombi in a 30-year-old recipient of a cadaveric renal allograft.[186] More recently, Van de Werf et al. reported successful lytic therapy of human coronary thrombi within 20–50 minutes in six of seven attempts with melanoma-derived tPA.[187] Since that time, several medical centers have instituted clinical trials of tPA in both the coronary circulation[163,164] and the peripheral circulation.[188,189]

Meyerovitz et al. in a recent communication published their results of a randomized prospective trial comparing the efficacy of rt-PA and urokinase in 32 patients with peripheral arterial or bypass graft occlusions.[190]

Sixteen patients were treated with rt-PA and the other 16 received urokinase infusion. The thrombus was initially lysed with 10ml of rt-PA, followed by infusion of 5mg/hr up to 24 hours. Patients treated with urokinase received 60,000 units into the thrombus followed by 240,000 units/hr for two hours, 120,000 units/hr per hour for two hours, and 60,000 units/hr up to 20 hours. All of them received systemic heparin and the end point was defined as 95% or greater clot lysis.

The results clearly indicate rapid lysis in patients in the rt-PA group. The clinical outcomes in the two groups of patients were similar. There were seven major bleeding episodes, five in the rt-PA group and two in the urokinase group.

The definition of major bleeding included infusion of two or more units of blood, surgery, or interruption of thrombolytic therapy. None of them experienced intracranial hemorrhage or died as a consequence of the infusion. The conclusions of the randomized trial are:

a. Similar clinical outcome in both groups.
b. The rate of thrombolysis is faster with rt-PA compared with urokinase; however, the 24 hour lysis rates are similar.
c. Complications secondary to bleeding tend to be higher in rt-PA groups.
d. The rate of decline of fibrinogen is greater in the rt-PA group compared to the urokinase group.[190]

Berridge reported his experience with 30 arterial thrombolyses in 28 patients. Low-dose intra-arterial rt-PA at a rate of 0.5mg/hour along with 250 units of intra-arterial heparin were administered. The overall limb salvage at 30 days was 83% (25 out of 30 limbs). Sixteen limbs (53%) required further intervention by percutaneous angioplasty.[191]

Minor complications included hematomas in four cases (13%); no major bleeding was seen. There were four deaths (13%) from myocardial infarction between 5 and 21 days after treatment. Rethrombosis occurred in four cases (13%).

The addition of low-dose heparin was of no significant benefit and might have prolonged the duration of therapy since it might have inhibited fibrinolysis by protecting the plasminogen and α_2-antiplasmins.

The authors concluded that rt-PA is a safe thrombolytic agent at much lower doses than are needed for other treatments.[191]

There is another potential agent for clinical fibrinolytic therapy. One of the vitamin K-dependent, hepatic-synthesized factors mentioned in earlier discussion of the basic coagulation cascade was protein C. Unlike the other factors, activated protein C has an anticoagulant effect. It inactivates the activated forms of factors V and VIII by limited proteolysis.[31,192] In addition, a stimulating effect of protein C on the fibrinolytic mechanism has been described, and apparently it is capable of increasing the levels of circulating plasminogen activator.[31] Future studies of this substance will determine its precise roles in inhibiting thrombus formation and in thrombolysis.

Acylated SK-plasminogen complex does not activate circulating plasminogen. Upon binding to fibrin, deacylation occurs and activator complexes activate fibrin-bound plasminogen. The result is selective clot lysis without a systemic lytic state.

Prourokinase offers potential as an endogenously administered fibrinolytic agent, because it has little or no activity while circulating, but it activates plasminogen in the presence of a fibrin clot.

Finally, a report by Bode et al. describes another important potential new avenue of therapeutic approach. The authors produced a highly specific fibrinolytic agent by covalently coupling urokinase to a fibrin-specific monoclonal antibody that did not cross-react with fibrinogen.[193] The newly created fibrinolytic agent showed a 100-fold increase in fibrinolysis over unmodified urokinase in vitro. This exciting new concept provides a means by which fibrin-specific action of the administered agent may be achieved while the systemic fibrinolytic state is avoided. Commercial laboratories are working on this murine antibody product.

SUMMARY

Fibrinolytic therapy is a tool increasingly utilized by the interventional angiographer. Its successful use depends on the cooperation of the angiographer, surgeon, nurses, and others involved in the total care of the patient. The techniques and agents are evolving rapidly, and it is incumbent on interventional radiologists to stay abreast of changes and to increase their participation in patient management.

References

1. Tillett WAS, Garner RL: The fibrinolytic activity of hemolytic streptococci. *J Exp Med* 1933;58:485
2. Sherry S: The fibrinolytic activity of streptokinase activated human plasmin. *J Clin Invest* 1954;33:1054
3. Welch WH: Thrombosis and embolism, in Albutt TC (ed): *A System of Medicine.* London, Macmillan and Co. Ltd, 1899, p 155
4. Moncada S, Vane JR: The discovery of prostacyclin: a fresh insight into arachidonic acid metabolism, in Kharasch K, Fried J (eds): *Biochemical Aspects of Prostaglandins and Thromboxanes.* New York, Academic Press, 1977, p 155
5. Bunting S, Gryglewski RJ, Moncada S, et al: Arterial walls generate from prostaglandin endoperoxides a substance (prostaglandin X) which relaxes strips of mesenteric and coeliac arteries and inhibits platelet aggregation. *Prostaglandins* 1976;12:897
6. Willis AL, Kuhn DC: A new potential mediator of arterial thrombosis whose biosynthesis is inhibited by aspirin. *Prostaglandins* 1973;4:127
7. Hamberg M, Samuelsson B: Detection and isolation of an endoperoxide intermediate in prostaglandin biosynthesis. *Proc Natl Acad Sci USA* 1973;70:899
8. Smith JB, Ingerman C, Kocsis JJ, et al: Formation of an intermediate in prostaglandin biosynthesis and its association with platelet release reaction. *J Clin Invest* 1974; 53:1468
9. Hamberg M, Svensson J, Samuelsson B: Thromboxanes: a new group of biologically active compounds derived from prostaglandin endoperoxides. *Proc Natl Acad Sci USA* 1975;72:2994
10. Bunting S, Moncada S, Vane JR: The effects of prostaglandin endoperoxides and thromboxane A_2 on strips of rabbit coeliac artery and other smooth muscle preparations. *Br J Pharmacol* 1976;57:462P
11. Smith EF III, Lefer AM, Nicolaou KC: Mechanism of coronary vasoconstriction induced by carbocyclic thromboxane A_2. *Am J Physiol* 1981;240:H493
12. Moncada S, Herman AG, Higgs EA, et al: Differential formation of prostacyclin (PGX or PGI_2) by layers of the arterial wall: an explanation for the anti-thrombotic properties of vascular endothelium. *Thromb Res* 1977;11:323

13. Glavind J, Hartmann S, Clemmesen J, et al: Studies on the role of lipoperoxides in human pathology: the presence of peroxidized lipids in the atherosclerotic aorta. *Acta Pathol Microbiol Scand* 1952;30:1

14. Moncada S, Gryglewski RJ, Bunting S, et al: A lipid peroxide inhibits the enzyme in blood vessel microsomes that generates from prostaglandin endoperoxides the substance (prostaglandin X) which prevents platelet aggregation. *Prostaglandins* 1976;12:715

15. D'Angelo V, Villa S, Mysliewic M, et al: Defective fibrinolytic and prostacyclin like activity in human atheromatous plaques. *Thromb Haemostas* 1978;39:535

16. Virchow R: *Cellular Pathology as Based upon Physiological and Pathological Histology.* London, Churchill, 1860, p 197

17. Beckering RE, Titus JL: Femoral-popliteal venous thrombosis and pulmonary embolism. *Am J Pathol* 1969;52:530

18. Paterson JC: The pathology of venous thrombi, in Sherry S, Brinkhous KM, Genton E, et al. (eds): *Thrombosis.* Washington, DC, US National Academy of Sciences, 1969, p 321

19. Sevitt S: The structure and growth of valve-pocket thrombi in femoral veins. *J Clin Pathol* 1974;27:517

20. Nicolaides AN, Kakkar VV, Renney JTG: The soleal sinuses. *Br J Surg* 1970;57:860

21. Nicolaides AN, Kakkar VV, Renney JTG: Soleal sinuses and stasis. *Br J Surg* 1971;58:307

22. McLachlin AD, McLachlin JA, Jory TA, et al: Venous stasis in the lower extremities. *Ann Surg* 1960;152:678

23. Astrup T, Permin PM: Fibrinolysis in animal organism. *Nature* 1947;159:681

24. Astrup T: The biological significance of fibrinolysis. *Lancet* 1956;2:565

25. Todd AS: The histological localization of fibrinolysin activator. *J Pathol Bacteriol* 1959;78:281

26. Rjken DC, Wijngaards G, Welbergen J: Relationship between tissue plasminogen activator and the activators in blood and vascular wall. *Thromb Res* 1980;18:815

27. Ljungner J, Holmberg L, Kjeldgaard A, et al: Immunological characterization of plasminogen activators in the human vessel wall. *J Clin Pathol* 1983;36:1046

28. Levin EG: Latent tissue plasminogen activator produced by human endothelial cells in culture: evidence for an enzyme–inhibitor complex. *Proc Natl Acad Sci USA* 1983;80:6804

29. Ljunger J, Bergqvist D: Decreased fibrinolytic activity in the bottom of human vein valve pockets. *Vasa* 1983;12:333

30. Ljunger J, Bergqvist D, von Hebel I, et al: Influence of major surgery on plasminogen activator activity in superficial hand veins. *Eur Surg Res* 1983;15:161

31. McKee PA: Disorders of blood coagulation, in Wyngaarden JB, Smith LH Jr (eds): *Cecil Textbook of Medicine.* Philadelphia, WB Saunders, 1985, p 1040

32. Bookstein JJ, Moser KM, Hougie C: Coagulative interventions during angiography. *CardioVasc Intervent Radiol* 1982;5:46

33. Loskutoff DJ, Edgington TS: An inhibitor of plasminogen activator in rabbit endothelial cells. *J Biol Chem* 1981;256:4142

34. Emeiss JJ, van Hinsbergh VMW, Verheijen JH, et al: Inhibition of tissue-type plasminogen activator by conditioned medium from cultured human and porcine vascular endothelial cells. *Biochem Biophys Res Commun* 1983;110:392

35. Chmielewska J, Ranby M, Wiman B: Evidence for a rapid inhibitor to tissue plasminogen activator in plasma. *Thromb Res* 1983;31:427

36. Kruithop EKO, Ransijn A, Bachmann F: Inhibition of tissue plasminogen activator by human plasma, in Davidson JF, Bachmann F, Bouvier CA, Kruithop EKO (eds): *Progress in Fibrinolysis.* Edinburgh, Churchill Livingstone, 1983, p 365

37. Verheijen JH, Chang GTG, Kluft C: Evidence for the occurrence of a fast-acting inhibitor for tissue-type plasminogen activator in human plasma. *Thromb Haemost* 1984;51:392

38. Aoki N, Moroi M, Sakata Y, et al: Abnormal plasminogen: a hereditary molecular abnormality found in a patient with recurrent thrombosis. *J Clin Invest* 1978;61:1186

39. Wohl RC, Summaria L, Robbins KC: Physiological activation of the human fibrinolytic system: isolation and characterization of human plasminogen variants, Chicago I and Chicago II. *J Biol Chem* 1979;254:9063

40. Johansson L, Hedner U, Nilsson IM: A family with thromboembolic disease associated with deficient fibrinolytic activity in vessel wall. *Acta Med Scand* 1978;203:477

41. Jorgensen M, Mortensen JZ, Madsen AG, et al: A family with reduced plasminogen activator activity in blood associated with recurrent venous thrombosis. *Scand J Haematol* 1982;29:217

42. Aoki N, Saito H, Kamiya T, et al: Congenital deficiency of alpha-2-plasmin inhibitor associated with severe hemorrhagic tendency. *J Clin Invest* 1979;63:877

43. Miles LA, Plow EF, Donnelly KJ, et al: A bleeding disorder due to deficiency of alpha-2-antiplasmin. *Blood* 1982;59:1246

44. Kluft C, Vallenga E, Brommer EJP, et al: A familial hemorrhagic diathesis in a Dutch family: an inherited deficiency of alpha-2-antiplasmin. *Blood* 1982;59:1169

45. Booth NA, Bennett B, Wijngaards G, et al: A new life-long hemorrhagic disorder due to excess plasminogen activator. *Blood* 1983;61:267

46. Alkjaersig N, Fletcher AP, Sherry S: The mechanism of clot dissolution by plasmin. *J Clin Invest* 1959;38:1086

47. Johnson AJ, McCarty WR: The lysis of artificially induced intravascular clots in man by intravenous infusions of streptokinase. *J Clin Invest* 1959;38:1627

48. Becker GJ: Local thrombolytic therapy: bridging the "generation gap." *AJR* 1983;140:403

49. Macfarlane RG, Pilling J: Observations on fibrinolysis: plasminogen, plasmin and antiplasmin content of human blood. *Lancet* 1946;2:562

50. Sherry S, Lindemeyer RI, Fletcher AP, Alkjaersig N: Studies on enhanced fibrinolytic activity in man. *J Clin Invest* 1959;38:810

51. Verstraete M, Vermylen J, Amery A, et al: Thrombolytic therapy with streptokinase using a standard dosage scheme. *Br Med J* 1966;1:454

52. Mattsson C, Nyberg–Arrhenius V, Wallen P: Dissolution of thrombi by tissue plasminogen activator, urokinase and streptokinase in an artificial circulating system. *Thromb Res* 1981;21:535

53. Becker GJ: Second-generation fibrinolytic therapy: state of the art. *Semin Intervent Radiol* 1985;2:409

54. Katzen BT: Mechanism and clinical application of fibrinolysis. *Proceedings of the Joint Meeting of the European and American Societies of Cardiovascular and Interventional Radiology,* 1987, p 10

55. Tennant SN, Dixon J, Venable TC, et al: Intracoronary thrombolysis in patients with acute myocardial infarction: comparison of the efficacy of urokinase with streptokinase. *Circulation* 1984;69:756

56. Browse NL, Thomas ML, Pim HP: Streptokinase and deep vein thrombosis. *Br Med J* 1968;4:421

57. Den Ottolander GJH, Craandjik A: Treatment of thrombosis of the central retinal vein with streptokinases. *Thromb Diath Haemorrh* 1968;20:41

58. Kakkar VV, Flanc C, Howe CT, et al: Treatment of deep vein thrombosis: a trial of heparin, streptokinase, and Arvin. *Br Med J* 1969;1:806

59. Ploug J, Kjeldgaard NO: Urokinase: an activator of plasminogen from human urine: isolation and properties. *Biochim Biophys Acta* 1957;24:278

60. Sasahara AA, Hyers TM, Cole CM, et al. (eds): The Urokinase Pulmonary Embolism Trial: a national cooperative study. *Circulation* 1973;47(suppl 2):161

61. Urokinase-Streptokinase Pulmonary Embolism Trial (Phase II): Results: a cooperative study. *JAMA* 1974;229:1606

62. Sharma GVRK, Burleson VA, Sasahara AA: Effect of thrombolytic therapy on pulmonary capillary blood volume in patients with pulmonary embolism. *N Engl J Med* 1980;303:842

63. Palaskas C, Totty WG, Gilula LA, Reinus WR: Complications of local intra-arterial fibrinolytic therapy. *Semin Intervent Radiol* 1985;2:396

64. Dotter CT, Rösch J, Seaman AJ: Selective clot lysis with low-dose streptokinase. *Radiology* 1974;111:31

65. Eskridge JM, Becker GJ, Rabe FE, et al: Catheter-related thrombosis and fibrinolytic therapy. *Radiology* 1983;149:429

66. Katzen BT, van Breda A: Low dose streptokinase in the treatment of arterial occlusions. *AJR* 1981;136:1171

67. Rentrop P, Blanke H, Karsch KR, et al: Acute myocardial infarction: intracoronary application of nitroglycerin and streptokinase. *Clin Cardiol* 1979;2:354

68. Totty WG, Gilula LA, McClennan BL, Ahmed P, Sherman L: Low-dose intravascular fibrinolytic therapy. *Radiology* 1982; 143:59

69. Becker GJ, Rabe FE, Richmond BD, et al: Low-dose fibrinolytic therapy: results and new concepts. *Radiology* 1982;148:663

70. Hess J, Ingrisch H, Mietaschk A, Rath H: Local low-dose thrombolytic therapy of peripheral arterial occlusions. *N Engl J Med* 1982;307:1627

71. Rabe FE, Becker GJ, Richmond BD, et al: Contrast extravasation through Dacron grafts: a sequela of low dose streptokinase therapy. *AJR* 1982;138:917

72. Graor RA, Risius B, Young JR, et al: Low-dose streptokinase for selective thrombolysis: systemic effects and complications. *Radiology* 1984;152:35

73. Dardik H, Sussman BC, Kahn M, et al: Lysis of arterial clot by intravenous or intra-arterial administration of streptokinase. *Surg Gynecol Obstet* 1984;158:137

74. Lang EK: Streptokinase therapy: complications of intra-arterial use. *Radiology* 1985;154:75

75. Mori KW, Bookstein JJ, Heeney DJ, et al: Selective streptokinase infusion: clinical and laboratory correlates. *Radiology* 1983;148:677

76. Tennant SN, Dixon J, Venable TC, et al: Intracoronary thrombolysis in patients with acute myocardial infarction: comparison of the efficacy of urokinase with streptokinase. *Circulation* 1984;69:756

77. McNamara TO, Fischer JR: Thrombolysis of peripheral arterial and graft occlusions: improved results using high-dose urokinase. *AJR* 1985;144:769

78. Bean WJ, Rodan BA, Thebaut AL: Leriche syndrome: treatment with streptokinase and angioplasty. *AJR* 1985; 144:1285

79. Lynch WA, Westcott JL: "Blind" femoral angiography. *Radiology* 1977;125:379

80. Dotter CT, Rösch J, Robinson M: Fluoroscopic guidance in femoral artery puncture. *Radiology* 1978;127:266

81. Sullivan KL, Gardiner GA, Shapiro MJ, Bonn J, Levin DC: Acceleration of thrombolysis with a high-dose transthrombus bolus technique. *Radiology* 1989;173:805–808

82. Strife JL, Ball WS, Towbin R, Keller MS, Dillon T: Arterial occlusions in neonates: use of fibrinolytic therapy. *Radiology* 1988;166;395–400

83. Motarjeme A: Thrombolytic therapy in arterial occlusion and graft thrombosis. *Semin Vasc Surg* 1989;2(3):155–178

84. Wilms GE, Verhaeghe RH, Pouillon MM, Dewaele D, Baert AL, Vermylen J, Verstraete M: Local thrombolysis in femoropopliteal occlusion: early and late results. *Cardiovasc Intervent Radiol* 1987;10:272–275

85. Lammer J, Pilger E, Neumayer K, Schreyer H: Intraarterial fibrinolysis: long-term results. *Radiology* 1986;161:159–163

86. Lupattelli L, Barzi F, Corneli P, Lemmi A, Mosca S: Selective thrombolysis with low-dose urokinase in chronic arteriosclerotic obstructions. *Cardiovasc Intervent Radiol* 1988;11:123–126

87. Hess H, Mietaschk A, Bruckl R: Peripheral arterial occlusions: A 6 year experience with low-dose thrombolytic therapy. *Radiology* 1987;163:753–758

88. Wolfson RH, Kumpe DA, Rutherford RB: Role of intra-arterial streptokinase in treatment of arterial thromboembolism. *Arch Surg* 1984;119:697

89. Gardiner GA, Koltun W, Kandarpa K, Whittemore A, Meyerovitz MF, Bettmann MA, Levin DC, Harrington DP: Thrombolysis of occluded femoropopliteal grafts. *AJR* 1986;147:621–626

90. Gardiner GA: Thrombolysis of occluded arterial bypass grafts. *Cardiovasc Intervent Radiol* 1988;11:S58–S59

91. Durham JD, Geller SC, Abbott WM, Shapiro H, Waltman AC, Walker TG, Brewster DC, Athanasoulis CA: Regional infusion of urokinase into occluded lower-extremity bypass grafts: long-term clinical results. *Radiology* 1989;172:83–87

92. Gardiner GA, Harrington DP, Koltun W, Whittemore A, Mannick JA, Levin DC: Salvage of occluded arterial bypass grafts by means of thrombolysis. *J Vasc Surg* 1989;9:426–431

93. McNamara TO: The use of lytic therapy with endovascular "repair" for the failed infrainguinal graft. *Semin Vasc Surg* 1990;3(1):59–65

94. Risius B, Graor RA, Geisinger MA, Zelch MG, Lucas FV, Young JR, Grossbard EB: Recombinant human tissue-type plasminogen activator for thrombolysis in peripheral arteries and bypass grafts. *Radiology* 1989;160:183–188

95. Tisnado J, Bartol DT, Cho S–R, et al: Low-dose fibrinolytic therapy in hand ischemia. *Radiology* 1984;150:375

96. Tisnado J, Cho S–R, Beachley MC, Vines FS: Low-dose fibrinolytic therapy in hand ischemia. *Semin Intervent Radiol* 1985;2:367

97. Gross WS, Flanigan DP, Kraft RO, et al: Chronic upper extremity arterial insufficiency: etiology, manifestations and operative management. *Arch Surg* 1978;113:419

98. Erlandson EE, Forrest ME, Shields JJ, et al: Discriminant arteriographic criteria in the management of forearm and hand ischemia. *Surgery* 1981;90:1025

99. Schmidt FE, Hewitt RL: Severe upper limb ischemia. *Arch Surg* 1980;115;1188

100. Baur GM, Porter JM, Bardana EJ Jr, et al: Rapid onset of hand ischemia of unknown etiology: clinical evaluation and follow-up in ten patients. *Ann Surg* 1977;186:184

101. Holleman JH, Hardy JD, Williamson JW, et al: Arterial surgery for arm ischemia: a survey of 136 patients. *Ann Surg* 1980;191:727

102. Taylor LM Jr, Baur GM, Porter JM: Finger gangrene caused by small artery occlusive disease. *Ann Surg* 1981;193:453

103. McNamara MF, Takaki HS, Yao JST, et al: A systemic approach to severe hand ischemia. *Surgery* 1978;83:191

104. Silcott GR, Polich VL: Palmar arch arterial reconstruction for the salvage of ischemic fingers. *Am J Surg* 1981;142:219

105. Slany J, Enzenhofer V, Karnik R: Local thrombolysis in arterial occlusive disease. *Angiology* 1984;35:231

106. Rapaport S, Glickman MG, Salomon JC, Cuono CB: Aggressive postoperative pharmacotherapy for vascular compromise of replanted digits. *AJR* 1985;144:1065

107. Widlus DM, Venbrux AC, Benenati JF, Mitchell SE, Lynch–Nyhan A, Cassidy FP, Osterman FA: Fibrinolytic therapy for upper-extremity arterial occlusions. *Radiology* 1990;175:393–399

108. Sullivan KL, Minken SL, White RI: Treatment of a case of thromboembolism resulting from thoracic outlet syndrome with intra-arterial urokinase infusion. *J Vasc Surg* 1988;7:568–571

109. Hunter DW: Personal communication.

110. Zeit RM: Clearing of clotted dialysis shunts by streptokinase injection at multiple sites. *AJR* 1983;141:1053

111. Rodkin RS, Bookstein JJ, Heeney DJ, Davis GB: Streptokinase and transluminal angioplasty in the treatment of acutely thrombosed hemodialysis access fistulas. *Radiology* 1983; 149:425

112. Davis GB, Dowd CF, Bookstein JJ, Maroney TP, Lang EV, Halasz N: Thrombosed dialysis grafts: efficacy of intrathrombic deposition of concentrated urokinase, clot maceration, and angioplasty. *AJR* 1987;149:177–181

113. Young AT, Hunter DW, Castañeda–Zúñiga WR, et al: Thrombosed synthetic hemodialysis access fistulas: failure of fibrinolytic therapy. *Radiology* 1985;154:639

114. Bookstein JJ, Fellmeth B, Roberts A, Valji K, et al: Pulsed spray pharmacomechanical thrombolysis: preliminary clinical results. *AJR* 1989;152:1097–1100

115. Kandarpa K, Drinker PA, Singer SJ, Caramore D: Forceful pulsatile local infusion of enzyme accelerates thrombolysis: in vivo evaluation of a new delivery system. *Radiology* 1988;168:739–744

116. Kaufman SL: Use of the EDM catheter for thrombolysis. Presented at the 1990 Annual Meeting of the Society of Cardiovascular and Interventional Radiology. Miami, FL, March 1990

117. Price C, Jacocks MA, Tytle T: Thrombolytic therapy in acute arterial thrombosis. *Am J Surg* 1988;156:488–491

118. Flickinger EG, Johnsrude IS, Ogburn NL, Weaver MD, Pories WJ: Local streptokinase infusion for superior mesenteric artery thromboembolism. *AJR* 1983;140:771

119. Pillari G, Doscher W, Fierstein J, Ross W, Loh G, Berkowitz BJ: Low-dose streptokinase in the treatment of celiac and superior mesenteric artery occlusion. *Arch Surg* 1983;118:1340

120. Ziessman HA, Juni JE, Gyves JW, Brady TM, Ensminger WD: Thrombosis and streptokinase lysis during hepatic intraarterial chemotherapy: the value of perfusion scintigraphy. *AJR* 1985;144:1067

121. Gormsen J: Thrombolytic therapy of acute phlebothrombosis, in Hiemeyer V, Schattauer FE (eds): *Therapeutische und Experimentelle Fibrinolyse.* Stuttgart, Verlag, 1969, p 267

122. Browse NL, Thomas ML, Pim HP: Streptokinase and deep vein thrombosis. *Br Med J* 1968;3:707

123. Robertson BR, Nillson IM, Nylander G: Value of streptokinase and heparin in therapy of acute deep vein thrombosis. *Acta Chir Scand* 1968;134:203

124. Robertson BR, Nillson IM, Nylander G: Thrombolytic effect of streptokinase as evaluated by phlebography of deep vein thrombosis of the leg. *Acta Chir Scand* 1970;136:173

125. Tsapogas MJ, Peabody RA, Wu KT, et al: Controlled study of thrombolytic therapy in deep vein thrombosis. *Surgery* 1973;74:973

126. Duckert F, Muller G, Nyman D, et al: Treatment of deep vein thrombosis with streptokinase. *Br Med J* 1975;1:479

127. Rösch JJ, Dotter CT, Seaman AJ, et al: Healing of deep vein thrombosis: venographic findings in a randomized study comparing streptokinase and heparin. *AJR* 1976;127:533

128. Marder VJ, Soulen RL, Atichartakarn V: Quantitative venographic assessment of deep vein thrombosis in the evaluation of streptokinase and heparin therapy. *J Lab Clin Med* 1977;89:1018

129. Arnesen H, Heilo A, Jakobsen E, et al: A prospective study of streptokinase and heparin in the treatment of venous thrombosis. *Acta Med Scand* 1978;203:457

130. Elliot MS, Immelman EJ, Jeffery P, et al: A comparative randomized trial of heparin versus streptokinase in the treatment of acute proximal venous thrombosis: an interim report of a prospective trial. *Br J Surg* 1979;66:838

131. Watz R, Savidge GF: Rapid thrombolysis and preservation of venous valvular function in high deep vein thrombosis. *Acta Med Scand* 1979;205:293

132. Greenwood LH, Yrizarry JM, Hallett JW Jr, Scoville GS Jr: Urokinase treatment of Budd–Chiari syndrome. *AJR* 1983;141:1057

133. Warren RL, Schlant RC, Wenger NK, Galambos JT: Treatment of Budd–Chiari syndrome with streptokinase. *Gastroenterology* 1972;62:200

134. Goldsmith JC, Lollar P, Hoak JC: Massive fatal pulmonary emboli with fibrinolytic therapy. *Circulation* 1982;64:1068

135. Herrera JL, Willis SM, Williams TH: Successful streptokinase therapy of acute idiopathic superior vena cava thrombosis. *Am Heart J* 1981;102:1063

136. Paget J: *Clinical Lectures and Essays.* London, Longmans Green and Co, 1875

137. Swinton NW, Edgett JW, Hall RJ: Primary subclavian–axillary vein thrombosis. *Circulation* 1968;38:737

138. Adams JT, McEvoy RK, DeWeese JA: Primary deep venous thrombosis of upper extremity. *Arch Surg* 1965;91:29

139. Becker GJ, Holden RW, Rabe FE, et al: Local thrombolytic therapy for subclavian and axillary vein thrombosis: treatment of the thoracic inlet syndrome. *Radiology* 1983; 149:419

140. Becker GK, Holden RW, Mail JT, Olson EW, Castañeda–Zúñiga WR: Local thrombolytic therapy for "thoracic inlet syndrome." *Semin Intervent Radiol* 1985;2:349

141. Hoshal VL Jr, Ause RG, Hoskins PA: Fibrin sleeve formation on indwelling subclavian central venous catheters. *Arch Surg* 1971;102:353

142. Peters WR, Bush WH Jr, McIntyre RD, Hill LD: The development of fibrin sheath on indwelling venous catheters. *Surg Gynecol Obstet* 1973;137:43

143. Zajko AB, Reilly JJ Jr, Bron KM, Desai R, Steed DL: Low-dose streptokinase for occluded Hickman catheters. *AJR* 1983;141:1311

144. Hurtubise MR, Bottino JC, Lawson M, McCredie KB: Restoring patency of occluded central venous catheters. *Arch Surg* 1980;115:212

145. Glynn MFX, Langer B, Jeejeebhoy KN: Therapy for thrombotic occlusion of long term intravenous alimentation catheters. *J Parent Enteral Nutr* 1980;4:387

146. Barbarena J: Intraarterial infusion of urokinase in the treat-

ment of acute pulmonary thromboembolism: preliminary observations. *AJR* 1983;140:883

147. Miller GAH, Sutton GC, Karr IH, Gibson RV, Honey M: Comparison of streptokinase and heparin in treatment of isolated acute massive pulmonary embolism. *Br Med J* 1971;2:681

148. Vujic I, Young JWR, Gobien RP, Dawson WT, Liebscher L, Shelley BE Jr: Massive pulmonary embolism: treatment with full heparinization and topical low-dose streptokinase. *Radiology* 1983;148:671

149. Risius B, Graor RA: Fibrinolytic therapy in pulmonary thromboembolic disease. *Semin Intervent Radiol* 1985,2:338

150. Holden RW, Becker GJ, Schauwecker DS, et al: Capillary blockade due to rapid clot lysis in an experimental rabbit pulmonary thromboembolism mode (poster session). Tenth Congress of the International Society on Thrombosis and Hemostasis, San Diego, CA, July 1985

151. DeWood MA, Spores J, Notske R, et al: Prevalence of total coronary occlusion during the early hours of transmural myocardial infarction. *N Engl J Med* 1980;303:897

152. Boucek RJ, Murphy WP Jr: Segmental perfusion of the coronary arteries with fibrinolysis in man following a myocardial infarction. *Am J Cardiol* 1960;6:525

153. Chazov EI, Mateeva LS, Mazaev AV, et al: Intracoronary administration of fibrinolysis in acute myocardial infarction. *Ter Arkh* 1976;48:8

154. Paulin S, Als AV: Thrombolytic therapy in coronary artery occlusion. *Semin Intervent Radiol* 1985;2:381

155. Terrosu P, Ibba GV, Contini GM, Franceschino V: Angiographic features of the coronary arteries during intracoronary thrombolysis. *Br Heart J* 1984;52:154

156. Tennant R, Wiggers C: The effect of coronary occlusion on myocardial contraction. *Am J Physiol* 1935;112:351

157. Blumgart H, Gilligan R, Schlesinger M: Experimental studies on the effect of temporary occlusion of coronary arteries. *Am Heart J* 1941;22:374

158. Jennings R, Summers J, Smyth G, et al: Myocardial necrosis induced by temporary occlusion of a coronary artery in the dog. *Arch Pathol* 1960;70:82

159. Braunwald E, Kloner RA: The stunned myocardium: prolonged, post-ischemic ventricular dysfunction. *Circulation* 1982;66: 1146

160. Silverman KJ, Becker LC, Bulkley BH, et al: Value of early thallium 201 scintigraphy for predicting mortality in patients with acute myocardial infarction. *Circulation* 1980;61:996

161. Kennedy JW, Ritchie JL, Davis KB, Fritz JK: Western Washington Randomized Trial of Intracoronary Streptokinase in Acute Myocardial Infarction. *N Engl J Med* 1983;309:1477

162. Schroder R, Biamino G, Von Leitner ER, Linderer TH: Intravenous streptokinase infusions in acute myocardial infarction. *Dtsch Med Wochenschr* 1981;106:294

163. Van de Werf F, Bergmann SR, Fox KAA, et al: Coronary thrombolysis with intravenously administered human tissue-type plasminogen activator produced by recombinant DNA technology. *Circulation* 1984;69:605

164. Gold HK, Fallon JT, Yasuda T, et al: Coronary thrombolysis with recombinant human tissue-type plasminogen activator. *Circulation* 1984;70:700

165. Blaisdell WF, Clauss RH, Galbraith JG, et al: Joint study of extracranial arterial occlusion: review of surgical complications. *JAMA* 1969;209:1889

166. Eskridge JM, Becker GJ, Rabe FE, Holden RW: Local fibrinolytic therapy for acute carotid occlusion in a canine model. *Semin Intervent Radiol* 1985;2:405

167. Narayan RK, Narayan TM, Katz DA, Kornblith PL, Murano

168. G: Lysis of intracranial hematomas with urokinase in a rabbit model. *J Neurosurg* 1985;62:580

168. Ramchandani P, Soulen RL: Laboratory monitoring in fibrinolytic therapy. *Semin Intervent Radiol* 1985;2:391

169. Marder VJ: The use of thrombolytic agents: choice of patient, drug administration, laboratory monitoring. *Ann Intern Med* 1979;90:802

170. Rutkowsky DM, Burkle WS: Advances in thrombolytic therapy. *Drug Intell Clin Pharm* 1982;96:115

171. Brogden RN, Speight TM, Avery GS: Streptokinase: review of its clinical pharmacology, mechanism of action and therapeutic uses. *Drugs* 1973;5:357

172. Feissinger JN, Aiach M, Vaysariat M, et al: Traitment thrombolytique des arteriopathies. *Ann Anesthesiol Fr* 1978;19:739

173. Feissinger JN, Vayssariat M, Juillet Y, et al: Local urokinase in arterial thromboembolism. *Angiology* 1980;31:715

174. Totty WG, Romano T, Benian G, et al: Serum sickness following streptokinase therapy. *AJR* 1982;138:143

175. Sicard GA, Schier JJ, Totty WG, et al: Thrombolytic therapy for acute arterial occlusion. *J Vasc Surg*, in press

176. Sherry S: Thrombolytic therapy in surgical patients. *Curr Surg* 1981;38:75

177. Pilla T, Tantana S, Peterson G, et al: A modified technique for the infusion of low-dose streptokinase. *AJR* 1984; 142:1213

178. Berkman WA, White RI Jr, Parandian BB: Lysis of a chronic arterial occlusion with streptokinase. *AJR* 1983;141:40

179. Martin M: *Streptokinase in Chronic Arterial Disease*. Boca Raton, FL, CRC Press, 1982

180. Becker GJ, Holden RW, Rabe FE: Contrast extravasation from a Gore–Tex graft: a complication of thrombolytic therapy. *AJR* 1984;142:573

181. Rosner NH, Doris PE: Contrast extravasation through a Gore–Tex graft: a sequela of low dose streptokinase therapy. *AJR* 1984;143:633

182. Matsuo O, Collen DC: Comparison of the relative fibrinogenolytic, fibrinolytic and thrombolytic properties of tissue plasminogen activator and urokinase in vitro. *Thromb Haemostas* 1981;45:225

183. Rijken DC, Wijngaards G, Zall–de Jong M, Welbergen J: Purification and partial characterization of plasminogen activator from human uterine tissue. *Biochim Biophys Acta* 1979;580:140

184. Rijken DC, Collen D: Purification and characterization of the plasminogen activator secreted by human melanoma cells in culture. *J Biol Chem* 1981;256:7035

185. Pennica D, Holmes WE, Kohr WJ, et al: Cloning and expression of human tissue-type plasminogen activator cDNA in E. coli. *Nature* 1983;301:214

186. Weimar W, Stibbe J, van Seyen AJ, Billiau A, Somer P, Collen D: Specific lysis of an iliofemoral thrombus by administration of extrinsic (tissue-type) plasminogen activator. *Lancet* 1981;2:1018

187. Van de Werf F, Ludbrook PA, Bergmann SR, et al: Coronary thrombolysis with tissue-type plasminogen activator in patients with evolving myocardial infarction. *N Engl J Med* 1984;310:609

188. Risius B, Graor RA, Geisinger MA, et al: Recombinant human tissue-type plasminogen activator for thrombolysis in peripheral arteries and bypass grafts. *Radiology* 1986;160;183

189. Graor RA, Risius B, Denny KM, et al: Local thrombolysis in the treatment of thrombosed arteries, bypass grafts and arteriovenous fistulas. *J Vasc Surg* 1985;2:406

190. Meyerovitz MF, Goldhaber SZ, Reagan K, Polak JF, Kan-

darpa K, Grassi CJ, Donovan BC, Bettmann MA, Harrington DP: Recombinant tissue-type plasminogen activator versus urokinase in peripheral arterial and graft occlusions: a randomized trial. *Radiology* 1990;175:75–78

191. Berridge DC, Gregson RHS, Makin GS, Hopkinson BR: Tissue plasminogen activator in peripheral arterial thrombolysis. *Br J Surg* 1990;77:179–181

192. Esmon CT: Protein-C biochemistry, physiology and clinical implications. *Blood* 1983;62:1155

193. Bode C, Matsueda GR, Hui KY, Haber E: Antibody-directed urokinase: a specific fibrinolytic agent. *Science* 1985;229:765

9

MECHANICAL THROMBECTOMY

—Wilfrido R. Castañeda–Zúñiga, M.D., M.Sc., Joseph W. Yedlicka, Jr., M.D., John E. Carlson, M.D., Ph.D., David W. Hunter, M.D., Eugenio Ponomar–Sulepov, M.D., S. Murthy Tadavarthy, M.D., Marcos A. Herrera, M.D., and Kurt Amplatz, M.D.

Mechanical removal of clot from acutely occluded vessels or grafts using balloon catheters has been shown to be a reliable method for prompt restoration of perfusion.[1,2] However, restoration of flow may be incomplete, due to distal location of thrombi or emboli, thrombus propagation beyond the reach of the catheter, and atherosclerotic obstruction that prevents passage of the catheter into occluded distal arteries.[1] Repeated futile attempts to remove thrombus under these circumstances may cause significant intimal damage and, on occasion, perforate the vessel wall.[1] Failure to restore distal circulation, rethrombosis, or hemorrhage into the soft tissues may ensue.[1]

Chemical fibrinolysis has recently become an effective treatment for vascular thrombosis, but potential drawbacks exist. First, chemical thrombolysis often requires prolonged infusion times and may be contraindicated when an immediate need to restore perfusion precludes a 24–48-hour trial of lytic therapy.[1] Second, prolonged infusion of these agents eventually produces a systemic lytic state with increased risk of bleeding.[1] Third, it is often difficult for the patient to maintain a supine position for up to 48 hours (when a femoral approach is used). Fourth, thrombolytic therapy may fail to achieve recanalization of the occluded vessel. Finally, currently used thrombolytic agents are expensive, as is the required stay in the intensive care unit during infusion.

Because of these limitations, several investigators have directed their attention to percutaneous mechanical rotational thrombectomy devices for clot removal or dissolution.[3-6] Theoretically, such devices can reduce or even completely remove thrombus from grafts or vessels, thereby obviating infusion or reducing thrombolytic infusion time. This approach may also be useful for thrombus

that is refractory to fibrinolytic therapy and should reduce overall patient morbidity as well as the cost of chemical thrombolysis.

Among the mechanical thrombectomy devices are:

—Transluminal extraction catheter;
—Amplatz mechanical thrombolysis catheter;
—Ponomar transjugular clot-trapper device;
—Günther aspiration thromboembolectomy catheter;
—Rotational thrombectomy catheter;
—Starck aspiration thromboembolectomy;
—Ultrasonic thrombolysis catheter;
—Rheolytic thrombectomy catheter.

References

1. Cohen LH, Kaplan M, Bernhard VM: Intraoperative streptokinase: an adjunct to mechanical thrombectomy in the management of acute ischemia. *Arch Surg* 1986;12(6):708–715
2. Fogarty TJ, Chin AK, Ollott C, Shoor PM, Zimmerman JJ, Garry MT: Combined thrombectomy and dilation for the treatment of acute lower extremity arterial thrombosis. *J Vasc Surg* 1989;10(5):530–534
3. Bildsoe MC, Moradian GP, Hunter DW, Castañeda-Zúñiga WR, Amplatz K: Mechanical clot dissolution: new concept. *Radiology* 1989;171:231–233
4. Hansen DD, Auth DC, Vracko R, Ritchie JL: Rotational thrombectomy in acute canine coronary thrombosis. *Int J Cardiol* 1989;22(l):13–19
5. Hansen DD, Auth DC, Vracko R, Ritchie JL: Mechanical thrombectomy: a comparison of two rotational devices and balloon angioplasty in subacute canine femoral thrombosis. *Am Heart J* 1987;114(5):1223–1231
6. Kensey KR, Nash JE, Abrahams C, Zarins CK: Recanalization of obstructed arteries with a flexible, rotating tip catheter. *Radiology* 1987;165:387–389

Part 1. Mechanical Thrombectomy with the Transluminal Extraction Catheter

—Joseph W. Yedlicka, Jr., M.D., John E. Carlson, M.D., Ph.D., David W. Hunter, M.D., Wilfrido R. Castañeda–Zúñiga, M.D., M.Sc., and Kurt Amplatz, M.D.

The transluminal extraction catheter (TEC) was originally designed for the percutaneous removal of atherosclerotic plaque. The catheter has, however, been successfully used by Yedlicka et al. for the removal of fresh and chronic thrombus in laboratory animals and in humans.[1]

MATERIALS AND METHODS

One-week-old thrombus was induced on 10cm-long Gore-Tex interpositional grafts placed to bypass surgically created occlusions of the right superficial femoral artery, and on the isolated contralateral femoral artery, whose branches were ligated. Prior to using the TEC device to mechanically remove the thrombus, the distal occlusive ties were removed. A 9Fr sheath was placed in the right carotid artery in each dog. Arteriograms of the proximal and distal aspects of the lower extremities were obtained, demonstrating thrombosis of the occluded grafts and arteries and

patency of the distal vascular bed reconstituted via collaterals (Fig. 9.1.1). Heparin (100 units/kg) was given intravenously. A 0.014-inch exchange-length guidewire was placed through a catheter into either the thrombosed graft or the thrombosed superficial femoral artery. The TEC endarterectomy device (Fig. 9.1.2) was inserted over the guidewire through the right carotid artery sheath and advanced under fluoroscopic guidance. The 2.0mm TEC catheter was used in the distal superficial femoral and popliteal arteries, the 2.3mm catheter in the mid-superficial femoral arteries and distal anastomoses, and a 3.0mm catheter in the proximal femoral arteries and proximal anastomoses. Each TEC catheter assembly (torque tube/cutter) is connected to the motorized catheter drive unit (CDU), which is driven by an accompanying battery pack (Fig. 9.1.3). The torque tube/cutter rotates at approximately 750 rpm. The disrupted thrombus is simultaneously aspirated through the torque tube and CDU into a vacuum bot-

Figure 9.1.1. Preprocedure angiogram demonstrating occlusion of the right Gore-Tex graft *(straight arrow)* and the left femoral artery *(curved arrow).*

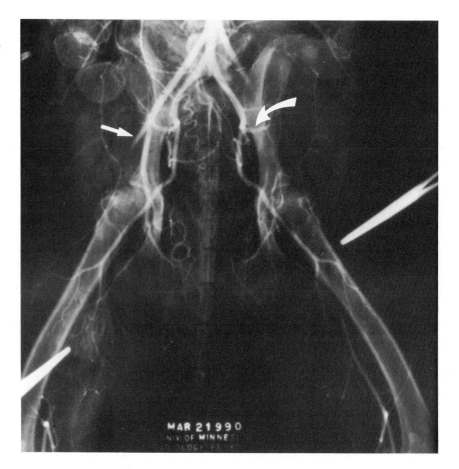

MAR 21990
NIV OF MINNE
LOGY

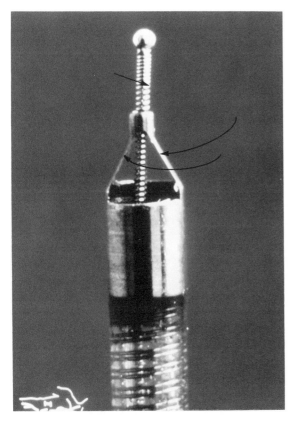

Figure 9.1.2. Close-up of cutter tip. The 0.014-inch guidewire *(straight arrow)*. Cutter tip *(curved arrows)*.

tle. The torque tube/cutter is advanced into the thrombus by means of a sliding control on the CDU. Following the TEC mechanical thrombectomy, angiography was performed to check patency of the treated arteries and the thrombectomy repeated if necessary. At the conclusion of the procedure, a final angiogram was obtained to check for vascular patency and to evaluate for possible distal embolization. The superficial femoral arteries were removed and sent to pathology for microscopic evaluation.

The device was also used in patients with superior vena cava (SVC) syndrome. The 3.0mm catheter was inserted through a 9Fr sheath in the right femoral vein over an 0.014-inch guidewire previously placed through the SVC thrombus. Mechanical thrombectomy of the SVC, left innominate vein, and right subclavian vein was performed.

RESULTS

The TEC device was successful at removing one-week old thrombus in five grafts and four native femoral arteries in five dogs (Fig. 9.1.4). A wound infection involving a native femoral artery in one dog precluded evaluation of this vessel. The thrombectomy was performed quickly and without complications in all dogs. No significant distal embolization was noted in any of the dogs on postprocedure arteriograms. Microscopic examination of the superficial femoral arteries demonstrated mild intimal disruption and no evidence of perforation.

This device was also used in a 63-year-old female with chronic renal failure who developed SVC syndrome with thrombosis of the SVC, left innominate, and right subcla-

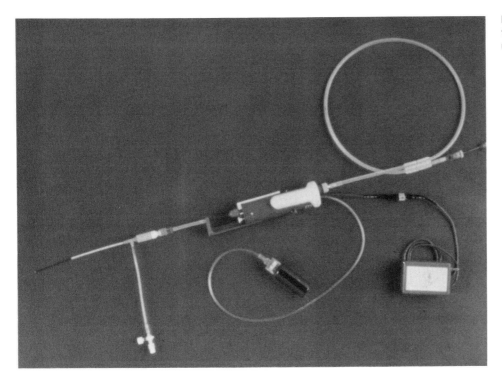

Figure 9.1.3. TEC endarterectomy system. Torque tube/cutter, catheter drive unit, battery pack, and vacuum bottle.

Figure 9.1.4. Postprocedure angiogram demonstrating patency following mechanical thrombectomy with the TEC system. Right Gore-Tex graft *(straight arrow).* Left femoral artery *(curved arrow).* Stenoses are present involving the proximal and distal graft anastomoses *(open arrows)* as well as the previously ligated area of the left superficial femoral artery *(small arrow).*

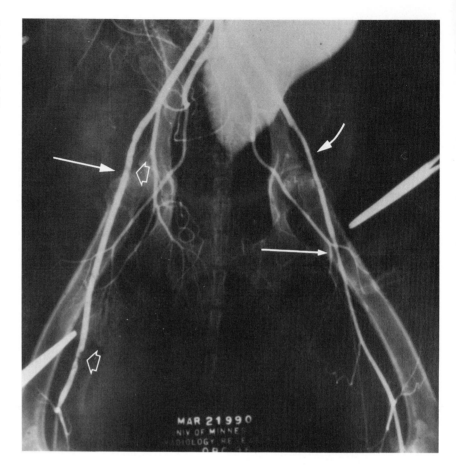

vian veins. Forty-eight hours of urokinase infusion into the thrombus failed to produce lysis of clot, in a patient considered a poor operative candidate (Fig. 9.1.5A,B). A 3.0mm TEC catheter (Fig. 9.1.5C,D) was introduced through the right femoral vein, and this device was able to remove the vast majority of the thrombus from these vessels (Fig. 9.1.5E). The patient's clinical symptoms dramatically improved within hours after the mechanical clot removal. She was maintained on systemic anticoagulation. Follow-up duplex sonography three months later demonstrated continued patency of the treated vessels.

In conclusion, the TEC endarterectomy system is a safe, convenient, and effective means of removing thrombus from grafts and arteries in experimental animals as well as from central veins in human subjects. We believe that this system will prove to be useful in treating thrombus refractory to thrombolytic therapy as well as in reducing overall fibrinolytic infusion time, by debulking thrombus.

Reference

1. Yedlicka JW Jr, Carlson J, Hunter DW, Castañeda–Zúñiga WR, Amplatz K. Thrombectomy with the TEC endarterectomy system: an experimental study. *JVIR,* in press

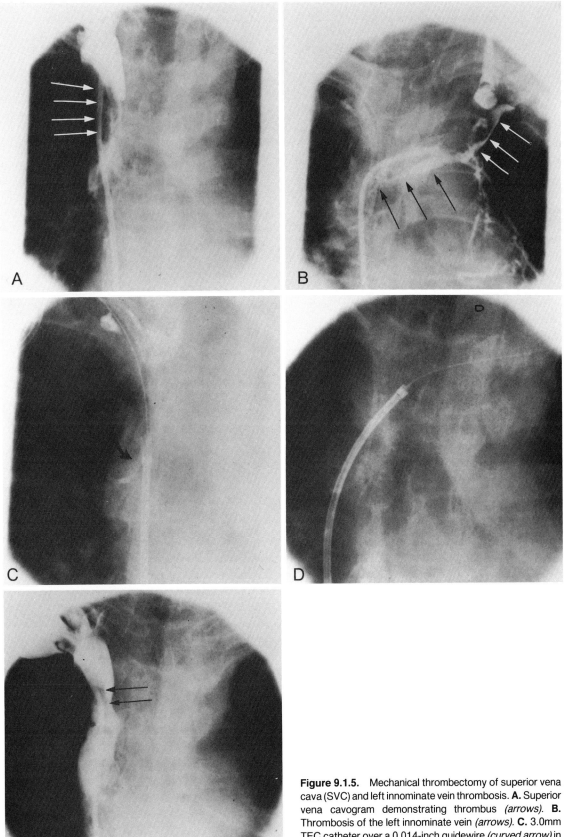

Figure 9.1.5. Mechanical thrombectomy of superior vena cava (SVC) and left innominate vein thrombosis. **A.** Superior vena cavogram demonstrating thrombus *(arrows).* **B.** Thrombosis of the left innominate vein *(arrows).* **C.** 3.0mm TEC catheter over a 0.014-inch guidewire *(curved arrow)* in the SVC. **D.** TEC in innominate vein. **E.** SVC one day after mechanical thrombectomy. Note the continued luminal patency and minimal residual thrombus *(arrows).*

Part 2. Amplatz Mechanical Thrombolysis Catheter

—Wilfrido R. Castañeda–Zúñiga, M.D., M.Sc., S. Murthy Tadavarthy, M.D., David W. Hunter, M.D., Joseph W. Yedlicka, Jr., M.D., and Kurt Amplatz, M.D.

Acute vascular thrombosis is a major complication of percutaneous interventional vascular and surgical vascular procedures. It occurs when endothelium is damaged, in low-flow states and during hypercoagulable conditions. Surgical treatment using balloon thromboembolectomy is the most invasive, but most definitive, therapy.[1,2] Medical treatment consists primarily of long-term anticoagulation. Currently, radiologic treatment of acute and subacute thrombosis involves intravascular delivery of thrombolytic agents. Such treatment is time-consuming, expensive, and has the potential for major hemorrhagic side effects. In addition, patients with mural cardiac or vascular thrombi are at additional risk of peripheral embolization when conventional thrombolytic agents are used. A safe, rapid, and relatively noninvasive means of thrombolysis is needed.

Moradian et al. presented preliminary data on in vitro mechanical thrombolysis utilizing a catheter which has a special housing enclosing a tiny spinning propeller.[3] Mechanical thrombolysis could potentially be used in any natural or synthetic vessel containing acute or subacute thrombosis with fewer complications and lower cost than traditional methods.

DESCRIPTION OF DEVICE

The prototype catheter is 100cm long, 8Fr in size, and made of polyurethane. At its distal tip is a 1cm-long, open-ended metal capsule with two side holes (Fig. 9.2.1). The capsule serves as the housing for a tiny propeller similar to the blade of a household mixer. The propeller is connected to a drive shaft which can be connected either to a high-speed electric or air-driven motor. Rotational speeds of 100,000 rpm can be achieved. The drive shaft extends through a "Y" connector at the proximal end of the catheter which allows the infusion of saline, contrast medium, or fibrinolytic solutions, any of which also serve to lubricate and cool the drive shaft.

RESULTS

The completeness of clot dissolution is directly related to both the duration and the speed of rotation of the propeller. It should be noted that by simply moving the catheter back and forth within the clot without rotation of the propeller, 50% clot disruption was achieved after two minutes. However, at 10,000 rpm, two minutes of application resulted in 95% dissolution. A similar degree of clot dissolution occurred after only 27 seconds at 60,000 rpm.

Finally, at 80,000 rpm, 97% dissolution was achieved after just 10 seconds.

The vast majority of the residue after fragmentation was normal-appearing red blood cells. In addition, there was a sparse scattering of inhomogeneous aggregates of amorphous, nonstaining material which contained basophilic clumps of material resembling disrupted white cell nuclei. The largest of these measured 208 μm in diameter. No fibrin fragments or other potentially embolic debris was seen.[3,4]

Plasma hemoglobin prior to clot formation was 159mg/dL (for our laboratory, normal is less than 15mg/dL). Following clot formation and mechanical lysis, plasma hemoglobin was 228mg/dL.[3,4]

DISCUSSION

The mechanism of this device is identical to that of a blender. A blender contains a cutting blade at the bottom of a vessel. The blade has a cutting edge and is slightly tilted (pitched). This allows for both the cutting of particles and for their recirculation. By recycling cut particles over and over again, particle size is progressively reduced. The effec-

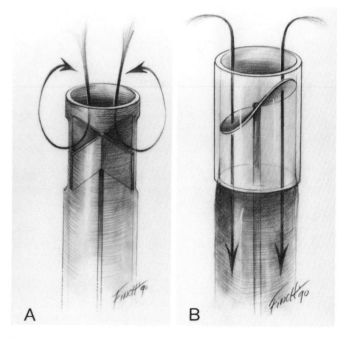

Figure 9.2.1. **A,B.** Schematic drawing of catheter tip with propeller in operational position demonstrating fluid circulation paths, allowing for recirculation of mechanically lysed clot during propeller rotation.

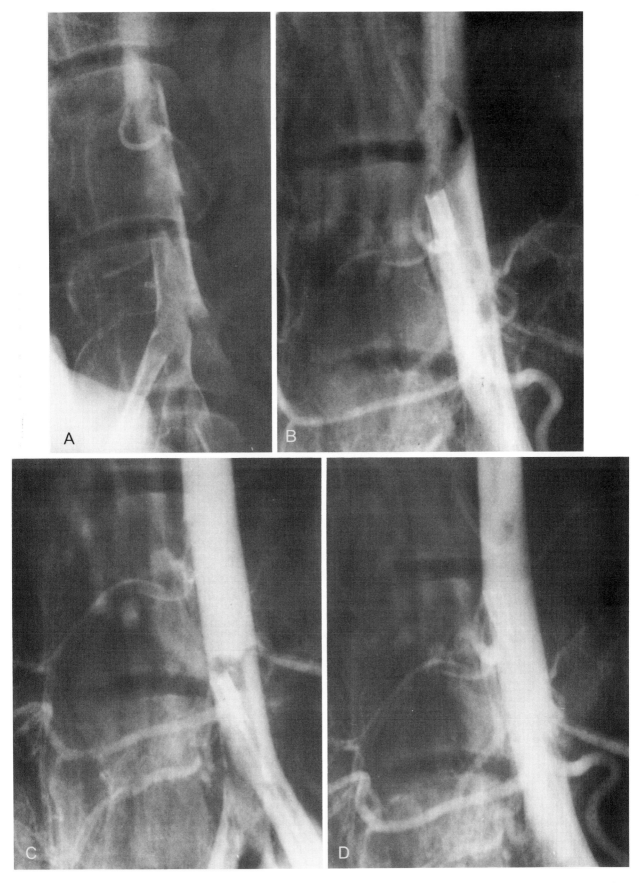

Figure 9.2.2. **A.** Thrombosed canine abdominal aorta. Proximal occlusion with balloon. **B,C.** Amplatz thrombectomy catheter fragmenting thrombus in abdominal aorta. **B.** High abdominal aorta. **C.** Low abdominal aorta. **D.** After completion of thrombectomy; no residual thrombus seen. No evidence of extravasation.

tiveness of a blender depends also on revolutions per minute and duration of application. The miniature version of a blender blade used in this design rotates in a small, metallic housing with two large side holes made to allow for material recycling. A nonencased, rapidly rotating turning blade would be dangerous if used in the vascular system. Consequently, the blade is recessed in the metal housing, preventing contact with the vessel wall.

The results obtained with the propeller catheter were surprising and far better than expected, especially since anticipated residues of fibrin were not found. Although there was nearly a 31% increase in plasma hemoglobin post-lysis, the total blood volume in the in vitro model was so much smaller than the total blood volume in a human that the in vivo human effect is expected to be much smaller and not likely to be clinically significant, even with larger clots. In vivo animal experimentation has verified this hypothesis (Fig. 9.2.2).[5]

The aged blood clots used in the experiments most closely resemble a venous or "red" thrombus which is primarily an admixture of red blood cells and fibrin, whereas an arterial or "white" thrombus is composed primarily of fibrin and platelets.[6]

Clinical application of this technique may be possible in both the venous and arterial systems. For example, deep vein thrombosis, particularly above the knee, has a significant potential for embolization.[7] Long-term oral anticoagulation necessitates several days of hospitalization and fails to protect against pulmonary emboli in as many as 28% of cases.[8] Mechanical thrombolysis immediately after placement of a retrievable inferior vena cava filter may prove to be a safe, rapid alternative means of treating such patients. Pulmonary embolus has been treated by percutaneous aspiration thromboembolectomy but requires a large catheter which is difficult to control.[9] Mechanical clot dissolution may be a more efficacious nonsurgical treatment.

Probably the most promising application of this new technique is the mechanical dissolution of clotted arterial bypass grafts. These thromboses are usually recent because they are immediately clinically evident. Therefore, clot dissolution can be expected to be similar to the in vitro experiments. Occlusion of the distal anastomosis or outflow vessels should not be necessary in order to prevent embolization. The extremely forceful, retrograde flow produced by the device should allow the clot to be dissolved from its proximal extent to its distal extent without any tendency to push or expel debris of any significant size distally. Mechanical dissolution may be accomplished in a few minutes compared to hours or days for enzymatic thrombolysis. The advantages of percutaneous mechanical dissolution over operative techniques (as in Fogarty procedures) include absence of a skin incision, lessened risk of infection, and the safety of continuous fluoroscopic control. In addition, the percutaneous technique probably will cause less endothelial damage and be less expensive. Advantages of mechanical dissolution over enzymatic thrombolysis are ones of time and expense since current thrombolytic regimens require intensive care unit monitoring, often for several days, multiple angiographic procedures to monitor the progress of thrombolysis and repeated laboratory tests such as the prothrombin time, partial thromboplastin time, thrombin time, and fibrinogen level.[10] In addition, the complications of enzymatic thrombolysis such as hematoma at the puncture site, internal bleeding, distal embolization of large particles (including remote mural thrombi sources), pericatheter thrombosis, graft extravasation, fever, and allergic reactions are eliminated.

Whether the mechanical catheter thrombolysis can become even more effective and faster when combined with the simultaneous administration of low-dose thrombolytic agents infused through the side port of the catheter currently remains to be demonstrated. One might expect that this would reduce the embolic potential of mechanical clot lysis. However, our present early results would indicate that simultaneous thrombolytic agent infusion may not appreciably diminish the number and size of particles, since tiny particles most likely represent combinations of cytoplasmic and nuclear cell fragments rather than fibrin.

References

1. Cohen LH, Kaplan M, Bernhard VM: Intraoperative streptokinase: an adjunct to mechanical thrombectomy in the management of acute ischemia. *Arch Surg* 1986;12(6):708–715

2. Fogarty TJ, Chin AK, Ollott C, Shoor PM, Zimmerman JJ, Garry MT: Combined thrombectomy and dilation for the treatment of acute lower extremity arterial thrombosis. *J Vasc Surg* 1989;10(5):530–534

3. Moradian GP, Bildsoe M, Hunter DW, Castañeda–Zúñiga WR, Amplatz K: In-vivo mechanical clot dissolution: experimental work in progress. *Radiology* 1988;169(suppl):366

4. Bildsoe MC, Moradian GP, Hunter DW, Castañeda–Zúñiga WR, Amplatz K: Mechanical clot dissolution: new concept. *Radiology* 1989;171:231–233

5. Carlson JE, Sunram SE, Kurisu Y, Yedlicka JW Jr, Hunter DW, Castañeda–Zúñiga WR, Amplatz K: New mechanical thrombectomy device. *Radiology* 1990;177(suppl):125

6. Robbin SL, Cotran RS (eds): Fluid and hemodynamic derangements, in *Pathologic Basis of Disease.* 2nd Ed. Philadelphia, W.B. Saunders, 1979, p 123

7. Moser KM, LeMoine JR: Is embolic risk conditioned by location of deep vein thrombosis? *Ann Intern Med* 1981;94:439–444

8. Bomalaski JS, Martin GJ, Hughes RL, Yao JST: Inferior vena cava interruption in the management of pulmonary embolism. *Chest* 1982;82:767–772

9. Greenfield LJ, Kimmell GO, McMurdy WC III: Transvenous removal of pulmonary emboli by vacuum-cup catheter technique. *J Surg Res* 1969;9:347–352

10. Klatte EC, Becker GJ, Holden RE, Yune HY: Fibrinolytic therapy. *Radiology* 1986;159:619–624

Part 3. Ponomar Transjugular Clot-trapper Device

—Eugenio Ponomar–Sulepov, M.D., Wilfrido R. Castañeda–Zúñiga, M.D., M.Sc., S. Murthy Tadavarthy, M.D., Joseph W. Yedlicka, Jr., M.D., David W. Hunter, M.D., Marcos A. Herrera, M.D., and Kurt Amplatz, M.D.

INTRODUCTION

Pulmonary embolism is a known complication of lower extremity and iliac vein thrombosis with an estimated non-fatal pulmonary embolism incidence in the United States

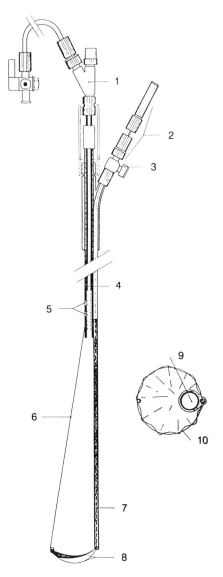

Figure 9.3.1. Diagram showing the different components of the clot-trapper device. Coaxial sheath (*1*), used to open and/or close side holes (*5*). Contrast medium can be injected through the sidearm adapter. Stainless-steel loop introducer which is used to open and/or close the funnel (*2*). Locking mechanism for holding the bag open and/or closed (*3*). Primary lumen of catheter (*4*) with side holes (*5*) and funnel attached to it (*6*). Second lumen of catheter (*7*) with stainless steel loop holding funnel open (*8*). Cross-section of end of funnel (*10*); cross-section of second lumen (*9*).

of 600,000 per year. Each year in the United States 140,000 patients die of pulmonary embolism.[1]

Most pulmonary emboli originate in the iliocaval (63.8%) and femoropopliteal segments (36.2%).[2] The presence of free-floating thrombus within the iliac veins and/or the inferior vena cava is a common indication for the placement of an inferior vena cava filter, but if the thrombus load is too large, patency of the inferior vena cava cannot be guaranteed after filter placement.

Recently, several devices have been described for the percutaneous removal of thrombus, predominantly on the arterial side, but with obvious applications on the venous side, including the thrombus aspiration catheters, and mechanical clot dissolution devices.[3–16] A mechanical device has also been used for thromboembolectomy in patients with pulmonary emboli.[17] All of these devices need to reach the level where the thrombus is lodged in order to either aspirate it or mechanically fragment it in situ. The risk with these methods is that a fragment of the thrombus might be dislodged and embolize into the pulmonary arteries. This is particularly risky in the presence of large free-floating thrombus in the inferior vena cava and/or iliac veins. The clot-trapper device (CTD) was developed for the removal of large amounts of thrombus from the iliac veins and from the inferior vena cava. The device can be used in conjunction with a mechanical thrombectomy device[3,8,10] to

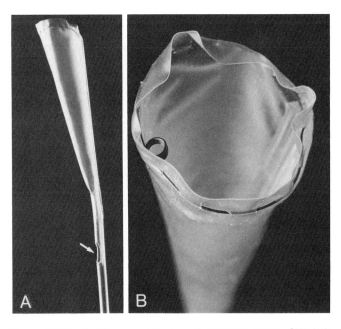

Figure 9.3.2. **A.** Close-up side view of Ponomar device. Side hole (*arrow*). **B.** Close-up view of open end of bag.

fragment the thrombus once this has been caught within the bag.

MATERIALS AND METHODS

The prototype CTD consists of a 12Fr double-lumen catheter (Fig. 9.3.1). The smaller lumen of the catheter is 15cm long in the distal end of the device and houses a stainless-steel wire whose distal end emerges as a spring loop at a 90° angle to the shaft. The loop is attached to the distal end of a 15cm long funnel-shaped polyvinyl bag (Fig. 9.3.2A,B). The proximal end of the bag is connected to the second lumen. The distal end of the bag can be opened or closed by advancing or retracting the wire. Adjustments on the size of the spring loop allow adaptation to different inferior vena cava (IVC) diameters.

In the proximal end of the large lumen there is a coaxial introducer with a check-flow valve and a side-arm flushing port. The forward movement of the introducer closes the side holes, made in the midsegment of the large lumen just above the connection of the large lumen with the proximal end of the bag.

The clot-trapper device for transjugular thrombectomy is introduced using a venous cut-down in the right internal jugular vein to place a 20Fr Teflon sheath. The CTD is then introduced through the sheath over a stiffening wire. Com-

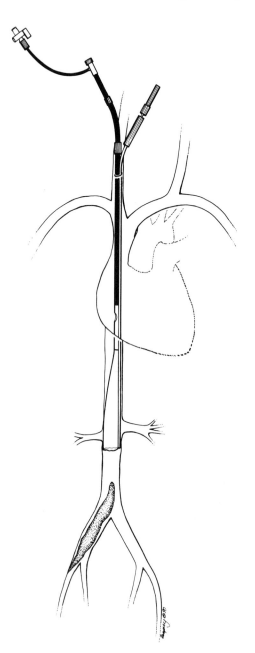

Figure 9.3.3.   Diagram illustrating the position of the clot-trapper device below the renal veins.

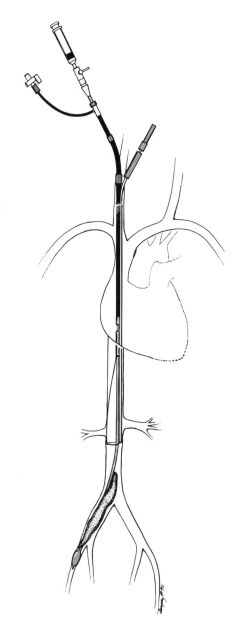

Figure 9.3.4.   A Medi-tech occlusion balloon has been passed beyond the location of the iliac vein thrombus which will be pulled back into the open end of the funnel.

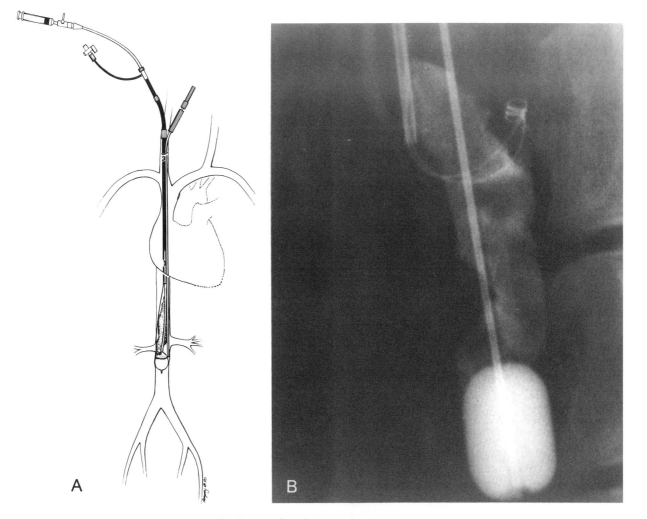

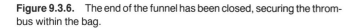

Figure 9.3.5. **A.** The iliac thrombus has been pulled into the funnel-shaped bag. **B.** A contrast-labeled thrombus injected into the common femoral vein of a mongrel dog is being pulled into the funnel by the balloon catheter.

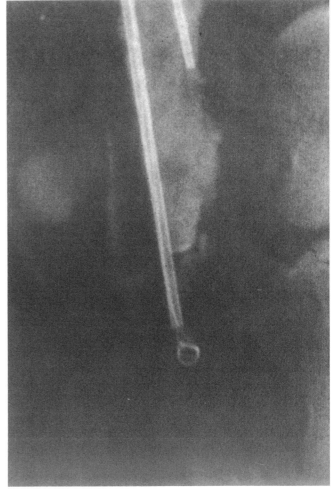

Figure 9.3.6. The end of the funnel has been closed, securing the thrombus within the bag.

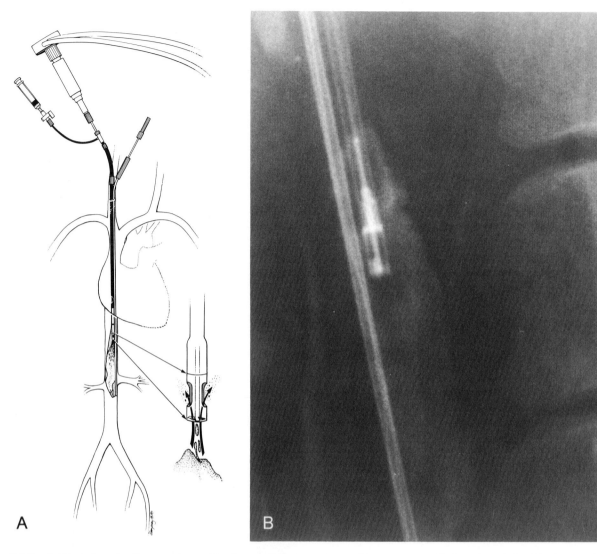

Figure 9.3.7. **A.** The balloon has been exchanged for the mechanical thrombectomy device, which is being used to fragment the clot within the closed bag. The close-up shows the thrombus being aspirated into the end of the mechanical thrombectomy device, where it is fragmented and the small fragments are spilled out through the side windows. **B.** Contrast-labeled thrombus trapped within the bag in a mongrel dog is being fragmented by the mechanical thrombectomy device (same dog as in Fig. 9.3.5).

monly, the distal end of the CTD is placed below the level of the renal veins in the inferior vena cava (Fig. 9.3.3). The bag is opened to allow the blood flow in the vena cava to pass through the bag and go out through the two side holes in the lateral wall of the large lumen, therefore preserving vena caval flow. A Medi-tech occlusion balloon catheter is introduced through the check-flow valve and is advanced over a guidewire into the iliac vein or inferior vena cava where the thrombus is lodged (Fig. 9.3.4). By injecting contrast medium in the iliac vein through the end hole of the catheter, the thrombus is localized; using the inflated balloon, the thrombus is pulled toward the opening of the bag (Fig. 9.3.5A,B). Once the thrombus is trapped in the bag, the check-flow introducer set is pushed forward to close the side holes. The injection of contrast material through

the side arm allows one to verify the presence of the thrombus in the bag. The balloon is deflated and withdrawn, and the entrance of the bag closed, effectively trapping the thrombus. Flow through the IVC is not blocked during this maneuver for more than a few seconds.

The CTD was first tested in an inferior vena cava simulator to determine its ability to trap in vitro-created thrombus. In all experiments, the Amplatz mechanical thrombectomy device (MTD) was used to destroy thrombus trapped in the bag. The MTD device consists of an 8Fr catheter with a rotating propeller enclosed in a metal housing. The distal open end allows flow into the housing, while two lateral windows allow flow out of the housing. The rotation of the propeller at 100,000 rpm produces suction, bringing thrombi against the open distal end and, therefore, into contact with the rotating propeller that fragments the thrombi into minuscule fragments.[3,8,10]

In 10 dogs, the CTD was placed below the level of the renal veins and the bag was opened. Thirty-six in vitro-created thrombi 10 × 100mm, incubated in contrast medium for 24 hours to render them radiopaque, were then injected into the iliac vein or the inferior vena cava through a 24Fr sheath placed in the right femoral vein. A balloon catheter was used to manipulate the thrombus into the bag. Once the thrombi were trapped in the bag, the distal end of the bag was closed (Fig. 9.3.6). Injection of contrast

material through the side arm allowed verification of the presence of thrombus in the bag. The balloon was withdrawn, and the MTD introduced to destroy the clot within the bag (Fig. 9.3.7*A,B*). The fragmentation occurs within the bag and thus minimizes or prevents embolization by the fragments. After successful fragmentation of the thrombus, the MTD was removed, the bag was emptied by suction through the side-arm flushing port (Fig. 9.3.8), and the CTD was removed through the access sheath. In addition, depending on the amount of thrombus trapped within the bag, the CTD with the intact clot can also be removed through the internal jugular vein access (Fig. 9.3.9*A,B*). In two dogs, semi-acute inferior vena cava thrombosis was produced by percutaneously placing a clip in the infrarenal segment of the inferior vena cava, approximately 5–10cm below the renal veins. After seven days, thrombosis of the inferior vena cava was confirmed by venography (Fig. 9.3.10*A*). The clip was removed after placing the CTD. The CTD, in combination with the MTD, was used immediately thereafter to remove the thrombus (Fig. 9.3.10*B*). The iliac vein and IVC of all dogs were resected at the end of the procedure and submitted for histopathologic examination.

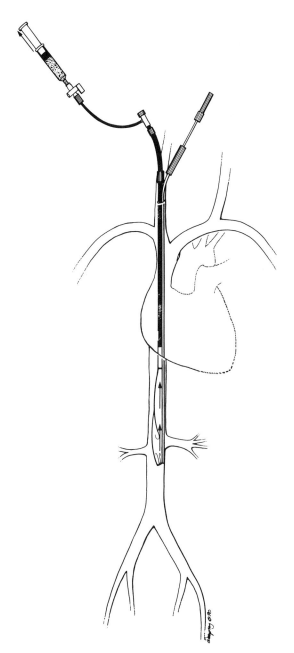

Figure 9.3.8. Diagram of bag being removed after in situ fragmentation.

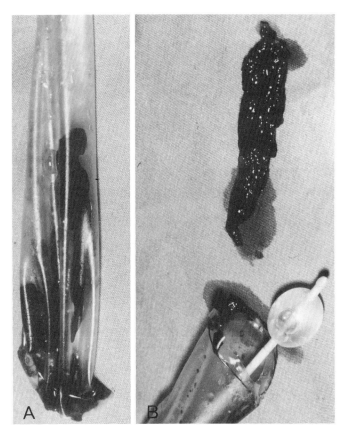

Figure 9.3.9. A,B. Photograph of the bag of the clot-trapper device with the trapped clot inside, which was removed intact through the access in the jugular vein. The bag measures 15cm in length.

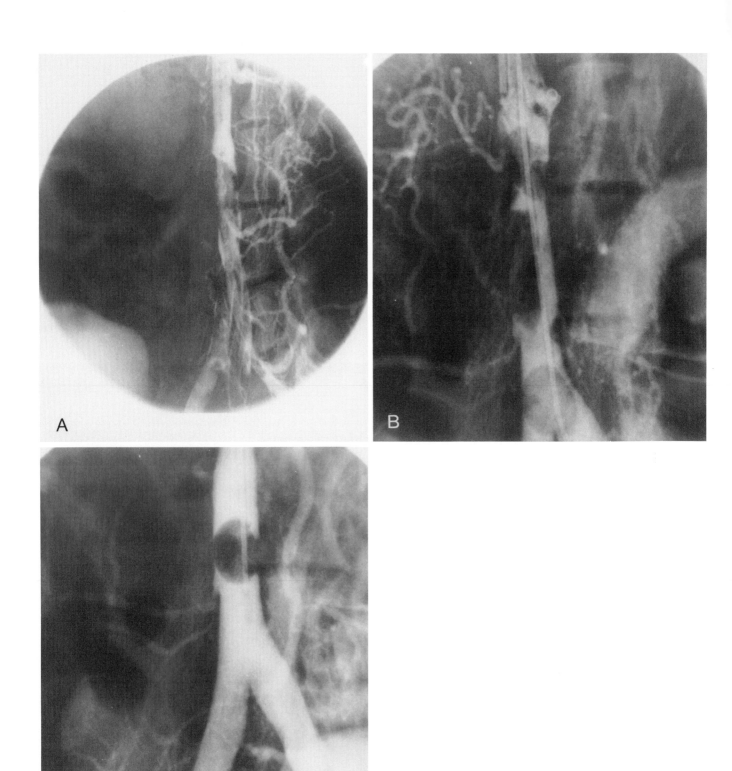

Figure 9.3.10. **A.** Extensive thrombosis of inferior vena cava one week post-clipping. **B.** Ponomar trapper device in place trapping thrombus. **C.** Inferior vena cavogram post-thrombus removal.

RESULTS

The CTD was tested in 10 acute experiments using 36 in vitro-created thrombi.[11] In the first two acute dogs, pulmonary embolism occurred after four contrast-labeled in vitro thrombi (two in each dog) were introduced into the iliac vein and the IVC and the CTD failed to trap them because there was a discrepancy between the IVC diameter and the diameter of the bag opening. After increasing the size of the loop and bag opening to match different inferior vena cava diameters forcing, therefore, all the blood flow into the bag, trapping of all the injected clot was possible in both acute and chronic experiments. In the following 8 acute dogs, 32 in vitro-created thrombi (16 contrast-labeled and 16 unlabeled) were introduced into the iliac vein and IVC and trapped successfully by the CTD. All the thrombi were then successfully fragmented by the MTD.

In two dogs, extensive semi-acute inferior vena cava thromboses produced by clipping of the infrarenal IVC were removed using the CTD in combination with the MTD.

Histopathologic examinations of the IVC after the use of the CTD showed endothelial desquamation. No evidence of perforation was found.

DISCUSSION

The management of acute iliofemoral venous thrombosis remains a difficult problem particularly if large floating thrombus is present in the IVC and/or iliac veins. Technological developments in recent times include several thrombus-removing devices. Günther reported that the aspiration catheter for percutaneous thrombectomy was not efficient in the venous system because of collapse of the vein during aspiration.[12] Several authors have reported the use of mechanical thrombectomy devices for the rapid removal of thrombus from arteries and/or veins.[3-16] All of these devices have the risk of embolization of the fragmented thrombus. This would be particularly dangerous in the presence of large free-floating thrombi in the IVC and/or iliac veins. The CTD was developed for the removal of large amounts of thrombus from the iliac veins and/or IVC.

Mechanical thrombus fragmentation inside the bag of the CTD where the clot is isolated reduces the possibility of embolism. Our preliminary in vitro and in vivo results are encouraging. CTD, used in combination with MTD, will enable the quick and effective removal of large venous thrombus from the IVC and the iliac veins. Large thrombus in the iliac vein or IVC can usually be fragmented and pulled into the bag. This was the situation in the two dogs with IVC clipping. Once the bag is filled, its end is closed prior to fragmentation with the MTD. If there is fear of migration of untrapped fragments, the bag can be left open, since the IVC blood flow will keep the trapped thrombus within the bag during fragmentation with the

MTD. The suction produced by the MTD further attracts the thrombus against the end of the device. Contrast medium can be injected through the lumen of the MTD to facilitate visualization of the trapped thrombus in the bag.

Further improvements in the technology will allow an easier introduction since, in its present prototype stage, the device requires a 20Fr size introducer sheath. The use of a 30mm universal diameter bag will allow, in most cases, a good match with the IVC diameter. The diameter of the IVC will be determined by inferior vena cavography. Oversize bags can be made available for large inferior venae cavae.

References

1. Dalen JE, Alpert JS: Natural history of pulmonary emboli. *Prog Cardiovasc Dis* 1975;17:259–270
2. Savelyev VS, Yablokov EG, Kirienko AI: Surgical prevention of pulmonary embolism. *World J Surg* 1980;4:709–716
3. Bildsoe MC, Moradian GP, Hunter DW, Castañeda–Zúñiga WR, Amplatz K: Mechanical clot dissolution: new concept. *Radiology* 1989;171:231–233
4. Hansen DD, Auth DC, Vracko R, Ritchie JL: Rotational thrombectomy in acute canine coronary thrombosis. *Int J Cardiol* 1989;22(l):13–19
5. Hansen DD, Auth DC, Vracko R, Ritchie JL: Mechanical thrombectomy: a comparison of two rotational devices and balloon angioplasty in subacute canine femoral thrombosis. *Am Heart J* 1987;114(5):1223–1231
6. Kensey KR, Nash JE, Abrahams C, Zarins CK: Recanalization of obstructed arteries with a flexible, rotating tip catheter. *Radiology* 1987;165:387–389
7. Yedlicka JW Jr, Carlson JE, Hunter DW, Castañeda–Zúñiga WR, Amplatz K: Thrombectomy with the TEC endarterectomy system: an experimental study. *JVIR*, in press
8. Moradian GP, Bildsoe M, Hunter DW, Castañeda-Zúñiga WR, Amplatz K: In-vivo mechanical clot dissolution. Experimental work in progress. *Radiology* 1988;169(suppl):366
9. Hawkins IF, Helms R, Spencer C, Hawkins MC: Mechanical spiral embolectomy catheter. *Semin Intervent Radiol* 1985;2(4):414–418:
10. Carlson JE, Sunram SE, Kurisu Y, Yedlicka JW Jr, Hunter DW, Castañeda–Zúñiga WR, Amplatz K: New mechanical thrombectomy device. *Radiology* 1990;177(suppl):125
11. Ponomar–Sulepov E, Carlson JE, Kindlund A, Pacho–Rodriguez J, Yedlicka JW Jr, Hunter DW, Castañeda-Zúñiga WR, Amplatz K: Clot trapper device for transjugular thrombectomy from the inferior vena cava. *Radiology* 1991;179(1):279–282
12. Günther RW, Vorwerk D: A new aspiration thromboembolectomy catheter with propeller-tipped rotating wire: an in-vitro study. *J Intervent Radiol* 1990;1:17–20
13. Günther RW, Vorwerk D: Aspiration catheter for percutaneous thrombectomy: clinical results. *Radiology* 1990;175:271–273
14. Starck EE, McDermott JC, Crummy AB: Percutaneous aspiration thromboembolectomy. *Radiology* 1985;156:61–66
15. Buxton DR Jr, Mueller CF: Removal of iatrogenic clot by transcatheter embolectomy. *Radiology* 1974;111:39–41
16. Sniderman KW, Bodner L, Saddekni S, Srur M, Sos TA: Percutaneous embolectomy by transcatheter aspiration. *Radiology* 1984;150:357–361
17. Greenfield LJ, Kimmell GO, McMurdy WC III: Transvenous removal of pulmonary emboli by vacuum-cup catheter technique. *J Surg Res* 1969;9:347–352

Part 4. Günther Aspiration Thromboembolectomy Catheter

—Wilfrido R. Castañeda–Zúñiga, M.D., M.Sc., Marcos A. Herrera, M.D., S. Murthy Tadavarthy, M.D., David W. Hunter, M.D., Joseph W. Yedlicka, Jr., M.D., and Kurt Amplatz, M.D.

A modification of the Amplatz propeller-tipped thromboembolectomy catheter[1-3] has been used by Günther in vitro and in clinical cases.[4,5] The new thrombectomy catheter consists of a 7Fr Teflon catheter with an inner lumen of 1.8mm. A 0.4mm rotating shaft is attached to a 1.2mm propeller. The propeller is encased within the distal end of the Teflon catheter (Fig. 9.4.1). The propeller/rotating shaft is driven by a waterproof 25-volt DC motor unit that can rotate the propeller at speeds up to 1000 rpm. Continuous suction is applied using a roller pump to transport the fragmented thrombus via a sidearm adapter to a reservoir. A recent modification of the device has the propeller enclosed inside of a basket, to allow fast, safe application, particularly for pulmonary embolism management.[6]

TECHNIQUE

Access is achieved using either an antegrade puncture for the femoral vessels or a retrograde puncture for the iliac arteries. A 7Fr check-flow sheath is placed. The thrombectomy catheter is advanced under fluoroscopic or roadmapping guidance until it reaches the level of the obstruction. With the tip of the catheter placed against the thrombus, the suction and the motor drive are started, with the propeller rotating at speeds of 500–1000 rpm. As the thrombus fragments and is aspirated, the catheter is slowly advanced, until all the obstructing material has been removed, as demonstrated by angiography.

RESULTS

In vitro experimentation proved the 7Fr catheter to be less effective than the 10Fr version. This is mostly related to clogging of the 7Fr propeller by fibrin winding around the distal end. There were only minimal fibrin deposits around the rotating shaft. These problems were not seen with the 10Fr catheter. Another significant difference between the two catheters was the time required for fragmentation, which was 6 times longer with the 7Fr design. Aspiration performance at different speeds of the propeller was not significantly different.[5]

The ability of the catheter to declot thrombosed caval filters was also tested in vitro; five clotted Günther filters (40g) were successfully declotted, without causing migration of thrombi.[5]

The 7Fr catheter has been successfully used in two out of three patients to fragment/aspirate thrombus. In one patient with a clotted polytetrafluoroethylene hemodialysis fistula, the procedure was only partially successful. Distal migration of thrombus was seen in one of the patients; incomplete removal of the migrated fragment was achieved by advancing the 7Fr catheter distally into the tibioperoneal trunk.[4]

DISCUSSION

The design of the catheter allows the safe removal of thrombus, although migration of breakaway fragments may occur. Vascular perforation has not been seen, and it is unlikely to occur due to the recessed location of the propeller within the catheter tip. Catheter obstruction by fibrin deposits winding around the wire or propeller can occur, particularly with the 7Fr catheter. The small size of the propeller and rotating shaft provides for overall flexibility of the catheter, facilitating its introduction into smaller vessels.

Preliminary results are encouraging with fast, effective removal of thrombus, making this technique an attractive alternative to thrombolytic therapy, with potential for tremendous cost savings.[7]

References

1. Bildsoe MC, Moradian GP, Hunter DW, Castañeda–Zúñiga WR, Amplatz K: Mechanical clot dissolution: new concept. *Radiology* 1989;171:231–233
2. Moradian GP, Bildsoe M, Hunter DW, Castañeda–Zúñiga WR, Amplatz K: In vivo mechanical clot dissolution: experimental work in progress. *Radiology* 1988;169(suppl):366
3. Carlson JE, Sunram SE, Kurisu Y, Yedlicka JW Jr, Hunter DW, Castañeda-Zúñiga WR, Amplatz K: New mechanical thrombectomy device. *Radiology* 1990;177(suppl):125
4. Günther RW, Vorwerk D: Aspiration catheter for percutaneous thrombectomy: clinical results. *Radiology* 1990;175:271–273

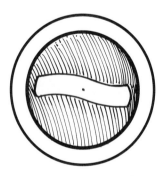

Figure 9.4.1. Diagrammatic representation of Günther propeller tip.

5. Günther RW, Vorwerk D: A new aspiration thromboembolectomy catheter with propeller-tipped rotating wire: an in-vitro study. *J Intervent Radiol* 1990;1:17–20

6. Schnitz–Rode T, Günther RW, Vorwerk D: A new device for percutaneous fragmentation of pulmonary emboli. Presented at the SCVIR Annual Meeting. San Francisco, CA, 1991

7. Dacey LJ, Dow R, McDaniel MD: Cost-effectiveness of intra-arterial thrombolysis. *Arch Surg* 1988;123:1218–1223

Part 5. Rotational Thrombectomy

—Wilfrido R. Castañeda–Zúñiga, M.D., M.Sc., Patricia E. Thorpe, M.D., S. Murthy Tadavarthy, M.D., Joseph W. Yedlicka, Jr., M.D., David W. Hunter, M.D., Marcos A. Herrera, M.D., and Kurt Amplatz, M.D.

A new thrombectomy catheter was described by Ritchie in 1986[1] consisting of a rotating guidewire capable of lysing acute arterial thrombus. The wire is an 0.008- or 0.006-inch diameter wire with a steerable 0.025-inch diameter platinum tip (Fig. 9.5.1). Rotation of the wire at 6000 rpm within the thrombus wraps fibrin tightly around the shaft. Cellular elements are released into the circulation and the clot is effectively lysed. Particle analysis of the liquefied thrombus showed only single red cells and clumps of red cells under 10 μm in diameter. Angioscopy revealed residual thrombus lining the arterial wall. Histology confirmed luminal thrombin.[2] The device was subsequently modified by Auth to more effectively fragment thrombus, by substituting the noncutting for a cutting rotating abrasive head, with a central, flexible 0.008-inch guidewire. The wire and the tip were designed to be advanced independently. The central guidewire serves to maintain the intraluminal position of the tip. The abrasive surface on the cutting head consists of 30–40 μm diameter diamond particles partially buried in a nickel substrate. Rotational speed was increased to 40,000 rpm.[3]

The cutting tip was found to be more effective than the non-cutting tip.[3]

References

1. Ritchie JL, Hansen DD, Vracko R, Auth DC: Mechanical thrombolysis: a new rotational catheter approach for acute thrombi. *Circulation* 1986;73(5):1006–1012

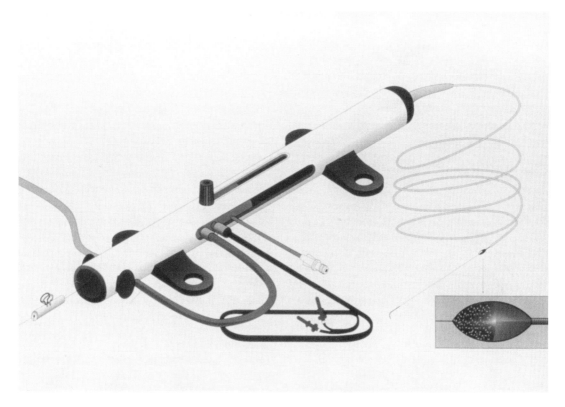

Figure 9.5.1. Rotablator thrombectomy system. Close-up of tip of device.

2. Ritchie JL, Hansen DD, Intlekofer R, Vracko R, Auth DC: Thrombolysis: a new rotational thrombectomy catheter and evaluation by angioscopy. International Symposium on Interventional Cardiology. 16th Annual Symposium of the Texas Heart Institute. September 1986

3. Hansen DD, Auth DC, Vracko R, Ritchie JL: Mechanical thrombectomy: a comparison of two rotational devices and balloon angioplasty in subacute canine femoral thrombosis. *Am Heart J* 1987;114(8):1223–1231

Part 6. Percutaneous Aspiration Thromboembolectomy

—Erhard Starck, M.D., and Hans–Joachim Wagner, M.D.

The principle of removing embolic material by aspiration was reported in 1960 by Greenfield using the transvenous aspiration of pulmonary emboli through a femoral venotomy.[1] In 1974, Buxton and Mueller reported successful removal of iatrogenic clot from a renal artery by catheter aspiration.[2] In 1978, Horvath suggested that emboli caused by balloon angioplasty might be removed by aspiration.[3] In 1984, Sniderman et al. published five successful removals of postangioplasty emboli, out of six patients.[4] In 1985, experience with the percutaneous aspiration thromboembolectomy (PAT) was reported.[5] The further development of PAT, the rotating aspiration thromboembolectomy (RAT), was published in 1988.[6]

Materials

Digital subtraction angiography with roadmapping capability is very useful to guide the aspiration. The material required for PAT is an 8Fr sheath, the aspiration catheter, a 50ml syringe, and guidewires. The hemostasis valve on the sheath must be removable, easy to clean of entrapped clot material, and adjustable to the diameters of the aspiration catheters and guidewires to prevent blood loss. The side port of the hemostasis valve serves for flushing and contrast medium injections.

A detachable hemostasis valve is necessary because large fragments of thrombus protruding from the tip of the aspiration catheter will be trapped at the valve level, and this needs to be taken apart to be cleaned. Clot aspiration can be performed with any catheter without side holes, but effectiveness of aspiration increases significantly with luminal width. Therefore, the specially designed aspiration catheters—available from 5 to 9Fr (Angiomed Corp; Germany)—are thin-walled and only minimally tapered. The different sites are used according to the treated vessel site; 7–8Fr in the femoral popliteal region, 5–6Fr in the tibial and pedal region.

Technique

The application of PAT depends upon the individual situation with respect to site, length, volume, consistency, and age of the occlusion. The basic technique is shown in Figure 9.6.1. The occluded vascular segment is first recanalized with a guidewire—preferably a flexible wire with hydrophilic coating (Glidewire, Terumo Corp.)—and a 5Fr Berenstein-type catheter (CE VI; Bald Corp., France). The initial wire and catheter passage serves for information about the consistency of the occlusive material. The aspiration catheter then is advanced over the wire to the site of occlusion. After removal of the wire, the catheter is advanced to obtain contact with the embolus. Digital subtraction arteriography (DSA)-roadmapping is useful. Negative pressure for aspiration is applied by hand with a 50ml syringe. Thrombotic firmer material will be engaged at the tip and needs to be extracted together with the catheter through the sheath, after disconnection of the hemostasis valve.

If blood readily enters the syringe during catheter extraction, the occlusive material either has cleared the catheter or has dropped distally. The syringe is removed and its contents are ejected over a gauze-draped basin. Particles present indicate the type of occlusive material removed. Blood filtered into the basin is an indicator of blood loss. The aspiration catheter is reintroduced and contrast material is then injected through the aspiration catheter to reassess the situation. Multiple aspirations can be performed as necessary.

The most important point concerning applicability of PAT is the age of the thrombus. Fresh, soft thrombus and embolus can be easily aspirated (Fig. 9.6.2). The harder the thrombus, the more passes will be required to remove the obstructing material. In chronic occlusions with firm thrombus, pretreatment is necessary to soften, loosen, or break apart the thrombus by local thrombolytic infusion, balloon dilatation, or rotating mechanical devices. Information about the age of the thrombus is gained from the patient's history and by the resistance felt during the initial wire and catheter passage.

PAT before Balloon Dilation in Fresh Thrombotic Occlusions

In fresh occlusions, the patient's history is short and the resistance during catheter passage is very low except at the

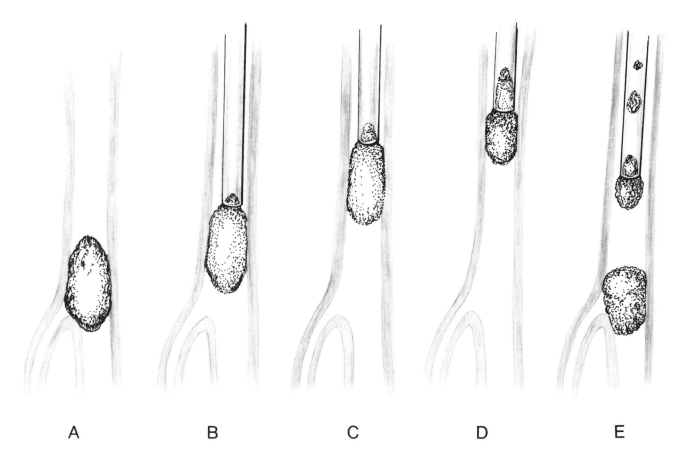

| A | B | C | D | E |

Figure 9.6.1. Basic technique of PAT. **A.** Embolus lodged in a vessel bifurcation. **B.** Aspiration catheter in contact moves the embolus. **C.** Catheter is withdrawn. **D.** Embolus remodels to the distal catheter lumen. **E.** The material becomes fragmented, small particles pass; firmer material is entrapped at the catheter tip and has to be extracted.

stenotic site (Fig. 9.6.3). In these cases, PAT before balloon dilatation serves two functions. The aspiration of soft thrombotic material minimizes the chances for distal embolization and also reduces procedure time significantly. After PAT, balloon dilatation can be used to treat the underlying stenosis which caused the thrombotic occlusion. In this situation, PAT also excludes the need for time-consuming local thrombolysis.

Bᴀʟʟᴏᴏɴ Dɪʟᴀᴛᴀᴛɪᴏɴ ʙᴇғᴏʀᴇ PAT

When a chronic occlusion with hard embolic material is present, the lesion is predilated (Fig. 9.6.4). Fragmentation of the material by balloon dilatation reduces the consistency of the occluding material, improving the ability to pass the aspiration catheter. This also decreases the need for local urokinase infusion. The increased contact surface for the lytic agent caused by mechanical fragmentation speeds the process enormously.[7,8] However, if the most distal part of an occlusion is dilated before PAT, the chances of distal embolization are increased. Distal embolization can be solved by further aspiration, although vascular wall trauma can occur. The fragmentation and detachment of firm thrombus with the rotating devices or the softening of hard thrombus with thrombolysis is a better alternative.

PAT ᴀɴᴅ Lᴏᴄᴀʟ Lʏsɪs

Local thrombolytic infusion of urokinase helps PAT by reducing the volume of occluding material. Fragmentation, loosening, and aspiration of the material through the catheter is facilitated.

PAT and local thrombolysis balance each other. As more lysis is used, the less PAT will be necessary and vice versa. So with PAT we not only improve the success rate but also decrease thrombolysis procedure time and the hemorrhagic complications related to thrombolysis. In our experience, lysis overnight is exceptional, with most intra-arterial thrombolytic infusions lasting a maximum of six hours. Most often, we finish the procedure within two to four hours by performing aspiration at intervals during lysis. Using this protocol, we are able to limit the dose of urokinase to 400,000 IU. In 65% of the cases, we do not use any lysis, and in 11% a minidose regimen is used. We use the regular dose of up to 700,000 units of urokinase in only 24% of patients.

The increased contact surface for the lytic agent caused by mechanical fragmentation enormously speeds the process.[7,8] Initially, however, we should not touch the most distal occlusion segment, because of the higher embolization risk.

Figure 9.6.2. Fresh thrombolytic occlusions, PAT application only. **A.** Diagnostic arteriogram. **B.** After first aspiration. **C.** After second aspiration. **D.** Final after several passes.

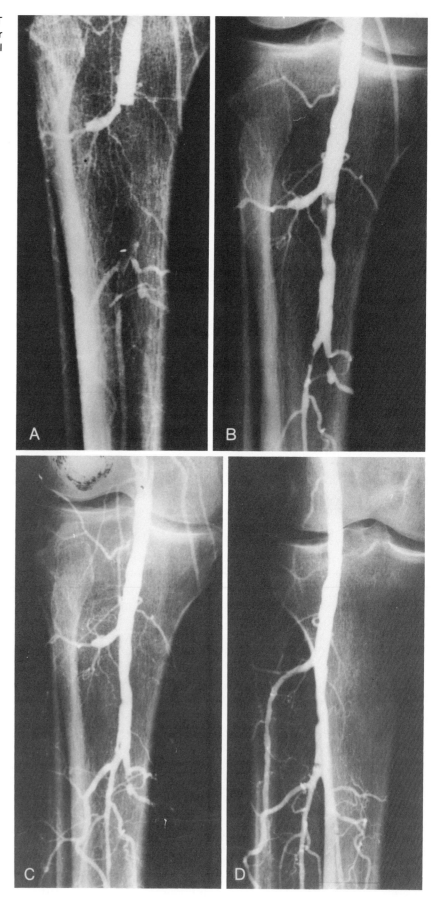

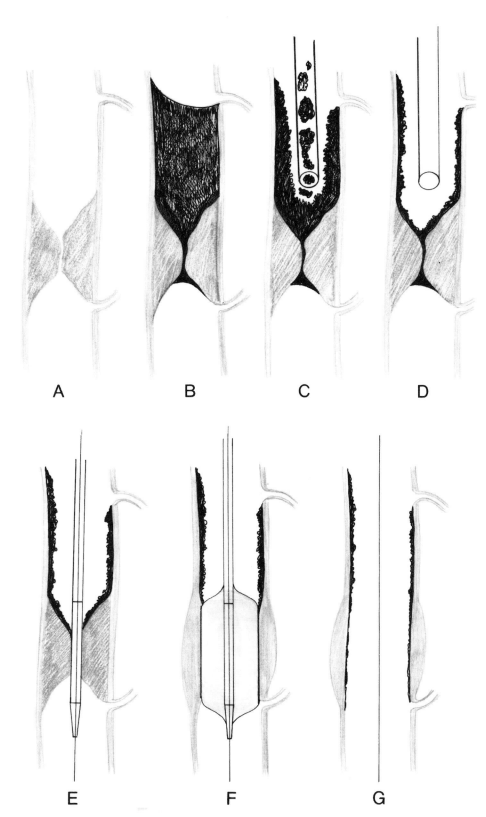

Figure 9.6.3. PAT before balloon dilatation in case of fresh thrombotic occlusion. **A.** High-grade stenosis. **B.** Subsequent thrombotic occlusion. **C.** Removal of thrombotic material by PAT. **D.** Stenosis uncovered. **E.** Balloon catheter placement. **F.** Dilatation to finish reopening. **G.** Final control angiography.

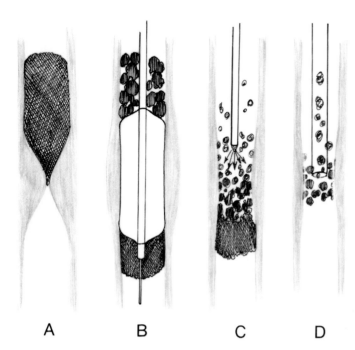

Figure 9.6.4. Accelerated thrombolysis with PAT. **A.** Thromboembolic occlusion. **B.** Fragmentation by balloon dilatation increasing the contact surface for the lytic agent. **C.** Local lytic infusion. **D.** PAT removes unlysable components, thus speeding the reopening significantly.

SPECIAL PAT PROCEDURES

Aspiration over a Wire

Aspiration over a wire can be useful to decrease the incidence of subintimal passage. The risk increases at curved vessel sites, for instance at the popliteal artery, when the catheter is moved against resistance, especially with aspiration. A wire in the aspiration channel requires a Tuohy–Borst adapter and reduces the effectiveness of aspiration by its size. It also prevents extraction of large fragments.

Small Vessel PAT

In small vessels, a wire is initially passed distally. A 5Fr aspiration catheter will follow. After removal of the wire, negative pressure is created and the catheter is withdrawn. If the aspiration catheter is advanced under aspiration into small vessels distally, the risk of subintimal passage is higher. Aspiration during catheter pullback excludes subintimal passage. The occlusion is then removed from distal to proximal; this unfortunately takes more time and sometimes proximal embolic particles migrate distally.

Cross-over PAT

Contralateral PAT presents the risk of embolization of the unaffected leg. In this situation, one needs to make sure that the aspirated material fits perfectly within the lumen of the aspiration catheter, so it can be withdrawn through the sheath without embolizing.

Thrombus Overload

Overload occurs when a large thrombus is aspirated only partially into the aspiration catheter and gets stuck in the distal portion of the sheath. The existence of this problem is signaled by the lack of backbleeding if the hemostasis valve is taken off. An attempt can be made to aspirate the material through the sheath with a 50ml syringe. If this fails, a Terumo wire is passed, while maintaining continuous suction through the side port of the repositioned hemostasis valve. If the wire pushes the thrombus fragment back into the artery, blood will enter the syringe immediately. If it does not, the sheath is removed under suction. The sheath is cleaned and repositioned over the wire. If the fragment has been pushed back, a second wire is inserted through the sheath. The sheath is then removed and reintroduced over one of the wires. The second wire remains outside the sheath functioning as a safety wire. If the fragment is caught during the next aspiration, it is pulled back into the sheath, and, after removal of the hemostasis valve, aspiration is performed or the sheath is removed, keeping the safety wire in place. PAT through the sheath is more effective because of the greater luminal width. During aspiration through the sheath, one has to avoid kinking of the sheath or manual pressure at the puncture site. The second wire serves for reintroduction of the sheath to reassess the situation angiographically.

Aspiration of intimal flap or plaque material is a rare but sometimes extremely difficult problem, because intimal flap or plaque material is less elastic and does not fit easily through the catheter lumen like clot material. It therefore cannot be fixed sufficiently for extraction. A spherical-tip spiral or a spherical-tip basket rotated by hand can be used to trap these hard fragments (Fig. 9.6.5).[6]

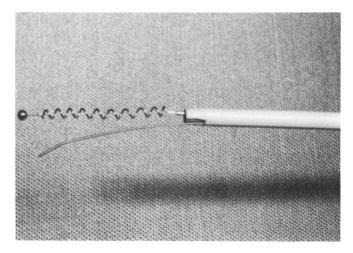

Figure 9.6.5. Spherical-tip spiral for rotating aspiration thromboembolectomy (RAT) together with the double lumen aspiration catheter for simultaneous thrombolytic contrast injection. The spiral also catches intimal flap material or emboli for extraction under aspiration.

GENERAL INDICATIONS

PAT below the inguinal ligament can be used in thrombotic and embolic occlusions causing clinical symptoms according to Fontaine classification IIb, III, and IV. The indications for PAT embolectomy were mainly emergency situations, in comparison to the balloon angioplasty group. Most of the embolizations treated not related to angioplasty were cardiogenic in origin (Fig. 9.6.6). Rare opportunities for PAT are renal or mesenteric embolizations. These patients need to be treated as fast as possible, because of the low ischemic tolerance of these organs. For PAT in these regions, a transaxillary approach is needed.

PAT is not recommended for thromboembolic occlusions of the abdominal aorta, pulmonary, and iliac arteries because of the large amount of material that has to be withdrawn through a relatively small catheter lumen. It is also nearly impossible to aspirate embolized material lying beside the sheath in retrograde femoral punctures. So, by far the main indication for PAT is below the inguinal ligament after antegrade punctures. Contralateral PAT is very exceptional, as mentioned earlier.

RESULTS

Since the first application in 1981, we have treated more than 400 patients with PAT, mainly in combination with other revascularization methods (Table. 9.6.1). The addition of the aspiration technique improved our clinical balloon dilatation results in the femoral-popliteal region from 59–75% to 91% of the first 156 treatments where PAT was applied.[9,10] In 50% of these, local lysis was employed as well.

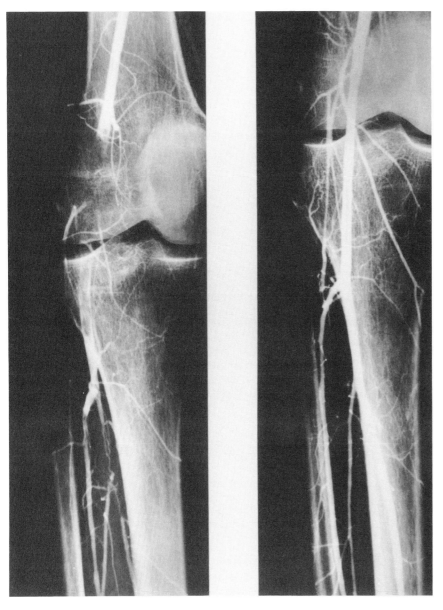

Figure 9.6.6. Acute cardiogenic, PAT application only. **A.** Diagnostic arteriogram. **B.** Follow-up arteriogram after a few aspirations.

Table 9.6.1. Additional Angioplastic Techniques in 82 PAT Patients[a]

Balloon dilatation	162 (61 × tibial)
Local thrombolysis	29 (35%)
RAT	7 (9%)
Endarterectomy (TEC)	2
Stent implantation	3

[a]Out of the total of 489 leg angioplasties in 1989.

Since the advent of PAT, we have not had significant embolization after angioplasty requiring surgical embolectomy.

In 1989, we had 489 patients with angioplasty of the legs. PAT was used on 82 (16%) of these patients. Of these, 43 (52%) were in Stage IIb, 7 (9%) in Stage III, and 32 (39%) in Stage IV, according to Fontaine, before the angioplasty treatment, not including the emergency situations because of distal embolization after balloon dilatation and/or local lysis.

Fifty-five percent of the PAT cases were performed in thrombotic occlusions, and 29% in embolic related to angioplasty, and in 16% of these embolic occlusions, the embolus was of cardiogenic origin. The overall clinical primary success was 92% (Table 9.6.2).

A lower clinical success (84%) with more complications was seen in the group of cardiogenic emboli. In spite of this, our results are superior to the published data for the Fogarty embolectomy.[10,11] In our department, all patients with acute embolic occlusions below the inguinal ligament are primarily treated by PAT embolectomy. Up to now, we also have had a chance to successfully treat 7 out of 7 mesenteric and 3 out of 4 renal cardiogenic embolizations. Two of the mesenteric arteries were operated on subsequently because the surgeons did not believe that sufficient perfusion had been reestablished. There was no bowel resection in any of these cases. One mycotic aneurysm after embolization caused by endocarditis was resected.

Starck improved the technique by developing three additional devices in 1988: 1) a double-lumen catheter to allow aspiration and injection of contrast or lytic substance with the wire in place; 2) a motor-driven, metal, round-tip spiral to remove firm unlysable occlusive material; and 3) a spherical-tip basket with soft, flexible branches to detach wall-adherent occlusive material. It also serves for fragmentation or fixation of firmer components for aspiration and extraction.[6]

Table 9.6.2. Material and Clinical Success of PAT in 1989

	Material Success	Clinical Success
Thrombotic occlusion	45 (55%)	41 (91%)
Embolic occlusion related to PTA	24 (29%	24 (100%)
Embolic occlusion unrelated to PTA	13 (16%)	11 (84%)
Total	82 patients	76 (92%)

COMPLICATIONS

There is only one PAT-specific complication, the antegrade dissection. The risk increases if the catheter is advanced against resistance under aspiration and at sites of previous balloon dilatation. Up to now, four antegrade dissections have occurred in over 400 procedures in the femoral-popliteal region. These dissections were treated by balloon dilatation. Subintimal passage and dissection is excluded if the catheter is advanced over a wire. After removal of the wire, aspiration is performed during catheter pullback.

In the 82 PAT patients in 1989, we had the following complications: one rupture of the artery after balloon dilatation without further treatment and one pseudoaneurysm had to be resected. Two compartment syndromes due to severe ischemia before successful angioplasty required fasciotomy and had a good clinical outcome. Two below-the-knee amputations were unavoidable. One patient from the cardiogenic embolic group of 13 (7.6%) died 24 hours after successful aspiration embolectomy because of the severe heart disease.

This figure for mortality in the embolic group unrelated to PTA is a little higher than the experience in more recent cases. But it is still far less than those published for surgery from 14 to 22% in the femoral and popliteal region.[11−13]

References

1. Greenfield LJ, Kimmell GO, McMurdy WC III: Transvenous removal of pulmonary emboli by vacuum-cup catheter technique. *J Surg Res* 1969;9:347–352
2. Buxton DR Jr, Mueller CF: Removal of iatrogenic clot by transcatheter embolectomy. *Radiology* 1974;111:39–41
3. Horvath L, Illes I, Varo J: Complications of the transluminal angioplasty excluding the puncture site complications, in Zeitler E, Grüntzig A, Schoop W (eds): *Percutaneous Vascular Recanalization.* Berlin, Springer–Verlag, 1978, pp 126–140
4. Sniderman KW, Bodner L, Saddekni S, Srur M, Sos TA: Percutaneous embolectomy by transcatheter aspiration. *Radiology* 1984;150:357–361
5. Starck EE, McDermott JC, Crummy AB: Percutaneous aspiration thromboembolectomy. *Radiology* 1985;156:61–66
6. Starck EE, McDermott JC: Rotating aspiration thromboembolectomy. *Radiology* 1988;169(P):366
7. Bookstein JJ, Saldinger E: Accelerated thrombolysis: in-vitro evaluation of agents and methods of administration. *Invest Radiol* 1985;20(5):731–735
8. Davis GB, Dowd CF, Bookstein JJ, Maroney TP, Lang EV, Halasz N: Thrombosed dialysis grafts: efficacy of intrathrombic deposition of concentrated urokinase, clot maceration, and angioplasty. *AJR* 1987;149:177–181
9. von Heydwolff A: Percutane transluminale Angioplastie. Dissertation, University of Frankfurt, 1986
10. Starck E, McDermott JC: Advantages of percutaneous aspiration thromboembolectomy, in Zeitler E, Seyferth W (eds): *Pros and Cons in PTA and Auxiliary Methods.* Berlin, Springer–Verlag 1989, pp 241–247
11. Abbott WM, Maloney RD, McCabe CC, Lee CE, Wirthlin LS: Arterial embolism: a 44-year perspective. *Am J Surg* 1982;143:460–474

12. Connett MC, Murray DH Jr, Wenneker WW: Peripheral arterial emboli. *Am J Surg* 1984;148:14–19
13. Elliott JR, Hageman JH, Szilagyi E, Ramakrishnan V, Bravo JJ, Smith RF: Arterial embolization: problems of source, multiplicity, recurrence and delayed treatment. *Surgery* 1980;88:833

Part 7. Sonic Thrombolysis

—Wilfrido R. Castañeda–Zúñiga, M.D., M.Sc., S. Murthy Tadavarthy, M.D., Joseph W. Yedlicka, Jr., M.D., David W. Hunter, M.D., and Kurt Amplatz, M.D.

Ultrasound wave energy has been used successfully in the management of urinary and gallbladder lithiasis with a wide safety margin.[1–5]

The use of ultrasound energy for dissolution of atherosclerotic plaque was suggested by Anschuetz in 1965,[6] and its applicability for mechanical thrombectomy was described in 1976 by Trubestein.[7] The studies of Siegel et al. showed that power, strength, and length of exposure to ultrasonic energy at the levels required to ablate atherosclerotic plaque resulted in insignificant damage to normal vascular endothelium.[8–10]

Trubestein noted that the viscosity of fluids can be reduced by ultrasound with breakdown of macromolecules in ultrasonic fields.[7] Based on these findings and his own experimental observations, Trubestein described the applicability of ultrasonic energy for mechanical thrombectomy.[7] Siegel, on the other hand, believes that the principal mechanism seems to be the mechanical effect caused by the longitudinal and transverse oscillations of the probe with an amplitude of 25 μm and a frequency of 20–25 kHz. The waves created are strong enough to disrupt and cause breakdown of rigid noncompliant atherosclerotic plaque, without damaging the more compliant, "normal" blood vessel wall.[11]

Four mechanisms of action have been described: direct mechanical effect, cavitation, thermal effects, and generation of microcurrents at the cellular level.[7,8,12]

The potential local thermal injury in the intravascular applications, resulting from the conversion of ultrasonic to thermal energy in the delivery system, can be minimized by the use of pulsed wave energy delivery and cool perfusates.[8] The probe initially used by Siegel had the disadvantage of lack of steering capability and its rigidity.[11] Rosenschein described a flexible, solid ultrasound transmission wire attached at its proximal end to a piezoelectric element vibrating at 20 kHz. The device used an external power generator. As with the device used by Siegel, the distal end of the ultrasound wire vibrates longitudinally with an amplitude of 150 $\pm$ 25 μm. The ultrasonic generator was operated in the pulsed mode with a 50% duty cycle to ensure resonance capture. Duration of pulse was 0.5 second with an interval of 0.5 second.[13]

In Trubestein's in vivo experience in 44 dogs, no significant changes were seen in the fibrinolytic system or the microscopic structure of the vessel wall after ultrasound.[7] In 1979 Trubestein described the application of the technique in a patient with a two-day-old femoral artery occlusion using a percutaneous approach. The thrombus was dissolved and the remnants aspirated through the hollow guide shaft.[14] Chae et al.'s in vitro and in vivo studies in a canine model of a venous thrombotic occlusion explored the efficacy of ultrasound on human blood clot disruption, the effects of clot age, and the size of the debris produced. They found that disruption of all thrombi present was achieved within two minutes for acute thrombi (one- to two-hour-old clot); and within four minutes for chronic thrombi (four to seven days). No arterial embolism, vascular perforation, or vasospasm was detected and 99.8% of particles were under 10 μm.[15] Rosenschein et al. reported the efficacy of ultrasonic energy for in vivo thrombolysis in 14 canine arteries. Procedure time was within two minutes and no damage to the arterial wall was found.[16] Monteverde et al., using a 22-kHz energy source transmitted through a ball-tipped wire probe, reported successful thrombolysis in 12 acute coronary artery thrombotic occlusions in a canine model. Procedure time varied from 8 to 10 seconds.[17]

Although technical limitations such as rigidity, diameter, and lack of steering capability of the ultrasonic probe at the present time limit the scope of applications of ultrasonic thrombectomy, the available data suggest that the technique may be a safe and effective alternative to fibrinolytic therapy.

References

1. Segura JW, LeRoy AJ: Percutaneous ultrasonic lithotripsy. *Urology* 1984;23:7–10
2. Marberger M, Stackl W, Hruby W, Krosis A: Late sequelae of ultrasonic lithotripsy of renal calculi. *J Urol* 1985;133:170–174
3. Chan KK, Watmough DJ, Hope DT, Moir K: A new motor-driven surgical probe and its in vitro comparison with the Cavitron ultrasonic surgical aspirator. *Ultrasound Med Biol* 1986;12:279–283
4. Hodgson WJB, DelGuercio LRM: Preliminary experience in liver surgery using the ultrasonic scalpel. *Surgery* 1984;95:230–234
5. Bown AH, Davies PG: Ultrasonic decalcification of calcified cardiac valves and annuli. *Br Med J* 1972;3:274–277

6. Anschuetz R, Bernard HR: Ultrasonic irradiation and atherosclerosis. *Surgery* 1965;57:549–553
7. Trubestein G, Engel C, Etzel F, et al: Thrombolysis by ultrasound. *Clin Sci Mol Med* 1976;51:697s–698s
8. Siegel RJ, Fishbein MC, Forrester J, et al: Ultrasonic plaque ablation: a new method for recanalization of partially or totally occluded arteries. *Circulation* 1988;78:1443–1448
9. Siegel RJ, DonMichael TA, DeCastro E, et al: In vivo recanalization of total atherosclerotic arterial occlusions: combined use of an ultrasonic probe and balloon angioplasty system (abstr). *J Am Coll Cardiol* 1989;13:195A
10. Siegel RJ, DeCastro E, Forrester JS, DonMichael TA: In-vivo ultrasonic recanalization of arterial occlusion (abstr). *Circulation* 1990;82(suppl III):III–2733
11. Siegel RJ, Myler RK, Cumberland DC, DonMichael TA: percutaneous ultrasonic angioplasty: initial clinical experience. *Lancet* 1989;772–774
12. Bhabredier T, Lemaire V, Louis V, Merchier PA, Montalescot G, Moussallem N: Elaboration d'un systeme a ultrasons

pour deobstuction des arteries coronaires. *Arch Mal Coeur* 1989;82:377–380
13. Rosenschein U, Bernstein JJ, DeSegni E, Kaplinsky E, Bernheim J, Rozenszajn LA: Experimental ultrasonic angioplasty: disruption of atherosclerotic plaques and thrombi in-vitro and arterial recanalization in-vivo. *J Am Coll Cardiol* 1990;15:711–717
14. Trubestein G: Ultrasonic thrombolysis. *J Acoust Soc Am* 1979;65:542–545
15. Chae JS, Hong AS, Dubin S, Lee S, Fishbein MC, Siegel RJ: Ultrasonic dissolution of human thrombi (abst). *J Am Coll Cardiol* 1990;15:65A
16. Rosenschein U, Bernstein JJ, Bakst A, DeSegni E, Kaplinsky E, Bernheim J, Rozenszajn LA: *Circulation* 1988;78(suppl II):II–270
17. Monteverde C, Velez M, Victoria R, Nava G, Alliger H, Borges J: Percutaneous ultrasonic angioplasty in totally occluded peripheral arteries. *Circulation* 1990;82(suppl III):III–2694

Part 8. A Rheolytic Catheter for Percutaneous Removal of Thrombus

—William J. Drasler, Ph.D., Mark L. Jenson, B.S., Joseph M. Thielen, Emmanuil I. Protonotarios, M.S., Robert G. Dutcher, M.S., and Zinon C. Possis, Bm.Ech.E.

INTRODUCTION

Thrombolytic therapy or Fogarty balloon embolization, alone or in combination with angioplasty or anticoagulation, is the accepted treatment for acute peripheral ischemia.[1,2] Various mechanical thrombectomy methods are being evaluated, including percutaneous aspiration,[3–7] Amplatz thrombectomy catheter,[8–10] Günther aspiration thromboembolectomy catheter,[4,11] transluminal extraction catheter (TEC) endarterectomy catheter,[12] Ponomar transjugular clot-trapper device,[13] the rotational thrombectomy catheter,[14–16] and the ultrasonic thrombolytic catheter,[17–21] as well as other catheter systems. These devices have been used either clinically or experimentally for thrombectomy. Most of these devices are limited in the size of the channel that can be recanalized, or are otherwise cumbersome due to size or stiffness. The rheolytic thrombectomy catheter (RTC) uses high-velocity saline jets to break up thrombus and allows withdrawal of the resulting debris via the same catheter. The RTC looks promising in the initial in vitro and in vivo experiments and may offer significant clinical advantages over other methods. Specifically, hemorrhagic complications associated with thrombolytic drug therapy and vascular wall damage associated with the Fogarty procedure are avoided. The design of the system, with the recirculation pattern provided by the saline jets, can lyse thrombus larger than the catheter, providing more effective treatment for large vessels. The present report describes the initial testing of the rheolytic

thrombectomy catheter and suggests some of the possible applications of this system.

METHODS

Device Construction

The rheolytic thrombectomy catheters were fabricated from 4–6Fr dual-lumen tubing (Fig. 9.8.1). The smaller lumen contains high-pressure stainless-steel tubing used to supply the saline jets; this lumen also is used as the inflation lumen for a latex balloon which serves to center the catheter tip in the vessel lumen. A second larger lumen provided for the evacuation of debris can also be used to inject drugs or contrast medium or to pass a guidewire. The stainless-steel tubing at the catheter tip has four to eight jet orifices 25–50μm (0.001–0.002 inch) in diameter. One jet is directed against the catheter's large lumen to promote the evacuation of debris; the remaining jets are oriented at a retrograde angle to avoid direct impact on the vessel wall, while providing, at the same time, the necessary mixing and recirculation for effective clot lysis (Figs. 9.8.2–9.8.7). A positive displacement pump supplies pressurized saline to the catheter and is activated by a foot switch by the catheter operator.

In Vitro Testing

Fresh animal blood was placed in woven polyester tubing and expanded polytetrafluoroethylene (E-PTFE) vas-

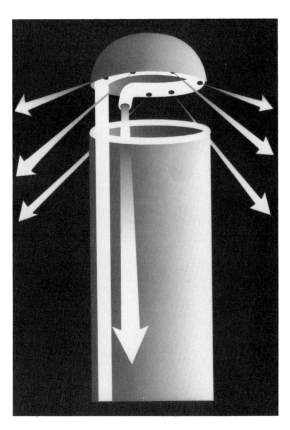

Figure 9.8.1. Diagram of rheolytic thrombectomy catheter double-lumen catheter; large lumen will allow passage over a 0.035-inch guidewire, and after removal of the guidewire the central jet creates a negative flow for removal of debris. The second lumen houses hypodermic tubing. A loop of hypodermic tubing at the distal end has multiple side holes whose size and direction can be modified. The distal end of the tubing directs a jet toward the large catheter lumen.

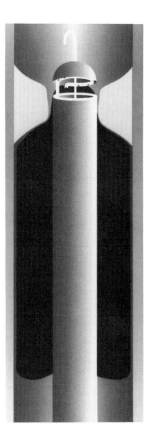

Figure 9.8.3. The rheolytic catheter has been advanced over the guidewire.

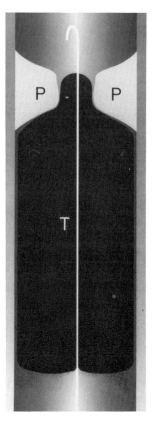

Figure 9.8.2. Diagram showing a 0.035-inch guidewire across a thrombus (*T*) superimposed on an area of atherosclerotic narrowing (*P*).

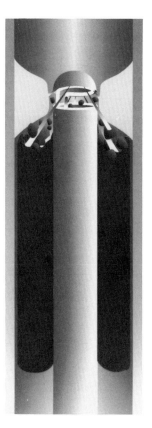

Figure 9.8.4. After removal of the guidewire, the fluid jets are turned on to begin fragmentation of the thrombus.

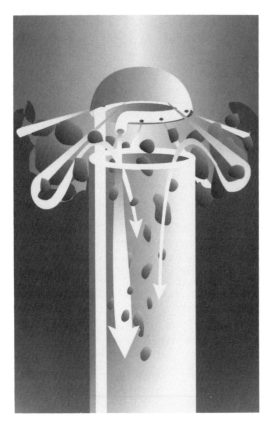

Figure 9.8.5. Close-up view showing the circulation of fluid and debris during fragmentation.

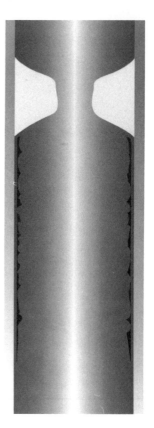

Figure 9.8.7. At the end of the procedure, a minimal amount of debris remains in the wall.

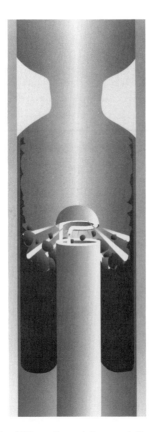

Figure 9.8.6. Midway through fragmentation of thrombus.

cular grafts and allowed to clot. The blood was forced through the pores to obtain better adhesion of the thrombus to the wall. After allowing the thrombus to age for one to seven days, the rheolytic thrombectomy catheter was used to lyse the clot. The RTC was advanced through the thrombus, and the evacuated debris was collected. The tubing or graft was opened longitudinally and photographed; balloon embolectomy on a similar model was used as a control. The debris evacuated by the RTC was examined microscopically for particle sizing.

In Vivo Testing

Bilateral E-PTFE interpositional grafts were placed in the superficial femoral arteries of 28–38kg canines. The grafts were 3–5cm long and 5mm in diameter. Small clamps were placed on the femoral arteries distal to the graft, and nearby vessel branches were ligated to ensure thrombosis in the graft and vessels. After three to seven days, a rheolytic thrombectomy catheter was inserted either directly into the femoral artery or graft or through a carotid artery and advanced into the femoral artery using a guiding catheter to place the RTC in the appropriate vessel under fluoroscopic guidance. The thrombus was lysed using the RTC at 10,000–15,000 psi. A balloon embolectomy/thrombectomy procedure was used on the contralateral vessel as a control, using either the femoral artery or the graft for access. Radiographic documentation of the results was obtained. Following the procedure, the vessels were excised and examined using light and electron microscopy. In one animal, the RTC was passed at 10,000 psi through undisturbed arteries to assess the presence or absence of vascular wall damage caused by the RTC, without the manipulations required for graft placement or clotting. In one case, the animal was kept alive for two weeks; the vessels were then restudied radiographically, excised, and stained to observe vessel healing and demonstrate patency.

RESULTS

In Vitro Testing

The rheolytic thrombectomy catheter lysed the thrombus in all cases.[23] Ten centimeter-long thrombus was lysed by the catheter at 10,000–13,000 psi in one minute. The RTC left very little remaining thrombus, less than that left by the Fogarty procedure. The RTC jets infused saline typically at a rate of 50ml/min, removing debris at the same rate through the evacuation lumen.

In Vivo Testing

The RTC was used to lyse and evacuate thrombus from eight vessels.[22] The average age of the thrombus was four days (range three to seven days); the average pressure used was 12,000 psi. The RTC successfully lysed thrombus and restored patency in all cases. Balloon thrombectomy procedures were used to declot four vessels. There appeared to be more residual thrombus seen on postprocedure radiographs using the balloon procedure than following the use of the RTC.

Excised vessels after thrombectomy using the RTC showed little damage; the excised graft and native vessels from the animals sacrificed two weeks following the thrombectomy procedure showed a lack of an endothelialized surface on the E-PTFE graft; the native femoral artery was free of thrombus and showed little wall trauma. Histological examination demonstrated no damage to the elastica in the vessels in which the RTC was used. The rheolytic catheter was capable of removing one-week-old thrombus from both the E-PTFE graft and the native vessel. In contrast, the vessels after balloon thrombectomy showed a pattern of damage consistent with the radial stress pattern expected using a balloon.

For most of the procedures, the RTC was introduced through a guiding catheter, which helped to position the device and allowed for contrast medium delivery; however, the flexibility of the RTC enabled it to follow a 0.014-inch guidewire when that was desired. No vessel dissection or perforations were evident in any of the experiments.

Debris collected from the evacuation lumen of the catheter consisted of clumps of platelets and red blood cells; effluent blood that was collected downstream of the thrombus during RTC thrombectomy consisted primarily of individual red blood cells with occasional clumping.

DISCUSSION

The ability of the rheolytic thrombectomy catheter to lyse clots at least one week old in vivo points to its potential usefulness in a variety of cases.

The RTC advantages over the Fogarty-type balloon embolectomy procedures include reduced vessel wall trauma, the percutaneous access combined with fluoroscopic guidance may allow the treatment of thrombi not easily treatable by balloon embolectomy. The removal of the thrombotic debris seems desirable, rather than the mere fragmentation of thrombus achieved by other devices,[4,8,12] although controlled studies of distal embolization have not been done using the RTC to verify the benefit of debris evacuation. Debris removal, combined with the jet action breaking the thrombus into small fragments, seems preferable to balloon embolectomy procedures and/or other mechanical thrombectomy devices.

Although heparin anticoagulation would likely be used perioperatively, the local action of the RTC may significantly reduce the incidence of bleeding complications compared with the thrombolytic agents. In addition, while thrombolytic drugs often require many hours for complete clot lysis, treatment using the RTC may provide rapid symptomatic relief in a matter of minutes.

The main shortcoming of other mechanical thrombectomy devices appears to have been addressed by the RTC system; that is the ability of the RTC to clear vessels much larger than the catheter diameter. In addition, the RTC may be able to lyse an entire lesion on a single pass of the device, thus avoiding the repeated withdrawal and reinsertion required with other devices.

By infusing radiologic contrast material via the evacuation lumen of the RTC, direct assessment of the vessel lumen may be obtained without the need to use a separate catheter.

The treatment of acute pulmonary emboli requires facing a variety of undesirable choices. Open vessel surgical embolectomy is associated with great operative risk; thrombolytic drug therapy is time-consuming and may be ineffective in addition to the risk of bleeding complications. The rapid treatment of large pulmonary emboli by a percutaneous device has been advocated; the RTC may offer fast, effective treatment and thus significantly reduce mortality and morbidity. In addition, it may be desirable to lyse any large thrombi found in the deep veins using the RTC immediately, to reduce the likelihood of recurrent pulmonary emboli.

The ability of the RTC to follow a guidewire and access coronary vessels suggests its possible use in acute myocardial infarction, after sufficient preclinical and clinical testing.

CONCLUSIONS

An effective system for the percutaneous lysing and removal of thrombus utilizing high-velocity saline jets has been presented. The ability of this rheolytic thrombectomy catheter system to lyse thrombus up to one week old has been demonstrated both in vitro and in vivo in canine arteries and in vascular grafts. Initial vessel examinations from short-term in vivo studies were favorable, and follow-up in one animal demonstrated patent vessels and E-PTFE vascular graft two weeks following thrombectomy using the RTC. The size and flexibility of the catheter, and its ability to follow a guidewire, suggest possible applications to the treatment of acute coronary thrombosis.

References

1. Cohen LH, Kaplan M, Bernhard VM: Intraoperative streptokinase: an adjunct to mechanical thrombectomy in the management of acute ischemia. *Arch Surg* 1986;12(6):708–715
2. Fogarty TJ, Chin AK, Ollott C, Shoor PM, Zimmerman JJ, Garry MT: Combined thrombectomy and dilation for the treatment of acute lower extremity arterial thrombosis. *J Vasc Surg* 1989;10(5):530–534
3. Greenfield LJ, Kimmell GO, McMurdy WC III: Transvenous removal of pulmonary emboli by vacuum-cup catheter technique. *J Surg Res* 1969;9:347–352
4. Günther RW, Vorwerk D: Aspiration catheter for percutaneous thrombectomy: clinical results. *Radiology* 1990; 175:271–273
5. Starck EE, McDermott JC, Crummy AB: Percutaneous aspiration thromboembolectomy. *Radiology* 1985;156:61–66
6. Buxton DR Jr, Mueller CF: Removal of iatrogenic clot by transcatheter embolectomy. *Radiology* 1974;111:39–41
7. Sniderman KW, Bodner L, Saddekni S, Srur M, Sos TA: Percutaneous embolectomy by transcatheter aspiration. *Radiology* 1984;150:357–361
8. Bildsoe MC, Moradian GP, Hunter DW, Castañeda–Zúñiga WR, Amplatz K: Mechanical clot dissolution: new concept. *Radiology* 1989;171:231–233
9. Moradian GP, Bildsoe M, Hunter DW, Castañeda–Zúñiga WR, Amplatz K: In-vivo mechanical clot dissolution: experimental work in progress. *Radiology* 1988;169(suppl):366
10. Carlson JE, Sunram SE, Kurisu Y, Yedlicka JW Jr, Hunter DW, Castañeda–Zúñiga WR, Amplatz K: New mechanical thrombectomy device. *Radiology* 1990;177(suppl):125
11. Günther RW, Vorwerk D: A new aspiration thromboembolectomy catheter with propeller-tipped rotating wire: an in-vitro study. *J Intervent Radiol* 1990;1:17–20
12. Yedlicka JW Jr, Carlson JE, Hunter DW, Castañeda–Zúñiga WR, Amplatz K: Thrombectomy with the TEC endarterectomy system: an experimental study. *JVIR*, in press.
13. Ponomar–Sulepov E, Carlson JE, Kindlund A, Pacho–Rodriguez J, Yedlicka JW Jr, Hunter DW, Castañeda–Zúñiga WR, Amplatz K: Clot trapper device for transjugular thrombectomy from the inferior vena cava. *Radiology* 1991; 179(1):279–282
14. Ritchie JL, Hansen DD, Vracko R, Auth DC: Mechanical thrombolysis: a new rotational catheter approach for acute thrombi. *Circulation* 1986;73(5):1006–1012
15. Ritchie JL, Hansen DD, Intlekofer R, Vracko R, Auth D: Thrombolysis: a new rotational thrombectomy catheter and evaluation by angioscopy. International Symposium on Interventional Cardiology. 16th Annual Symposium of the Texas Heart Institute, September 1986
16. Hansen DD, Auth DC, Vracko R, Ritchie JL: Mechanical thrombectomy: a comparison of two rotational devices and balloon angioplasty in subacute canine femoral thrombosis. *Am Heart J* 1987;114(8):1223–1231
17. Rosenschein U, Bernstein JJ, DeSegni E, Kaplinsky E, Bernheim J, Rozenszajn LA: Experimental ultrasonic angioplasty: disruption of atherosclerotic plaques and thrombi in-vitro and arterial recanalization in-vivo. *J Am Coll Cardiol* 1990;15:711–717
18. Trubestein G: Ultrasonic thrombolysis. *J Acoust Soc Am* 1979;65:542–545
19. Chae JS, Hong AS, Dubin S, Lee S, Fishbein MC, Siegel RJ: Ultrasonic dissolution of human thrombi. *J Am Coll Cardiol* 1990;15(2):65A
20. Rosenschein U, Bernstein JJ, DeSegni E, Kaplinsky E, Bernheim J, Rozenszajn LA: Experimental ultrasonic angioplasty: disruption of atherosclerotic plaques and thrombi in vitro and arterial recanalization in vivo. *J Am Coll Cardiol* 1990;1:15(3):711–717
21. Monteverde C, Velez M, Victoria R, Nava G, Alliger H, Borges J: Percutaneous ultrasonic angioplasty in totally occluded peripheral arteries. *Circulation* 1990;82(suppl III):III–2694
22. Drassler WJ, Jenson ML, Thielen JM, et al: A rheolytic catheter for percutaneous removal of thrombus. *Circulation*, submitted for publication

10

INFERIOR VENA CAVA FILTERS

Part 1. Mobin–Uddin, Greenfield, Hunter–Sessions, Amplatz, Günther, Bird's Nest, Simon Nitinol, and Temporary Filters

—Marcos A. Herrera, M.D., S. Murthy Tadavarthy, M.D., Joseph W. Yedlicka, Jr., M.D., Carol C. Coleman, M.D., Flavio Castañeda, M.D., David W. Hunter, M.D., Kurt Amplatz, M.D., and Wilfrido R. Castañeda–Zúñiga, M.D., M.Sc.

Pulmonary embolism is one of the principal causes of hospital morbidity and mortality and accounts for approximately 200,000 deaths annually in the United States.[1] In another series, it was reported that 140,000 patients per year suffer fatal pulmonary embolism, and nonlethal embolism was estimated to occur in 570,000 patients per year.[2]

In most cases, pulmonary embolism is effectively treated by heparin. However, certain situations do require mechanical interruption of the inferior vena cava. For example, in patients whose response to anticoagulants has been inadequate, or in patients in whom anticoagulation is contraindicated, the placement of an inferior vena cava filter is an effective alternative. The inferior vena cava is interrupted because in 75–90% of the cases pulmonary emboli originate in the legs and pelvis. The other sources of pulmonary emboli are the arms and the right atrium, and these emboli probably account for some of the apparent failures of filter placement.

Surgical techniques to prevent pulmonary emboli include inferior vena cava ligation and clipping,[3–9] which are major procedures necessitating extensive extraperitoneal dissection. Less drastic surgical procedures, such as ligation of the superficial and common femoral veins, are ineffective, being associated with a 10–26% incidence of recurrent pulmonary emboli and complications attributable to venous stasis.[10] Furthermore, open operations have a 10–15% mortality rate,[11] and emboli recur in 5.9% of patients.[12]

To decrease the mortality rate and avoid general anesthesia in patients with severely compromised cardiac and pulmonary reserves, several transluminal approaches to interruption of the inferior vena cava have been used.[13–19] The Eichelter sieve[15] and the Moser balloon[16] offered temporary protection but had significant drawbacks, namely dislodgment and migration of trapped emboli at the time of catheter removal. Another group of devices is the detachable type, including the Pate clip,[17] the Hunter balloon,[18] the Mobin–Uddin (MU) umbrella filter,[19] and the Kimray–Greenfield (KG) filter.[13,14] In most institutions, the popular MU and KG filters are placed under local anesthesia through a venotomy in either the jugular or the femoral vein.

Placement through a venous cutdown under local anesthesia avoids major operations that require extensive retroperitoneal dissection. A mortality rate of 4% for the surgical placement of filters has been reported, with deaths being related to the underlying disease rather than to the placement of filters.[11] This is a striking improvement over the 10–15% operative mortality rate for vena caval ligation and the 8% rate for partial interruption.[11,20,21] Techniques for percutaneous introduction of the MU and KG filters, developed at the University of Minnesota,[22–24] further reduced morbidity and mortality rates.[24,25] However, the principal drawback of these methods was the need to use large dilators to enlarge the venipuncture in order to introduce the filters. Continued research for new alternatives has led to the development of several new devices,[26–32] which will be discussed later in this chapter. In recent years, in part due to the development of several highly effective filters, the indications for filter placement have expanded significantly, not only for the management of symptomatic patients, but also to include the prophylactic placement of filters in high-risk patients.[33]

INFERIOR VENACAVOGRAPHY

Before operative or percutaneous placement of inferior vena cava filters, inferior venacavography should be performed to demonstrate the size of the vessel, any anatomic variations, and the location of the renal veins.[34] The position of the latter is marked with a metallic marker in the lumbar area with reference to the lumbar vertebral bodies. Filters can then be placed below the level of the renal veins by placing them at the level of the metallic marker, thus minimizing interference with renal venous return. An alternative technique for accurate placement of the filter utilizes a radiopaque ruler placed on the table at the time the inferior vena cavogram is performed; in this manner the exact placement site can be decided by relating the level of the renal veins to the radiopaque marks. The size of the inferior vena cava (IVC) is determined directly from the angiogram, the transverse diameter of the vessel below the renal veins being measured with correction for magnification (Fig. 10.1.1). The ruler can also be used to determine the real diameter of the IVC. Accurate measurement is essential, because if the vena cava is larger than the transverse diameter of the filter, secure placement is unlikely. If the vena cava is larger than the available filters (Greenfield, titanium Greenfield, Simon, Vena-Tech), one of these filters can be placed in each iliac vein or, preferably, a bird's nest filter can be safely placed in large venae cavae. Surgical interruption can also be considered.

The presence of iliac or low inferior vena caval thrombi is a contraindication to the placement of the filter by the femoral approach. An internal jugular vein entry is the only effective route in these cases, although low-profile new filters have been placed through the femoral vein in some cases, particularly when no other access is available.

Anomalies of the Vena Cava

Several congenital anomalies of the inferior vena cava can interfere with the placement of filters:

1. Double inferior vena cava;
2. Circumaortic left renal vein;
3. Retroaortic left renal vein;
4. Left-sided inferior vena cava;
5. Interrupted IVC with azygous or hemiazygous continuation;
6. Acquired abnormalities of the inferior vena cava.

DOUBLE INFERIOR VENA CAVA

Embryologic persistence of the right and left cardinal veins results in a double inferior vena cava.[35] The two vessels may be the same size, but more commonly the left is smaller than the right. After joining with the left renal vein, the left vena cava passes in front of the aorta to join the right inferior vena cava (Fig. 10.1.2). This anomaly is seen in 0.2 to 3.0%.[36]

CIRCUMAORTIC LEFT RENAL VEIN

A circumaortic left renal vein is seen in 8.7% of the population.[35] The anterior half ring of the left renal vein joins

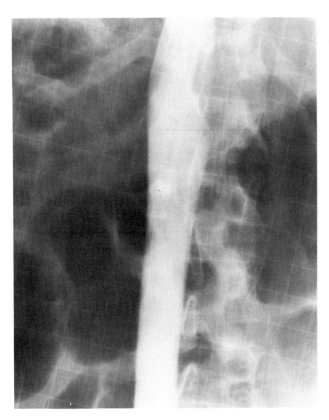

Figure 10.1.1. Inferior venacavography performed with grid for determining magnification prior to filter placement.

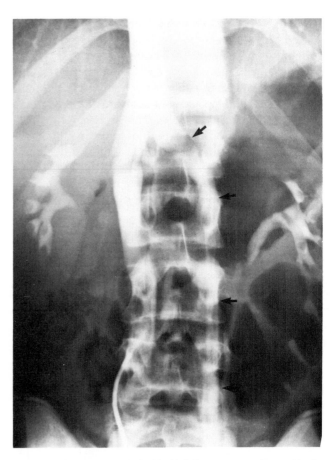

Figure 10.1.2. Persistent left-sided inferior vena cava *(arrows)* is demonstrated following Valsalva maneuver during inferior vena cavogram.

the inferior vena cava at the usual level, whereas the posterior half follows a right downward course posterior to the aorta to join the inferior vena cava at a lower level. Location of the posterior branch is important, because the filter should be placed below the ostium of both renal veins.

RETROAORTIC LEFT RENAL VEIN

The retroaortic left renal vein occurs with an incidence of 1.8 to 2.4%. The anomalous renal vein enters the IVC below the usual level and, therefore, requires the placement of a filter at a lower level than usual.[36]

LEFT-SIDED INFERIOR VENA CAVA

A left-sided inferior vena cava occurs with an incidence of 0.2–0.5%.[2,35] The vessel courses along the left side of the lumbar spine, and, after receiving the left renal vein, it crosses in front of the spine to the right and then continues upward in the normal location of the inferior vena cava. The placement of KG or MU filters in a left-sided infrarenal vena cava is practically impossible from a jugular approach because of the stiffness of the introducing systems. The bulky capsules that carry the filters may not be able to angle to the left despite preshaping of the introducer. Forceful advancement should be avoided, because the inferior vena cava may be perforated at the site where the intrahepatic straight segment of the vessel joins the transverse segment of the left vena cava. With the KG filter, advancement of a stiff leading guidewire may help to advance the system toward the left. This obviously cannot be done with the MU filter, because it does not admit a wire. In this situation, placement of the KG filter[24] or the modified MU filter[22] via the left groin is the most logical approach.

INTERRUPTED VENA CAVA WITH AZYGOUS OR HEMIAZYGOUS CONTINUATION

This occurs with an incidence of 0.6%[36] and may preclude filter placement in the IVC, but placement could be done in the azygous or hemiazygous vein.

ACQUIRED ABNORMALITIES OF THE INFERIOR VENA CAVA

Acquired abnormalities may also affect the IVC anatomy. The incidence of these abnormalities is difficult to determine because of the large variability associated with different patient populations. Acquired abnormalities include:

1. Megacava, a dilated IVC, is of significance because most of the filters available have a limited diameter. Filters cannot be placed in an IVC with a diameter over 30mm, with the exception of the bird's nest filter, although the effectiveness of this filter might decrease in this situation because of the wider separation between the wires caused by the large diameter of the cava.
2. Severe narrowing of the intrahepatic vena cava. Filter placement in these patients requires a femoral approach.

3. Presence of collateral drainage bypassing the inferior vena cava obstruction. These large collateral channels allow different pathways for embolus to travel. Collateral channels are better visualized by injecting in the common femoral or external iliac vein.
4. Intraluminal thrombus in the IVC. The presence of thrombus in the IVC mandates careful manipulations proximal to the thrombus to avoid embolization when using a femoral approach. Preferably, a transjugular approach should be used.

Diagnosis of congenital and acquired abnormalities of the inferior vena cava can be obtained by different diagnostic methods including sonography, computed tomography, and magnetic resonance imaging, in addition to inferior venacavography. All can be useful; however, inferior vena cavography is considered the gold standard for vena cava imaging despite its invasiveness.

Postprocedure Films

Venacavography after filter placement is helpful in the diagnosis of complications such as perforation or filter migration and, later, in the evaluation of the source of recurrent embolism. For example, a large left ovarian or prevertebral vein may serve as a conduit for emboli in spite of an adequately positioned filter.

INDICATIONS FOR INTRALUMINAL INTERRUPTION OF THE INFERIOR VENA CAVA

Contraindications to Anticoagulants

Patients with pulmonary emboli associated with bleeding peptic ulcer, intracranial hemorrhage, or recent major operation cannot be given anticoagulants. Also, there is a 50% risk of hemorrhagic complications if women older than 60 years receive anticoagulants.[37] Such contraindications to anticoagulants are one of the principal indications for transluminal interruption of the inferior vena cava by a mechanical device.[14,37]

Documented Recurrent Thromboembolism in Patients Adequately Treated with Anticoagulants

In patients who have received adequate anticoagulation, there is an 18% incidence of recurrent emboli, half of which are fatal.[2,38] This incidence is not surprising if one remembers that heparin is only thrombostatic and that final lysis of clots already formed depends on natural fibrinolytic activity. Inferior vena cava interruption is indicated in patients who have recurrent pulmonary embolism in spite of adequate anticoagulation.[14,37,39] This is a common problem in patients with congestive heart failure.[37]

Complications of Anticoagulation

Patients with such complications as intracerebral or retroperitoneal hemorrhage or severe oozing from a recent incision require discontinuation of anticoagulants. These patients are typical candidates for intraluminal interruption with filters.

Chronic Pulmonary Hypertension

Pulmonary hypertension can have many causes, such as left-to-right intracardiac shunts, left-sided intracardiac obstruction such as that caused by mitral stenosis, recurrent pulmonary emboli, and hypoxic states of the lung. Primary pulmonary hypertension has no demonstrable cause. All of these patients have poor prognoses, often dying within two to three years of complications such as right-sided heart failure or recurrent embolism. These patients can be managed prophylactically with anticoagulants and inferior vena cava interruption with devices such as filters.[40] There are no large-scale trials of filters with long-term follow-up and comparison with control groups, but the inability of many of these patients to tolerate even a single episode of pulmonary embolism suggests the advisability of filter placement.

Septic Thromboemboli

The conventional treatment for septic thromboemboli has been ligation of the inferior vena cava to prevent migration of emboli to the lungs. In dog experiments, KG filter placement plus antibiotic administration proved superior to vena caval ligation, because the former treatment prevented the infected emboli from reaching the lungs while the antibiotics sterilized the clots trapped within the KG device.[41]

Postembolectomy

After surgical or catheter pulmonary embolectomy, further episodes of pulmonary emboli can be prevented by placing filters in the infrarenal segment of the inferior vena cava.

Prophylactic Interruption of the IVC in Patients with Iliocaval Thrombus

In patients with documented iliofemoral venous thrombi loosely adherent to the walls or free floating in the iliac veins or lower inferior vena cava, prophylactic filter placement may well be warranted.[2,14,39] Free-floating clots that are loosely attached to the inferior vena cava have a higher chance of detachment than do thrombotic clots and may result in fatal complications. Anticoagulation probably will not prevent detachment and migration of such clots.[37]

Prophylactic Interruption of the IVC in High-risk Patients without Current Iliocaval Thrombus

The population requiring the prophylactic placement of an IVC filter include neurosurgical trauma, oncologic, and elderly orthopedic patients.[33,42] In Tobin's series, 57% of their filter placements were prophylactic in high-risk patients.[33] In the same series 18% were placed in patients without pulmonary emboli, but with iliocaval thrombus.[33] In Golueke's series 76.2% of filter placements were undertaken because of a significant history of deep venous thrombosis and 14% as protection from additional cardiopulmonary compromise.[42] Jarrell reported a 62% incidence of deep vein thrombosis in patients with spinal cord injury treated with prophylactic heparinization upon admission. Filter placement was, however, used only in 16% of all the patients with documented deep vein thrombosis.[43] Fatal pulmonary embolism has been reported following total hip replacement in 2.3% of patients not protected with heparinization in a series of 1174 patients.[44] In anticoagulated patients the incidence drops to 0.6–1.0%.[45,46] Bleeding is, however, a significant risk in these patients. Woolson described the prophylactic use of Greenfield filters in five patients for the prevention of pulmonary embolism.[47] Vaughn, in 1989, described the prophylactic use of the Greenfield filter in 42 of 4000 patients who were to undergo total hip or knee replacement.[48] The main objection to the prophylactic placement of IVC filters has been the permanent placement of a foreign body in an "asymptomatic" patient without pulmonary emboli. To eliminate this objection, Darcy reported the use of the Amplatz/Lund retrievable filter which was used for the short-term prophylaxis.[49] Maynar also reported a series of patients treated with the Amplatz/Lund filter prophylactically.[50]

Elderly Persons with Recurrent Thromboemboli

Filters may be superior to anticoagulation in this group.[12] Indeed, this is the third most common indication for filter insertion, accounting for 18% of procedures in one series.[14]

TYPES OF DEVICES AND THEIR USE

Mobin–Uddin Umbrella Filter

One of the earliest devices to filter the inferior vena caval blood is the MU filter, which was released for clinical use in 1970.[51] It was designed for introduction through a venotomy under local anesthesia,[2,5,37,38,51,52] and its use reduced the prohibitive operative mortality rate of 5–39%[38] to 0.[51] Up to 1982, it was estimated that approximately 10,000 MU filters had been implanted.[51] At present, only a 28mm umbrella filter impregnated with heparin is available, the 23mm filter having been discontinued because of its high migration rate.

Patency rates of the inferior vena cava ranging from 33–40%[52] to 60–68%[51,53] have been reported with the MU filter. The heparin reportedly inhibits thrombus formation on the undersurface of the device, and within 6–8 weeks, endothelialization can occur.[51] Migration has been reported in 0.4% of patients and recurrent pulmonary emboli in 0.5%.[38,51] Leg edema and stasis complications such as dermatitis and ulcerations have occurred in 16–75% of patients.[53] The incidence of leg edema was reported to be as high as 50% even in patients with a patent inferior vena cava,[54] so this is a highly controversial complication. Some authors maintain this problem is not a complication of Mobin–Uddin filter placement but rather a consequence of pre-existing thrombi in the leg veins and of poor development of collateral vessels after filter placement.[38]

DESIGN OF THE MU FILTER

The MU filter consists of a central hub, from which six cobalt–chromium spokes radiate (Fig. 10.1.3). This framework makes the device visible on plain radiographs (Fig. 10.1.4). A thin layer of silicone rubber covers each side of the metallic spokes and extends like a web, leaving only the distal 2mm of the spokes bare. By its design, the uncovered 2mm of the sharp spokes limit their penetration of the inferior vena cava to about 1–2mm. There are eighteen 3mm perforations in the silicone webbing to maintain blood flow through the inferior vena cava. The Silastic covering is bonded to a heparin coating to minimize clotting and to augment endothelialization.

The center of the hub has a 1mm hole to receive the threaded tip of the stylet. The filter is loaded on either a 90cm-long regular applicator or the modified angiography applicator-catheter. The modified carrier capsule has a sideport for injection of contrast medium, and the capsule is designed with perforations so that contrast escapes at the base, allowing performance of an inferior vena cavogram before and after the delivery of the filter without need to resort to a conventional angiographic catheter. The capsule is 32mm long and 7mm wide, with a bullet "nose" for easier insertion through small hypoplastic jugular veins. The stiff nylon catheter, along with the stylet, has good torque control and can be bent sideways to negotiate prominent eustachian valves. This maneuver avoids repeated entry of the applicator into the hepatic or renal veins.

If it proves difficult to advance the carrier capsule from the right atrium, the patient can be turned to the left lateral

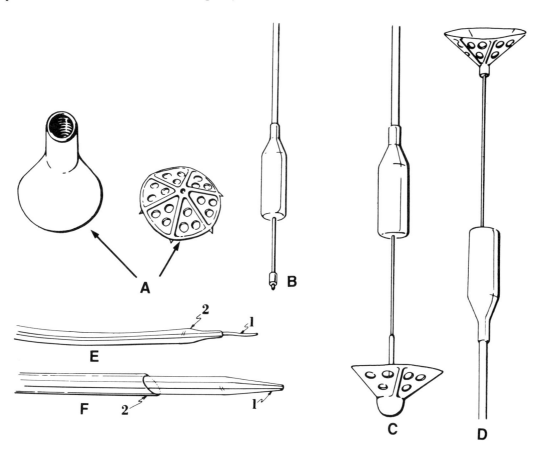

Figure 10.1.3. Mobin–Uddin filter. **A.** Filter and loading cone for femoral introduction. **B.** Introducer capsule with stylet. **C.** Filter mounted on stylet for transjugular approach. **D.** Filter mounted on stylet for transfemoral introduction. **E.** 8Fr (*1*) and 24Fr (*2*) Teflon dilators. **F.** 24Fr dilator (*1*) with Teflon sleeve (*2*) for percutaneous introduction through either transjugular or transfemoral approach.

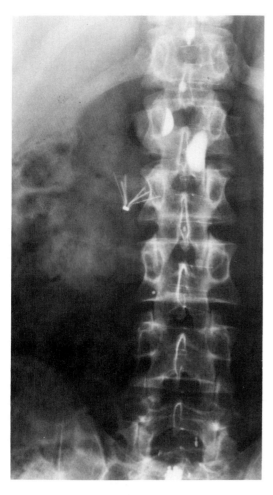

Figure 10.1.4. Mobin–Uddin filter placed below renal veins. Observe tilting due to discrepancy between diameters of inferior vena cava and filter.

decubitus position to free the tip of the capsule from the right atrial wall. The capsule can then be manipulated into the inferior vena cava.

LOADING AND INSERTION OF THE MU FILTER THROUGH THE JUGULAR VEIN

The stylet pin vise is retracted 5–6cm away from the Luer-Lok hub and retightened, and the stylet is advanced until the pin vise is flush with the hub. The protruding stylet tip is then screwed onto the receiving end of the filter. The stylet is turned counterclockwise one-half turn to facilitate detachment of the filter and to ensure that the threads are not stripped.

Before collapsing the filter, the operator lubricates the inner surface of the loading cone and the filter adequately with either K-Y Jelly (Johnson & Johnson) or Lubafax (Burroughs–Wellcome). The filter should be loaded into the capsule gently, without damaging the spokes or the Silastic web. With an assistant holding the stylet catheter along with the mounted filter, the operator aligns the loading cone axially and, by gentle thrusts, collapses the filter. The carrier capsule is advanced by the assistant onto the load-

ing cone, and the operator pulls the stylet backward, thereby loading the filter. The previously retracted pin vise is loosened, moved forward until it is flush with the Luer-Lok, and retightened. This final step prevents accidental premature ejection of the filter. The loaded carrier catheter is advanced through the venotomy under fluoroscopic guidance across the right atrium into the inferior vena cava.

This filter device should always be placed below the renal veins, the level of which is determined from the inferior vena cavogram as previously described. The carrier catheter is advanced distally into the lower inferior vena cava or, preferably, into the iliac veins to prevent accidental ejection of the filter into a vertically oriented renal vein. The applicator catheter is then retracted until the proximal end is at the level of the more inferiorly located renal vein. The stylet pin vise is loosened, moved 2–3cm away from the Luer-Lok, and retightened. The applicator catheter is held firmly by the assistant or the operator, and the filter is ejected by pushing the stylet pin vise. The springing of the filter is watched under fluoroscopy, and the filter is secured to the inferior vena caval wall by gently tugging on the stylet several times. After the filter firmly engages the wall, constant traction is applied to the stylet while it is turned counterclockwise to detach the filter. If accidental premature ejection occurs, the filter can be advanced to a level inferior to the renal veins with the engaged stylet.[51] The carrier catheter and the capsule are removed, and the venotomy incision is closed.

If the clinical situation permits, anticoagulants can be resumed in 12 hours[5] and continued for 3–6 months to diminish thrombus formation on the filter. However, in most cases, the filters are placed in lieu of anticoagulation, so that combined treatment of the filter with anticoagulants is not practical.

PERCUTANEOUS INTRODUCTION OF THE MU FILTER THROUGH THE FEMORAL VEIN

A method was proposed by Knight, Rizk, and Amplatz for introducing the Mobin–Uddin umbrella filter percutaneously by the femoral route.[25,55,56] When the internal jugular vein cannot be approached because of infection, trauma, abscess secondary to surgical resection, congenital hypoplasia, or recent thrombosis of the superior vena cava, the femoral approach is an effective alternate route.

The antegrade approach from the femoral vein is accomplished by modifying the commercially available filter set as follows:

1. The cylindrical end of the loading cone is opened (Fig. 10.1.3A).
2. The central hole in the umbrella is extended through and through.
3. The stylet tip is shortened (Fig. 10.1.3B).

These three modifications allow mounting and loading of the capsule in a retrograde fashion (Fig. 10.1.3C).

In 1978, a warning was published in a bulletin from American Edwards Laboratories against inserting the MU filter from the femoral approach, with the contention that the filter could not be secured properly if ejected in the inverted position.[57] Several published and unpublished cases belie this claim.[25,55,56]

To insert the MU filter via the femoral vein, an inferior vena cavogram is obtained by introducing the catheter through the femoral vein by the Seldinger technique. The presence or absence of thrombi in the femoral and iliac veins and the lower inferior vena cava is ascertained; if thrombi are found, this approach is not appropriate, because the introduction of dilators and catheters can dislodge the clots.

The filter is mounted on the carrier catheter as follows:

1. The open loading cone is held upright (so the flared end points upward).
2. A small amount of lubricant is applied to the inside of the cone and to the capsule and the modified filter.
3. The modified filter with its through-and-through hole in the center of the hub is placed on top of the flared end of the loading cone.
4. The shortened stylet is introduced through the narrow end of the cone and screwed onto the filter by clockwise rotation.
5. After the stylet is tightened, it is rotated counterclockwise one-half turn so the filter can be disengaged more easily after it is securely placed.
6. The stylet is pulled backward so that the filter collapses as it traverses the narrow segment of the cone. As it is collapsing, the filter is gently withdrawn into the capsule while central axial pressure is maintained.

With this technique, the filter nicely forces itself into the capsule. One should make sure the spokes are not protruding beyond the capsule edge.

Through the angiographic catheter used for the inferior vena cavogram, a guidewire is introduced up to the junction of the inferior vena cava and the right atrium. Over the guidewire, a long 8Fr Teflon dilator is introduced. Over the dilator, the puncture site in the femoral vein are sequentially dilated to 24Fr (Fig. 10.1.3*E*) after the skin and subcutaneous tissues have been anesthetized liberally. (The subcutaneous planes are spread apart with a hemostat.)

After dilatation to 24Fr is completed, the working sheath that comes with the filter set is advanced into the low inferior vena cava (Fig. 10.1.3*F*). One should make sure that the tip of the working sheath reaches the lower inferior vena cava; otherwise, the filter capsule is difficult to advance. If the working sheath provided does not reach far enough, one of the longer commercially available working sheaths is used. During placement of the filter, hemostasis is achieved by placing a rubber stopper on the working sheath. Through the working sheath, the carrier capsule is advanced until it is below the renal veins (Fig. 10.1.4), and

the stylet is advanced to release the filter, as in the conventional jugular approach. The filter is secured to the inferior vena caval wall by tugging on the catheter, and the stylet is released by counterclockwise rotation.

Hemostasis is secured by manual compression at the femoral puncture site for 5–10 minutes, and a pressure bandage is applied. Placing the patient in a slight Trendelenburg position lowers the femoral vein pressure to zero so that effective hemostasis is secured rapidly.

Kimray–Greenfield Filter

This filter is a cone-shaped stainless-steel device with six limbs, each with a terminal curved hook that assures fixation to the inferior vena caval wall (Fig. 10.1.5). The KG filter measures 45mm from apex to base, with a maximum span at its base of 30mm.

The principal advantage of this filter is that, even with 80% of the cone filled with clot, the cross-sectional area is reduced by only 64%.[10,13,58] By design, a properly positioned filter should trap emboli >3–4.5mm. However, if the central axis of the filter is tilted out of alignment with the axis of the inferior vena cava, larger clots can bypass the filter through the wider spaces between the limbs (Fig. 10.1.6).

The filter should be placed straight up without any tilting and should be parallel to the central axis of the inferior vena cava. In a deviated vena cava, the filter may look misaligned without affecting filtration, if in reality it is parallel to the lumen. A truly off-axis position may cause several undesired effects:

1. Passage of larger clots;
2. Propagation of clots trapped in the apex of the filter;

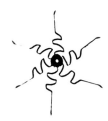

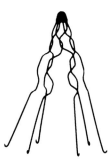

Figure 10.1.5. Greenfield filter: top and frontal views.

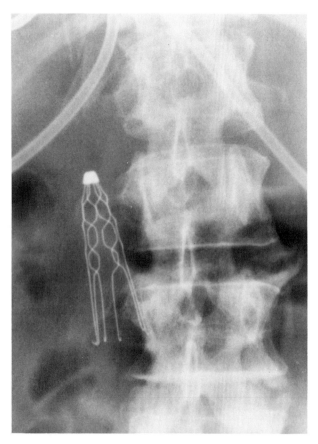

Figure 10.1.6. Spot film of abdomen showing slightly tilted Greenfield filter within inferior vena cava.

3. Penetration, with subsequent perforation of the inferior vena cava because of undue pressure on one of the walls.

Because of its cone shape, the filter preserves laminar peripheral flow of blood around the entrapped clots, and this continuous flow permits lysis of the entrapped clots and, therefore, prevents complete occlusion of the vena cava. The reported 95–98% patency rate of the inferior vena cava in patients with the KG filter[12,14] has been attributed to this cone-shaped design that allows central retention of clots while maintaining the circumferential laminar blood flow.[10]

Because of their high patency rates, the KG filter and some of the newer designs such as the Amplatz–Lund, Günther, bird's nest, Simon, and Vena-Tech are best suited for placement above the renal veins when an infrarenal position is not possible or when suprarenal filtration is desirable. Suprarenal placement of Greenfield filters was carried out in 11 patients below the eustachian valve without any serious sequelae.[59] Suprarenal placement is desirable when the sources of emboli are the renal veins, ovarian veins functioning as collaterals after infrarenal caval ligation, thrombi extending along the inferior vena cava up to and beyond the renal veins and recurrent thrombi despite infrarenal caval ligation with adequate anticoagulation.[59]

Thirty-five patients with a filter placement above the renal veins have been reported in the English literature.[60] Of the reported patients, no instances of caval occlusions were reported and the renal function remained unchanged in all patients.[60] Suprarenal placement of the filter probably will be required in <20% of cases.[59]

To avoid the placement of a suprarenal Greenfield filter, Günther described a technique to displace the caval thrombus downward, with the help of a modified Dormia basket inserted via the transfemoral access to pull the thrombus down while the Greenfield filter is introduced from a transjugular approach and placed in an infrarenal position. Once the Greenfield is placed in an infrarenal position, the basket is removed leaving the thrombus free. The technique was used in two patients.[61]

When the source of thromboembolism is in the upper extremities, a filter might need to be placed in the superior vena cava as prophylaxis against embolism in those patients in whom anticoagulation therapy is contraindicated.[62]

Experimental work by Langham et al. involving superior vena cava filter placement in dogs showed patency of the superior vena cava in 100% of 11 dogs studied after three months.[63] For a femoral insertion a jugular vein assembly must be used to orient the superior vena cava filter correctly. Positioning of the superior vena cava filter is critical. Releasing the filter from the assembly when it is positioned too low could result in the filter being placed into the right atrium or right ventricle with the risk of perforation or tamponade. Placing the filter too high into the brachiocephalic or jugular vein may render the filter ineffective or may increase the risk of venous obstruction. Therefore, exact placement of the filter is necessary.

The patency rate of the KG filter surpasses that of the MU filter, because the former design allows circumferential flow past the device.[11–14,20] Stasis complications occur in 38% of patients with the KG filter, compared with 75% with the MU filters. The lower rate of complications may be a consequence of caval patency.[20]

INTRODUCTION OF THE KG FILTER FROM THE JUGULAR VEIN THROUGH A SURGICAL VENOTOMY

Venacavography before filter placement is obligatory, because caval size and abnormalities, as well as extension of thrombi, should be evaluated to permit correct filter placement.

A right internal jugular vein approach is generally preferred, because of its straighter course and direct alignment in the vertical plane with the right atrium and the inferior vena cava, unless the vein is not accessible because of hematoma, infection, or thrombosis. The large carrier capsules of the KG and MU filters are difficult to advance through the left internal jugular and innominate vein into the superior vena cava and right atrium, and complications such as perforation or mediastinal hemorrhage have been reported with this approach.[64]

A horizontal incision is made above the clavicle, and the

internal jugular vein is dissected out. After proper control of the vein has been gained, a small venotomy is created. Initially, routine dilatation of the junction of the internal jugular with the subclavian vein with a Fogarty balloon catheter was recommended, but this probably is not necessary in every case.[12] The use of guidewires makes for easier advancement of the carrier capsules through the eustachian valve.[65]

Before introduction the guidewire and pusher stylet are retracted fully. After full retraction of the pusher stylet, it is locked by tightening the stylet seal to prevent premature ejection of the filter (Fig. 10.1.7A).

With the help of the loading tool, the tip of the filter is advanced into the carrier capsule until the hooks are a few millimeters from the edge of the capsule (Fig. 10.1.7B). The hooks are then gathered with the concave end of the loading tool and advanced fully into the capsule (Fig. 10.1.7C). One must make sure that the "legs" of the filter are not crossed during loading (Fig. 10.1.7E); if they are crossed, all the steps will have to be repeated. Alternatively, a loading cone can be used to load the filter into the capsule (Fig. 10.1.7F). The cone is also used for loading of the filter into the modified capsule for femoral approach (Fig. 10.1.7G,H).

The present design has two side holes, one for flushing or guidewire introduction, the other for flushing of the carrier capsule that houses the filter. Flushing of the capsule prevents clot formation between the legs and apex of the filter, which might prevent complete expansion upon ejection. Incomplete expansion can result in a tilted position, with consequent poor filtration.[66]

If the carrier capsule cannot be advanced across the eustachian valve easily, insertion can be successfully completed either by curving the stylet to redirect the capsule[65] or by advancing the capsule over a prepositioned guidewire. Advancement over a guidewire also prevents persistent entry of the carrier capsule into the hepatic or right renal vein. In another maneuver to solve this problem, the patient is placed in the left lateral decubitus position; the weight of the capsule will then force it into the more dependent position away from the vein orifices.[65–67] The capsule can then be advanced to the desired location. Dislodgment of the filter into the right renal vein can be prevented by initially advancing the carrier capsule distally into the iliac vein and subsequently pulling it back into the inferior vena cava to the desired location.[12]

The filter is released by withdrawing the capsule while holding the filter in place (Fig. 10.1.8) rather than by advancing the pusher stylet, because the latter maneuver may place the filter further distally than desired. After capsule withdrawal, the apex of the filter is placed at the desired location, below the renal veins at the level determined by the metallic marker placed on the lumbar area or in respect to the radiopaque ruler as described earlier. Other radiologists prefer to leave a catheter in the lowermost renal vein to serve as a marker; it is removed along with the catheter assembly through the venotomy.[24,68]

Percutaneous Introduction

Percutaneous introduction is performed under fluoroscopy guidance and local anesthesia without venotomy. Introduction can be accomplished only through the right

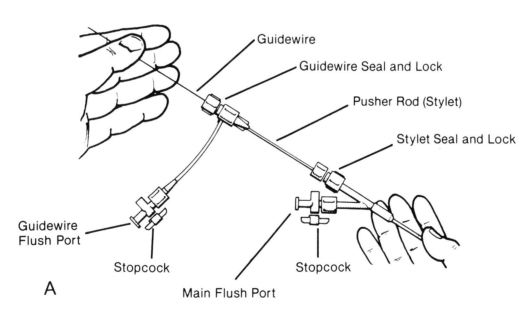

Figure 10.1.7. Preparation of Greenfield filter. **A.** Proximal end of introducer catheter. **B.** Narrowed end of loading tool is used to advance filter into capsule until hooks are approximately 3–5mm away from the capsule edge. **C.** Hooks are gathered with concave end of loading tool, which is then used to advance filter fully into the capsule. **D.** Cross-section of capsule with loaded Greenfield filter shows adequate position of struts. **E.** Crossing of struts within capsule will cause inadequate placement. **F.** Loading cone and tool being used to advance filter into capsule for jugular approach. **G.** Loading cone used to advance filter into capsule for femoral approach. **H.** Filter loaded into capsule modified for femoral approach. (Courtesy of Medi–tech, Inc.)

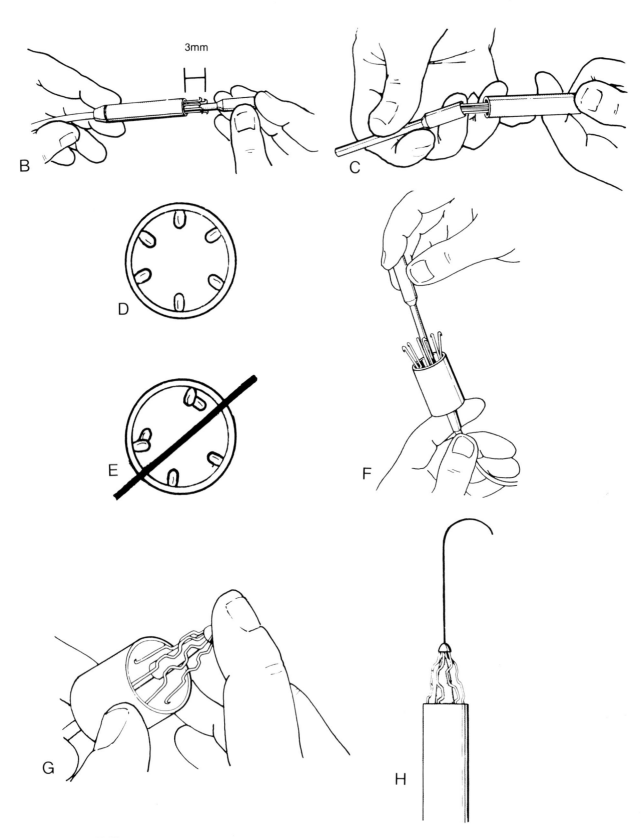

Figure 10.1.7 (B–H).

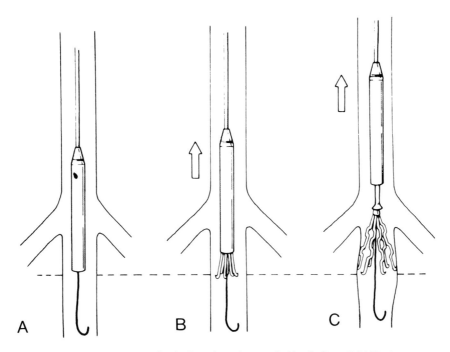

Figure 10.1.8. Introduction of Greenfield filter. **A.** Most distal edge of introducer capsule has been placed at level where filter will be released. **B.** While stylet is held in place, capsule is pulled back. **C.** After capsule has been pulled back, Greenfield filter has re-expanded; legs are fixed to wall by gently pulling back on stylet. (Courtesy of Medi–tech, Inc.)

internal jugular vein, because it involves the introduction of semirigid dilators and a 24Fr working sheath, and the tortuous course of the left internal jugular vein will not permit such manipulation without a high risk of perforation. The right internal jugular vein approach is preferred to the femoral vein approach because of the straighter venous course of the jugular vein, which facilitates the passage of dilators and sheaths. Moreover, the filter will sit better within the lumen of the vena cava when introduced from above, thereby minimizing or avoiding off-axial seating and subsequent poor filtering.[24]

Filter Insertion by the Jugular Vein Approach

The patient is placed in the supine position with the head turned to the left side. The shoulders are elevated by placing a pillow between the scapulae posteriorly. The skin is infiltrated with local anesthetic approximately five fingerbreadths (10cm) above the clavicle and lateral to the carotid artery.[69] The internal jugular vein is immediately posterior to the belly of the sternocleidomastoid muscle. The needle is directed toward the jugular notch at the medial end of the clavicle while the patient performs the Valsalva maneuver to distend the vein. The internal jugular vein is punctured high to avoid puncturing the apex of the lung and subsequent pneumothorax formation.

Following the puncture of the vein, a guidewire is passed through the needle and advanced into the inferior vena cava. Liberal amounts of lidocaine are then infiltrated into the subcutaneous tissues along the needle track. Over the guidewire, the 8Fr Teflon guiding catheter of the Amplatz coaxial dilator system is advanced into the infra-

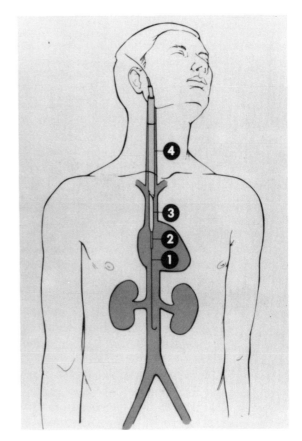

Figure 10.1.9. Dilatation of jugular vein with Amplatz renal dilators and placement of Teflon sheath tip (*4*) within superior vena cava; 24Fr dilator (*3*); 8Fr dilator (*2*); guidewire (*1*). (Reproduced from Tadavarthy SM, Castañeda–Zúñiga WR, Salomonowitz E, et al: Kimray–Greenfield vena cava filter: percutaneous introduction. *Radiology* 1984;151:525–526.)

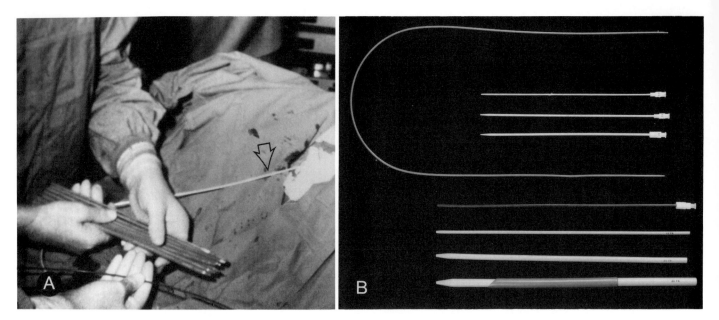

Figure 10.1.10. Transjugular approach. **A.** Pigtail catheter passed through jugular puncture *(arrow)*. Operator shows set of Amplatz renal dilators prior to dilatation. **B.** Amplatz dilator set with Teflon sheath over 24Fr dilator for percutaneous placement of Greenfield filter.

renal inferior vena cava (Fig. 10.1.9).[24,70] The subcutaneous tract is loosened with a hemostat, and the tract is dilated sequentially to 24Fr (Figs. 10.1.10 and 10.1.11). A 28Fr working sheath is then advanced over the 24Fr dilator into the superior vena cava.

Before the dilators and guidewire are removed from the sheath, the patient is instructed to hold his/her breath or to perform a Valsalva maneuver to increase the intrathoracic pressure. A gush of blood will be noticed through the working sheath upon removal of the dilators. These measures are not required if the venous pressure is high secondary to pulmonary hypertension or if the patient is placed in the Trendelenburg position.

After removal of the dilators, the carrier capsule is immediately advanced through the working sheath (Figs. 10.1.12 and 10.1.13). If time elapses between dilator removal and carrier advancement, large amounts of air can be aspirated through the sheath, resulting in severe air embolism. To decrease bleeding upon removal of the dilator as well as to decrease the risk of air embolism, a modification of the Teflon sheath by adding a segment of latex tubing to the end of the sheath was proposed by Coons.[71] After removal of the dilator, the latex tubing is collapsed either manually or with forceps. The filter is then advanced over the wire and into the latex tubing until it reaches the forceps, which are then removed. As soon as the carrier capsule exits from the working sheath into the vein, the sheath is retracted (Fig. 10.1.14), and hemostasis is secured at the puncture site by manual compression over the catheter. While the assistant holds the puncture site, the catheter assembly is advanced under fluoroscopy into the infrarenal inferior vena cava, and the filter is released as discussed previously.

After filter placement, the catheter is removed, and the patient's upper body is elevated 20–30° above the horizontal level with a wedge. Because of the negative pressure in the internal jugular vein, there is no oozing of blood at the puncture site. The incision is closed with No. 4 or No. 5 suture material. The patient's head is kept elevated for 1–2 hours.[24]

Filter Insertion by the Femoral Vein Approach

Introduction through the femoral vein approach carries the risk of dislodgment of any iliac vein or lower inferior vena cava thrombi. Therefore, iliac venography and inferior vena cavography should be performed first.

For femoral insertion, the carrier was redesigned by shortening the capsule (Fig. 10.1.15). As in the jugular carrier, there are two side ports, one for guidewire introduction and the other to flush the carrier capsule. The pusher stylet is advanced by unlocking the stylet seal. The loading cone is placed over the carrier capsule, and the base of the filter is inserted slowly into the capsule by gently pushing on the nose. The pusher stylet is then locked, to prevent accidental dislodgments. Guidewire motion is checked, after unlocking the guidewire seal, by advancing the wire through the pusher stylet out through the nose of the filter.

For insertion via a femoral access, the carrier capsule and catheter assembly are advanced over the guidewire across the iliac system into the inferior vena cava (Fig. 10.1.16). During introduction, the guidewire and the main flush ports are flushed with heparinized saline to prevent clotting on the filter. When the desired position below the renal veins is reached, the shaft is held firmly, the pusher stylet is unlocked, and the filter is uncovered by withdrawing the capsule toward the groin. In this fashion, the filter

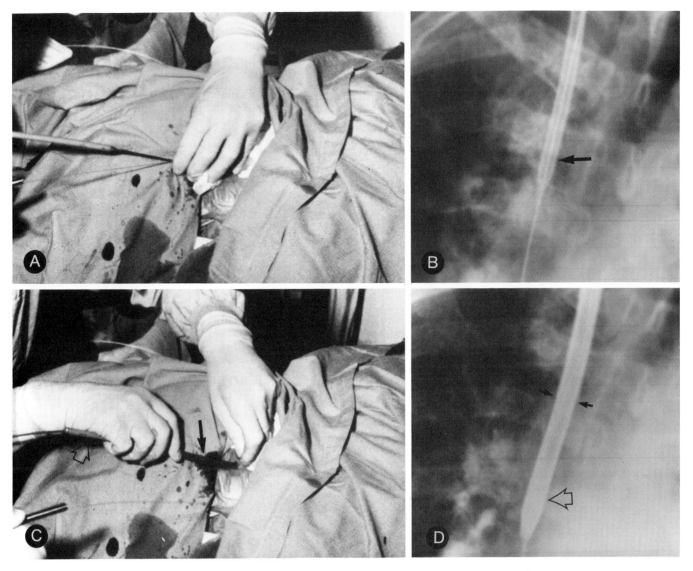

Figure 10.1.11. Transjugular approach (see Fig. 10.1.10). **A.** 20Fr dilator being advanced over guiding 8Fr catheter and guidewire. B. Spot film shows 20Fr dilator *(arrow)* with its tip within superior vena cava. **C.** Teflon sheath *(arrow)* being advanced over 24Fr dilator *(open arrow)* across puncture site. **D.** Spot film shows position of 24Fr dilator *(open arrow)* within superior vena cava during advancement of Teflon sheath, the edge of which is faintly visible *(small arrows).*

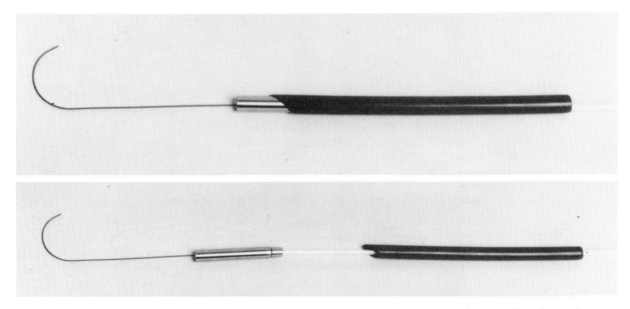

Figure 10.1.12. Introducer catheter with capsule passed through Teflon sheath. Observe guidewire in lumen of introducer catheter.

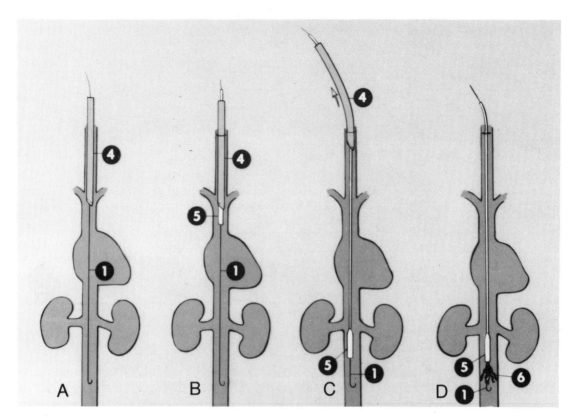

Figure 10.1.13. Percutaneous introduction of Greenfield filter. **A.** Teflon sheath (4) in place with tip in superior vena cava. 1 = guidewire. **B.** Greenfield filter loaded in capsule (5) being introduced through Teflon sheath. **C.** Once capsule has been passed into superior vena cava, Teflon sheath is removed. **D.** Then, with manual compression of puncture site, Green-

field filter (6) is positioned below renal veins. (Reproduced from Tadavarthy SM, Castañeda–Zúñiga WR, Salomonowitz E, et al: Kimray–Greenfield vena cava filter: percutaneous introduction. *Radiology* 1984; 151:525–526.)

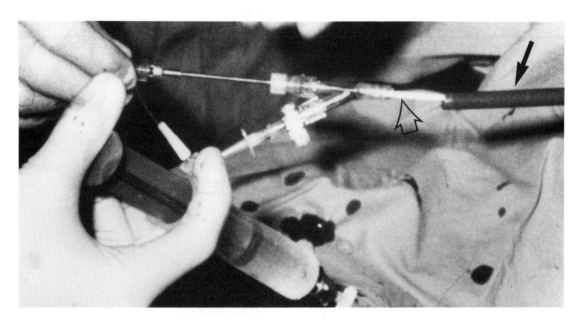

Figure 10.1.14. After introduction of capsule, Teflon sheath has been pulled back *(black arrow)* over shaft of introducing catheter *(open arrow).* Contrast medium is being injected through sidearm fitting to verify position of capsule within inferior vena cava.

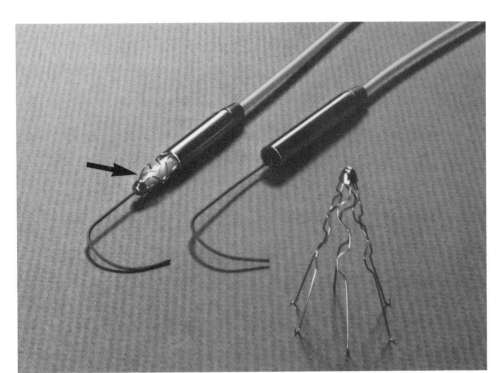

Figure 10.1.15. Greenfield filter loaded in capsule for transfemoral placement *(arrow).*

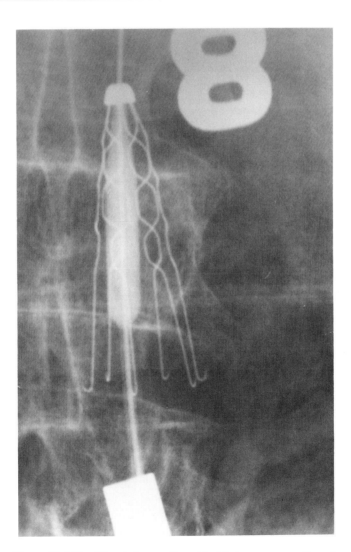

Figure 10.1.16. Filter being positioned in inferior vena cava through femoral approach.

is held in position by the tapered pusher. No further manipulation is required.

In most older patients, the carrier capsule, in spite of its redesign, is difficult to advance through the iliac system. The use of heavy-duty guidewires, such as the Lunderquist, the Lunderquist–Ring, or the Amplatz stiffening wire, is recommended. Usually, the carrier capsule is caught where the distal right iliac vein joins the inferior vena cava; at this site, the iliac artery crosses the iliac vein anteriorly and courses toward the right side of the pelvis. Forceful advancement, even over the guidewire, is not advisable because the iliac veins can be perforated easily.

To minimize problems in these older patients, the puncture site in the femoral vein is dilated to 24Fr with the coaxial dilator system, and a long Teflon sheath is advanced until its tip is located high in the distal iliac vein or in the lower inferior vena cava.[24] Through this working sheath, the carrier capsule can then be advanced and the filter uncovered in the usual fashion. Simple manual pressure over the puncture site secures hemostasis, despite the large hole in the femoral vein, because of the low venous pressure.

To expedite and decrease the incidence of iatrogenic changes at the venotomy site, Shetty described the use of balloon dilatation of the venous access.[72] Dorfman supported this approach with experimental and clinical data in 68 patients following percutaneous Greenfield filter placement.[73] Thrombus developed in 14.3% of patients at the puncture site.[74] Asymptomatic thromboses have been reported in up to 41% of patients,[75] while symptomatic thrombosis occurred in 1.8–24% of patients.[76–81]

Titanium Greenfield Vena Cava Filter (TGF)

To facilitate insertion and decrease the incidence of puncture site complications associated with the percuta-

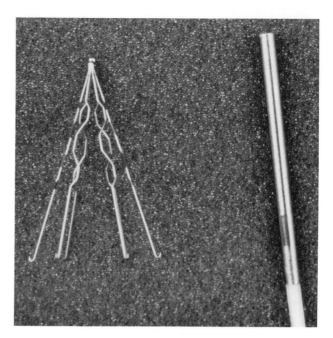

Fig. 10.1.17. Titanium Greenfield filter.

neous insertion of the Greenfield filter (GF), a titanium alloy model of the Greenfield filter was developed[82] (Fig. 10.1.17).

The titanium Greenfield filter utilizes the elastic properties of titanium, allowing its introduction through a 12Fr capsule. The TGF is larger (47mm vs. 44mm) than the GF; and its base is also broader (38mm vs. 30mm). Its trapping and fixation capabilities were found to be similar to those of the GF.[82]

TECHNIQUE

A 14Fr sheath is used for introduction (Fig. 10.1.18). The sheath is placed using either a right internal jugular or femoral vein approach, advancing the dilator/sheath over

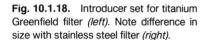

Fig. 10.1.18. Introducer set for titanium Greenfield filter *(left)*. Note difference in size with stainless steel filter *(right)*.

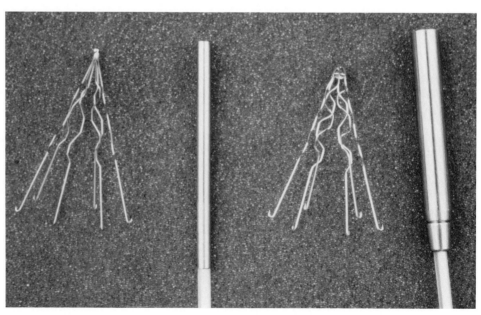

the guidewire until it reaches the predetermined level for filter placement. The dilator and wire are withdrawn and the TGF is advanced until the tip of the filter reaches the level of placement. The carrier is then pulled back while holding the filter fixed at the desired location.

RESULTS

The initial results reported by Greenfield in 40 patients showed that in 24 patients the TGF was placed from the right femoral vein, in 11 from the left femoral vein, and in 2 from the right internal jugular vein. Three filters were placed using a surgical cutdown. Insertion was successful in 39 of 40; femoral vein thrombosis occurred in one of 35 (3%). Distal filter migration was seen in three cases (7.5%) and there was no proximal migration.[82] Teitelbaum reported three cases of inferior vena cava wall perforation by the TGF. In all three cases the TGF had a tilt of 30–36°, caudal displacement of 18–21mm and a filter span varying from 35–49mm.[83] Perforation of the caval wall was confirmed by computed tomography in all three cases, and in one case perforation of the abdominal aorta was also shown. All patients complained of flank pain.[83] Differences between the GF and the TGF were found by Teitelbaum in leg length (43mm vs. 49mm), filter span (28mm vs. 38.5mm), hook angle (23.5° vs. 41°) and flexibility of the TGF, which was found to be 7-fold greater than that of the GF. Because of this increased propensity to perforate the caval wall, the filter was removed from the market. Modifications to the hook design improved the safety of this device and in a subsequent series of 150 patients, no evidence of caval wall perforation was found.[83] The TGF filter has received FDA approval for clinical applications recently.

Hunter–Sessions Transvenous Balloon Occlusion

Hunter et al. developed a balloon catheter for percutaneous inferior vena caval occlusion.[35,84–86] Excellent long-term results, with follow-up as long as 13 years, were reported.[84]

The shaft of the catheter is 17Fr and 75cm long. The balloon is attached to the catheter by a collar, so it can be detached easily. The balloon was devised with six principles in mind[35,84–86]:

1. Avoidance of vessel trauma. The balloon has no hooks or pins to traumatize or penetrate the vena caval wall. Therefore, retroperitoneal hemorrhage and trauma to nearby organs such as the ureter and duodenum are avoided, as is migration of the device into the peritoneum.
2. Facilitation of radiologic studies. Venograms can be obtained by instilling contrast medium through the catheter shaft, thus facilitating positioning of the balloon. Postocclusion venography is necessary to confirm proper position.
3. Avoidance of general anesthesia and laparotomy. Balloon occlusion of the inferior vena cava can be accomplished under local anesthesia through a jugular venotomy.
4. Precise fit of the device to the blood vessel. The balloon can be inflated under fluoroscopy with diluted contrast medium so that it adapts to the dimensions of the inferior vena cava. The balloon usually remains inflated for 1–2 years.
5. Ability to use anticoagulants safely. Balloon occlusion of the inferior vena cava permits simultaneous administration of anticoagulants. Because the balloon does not penetrate the vessel wall, there is no risk of retroperitoneal hemorrhage. The combination of balloon occlusion and anticoagulants expedites clot resolution in the legs, thereby minimizing stasis sequelae.
6. Avoidance of thrombosis. Complete occlusion of the inferior vena cava is required to prevent recurrent pulmonary emboli, and this can be accomplished without laparotomy by the balloon technique.

Balloon occlusion usually is well tolerated even by very sick patients. No periprocedural deaths have been reported. In about 5% of cases, however, acute balloon occlusion is not well tolerated and causes hypovolemia and shock, which may create problems in patients with minimal cardiopulmonary reserve.[37] Hypotension is treated by deflation of the balloon, administration of fluids, and reinflation of the device.[37]

The balloon is placed through a venotomy under fluoroscopy guidance and inflated with 25% Hypaque (average volume: 17 ml).[37] Fluoroscopy and traction on the balloon ensure correct position. The balloon gradually deflates within two years; commonly the inferior vena cava fibroses around the deflated balloon, and permanent complete occlusion is achieved.

Long-term results at 18 years were recently reported in 191 patients. Ninety-four patients are dead; 95 are alive and 2 were lost to follow-up. No patients had recurrent pulmonary embolism while in the hospital and no patients died of pulmonary embolism during the follow-up. Late minor pulmonary embolism occurred in three patients. There was no evidence of balloon migration or malfunction. At last follow-up 75% of patients had legs free of edema and 25% had need for elastic stockings.[87]

GENERAL CONSIDERATIONS IN THE DESIGN OF NEWER FILTERS

The authors' in vitro testing showed that the available filters have certain limitations and drawbacks. For example, filtration with the KG device is highly dependent on filter position. If the filter is off center, it does not filter some of the caval flow adequately and therefore, it may allow larger clots to pass.[32] In vitro, the KG filter is gravity-dependent. Clots pass along the dependent part of the vena cava model, especially if the filter is not aligned with the vessel axis. Whereas the KG filter offers minimal resistance to the flow of blood, the design of the MU filter offers higher resistance that may ultimately lead to thrombosis of the inferior vena cava.

Because of the shortcomings of the available occlusion devices, newer designs for caval filters have been developed. The ideal filter would have these characteristics:

1. It would be small (8–14Fr), allowing introduction using Seldinger technique through either the femoral or jugular veins.[26,27,32] Catheters and capsules of this size avoid the complications of air embolism.[32]
2. It would not migrate or damage the surrounding tissues.
3. If the filter is not in the correct position after release, it would be possible to make adjustments until the correct position is achieved.

4. The device would be removable percutaneously so that it could be inserted for prophylaxis and removed after the crisis to avoid the long-term complications of occlusion of the inferior vena cava.
5. Its material would be biocompatible, stress resistant, and nonthrombogenic.[26,27,32]
6. It would trap small emboli while maintaining the physiologic flow in the inferior vena cava.

These features are desirable to prevent complications such as thrombosis, leg edema, and stasis.

Several newer designs, such as the Simon nitinol,[26] Vena-Tech, bird's nest,[28–30] Lund–Amplatz retrievable,[32] and helix[31] filters are undergoing experimental and clinical evaluation. Some of these filters are promising to satisfy some or all of the above criteria.

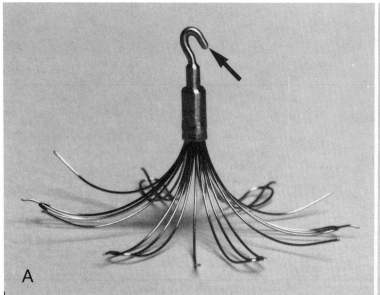

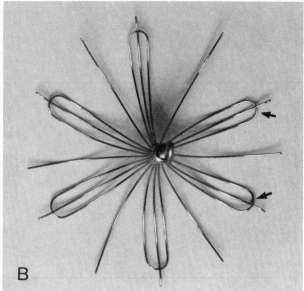

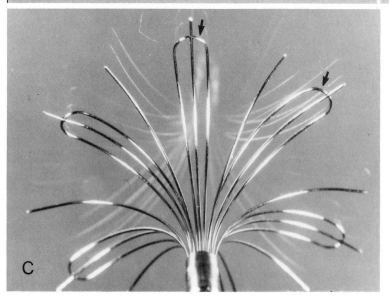

Figure 10.1.19. Lund–Amplatz retrievable filter. **A.** Profile; observe hook for retrieval *(arrow).* **B.** Filter seen from top to show spaces between legs as well as stoppers *(arrows)* that restrict penetration of vena caval wall. **C.** Close-up view shows stoppers to better advantage *(arrows)* as well as decreasing size of spaces toward center of filter. (Reproduced from Lund G, Castañeda-Zúñiga WR, Amplatz, K: Retrievable vena caval filter percutaneously introduced. *Radiology* 1985;155(3):831.)

Lund–Amplatz Filter

A newer design and material were chosen for this filter. It is shaped in the form of an umbrella ("spider" design) and is made from MP35 alloy (35% nickel, 35% cobalt, 20% chromium, and 10% molybdenum),[32] which is a biocompatible, corrosion-resistant material with higher fatigue resistance. It also is used in the production of endocardial pacer wires.[88]

The spider filter has a central stem that has a retrieval hook at one end and an attachment for a threaded cable wire at the other (Fig. 10.1.19A,B). Fixation of the filter is accomplished by pointed wires that pierce the caval wall; wire loops prevent the prongs from penetrating the wall more than 2mm (Fig. 10.1.19C). The filter is attached to a threaded guidewire and inserted through a 14Fr catheter. The prongs are compressed during passage through the catheter (Fig. 10.1.20A) and spring open (Fig. 10.1.20B) when extruded in the infrarenal vena cava. The filter is secured by gently pulling back (in the transjugular approach) or gently pushing forward (in the transfemoral approach) on the wire to engage the prongs firmly in the caval wall. The threaded guide is subsequently unscrewed, and all the introducing catheters are removed.

Percutaneous retrieval is accomplished through the femoral vein. The hook on the caudal end of the filter is engaged by a snare (Fig. 10.1.21A–C), and the filter is held securely in position while the 14Fr removing Teflon sheath is advanced over it. The sheath compresses the prongs, freeing them from the wall of the vena cava (Fig. 10.1.22). Once the filter is completely inside the sheath, the sheath and filter are removed through the femoral vein as a single unit. The filter should not be pulled back into the sheath, because this would cause extensive laceration of the caval wall.

The present design of this filter is very effective in trapping all small and large clots (Fig. 10.1.23). As was proved in the authors' in vitro experiments, the filter is not gravity-dependent. After uneventful testing in dogs, the filter has been placed in patients. In dogs, retrieval with the snare 2–3 weeks after placement was successful in most cases. Successful retrieval has been achieved recently in human beings.

Long-term results in 52 patients were reported by Epstein. No deaths occurred as a result of filter placement. Follow-up in 42 patients (81%) by inferior vena cavography in 31, by computed tomography (CT) in 4, by duplex ultrasound in 4, and by autopsy in 3 revealed inferior vena cava thrombosis in seven of 40 (17.5%) previously nonobstructed vena cavae studied. Two patients with caval

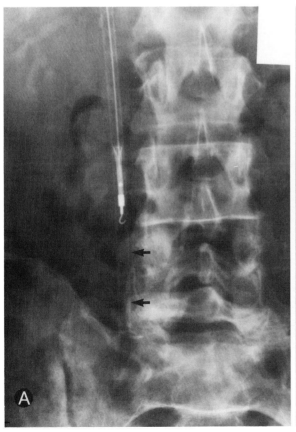
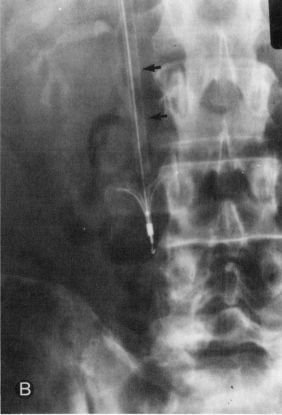

Figure 10.1.20. Introduction of Lund–Amplatz filter. **A.** Long Teflon sleeve *(arrows)* has been advanced to level of right common iliac vein. **B.** After placement of filter at desired level, Teflon sheath *(arrows)* is gently pulled back until filter is released.

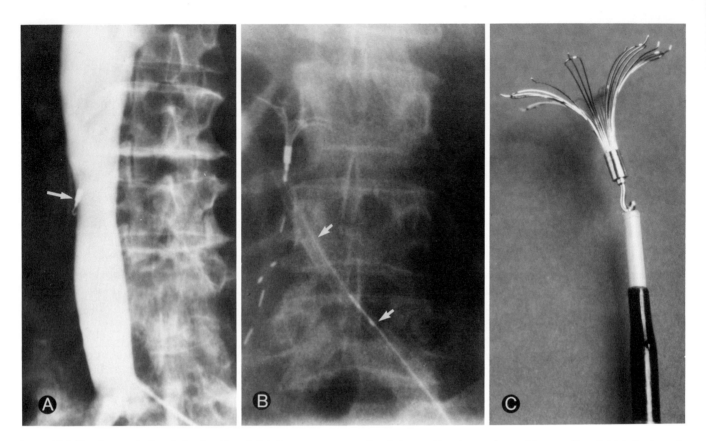

Figure 10.1.21. Removal of Lund–Amplatz filter. **A.** Inferior vena cavogram performed through left femoral vein shows tilting of filter *(arrow)* within vessel lumen. Hook appears to be embedded in caval wall, but this proved to be an artifact due to layering of contrast medium. **B.** Teflon sheath *(arrows)* has been advanced to a position distal to hook, and a snare has trapped hook. Teflon sheath is slowly advanced over filter to close legs. **C.** Snare and catheter for percutaneous retrieval of Lund–Amplatz filter.

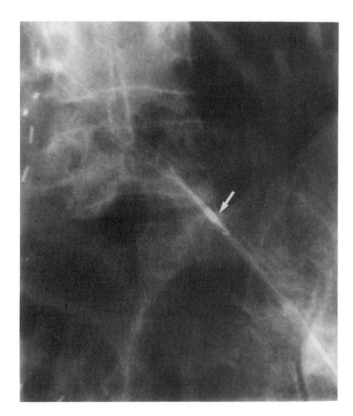

Figure 10.1.22. Filter *(arrow)* has been disengaged from the caval wall and is withdrawn slowly through the Teflon sheath.

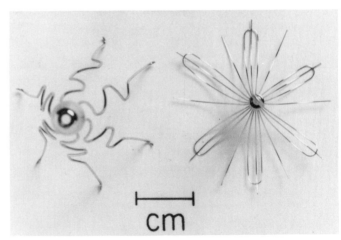

Figure 10.1.23. View from above of Greenfield and Lund–Amplatz filters showing slightly smaller spaces between struts of the latter.

thrombosis required placement of a second filter to prevent embolization of thrombus extending proximal to the filter. No clinical pulmonary emboli were recorded. Six filters were successfully retrieved percutaneously.[89] McCowan reported recurrent pulmonary embolism in two of 30 (7%), caval thrombosis in seven of 30 (23%), caval wall penetration in two of 20 (10%), caval stenosis in one of 20 (5%); and no migration was noted.[90]

The higher rate of caval thrombosis found with this filter can be related to the high trapping efficiency of small and large thrombus found for this filter.[91,92] The Lund–Amplatz filter was found to be second only to the Mobin–Uddin filter in in vitro testing.[91] Another factor predisposing to caval thrombosis could be the flow disturbances caused by the geometric design of the filter.[91,92] Its inverted cone orientation, while necessary for transfemoral retrieval, results in diversion of emboli to the periphery of the caval lumen where the presumably slower peripheral or para-axial flow would result in reduced spontaneous clot dissolution.[89]

Basket (Günther) Filter

This filter consists of two segments, the proximal in the shape of a basket and the distal composed of anchoring limbs.[93] The tips of the limbs form tiny balls, limiting penetration of the vessel wall. The two segments of the filter are constructed from 12 single pieces of 0.2mm-diameter stainless-steel wires with no soldering, thereby avoiding breakage points between the segments. The total filter length is 7.5cm, the diameter of the basket is 2.5cm, and the anchoring limbs encompass a circle of 3.0cm (Fig. 10.1.24). By virtue of its design, the basket traps emboli at three levels: the distal end outside the basket, inside the basket, and between the anchoring limbs and the basket.

In vitro and in vivo (canine) testing proved that the Günther filter captures tiny (15 × 2 × 2mm) emboli. The filter also effectively maintained its position. Unlike the KG filter,[61] it stayed parallel to the central axis of the inferior vena cava without tilting, because of the presence of the proximal basket and of the distal anchoring segments. Filter position was stable, without migration, and only a 5mm Hg gradient was noted across the filter after the capture of several clots. On postmortem examination of the dogs, the inferior vena cava demonstrated tiny nodular fibrotic changes, indicating a mild inflammatory reaction.[93]

The method of introduction is simple. The filter is first inserted into a loading cartridge and then advanced by a stylet through a 10Fr catheter from either the femoral or jugular vein approach (Fig. 10.1.24). The device can be retrieved within 1–2 weeks without undue damage to the vessel wall.[93]

Fobbe reported the use of this device in 59 patients with no complications at the puncture site. At 21 months' follow-up, caudal migration occurred in 70%, but it rarely exceeded 2cm. No cranial migration was seen and three fil-

ters occluded (7%).[94] Schneider reported downward migration of more than 2cm in two patients, to the level of the iliocaval junction, compromising the trapping efficiency of the filter and requiring, therefore, the placement of a second filter.[95] Upward migration of the filter has been seen in some patients when a large amount of thrombus has been trapped by the filter, causing an increase in the intracaval pressure to a degree that it overcomes the fixation capability of the anchoring limbs, which become inverted.[96] Although the design of the filter allows its percutaneous retrieval after its prophylactic placement, this application has not been reported. Günther reported that filter retrieval is recommended only in those cases where the filter is malpositioned.[93] Attempts to remove a prophylactically placed filter failed because the tip of the basket became adherent at the iliac bifurcation.[97] Günther recommends heparinization for one to two weeks to allow endothelialization of the basket wires reducing, therefore, the thrombogenicity of the wires.[97] Because of several reported complications, the filter has been recently removed from the European market. It was never used in the United States.

Bird's Nest Filter

The bird's nest filter is composed of four 25cm-long stainless-steel wires 0.18mm in diameter with two short angled hooks at each end for venous fixation (Fig. 10.1.25).[28] It is shaped into a nonmatching mesh with gaps no larger than 3–4mm (Fig. 10.1.26) and effectively traps emboli as small as 1–2mm.[30]

The filter is designed to be introduced percutaneously by the Seldinger technique through an 8Fr catheter, thereby eliminating the venotomy and the need for bulkier capsules.[28,29] The wire mesh is loaded into an 8Fr Teflon catheter and introduced through a femoral or jugular sheath. The filter is positioned in the infrarenal vena cava with a detachable wire pusher (Fig. 10.1.27).[28,29] After ejection and clockwise rotation, the filter assumes its configuration and is fixed to the vessel wall (Fig. 10.1.28).[28,29] The wire pusher is detached, and the Teflon catheter and sheath are removed together.

Roehm reported follow-up of six months or more in 568 patients following placement of the bird's nest filter.[98]

The bird's nest filter is inserted through an 8Fr catheter. A transfemoral approach was used in 513 cases (93.4%), and a transjugular approach in 28 cases (5.1%).

The prevalence of clinically suspected recurrent pulmonary thromboembolism was 2.7%. Inferior vena cava occlusion was seen in 2.9%, most likely related to the massive volume of embolic material trapped in the bird's nest filter. With the initial filter design, filter migration occurred in five patients. No migration has occurred after the filter was modified, improving the anchoring system.[98]

If the inferior vena cava diameter is greater than 28mm, this is considered as a contraindication for the placement

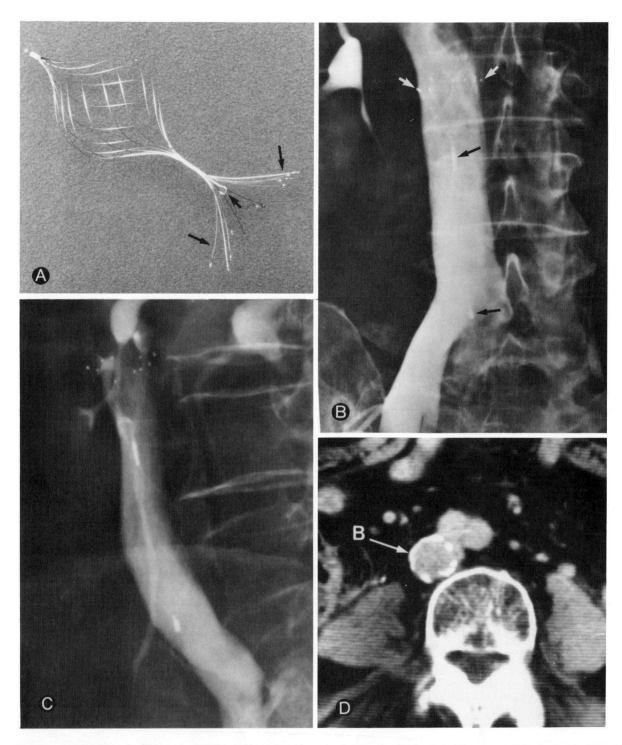

Figure 10.1.24. Günther filter. **A.** Observe basket-like configuration of filter with a spider *(long arrows)* attached to one of its ends for fixation to caval wall. A hook is also placed in center of spider for percutaneous introduction and removal *(short arrow)*. **B.** Inferior vena cavogram in anteroposterior projection shows filter low in vessel *(black arrows)*. Fixation hooks pierce wall of vein *(white arrows)*. **C.** Lateral projection of inferior vena cavogram shows filter centered in lumen. **D.** CT scan shows basket wires in filter midsection (*B*) braced against venous wall. (Reproduced from Günther RW, Schild M, Fries A, et al: Basket filter for prevention of pulmonary embolism. *Semin Intervent Radiol* 1986;3:220–226.)

of the Greenfield, Vena-Tech, and Simon filters, necessitating bi-iliac placement of these filters. Alternatively, the bird's nest filter, with a span of 60mm, can be used in an oversized vena cavae. Sixteen filters were placed in oversized vena cavae; all of them were successfully placed except one. In this case, the inferior vena cava measured 36mm in diameter and the filter hooks failed to engage the caval wall.[99] In a comparison study by Denny et al., the bird's nest was found to be equally effective as the Greenfield filter in preventing pulmonary embolus. In addition,

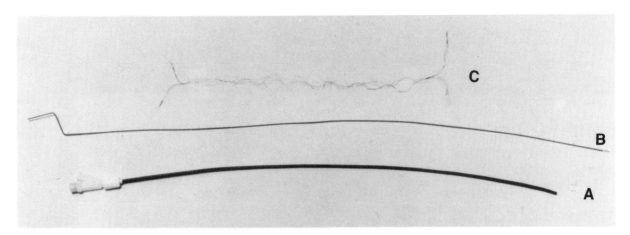

Figure 10.1.25. Unassembled set of Gianturco bird's nest filter showing introducing catheter (*A*), fixation stylet (*B*), and filter (*C*).

the bird's nest was found to be easier to insert and to have a lower complication rate.[100]

Nitinol Filters

Nitinol is a unique alloy of nickel and titanium that has a thermal-dependent memory.[26,27] The design of the filter is embodied in the wire at the time of annealing at high temperature[26,27]; by cooling, the wire can be made pliable and straight. In this condition, the nitinol wire can be introduced through small catheters by the Seldinger technique.[27]

PALESTRANT/SIMON FILTER

Palestrant et al. described a nitinol inferior vena cava filter and tested it in vitro.[26] The filter has two components, one a filter mesh and the other with six anchoring limbs with terminal hooks that penetrate the vena caval wall up

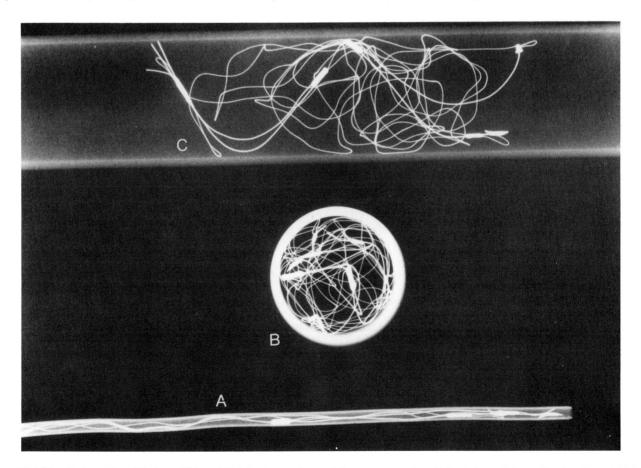

Figure 10.1.26. Radiographs of bird's nest filter within introducer catheter (*A*) and cross-sectional (*B*) and longitudinal (*C*) views of filter within inferior vena caval model illustrate mesh formed by the wires, which helps prevent migration of embolus.

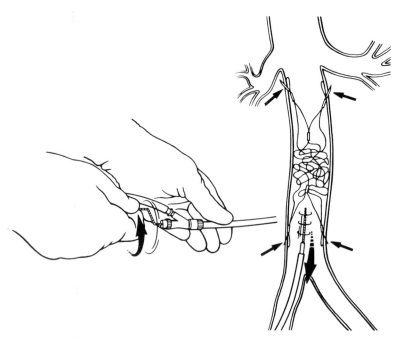

Figure 10.1.27. Placement of bird's nest filter below renal veins. Proximal and distal fixation points *(arrows)* have been anchored to caval wall, and stylet has been removed by gentle unscrewing. (Courtesy of Cook, Inc.)

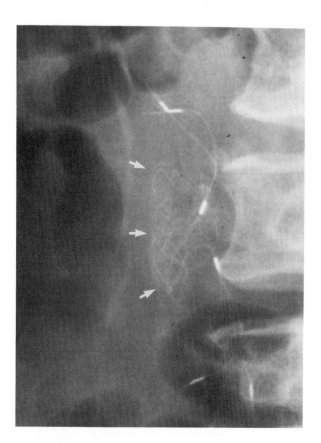

Figure 10.1.28. Lateral view of abdomen showing bird's nest filter positioned in inferior vena cava *(arrows).*

to 1mm, thus securing the device (Fig. 10.1.29). The filter limbs span as much as 32mm, and the filter mesh spans up to 25mm with nonoverlapping loops formed by a set of seven wires. The design allows the filter to be centered in the inferior vena cava lumen; the anchoring limbs and filter mesh can capture all emboli >5mm.[26] During in vitro testing, the filter was highly effective, allowing only 3% of small emboli to escape capture.[26] The gradient across the filter after clot capture was no greater than 5cm H_2O.[26]

An initial report by Simon included 103 patients.[101] Follow-up studies included plain film radiography, ultrasonography, magnetic resonance imaging, and clinical evaluation. Symptomatic occlusions occurred in 7–9%. No filter migration or perforation occurred. Just one case of symptomatic recurrent pulmonary embolism and two cases of asymptomatic pulmonary embolism were found. There were seven cases of confirmed symptomatic IVC occlusion and two possible IVC occlusions detected on the basis of clinical findings alone.[101]

Ultrasound studies of the puncture site in 18 patients revealed local thrombosis in 27%. Penetration of the vena cava wall by the filter legs did not occur. No evidence of retroperitoneal hemorrhage was found. The symptomatic IVC occlusion rate was 7–11%. Two-hundred fifty-six patients with a six month follow-up in 180 patients was reported by Kim in 1990.[102] Recurrent pulmonary embolism was seen in 1.8%, occlusion of the inferior vena cava in 7.5–9.4%, and no migration. Tilting of the dome was found in 25% of the cases, with nonsignificant filter dysfunction.[102] The filter has been approved by the FDA for clinical use in the United States.

5. It is less thrombogenic because of the smaller amount of wire.[27]
6. As with the KG filter, the apex of the Cragg filter is oriented superiorly and the spiral distends the inferior vena cava wall (Fig. 10.1.31). The emboli are trapped at the apex of the spiral sieve and, therefore, occlude less of the caval lumen, maintaining para-axial flow. This filter has not been used clinically.

TEMPORARY FILTERS

Thery et al. reported the use of a temporary vena cava filter percutaneously introduced to eliminate the risk of pulmonary embolism during thrombolytic therapy in patients with threatening venous thrombosis.[103] In patients at risk, but in whom a permanent implantable device is not desirable, the temporary device is a reasonable solution to filter and stop blood clots during thrombolytic therapy.

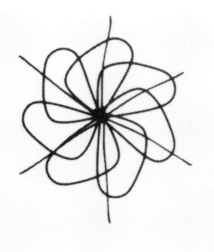

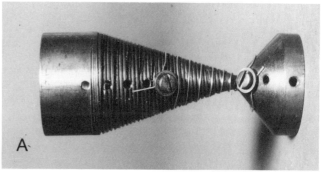

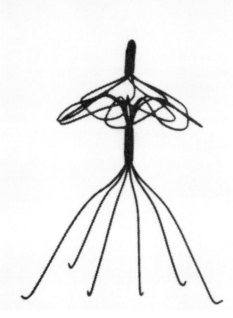

Figure 10.1.29. Palestrant nitinol filter.

CRAGG FILTER

Cragg et al. developed a simple spiral nitinol filter that can stop clots effectively without restricting blood flow (Fig. 10.1.30).[27] The spiral design has several advantages:

1. It can be introduced through an 8Fr angiographic catheter.
2. It can be repositioned easily.
3. It allows easier adjustments in size by tightening or loosening the spiral, allowing the filter to be effective in many sizes of vena cava.
4. The loop maintains proper orientation of the filter in the caval lumen.

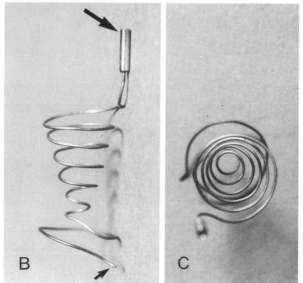

Figure 10.1.30. Cragg filter. **A.** Nitinol wire is tightly wound around cone-shaped stainless-steel barrel for thermal shaping. Lateral (**B**) and frontal (**C**) views of filter show its cone-shaped configuration with distal prong *(small arrow)* for fixation and proximal screw-carrying capsule for introduction and release *(large arrow)*. (Reproduced from Cragg A, Lund G, Salomonowitz E, et al: A new percutaneous vena cava filter. *AJR* 1983;141:601–604.)

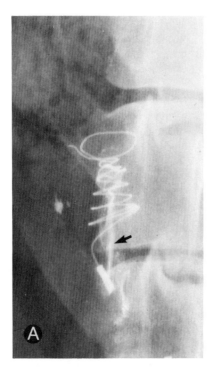
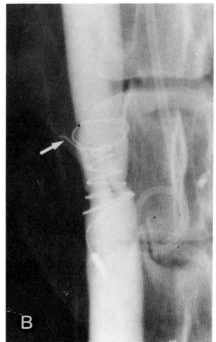

Figure 10.1.31. Experimental use of Cragg filter. **A.** Spot film shows filter of proper size placed within inferior vena cava of dog after injection of radiopaque autologous clot *(arrow)*. **B.** Superior vena cavogram six weeks after placement shows patent caval lumen with some filling defects within filter representing trapped embolus. Distal prong has perforated venous wall *(arrow)*.

The device is easy to insert and remove and does not damage the caval wall. The device (Prothia, Montrouge, France) consists of a 7Fr catheter provided with a two-way hub to allow injection of contrast medium, thrombolytics, or heparin (Fig. 10.1.32*A,B*). The temporary filter is passed through the catheter and consists of an eight-wire spiral basket which is pulled back into the catheter for introduction and removal purposes (Fig. 10.1.32*C,D*). The filter was used in 65 patients: 42 were cases of pulmonary embolism with threatening venous thrombosis; and 23 were cases of deep vein thrombosis with associated iliocaval thrombosis but without pulmonary embolism. The filter was introduced transfemorally in 38 cases, and 26 times transjugularly. In 16 cases thrombus fragments detached from the main iliocaval thrombus were caught by the filter and subsequently lysed with thrombolytics. The filter remained in place an average of 4.5 ± 1.2 days. No pulmonary embolism occurred after filter removal as proved by lung scan.[103]

COMPLICATIONS OF INTRALUMINAL FILTER DEVICES

Misplacement

Misplacement of the filter is one of the most common complications, although the frequency decreases with experience. Routine preoperative venography and adequate determination of renal vein position with metallic markers or a radiopaque ruler minimizes the frequency of misplacement.

Misplacement of filters most often involves the right side of the heart, the right renal vein, and the iliac veins. The right renal vein can easily be involved if the kidney is ptotic or if the renal vein is vertical and parallel to the inferior vena cava. Initial advancement of the filter capsule into the iliac vein under fluoroscopy guidance, before final ejection at the infrarenal position, minimizes the incidence of accidental misplacement into the hepatic, iliac, or renal veins.[104]

Inadvertent placement of MU filters into the right renal vein has been reported[2,39,51] and was corrected by operative removal and repair of the vein.[62] Misplacement into the right iliac vein[2] and perforation of the hepatic vein with filter extrusion into the retroperitoneal space also have been reported.[105] Other, rare, sites of misplacement include the right atrium, right ventricle, and suprarenal inferior vena cava.[105]

Deutsch described the percutaneous removal of a Greenfield filter from the right atrium.[106] For removal, a 7Fr loop snare was introduced into the right atrium and used to fix the Kimray–Greenfield filter and to see if the filter was partially mobile. The 7Fr vascular access sheath was replaced for a 24Fr Amplatz sheath and the snare wire was placed around the struts of the Kimray–Greenfield filter (Fig. 10.1.33). By closing the snare, the filter was fixed. The sheath was then advanced over the filter by using the snare to provide immobilization and guide advancement of

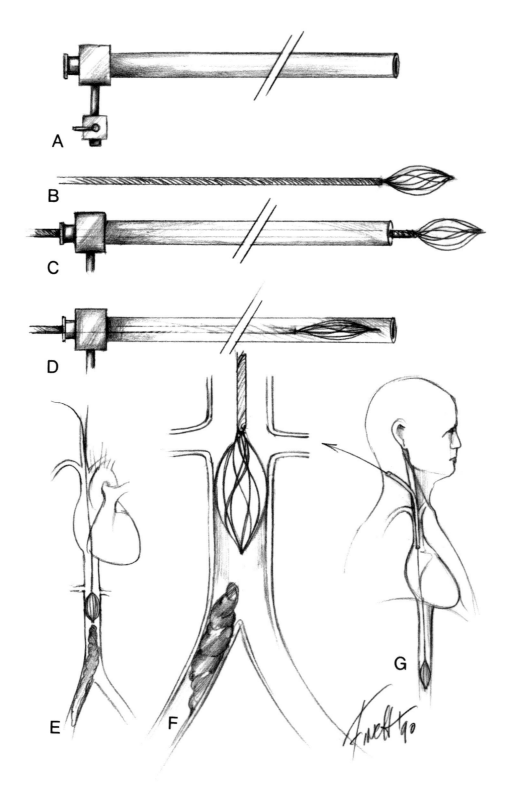

Fig. 10.1.32. Thery temporary filter placed during lysis of free-floating thrombus. **A.** 7Fr catheter. **B.** 8-wire basket/filter. **C.** Basket filter through 7Fr catheter—in open position. **D.** Basket filter through 7Fr catheter—in closed position. **E–G.** Position of filter below renal veins. Free-floating thrombus in right iliac vein.

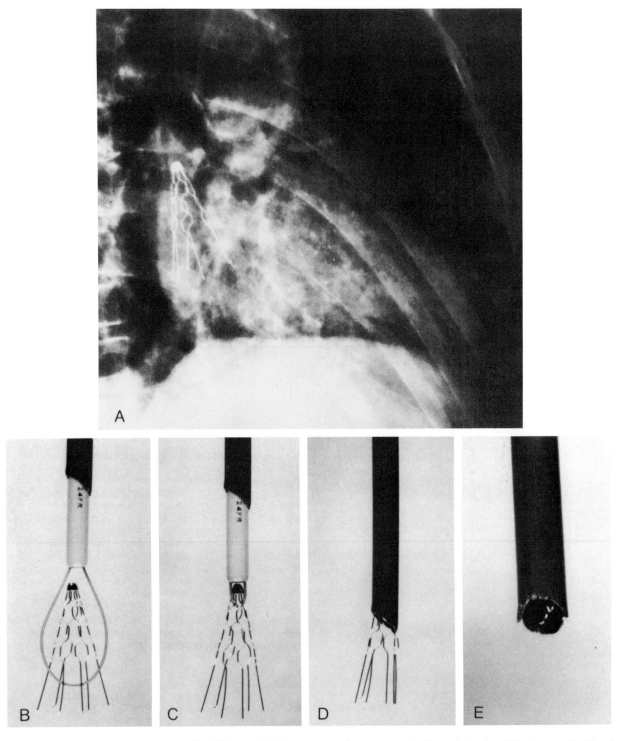

Fig. 10.1.33.   A. Greenfield filter in right atrium. **B.** 0.038-inch (0.096cm) guidewire loop snare through a 24Fr Amplatz sheath and dilator, with loop through Greenfield filter. **C.** Loop snare tightened to provide immobilizing counteraction on filter. **D.** Amplatz sheath is advanced over immobilized filter, partially collapsing it. **E.** Retention hooks completely surrounded by sheath; note ragged edges of sheath which developed while advancing sheath over filter. (Reproduced with permission from Deutsch LS: Percutaneous removal of intracardiac Greenfield vena caval filter. *AJR* 1988;151:677–679.)

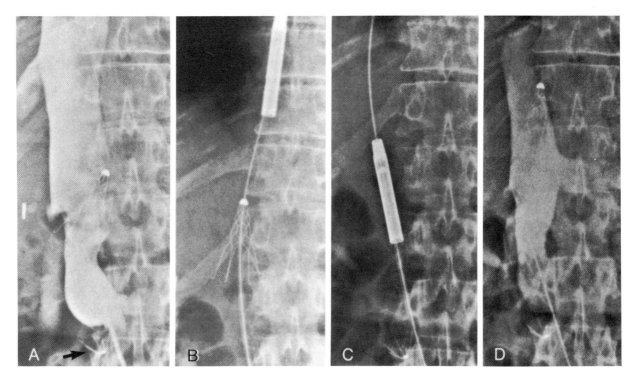

Fig. 10.1.34. A. Greenfield filter at level of L1-L2 with extreme obliquity below right renal vein. Mobin–Uddin at a lower level *(arrow)*. **B.** A guidewire has been passed through the central hole of the filter. The wire has been snared from above and pulled out through the jugular puncture. The carrier of the Greenfield filter is advanced from above over the wire. **C.** The carrier has been advanced over the filter, pushing the filter with the cath-eter advanced in a cephalic direction over the wire as the carrier surrounds the collapsed filter from above. **D.** Inferior vena cavogram shows a better position of the filter at T12-L1 above the renal veins. (Reproduced from Guthaner DF, Wyatt JO, Mehigan JT, Wright AM, Breen JF, Wexler L: Monorail system for percutaneous repositioning of the Greenfield filter. *Radiology* 1990;176:872–874.)

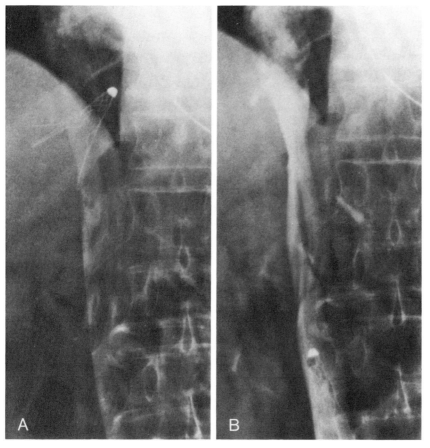

Fig. 10.1.35. A. Misplaced Greenfield filter in high IVC protruding into right atrium. **B.** After repositioning of filter into the IVC below the renal veins. (Reproduced from Guthaner DF, Wyatt JO, Mehigan JT, Wright AM, Breen JF, Wexler L: Monorail system for percutaneous repositioning of the Greenfield filter. *Radiology* 1990;176:872–874.)

Figure 10.1.36. Chest radiograph showing migrating Mobin–Uddin filter lodged in right pulmonary artery *(arrows).*

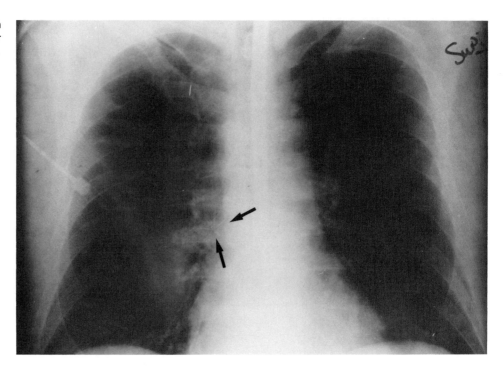

the sheath. Once the sheath had been advanced over the filter retention hooks, the whole assembly was withdrawn. A postprocedural electrocardiogram confirmed an atraumatic removal of the filter from the right atrium.[106]

Persistent entry of the capsule into the right renal vein can be prevented by blocking this vein with a Fogarty balloon catheter advanced through the venotomy.[107] Repositioning of misplaced Kimray–Greenfield filters by first passing a wire across the central hole of the cone from a femoral approach, followed by advancement of the carrier capsule over the wire to collapse the filter, and subsequently reposition it (Figs. 10.1.34 and 10.1.35) was described by Wexler.[108]

Migration

This complication can happen if there is a mismatch between the diameter of the filter device and the inferior vena cava. The size of the inferior vena cava can be assessed easily from an inferior vena cavogram and is not related to the age, sex, body habitus, or weight of the patient. The width of the inferior vena cava in normal adults is usually between 15 and 28mm. Megacava may occur in persons with chronic pulmonary hypertension, congestive heart failure, or tricuspid insufficiency and, rarely, as a congenital anomaly. Filters also can migrate if their limbs are not properly engaged in the caval wall prior to release.

With the 23mm MU filter, migration was reported in 22 patients (0.9%) of a large series and was fatal in 14 (0.6%).[11,52] With the latest design of 28mm MU filters, the migration incidence was decreased to 0.4% in a series of 300,333 patients.[109] The 2mm (extended length) prongs from the 28mm filter ensure secure seating of the device in the infrarenal inferior vena cava in most patients.

Migration of the MU filter to the right atrium or ventricle or to the pulmonary artery has been reported (Fig. 10.1.36).[105,110,111] Although less common, migration also has been reported with the KG filter (Fig. 10.1.37).[112] Other complications reported with this type of filter

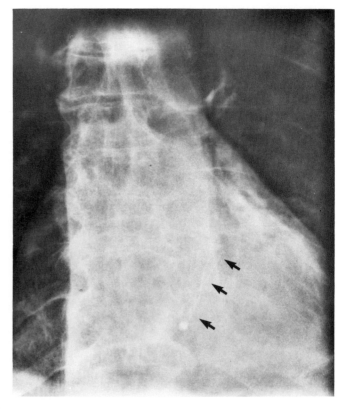

Figure 10.1.37. Close-up of heart shows Greenfield filter that has migrated into right ventricle *(arrows).*

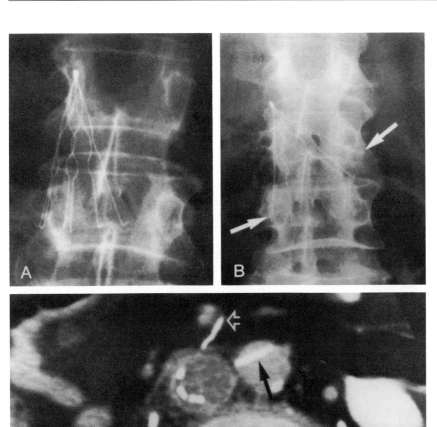

Fig. 10.1.38. A. Titanium Greenfield filter in position after deployment below the level of the renal veins. **B.** Follow-up plain film of the abdomen reveals wide splaying of the filter legs *(arrows)*. **C.** CT shows perforation of the caval wall by two of the filter struts. One of the struts has perforated through the aortic wall. (Reproduced from Teitelbaum GP, Jones DL, van Breda A, et al: Vena cava filter splaying: potential complication of use of the titanium Greenfield filter. *Radiology* 1989;173:809–814.)

include locking of the struts, which results in incomplete, asymmetrical opening of the filter,[113] perforation of the inferior vena cava,[114–116] (Fig. 10.1.38) misplacement,[115,117–119] distal migration,[120] and premature ejection into the right atrium.[113,114,117]

An unusual complication of the Greenfield filter was reported by Alexander with fracture and migration of the filter struts due to unrecognized operative manipulation in a patient during cholecystectomy. The presence of an intracaval device should be recognized preoperatively and manipulations of the device should be carefully avoided, especially during retroperitoneum dissections.[121]

Two cases of spontaneous fracture of the Kimray–Greenfield filter struts have been reported.[122] In one case the filter showed migration after three years of placement; in the second case migration was noticed four years after insertion, and eight years after the insertion, a CT scan of the abdomen confirmed that three legs of the filter had penetrated the caval wall. The patients remained asymptomatic.[122]

An unusual complication after suprarenal placement of a Greenfield filter with spreading of the filter struts and perforation of the inferior vena caval wall and penetration of the aortic wall and a vertebral body followed by fracture of one of the struts was reported by Kim et al.[123] The complication was discovered three months after suprarenal placement of a Greenfield filter and was demonstrated by a CT scan. The modifications in the filter's position, the penetration of the aorta and fracture of the struts were said to be possibly due to respiratory and cardiac motion, postural changes, or surgical manipulations.[123]

PUNCTURE SITE COMPLICATIONS

Two cases of arteriovenous fistula formation were reported by Grassi in 2 of 65 patients following Greenfield filter placement using a femoral approach.[124] Thrombosis at the puncture site was reported by Dorfman in 14.3%.[74] Asymptomatic thrombosis has been reported in up to 41%

of patients,[75] while symptomatic thrombosis occurred in 1.8–24% of patients following percutaneous Greenfield filter placement.[76–81] Mewissen reported a decrease in the incidence of thrombosis at the puncture site using balloon dilatation of the venotomy site from 24 to 10%.[125] A significant difference was also noted in the incidence of local thrombosis when using the femoral vein in comparison to the internal jugular vein.[125]

References

1. Dalen JE, Alpert JS: Natural history of pulmonary embolism. *Prog Cardiovasc Dis* 1975;17:259
2. Mobin–Uddin K, Utley JR, Bryant LR: The inferior vena cava umbrella filter. *Prog Cardiovasc Dis* 1975;17:391
3. Ochsner A, Ochsner JL, Sanders HS: Prevention of pulmonary embolism by caval ligation. *Ann Surg* 1970;171:923
4. Spencer FC, Quattlebaum JK, Quattlebaum JK Jr, Sharp EH, Jude JR: Plication of the inferior vena cava for pulmonary embolism. *Ann Surg* 1962;155:827
5. Sensenig DM, Achar BG, Serlin O: Plication of the inferior vena cava with staples. *Am J Surg* 1965;109:679
6. Moretz WH, Still MJ Jr, Griffin LH, Jennings WD, Wray CH: Partial occlusion of the inferior vena cava with a smooth Teflon clip: analysis of long-term results. *Surgery* 1972;71:710
7. Miles RM, Chappell F, Renner O: A partially occluding vena caval clip for the prevention of pulmonary embolism. *Am Surg* 1964;30:40
8. Adams JT, Deweese JA: Partial interruption of the inferior vena cava with a new plastic clip. *Surg Gynecol Obstet* 1966;123:1087
9. Deweese JA, Hunter JR: Vena cava filter for the prevention of pulmonary embolism: five years' clinical experience. *Arch Surg* 1963;86:852
10. Schroeder TM, Elkins RC, Greenfield LJ: Entrapment of sized emboli by the KMA-Greenfield intracaval filter. *Surgery* 1978;83:435
11. Cimochowski GE, Evans RH, Zarins CK, Lu C–T, DeMeester TR: Greenfield filter versus Mobin–Uddin umbrella: the continuing quest for the ideal method of vena caval interruption. *J Thorac Cardiovasc Surg* 1980;79:358
12. Gomez GA, Curler BS, Wheeler HB: Transvenous interruption of the inferior vena cava. *Surgery* 1983;93:612
13. Greenfield LF, McCurdy JR, Brown PP: A new intracava filter permitting continued flow and resolution of emboli. *Surgery* 1973;73:599
14. Greenfield LF: Current indications for and results of Greenfield filter placement. *J Vasc Surg* 1984;1:502
15. Eichelter P, Schenk WG Jr: Prophylaxis of pulmonary embolism: a new experimental approach with initial results. *Arch Surg* 1968;97:348
16. Moser KM, Harsany PG, Harvey–Smith W, Durante P, Gursan M: Reversible interruption of inferior vena cava by means of a balloon catheter: preliminary report. *J Thorac Cardiovasc Surg* 1971;62:205
17. Pate JW, Melvin D, Cheek RC: A new form of vena caval interruption. *Ann Surg* 1969;169:873
18. Hunter JA, Sessions R, Buenger R: Experimental balloon obstruction of the inferior vena cava. *Ann Surg* 1970;171:315
19. Mobin–Uddin K, McLean R, Bolooki H, Jude JR: Caval interruption for prevention of pulmonary embolism: long-term results of a new method. *Arch Surg* 1969;99:711
20. Wingerd M, Bernhard VM, Maddison F, Towne JB: Comparison of caval filters in the management of venous thromboembolism. *Arch Surg* 1978;113:1264
21. Bernstein E: The place of venous interruption in the treatment of pulmonary thromboembolism, in Moser K, Stein M (eds): *Pulmonary Thromboembolism.* Chicago, Year Book Medical Publishers, 1973, p 312
22. Rizk GK, Amplatz K: A percutaneous method of introducing the caval umbrella. *AJR* 1973;117:903
23. Knight L, Amplatz K, Nicoloff DM: Alternate method for introduction of IVC filters. *Surg Gynecol Obstet* 1974;138:763.
24. Tadavarthy SM, Castañeda–Zúñiga WR, Salomonowitz E, et al: Kimray–Greenfield vena cava filter: percutaneous introduction. *Radiology* 1984;151:525
25. Formanek A, Castañeda–Zúñiga WR, Knight L, Amplatz K: Three year experience with percutaneous introduction of inferior vena cava filter. *Rev Interam Radiol* 1977;2:171
26. Palestrant AM, Prince M, Simon M: Comparative in vitro evaluation of the Nitinol inferior vena cava filter. *Radiology* 1982;145:351
27. Cragg A, Lund G, Salomonowitz E, et al: A new percutaneous vena cava filter. *AJR* 1983;141:601
28. Roehm JO Jr: The bird's nest filter: a new percutaneous transcatheter inferior vena cava filter. *J Vasc Surg* 1984;1:498
29. Roehm JO Jr, Gianturco C, Barth MH, Wright KC: Percutaneous transcatheter filter for the inferior vena cava: a new device for treatment of patients with pulmonary embolism. *Radiology* 1984;150:255
30. Gianturco C, Anderson JH, Wallace S: A new vena cava filter: experimental animal evaluation. *Radiology* 1980;137:835
31. Maass D, Demierre D, Wallsten H, Senning A: The helix filter: a new vena caval filter for the prevention of pulmonary embolism. *J Cardiovasc Surg (Torino)* 1985;26:116
32. Lund G, Rysavy JA, Salomonowitz E, et al: A new caval filter for percutaneous placement and retrieval: experimental study. *Radiology* 1984;152:369
33. Tobin KD, Pais SO, Austin CB: Reevaluation of indications for percutaneous placement of the Greenfield filter. *Invest Radiol* 1989;24(2):115
34. Gray RK, Buckberg GD, Grollman JH Jr: The importance of inferior vena cavography in placement of the Mobin–Uddin vena caval filter. *Radiology* 1973;106:277
35. Ferris EJ: The inferior vena cava, in Abrams H (ed): *Abrams Angiography,* ed 3. Boston, Little, Brown, p 939
36. Mejia EA, Saroyan M, Balkin PW, Kerstein MD: Analysis of inferior venacavography before Greenfield filter placement. *Ann Vasc Surg* 1989;3(3):232
37. Stansel MC: Vena cava interruption: three points of view. *Contemp Surg* 1982;20:63
38. Santos GH, Lansman S: Prevention of pulmonary embolism with use of Mobin–Uddin filter. *NY State J Med* 1982;82:185
39. Mobin–Uddin K: Invited commentary. *World J Surg* 1978;2:55
40. Greenfield LJ, Scher LA, Elkins RC: KMA–Greenfield filter placement for chronic pulmonary hypertension. *Ann Surg* 1979;189:560
41. Peyton JW, Hylemon MB, Greenfield LJ, Crute SL, Sugerman HJ, Quershi GD: Comparison of Greenfield filter and vena caval ligation for experimental septic thromboembolism. *Surgery* 1983;93:533
42. Golueke PJ, Garrett WV, Thompson JE, Smith BL, Talkington CM: Interruption of the vena cava by means of the Greenfield filter: expanding the indications. *Surgery* 1988;103:111
43. Jarrell BE, Posuniak E, Roberts J, Osterholm J, Cotler J,

Ditunno J: A new method of management using the Kimray–Greenfield filter for deep venous thrombosis and pulmonary embolism in spinal cord injury. *Surg Gynecol Obstet* 1983;157:316

44. Johnson R, Green JA, Charnley J: Pulmonary embolism following the Charnley hip replacement and its prophylaxis. *Clin Orthop* 1977;127:123

45. Coventry MB, Beckenbaugh RD, Nolan DR, Ilstrup DM: 2,012 total hip arthroplasties: a study of postoperative course and early complications. *J Bone Joint Surg* 1974; 56A:273

46. Salzman EW, Harris WH: Prevention of venous thromboembolism in orthopaedic patients. *J Bone Joint Surg* 1976;58A:903

47. Woolson ST, Harris WH: Greenfield vena caval filter for management of selected cases of venous thromboembolic disease following hip surgery—a report of five cases. *Clin Orthop* 1986;204:201

48. Vaughn BK, Knezevich S, Lombardi AV Jr, Mallory TH: Use of the Greenfield filter to prevent fatal pulmonary embolism associated with total hip and knee arthroplasty. *J Bone Joint Surg (Am)* 1989;71(10):1542

49. Darcy MD, Smith TP, Hunter DW, Castañeda–Zúñiga WR, Lund G, Amplatz K: Short-term prophylaxis of pulmonary embolism by using a retrievable vena cava filter. *AJR* 1986;147:836

50. Maynar M, Reyes R, Pulido–Duque JM, Casal G: Experience with the Amplatz Retrievable Filter. *Cardiovasc Intervent Radiol* 1987;14:221

51. Mobin–Uddin K, Callarda M, Bolooko M, Rubinson R, Michie D, Jude JR: Transvenous caval interruption with umbrella filters. *N Engl J Med* 1972;286:255

52. Mensoian JO, LoGerfo FW, Weitzman AF, Ezpeleta M, Sequeira JC: Clinical experience with the Mobin–Uddin vena cava umbrella filter. *Arch Surg* 1980;115:1179

53. McIntyre AB, McCready RA, Hyde GL, Mattingly W: A ten year follow-up study of the Mobin–Uddin filter for vena cava interruption. *Surg Gynecol Obstet* 1984;158:513

54. Wingerd M, Bernhard VM, Maddison F, Towne JB: Comparison of caval filters in the management of venous thromboembolism. *Arch Surg* 1978;113:1264

55. Knight L, Amplatz K, Nicoloff DM: Alternate method for introduction of IVC filters. *Surg Gynecol Obstet* 1974; 138:763

56. Rizk GK, Amplatz K: A percutaneous method of introducing the caval umbrella. *AJR* 1973;117:903

57. Greenfield LJ, Crute SL: Retrieval of the Greenfield vena caval filter. *Surgery* 1980;88:719

58. Stewart JR, Greenfield LJ: Transvenous vena caval filtration and pulmonary embolectomy. *Surg Clin North Am* 1982;62:411

59. Orsini RA, Jarrell BE: Suprarenal placement of vena caval filters: indications, techniques, and results. *J Vasc Surg* 1984;1:124

60. Kanter B, Moser KM: The Greenfield vena cava filter. *Chest* 1988;93(1):170

61. Günther RW, Bohndorf K, Schuster CJ, Steffens M: A new technique to avoid suprarenal placement of Kimray–Greenfield filters: technical note. *Cardiovasc Intervent Radiol* 1989;12(3):166

62. Langham MR, Etheridge JC, Crute SL, Greenfield LJ: Experimental superior vena cava placement of the Greenfield filter. *J Vasc Surg* 1985;2:794

63. Pais SO, De Orchis DF, Mirvis SE: Superior vena caval placement of a Kimray–Greenfield filter. *Radiology* 1987;165:385

64. Novelline RA: Practical points on transvenous insertion of inferior vena cava filters. *Cardiovasc Intervent Radiol* 1980;3:319

65. Greenfield LJ, Stewart JR, Crute S: Improved technique for insertion of Greenfield vena caval filter. *Surg Gynecol Obstet* 1983;156:217

66. Leiter B, Sequeira J, Weitzman R, Menzoian J: A complication following Kimray–Greenfield filter insertion. *Cardiovasc Intervent Radiol* 1981;4:215

67. Menzoian JO, Logerfo FW, Doyle JE, Weitzman AF, Sequeira JC: Technical modifications in the placement of inferior vena caval filter devices. *Am J Surg* 1981;142:216

68. Sequeira JC, Sacks BA, Tata J, Simon M: A safe technique for introduction of the Kimray–Greenfield filter. *Radiology* 1979;133:799

69. Gonzalez R, Narayan P, Castañeda–Zúñiga WR, Amplatz K: Transvenous embolization of the internal spermatic veins for the treatment of varicocele scroti. *Urol Clin North Am* 1982;9:17

70. Rusnak B, Castañeda–Zúñiga WR, Kotula F, Herrera M, Amplatz K: An improved dilator system for percutaneous nephrostomies. *Radiology* 1982;144:174

71. Coons H: Personal communication, 1985. Sharp Memorial Hospital, San Diego, CA

72. Shetty PC, Bok LR, Burke MW, Sharma RP: Balloon dilation of the femoral vein expediting percutaneous Greenfield vena caval filter placement. *Radiology* 1986;161:275

73. Dorfman GS, Esparaza AR, Cronan JJ: Percutaneous large bore venotomy and tract creation: comparison of sequential dilator and angioplasty balloon methods in a porcine model—preliminary report. *Invest Radiol* 1988;23:441

74. Dorfman GS, Cronan JJ, Paolella LP, Lambiase RE, Hass RA, Scola FH, Schepps B: Iatrogenic changes at the venotomy site after percutaneous placement of the Greenfield filter. *Radiology* 1989;173:159

75. Kantor A, Glanz S, Gordon DH, Sclafani SJA: Percutaneous insertion of the Kimray–Greenfield filter: incidence of femoral vein thrombosis. *AJR* 1987;149:1065

76. Pais SO, Tobin KD, Austin CB, Queral L: Percutaneous insertion of the Greenfield inferior vena cava filter: experience with ninety-six patients. *J Vasc Surg* 1988;8:460

77. Denny DF, Cronan JJ, Dorfman GS, Esplin C: Percutaneous Kimray–Greenfield filter placement by femoral vein puncture. *AJR* 1985;145:827

78. Denny DF, Dorfman GS, Cronan JJ, Greenwood LH, Morse SS, Yoselevitz M: Percutaneous Greenfield inferior vena cava filter placement: experience in 50 patients. *AJR* 1988;150:427

79. Rose BS, Simon DC, Hess ML, Van Aman ME: Percutaneous transfemoral placement of the Kimray–Greenfield vena cava filter. *Radiology* 1987;165:373

80. Pais SO, Mirvis SE, DeOrchis DF: Percutaneous insertion of the Kimray–Greenfield filter: technical considerations and problems. *Radiology* 1987;165:377

81. Welch TJ, Stanson AW, Sheedy PF II, Johnson CM, Miller WE, Johnson CD: Percutaneous placement of the Greenfield vena caval filter. *Mayo Clin Proc* 1988;63:343

82. Greenfield LJ, Cho KJ, Pais SO, Van Aman M: Preliminary clinical experience with the titanium Greenfield vena cava filter. *Arch Surg* 1989;124:657

83. Teitelbaum GT, Jones DJ, van Breda A, Matsumoto AH, Fellmeth BD, Chespak LW, Barth K: Vena caval filter splaying: potential complication of use of the titanium Greenfield filter. *Radiology* 1989;173:809

84. Hunter JA, DeLaria GA: Hunter vena cava balloon: rationale and results. *J Vasc Surg* 1984;1:491

85. Hunter JA, Dye WS, Javid H, Najafi H, Golding MD, Serry C: Permanent transvenous balloon occlusion of the inferior

vena cava: experience with 60 patients. *Ann Surg* 1977;186:491

86. Stiegel D, Duesman JF: Experience with the Hunter–Sessions inferior vena cava balloon occluder. *Arch Surg* 1979;114:746

87. Hunter JA, Delaria GA, Goldin MD, Serry C, Monson DO, DaValle MJ, Najafi H: Inferior vena cava interruption with the Hunter–Sessions balloon: eighteen years' experience in 191 cases. *J Vasc Surg* 1989;10:450

88. Williams DF: Implantable prostheses. *Phys Med Biol* 1980;25:611

89. Epstein DH, Darcy MD, Hunter DW, Coleman CC, Tadavarthy SM, Murray PD, Castañeda–Zúñiga WR, Amplatz K: Experience with the Amplatz retrievable vena cava filter. *Radiology* 1989;172:105

90. McCowan TC, Ferris EJ, Carver DK, Baker ML: Amplatz vena caval filter: clinical experience in 30 patients. *AJR* 1990;155(1):177

91. Robinson JD, Hunter DW, Castañeda–Zúñiga WR, Amplatz K: In-vitro evaluation of caval filters. *Cardiovasc Intervent Radiol* 1988;11(6):346

92. Katsamouris AA, Waltman AC, Delichatsios MA, Athanasoulis CA: Inferior vena cava filters: in-vitro comparison of clot trapping and flow dynamics. *Radiology* 1988;166:361

93. Günther RW, Schild M, Fries A, Storkel S: Vena caval filter to prevent pulmonary embolism: experimental study. *Radiology* 1985;156:315

94. Fobbe F, Dietzel M, Korth R, Felsenberg D, Bender S, Hamed M, Laass C, Sörensen R: Günther vena caval filter: results of long-term follow-up. *AJR* 1988;151:1031

95. Schneider PA, Parmeggiani L, Piguet JC, Bounameaux H: Caudal migration of the Günther vena caval filter. *Radiology* 1989;173(2):465

96. Martin–Santos, L: Personal communication, 1984. Hospital Seguridad Social, Sevilla, Spain

97. Günther RW, Schild H, Hollman JP, Vorwerk D: First clinical results with a new caval filter. *Cardiovasc Intervent Radiol* 1987;10:104

98. Roehm JOF Jr, Johnsrude IS, Barth MH, Gianturco C: The bird's nest inferior vena cava filter: progress report. *Radiology* 1988;168:745

99. Reed RA, Teitelbaum GP, Taylor FC, Kennedy TF, Pais OS, Roehm JO: Use of the bird's nest filter in the oversized inferior vena cava to avoid biiliac filter placement. *Radiology* 1990;177(suppl):220 (Abstr. 810)

100. Denny DF, Markowitz DM, Yoselevitz M, Pollak J, Wilkinson A: Comparison of percutaneously placed Greenfield and bird's nest inferior vena cava filters. *Radiology* 1990;177(suppl):220 (Abstr. 809)

101. Simon M, Athanasoulis CA, Kim D, Steinberg FL, Porter DH, Byse BH, Kleshinski S, Geller S, Orron DE, Waltman AC: Simon nitinol inferior vena cava filter: initial clinical experience—work in progress. *Radiology* 1989;172:99

102. Kim D, Grassi CJ, Porter DH, Siegel JB, Kleshinski S, Simon M: Simon nitinol filter clinical trial: final results. *Radiology* 1990;177(suppl):220 (Abstr. 807)

103. Thery C, Asseman P, Amrouni N, Becquart J, Pruvost P, Lesenne M, Legghe R, Marache P: Use of a new removable vena cava filter in order to prevent pulmonary embolism in patients submitted to thrombolysis. *Eur Heart J* 1990;11:334

104. Fee HJ, McAvoy JH, O'Connell TX: Treatment and prevention of Mobin–Uddin umbrella misplacement. *Arch Surg* 1978;113:331

105. Isch JH, Shumacker HB Jr: Embolization of caval umbrella: discussion and report of successful removal from the right ventricle. *J Thorac Cardiovasc Surg* 1976;72:256

106. Deutsch LS: Percutaneous removal of intracardiac Greenfield vena caval filter. *AJR* 1988;151:677

107. Edoga JK, Widmann WD: Avoiding renal vein entry when implanting the Mobin–Uddin vena cava umbrella filter. *Arch Surg* 1979;144:752

108. Guthaner DF, Wyatt JO, Mehigan JT, Wright AM, Breen JF, Wexler L: Monorail system for percutaneous repositioning of the Greenfield vena cava filter. *Radiology* 1990;176:872

109. Mobin–Uddin K: Vena cava interruption: three points of view. *Contemp Surg* 1982;20:43

110. Nevin WS: Migration of vena cava filter. *JAMA* 1972;222:88

111. Flores L, Caldera F, Lotlikar U, et al: Arterial thromboembolism: a complication after insertion of Mobin–Uddin vena cava filter. *NY State J Med* 1982;82:1588

112. Castañeda F, Herrera M, Cragg AH, et al: Migration of a Kimray–Greenfield filter to the right ventricle. *Radiology* 1983;149:690

113. Leiter B, Sequeira J, Weitzman AF, Menzoian J: A complication following Kimray–Greenfield filter insertion. *Cardiovasc Intervent Radiol* 1981;4:215

114. Simon M, Palestrant AM: Transvenous devices for the management of pulmonary embolism. *Cardiovasc Intervent Radiol* 1980;3:308

115. Sequeira JC, Sacks BA, Tata J, Simon M: A safe technique for introduction of the Kimray–Greenfield filter. *Radiology* 1979;133:799

116. Phillips MR, Widrich WC, Johnson WC: Perforation of the inferior vena cava by the Kimray–Greenfield filter. *Surgery* 1980;87:233

117. Greenfield LJ, Crute SL: Retrieval of the Greenfield vena caval filter. *Surgery* 1980;88:719

118. Akins CW, Thurer RL, Waltman AC, Margolies MN, Schneider RC: A misplaced caval filter: its removal from the heart without cardiopulmonary bypass. *Arch Surg* 1980;115:1133

119. Allen MA, Cisterninos J, Otteseno E, Queral L, Dagher F: The Kimray–Greenfield filter: a case of unusual misplacement. *Cardiovasc Intervent Radiol* 1982;5:82

120. Berland LL, Maddison FE, Bernhard VM: Radiologic follow-up of vena cava filter devices. *AJR* 1980;134:1047

121. Alexander JJ, Gewertz BL, Zarins CK: Intraoperative disruption of a Greenfield vena cava filter. *J Cardiovasc Surg* 1989;30(1):130

122. Lang W, Schweiger H, Fietkau R, Hofman–Preiss K: Spontaneous disruption of two Greenfield vena caval filters. *Radiology* 1990;174:445

123. Kim D, Porter DH, Siegel JB, Simon M: Perforation of the inferior vena cava with aortic and vertebral penetration by a suprarenal Greenfield filter. *Radiology* 1989;172:721

124. Grassi CJ, Bettmann MA, Rogoff P, Reagan K, Harrington DP: Femoral arteriovenous fistula after placement of a Kimray–Greenfield filter. *AJR* 1988;151:681

125. Mewissen MW, Erickson SJ, Foley WD, Lipchik EO, Olson DL, McCann KM, Schreiber ER: Thrombosis at venous insertion sites after inferior vena caval filter placement. *Radiology* 1989;173:155

Part 2. Vena-Tech Filter

—Harvey A. Koolpe, M.D., and Robert M. Zeit, M.D.

INTRODUCTION

In 1973, Lazar Greenfield introduced the first practical device for mechanical protection from massive pulmonary embolism.[1] While other techniques predated the Kimray–Greenfield (KG) filter (Medi-tech, Incorporated, Watertown, MA), each had significant complications. Surgical interruption of the inferior vena cava frequently led to the development of lower extremity edema which was often debilitating.[1] In addition, large collateral vessels developed which were capable of transmitting life-threatening emboli from the pelvis and lower extremities to the lungs, thereby negating the surgical goal.[2] Although vena cava plication techniques held the promise of long-term patency without the development of collaterals, major open abdominal surgery was involved.[3] Subsequently, clips of various designs were utilized to achieve the same result. However, laparotomy was still required.[4] This was considered undesirable since the patients most in need of the procedure were those morbidly ill from recent massive or submassive pulmonary embolism.

Although mechanical transvenous filters used before the KG avoided general anesthesia and laparotomy, they often produced unsatisfactory results. The Mobin–Uddin umbrella had to be introduced by jugular cutdown, resulted in a high rate of inferior vena cava thrombosis,[6,7] and was associated with several dislodgements, some with serious sequelae. Another transvenous device, the Hunter–Sessions balloon, was designed to completely occlude the inferior vena cava. This resulted in the same long-term problems as the original surgical ligation methods.[5]

Greenfield's cone-shaped wire filter was a conceptual advance because it avoided total occlusion of the vena cava, but effectively filtered major emboli. Large emboli were carried into its centrally positioned cone. This conical geometry allowed large volumes of thrombus to be trapped without occluding the inferior vena cava. Gradual lysis of the trapped thrombi could then occur. The device is described in detail in Chapter 10, Part 1, and the reader is directed to that section for an analysis of the principles of this device. In summary, the KG filter has offered a low complication rate when inserted by either surgical or percutaneous technique, as long as meticulous attention to detail is paid. Its long-term effectiveness and safety have been borne out over 17 years of use.[6] Because of its favorable risk:benefit ratio, the indications for caval filtration have expanded.[7] The only remaining drawback to the KG device is its large size, which necessitates either surgical

exposure of the jugular or femoral vein or, more recently, percutaneous dilatation of these access routes to 24Fr with a long sheath.[8] If the latter technique is chosen, this large venotomy necessitates the use of a subcuticular suture at the femoral site in order to avoid delayed hemorrhage.

Several manufacturers have recently offered mechanical filters which can be introduced to the vena cava through smaller sheaths using the same principle. The one which has been most frequently utilized at Albert Einstein Medical Center has been the Vena-Tech filter (L.G. Medical, Chasseneuil, France, imported by Vena-Tech Corporation, Evanston, IL). It most nearly approximates the original principles described by Greenfield.

THE DEVICE

The original KG filter geometry was based upon the premise that a cone-shaped wire structure would cause minimal disruption of flow as it accumulated thrombus within the central portion of the inferior vena cava.[9] The Vena-Tech (VT) filter is a device that attempts to maintain the same geometry yet can be inserted through a smaller hole than the original KG filter.[10] The VT filter is constructed of two different metals, fashioned in the form of a cone. The filter is anchored in the inferior vena cava by metallic struts bonded to the cone at its base. The possible significance of this bimetallic construction will be discussed below. Each of these struts has multiple small hooks, which anchor the device to the caval wall and prevent migration (Fig. 10.2.1). This differs from the KG filter, which anchors by hooks at the base of the cone itself. Because of the struts, and the flat wire from which it is made, the VT filter presents a larger, potentially more thrombogenic surface to the blood flowing in the inferior vena cava than does the KG filter. However, it is less likely to penetrate through the vena cava wall because of the greater surface area pressing against the venous intima, and because the struts themselves serve to limit caval penetration.

As with the KG, the VT filter is meant to be positioned axially within the lumen and is ideally placed just below the renal veins, where the increased blood flow may help to keep thrombus from developing on the apex of the cone (Fig. 10.2.2). Each VT kit contains, along with the filter, a dedicated introducing system allowing placement from either the right common femoral or right internal jugular veins. Because of the length of the filter, this device is specifically not recommended for introduction from the left internal jugular or left common femoral veins.

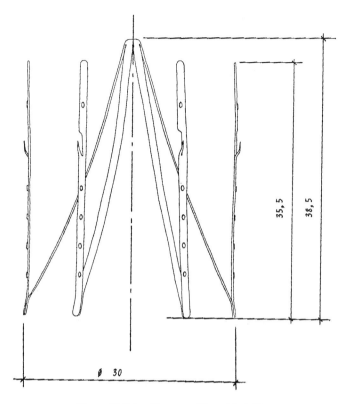

Figure 10.2.1. Diagram of Vena-Tech filter.

TECHNIQUE OF INTRODUCTION

Transfemoral

In our hands, the femoral route has been used for approximately 80% of the cases where the VT filter is placed. Cardiovascular monitoring is used for all vena cava filter insertions from either venous route. A slightly larger area is infiltrated with local anesthetic than for simple inferior venacavography, because a 12Fr introducer sheath is used. The manufacturer provides a complete, self-sufficient kit, containing a venotomy needle, guidewire, the filter, and the combined introduction sheath/fascial dilator. However, as described below, additional dilatation may be desirable.

Either the materials supplied or an ordinary 18-gauge one-wall arterial needle may be used to enter the common femoral vein, after which the introducer sheath with its dilator may be advanced to the lower portion of the inferior vena cava without the use of preliminary dilating catheters. The dilator is then removed and the radiolucent sheath connected to a continuous intravenous infusion with a three-way stopcock. Following a test injection of contrast, either conventional cut-film inferior venacavography or digital subtraction imaging is performed, using vertical metallic markers on the abdomen to identify the renal vein level and metal "BBs" placed transversely 28mm apart to assess vena caval size. This is critical because, like the KG filter, the VT device is not recommended if the vena caval diameter is greater than 28mm.

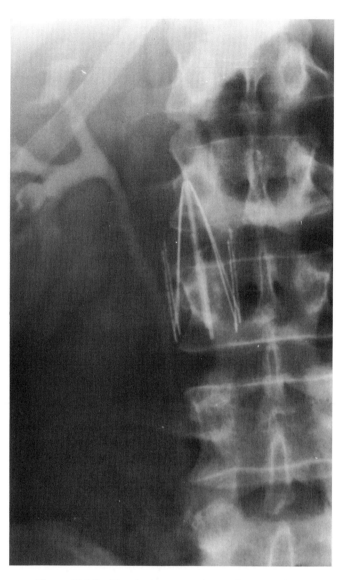

Figure 10.2.2. Usual appearance of properly opened filter.

The introducing apparatus with the dilator is then advanced over a guidewire to the desired level, usually below the renal veins. A radiopaque marker connects the radiolucent dilator tip and shaft by threaded screw connections. This construction creates the potential for separation of the dilator tip from the shaft, as will be described below. This radiopaque marker identifies the location of the tip of the introducing sheath, which defines the position of the filter at the end of the sheath just prior to release. The filter is furnished inside a loading carrier, which is screwed into the base of the sheath and the filter is injected into the sheath. The "filter pusher" is then used to move the device to the end of the insertion sheath *but not beyond it*. It is important to emphasize that release of the filter is performed by pulling the sheath back briskly to the hub of the pusher. The necessity for this, especially in jugular insertions, will be discussed. Brisk withdrawal assures that the filter will be discharged quickly and will align itself with the vena cava most satisfactorily. If the filter is inadvertently pushed beyond the end of the sheath, anchoring will be at a higher level than intended. Moreover, the filter may become tilted or not open fully. Following release, the apparatus is withdrawn and digital hemostasis usually easily obtained.

Transjugular

The two major indications for the use of the jugular approach have been iliofemoral thrombosis, often with extension to the inferior vena cava, and coagulopathy. Iliofemoral thrombosis creates the possibility that femoral introduction of the device might dislodge a potentially life-threatening thrombus. The existence of a coagulopathy suggests the use of the jugular approach because hemostasis is more easily obtained at this site than in the groin. The jugular venotomy seals quickly and reliably when the head and shoulders are elevated just after removal of the introducer sheath. Also, compression is quite easy and there is virtually no chance of occult hemorrhage.

Jugular filter placement begins with placing the patient in the Trendelenburg position, with the patient's head down 10–15°. This is usually sufficient to distend the jugular vein and to reduce the risk of possible air embolism during catheter exchanges and filter insertion.

The course of the common carotid artery is palpated, and a local anesthetic wheal is infiltrated approximately 1cm lateral to the most cephalad point at which the carotid is clearly identified. This is usually just lateral to the sternocleidomastoid muscle. Deeper infiltration of anesthesia is then directed caudad and slightly medial, with careful aspiration to avoid intracarotid injection of local anesthetic. The skin and subcutaneous tissues are gently spread with a hemostat, after which a 21-gauge, 5cm-long one-wall arterial needle is introduced with its tip directed lateral to the carotid artery and in the direction of the sternoclavicular joint. A syringe filled with local anesthetic attached to the needle is used for continuous suction, as well as deeper infiltration of anesthetic should the patient experience any discomfort.

When blood is freely aspirated, the 0.018-inch diameter platinum tipped guidewire is introduced through the needle, coaxial dilatation is performed and a 0.038-inch diameter heavy duty guidewire with a 3mm diameter J curve is advanced through the larger sheath and its tip is directed towards the inferior vena cava. The jugular introducer sheath and dilator are then passed over the wire with fluoroscopy to guide the tip of the wire and dilator to the inferior vena cava at the level of the confluence of the common iliac veins. If there is a question of vena caval thrombus, the guidewire may be removed at any stage, and contrast injected through the dilator. If difficulty is encountered negotiating the eustachian opening at the thoraco-abdominal junction, a steerable guidewire may be inserted through the VT dilator to gain access to the inferior vena cava. If this fails, the dilator may be removed over a guidewire and further attempts using a steerable catheter/guidewire combination of the operator's choice will usually be successful in entering the inferior vena cava.

Following placement of the sheath in the inferior vena cava, the procedure used for the transfemoral approach is followed for inferior vena cavography and identification of renal veins. The sheath may be withdrawn to the level of the renal veins without the dilator. However, the sheath is not radiopaque, and this must be done with contrast material in the sheath to mark its position. The filter is then engaged, and the same dilator that is used to place the working sheath is then used to push the filter to the end of the sheath. This use of the same dilator to advance the filter is the only major difference in the apparatus from the transfemoral kit, which contains a separate filter pusher.

When the filter is at the end of the sheath, a mark on the dilator will indicate that release of the filter is imminent. The sheath is then briskly pulled back, and the filter will be released, usually more caudad than initially anticipated. If the release is performed more slowly, the struts at the base of the filter may not separate fully, and the filter then assumes a rhomboid configuration (Fig. 10.2.3). This phenomenon has been termed ''coning,'' and occurs much more frequently from the jugular than from the femoral approach.[11] The authors have been assured by a company representative that the company has cured this problem by lengthening the support struts on newer filters.[12] The sheath may be used for follow-up inferior vena cavography, after which it is withdrawn, and the patient's head and shoulders are elevated. Hemostasis is usually immediate.

CLINICAL EXPERIENCE

Since December 1989 we have inserted 75 VT filters at the Albert Einstein Medical Center. Of these, 56 were from the femoral approach and the remainder from the jugular route. We prefer the femoral access because in our hands it is simpler, maintenance of a sterile field is less of a problem, it is unnecessary to partially or fully drape the patients' heads and faces, and the patients are not forced to keep their heads in an abnormal posture throughout the procedure.

COMPLICATIONS

We have encountered three types of complications with the Vena-Tech filter, and a fourth has been reported. In our experience the commonest complication is ''coning,'' the failure of the base of the cone to open when the filter is inserted via the jugular vein, as discussed above.[11-13] Coning occurred in 3 of our jugular filter insertions (3 of 19). Occasionally, we have felt it necessary to insert a second filter proximal to the unopened one (Fig. 10.2.3).

Thrombosis of the inferior vena cava has occurred once

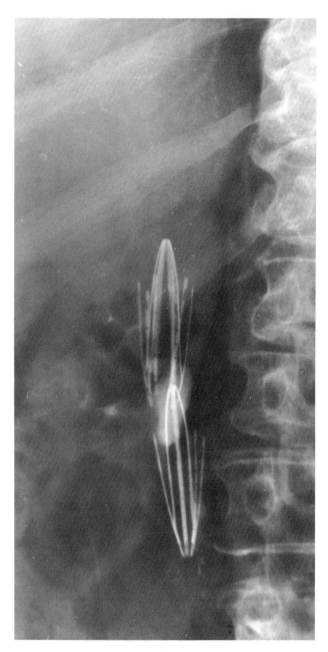

Figure 10.2.3. "Coned" filter, in which base has not opened. Second filter placed cephalad to unopened one using same jugular introducer.

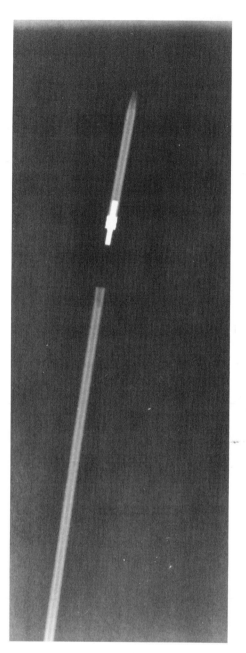

Figure 10.2.4. Radiograph of separated introducer tip after removal from patient.

in our series after insertion of the VT filter by the femoral route, and has also been reported by others.[11]

We have recently experienced a most disquieting event, in which the dilator tip unscrewed from the dilator shaft during a jugular filter insertion. The patient had considerable scar tissue in the area from previous jugular cannulations, and the dilator was rotated several times during attempted advancement. When the dilator and sheath were removed over a guidewire, only the dilator shaft was withdrawn from the skin. Fluoroscopy revealed that the tip of the dilator remained inside the patient, still on the guidewire. Puncture of the left groin was then performed and

the tip of the guidewire was snared from the left femoral vein by a Curry snare (Cook, Inc., Bloomington, IN). The end of the guidewire was then brought out of the left femoral vein through a sheath, and the tip of the dilator was then pushed along the guidewire until it exited the sheath.

Subsequent investigation revealed that the radiopaque screw holding the dilator tip to the shaft will unscrew after 10 turns, separating the tip from the shaft. Thus, it may be prudent to overdilate the tract slightly before attempting to insert the VT introducer system, and to avoid counterclockwise rotation of the dilator shaft (Fig. 10.2.4).

Finally, the bimetallic construction of the VT filter may

theoretically lead to separation of the components some time after implantation. However, this has not occurred in our series.

Conclusions

The Vena-Tech filter is a useful vena cava filtering device. However, in inserting the filter, it is essential to avoid counterclockwise rotation of the dilator. This is not mentioned in the instruction booklet. It remains to be seen if modifications to the carrier indeed eliminate the "coning" problem. The VT filter has not been in use long enough to assess long-term caval patency rates and the possibility of eventual filter fracture because of the bimetallic construction. Its advantages are ease of use and reliable positioning.

References

1. Greenfield LJ, McCurdy JR, Brown PP, et al: A new intracaval filter permitting continued flow and resolution of emboli. *Surgery* 1973;73:599
2. Piccone VA, Vidal E, Yarnoz M, et al: The late results of caval ligation. *Surgery* 1970;68:980
3. Gurewich V, Thomas DP, Rabinov KR: Pulmonary emboli after ligation of the inferior vena cava. *N Engl J Med* 1966;274:1350
4. Spencer FC, Quattlebaum JR, Quattlebaum JK Jr, et al: Plication of the inferior vena cava for pulmonary embolism: a report of 20 cases. *Ann Surg* 1962;155:827
5. Miles RM, Chappell F, Renner O: A partially occluding vena caval clip for prevention of pulmonary embolism. *Am Surg* 1964;30:40
6. Mobin–Uddin K, Utley JR, Bryant LR: The inferior vena cava umbrella filter. *Prog Cardiovasc Dis* 1975;17:391
7. Friedman SA, Cerruti MM, Berger N, et al: Thromboembolism with the intracaval filter. *Am Heart J* 1972;84:537
8. Hunter JA, Sessions R, Buenger R: Experimental balloon obstruction of the inferior vena cava. *Ann Surg* 1970;171:315
9. Greenfield L: Current indications for and results of Greenfield filter placement. *J Vasc Surg* 1984;1:502
10. Rohrer J, Scheidler MG, Wheeler HB, et al: Extended indications for placement of an inferior vena cava filter. *J Vasc Surg* 1989;10:44
11. Hunter DW, Juravsky L, Fernando CC, et al: Vena-Tech filter. Presented at the 1990 Society of Cardiovascular and Interventional Radiology Meeting, March 24, 1990
12. O'Connell P: Vena-Tech Co. Oral communication, November 12, 1990
13. Ricco JB, Crochet D, Sebilotte P, et al: Percutaneous transvenous caval interruption with the "LGM" filter: early results of a multicenter trial. *Ann Vasc Surg* 1988;3:242

INDEX

Page numbers followed by "f" denote figures; those followed by "t" denote tables. Boldface entries indicate major discussions.

type of lesion at restenosis site,
452–453, 453f–456f
relation to peripheral restenosis,
457–459
type of lesion at, 452–453, 453f–456f
of failing direct arteriovenous fistulae for
hemodialysis access, 443f–444f,
444–445, 445f
failure, intraluminal stents as mechanical
solution to, 553
laser-assisted, 481f, **481–482**
long-term results of, 489
for peripheral pulmonary artery stenosis,
746–748, 747f
for pulmonary venous obstructions, 748
restenosis after, treatment of, 459, 459f
for systemic venous obstruction, 748–
749
technology of, **345–350**
thrombi due to, thrombolytic therapy for,
608–609
for vena caval obstruction, 748
Balloon atrial septostomy, **737–738**
complications of, 737–738
technique for, 737, 738f
Balloon catheter(s), 35, **37–38**
for angioplasty, 383
with calibrated leak, 38
history of, 9
with debris protection, 349f, 349
dilating force, 346–347, 347f
and balloon compliance, 348–350
versus balloon pressure, 347
versus degree of stenosis, 348
versus stenosis area, 347–348
double-lumen, 37, 38f
for drug delivery, 349, 349f
for embolotherapy, 111
historical aspects of, 9, 111
hoop stress, 346–347
for iliac angioplasty, insertion and
removal of, 394, 394f
in intravascular foreign body removal,
708
in lower genitourinary tract interventions,
1028
low-profile, in management of arterial
occlusive disease below the knee,
409
in prevention of embolic reflux, 11, 13,
16, 26, 37, 58, 136–137, 140
for renal angioplasty, 365–370
retrograde transurethral prostatic
urethroplasty with
experimental work, **1016–1020**
human experience, **1020–1027**
single-lumen, 37–38
in thrombectomy, 635
for transluminal angioplasty, 249–251,
345–350
crossability, 346
high-pressure, 348
historical perspective on, 345–346
improved designs of, 349
low profile, 348
monorail, 348, 349f
no tip, 348, 349f

pre-curved, 348–349
with proximal or distal side holes, 348–
349
pushability, 346
short tip, 348
tapered, 348–349
trackability, 346
Balloon dilation
of achalasia, 1232–1233, 1234f, 1234,
1241f
of anastomotic strictures, **1246–1252**
of antral strictures, **1244–1246**
of duodenal strictures, 1246, 1247f
of enteric strictures, **1238–1253**
of esophageal strictures, 1234–1237,
1238–1244
of external urethral sphincter, 1034–
1035, 1035f
for nephrostolithotomy, 933–934, 935f–
936f
of pyloric strictures, **1244–1246**
of ureteral strictures, 893, 894f–895f
in renal allograft recipient, 856–857,
863f–865f
Balloon dilation valvuloplasty, **738–744**
for aortic stenosis, 741–743, 742f
applications of, 738–739
for mitral stenosis, 743–744
for pulmonic stenosis, 739–741, 739f–
741f
Balloon dilators
for anastomotic strictures, selection of
balloon size, 1252, 1252f
for antral strictures, selection of balloon
size, 1246
for biliary tract, 1070, 1073
for esophageal strictures, 1230, 1230f
selection of balloon size, 1239–1242
for nephrostomy tracts, **808**, 808f
for pyloric strictures, selection of balloon
size, 1246
Balloon embolotherapy. *See also* Detachable
balloons
backfolding of balloon in, 125–126
extracranial, **111–134**
of hepatic artery lesions, 125f, 125–
126
histologic effects of, 112, 113f
indications for, 119–134
nonvascular, 119–121
of pelvic artery lesions, 128
principles of, 111–112
of pulmonary arteriovenous
malformations, 120f–121f, **121–
125**
of renal artery lesions, 126f–127f, 126–
128
of retroperitoneal arterial lesions, 128
of splenic artery lesions, 126
of systemic arteriovenous fistulae, **125–
128**
of systemic arteriovenous malformations,
128
of systemic false aneurysms, **125–128**
systems available for, 111, 112f, **113–
117**
for ureteral fistulae, 886–890

Balloon-expandable tantalum stent, for
prostatic stenting, **1039**, 1041f
Balloon occlusion
for bleeding in pancreatic disease, 237f,
240
of splenic artery, preoperative, 241, 241f
Balloon-on-a-wire, 348, 348f
Baltaxe–Mitty–Pollack needle, **808–809**,
809f
Balt balloon. *See also* Detachable balloons
source of, 157
Bannayan's syndrome, 154
Bard rotary atherectomy system, xxx1, 490,
520–527
advantages of, 527
complications with, 522
efficacy of, alone and in combination
with angioplasty, 522, 524f–525f
materials and methods for, 521–522
mechanism of action, 521–522
patency rate with, related to bulk of
atheroma removed, 522
patient demographics, 522
periprocedure radiography, 522
pharmacologic therapy used with, 522
restenosis after, 522
results with, 522
technical description of, 520–521, 521f
BAS. *See* Balloon atrial septostomy
Basilic vein, 328, 329f
Basket (Günther) filter, placement of, 672,
685, 686f
Baskets. *See also* Stone baskets
for removal of intravascular foreign
body, 706f, 706–707, 707f
BDA. *See* Balloon dilation angioplasty
BDV. *See* Balloon dilation valvuloplasty
Becton Dickinson balloon. *See also*
Detachable balloons
source of, 157
Benign prostatic hyperplasia
clinical evaluation of, 1020
hyperthermia treatment of, 1041
incidence of, 1015
management of, xxxiv, 1028, 1038
current techniques, 1016. *See also*
Transurethral resection of prostate
historical perspective on, 1015
stents for, 1038–1039
of middle lobe, 1021, 1021f–1022f
Bentson wire, 804, **1069**, 1128
Bile
gallbladder needle aspiration of, **1190**
infected
with choledocholithiasis, incidence of,
1054, 1058
with malignant biliary obstruction,
incidence of, 1054, 1058
microorganisms in, 1054
subhepatic collection of, after
percutaneous removal of biliary
stones, 1178
Bile duct(s). *See also* Common bile duct
extrahepatic, ultrasound of, 1079, 1079f
intraluminal lesions, biopsy of, 1277,
1281f
left-sided, imaging of, **1082–1084**, 1083f

for coaxial and modified coaxial
techniques, 1260–1262
cutting-type, 1257, 1259, 1266
larger-caliber, 1259–1260
nonferromagnetic, 1260
for percutaneous fine-needle aspiration
of lung nodules, 1359, 1360t–
1362t
screw type, 1257, 1266
spring-loaded systems, 1262, 1265f, 1267
Biopsy transducer, 1082f
Biopty Gun, 1262
for breast biopsy, 1300–1302, 1301f–
1302f
Bird's nest filter, **685–687**, 687f–688f
placement of, 672
Bladder, anatomy of, 1316f, 1318f, 1321f–
1322f
Bladder hemorrhage, in radiation cystitis,
embolotherapy, 58, 59f
Bladder outlet obstruction, from benign
prostatic hyperplasia, balloon
dilatation for
experimental work, **1016–1020**
human experience, **1020–1027**
Bladder tumors, embolotherapy, 58–60
Bleeding, with biliary drainage, 1075
frequency of, 1120
management of, 1179
Blood flow
color Doppler imaging of, 302
Doppler flowmetry, 298, 300
spectral analysis, 300–302, 302f
hemodynamics of, 309–310
Blood-forming organs, maximum
permissible dose equivalent for, 2t
Blood pressure. *See also* Ankle-brachial
pressure measurement;
Hypertension
monitoring, after renal angioplasty, 370
Blood urea nitrogen tests, before
percutaneous biliary drainage,
1075
Blue digit syndrome, **387–389**
directional atherectomy in, **534**, 534f
etiology of, 388
pathology of, 387–388
treatment of, 388–389
Blue toe syndrome, etiology of, 388
Bone, attenuation by, 3f
Bone cysts, aneurysmal, embolotherapy, 60
Bone tumors, blood loss from,
embolotherapy, 60, 62f
Boren–McKinney retriever set, 706f
Bowel infarction
with embolotherapy of colon, 218
with pancreatitis, 234
BPH. *See* Benign prostatic hyperplasia
Brachial artery, occlusion, fibrinolytic
therapy for, 612–613
Brachial vein(s), 328, 329f
Brachiocephalic branch, nitinol stent
placement in, 577t, 579
Brain stem auditory evoked potentials,
monitoring, during neurosurgery,
176
Branch pads, 244

BRAS. *See* Bard rotary atherectomy system
Breast
carcinoma
diagnosis of, 1292–1293, 1301–1302,
1302f
treatment of, potential for
interventional radiology in, 1308
papillomas, diagnosis of, 1292f, 1292–
1293
pericannicular fibroadenoma, diagnosis
of, 1301, 1302f
Breast abscess, drainage, **1291**
Breast biopsy, large-core, **1300–1305**,
1302f–1307f, 1308
automated biopsy guns for, 1300–1302,
1301f–1302f
stereotactic automated technique, 1302,
1303f–1306f, 1308
ultrasound-guided automated technique,
1302–1305, 1306f–1307f
Breast cyst(s)
aspiration, **1289–1291**
indications for, 1289–1290
technique, 1290
ultrasound guidance, 1290f, 1290–
1291, 1291f
vacutainer needle for, 1291
etiology of, 1289
Breast lesions
biopsy and definitive surgery of, one-
and two-stage procedures, 1296–
1297
cancer yield in, 1296
equipment, 1293–1294, 1293f–1294f
fine-needle aspiration biopsy of, **1299–
1300**, 1301f, 1308
hookwires, 1293, 1293f
needle localization of, 1293–1295
contrast material instillation, 1295
guidance modalities, 1294–1295, 1295f
specimen radiography with, 1295,
1296f
surgical excision biopsy with, 1294,
1294f
percutaneous needle biopsy, **1295–1299**,
1305
large-core technique, **1300–1305**,
1302f–1307f
mammographic guidance, 1297, 1297f
stereotactic
adapted standard mammography
units for, 1297–1298, 1298f
dedicated stereotactic mammography
units for, 1298–1299, 1299f–1300f
surgical biopsy, 1296–1297, 1305
Brescia–Cimino fistula, 425–426, 438, **441–
442**
complications of, 425f–427f, 426, 441–
442, 442f
failing, venous fistulogram for evaluation
of, 442–443
Bristle brushes, as embolic agents, **32**
Bronchial arteries
aberrant, 38
anatomic relations of, 203
anatomy of, 38–39
embolotherapy, 38–41

with absolute ethanol, **148**
angiography after, 39, 40f
for bronchopulmonary disease, 41
catheters for, 39
complications of, 41
contraindications to, 148
in cystic fibrosis, 39–41
indications for, 39–41
with isobutyl 2-cyanoacrylate, 148
in pneumoconiosis, 41
for post-thoracotomy bleeding, 41
technique, 39
in tuberculosis, 41
with unresectable malignant
tumor, 41
Bronchial arteriography, before
embolotherapy, 38–39
Bronchiectasis, hemoptysis with, 38
Bronchopulmonary neoplasm, hemoptysis
with, 38
Bucrylate. *See* Isobutyl 2-cyanoacrylate
Budd–Chiari syndrome
inferior vena cava compression/occlusion
in
Maass double-helix stent for, 589, 591f
thrombolytic therapy for, 617
ultrasound findings in, 334
BUD Percuflex catheter, 789f
Bulbourethral artery(ies), 764
Bullae, infected, percutaneous aspiration
and drainage of, 1375–1377, 1376f
Bullet fragment, intravascular, retrieval,
712
Burhenne catheter, in nephrostolithotomy,
958–960, 961f
N-Butyl cyanoacrylate
as embolic agent, **157**
embolotherapy
for intracranial arteriovenous fistula(s),
177
for intracranial arteriovenous
malformations, 177
for management of ureteral fistulae,
886
for spinal dural arteriovenous fistula(s),
184
of varicocele, **73–100**
polymerization, in embolization of
varicocele, 76–85
source of, 157
Bypass grafts, emboli from, blue digit
syndrome caused by, 388

Caged balloon catheter, for percutaneous
transluminal angioplasty, xxix,
249, 250f, 378
Calf veins
anatomy of, 321–322, 322f
ultrasound examination of, 323–324
Cancer. *See also* Carcinoma; Lung cancer;
Prostate cancer
embolotherapy in, **53–63**
complications of, 60–63
embolic agents for, 60
Canine gallbladder, percutaneous ablation
of, 1199, 1200f
Capillary hemangioma, 154

eye exposure limits, 2t
  recommendations on radiation
    protection, 2
International Council on Radiation
  Protection and Units,
    recommendations on radiation
    protection, 2
Interventional radiology, future of, xxxv
Intestinal angina, 359
Intimal flap
  elevation of, in percutaneous
    transluminal angioplasty, 414f, 414
  postangioplasty
    directional atherectomy of, **535**, 536f–
      537f
    management of, 344
    nonobstructive, 535
    obstructive, 535, 536f, 572
Intimal hyperplasia
  in arteriosclerosis, endosonography of,
    342, 343f
  in carotid artery, recurrent postsurgical
    stenosis due to, 353, 355f, 356
  with hemodialysis access, 424
  after percutaneous transluminal
    angioplasty, 258, 261–262, 263f,
      264–265
  and restenosis, 279, 567
  in restenosis after coronary balloon
    angioplasty, 452t, 452–453, 453f–
      455f, **455–457**
  in restenosis after peripheral balloon
    angioplasty, 459
  venous, with Brescia–Cimino fistula, 426,
    427f
Intimal thickenings, arterial, 244
Intra-abdominal hemorrhage, and biliary
  drainage, 1179
Intra-arterial digital subtraction
  angiography, in children, 717
Intracanalicular irradiation, percutaneous,
  biliary stents for, **1156**
Intracolic space, anatomy of, 1319
Intracranial hemorrhage, in neonate, 608
Intrahepatic hemorrhage, and biliary
  drainage, 1179
Intrahepatic obstruction(s)
  multiple, and percutaneous transhepatic
    biliary drainage, 1075
  and percutaneous transhepatic biliary
    drainage, 1075
Intrahepatic stones, removal of, 1178
Intramuscular hemangioma, 153
Intramuscular venous malformations. See
  Venous malformations,
    intramuscular
Intravascular foreign body, removal. See
  Foreign body, intravascular,
    removal
Intravascular ultrasound. See Ultrasound,
  intravascular
Intravenous digital subtraction
  angiography, in children, 717
Intravenous urogram, in trauma patient,
  44–45
Inverse-square law, reduction of radiation
  intensity according to, 1, 2f

Iodine allergy, and nephrostolithotomy,
  902
Iothalamate sodium, 107
Ischemic necrosis, after embolotherapy,
  factors influencing, 10–11
Isobutyl 2-cyanoacrylate
  bronchial artery embolization with, 148
  as embolic agent, xxxii, 10, **22–25, 157**
    for bronchial arteries, 39
    in cancer, 60
    catheters for, 35–37
    foreign body-type reaction to, 25
    introduction technique, 22–25
    for liver, 46
    for peripheral pseudoaneurysms, 63
    for postbiopsy renal AV fistula, 44
    precautions with, 25
    for renal ablation, 53
    for renal carcinoma, 58
    for varicocele, 107
  embolotherapy
    of arteriovenous fistula(s), 165
    for bleeding esophageal varices, 205–
      206
    of esophageal varices, 205–206
    for intracranial arteriovenous fistula(s),
      177
    for intracranial arteriovenous
      malformations, 177
    for spinal dural arteriovenous fistula(s),
      184
    of varicocele, 73
  polymerization, 22, 25
  source of, 157
Ivalon. See Polyvinyl alcohol foam
IVM. See Venous malformations,
  intramuscular
IVUS. See Ultrasound, intravascular

Jaundice. See also Obstructive jaundice
  differential diagnosis of, 1053
Jejunostomy, through percutaneous
  gastrostomy, **1222–1224**
Jejunum, anatomy of, 1316f
Jugular technique
  for spermatic venography, 103, 104f–
    105f
  for Vena-Tech filter placement, 701
Jugular vein(s)
  for hemodialysis access, 447–449, 448f
  internal, 329f
    ultrasound examination of, 329
  Mobin–Uddin umbrella filter placement
    through, 670
  percutaneous introduction of Kimray–
    Greenfield filter through, 675–
      676, 675f–678f
  placement of Kimray–Greenfield filter
    from, through surgical venotomy,
      672–673, 673f–675f
J-wires, 1069

Kaliman atherectomy catheter, 490, **552**
Kasabach–Merritt syndrome, 159
Kast syndrome, 154

Kaye tamponade catheter, for nephrostomy
  drainage after nephrostolithotomy,
    placement of, 971, 972f
Kensey dynamic angioplasty catheter, xxx,
  490, **497–503**
  clinical results with, 503
  current status of, 503
  description of, 497, 498f
  diameter of recanalized channel, 501–
    503, 502f
  extravasation of dye with, 500, 500f
  guidelines for use of, 500–501
  guidewires used with, 500, 501f
  mechanism of action, theories of, 501–
    503
  operating principles, 497–498
  path of least resistance, 499–500, 499f–
    500f
  pressurized fluid jets, 498–499, 499f
  recommended speeds and fluid pressures
    for, 500–501
  rotating cam of, 498, 498f
  technical results with, 503
  use with calcific tissue, 501–503, 502f
Kensey–Nash lithotrite, **1197**, 1198f–1199f
KG filter. See Kimray–Greenfield filter
Kidney(s). See also Horseshoe kidney; Renal
  anatomy of, **777–787**, 1316f–1317f,
    1348f
    anomalous, and nephrostolithotomy,
      902
    arterial, 783–785, 785f–787f
      and nephrostomy puncture, 818,
        821f
    after extracorporeal shock wave
      lithotripsy, 1003
    lobar, 783, 784f
    position of, 777, 778f
    relations to adjacent organs and
      structures, 781–783, 781f–783f
    relations to pleura and ribs, 779–781,
      780f
    retroperitoneal relations, 777–778,
      779f–780f
    for ultrasound-guided nephrostomy
      puncture, 814f–816f
    vascular, 783–787, 785f–788f
    venous, 785–787, 788f
  Brödel type, 784f, 904f
  calices, 783, 784f
    position of, variations in, 833, 834f
  embryology of, 783
  Hodson type, 784f, 904f
  lobes of, 783
  malrotated, and nephrostolithotomy, 909,
    909f
  papillae, 783
  percutaneous biopsy of, **1270**, 1273f
    arteriovenous fistula formed after,
      embolotherapy, 43f, 43–44
    complications of, 1278
  percutaneous interventional techniques
    for, xxxiii–xxxiv
  plane of arterial division, 787f
  septal cortex, 783
  solitary
    etiology of, 1006

TEC. *See* Transluminal extraction (endarterectomy) catheter
Teflon. *See also* Polytetrafluoroethylene catheters
    for embolotherapy, 35
    for percutaneous nephrostomy, **790**, 790f
Teflon (coaxial) dilators, xxix, **805**, 806f, 893, 1070–1072
Teflonized J-wire, 804
Teflon stents, for internal biliary drainage, 1110
    placement of, 1110, 1111f–1112f
Tegtmeyer catheter, 790
Tegwire angioplasty catheter, 367
Temporalis muscle, intramuscular venous malformation, embolotherapy, 171, 174f
Terlipressin, for bleeding esophageal varices, 205
Terminal ileum, anatomy of, 1316f
Terumo glidewire, 1128
Tetralogy of Fallot, preoperative thoracic vascular embolization with, 750
TGF. *See* Transforming growth factor-α; Transforming growth factor-β
Thalassemia major, splenic embolization in, 48
THC. *See* Cholangiography, percutaneous transhepatic
Thermal balloons, 349–350
Thermoluminescent dosimeters, 3
Thoracic aorta
    aneurysm, embolotherapy, 63
    false aneurysms in, blue digit syndrome caused by, 388
    transluminal angioplasty
        in atherosclerotic rabbits, 270–275
        morphology of vasa vasorum after, 275–277
Thoracic inlet syndrome, 618–619, 619f
Thoracic outlet syndrome, 388
    subclavian vessel thrombosis with, fibrinolytic therapy for, 614
Thoracic vascular embolization, for children, 750–752
Thoracolumbar fascia, 779, 780f
Thrombectomy
    mechanical, xxxii, **635–664**. *See also* Sonic thrombolysis
        advantages of, 635, 642
        devices for, 635, 660. *See also* Amplatz mechanical thrombolysis catheter; Ponomar transjugular clot-trapper device; Rheolytic thrombectomy catheter; Transluminal extraction catheter
    percutaneous. *See also* Percutaneous aspiration thromboembolectomy; Thrombectomy, mechanical with transluminal endarterectomy catheter, 545
    rheolytic, **660–664**
    rotational, **651**
Thrombi. *See* Thrombosis; Thrombus
Thrombin, 600
    and clot lysis, 12
    as embolic agent, **12**

for peripheral pseudoaneurysms, 63
Thrombocytopenia, splenic embolization for, 48–49
Thromboembolism
    recurrent
        with anticoagulation, as indication for IVC interruption, 667
        in elderly, as indication for IVC filter placement, 668
        septic, as indication for IVC interruption, 668
Thrombolysis, xxxi–xxxii. *See also* Sonic thrombolysis
    accelerated, 616
        with percutaneous aspiration thromboembolectomy, 653, 656f
    in chronic occlusion, **608–609**
    definition of, 599
    with multiple sidehole infusion catheter, 616
    pulsed spray pharmacomechanical method, **615–616**
    in recanalization of occluded common iliac artery, 399, 400f
    in salvage of hemodialysis access, 431–432
        complications of, 432
        economic considerations, 433–434
Thrombolytic therapy. *See also* Fibrinolytic therapy
    chemical, compared to mechanical thrombectomy, 642
    for deep vein thrombosis, 321
    drawbacks of, 635, 640
    for graft occlusions, **609–612**, 610f–611f
    pulmonary embolism in, 617
    for renal artery thrombus, 372
    for superior mesenteric artery thrombus, 362f, 363
    for superior vena cava thrombosis, 617
    temporary IVC filter placement during, 689–690, 691f
Thromboplastin, 600
Thrombosis. *See also* Deep vein thrombosis; Thrombus
    acute
        management of, 640. *See also* Thrombectomy, mechanical
        postangioplasty, 416, 416f
    from angiographic or interventional procedures, in children, fibrinolytic therapy for, 721–724
    arterial
        with atherosclerotic plaques, 246, 247f
        pathophysiology of, 599
    definition of, 599
    of hemodialysis access, 424–425, 425f, 441
        in direct arteriovenous fistulae, **444–445**
        early warning signs of, **429–430**
    with inferior vena cava filters, 682, 685, 688
    at Kimray–Greenfield filter puncture site, 695–696
    pathophysiology of, 599–600
    with Scribner shunt, 423

with self-expandable intravascular stent, 566–568, 567f
    venous, pathophysiology of, 600
Thrombostat. *See* Thrombin
Thromboxane A₂, 599
    and arterial wall biology, 283, 283f
    inhibitor, and transluminal angioplasty, 286–287
    in intimal hyperplasia after balloon angioplasty, 455
    and transluminal angioplasty, 285–287
Thrombus. *See also* Thrombosis
    as anatomic contraindication to angioplasty, 380
    arterial (white), components of, 642
    definition of, 599
    in extremities, from atherosclerotic lesions in aorta, iliac, or femoral vessels, 388
    formation, after transluminal angioplasty, 264, 268
    neovascularization, 246
    organization of, 246, 247f
    recanalization, 246, 247f
    venous (red), components of, 642
Through-and-through guidewire, for nephrostomy tract, establishment, endofluoroscopic technique for, 1000, 1000f
Thyroid nodules, ablation, with absolute ethanol, **149**
Tibial artery(ies), 310
    angioplasty of
        anatomic contraindications to, 379
        lesions ideal for, 380
    anterior, stenosis, laser-assisted angioplasty of, 482, 483f
    distal occlusion, transluminal angioplasty, **410–411**
    spasm, in transluminal angioplasty, 382–383
Tibial vein(s)
    anterior, 322, 322f
    posterior, 322, 322f
    ultrasound examination of, 324
Tibioperoneal run-off system, atherosclerotic involvement in, 310
Time of flight angiography, 319
Tissue adhesive. *See also* N-Butyl cyanoacrylate; Isobutyl 2-cyanoacrylate
    as embolic agent, **157**
Tissue plasminogen activator, 600–602
    recombinant, as thrombolytic agent, 611–612, 628–629
    as thrombolytic agent, xxxii, 628, 722
        for coronary occlusion, 623
        efficacy of, compared to urokinase, 628–629
        mechanism of action, 628, 628f
Titanium Greenfield vena cava filter, 680f, **680–681**
    complications with, 695, 695f
T-lymphocytes, in atherogenesis, 247–248
Toe pressure, measurement, 317–318
Tolazoline, for angioplasty patient, 382–383